Grant's
Atlas of Anatomy

Edition
16

Grant's
Atlas of Anatomy

Edition 16

Anne M. R. Agur, BSc (OT), MSc, PhD, FAAA
Professor, Division of Anatomy, Department of Surgery, Faculty of Medicine
Division of Physical Medicine and Rehabilitation, Department of Medicine
Department of Physical Therapy
Department of Occupational Science and Occupational Therapy
Division of Biomedical Communications, Institute of Medical Science
Rehabilitation Sciences Institute, Graduate Department of Dentistry
University of Toronto
Toronto, Ontario, Canada

Arthur F. Dalley II, PhD, FAAA
Professor Emeritus, Department of Cell and Developmental Biology
Former Director, Medical Gross Anatomy and
Co-Director, Brain, Behavior, and Movement
Former Adjunct Professor, Department of Orthopaedic Surgery and Rehabilitation
Vanderbilt University School of Medicine
Former Adjunct Professor for Anatomy
Belmont University School of Physical Therapy
Nashville, Tennessee

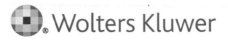

Philadelphia • Baltimore • New York • London
Buenos Aires • Hong Kong • Sydney • Tokyo

Acquisitions Editor: Crystal Taylor
Development Editors: Greg Nicholl (freelance), Amy Millholen
Editorial Coordinator: Marisa Solorzano-Taylor
Editorial Assistant: Parisa Saranj
Marketing Manager: Danielle Klahr
Production Project Manager: Bridgett Dougherty
Design Coordinator: Stephen Druding
Art Director: Jennifer Clements
Artists: Imagineeringart.com, Inc.; Dragonfly Media Group
Manufacturing Coordinator: Margie Orzech
Prepress Vendor: Absolute Service, Inc.

Sixteenth Edition

Library of Congress Cataloging-in-Publication Data

Names: Agur, A. M. R. author. | Dalley, Arthur F., II, author.
Title: Grant's atlas of anatomy / Anne M.R. Agur, Arthur F. Dalley II.
Other titles: Atlas of anatomy
Description: Edition 16th. | Philadelphia : Wolters Kluwer, [2025] |
   Includes bibliographical references and index.
Identifiers: LCCN 2023037047 (print) | LCCN 2023037048 (ebook) | ISBN
   9781975193430 (paperback) | ISBN 9781975193454 | ISBN 9781975193461
Subjects: MESH: Anatomy | Atlas | BISAC: MEDICAL / Anatomy
Classification: LCC QM25 (print) | LCC QM25 (ebook) | NLM QS 17 | DDC
   611.0022/2--dc23/eng/20231004
LC record available at https://lccn.loc.gov/2023037047
LC ebook record available at https://lccn.loc.gov/2023037048

shop.lww.com

QUADM1223

To my husband Enno and to my family Kristina, Erik, and Amy for their support and encouragement

(A.M.R.A.)

In loving memory of Muriel
My bride of 50 years and
devoted mother and grandmother
And to my family
Tristan and Lana, Elijah, Finley, Sawyer, and Dashiell;
Denver and Samantha, Olin and Anderson; and
Skyler and Sara, Dawson, Willa, and Foster
With great appreciation for their love, support, humor, and patience

(A.F.D.)

And with sincere appreciation for the anatomical donors and their supporting families
Without whom our studies would not be possible

DR. JOHN CHARLES BOILEAU GRANT (1886–1973)

by Dr. Carlton G. Smith, MD, PhD (1905–2003)
Professor Emeritus, Division of Anatomy, Department of Surgery
Faculty of Medicine, University of Toronto, Toronto, Ontario, Canada

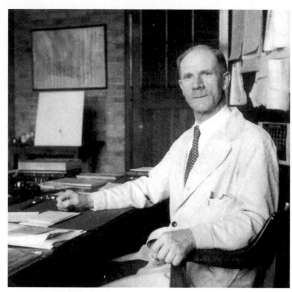

Dr. J. C. Boileau Grant in his office, McMurrich Building, University of Toronto, 1946. Through his textbooks, Dr. Grant made an indelible impression on the teaching of anatomy throughout the world. (Courtesy of Dr. C. G. Smith.)

The life of Dr. J. C. Boileau Grant has been likened to the course of the seventh cranial nerve as it passes out of the skull: complicated but purposeful.[1] He was born in the parish of Lasswade in Edinburgh, Scotland, on February 6, 1886. Dr. Grant studied medicine at the University of Edinburgh from 1903 to 1908. Here, his skill as a dissector in the laboratory of the renowned anatomist, Dr. Daniel John Cunningham (1850–1909), earned him a number of awards.

Following graduation, Dr. Grant was appointed the resident house officer at the Infirmary in Whitehaven, Cumberland. From 1909 to 1911, Dr. Grant demonstrated anatomy in the University of Edinburgh, followed by 2 years at the University of Durham, at Newcastle-on-Tyne in England, in the laboratory of Professor Robert Howden, editor of *Gray's Anatomy*.

With the outbreak of World War I in 1914, Dr. Grant joined the Royal Army Medical Corps and served with distinction. He was mentioned in dispatches in September 1916, received the Military Cross in September 1917 for "conspicuous gallantry and devotion to duty during attack," and received a bar to the Military Cross in August 1918.[1]

In October 1919, released from the Royal Army, he accepted the position of Professor of Anatomy at the University of Manitoba in Winnipeg, Canada. With the frontline medical practitioner in mind, he endeavored to "bring up a generation of surgeons who knew exactly what they were doing once an operation had begun."[1] Devoted to research and learning, Dr. Grant took interest in other projects, such as performing anthropometric studies of Indian tribes in northern Manitoba during the 1920s. In Winnipeg, Dr. Grant met Catriona Christie, whom he married in 1922.

Dr. Grant was known for his reliance on logic, analysis, and deduction as opposed to rote memory. While at the University of Manitoba, Dr. Grant began writing *A Method of Anatomy, Descriptive and Deductive*, which was published in 1937.[2]

In 1930, Dr. Grant accepted the position of Chair of Anatomy at the University of Toronto. He stressed the value of a "clean" dissection, with the structures well defined. This required the delicate touch of a sharp scalpel, and students soon learned that a dull tool was anathema. Instructive dissections were made available in the Anatomy Museum, a means of student review on which Dr. Grant placed a high priority. Illustrations of these actual dissections are included in *Grant's Atlas of Anatomy*.

The first edition of the Atlas, published in 1943, was the first anatomical atlas to be published in North America.[3] *Grant's Dissector* preceded the *Atlas* in 1940.[4]

Dr. Grant remained at the University of Toronto until his retirement in 1956. At that time, he became Curator of the Anatomy Museum in the University. He also served as Visiting Professor of Anatomy at the University of California at Los Angeles, where he taught for 10 years.

Dr. Grant died in 1973 of cancer. Through his teaching method, still presented in the Grant's textbooks, Dr. Grant's life interest—human anatomy—lives on. In their eulogy, colleagues and friends Ross MacKenzie and J. S. Thompson said, "Dr. Grant's knowledge of anatomical fact was encyclopedic, and he enjoyed nothing better than sharing his knowledge with others, whether they were junior students or senior staff. While somewhat strict as a teacher, his quiet wit and boundless humanity never failed to impress. He was, in the very finest sense, a scholar and a gentleman."[1]

1 Robinson C. *Canadian Medical Lives: J. C. Boileau Grant: Anatomist Extraordinary*. Ontario, Canada: Associated Medical Services Inc/Fitzhenry & Whiteside, 1993.

2 Grant JCB. *A Method of Anatomy: Descriptive and Deductive*. Baltimore, MD: Williams & Wilkins Co, 1937.
3 Grant JCB. *Grant's Atlas of Anatomy*. Baltimore, MD: Williams & Wilkins Co, 1943.
4 Grant JCB, Cates HA. *Grant's Dissector (A Handbook for Dissectors)*. Baltimore, MD: Williams & Wilkins Co, 1940.

RADIOLOGIC FIGURE CONTRIBUTORS

Joel A. Vilensky, PhD
Professor Emeritus of Anatomy and Cell Biology
Indiana University School of Medicine
Fort Wayne, Indiana

Edward C. Weber, DO
The Imaging Center
Fort Wayne, Indiana

FACULTY REVIEWERS

Abduelmenem Alashkham, PhD, MSc (Distinction), MBBCh
Anatomy, School of Biomedical Sciences
University of Edinburgh
Edinburgh, Scotland, United Kingdom

William S. Brooks, PhD
Marnix E. Heersink School of Medicine
University of Alabama at Birmingham
Birmingham, Alabama

Sandra J. Colello, PhD
School of Medicine
Virginia Commonwealth University
Richmond, Virginia

Alan J. Detton, PhD
Department of Pathology and Cell Biology
Columbia University Irving Medical Center
Vagelos College of Physicians and Surgeons
Columbia University
New York, New York

James D. Foster, PhD
Alabama College of Osteopathic Medicine
Dothan, Alabama

Nicole R. Herring, PhD
Department of Anatomical Sciences and Neurobiology
University of Louisville
Louisville, Kentucky

Ryan Splittgerber, PhD
Vanderbilt University Medical Center
Vanderbilt University School of Medicine
Nashville, Tennessee

Brent J. Thompson, PhD
DeBusk College of Osteopathic Medicine
Lincoln Memorial University-Knoxville
Knoxville, Tennessee

STUDENT REVIEWERS

Aryan Hemani
Spartan Health Sciences University

Dr. Shaily Singh
Ganesh Shanker Vidyarthi Memorial College
Lala Lajpat Rai Hospital

This edition of *Grant's Atlas* has, like its predecessors, required intense research, market input, and creativity. It is not enough to rely on a solid reputation; with each new edition, we have adapted and changed many aspects of the *Atlas* while maintaining the commitment to pedagogical excellence and anatomical realism that has enriched its long history. Medical and health sciences education, and the role of anatomy instruction and application within it, continually evolve to reflect new teaching approaches and educational models. The health care system itself is changing, and the skills and knowledge that future health care practitioners must master are changing along with it. Finally, technologic advances in publishing, particularly in online resources and electronic media, have transformed the way students access content and the methods by which educators teach content. All of these developments have shaped the vision and directed the execution of this sixteenth edition of *Grant's Atlas*, as evidenced by the following key features.

New and expanded content of the female perineum. New illustrations of erectile tissues have been added. There is now a balanced focus on both female and male anatomy.

Expanded diversity. Surface anatomy photography, clinical procedures, and anatomical illustrations have been updated and revised with the aim of reflecting the diversity of those using the textbook and the patients they will be treating.

Recolorization of the original carbon-dust *Grant's Atlas* images from high-resolution scans. The entire collection of carbon-dust illustrations were remastered and recolored for the fourteenth edition using a vibrant new palette. The stunning detail and contrast of the original Grant's art was maintained while adding a new level of luminosity of organs and especially transparency of tissues, enabling demonstrations of deeper relationships not possible with merely recolored grayscale illustrations, thereby enhancing the student learning experience. The student is able to visualize and appreciate clearly the newly revealed relationships between structures, enabling the formation of three-dimensional (3D) constructs for each region of the body. The recolorization, enabled by modern image processing, allows reproduction and viewing of the images—both in print and electronically—with unprecedented high resolution and fidelity, continuing their vital role informing future generations of medical and health care providers about the structure and function of the human body.

A unique feature of *Grant's Atlas* is that rather than providing an idealized view of human anatomy, the classic illustrations represent actual dissections that the student can directly compare with specimens in the lab. Because the original models used for these illustrations were real cadavers, the accuracy of these illustrations is unparalleled, offering students the best introduction to anatomy possible.

Schematic illustrations. Updated for the sixteenth edition with a modern uniform style and consistent color palette, the full-color schematic illustrations and orientation figures supplement the dissection figures to clarify anatomical concepts, show the relationships of structures, and give an overview of the body region being studied.

The illustrations conform to Dr. Grant's admonition to "keep it simple": Extraneous labels were deleted, and some labels were added to identify key structures and make the illustrations as useful as possible to students.

Legends with easy-to-find clinical applications. Admittedly, artwork is the focus of any atlas; however, the *Grant's* legends have long been considered a unique and valuable feature of the *Atlas*. The observations and comments that accompany the illustrations assist orientation and draw attention to salient points and significant structures that might otherwise escape notice. Their purpose is to interpret the illustrations without providing exhaustive description. Readability, clarity, and practicality were emphasized in the editing of this edition. Clinical comments, which deliver practical "pearls" that link anatomical features with their significance in health care practice, appear in blue text within the figure legends. New clinical comments based on current practices have been added in this edition, providing even more relevance for students searching for medical application of anatomical concepts.

Enhanced diagnostic imaging and surface anatomy. Because medical imaging has taken on increased importance in the diagnosis and treatment of injuries and illnesses, diagnostic images are used liberally throughout and at the end of each chapter. Over 100 clinically significant magnetic resonance images (MRIs), computed tomography (CT) scans, ultrasound scans, and corresponding orientation drawings are included, many of which are new to or updated for this edition. Labeled surface anatomy photographs, which, like the illustrations, feature ethnic diversity, continue to be an important feature in this new edition. All of the surface anatomy figures showing the musculature *in situ* have been replaced with new images providing an enhanced learning experience.

Updated and improved tables. Tables help students organize complex information in an easy-to-use format ideal for review and study. In addition to muscles, tables summarizing nerves, arteries, and other relevant structures are included. Tables are made more meaningful with illustrations strategically placed on the same page, demonstrating the structures and relationships described in the tables.

Improved directional orientation. Orientation guides have been added to many more illustrations and medical images to augment the viewpoints provided for all figures.

Logical organization and layout. The organization and layout of the *Atlas* have always been determined with ease of use as the goal. To facilitate dissection, the body regions have been ordered in the same sequence as the current edition of *Grant's Dissector*. The order of plates within every chapter was scrutinized to ensure that it is logical and pedagogically effective.

In preparing this revision, we have worked closely with Dr. Alan Denton to assure consistency in approach, content, and terminology between the *Atlas* and the *Dissector*. We hope that you enjoy using this sixteenth edition of *Grant's Atlas* and that it becomes a trusted partner in your educational experience. We believe that this new edition safeguards the *Atlas's* historical strengths while enhancing its usefulness to today's students.

Anne M. R. Agur
Arthur F. Dalley II

ACKNOWLEDGMENTS

Starting with the first edition of *Grant's Atlas of Anatomy* published in 1943, many people have given generously of their talents and expertise and we acknowledge their participation with heartfelt gratitude. Most of the original carbon-dust halftones on which this book is based were created by Dorothy Foster Chubb, a pupil of Max Brödel and one of Canada's first professionally trained medical illustrators. She was later joined by Nancy Joy. Mrs. Chubb was mainly responsible for the artwork of the first two editions and the sixth edition; Professor Joy, for those in between. In subsequent editions, additional line and halftone illustrations by Elizabeth Blackstock, Elia Hopper Ross, and Marguerite Drummond were added.

Medical illustrators have continued to update and create new illustrations to improve the *Atlas*: D. Mazierski, S. Mader, V. Oxorn, K. Yu, B. Vallecoccia, S. O'Sullivan, D. Rini, C. Sandone, C. Duckwall, and R. Duckwall. The photography of Anne Rayner of Vanderbilt University Medical Center's Medical Art Group has enhanced the surface anatomy photographs throughout the atlas. We extend our gratitude to Professors Nick Woolridge and David Mazerski who developed the carbon-dust recolorization process and along with Nicole Clough and Marissa Webber who recolorized all of the carbon-dust images for the fourteenth edition.

Much credit is due to Charles E. Storton for his role in the preparation of the majority of the original dissections and preliminary photographic work. We wish to acknowledge the work of Dr. James Anderson, a pupil of Dr. Grant, under whose stewardship the seventh and eighth editions were published. The work of Dr. C. G. Smith must also be acknowledged for illustrations of the human brain based on the neuroanatomical dissections.

SIXTEENTH EDITION

We are indebted to our students, colleagues, and former professors for their encouragement and invaluable input.

We would also like to acknowledge Jennifer Clements, Art Director at Wolters Kluwer, who managed the art program for this edition. Special thanks go to everyone at Wolters Kluwer—especially Crystal Taylor, Senior Acquisitions Editor, and Greg Nicholl, Freelance Development Editor. We also thank Amy Millholen, Senior Development Editor. All of your efforts and expertise are much appreciated.

We would like to thank the hundreds of instructors and students who have over the years communicated via the publisher and directly with the editor their suggestions for how this *Atlas* might be improved. Finally, we would like to acknowledge the reviewers who reviewed previous editions of the *Atlas* as well as the reviewers who reviewed the fifteenth edition and provided expert advice on the development of this edition.

CONTENTS

LIST OF TABLES

FIGURE CREDITS

The following figures have been modified from content in either Dalley AF, Agur AMR. *Moore's Clinically Oriented Anatomy*. 9th ed. Wolters Kluwer; 2023, or Agur AMR, Dalley AF. *Moore's Essential Clinical Anatomy*. 7th ed. Wolters Kluwer; 2024. (See below for additional credits from other sources.)

CHAPTER 1
BACK

Figures 1.2A&C, 1.3D&E, 1.4, 1.6B&D, 1.7A–E, 1.9A,B,D,&E, 1.13B&H, 1.14B, 1.15C, 1.17B, 1.18A–C, 1.19A&B, 1.21A&B, 1.33A–E, 1.34A–D, 1.40C, 1.43A,B,&D, 1.44A&B, 1.47D, 1.48A–E, 1.49, 1.50, and 1.51A&B.

CHAPTER 2
UPPER LIMB

Figures 2.3A–E&G, 2.8A&B, 2.9, 2.11A&H–J, 2.12A&B, 2.13A&B, 2.15A&B, 2.16A–D, 2.22, 2.25B, 2.26B&C, 2.27A&B, 2.28B, 2.32B, 2.36A–F, 2.38F, 2.40C, 2.48B, 2.49C, 2.51B&D, 2.52B, 2.57A,B,&D, 2.58A&D, 2.63, 2.65A&B, 2.70A&C, 2.71B, 2.72B, 2.73A&B, 2.74B, 2.76D, 2.77, 2.79B, 2.80A (*detail*), 2.84, 2.85A&B, 2.90C&D, 2.91D, 2.94E, 2.101A, and 2.102A (*illustration*).

CHAPTER 3
THORAX

Figures 3.4B, 3.7B&C, 3.14A–C, 3.15A&B, 3.19, 3.20A–C, 3.27A–C, 3.28A–D, 3.29A&B, 3.34B–F, 3.37C, 3.41A&B, 3.42A–C, 3.43C, 3.48A–C, 3.49A,B,&D, 3.50A&C, 3.51A&C–E, 3.52A&B, 3.53A–D, 3.54B, 3.55, 3.56A–C, 3.57C, 3.58B, 3.60C, 3.64C–F, 3.65A–C, 3.69C, 3.70, 3.71A&B, 3.72B, 3.78E, and 3.79F&H.

CHAPTER 4
ABDOMEN

Figures 4.5A, 4.7, 4.10A,B,D,&E, 4.17A–E, 4.18, 4.20C, 4.22B, 4.24A–C, 4.27B, 4.31A–C, 4.32A, 4.33A, 4.35A, 4.43B, 4.44 (*insets*), 4.51B&C, 4.54A–E, 4.55, 4.58B–D, 4.62A–H, 4.63B, 4.66A, 4.68B, 4.72A, 4.73A,B,&D–F, 4.76B, 4.79C, 4.80B–D, 4.81, 4.83A&B, 4.84B, 4.85A–C, 4.87A, 4.89A,B,&D–F, 4.91A&C, 4.92D, and 4.93A–C (*illustrations*).

CHAPTER 5
PELVIS AND PERINEUM

Figures 5.3C, 5.4B&C, 5.9B, 5.10B, 5.16B–D, 5.18A–D, 5.19, 5.21E&G, 5.24A–C, 5.29A&B, 5.30A–D, 5.31, 5.32, 5.41C, 5.42A&B, 5.43A–D, 5.44A&B, 5.48A–F, 5.50A, 5.51B, 5.52C, 5.56B&D, 5.57, 5.59B, 5.60B&C, and 5.62C.

CHAPTER 6
LOWER LIMB

Figures 6.2A&B, 6.10A, 6.12A&F, 6.16A–C, 6.18A–E, 6.20B, 6.22C, 6.25F&G, 6.27B&C, 6.32A&B, 6.33A&B, 6.34B, 6.35B&C, 6.36B, 6.41A, 6.51B&C, 6.56A,D,&F, 6.61A&B, 6.62A&E, 6.64A&B, 6.66D, 6.68A, 6.69D, 6.70B&E, 6.71B, 6.74A&B, 6.75A–C, 6.76C, 6.77A, 6.78A, 6.79A, 6.80A, 6.83B&C, 6.84D, 6.90A, 6.95C, and 6.97 (*orientation*).

CHAPTER 7
NECK

Figures 7.2A–C, 7.3A, 7.4A&B, 7.5A&C–H, 7.6A–C, 7.8B,D,&E, 7.9B, 7.12B, 7.15A–C, 7.17B, 7.19A, 7.22B–E, 7.23A, 7.26A–C (*schematics*), 7.27A, 7.28C, 7.33C–F, H–J, 7.34D, and 7.36.

CHAPTER 8
HEAD

Figures 8.3C, 8.6B, 8.12B–D, 8.14A, 8.15A&B, 8.17A&B, 8.18A&B, 8.19, 8.20A&B, 8.21A–C, 8.22A–D, 8.24B, 8.25A&B, 8.29, 8.30C, 8.31B, 8.33B&C, 8.38B, 8.39B,C,&E, 8.41A&B, 8.42A&B, 8.43A–E, 8.44A&B, 8.45B&D, 8.46B, 8.48A&D, 8.51, 8.52A&B, 8.55B&C, 8.56A–C&F, 8.57A–D, 8.58A&B, 8.59C, 8.60B, 8.63C, 8.64A&C, 8.65A, 8.70A–C, 8.74A&B, 8.75A&B, 8.76A (*top*), 8.82C, 8.83D&E, 8.86A&B, 8.89A, 8.90A, 8.93B, 8.94D&E, 8.95A&B, 8.96A–D, and 8.102A&C.

CHAPTER 9
CRANIAL NERVES

Figures 9.3, 9.5A&B, 9.6A–C, 9.7, 9.8C&D, 9.9A&B, 9.10A, 9.11A&B, 9.13B–F, 9.14A, 9.15C, 9.16B–D, 9.17A,B,D,&E, 9.18A,B,&D, 9.19A, 9.20B, and 9.21.

Additional credits include the following:

CHAPTER 1
BACK

Figure 1.8A&B. Courtesy of J. Heslin, University of Toronto, Ontario, Canada.

Figure 1.8C&D. Courtesy of D. Armstrong, University of Toronto, Ontario, Canada.

Figure 1.9C. Courtesy of D. Salonen, University of Toronto, Ontario, Canada.

Figure 1.21C&D. Courtesy of E. Becker, University of Toronto, Ontario, Canada.

Figure 1.22G. Courtesy of E. Becker, University of Toronto, Ontario, Canada.

Figure 1.23. Modified from Gest TR. *Lippincott Atlas of Anatomy*. 2nd ed. Wolters Kluwer; 2020.

Figure 1.45A–E. Modified from Gest TR. *Lippincott Atlas of Anatomy*. 2nd ed. Wolters Kluwer; 2020.

Figure 1.47A. Based on Foerster O. The dermatomes in man. *Brain*. 1933;56(1):1–39.

Figure 1.52A. Courtesy of The Visible Human Project. National Library of Medicine; Visible Man, 1168.

Figure 1.52B. Dean D, Herbener TE. *Cross-Sectional Human Anatomy*. Lippincott Williams & Wilkins; 2007.

Figure 1.52C. Courtesy of D. Armstrong, University of Toronto, Ontario, Canada.

Figure 1.53A. Courtesy of The Visible Human Project. National Library of Medicine; Visible Man, 1715.

Figure 1.53B. Dean D, Herbener TE. *Cross-Sectional Human Anatomy*. Lippincott Williams & Wilkins; 2007.

Figure 1.54A. Courtesy of The Visible Human Project. National Library of Medicine; Visible Man, 1805.

Figure 1.54B. Dean D, Herbener TE. *Cross-Sectional Human Anatomy.* Lippincott Williams & Wilkins; 2007.

Figure 1.55A–D. Courtesy of D. Salonen, University of Toronto, Ontario, Canada.

CHAPTER 2
UPPER LIMB

Figure 2.2L. Courtesy of D. Armstrong, University of Toronto, Ontario, Canada.

Figure 2.4A–D. Modified from Gest TR. *Lippincott Atlas of Anatomy.* 2nd ed. Wolters Kluwer; 2020.

Figure 2.5A&B. Modified from Gest TR. *Lippincott Atlas of Anatomy.* 2nd ed. Wolters Kluwer; 2020.

Figure 2.6A&B. Modified from Gest TR. *Lippincott Atlas of Anatomy.* 2nd ed. Wolters Kluwer; 2020.

Figure 2.7A&B. Modified from Gest TR. *Lippincott Atlas of Anatomy.* 2nd ed. Wolters Kluwer; 2020.

Figure 2.10A&B. Based on Foerster O. The dermatomes in man. *Brain.* 1933;56(1):1–39.

Figure 2.10C&D. Based on Keegan JJ, Garrett FD. The segmental distribution of the cutaneous nerves in the limbs of man. *Anat Rec.* 1948;102(4):409–437.

Figure 2.27C. Courtesy of D. Armstrong, University of Toronto, Ontario, Canada.

Figure 2.52C. Courtesy of D. Salonen, University of Toronto, Ontario, Canada.

Figure 2.52D. Courtesy of R. Leekam, University of Toronto and West End Diagnostic Imaging, Toronto, Ontario, Canada.

Figure 2.58B&C. Courtesy of J. Heslin, University of Toronto, Ontario, Canada.

Figure 2.59B. Courtesy of D. Salonen, University of Toronto, Ontario, Canada.

Figure 2.64A. Courtesy of K. Sniderman, University of Toronto, Ontario, Canada.

Figure 2.73C. Shutterstock (Zay Nyi Nyi).

Figure 2.83C. Courtesy of D. Armstrong, University of Toronto, Ontario, Canada.

Figure 2.94C&F. Courtesy of D. Armstrong, University of Toronto, Ontario, Canada.

Figure 2.94D. Courtesy of E. Becker, University of Toronto, Ontario, Canada.

Figure 2.100A–C. Courtesy of D. Salonen, University of Toronto, Ontario, Canada.

Figure 2.101B–D. Courtesy of D. Salonen, University of Toronto, Ontario, Canada.

Figure 2.102A–C. Courtesy of D. Salonen, University of Toronto, Ontario, Canada.

Figure 2.103B. Courtesy of R. Leekam, University of Toronto and West End Diagnostic Imaging, Toronto, Ontario, Canada.

CHAPTER 3
THORAX

Figure 3.5C. Kopans DB. *Breast Imaging.* 3rd ed. Lippincott Williams & Wilkins; 2007.

Figure 3.6C. Kopans DB. *Breast Imaging.* 3rd ed. Lippincott Williams & Wilkins; 2007.

Figure 3.36B. Based on *Stedman's Medical Dictionary.* 28th ed. Lippincott Williams & Wilkins; 2006.

Figure 3.38. Courtesy of I. Verschuur, Joint Department of Medical Imaging, UHN/Mount Sinai Hospital, Toronto, Ontario, Canada.

Figure 3.42D&E. Modified from Bickley LS. *Bates' Guide to Physical Examination and History Taking.* 13th ed. Wolters Kluwer; 2021.

Figure 3.43B&E. Courtesy of I. Verschuur, Joint Department of Medical Imaging, UHN/Mount Sinai Hospital, Toronto, Ontario, Canada.

Figure 3.49C. Courtesy of I. Verschuur, Joint Department of Medical Imaging, UHN/Mount Sinai Hospital, Toronto, Ontario, Canada.

Figure 3.50B&D. Courtesy of I. Morrow, University of Manitoba, Canada.

Figure 3.51B. Courtesy of J. Heslin, University of Toronto, Ontario, Canada.

Figure 3.52C. Feigenbaum H, Armstrong WF, Ryan T. *Feigenbaum's Echocardiography.* 5th ed. Lippincott Williams & Wilkins; 2005.

Figure 3.57B. Courtesy of I. Verschuur, Joint Department of Medical Imaging, UHN/Mount Sinai Hospital, Toronto, Ontario, Canada.

Figure 3.64B. Courtesy of E. L. Lansdown, University of Toronto, Ontario, Canada.

Figure 3.80A–E. Courtesy of M. A. Haider, University of Toronto, Ontario, Canada.

Figure 3.81A&B. Courtesy of M. A. Haider, University of Toronto, Ontario, Canada.

Figure 3.82A&B. Courtesy of M. A. Haider, University of Toronto, Ontario, Canada.

Figure 3.83A–E. Courtesy of I. Verschuur, Joint Department of Medical Imaging, UHN/Mount Sinai Hospital, Toronto, Ontario, Canada.

CHAPTER 4
ABDOMEN

Figure 4.32C (*photo*). Mills SE. *Histology for Pathologists.* 5th ed. Wolters Kluwer; 2020.

Figure 4.34A. Dudek RW. *High-Yield Gross Anatomy.* 5th ed. Lippincott Williams & Wilkins; 2015.

Figure 4.34B. Courtesy of J. Heslin, Toronto, Ontario, Canada.

Figure 4.34C&D. Courtesy of E. L. Lansdown, University of Toronto, Ontario, Canada.

Figure 4.36. Courtesy of J. Heslin, Toronto, Ontario, Canada.

Figure 4.42A. Courtesy of E. L. Lansdown, University of Toronto, Ontario, Canada.

Figure 4.42B. Courtesy of C. S. Ho, University of Toronto, Ontario, Canada.

Figure 4.42C&E. Based on *Stedman's Medical Dictionary.* 28th ed. Lippincott Williams & Wilkins; 2006.

Figure 4.42D. Courtesy of Schiller KFR, et al. *A Colour Atlas of Gastrointestinal Endoscopy.* London, United Kingdom: Elsevier, 1986.

Figure 4.45A. Courtesy of E. L. Lansdown, University of Toronto, Ontario, Canada.

Figure 4.45B. Courtesy of J. Heslin, Toronto, Ontario, Canada.

Figure 4.47. Courtesy of K. Sniderman, University of Toronto, Ontario, Canada.

Figure 4.53B. Courtesy of A. M. Arenson, University of Toronto, Ontario, Canada.

Figure 4.61A&B. Courtesy of J. Heslin, Toronto, Ontario, Canada.

Figure 4.63A&C. Courtesy of G. B. Haber, University of Toronto, Ontario, Canada.

Figure 4.66B (*MRI*). Courtesy of E. L. Lansdown, University of Toronto, Ontario, Canada.

Figure 4.66B (*photo*). Courtesy of Mission Hospital Regional Center, Mission Viejo, California.

Figure 4.70D (*MRI*). Schrier RW. *Diseases of the Kidney and Urinary Tract* (Vol. 3). 8th ed. Lippincott Williams & Wilkins; 2007.

Figure 4.70D (*illustration*). Based on Pham PTT, Pham PCT. *Quick Guide to Kidney Transplantation: From Initial Evaluation to Long-Term Post-Transplant Care.* Wolters Kluwer; 2020.

Figure 4.72B. Courtesy of E. L. Lansdown, University of Toronto, Ontario, Canada.

Figure 4.73C. Courtesy of M. Asch, University of Toronto, Ontario, Canada.

Figure 4.90A&C–G. Courtesy of M. A. Haider, University of Toronto, Ontario, Canada.

Figure 4.90B. Courtesy of The Visible Human Project. National Library of Medicine; Visible Man, 1499.

Figure 4.90H. Courtesy of The Visible Human Project. National Library of Medicine; Visible Man, 1625.

Figure 4.91B&D. Courtesy of M. A. Haider, University of Toronto, Ontario, Canada.

Figure 4.92A&C. Courtesy of M. A. Haider, University of Toronto, Ontario, Canada.

Figure 4.92B. Dean D, Herbener TE. *Cross-Sectional Human*. Lippincott Williams & Wilkins; 2007.

Figure 4.93A–C (*ultrasounds*). Courtesy of A. M. Arenson, University of Toronto, Ontario, Canada.

Figure 4.93D&E. J. Lai, University of Toronto, Ontario, Canada.

Figure 4.93F. Dean D, Herbener TE. *Cross-Sectional Human*. Lippincott Williams & Wilkins; 2007.

CHAPTER 5
PELVIS AND PERINEUM

Figure 5.7A&B. Wineski LE. *Snell's Clinical Anatomy by Regions*. 10th ed. Wolters Kluwer; 2019.

Figure 5.21B. Courtesy of M. A. Haider, University of Toronto, Ontario, Canada.

Figure 5.21C. Courtesy of A. M. Arenson, University of Toronto, Ontario, Canada.

Figure 5.21F. With permission from R. E. Bristow.

Figure 5.25A–C. Courtesy of A. M. Arenson, University of Toronto, Ontario, Canada.

Figure 5.25D. Courtesy of Donald R. Cahill, Department of Anatomy, Mayo Medical School, Rochester, MN.

Figure 5.26B. Wineski LE. *Snell's Clinical Anatomy by Regions*. 10th ed. Wolters Kluwer; 2019.

Figure 5.26D. Doubilet PM, Benson CB, Benacerraf BR. *Atlas of Ultrasound in Obstetrics and Gynecology*. 3rd ed. Wolters Kluwer; 2019.

Figure 5.27C. Courtesy of J. Heslin, University of Toronto, Ontario, Canada.

Figure 5.27D. Sadler TW. *Langman's Medical Embryology*. 15th ed. Wolters Kluwer; 2024.

Figure 5.34B. Courtesy of M. A. Haider, University of Toronto, Ontario, Canada.

Figure 5.34C. Courtesy of The Visible Human Project. National Library of Medicine; Visible Woman, 1870.

Figure 5.39B&D. Courtesy of M. A. Haider, University of Toronto, Ontario, Canada.

Figure 5.39E. Modified from Bickley LS. *Bates' Guide to Physical Examination and History Taking*. 13th ed. Wolters Kluwer; 2021.

Figure 5.40B. Courtesy of A. Toi, University of Toronto, Ontario, Canada.

Figure 5.40D. Courtesy of A. M. Arenson, University of Toronto, Ontario, Canada.

Figure 5.55A–D,F,&H. Courtesy of M. A. Haider, University of Toronto, Ontario, Canada.

Figure 5.65B&E–H. Courtesy of Dr. M. A. Haider, University of Toronto, Ontario, Canada.

Figure 5.65C. Courtesy of The Visible Human Project. National Library of Medicine; Visible Man, 1940.

Figure 5.66. Courtesy of J. Heslin, University of Toronto, Ontario, Canada.

CHAPTER 6
LOWER LIMB

Figure 6.3A. Courtesy of P. Babyn, University of Toronto, Ontario, Canada.

Figure 6.3C. Reprinted with permission from Dean D, Herbener TE. *Cross-Sectional Human Anatomy*. Lippincott Williams & Wilkins; 2007.

Figure 6.5A&C. Modified from Gest TR. *Lippincott Atlas of Anatomy*. 2nd ed. Wolters Kluwer; 2020.

Figure 6.6A&C. Modified from Gest TR. *Lippincott Atlas of Anatomy*. 2nd ed. Wolters Kluwer; 2020.

Figure 6.7A–C. Modified from Gest TR. *Lippincott Atlas of Anatomy*. 2nd ed. Wolters Kluwer; 2020.

Figure 6.8A–C. Modified from Gest TR. *Lippincott Atlas of Anatomy*. 2nd ed. Wolters Kluwer; 2020.

Figure 6.9A&B. Based on Foerster O. The dermatomes in man. *Brain*. 1933;56(1):1–39.

Figure 6.9C&D. Based on Keegan JJ, Garrett FD. The segmental distribution of the cutaneous nerves in the limbs of man. *Anat Rec*. 1948;102(4):409–437.

Figure 6.10B&C. Modified from Bickley LS. *Bates' Guide to Physical Examination and History Taking*. 13th ed. Wolters Kluwer; 2021.

Figure 6.12C. Modified from Bickley LS. *Bates' Guide to Physical Examination and History Taking*. 13th ed. Wolters Kluwer; 2021.

Figure 6.15D. Modified from *Stedman's Medical Dictionary*. 28th ed. Lippincott Williams & Wilkins; 2006.

Figure 6.17B. Courtesy of E. L. Lansdown, University of Toronto, Ontario, Canada.

Figure 6.37A&B. Modified from Gest TR. *Lippincott Atlas of Anatomy*. 2nd ed. Wolters Kluwer; 2020.

Figure 6.42A. Courtesy of E. Becker, University of Toronto, Ontario, Canada.

Figure 6.42C. Courtesy of D. Salonen, University of Toronto, Ontario, Canada.

Figure 6.52C. *Stedman's Medical Dictionary*. 28th ed. Lippincott Williams & Wilkins; 2006.

Figure 6.59B. Courtesy of P. Bobechko, University of Toronto, Ontario, Canada.

Figure 6.59C&D. Courtesy of D. Salonen, University of Toronto, Ontario, Canada.

Figure 6.68B. Reprinted with permission from Cordasco FA, Green DW, eds. *Pediatric and Adolescent Knee Surgery*. Wolters Kluwer; 2015.

Figure 6.73A. Courtesy of D. K. Sniderman, University of Toronto, Ontario, Canada.

Figure 6.85B. Courtesy of E. Becker, University of Toronto, Ontario, Canada.

Figure 6.88B. Courtesy of W. Kucharczyk, University of Toronto, Ontario, Canada.

Figure 6.89B. Courtesy of W. Kucharczyk, University of Toronto, Ontario, Canada.

Figure 6.92B. Weber JR, Kelley JH. *Health Assessment in Nursing*. 7th ed. Wolters Kluwer; 2022.

Figure 6.93E. Courtesy of P. Bobechko, University of Toronto, Ontario, Canada.

Figure 6.95B&D–F. Courtesy of D. Salonen, University of Toronto, Ontario, Canada.

Figure 6.97A–D. Courtesy of D. Salonen, University of Toronto, Ontario, Canada.

CHAPTER 7
NECK

Figure 7.5B. Courtesy of J. Heslin, University of Toronto, Ontario, Canada.

Figure 7.15D. Courtesy of D. Armstrong, University of Toronto, Ontario, Canada.

Figure 7.28A. Modified from Gest TR. *Lippincott Atlas of Anatomy*. 2nd ed. Wolters Kluwer; 2020.

Figure 7.34A. Rohen JW, Yokochi C, Lütjen-Drecoll E. *Photographic Atlas of Anatomy*. 9th ed. Wolters Kluwer; 2022.

Figure 7.34C. Courtesy of D. Salonen, University of Toronto, Ontario, Canada.

Figure 7.37A–C. Courtesy of D. Salonen, University of Toronto, Ontario, Canada.

Figure 7.39A. Courtesy of E. Becker, University of Toronto, Ontario, Canada.

Figure 7.40A. Siemens Medical Solutions USA, Inc.

Figure 7.40B. Modified from Gest TR. *Lippincott Atlas of Anatomy*. 2nd ed. Wolters Kluwer; 2020.

Figure 7.41A–D. Courtesy of R. Leekam, University of Toronto and West End Diagnostic Imaging, Toronto, Ontario, Canada.

CHAPTER 8

HEAD

Figure 8.1B,E,&F. Courtesy of D. Armstrong, University of Toronto, Ontario, Canada.

Figure 8.15A. Based on Tank PW, Gest TR. *Lippincott Williams & Wilkins Atlas of Anatomy*. Lippincott Williams & Wilkins; 2009.

Figure 8.15B. Based on Gest TR. *Lippincott Atlas of Anatomy*. 2nd ed. Wolters Kluwer; 2020.

Figure 8.34A–C. Courtesy of D. Armstrong, University of Toronto, Ontario, Canada.

Figure 8.35A&B. Courtesy of W. Kucharczyk, University of Toronto, Ontario, Canada.

Figure 8.38D. Courtesy of W. Kucharczyk, University of Toronto, Ontario, Canada.

Figure 8.39D. Courtesy of W. Kucharczyk, University of Toronto, Ontario, Canada.

Figure 8.46A. Courtesy of J. R. Buncic, University of Toronto, Ontario, Canada.

Figure 8.56D&E. Courtesy of Susanne Perschbacher.

Figure 8.56F (*radiography*). Courtesy of Teodora-Iunia Gheorghe.

Figure 8.59A. Modified from Gest TR. *Lippincott Atlas of Anatomy*. 2nd ed. Wolters Kluwer; 2020.

Figure 8.65B. Courtesy of Teodora-Iunia Gheorghe.

Figure 8.68B&D. Courtesy of Teodora-Iunia Gheorghe.

Figure 8.69E. Courtesy of B. Libgott, Division of Anatomy/Department of Surgery, University of Toronto, Ontario, Canada.

Figure 8.80B. Courtesy of D. Armstrong, University of Toronto, Ontario, Canada.

Figure 8.80C. Courtesy of E. Becker, University of Toronto, Ontario, Canada.

Figure 8.81B. Courtesy of E. Becker, University of Toronto, Ontario, Canada.

Figure 8.88D. *Stedman's Medical Dictionary*. 28th ed. Lippincott Williams & Wilkins; 2006.

Figure 8.98B&C. Courtesy of W. Kucharczyk, University of Toronto, Ontario, Canada.

Figure 8.99B. Courtesy of W. Kucharczyk, University of Toronto, Ontario, Canada.

Figure 8.100A. Courtesy of The Visible Human Project. National Library of Medicine; Visible Man, 1007.

Figure 8.100C. Courtesy of The Visible Human Project. National Library of Medicine; Visible Man, 1068.

Figure 8.100B&D. Dean D, Herbener TE. *Cross-Sectional Human*. Lippincott Williams & Wilkins; 2007.

Figure 8.103A–F. Colorized from photographs provided courtesy of Dr. C. G. Smith, which appears in Smith CG. *Serial Dissections of the Human Brain*. Urban & Schwarzenberg Inc/Gage Publishing Ltd; 1981. (© Carlton G. Smith)

Figure 8.104A–E. Colorized from photographs provided courtesy of Dr. C. G. Smith, which appears in Smith CG. *Serial Dissections of the Human Brain*. Urban & Schwarzenberg Inc/Gage Publishing Ltd; 1981. (© Carlton G. Smith)

Figure 8.105A&B. Colorized from photographs provided courtesy of Dr. C. G. Smith, which appears in Smith CG. *Serial Dissections of the Human Brain*. Urban & Schwarzenberg Inc/Gage Publishing Ltd; 1981. (© Carlton G. Smith)

Figure 8.106A&B. Colorized from photographs provided courtesy of Dr. C. G. Smith, which appears in Smith CG. *Serial Dissections of the Human Brain*. Urban & Schwarzenberg Inc/Gage Publishing Ltd; 1981. (© Carlton G. Smith)

Figure 8.108A–C. Colorized from photographs provided courtesy of Dr. C. G. Smith, which appears in Smith CG. *Serial Dissections of the Human Brain*. Urban & Schwarzenberg Inc/Gage Publishing Ltd; 1981. (© Carlton G. Smith)

Figure 8.109A–C. Colorized from photographs provided courtesy of Dr. C. G. Smith, which appears in Smith CG. *Serial Dissections of the Human Brain*. Urban & Schwarzenberg Inc/Gage Publishing Ltd; 1981. (© Carlton G. Smith)

Figure 8.110A–D. Colorized from photographs provided courtesy of Dr. C. G. Smith, which appears in Smith CG. *Serial Dissections of the Human Brain*. Urban & Schwarzenberg Inc/Gage Publishing Ltd; 1981. (© Carlton G. Smith)

Figure 8.111A–E (*MRIs*). Courtesy of D. Armstrong, University of Toronto, Ontario, Canada.

Figure 8.112A–F. Courtesy of D. Armstrong, University of Toronto, Ontario, Canada.

Figure 8.112G&H. Colorized from photographs provided courtesy of Dr. C. G. Smith, which appears in Smith CG. *Serial Dissections of the Human Brain*. Urban & Schwarzenberg Inc/Gage Publishing Ltd; 1981. (© Carlton G. Smith)

Figure 8.113A–C. Courtesy of D. Armstrong, University of Toronto, Ontario, Canada.

CHAPTER 9

CRANIAL NERVES

Figure 9.10B. Based on Melloni JL. *Melloni's Illustrated Review of Human Anatomy: By Structures—Arteries, Bones, Muscles, Nerves, Veins*. Lippincott Williams & Wilkins; 1988.

Figure 9.15B. Based on Gest TR. *Lippincott Atlas of Anatomy*. 2nd ed. Wolters Kluwer; 2020.

Figure 9.22C. Bickley LS. *Bates' Guide to Physical Examination and History Taking*. 13th ed. Wolters Kluwer; 2021.

Figure 9.22D. Weber J, Kelley JH. *Health Assessment in Nursing*. 4th ed. Wolters Kluwer Health, 2010.

Figure 9.22F. Modified from Campbell WW, Barohn RJ. *DeJong's The Neurologic Examination*. 8th ed. Wolters Kluwer; 2020.

Figure 9.23A–F. Courtesy of W. Kucharczyk, University of Toronto, Ontario, Canada.

Figure 9.24A–C. Courtesy of W. Kucharczyk, University of Toronto, Ontario, Canada.

REFERENCES

CHAPTER 1
Foerster O. The dermatomes in man. *Brain*. 1933;56(1):1–39.

CHAPTER 2
Foerster O. The dermatomes in man. *Brain*. 1933;56(1):1–39.
Keegan JJ, Garrett FD. The segmental distribution of the cutaneous nerves in the limbs of man. *Anat Rec*. 1948;102(4):409–437.

CHAPTER 3
Sadler TW. *Langman's Medical Embryology*. 15th ed. Wolters Kluwer; 2024.

CHAPTER 6
Foerster O. The dermatomes in man. *Brain*. 1933;56(1):1–39.
Keegan JJ, Garrett FD. The segmental distribution of the cutaneous nerves in the limbs of man. *Anat Rec*. 1948;102(4):409–437.

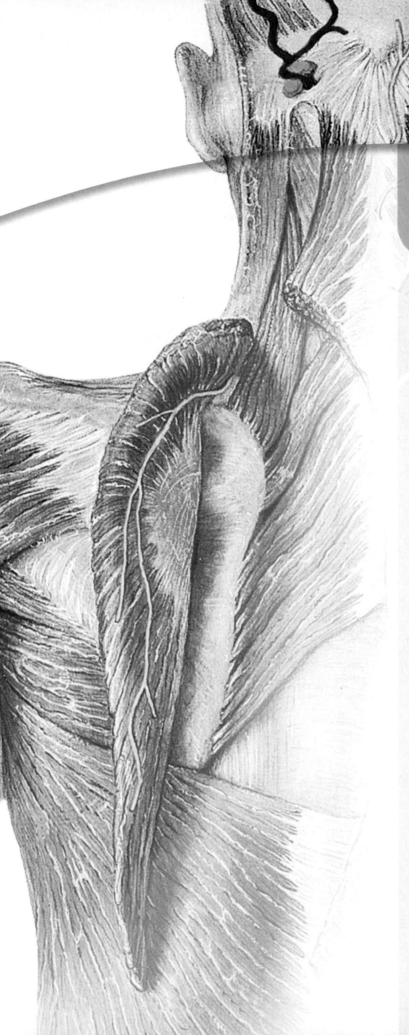

CHAPTER 1

BACK

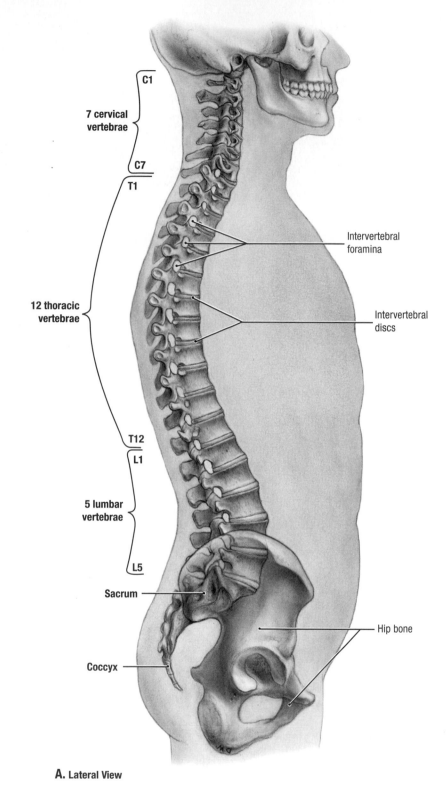

A. Lateral View

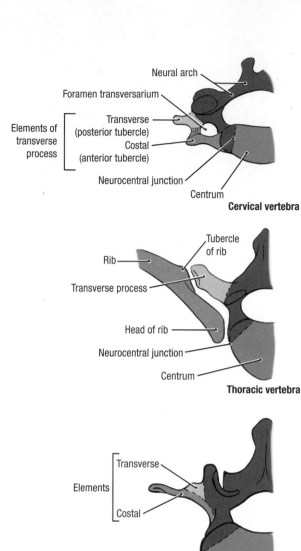

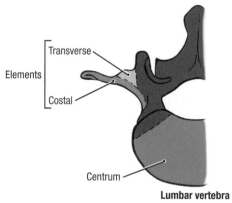

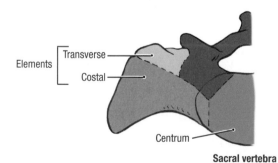

B. Superior Views

1.1   Overview of Vertebral Column

A. Vertebral column articulating with cranium and pelvic girdle.

- The vertebral column usually consists of 24 separate (presacral) vertebrae, 5 fused vertebrae in the sacrum, and 4 variably fused or separated coccygeal vertebrae. Of the 24 separate vertebrae, 7 are in the neck (cervical vertebrae), 12 support the ribs (thoracic vertebrae), and 5 are in the lower back (lumbar vertebrae).

- The spinal nerves exit the vertebral (spinal) canal via the intervertebral (IV) foramina.

B. Homologous parts of vertebrae. A rib is a free costal element in the thoracic region; in the cervical and lumbar regions, it is represented by the anterior part of a transverse process, and in the sacrum, by the anterior part of the lateral mass.

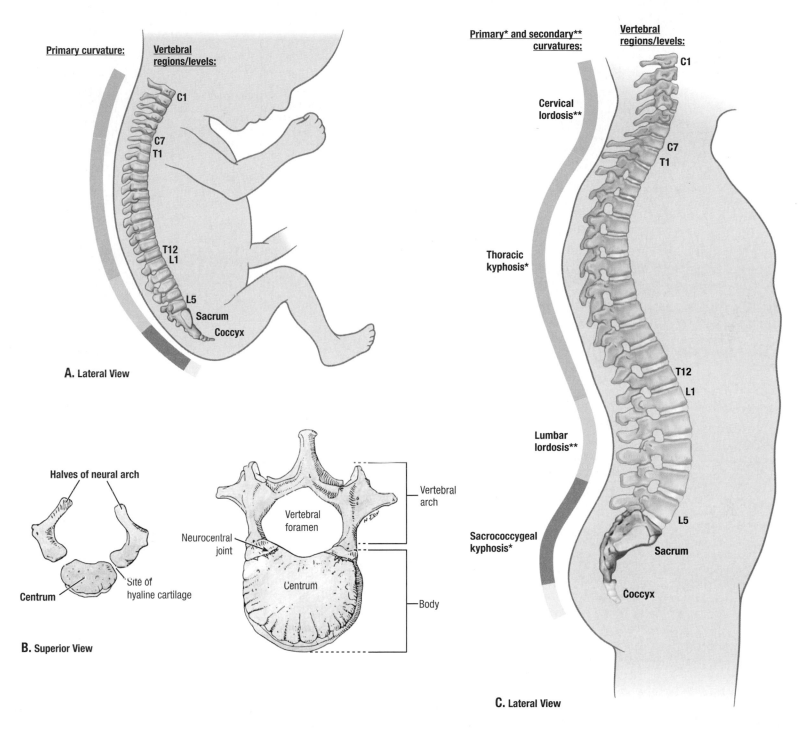

Primary curvature:

Vertebral regions/levels:

C1

C7
T1

T12
L1

L5

Sacrum

Coccyx

A. Lateral View

Halves of neural arch

Centrum

Site of hyaline cartilage

B. Superior View

Neurocentral joint

Vertebral foramen

Centrum

Vertebral arch

Body

Primary* and secondary** curvatures:

Vertebral regions/levels:

C1

Cervical lordosis**

C7
T1

Thoracic kyphosis*

T12
L1

Lumbar lordosis**

Sacrococcygeal kyphosis*

L5

Sacrum

Coccyx

C. Lateral View

Curvatures of Vertebral Column

1.2

A. Fetus. Note the C-shaped curvature of the fetal spine, which is concave anteriorly over its entire length. **B. Development of vertebrae.** At birth, a vertebra consists of three bony parts (two halves of the neural arch and the centrum) united by hyaline cartilage. At age 2, the halves of each neural arch begin to fuse, proceeding from the lumbar to the cervical region; at approximately age 7, the arches begin to fuse to the centrum, proceeding from the cervical to lumbar regions. **C. Adult.** The four curvatures of the adult vertebral column include the cervical lordosis, which is convex anteriorly and lies between vertebrae C1 and T2; the thoracic

kyphosis, which is concave anteriorly and lies between vertebrae T2 and T12; the lumbar lordosis, which is convex anteriorly and lies between T12 and the lumbosacral joint; and the sacrococcygeal kyphosis, which is concave anteriorly and spans from the lumbosacral joint to the tip of the coccyx. The anteriorly concave thoracic kyphosis and sacrococcygeal kyphosis are primary curves, and the anteriorly convex cervical lordosis and lumbar lordosis are secondary curves that develop after birth. The cervical lordosis develops when the child begins to hold the head up, and the lumbar kyphosis develops when the child begins to walk.

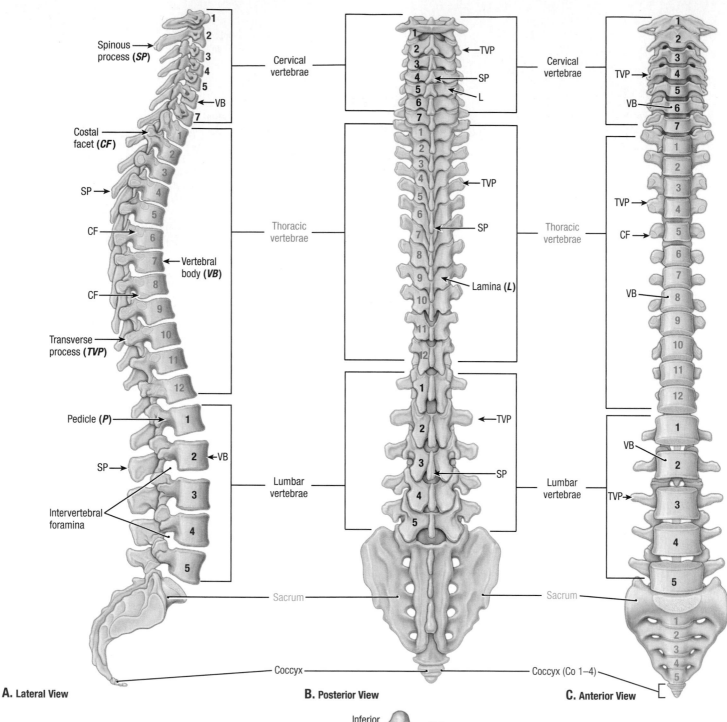

Spinous process (*SP*)

Costal facet (*CF*)

SP

CF

Vertebral body (*VB*)

CF

Transverse process (*TVP*)

Pedicle (*P*)

SP

Intervertebral foramina

VB

A. Lateral View

Cervical vertebrae

Thoracic vertebrae

Lumbar vertebrae

Sacrum

Coccyx

TVP

SP

L

TVP

SP

Lamina (*L*)

TVP

SP

Coccyx (Co 1–4)

B. Posterior View

Cervical vertebrae

Thoracic vertebrae

Lumbar vertebrae

Sacrum

TVP

VB

TVP

CF

VB

VB

TVP

C. Anterior View

1.3 Aspects and Parts of Vertebral Column

A. Lateral aspect. Intervertebral foramina provide exit for spinal nerves. **B. Posterior aspect.** Thoracic spinous processes overlap vertebra below. **C. Anterior aspect.** Intervertebral discs are located where gaps appear between the vertebral bodies (as in *Part A*). **D.** and **E.** Parts of a typical **vertebra** (e.g., the 2nd lumbar vertebra).

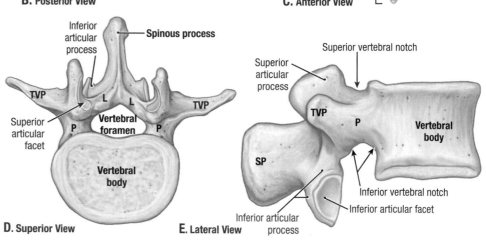

Inferior articular process

Spinous process

TVP

Superior articular facet

P

L   L

TVP

P

Vertebral foramen

Vertebral body

D. Superior View

Superior vertebral notch

Superior articular process

TVP

P

SP

Vertebral body

Inferior vertebral notch

Inferior articular facet

Inferior articular process

E. Lateral View

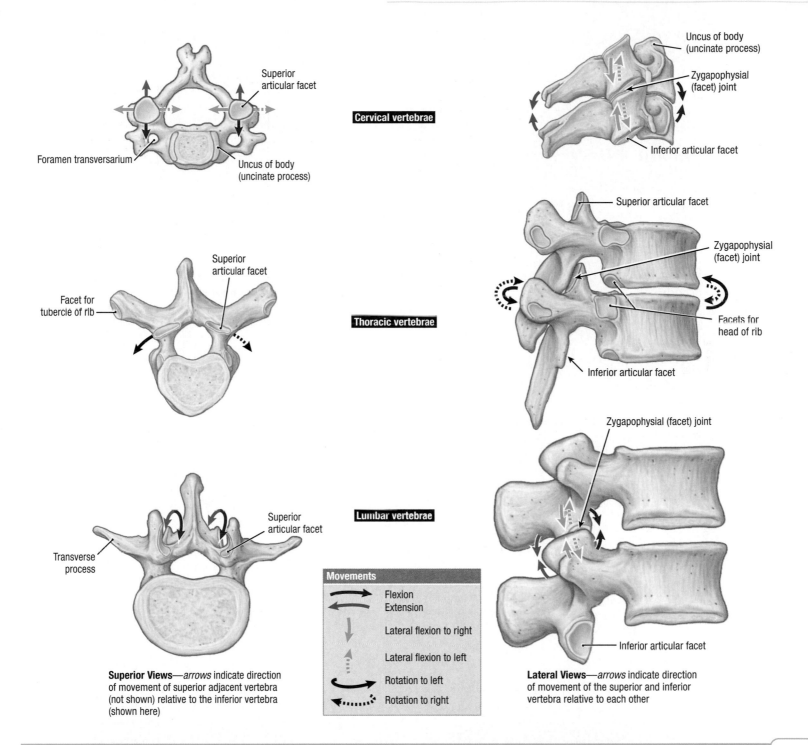

Cervical vertebrae

Superior articular facet

Foramen transversarium

Uncus of body (uncinate process)

Uncus of body (uncinate process)

Zygapophysial (facet) joint

Inferior articular facet

Thoracic vertebrae

Superior articular facet

Facet for tubercle of rib

Superior articular facet

Zygapophysial (facet) joint

Facets for head of rib

Inferior articular facet

Lumbar vertebrae

Transverse process

Superior articular facet

Zygapophysial (facet) joint

Inferior articular facet

Movements

Flexion
Extension

Lateral flexion to right

Lateral flexion to left

Rotation to left

Rotation to right

Superior Views—*arrows* indicate direction of movement of superior adjacent vertebra (not shown) relative to the inferior vertebra (shown here)

Lateral Views—*arrows* indicate direction of movement of the superior and inferior vertebra relative to each other

Vertebral Features and Movements

1.4

- In the thoracic and lumbar regions, the articular processes/facets lie posterior to the vertebral bodies and in the cervical region posterolateral to the bodies. Superior articular facets in the cervical region face mainly superiorly; in the thoracic region, mainly posteriorly; and in the lumbar region, mainly medially. The change in direction is gradual from cervical to thoracic but abrupt from thoracic to lumbar.
- Although movements between adjacent vertebrae are relatively small, the summation of all the small movements produces a considerable range of movement of the vertebral column as a whole.

- Movements of the vertebral column are freer (have greater range of motion) in the cervical and lumbar regions than in the thoracic region. Lateral bending is freest in the cervical and lumbar regions; flexion is greatest in the cervical region; extension is most marked in the lumbar region, but the interlocking articular processes prevent rotation.
- The thoracic region is the most stable because of the external support gained from the articulations of the ribs and costal cartilages with the sternum. The direction of the articular facets permits rotation, but flexion, extension, and lateral bending are severely restricted.

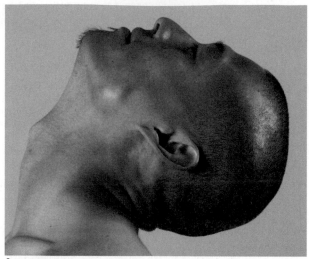

A. Lateral View

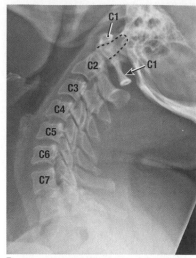

B. Lateral Radiograph

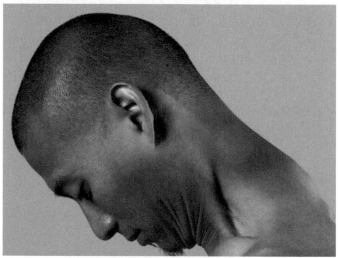

C. Lateral View

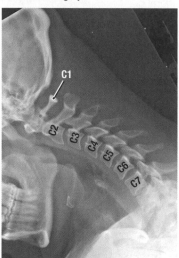

D. Lateral Radiograph

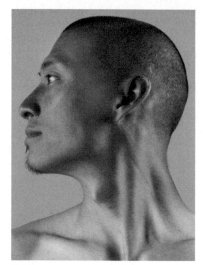

E. Anterior View, Head Rotated to Right

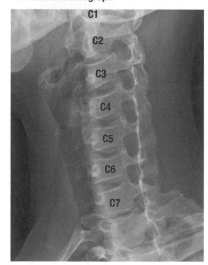

F. Oblique Radiograph

1.5 **Surface Anatomy with Radiographic Correlation of Selected Movements of Cervical Spine**

A. Extension of neck. **B.** Radiograph of extended cervical spine. (*Dashed line,* den of axis.) **C.** Flexion of neck. **D.** Radiograph of flexed cervical spine. **E.** Head rotated to right. **F.** Radiograph of cervical spine rotated to left.

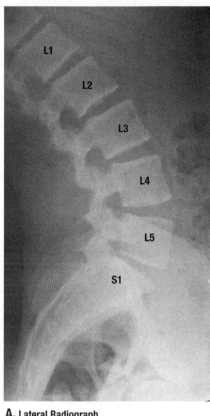

A. Lateral Radiograph

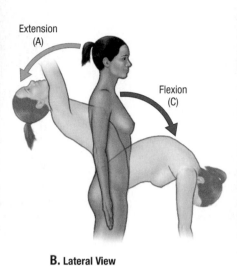

Extension
(A)

Flexion
(C)

B. Lateral View

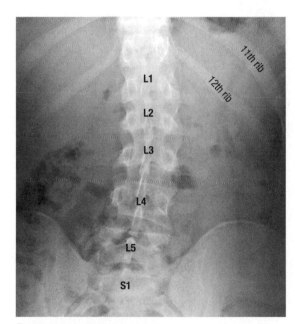

C. Lateral Radiograph

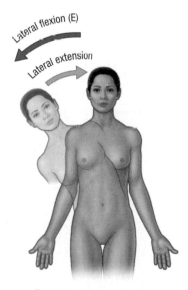

Lateral flexion (E)

Lateral extension

D. Anterior View

E. Anteroposterior Radiograph

Surface Anatomy with Radiographic Correlation of Selected Movements of Lumbar Spine   **1.6**

A. Extended lumbar spine. **B.** Schematic of flexion and extension of trunk. **C.** Flexed lumbar spine. **D.** Schematic of lateral (sideways bending) flexion of trunk. **E.** Lumbar spine during lateral bending.

The range of movement of the vertebral column is limited by the thickness, elasticity, and compressibility of the IV discs; the shape and orientation of the zygapophysial joints; tension of the joint capsules of the zygapophysial joints; resistance of the ligaments and back muscles; connection to thoracic (rib) cage; and bulk of surrounding tissue.

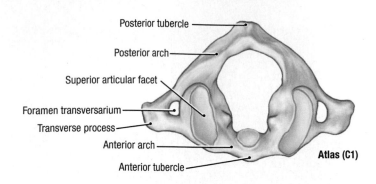

Atlas (C1)

Posterior tubercle
Posterior arch
Superior articular facet
Foramen transversarium
Transverse process
Anterior arch
Anterior tubercle

1.7 Cervical Spine

A. Disarticulated cervical vertebrae. The bodies of the cervical vertebrae can be dislocated in neck injuries with less force than is required to fracture them. Because of the large vertebral canal in the cervical region, some dislocation can occur without damaging the spinal cord. When a cervical vertebra is severely dislocated, it injures the spinal cord. If the dislocation does not result in "facet jumping" with locking of the displaced articular processes, the cervical vertebrae may self-reduce ("slip back into place") so that a radiograph may not indicate that the cord has been injured. Magnetic resonance imaging (MRI) may reveal the resulting soft tissue damage.

Aging of the IV disc combined with the changing shape of the vertebrae results in an increase in compressive forces at the periphery of the vertebral bodies, where the disc attaches. In response, *osteophytes* (bony spurs) commonly develop around the margins of the vertebral body, especially along the outer attachment of the IV disc. Similarly, as altered mechanics place greater stresses on the zygapophysial joints, osteophytes develop along the attachments of the joint capsules, especially those of the superior articular process.

TABLE 1.1	Typical Cervical Vertebrae (C3–C6)[a]
Part	**Distinctive Characteristics**
Body	Small and wider from side to side than anteroposteriorly; superior surface is concave with an uncus of body (uncinate process bilaterally); inferior surface is convex
Vertebral foramen	Large and triangular
Transverse processes	Foramina transversaria small or absent in vertebra C7; vertebral arteries and accompanying venous and sympathetic plexuses pass through foramina, except C7 foramina, which transmits only small accessory vertebral veins; anterior and posterior tubercles separated by groove for spinal nerve
Articular processes	Superior articular facets directed superoposteriorly; inferior articular facets directed inferoanteriorly; obliquely placed facets are most nearly horizontal in this region
Spinous process	Short (C3–C5) and bifid, only in Caucasians (C3–C5); process of C6 is long but that of C7 is longer; C7 is called "vertebra prominens"

 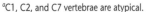
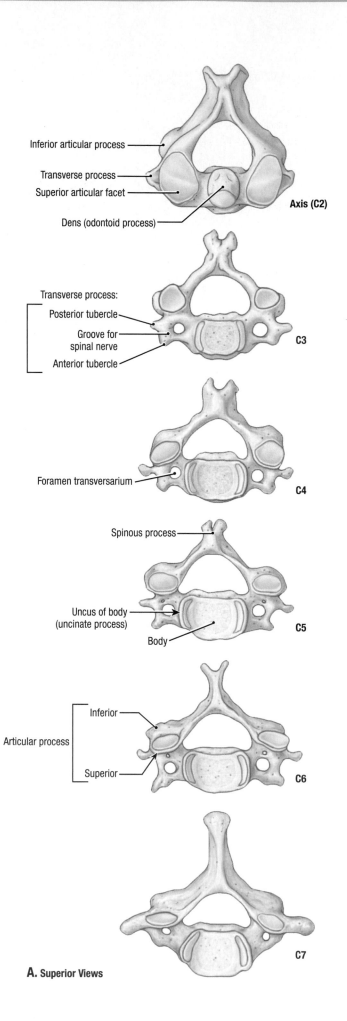

Axis (C2)

Inferior articular process
Transverse process
Superior articular facet
Dens (odontoid process)

Transverse process:
  Posterior tubercle
  Groove for spinal nerve
  Anterior tubercle
C3

Foramen transversarium
C4

Spinous process
Uncus of body (uncinate process)
Body
C5

Articular process
  Inferior
  Superior
C6

C7

A. Superior Views

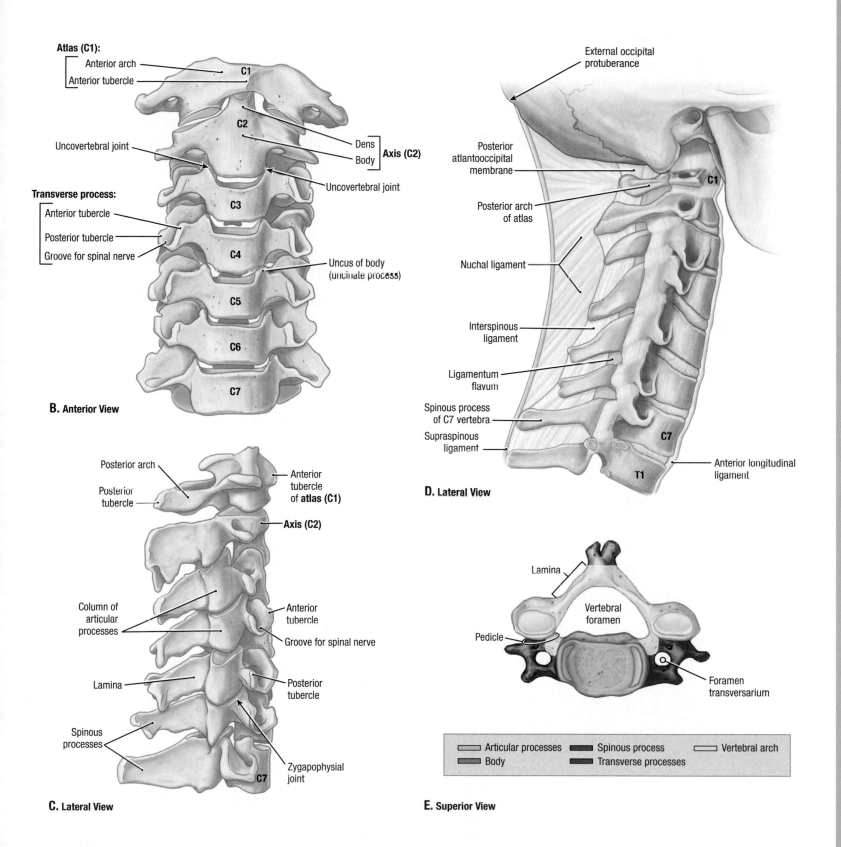

B. Anterior View

C. Lateral View

D. Lateral View

E. Superior View

Atlas (C1):
- Anterior arch
- Anterior tubercle

C1

C2

Uncovertebral joint

Dens
Body
Axis (C2)

Uncovertebral joint

Transverse process:
- Anterior tubercle
- Posterior tubercle
- Groove for spinal nerve

C3

C4

Uncus of body
(uncinate process)

C5

C6

C7

Posterior arch

Posterior tubercle

Anterior tubercle of **atlas (C1)**

Axis (C2)

Column of articular processes

Anterior tubercle

Groove for spinal nerve

Lamina

Posterior tubercle

Spinous processes

Zygapophysial joint

C7

External occipital protuberance

Posterior atlantooccipital membrane

C1

Posterior arch of atlas

Nuchal ligament

Interspinous ligament

Ligamentum flavum

Spinous process of C7 vertebra

Supraspinous ligament

C7

T1

Anterior longitudinal ligament

Lamina

Vertebral foramen

Pedicle

Foramen transversarium

Articular processes   Spinous process   Vertebral arch
Body   Transverse processes

Cervical Spine (continued)   **1.7**

B. and **C.** Articulated cervical vertebrae. **D.** Ligaments. **E.** Parts of a typical cervical vertebra.

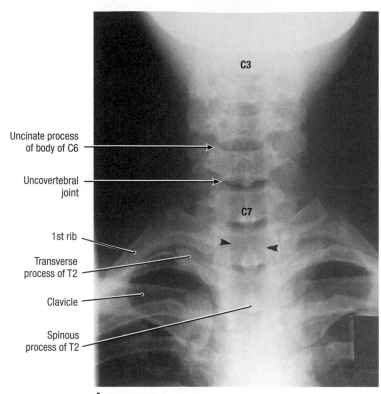

Uncinate process of body of C6

Uncovertebral joint

1st rib

Transverse process of T2

Clavicle

Spinous process of T2

A. Anteroposterior Radiograph

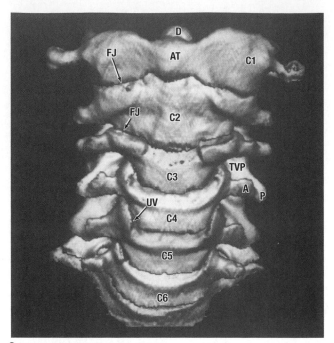

C. 3D CT Reconstruction, Anterior View

A	Anterior tubercle of transverse process	**PA**	Posterior arch of C1
AA	Anterior arch of C1	**PT**	Posterior tubercle of C1
AT	Anterior tubercle of C1	**SF**	Superior articular facet of C1
C1–C7	Vertebrae	**SP**	Spinous process
D	Dens (odontoid) process of C2	**T**	Foramen transversarium
FJ	Zygapophysial (facet) joint	**TVP**	Transverse process
La	Lamina	**UV**	Uncovertebral joint
P	Posterior tubercle of transverse process	**VC**	Vertebral canal

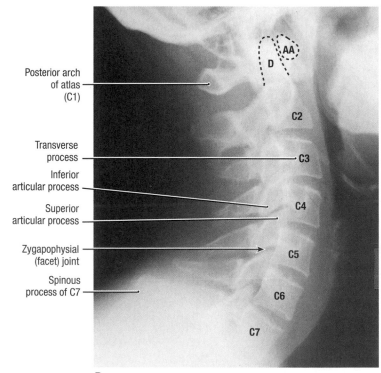

Posterior arch of atlas (C1)

Transverse process

Inferior articular process

Superior articular process

Zygapophysial (facet) joint

Spinous process of C7

B. Lateral Radiograph

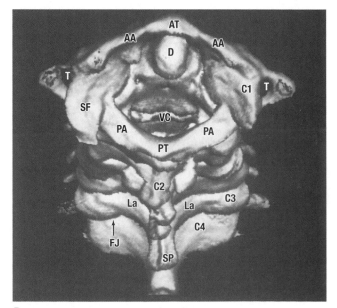

D. 3D CT Reconstruction, Posterosuperior View

1.8 **Imaging of Cervical Spine**

A. and **B. Radiographs.** The *arrowheads* demarcate the margins of the (*black*) column of air in the trachea. **C.** and **D.** Three-dimensional reconstructed computed tomographic (CT) images.

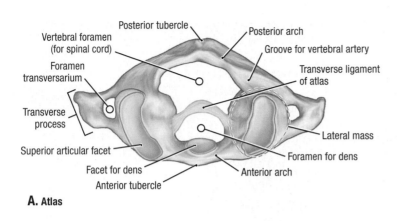

A. Atlas

Posterior tubercle

Posterior arch

Vertebral foramen (for spinal cord)

Groove for vertebral artery

Foramen transversarium

Transverse ligament of atlas

Transverse process

Lateral mass

Superior articular facet

Foramen for dens

Facet for dens

Anterior arch

Anterior tubercle

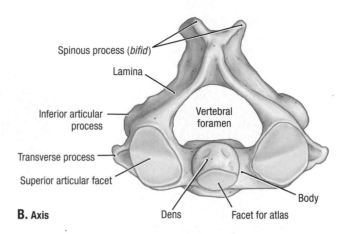

B. Axis

Spinous process (*bifid*)

Lamina

Inferior articular process

Vertebral foramen

Transverse process

Superior articular facet

Dens

Facet for atlas

Body

Superior Views

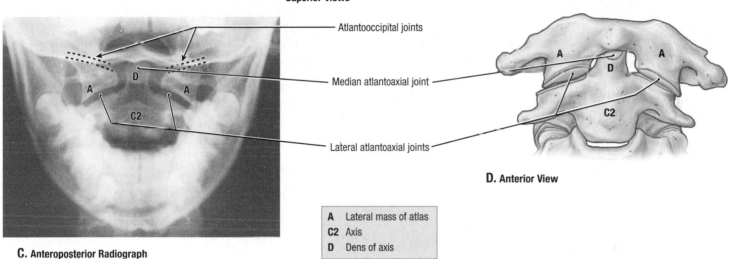

C. Anteroposterior Radiograph

Atlantooccipital joints

Median atlantoaxial joint

Lateral atlantoaxial joints

D. Anterior View

A	Lateral mass of atlas
C2	Axis
D	Dens of axis

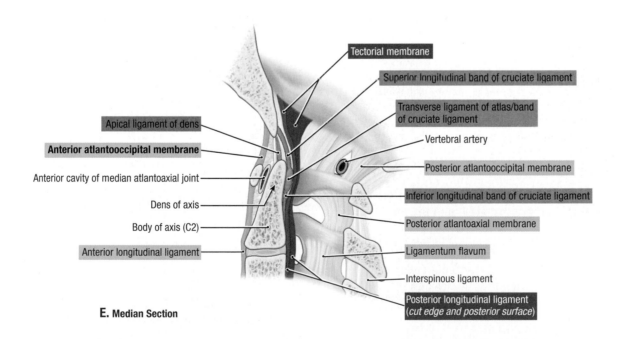

E. Median Section

Tectorial membrane

Superior longitudinal band of cruciate ligament

Apical ligament of dens

Transverse ligament of atlas/band of cruciate ligament

Anterior atlantooccipital membrane

Vertebral artery

Anterior cavity of median atlantoaxial joint

Posterior atlantooccipital membrane

Dens of axis

Inferior longitudinal band of cruciate ligament

Body of axis (C2)

Posterior atlantoaxial membrane

Anterior longitudinal ligament

Ligamentum flavum

Interspinous ligament

Posterior longitudinal ligament (*cut edge and posterior surface*)

Atlas and Axis and Atlantoaxial Joints

A. Atlas. **B.** Axis. **C.** Atlantoaxial joints in vivo (via open mouth). **D.** Articulated atlas and axis. **E.** Median section with ligaments (structures highlighted in same color are continuous).

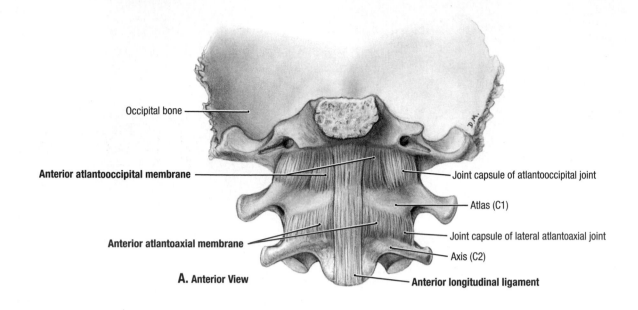

Occipital bone

Anterior atlantooccipital membrane

Joint capsule of atlantooccipital joint

Atlas (C1)

Joint capsule of lateral atlantoaxial joint

Anterior atlantoaxial membrane

Axis (C2)

A. Anterior View

Anterior longitudinal ligament

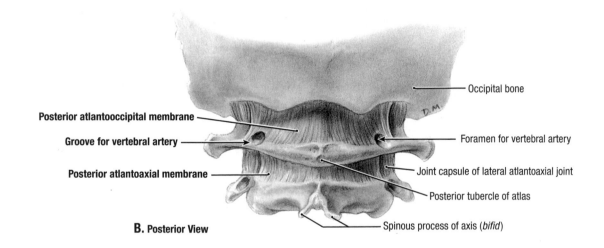

Occipital bone

Posterior atlantooccipital membrane

Groove for vertebral artery

Foramen for vertebral artery

Posterior atlantoaxial membrane

Joint capsule of lateral atlantoaxial joint

Posterior tubercle of atlas

B. Posterior View

Spinous process of axis (*bifid*)

1.10   Craniovertebral Joints and Vertebral Artery

A. Anterior atlantoaxial and atlantooccipital membranes.
The anterior longitudinal ligament ascends to blend with, and
form a central thickening in, the anterior atlantoaxial and atlantooccipital membranes. **B. Posterior atlantoaxial and atlantooccipital membranes.** Inferior to the axis (C2 vertebra), ligamenta
flava occur in this position. **C. Tectorial membrane and vertebral artery.** The tectorial membrane is a superior continuation
of the posterior longitudinal ligament superior to the body of
the axis. After coursing through the foramina transversaria of
vertebrae C6–C1, the vertebral arteries turn medially, grooving
the superior aspect of the posterior arch of the atlas and piercing
the posterior atlantooccipital membrane (*Part B*). The right and
left vertebral arteries traverse the foramen magnum and merge
intracranially, forming the basilar artery.

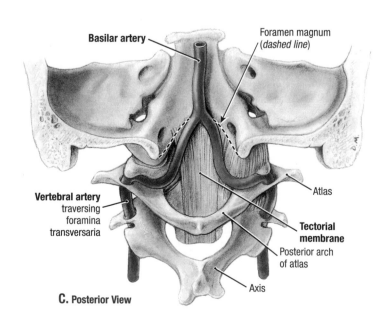

Basilar artery

Foramen magnum
(*dashed line*)

Vertebral artery
traversing
foramina
transversaria

Atlas

**Tectorial
membrane**

Posterior arch
of atlas

Axis

C. Posterior View

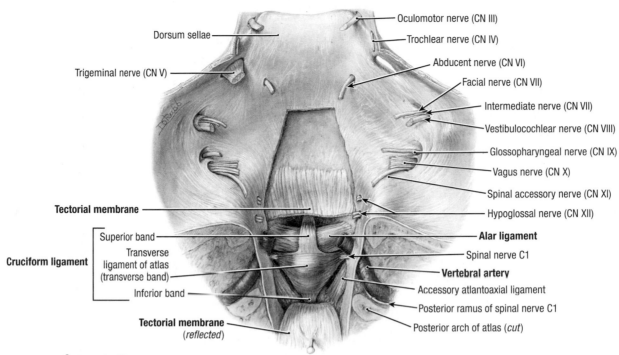

Dorsum sellae
Trigeminal nerve (CN V)
Oculomotor nerve (CN III)
Trochlear nerve (CN IV)
Abducent nerve (CN VI)
Facial nerve (CN VII)
Intermediate nerve (CN VII)
Vestibulocochlear nerve (CN VIII)
Glossopharyngeal nerve (CN IX)
Vagus nerve (CN X)
Spinal accessory nerve (CN XI)
Hypoglossal nerve (CN XII)
Tectorial membrane
Cruciform ligament
— Superior band
— Transverse ligament of atlas (transverse band)
— Inferior band
Alar ligament
Spinal nerve C1
Vertebral artery
Accessory atlantoaxial ligament
Posterior ramus of spinal nerve C1
Posterior arch of atlas (*cut*)
Tectorial membrane (*reflected*)

A. Posterior View

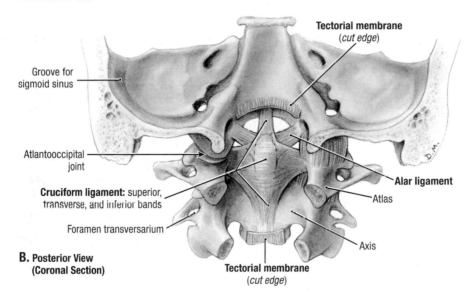

Tectorial membrane (*cut edge*)
Groove for sigmoid sinus
Atlantooccipital joint
Cruciform ligament: superior, transverse, and inferior bands
Foramen transversarium
Alar ligament
Atlas
Axis
Tectorial membrane (*cut edge*)

B. Posterior View (Coronal Section)

Anterior tubercle of atlas
Dens of axis
Articular cavity of median atlantoaxial joint
Foramen transversarium
Superior articular facet of atlas
Groove for vertebral artery
Transverse ligament of atlas
Vertebral canal
Posterior tubercle of atlas
Spinous process of axis

C. Superior View

Thoracic Vertebrae Ligaments of Atlantooccipital and Atlantoaxial Joints

1.11

A. Cranial nerves and dura mater of posterior cranial fossa. The dura mater and tentorial membrane have been incised and removed to reveal the medial atlantoaxial joint. The alar ligaments serve as check ligaments for the rotary movements of the atlantoaxial joints. **B.** and **C. Transverse ligament of atlas.** The transverse band of the cruciform ligament forms the posterior wall of a socket that receives the dens of the axis, forming a pivot joint.

Fracture of atlas. The atlas is a bony ring, with two wedge-shaped lateral masses, connected by relatively thin anterior and posterior arches and the transverse ligament of the atlas (see Figs. 1.12A & C). Vertical forces (e.g., striking the head on bottom of pool) may force the lateral masses apart fracturing one or both of the anterior or posterior arches. If the force is sufficient, rupture of the transverse ligament of the atlas will also occur.

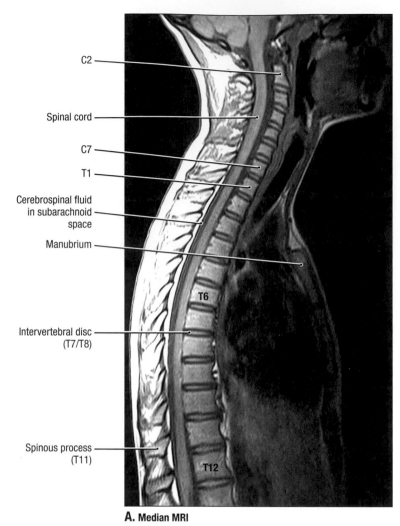

A. Median MRI

C2

Spinal cord

C7

T1

Cerebrospinal fluid
in subarachnoid
space

Manubrium

T6

Intervertebral disc
(T7/T8)

Spinous process
(T11)

T12

1.12 Thoracic Vertebrae

A. MRI of thoracic spine. **B.** Features.

Fracture of thoracic vertebrae. Although the characteristics of the superior aspect of vertebra T12 are distinctly thoracic, its inferior aspect has lumbar characteristics for articulation with vertebra L1. The abrupt transition allowing primarily rotational movements with vertebra T11 while disallowing rotational movements with vertebral L1 makes vertebra T12 especially susceptible to fracture.

TABLE 1.2	Thoracic Vertebrae
Part	**Distinctive Characteristics**
Body	Heart-shaped; has one or two costal facets for articulation with head of rib
Vertebral foramen	Circular and smaller than those of cervical and lumbar vertebrae
Transverse processes	Long and extend posterolaterally; length diminishes from T1 to T12; T1–T10 have transverse costal facets for articulation with a tubercle of ribs 1–10 (ribs 11 and 12 have no tubercle and do not articulate with a transverse process)
Articular processes	Superior articular facets directed posteriorly and slightly laterally; inferior articular facets directed anteriorly and slightly medially
Spinous process	Long and slopes posteroinferiorly; tip extends to level of vertebral body below

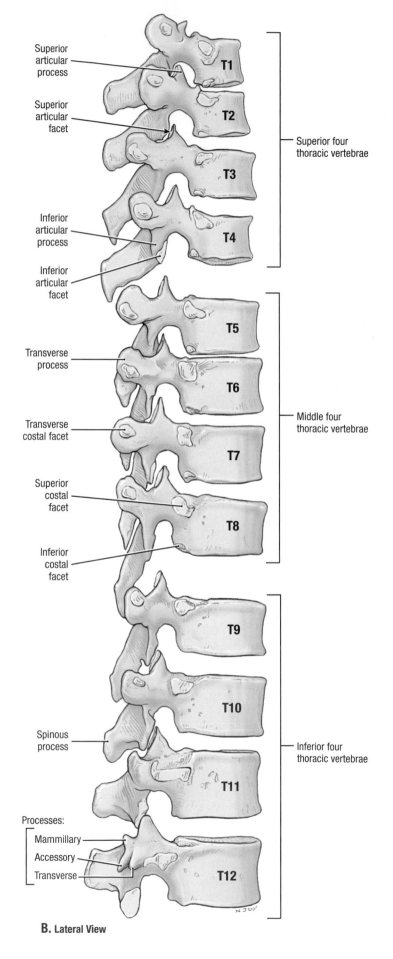

Superior
articular
process — T1

Superior
articular
facet — T2

T3

Superior four
thoracic vertebrae

Inferior
articular
process — T4

Inferior
articular
facet

T5

Transverse
process

T6

Middle four
thoracic vertebrae

Transverse
costal facet

T7

Superior
costal
facet

T8

Inferior
costal
facet

T9

T10

Spinous
process

Inferior four
thoracic vertebrae

T11

Processes:

Mammillary

Accessory

Transverse — T12

B. Lateral View

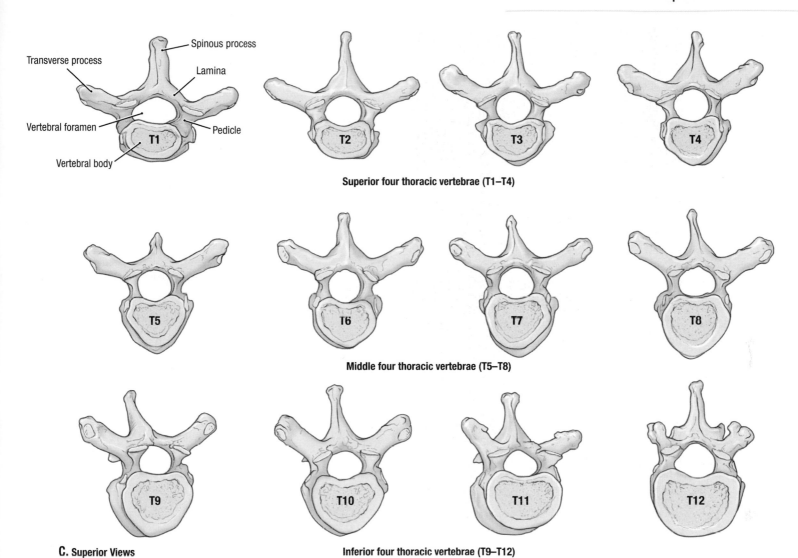

Transverse process

Spinous process

Lamina

Vertebral foramen

Pedicle

Vertebral body

T1

T2

T3

T4

Superior four thoracic vertebrae (T1–T4)

T5

T6

T7

T8

Middle four thoracic vertebrae (T5–T8)

T9

T10

T11

T12

C. Superior Views

Inferior four thoracic vertebrae (T9–T12)

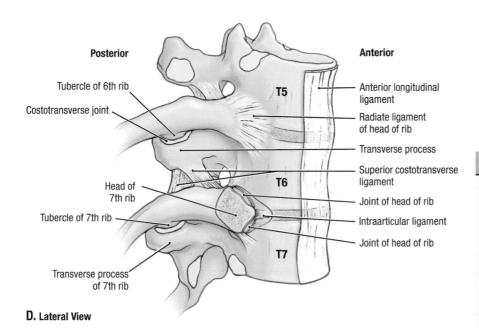

Posterior

Anterior

Tubercle of 6th rib

Costotransverse joint

Head of
7th rib

Tubercle of 7th rib

Transverse process
of 7th rib

D. Lateral View

T5

Anterior longitudinal
ligament

Radiate ligament
of head of rib

Transverse process

Superior costotransverse
ligament

T6

Joint of head of rib

Intraarticular ligament

Joint of head of rib

T7

Thoracic Vertebrae (continued) | 1.12

C. Disarticulated thoracic vertebrae. The vertebral bodies increase in size as the vertebral column descends, each bearing an increasing amount of weight transferred by the vertebra above. **D. Intraarticular and extraarticular ligaments of costovertebral articulations.** Typically, the head of each rib articulates with the bodies of two adjacent vertebrae and the IV disc between them, and the tubercle of the rib articulates with the transverse process of the inferior vertebra.

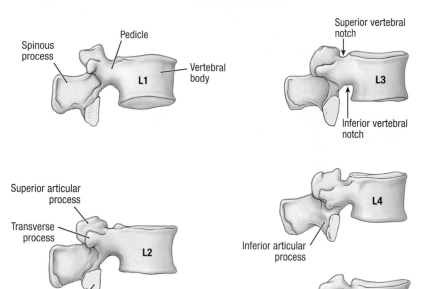

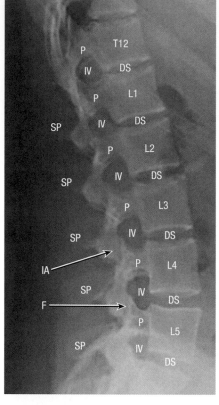

A. Lateral Views

C. Lateral Radiograph

Parts:

- Spinous process (1)
- Transverse process (2)
- Articular processes (4)
- Vertebral arch
- Vertebral body

Functions:

- Muscle attachment and movement
- Restriction of movement
- Protection of spinal cord
- Support of body weight

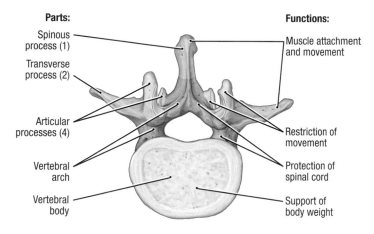

B. Superior View

1.13   Lumbar Vertebrae

A, B, E, and **F.** Features. **C, D,** and **G.** Radiographs.
H. Laminectomy.

TABLE 1.3	**Lumbar Vertebrae**
Part	**Distinctive Characteristics**
Body	Massive; kidney-shaped when viewed superiorly
Vertebral	Triangular; larger than in thoracic vertebrae and foramen smaller than in cervical vertebrae
Transverse	Long and slender; accessory process on posterior surface of base of each transverse process
Articular processes	Superior articular facets directed posteromedially (or medially); inferior articular facets directed anterolaterally (or laterally); mammillary process on posterior surface of each superior articular process
Spinous process	Short and sturdy; thick, broad, and rectangular

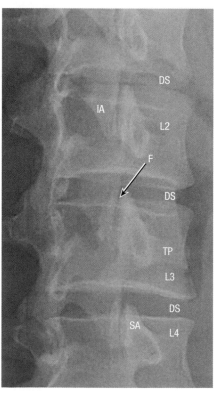

D. Right Anterior Oblique Radiograph

Key for C, D, and G			
DS	Intervertebral disc space	**P**	Pedicle
F	Zygapophysial (facet) joint	**SA**	Superior articular process
IA	Inferior articular process	**SP**	Spinous process
IV	Intervertebral foramen	**T12–L5**	Vertebral bodies
L	Lamina	**TP**	Transverse process

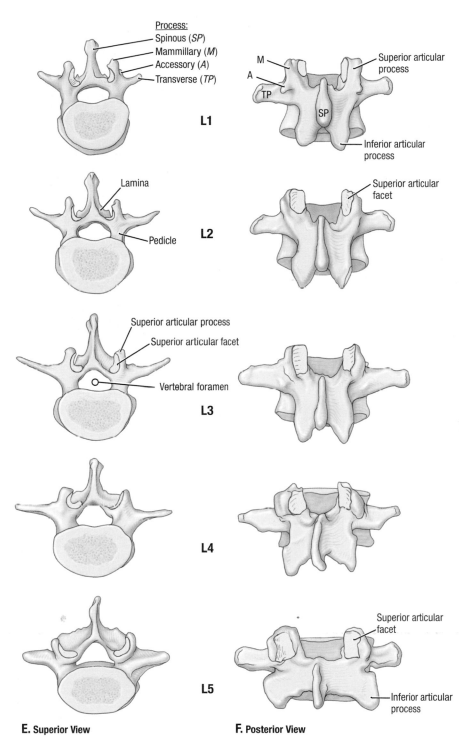

E. Superior View

F. Posterior View

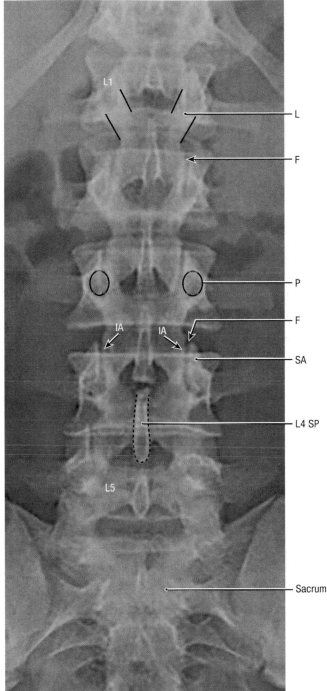

G. Anteroposterior Radiograph

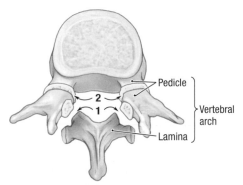

H. Superior View, Sites of Laminectomy (*1* and *2*)

Lumbar Vertebrae (*continued*)   1.13

A **laminectomy** is the surgical excision of one or more spinous processes and their supporting laminae in a particular region of the vertebral column by transecting the interarticular part (Fig. 1.13H, *1*). The term is also commonly used to denote the removal of most of the vertebral arch by transecting the pedicles (Fig. 1.13H, *2*). Laminectomies provide access to the vertebral canal to relieve pressure on the spinal cord or nerve roots, commonly caused by a tumor or herniated IV disc.

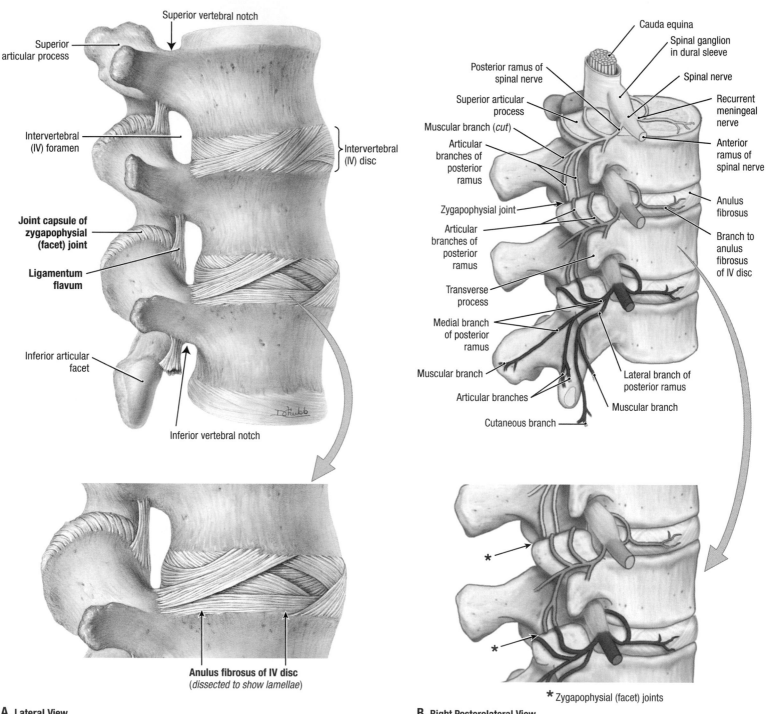

Superior vertebral notch

Superior articular process

Intervertebral (IV) foramen

Intervertebral (IV) disc

Joint capsule of zygapophysial (facet) joint

Ligamentum flavum

Inferior articular facet

Inferior vertebral notch

Anulus fibrosus of IV disc (*dissected to show lamellae*)

A. Lateral View

Cauda equina

Spinal ganglion in dural sleeve

Posterior ramus of spinal nerve

Spinal nerve

Superior articular process

Recurrent meningeal nerve

Muscular branch (*cut*)

Anterior ramus of spinal nerve

Articular branches of posterior ramus

Zygapophysial joint

Anulus fibrosus

Articular branches of posterior ramus

Branch to anulus fibrosus of IV disc

Transverse process

Medial branch of posterior ramus

Muscular branch

Lateral branch of posterior ramus

Articular branches

Muscular branch

Cutaneous branch

* Zygapophysial (facet) joints

B. Right Posterolateral View

1.14   Structure and Innervation of Intervertebral Discs and Zygapophysial Joints

A. Intervertebral discs and intervertebral foramen. Sections have been removed from the superficial layers of the anulus fibrosus of the inferior IV disc to show the change in direction of the fibers in the concentric layers of the anulus. Note that the IV discs form the inferior half of the anterior boundary of the IV foramen. **B. Innervation of zygapophysial joints and anulus fibrosus of IV discs.**

When the **zygapophysial joints are injured** or develop osteophytes during aging (*osteoarthritis*), the related spinal nerves are affected. This causes pain along the distribution pattern of the dermatomes and spasm in the muscles derived from the associated myotomes. Denervation of lumbar zygapophysial joints is a procedure that may be used for treatment of back pain caused by disease of these joints. The denervation process is directed at the articular branches of two adjacent posterior rami of the spinal nerves because each joint receives innervation from both the nerve exiting that level and the superjacent nerve.

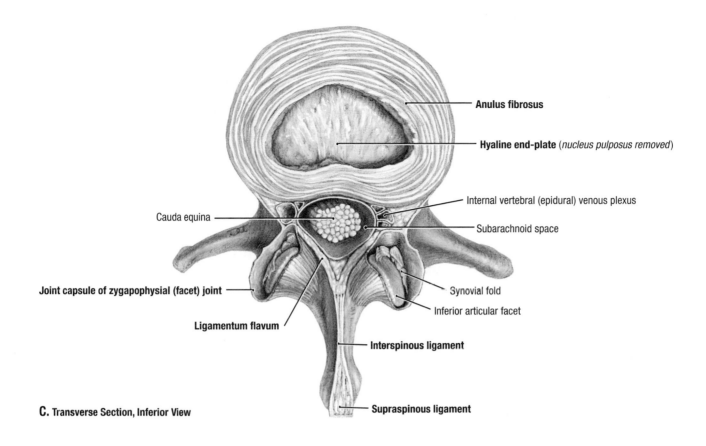

Anulus fibrosus

Hyaline end-plate (*nucleus pulposus removed*)

Internal vertebral (epidural) venous plexus

Cauda equina

Subarachnoid space

Joint capsule of zygapophysial (facet) joint

Synovial fold

Inferior articular facet

Ligamentum flavum

Interspinous ligament

Supraspinous ligament

C. Transverse Section, Inferior View

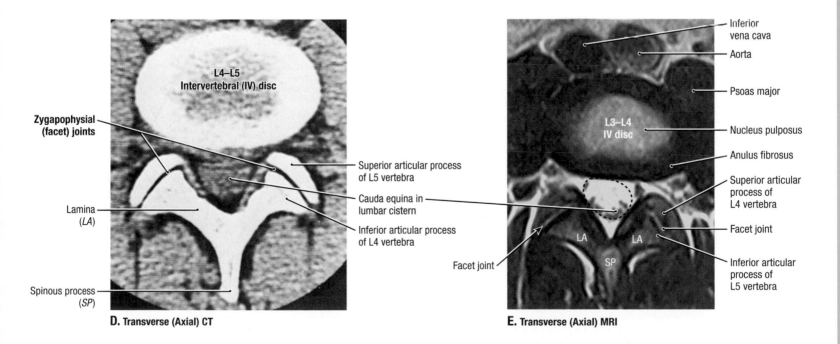

L4–L5
Intervertebral (IV) disc

**Zygapophysial
(facet) joints**

Superior articular process
of L5 vertebra

Cauda equina in
lumbar cistern

Inferior articular process
of L4 vertebra

Lamina
(*LA*)

Spinous process
(*SP*)

D. Transverse (Axial) CT

Inferior
vena cava

Aorta

Psoas major

L3–L4
IV disc

Nucleus pulposus

Anulus fibrosus

Superior articular
process of
L4 vertebra

LA   LA

SP

Facet joint

Facet joint

Inferior articular
process of
L5 vertebra

E. Transverse (Axial) MRI

Structure and Innervation of Intervertebral Discs and Zygapophysial Joints (*continued*)   **1.14**

C. Internal structure of discs and joints. The nucleus pulposus has been removed and the cartilaginous epiphysial plate exposed. There are fewer rings of the anulus fibrosus posteriorly, and consequently, this portion of the anulus fibrosus is thinner. The ligamentum flavum, interspinous, and supraspinous ligaments are continuous. **D.** CT image of L4/L5 IV disc. **E.** MRI of L3/L4 IV disc.

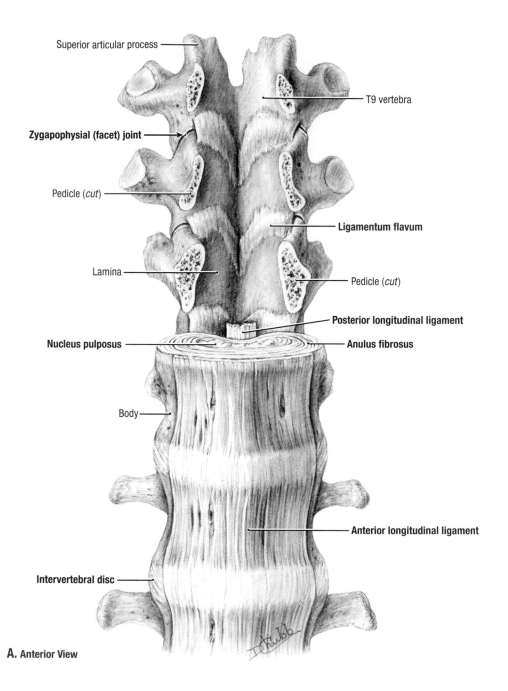

Superior articular process

T9 vertebra

Zygapophysial (facet) joint

Pedicle (*cut*)

Ligamentum flavum

Lamina

Pedicle (*cut*)

Posterior longitudinal ligament

Nucleus pulposus

Anulus fibrosus

Body

Anterior longitudinal ligament

Intervertebral disc

A. Anterior View

1.15   **Intervertebral Discs: Ligaments and Movements**

A. Anterior longitudinal ligament and ligamenta flava. The pedicles of the superior vertebrae were sawed through to show the ligamenta flava.

- The anterior and posterior longitudinal ligaments are ligaments of the vertebral bodies; the ligamenta flava are ligaments of the vertebral arches.
- The anterior longitudinal ligament consists of broad, strong, fibrous bands that are attached to the IV discs and vertebral

bodies anteriorly and are perforated by the foramina for arteries and veins passing to and from the vertebral bodies.

- The ligamenta flava, composed of elastic fibers, extend between adjacent laminae and converge in the median plane. They extend laterally to blend with the joint capsule of the zygapophysial joints.

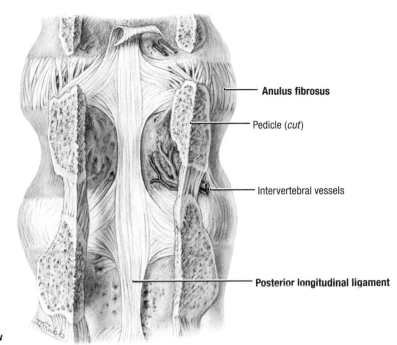

B. Posterior View

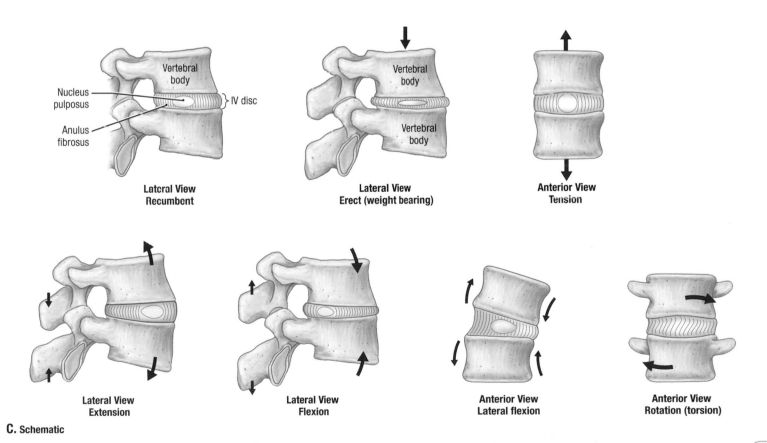

C. Schematic

Intervertebral Discs: Ligaments and Movements *(continued)*

B. Posterior longitudinal ligament. The pedicles of vertebrae T9–T11 were sawed through and the vertebral arch removed to show the posterior aspect of the vertebral bodies. The posterior longitudinal ligament is a narrow band passing from disc to disc, spanning the posterior surfaces of the vertebral bodies. **C. IV disc during loading and movement.** The movement or loading of the IV disc changes its shape and the position of the nucleus pulposus. *Red arrows* indicate the direction of movement.

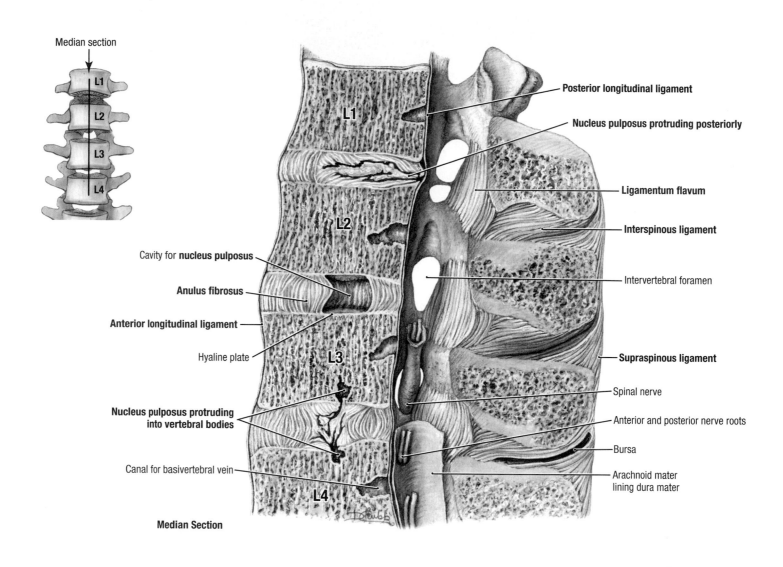

Median section

L1
L2
L3
L4

L1

L2

Cavity for **nucleus pulposus**

Anulus fibrosus

Anterior longitudinal ligament

Hyaline plate

L3

Nucleus pulposus protruding into vertebral bodies

Canal for basivertebral vein

L4

Median Section

Posterior longitudinal ligament

Nucleus pulposus protruding posteriorly

Ligamentum flavum

Interspinous ligament

Intervertebral foramen

Supraspinous ligament

Spinal nerve

Anterior and posterior nerve roots

Bursa

Arachnoid mater lining dura mater

1.16   **Lumbar Region of Vertebral Column**

Normal and degenerated (age and wear) IV discs. The nucleus pulposus of the normal disc between vertebrae L2 and L3 has been removed from the enclosing anulus fibrosus. The bursa between L3 and L4 spines is presumably the result of habitual hyperextension, which brings the lumbar spines into contact.

The nucleus pulposus of the disc between L1 and L2 has herniated posteriorly through the anulus. **Herniation** or **protrusion of the gelatinous nucleus pulposus** into or through

the anulus fibrosus is a well-recognized cause of low back and lower limb pain. If degeneration of the posterior longitudinal ligament and wearing of the anulus fibrosus has occurred, the nucleus pulposus may herniate into the vertebral canal and compress the spinal cord or nerve roots of spinal nerves in the cauda equina. Herniations usually occur posterolaterally, where the anulus is relatively thin and does not receive support from the ligaments.

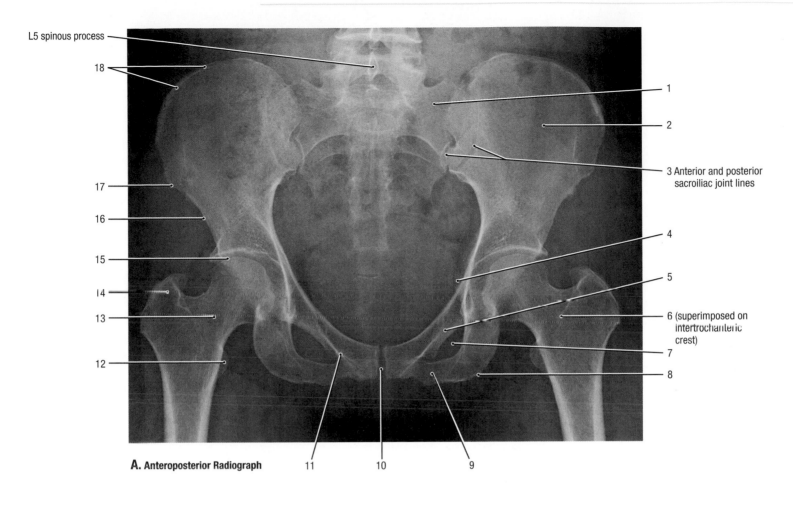

L5 spinous process

18

17

16

15

14

13

12

1

2

3 Anterior and posterior
   sacroiliac joint lines

4

5

6 (superimposed on
   intertrochanteric
   crest)

7

8

A. Anteroposterior Radiograph   11   10   9

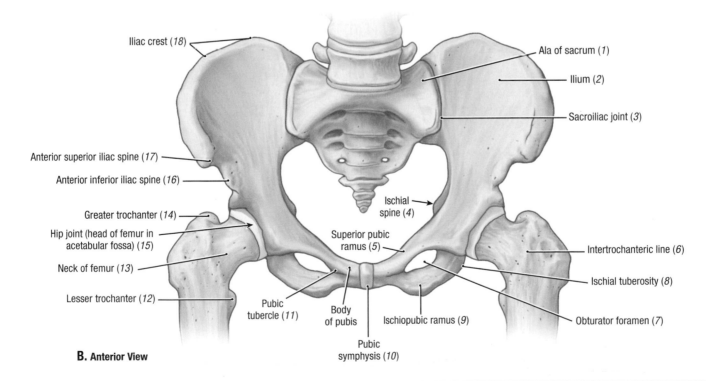

Iliac crest (*18*)

Anterior superior iliac spine (*17*)

Anterior inferior iliac spine (*16*)

Greater trochanter (*14*)

Hip joint (head of femur in
acetabular fossa) (*15*)

Neck of femur (*13*)

Lesser trochanter (*12*)

Pubic
tubercle (*11*)

Body
of pubis

Pubic
symphysis (*10*)

Ala of sacrum (*1*)

Ilium (*2*)

Sacroiliac joint (*3*)

Ischial
spine (*4*)

Superior pubic
ramus (*5*)

Intertrochanteric line (*6*)

Ischial tuberosity (*8*)

Ischiopubic ramus (*9*)

Obturator foramen (*7*)

B. Anterior View

Pelvic Girdle (Bony Pelvis)   **1.17**

A. Radiograph of male pelvis. **B.** Bony male pelvis with articulated femora.

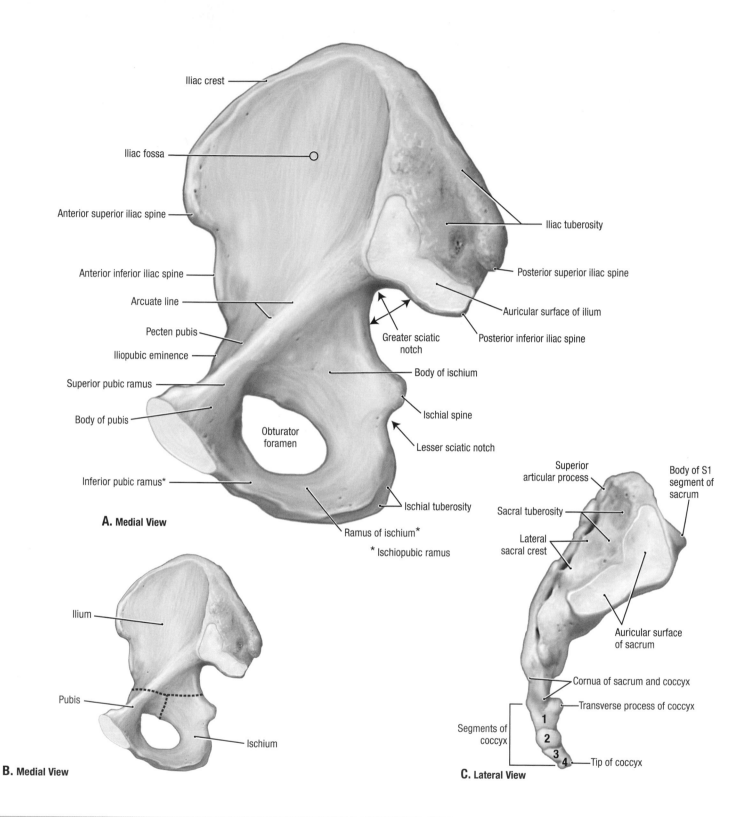

Iliac crest

Iliac fossa

Anterior superior iliac spine

Anterior inferior iliac spine

Arcuate line

Pecten pubis

Iliopubic eminence

Superior pubic ramus

Body of pubis

Inferior pubic ramus*

Obturator foramen

A. Medial View

Iliac tuberosity

Posterior superior iliac spine

Auricular surface of ilium

Posterior inferior iliac spine

Greater sciatic notch

Body of ischium

Ischial spine

Lesser sciatic notch

Ischial tuberosity

Ramus of ischium*

* Ischiopubic ramus

Ilium

Pubis

Ischium

B. Medial View

Superior articular process

Body of S1 segment of sacrum

Sacral tuberosity

Lateral sacral crest

Auricular surface of sacrum

Cornua of sacrum and coccyx

Transverse process of coccyx

1
2
3 4

Segments of coccyx

Tip of coccyx

C. Lateral View

1.18 **Hip Bone, Sacrum, and Coccyx**

A. Features of hip bone. **B.** Ilium, ischium, and pubis. **C.** Sacrum and coccyx.

- Each hip bone consists of three bones: ilium, ischium, and pubis.
- Anterosuperiorly, the auricular, ear-shaped surface of the sacrum articulates with the auricular surface of the ilium; the sacral and iliac tuberosities are for the attachment of the posterior sacroiliac and interosseous sacroiliac ligaments.
- The five sacral vertebrae are fused to form the sacrum.
- Distal coccygeal vertebrae may fuse.

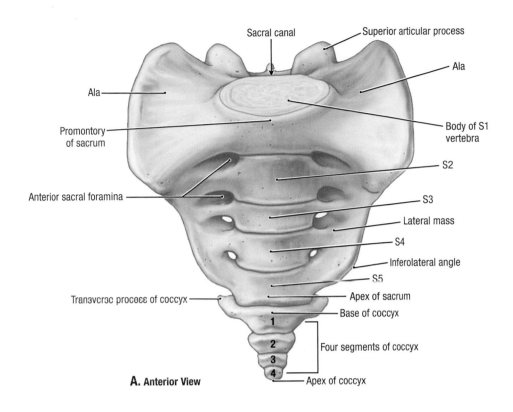

Sacral canal

Superior articular process

Ala

Ala

Promontory of sacrum

Body of S1 vertebra

S2

Anterior sacral foramina

S3

Lateral mass

S4

Inferolateral angle

S5

Transverse process of coccyx

Apex of sacrum

Base of coccyx

1
2
3
4

Four segments of coccyx

Apex of coccyx

A. Anterior View

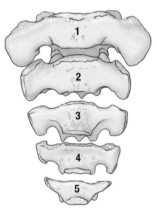

C. Anterior View, Sacral Vertebrae (1–5)

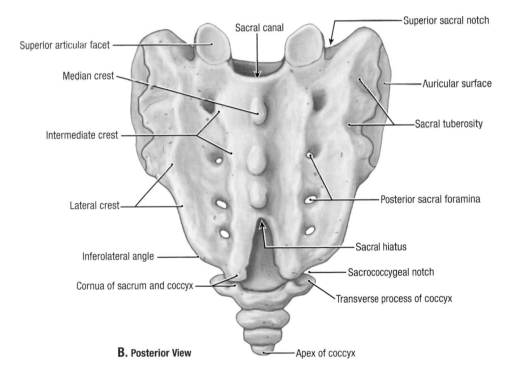

Sacral canal

Superior sacral notch

Superior articular facet

Median crest

Auricular surface

Intermediate crest

Sacral tuberosity

Lateral crest

Posterior sacral foramina

Inferolateral angle

Sacral hiatus

Cornua of sacrum and coccyx

Sacrococcygeal notch

Transverse process of coccyx

Apex of coccyx

B. Posterior View

Sacrum and Coccyx

1.19

A. Pelvic (anterior) surface. **B.** Dorsal (posterior) surface. **C.** Sacrum in youth.

- The bodies of the five sacral vertebrae are demarcated in the mature sacrum by four transverse lines ending laterally in four pairs of anterior sacral foramina (*Part A*). The coccyx has four

vertebrae (segments)—the first having a pair of transverse processes and a pair of cornua (horns).

- The ossification and fusion of the sacral vertebrae may not be complete until age 35.

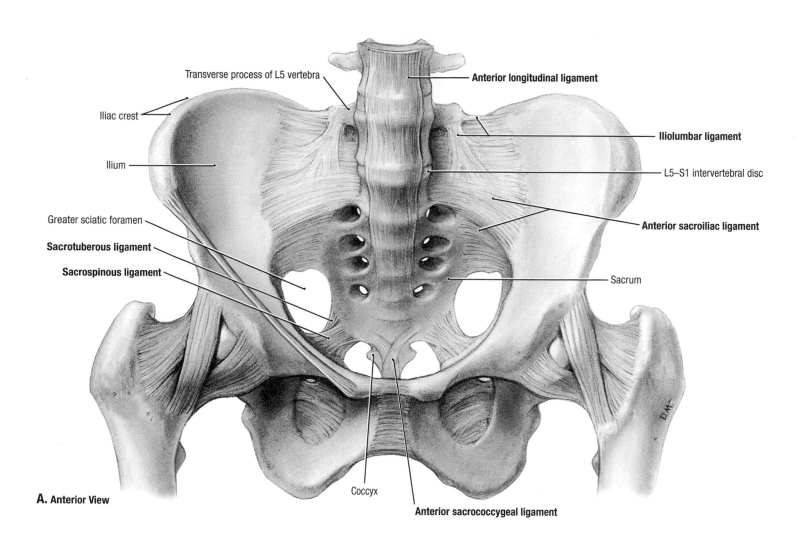

Transverse process of L5 vertebra

Anterior longitudinal ligament

Iliac crest

Iliolumbar ligament

Ilium

L5–S1 intervertebral disc

Greater sciatic foramen

Anterior sacroiliac ligament

Sacrotuberous ligament

Sacrospinous ligament

Sacrum

A. Anterior View

Coccyx

Anterior sacrococcygeal ligament

1.20   Lumbar and Pelvic Ligaments

A. Anterior aspect.

The anterior sacroiliac ligament is part of the fibrous capsule of the sacroiliac joint anteriorly and spans between the lateral aspect of the sacrum and the ilium, anterior to the auricular surfaces.

During **pregnancy**, the pelvic joints and ligaments relax and pelvic movements increase. The sacroiliac interlocking mechanism is less effective because the relaxation permits greater rotation of the pelvis and contributes to the lordotic posture often assumed during pregnancy with the change in the center of gravity. Relaxation of the sacroiliac joints and pubic symphysis permits as much as 10% to 15% increase in diameters (mostly transverse), facilitating passage of the fetus through the pelvic canal. The coccyx is also allowed to move posteriorly.

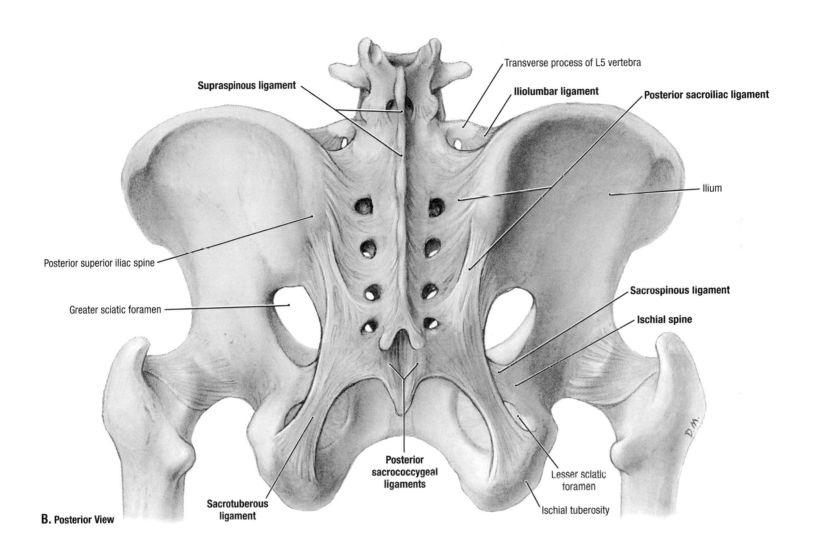

Transverse process of L5 vertebra

Supraspinous ligament

Iliolumbar ligament

Posterior sacroiliac ligament

Ilium

Posterior superior iliac spine

Sacrospinous ligament

Greater sciatic foramen

Ischial spine

Posterior sacrococcygeal ligaments

Lesser sciatic foramen

Sacrotuberous ligament

Ischial tuberosity

B. Posterior View

Lumbar and Pelvic Ligaments *(continued)*   **1.20**

B. Posterior aspect.
- The sacrotuberous ligaments attach the sacrum, ilium, and coccyx to the ischial tuberosity; the sacrospinous ligaments unite the sacrum and coccyx to the ischial spine. The sacrotuberous and sacrospinous ligaments convert the sciatic notches of the hip bones into greater and lesser sciatic foramina.
- The fibers of the posterior sacroiliac ligament vary in obliquity; the superior fibers are shorter and lie between the ilium and superior part of the sacrum; the longer, obliquely oriented inferior fibers span between the posterior superior iliac spine and the inferior part of the sacrum.
- The iliolumbar ligaments unite the ilia and transverse processes of L5.

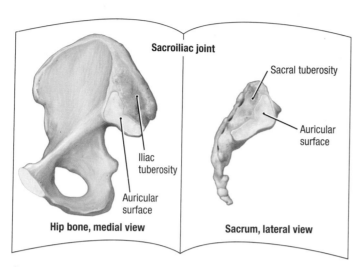

A. Open-Book View

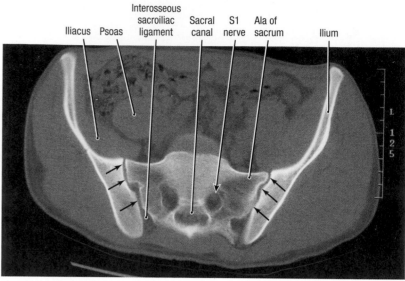

C. Transverse (Axial) CT

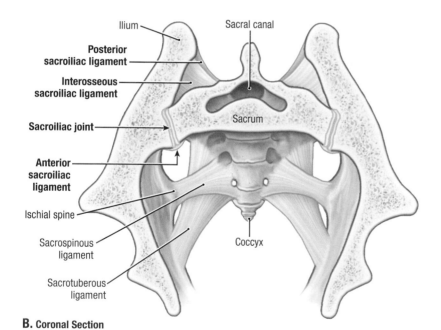

B. Coronal Section

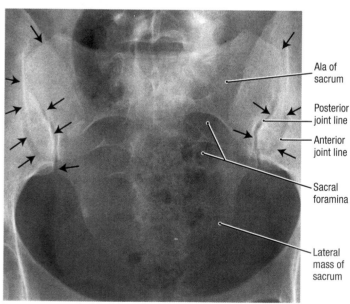

D. Anteroposterior Radiograph

| 1.21 | **Articular Surfaces of Sacroiliac Joint and Ligaments** |

A. Articular surfaces. Note the auricular surface (*blue*) of the sacrum and hip bone and the roughened areas superior and posterior to the auricular areas for the attachment of the interosseous sacroiliac ligament. **B. Sacroiliac ligaments.** The interosseous sacroiliac ligament consists of short fibers connecting the sacral tuberosity to the iliac tuberosity. **C. CT image.** The sacroiliac joint is indicated (*arrows*). Note that the articular surfaces of the ilium and sacrum have irregular shapes that result in partial interlocking of the bones. **D. Radiographic appearance of sacroiliac joints.** Due to the oblique placement of the sacroiliac joints, the anterior and posterior joint lines appear separately (*arrows*).

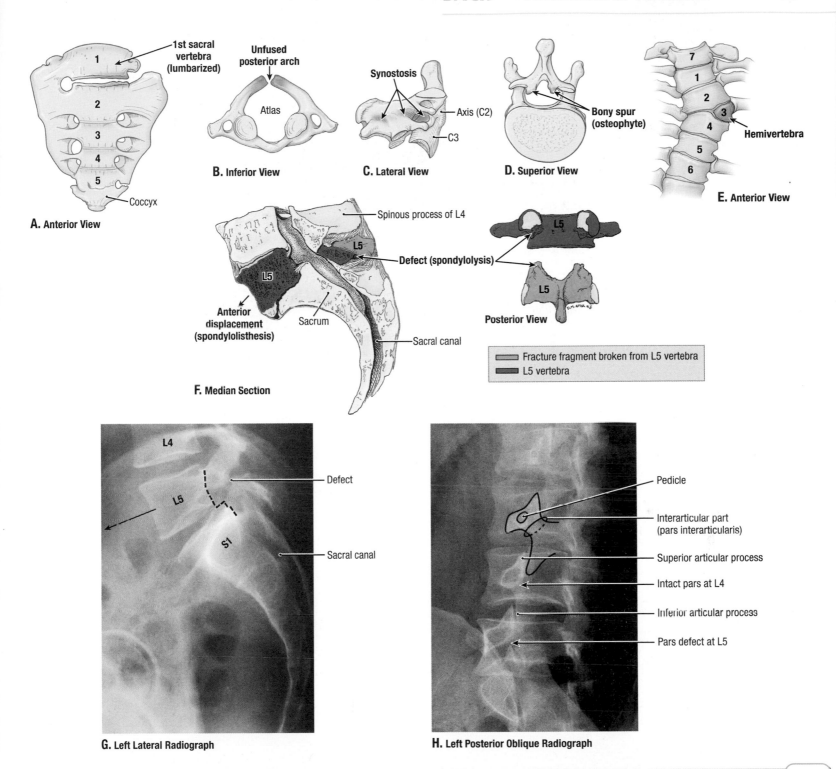

A. Anterior View

B. Inferior View

C. Lateral View

D. Superior View

E. Anterior View

F. Median Section

- Fracture fragment broken from L5 vertebra
- L5 vertebra

G. Left Lateral Radiograph

H. Left Posterior Oblique Radiograph

Anomalies of Vertebrae and Spondylolysis and Spondylolisthesis   **1.22**

A. Transitional lumbosacral vertebra. Here, the 1st sacral vertebra is partly free (lumbarized). Not uncommonly, the 5th lumbar vertebra may be partly fused to the sacrum (sacralized). **B. Unfused posterior arch of atlas. C. Synostosis (fusion) of vertebrae C2 (axis) and C3. D. Bony spurs.** Sharp bony spurs may grow from the laminae inferiorly into the ligamenta flava. **E. Hemivertebra.** The entire right half of vertebra T3 and the corresponding rib are absent. The left lamina and the spine are fused with those of T4, and the left IV foramen is reduced in size. Observe the associated scoliosis (lateral curvature of the spine). **F. Articulated and isolated spondylolytic L5 vertebra.**

The vertebra has an oblique defect (spondylolysis) through the interarticular part (pars interarticularis). Also, the vertebral body of L5 has slipped anteriorly (spondylolisthesis). **G.** and **H. Radiographs.** The posterior vertebral margins of L5 and the sacrum (*dashed line*) show the anterior displacement of L5 (*arrow*)—the **spondylolisthesis** (*Part G*). Note the superimposed outline of a dog (*Part H*): The nose is the transverse process, the eye is the pedicle, the neck is the interarticular part, and the ear is the superior articular process. The lucent (*dark*) cleft due to a fractured interarticular part (the "broken neck" of the dog) is the **spondylolysis**.

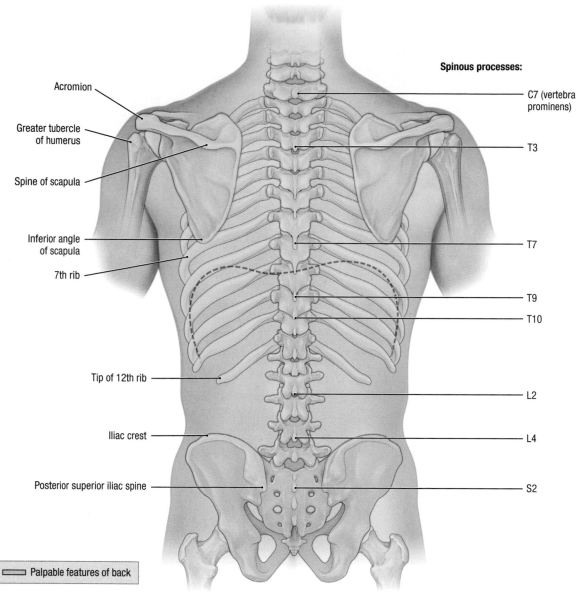

Acromion

Greater tubercle
of humerus

Spine of scapula

Inferior angle
of scapula

7th rib

Tip of 12th rib

Iliac crest

Posterior superior iliac spine

Spinous processes:

C7 (vertebra
prominens)

T3

T7

T9

T10

L2

L4

S2

☐ Palpable features of back

Posterior View

1.23 **Surface Anatomy of Back: Palpable Features and Landmarks**

TABLE 1.4	Relationships of Palpable Landmarks, Spinous Processes, and Significant Structures	
Palpable Landmark	**Spinous Process**	**Significance (Approximations)**
Vertebra prominens	C7	Apex of lungs, thyroid isthmus
Spine of scapula	T3	Formation of superior vena cava
	T4	T4–T5 IV disc; transverse thoracic plane (intersects: sternal angle, aortic arch, bifurcation of trachea, arch of azygos vein)
Inferior angle of scapula	T7	Level of nipple on anterior thoracic wall
	T9–T10	Central tendon of diaphragm; base of lungs
Tip of 12th rib	L2	Inferior end of spinal cord
Iliac crest	L4	Bifurcation of aorta; commonly lumbar puncture performed between laminae of the 4th and 5th lumbar vertebrae
Dimple overlying posterior superior iliac spine	S2	Inferior extent of dural sac/subarachnoid space

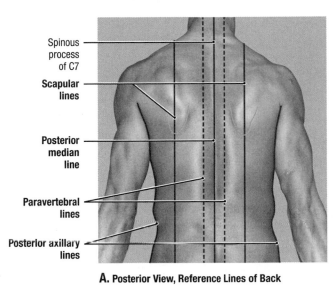

Spinous process of C7

Scapular lines

Posterior median line

Paravertebral lines

Posterior axillary lines

A. Posterior View, Reference Lines of Back

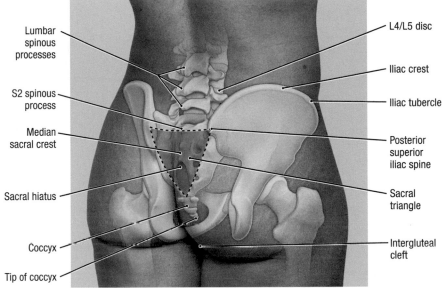

Lumbar spinous processes

S2 spinous process

Median sacral crest

Sacral hiatus

Coccyx

Tip of coccyx

L4/L5 disc

Iliac crest

Iliac tubercle

Posterior superior iliac spine

Sacral triangle

Intergluteal cleft

B. Right Posterolateral View, Anatomical Position

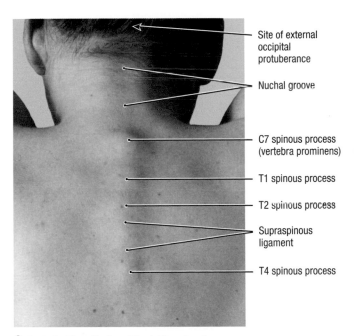

Site of external occipital protuberance

Nuchal groove

C7 spinous process (vertebra prominens)

T1 spinous process

T2 spinous process

Supraspinous ligament

T4 spinous process

C. Posterior View, Neck and Back Flexed and Scapulae Protracted

POSTERIOR

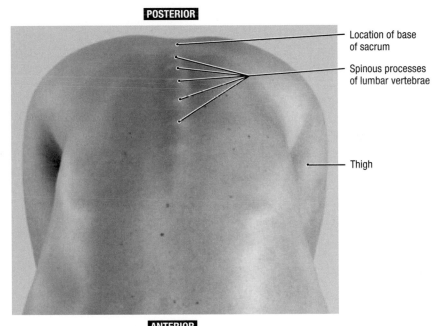

Location of base of sacrum

Spinous processes of lumbar vertebrae

Thigh

ANTERIOR

D. Anterior View, Hips and Back Fully Flexed

Surface Anatomy of Back: Reference Lines and Examination Maneuvers   1.24

A. Reference lines of back. *Vertical lines* are extrapolated from anatomical landmarks: The posterior median line overlies the spinous processes, the paravertebral lines overlie the transverse processes, the scapular lines intersect the inferior scapular angles (*green*), and the posterior axillary lines run vertically downward from the posterior axillary folds. **B. Pelvis** *in situ*. Changing the angle of view may enhance viewing of the surface features. **C.** and **D. Surface anatomy during flexion.** Flexion of the back in combination with flexion of the upper limbs makes the spinous processes more prominent.

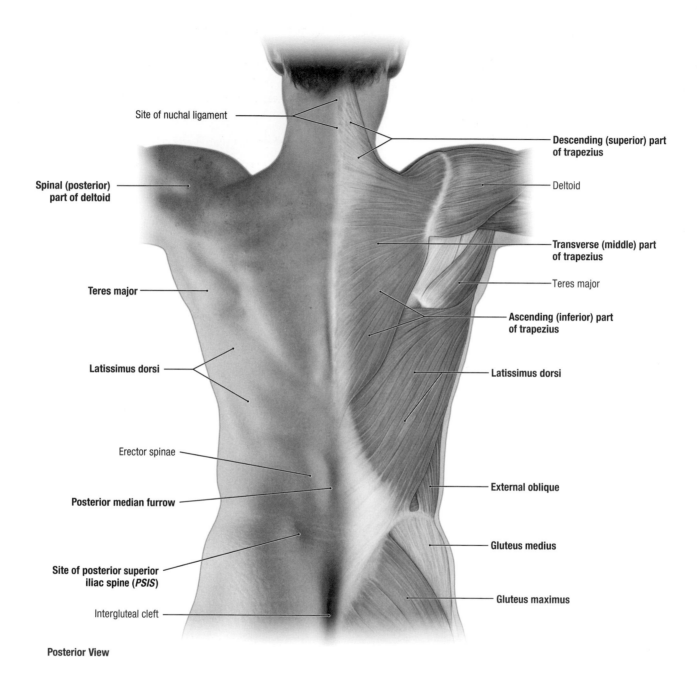

Site of nuchal ligament

**Descending (superior) part
of trapezius**

**Spinal (posterior)
part of deltoid**

Deltoid

**Transverse (middle) part
of trapezius**

Teres major

Teres major

**Ascending (inferior) part
of trapezius**

Latissimus dorsi

Latissimus dorsi

Erector spinae

External oblique

Posterior median furrow

Gluteus medius

**Site of posterior superior
iliac spine (*PSIS*)**

Intergluteal cleft

Gluteus maximus

Posterior View

1.25   **Surface Anatomy of Back: Muscles of Back**

- The arms are abducted, so the scapulae have rotated superiorly on the thoracic wall.
- The latissimus dorsi and teres major muscles form the posterior axillary fold.
- The trapezius muscle has three parts: descending, transverse, and ascending.

- The deep median furrow separates the longitudinal bulges formed by the contracted erector spinae group of muscles.
- Dimples (depressions) indicate the site of the posterior superior iliac spines, which usually lie at the level of the sacroiliac joints.

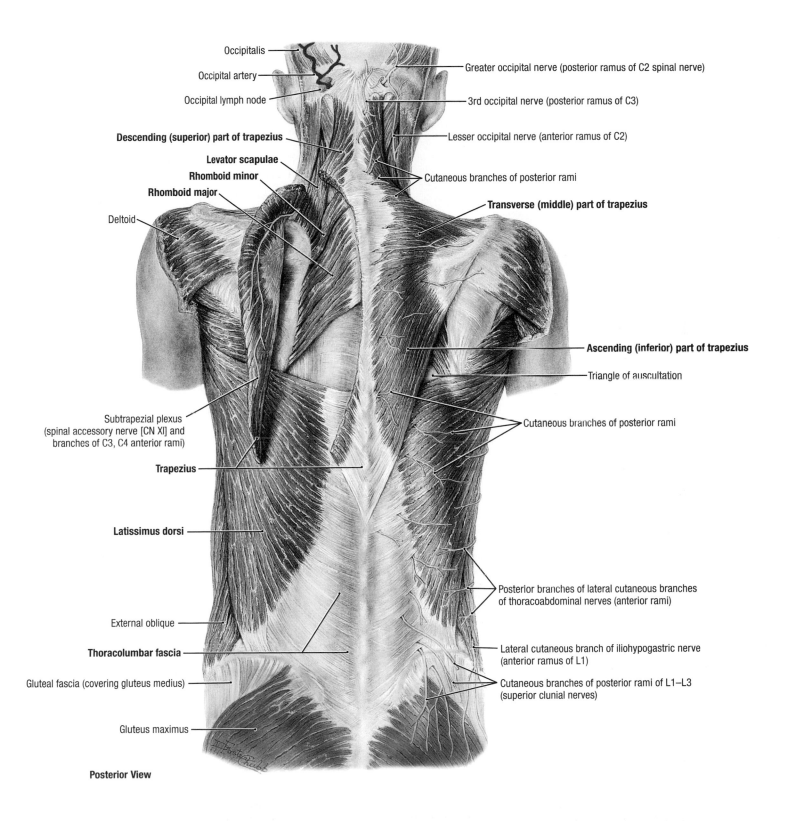

Occipitalis

Occipital artery

Occipital lymph node

Descending (superior) part of trapezius

Levator scapulae

Rhomboid minor

Rhomboid major

Deltoid

Subtrapezial plexus
(spinal accessory nerve [CN XI] and
branches of C3, C4 anterior rami)

Trapezius

Latissimus dorsi

External oblique

Thoracolumbar fascia

Gluteal fascia (covering gluteus medius)

Gluteus maximus

Posterior View

Greater occipital nerve (posterior ramus of C2 spinal nerve)

3rd occipital nerve (posterior ramus of C3)

Lesser occipital nerve (anterior ramus of C2)

Cutaneous branches of posterior rami

Transverse (middle) part of trapezius

Ascending (inferior) part of trapezius

Triangle of auscultation

Cutaneous branches of posterior rami

Posterior branches of lateral cutaneous branches
of thoracoabdominal nerves (anterior rami)

Lateral cutaneous branch of iliohypogastric nerve
(anterior ramus of L1)

Cutaneous branches of posterior rami of L1–L3
(superior clunial nerves)

Superficial Muscles of Back — **1.26**

The left trapezius muscle is reflected. Observe two layers: (1) the trapezius and latissimus dorsi muscles and (2) the levator scapulae and rhomboids minor and major. These axio-appendicular muscles help attach the upper limb to the trunk.

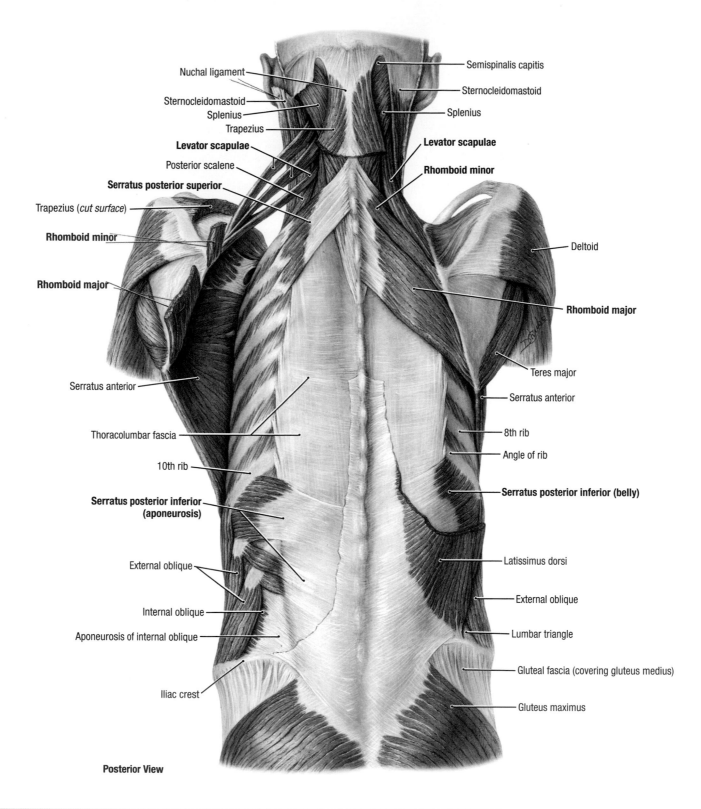

Nuchal ligament

Sternocleidomastoid
Splenius
Trapezius

Levator scapulae

Posterior scalene

Serratus posterior superior

Trapezius (*cut surface*)

Rhomboid minor

Rhomboid major

Serratus anterior

Thoracolumbar fascia

10th rib

Serratus posterior inferior (aponeurosis)

External oblique

Internal oblique

Aponeurosis of internal oblique

Iliac crest

Semispinalis capitis

Sternocleidomastoid

Splenius

Levator scapulae

Rhomboid minor

Deltoid

Rhomboid major

Teres major

Serratus anterior

8th rib

Angle of rib

Serratus posterior inferior (belly)

Latissimus dorsi

External oblique

Lumbar triangle

Gluteal fascia (covering gluteus medius)

Gluteus maximus

Posterior View

| **1.27** | **Intermediate Muscles of Back** |

The trapezius and latissimus dorsi muscles are largely cut away on both sides. The left rhomboid muscles have been reflected, allowing the vertebral border of the scapula to be raised from the thoracic wall. The serratus posterior superior and inferior form the intermediate layer of muscles, passing from the vertebral spines to the ribs; the two muscles slope in opposite directions and are accessory muscles of respiration. The thoracolumbar fascia extends laterally to the angles of the ribs, becoming thin superiorly and passing deep to the serratus posterior superior muscle. The fascia gives attachment to the latissimus dorsi and serratus posterior inferior muscles (see Fig. 1.32).

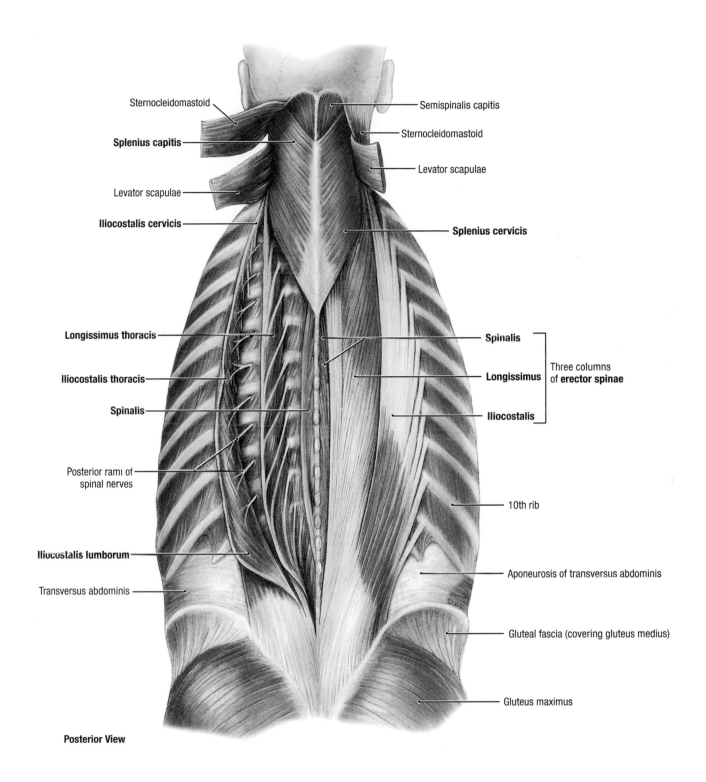

Sternocleidomastoid

Splenius capitis

Levator scapulae

Iliocostalis cervicis

Longissimus thoracis

Iliocostalis thoracis

Spinalis

Posterior rami of spinal nerves

Iliocostalis lumborum

Transversus abdominis

Semispinalis capitis

Sternocleidomastoid

Levator scapulae

Splenius cervicis

Spinalis

Longissimus

Iliocostalis

} Three columns of **erector spinae**

10th rib

Aponeurosis of transversus abdominis

Gluteal fascia (covering gluteus medius)

Gluteus maximus

Posterior View

Deep Muscles of Back: Splenius and Erector Spinae   **1.28**

The right erector spinae muscles are *in situ*, lying between the spinous processes medially and the angles of the ribs laterally. The erector spinae are split into three longitudinal columns: ilio-costalis laterally, longissimus in the middle, and spinalis medially.

The left longissimus muscle is pulled laterally to show the insertion into the transverse processes and ribs. Not shown here are its extensions to the neck and head: the longissimus cervicis and capitis.

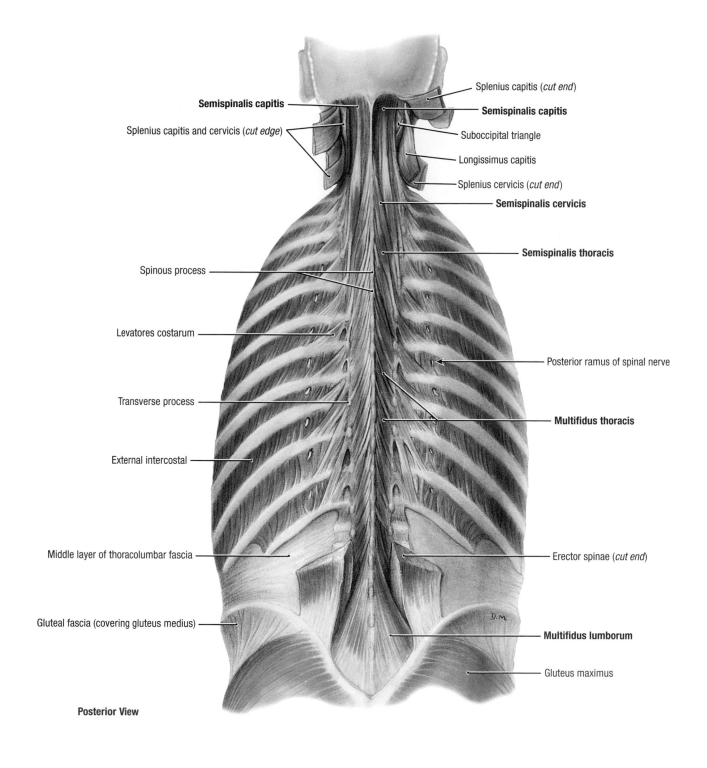

Semispinalis capitis

Splenius capitis and cervicis (*cut edge*)

Spinous process

Levatores costarum

Transverse process

External intercostal

Middle layer of thoracolumbar fascia

Gluteal fascia (covering gluteus medius)

Posterior View

Splenius capitis (*cut end*)

Semispinalis capitis

Suboccipital triangle

Longissimus capitis

Splenius cervicis (*cut end*)

Semispinalis cervicis

Semispinalis thoracis

Posterior ramus of spinal nerve

Multifidus thoracis

Erector spinae (*cut end*)

Multifidus lumborum

Gluteus maximus

D. M.

| 1.29 | **Deep Muscles of Back: Semispinalis and Multifidus** |

- The semispinalis, multifidus, and rotatores muscles constitute the transversospinalis group of deep muscles. In general, their bundles pass obliquely in a superomedial direction, from transverse processes to spinous processes in successively deeper layers. The bundles of semispinalis span approximately five interspaces, those of multifidus, approximately three, and those of rotatores, one or two.

- The semispinalis (thoracis, cervicis, and capitis) muscles span the lower thoracic region to the cranium.
- The multifidus muscle extends from the sacrum to the spinous process of the axis. In the lumbosacral region, it emerges from the aponeurosis of the erector spinae and extends from the sacrum, and mammillary processes of the lumbar vertebrae, to insert into spinous processes approximately three segments higher.

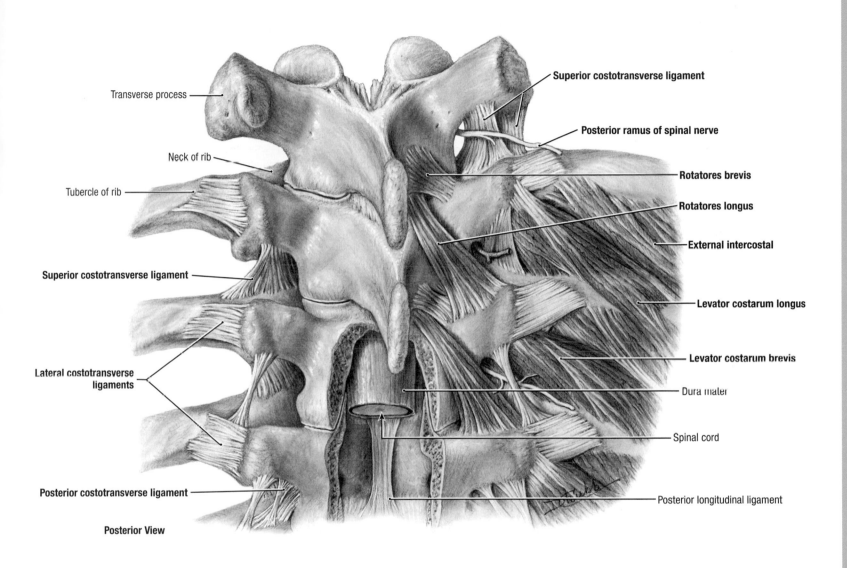

Transverse process

Neck of rib

Tubercle of rib

Superior costotransverse ligament

Lateral costotransverse ligaments

Posterior costotransverse ligament

Posterior View

Superior costotransverse ligament

Posterior ramus of spinal nerve

Rotatores brevis

Rotatores longus

External intercostal

Levator costarum longus

Levator costarum brevis

Dura mater

Spinal cord

Posterior longitudinal ligament

Rotatores and Costotransverse Ligaments   1.30

- Of the three layers of transversospinalis muscles, the rotatores are the deepest and shortest. They pass from the root of one transverse process superomedially to the junction of the transverse process and lamina of the vertebra above. Rotatores longi span two vertebrae.
- The levatores costarum pass from the tip of one transverse process inferiorly to the rib below (brevis); some span two ribs (longus).

- The posterior ramus passes posterior to the superior costotransverse ligament.
- The lateral costotransverse ligament is strong and joins the tubercle of the rib to the tip of the transverse process. It forms the posterior aspect of the joint capsule of the costotransverse joint.

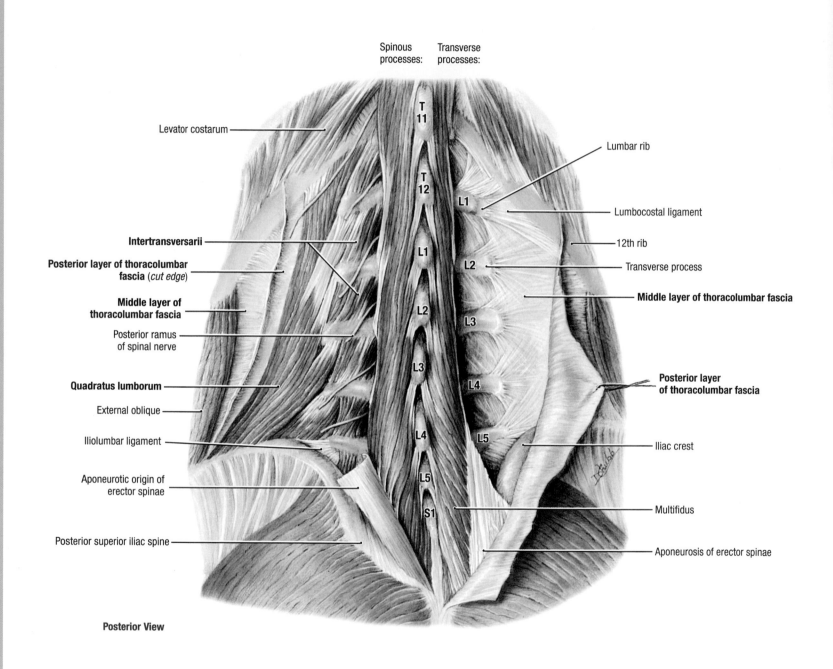

Spinous processes:

Transverse processes:

Levator costarum

T 11

T 12

L1

Lumbar rib

Lumbocostal ligament

12th rib

Transverse process

L1

Intertransversarii

Middle layer of thoracolumbar fascia

Posterior layer of thoracolumbar fascia (cut edge)

L2

Middle layer of thoracolumbar fascia

Middle layer of thoracolumbar fascia

Posterior ramus of spinal nerve

L2

L3

Quadratus lumborum

L3

Posterior layer of thoracolumbar fascia

L4

External oblique

Iliolumbar ligament

L4

L5

Iliac crest

Aponeurotic origin of erector spinae

L5

Multifidus

S1

Posterior superior iliac spine

Aponeurosis of erector spinae

Posterior View

1.31 **Back: Multifidus, Quadratus Lumborum, and Thoracolumbar Fascia**

After removal of right erector spinae at the L1 level, the middle layer of thoracolumbar fascia is seen to extend from the tip of each lumbar transverse process in a fan-shaped manner. A short lumbar rib is present at the level of L1.

After removal of the left posterior and middle layers of thoracolumbar fascia, the lateral border of the quadratus lumborum muscle is oblique, and the medial border is in continuity with the intertransversarii.

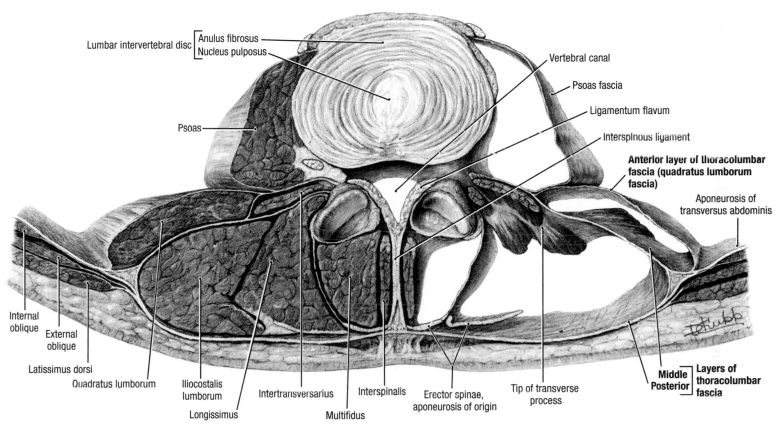

Lumbar intervertebral disc [Anulus fibrosus
Nucleus pulposus

Psoas

Vertebral canal

Psoas fascia

Ligamentum flavum

Interspinous ligament

Anterior layer of thoracolumbar fascia (quadratus lumborum fascia)

Aponeurosis of transversus abdominis

Internal oblique

External oblique

Latissimus dorsi

Quadratus lumborum

Iliocostalis lumborum

Longissimus

Intertransversarius

Interspinalis

Multifidus

Erector spinae, aponeurosis of origin

Tip of transverse process

Middle Posterior [**Layers of thoracolumbar fascia**

Transverse Section (Dissected), Superior View

Transverse Section of Back Muscles and Thoracolumbar Fascia   **1.32**

- The left muscles are seen in their fascial sheaths or compartments; the right muscles have been removed from their sheaths.
- The aponeurosis of transversus abdominis and posterior aponeurosis of internal oblique muscles split into two strong sheets, the middle and posterior layers of thoracolumbar fascia. The anterior layer of thoracolumbar fascia is the deep fascia of the quadratus lumborum (quadratus lumborum fascia). The posterior layer of the thoracolumbar fascia provides proximal attachment for the latissimus dorsi muscle and, at a higher level, the serratus posterior inferior muscle.

Back strain is a common back problem that usually results from extreme movements of the vertebral column, such as extension or rotation. Back strain refers to some stretching or microscopic tearing of muscle fibers and/or ligaments of the back. The muscles usually involved are those producing movements of the lumbar IV joints.

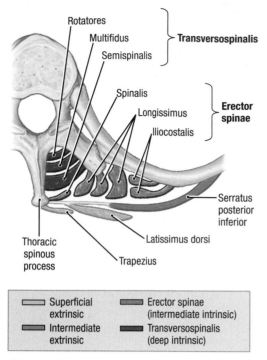

A. Transverse Section

Rotatores
Multifidus
Semispinalis
Transversospinalis

Spinalis
Longissimus
Iliocostalis
Erector spinae

Serratus posterior inferior

Thoracic spinous process
Trapezius
Latissimus dorsi

Legend:
- Superficial extrinsic
- Intermediate extrinsic
- Erector spinae (intermediate intrinsic)
- Transversospinalis (deep intrinsic)

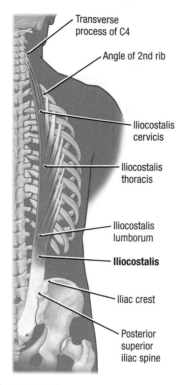

B. Posterior View

Transverse process of C4
Angle of 2nd rib
Iliocostalis cervicis
Iliocostalis thoracis
Iliocostalis lumborum
Iliocostalis
Iliac crest
Posterior superior iliac spine

C. Posterior View

Mastoid process
Longissimus capitis and cervicis
Angle of rib
Longissimus thoracis
Longissimus

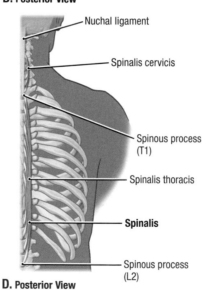

D. Posterior View

Nuchal ligament
Spinalis cervicis
Spinous process (T1)
Spinalis thoracis
Spinalis
Spinous process (L2)

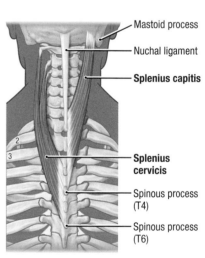

E. Posterior View

Mastoid process
Nuchal ligament
Splenius capitis
Splenius cervicis
Spinous process (T4)
Spinous process (T6)

1.33 **Superficial and Intermediate Layers of Intrinsic Back Muscles**

A. Erector spinae (three columns) and transverso-spinalis (three layers). **B–D.** Layers of erector spinae. **E.** Splenius capitis and cervicis.

TABLE 1.5	Superficial and Intermediate Layers of Intrinsic Back Muscles			
Muscles	**Inferior Attachment**	**Superior Attachment**	**Nerve Supply**	**Main Actions**
Superficial layer Splenius	Nuchal ligament and spinous processes of C7–T6 vertebrae	*Splenius capitis:* fibers run superolaterally to mastoid process of temporal bone and lateral third of superior nuchal line of occipital bone *Splenius cervicis:* posterior tubercles of transverse processes of C1–C3/C4 vertebrae	Posterior rami of spinal nerves	*Acting unilaterally:* laterally flex neck and rotate head ipsilaterally (to side of active muscles contraction) *Acting bilaterally:* extend head and neck
Intermediate layer Erector spinae	Arises by a broad tendon from posterior part of iliac crest, posterior surface of sacrum, sacral and inferior lumbar spinous processes, and supraspinous ligament	*Iliocostalis (lumborum, thoracis, and cervicis):* fibers run superiorly to angles of lower ribs and cervical transverse processes *Longissimus (thoracis, cervicis, and capitis):* fibers run superiorly to ribs between tubercles and angles to transverse processes in thoracic and cervical regions, and to mastoid process of temporal bone *Spinalis (thoracis, cervicis, and capitis):* fibers run superiorly to spinous processes in the upper thoracic region and to skull		*Acting unilaterally:* laterally bend vertebral column ipsilaterally *Acting bilaterally:* extend vertebral column and head; as back is flexed, control movement by gradually lengthening their fibers

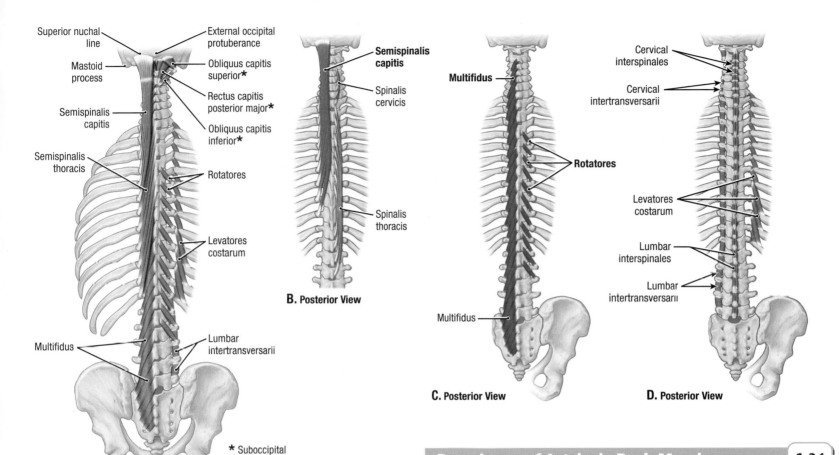

A. Posterior View

Superior nuchal line
Mastoid process
Semispinalis capitis
Semispinalis thoracis
Multifidus
External occipital protuberance
Obliquus capitis superior*
Rectus capitis posterior major*
Obliquus capitis inferior*
Rotatores
Levatores costarum
Lumbar intertransversarii
* Suboccipital muscles

B. Posterior View

Semispinalis capitis
Spinalis cervicis
Spinalis thoracis

C. Posterior View

Multifidus
Rotatores
Multifidus

D. Posterior View

Cervical interspinales
Cervical intertransversarii
Levatores costarum
Lumbar interspinales
Lumbar intertransversarii

Deep Layer of Intrinsic Back Muscles 1.34

A. Overview. **B.** Semispinalis. **C.** Multifidus and rotatores.
D. Interspinalis, intertransversarii, and levatores costarum.

TABLE 1.6 Deep Layers of Intrinsic Back Muscles

Muscles	Inferior Attachment	Superior Attachment	Nerve Supply[a]	Main Actions
Deep layer Transversospinalis	*Semispinalis:* arises from thoracic and cervical transverse processes *Multifidus:* arises from sacrum and ilium, transverse processes of T1–L5, and articular processes of C4–C7 *Rotatores:* arise from transverse processes of vertebrae; best developed in thoracic region	*Semispinalis:* thoracis, cervicis, and capitis: fibers run superomedially and attach to occipital bone and spinous processes in thoracic and cervical regions, spanning four to six segments *Multifidus (lumborum, thoracis, and cervicis):* fibers pass superomedially to spinous processes, spanning two to four segments *Rotatores (thoracis and cervicis):* fibers pass superomedially and attach to junction of lamina and transverse process of vertebra of origin or into spinous process above their origin, spanning one to two segments	Posterior rami of spinal nerves	**Extension** *Semispinalis:* extends head and thoracic and cervical regions of vertebral column and rotates them contralaterally *Multifidus:* stabilizes vertebrae during local movement of vertebral column *Rotatores:* stabilize vertebrae and assist with local extension and rotary movements of vertebral column; may function as organ of proprioception
Minor deep layer Interspinales	Superior surfaces of spinous processes of cervical and lumbar vertebrae	Inferior surfaces of spinous processes of vertebrae superior to vertebrae of origin		Aid in extension and rotation of vertebral column
Intertransversarii	Transverse processes of cervical and lumbar vertebrae	Transverse processes of adjacent vertebrae	Posterior and anterior rami of spinal nerves	Aid in lateral flexion of vertebral column *Acting bilaterally:* stabilize vertebral column
Levatores costarum	**Medial attachment:** tips of transverse processes of C7 and T1–T11 vertebrae	**Lateral attachment:** pass inferolaterally and insert on rib between its tubercle and angle	Posterior rami of C8–T11 spinal nerves	Elevate ribs, assisting inspiration Assist with lateral flexion of vertebral column

[a]Most back muscles are innervated by posterior rami of spinal nerves, but a few are innervated by anterior and posterior rami.

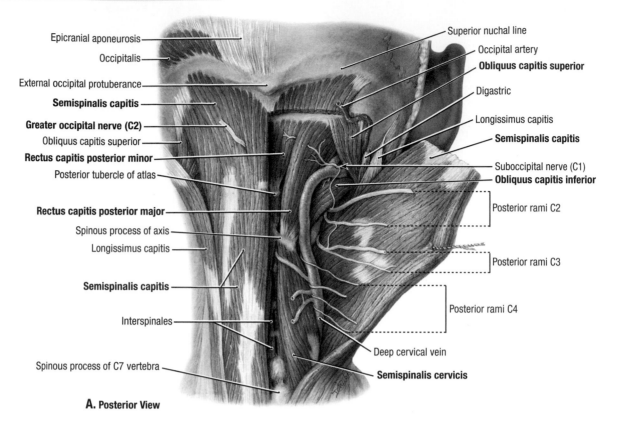

Epicranial aponeurosis

Occipitalis

External occipital protuberance

Semispinalis capitis

Greater occipital nerve (C2)

Obliquus capitis superior

Rectus capitis posterior minor

Posterior tubercle of atlas

Rectus capitis posterior major

Spinous process of axis

Longissimus capitis

Semispinalis capitis

Interspinales

Spinous process of C7 vertebra

Superior nuchal line

Occipital artery

Obliquus capitis superior

Digastric

Longissimus capitis

Semispinalis capitis

Suboccipital nerve (C1)

Obliquus capitis inferior

Posterior rami C2

Posterior rami C3

Posterior rami C4

Deep cervical vein

Semispinalis cervicis

A. Posterior View

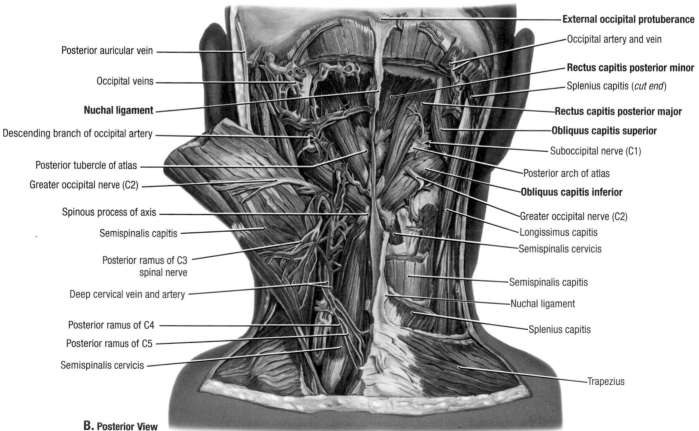

Posterior auricular vein

Occipital veins

Nuchal ligament

Descending branch of occipital artery

Posterior tubercle of atlas

Greater occipital nerve (C2)

Spinous process of axis

Semispinalis capitis

Posterior ramus of C3 spinal nerve

Deep cervical vein and artery

Posterior ramus of C4

Posterior ramus of C5

Semispinalis cervicis

External occipital protuberance

Occipital artery and vein

Rectus capitis posterior minor

Splenius capitis (cut end)

Rectus capitis posterior major

Obliquus capitis superior

Suboccipital nerve (C1)

Posterior arch of atlas

Obliquus capitis inferior

Greater occipital nerve (C2)

Longissimus capitis

Semispinalis cervicis

Semispinalis capitis

Nuchal ligament

Splenius capitis

Trapezius

B. Posterior View

1.35 **Suboccipital Region (I)**

A. Superficial dissection. **B.** Deep dissection.

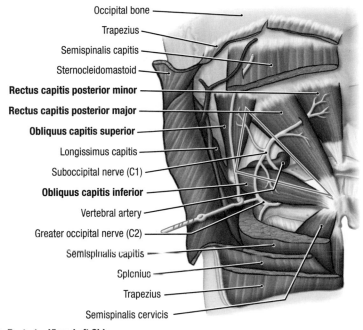

Occipital bone
Trapezius
Semispinalis capitis
Sternocleidomastoid
Rectus capitis posterior minor
Rectus capitis posterior major
Obliquus capitis superior
Longissimus capitis
Suboccipital nerve (C1)
Obliquus capitis inferior
Vertebral artery
Greater occipital nerve (C2)
Semispinalis capitis
Splenius
Trapezius
Semispinalis cervicis

A. Posterior View, Left Side

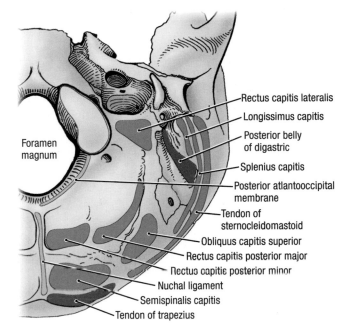

Foramen magnum
Rectus capitis lateralis
Longissimus capitis
Posterior belly of digastric
Splenius capitis
Posterior atlantooccipital membrane
Tendon of sternocleidomastoid
Obliquus capitis superior
Rectus capitis posterior major
Rectus capitis posterior minor
Nuchal ligament
Semispinalis capitis
Tendon of trapezius

B. Inferior View

Suboccipital Region (II) 1.36

A. Suboccipital triangle. **B.** Muscle attachments on inferior aspect of cranium.

TABLE 1.7 Muscles of Posterior Cervical Region

Muscle	Origin	Insertion	Innervation	Main Action
Intrinsic muscles of back—superficial layer (See Table 1.5.)				
Intrinsic muscles of back—intermediate layer (cervical/capitis parts)				
Longissimus	Transverse processes of T1–T5 vertebrae	*Longissimus capitis*: posterior mastoid process *Longissimus cervicis*: transverse processes of C2–C8	Posterior rami of spinal nerves	Extends neck; *acting unilaterally*: longissimus capitis rotates head to side of active muscle
Intrinsic muscles of back—deep layer (cervical/capitis parts)				
Semispinalis	Transverse processes of C4–T5 vertebrae	*Semispinalis capitis*: superior nuchal line of occipital bone *Semispinalis cervicis*: spinous processes of cervical vertebrae	Posterior rami of spinal nerves	*Acting unilaterally*: contributes to contra lateral rotation *Acting bilaterally*: extends head and neck
Multifidus	Transverse processes of T1–T3 Articular processes of C4–C7 vertebrae	Spinous processes two to four segments inferior to attachment		Stabilizes vertebrae during local movements of vertebral column
Rotatores	Transverse processes	Junction of lamina and transverse process or spinous process of vertebra immediately (brevis) or two segments (longus) superior to origin		Stabilize and assist with local extension and rotatory movements; may function as proprioceptive organ
Suboccipital muscles				
Rectus capitis posterior major	Spinous process of C2	Lateral part of inferior nuchal line	Suboccipital nerve (posterior ramus of C1)	Act on head directly or indirectly by extending it on C1 vertebra and rotating it on C1 and C2 vertebrae
Rectus capitis posterior minor	Posterior tubercle of C1	Medial part of inferior nuchal line		
Obliquus capitis inferior	Spinous process of C2 vertebra	Transverse process of C1 vertebra		
Obliquus capitis superior	Transverse process of C1 vertebra	Occipital bone between superior and inferior nuchal lines		

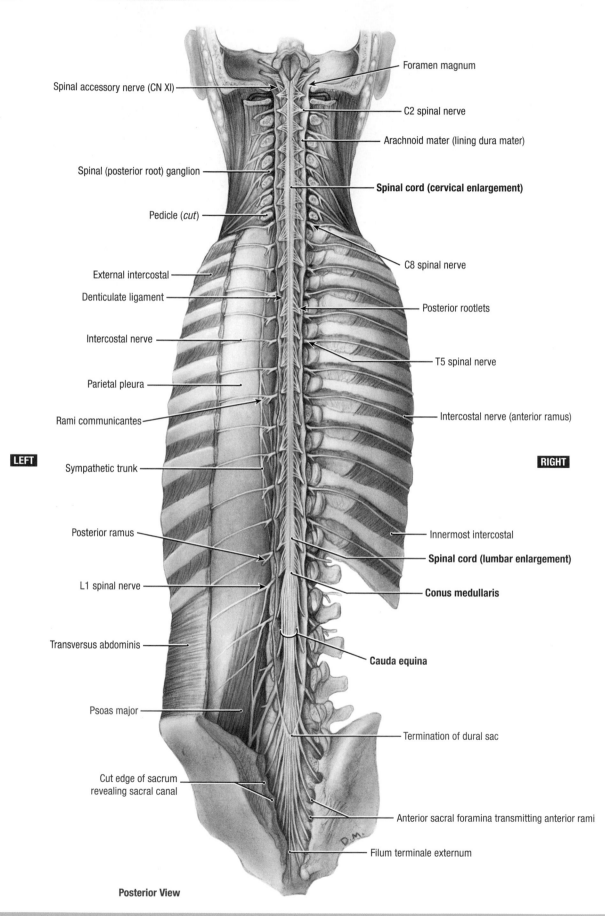

Foramen magnum

Spinal accessory nerve (CN XI)

C2 spinal nerve

Arachnoid mater (lining dura mater)

Spinal (posterior root) ganglion

Spinal cord (cervical enlargement)

Pedicle (*cut*)

C8 spinal nerve

External intercostal

Denticulate ligament

Posterior rootlets

Intercostal nerve

T5 spinal nerve

Parietal pleura

Rami communicantes

LEFT

RIGHT

Intercostal nerve (anterior ramus)

Sympathetic trunk

Posterior ramus

Innermost intercostal

Spinal cord (lumbar enlargement)

L1 spinal nerve

Conus medullaris

Transversus abdominis

Cauda equina

Psoas major

Termination of dural sac

Cut edge of sacrum revealing sacral canal

Anterior sacral foramina transmitting anterior rami

Filum terminale externum

Posterior View

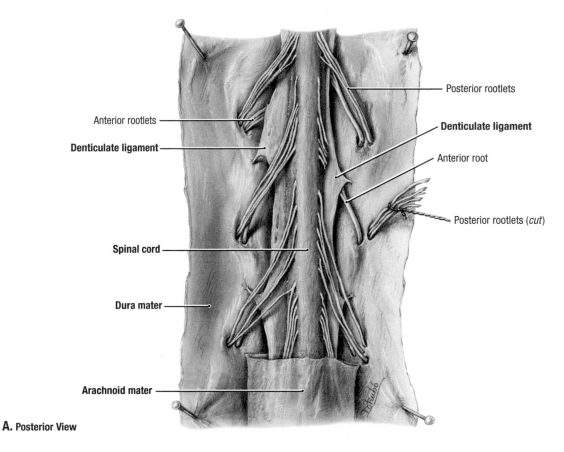

Posterior rootlets

Anterior rootlets

Denticulate ligament

Denticulate ligament

Anterior root

Posterior rootlets (*cut*)

Spinal cord

Dura mater

Arachnoid mater

A. Posterior View

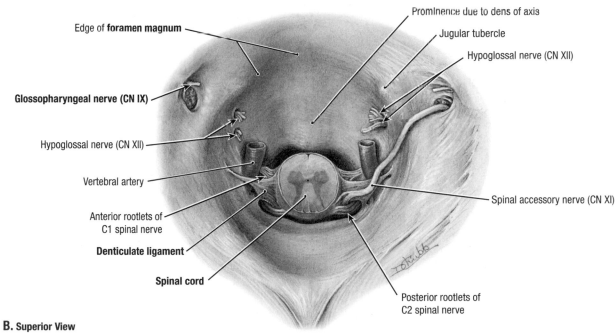

Prominence due to dens of axis

Edge of **foramen magnum**

Jugular tubercle

Hypoglossal nerve (CN XII)

Glossopharyngeal nerve (CN IX)

Hypoglossal nerve (CN XII)

Vertebral artery

Spinal accessory nerve (CN XI)

Anterior rootlets of
C1 spinal nerve

Denticulate ligament

Spinal cord

Posterior rootlets of
C2 spinal nerve

B. Superior View

Spinal Cord and Meninges

1.38

A. Dural sac cut open. The denticulate ligament anchors the cord to the dural sac between successive nerve roots by means of strong, toothlike processes. The anterior nerve roots (rootlets) lie anterior to the denticulate ligament, and the posterior nerve roots (rootlets) lie posterior to the ligament. **B. Structures of vertebral canal seen through foramen magnum.** The spinal cord, vertebral arteries, spinal accessory nerve (CN XI), and most superior part of the denticulate ligament pass through the foramen magnum within the meninges.

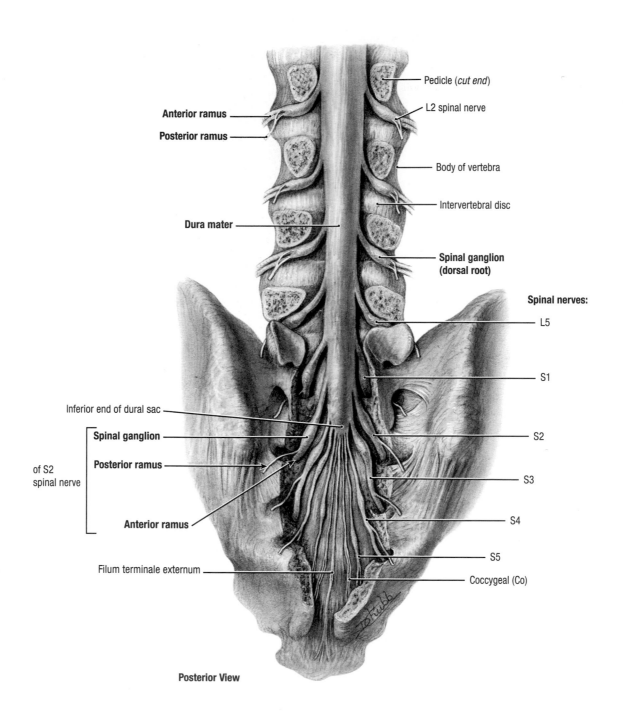

Pedicle (*cut end*)

Anterior ramus

L2 spinal nerve

Posterior ramus

Body of vertebra

Intervertebral disc

Dura mater

Spinal ganglion (dorsal root)

Spinal nerves:

L5

S1

Inferior end of dural sac

S2

Spinal ganglion

Posterior ramus

of S2 spinal nerve

S3

Anterior ramus

S4

S5

Filum terminale externum

Coccygeal (Co)

Posterior View

| 1.39 | **Inferior End of Dural Sac (I)** |

The posterior parts of the lumbar vertebrae and sacrum were removed, along with the fat and internal (epidural) venous plexus that occupy the epidural space. Note that the inferior limit of the dural sac is at the level of the posterior superior iliac spine (body of 2nd sacral vertebra); the dura continues as the filum terminale externum.

Epidural anesthesia (block). An anesthetic can be injected into the extradural space. The anesthetic has direct effect on the spinal nerve roots in the epidural space. The patient loses sensation inferior to the level of the block (see Fig. 1.40C).

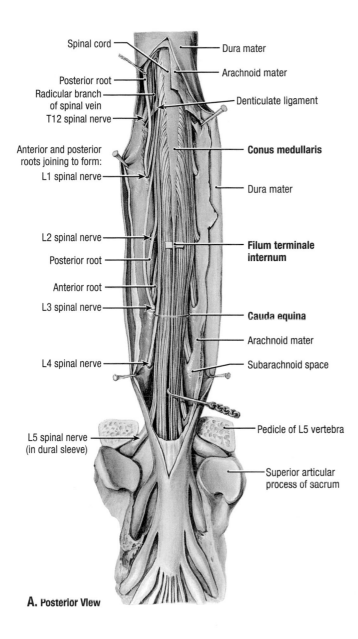

Spinal cord

Dura mater

Posterior root

Arachnoid mater

Radicular branch of spinal vein

T12 spinal nerve

Denticulate ligament

Anterior and posterior roots joining to form:

Conus medullaris

L1 spinal nerve

Dura mater

L2 spinal nerve

Filum terminale internum

Posterior root

Anterior root

L3 spinal nerve

Cauda equina

Arachnoid mater

L4 spinal nerve

Subarachnoid space

L5 spinal nerve (in dural sleeve)

Pedicle of L5 vertebra

Superior articular process of sacrum

A. Posterior View

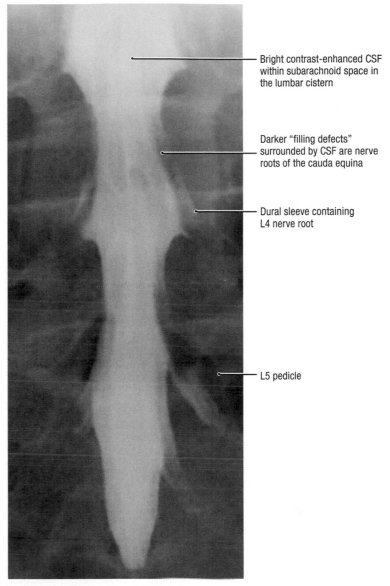

Bright contrast-enhanced CSF within subarachnoid space in the lumbar cistern

Darker "filling defects" surrounded by CSF are nerve roots of the cauda equina

Dural sleeve containing L4 nerve root

L5 pedicle

B. Frontal Myelogram

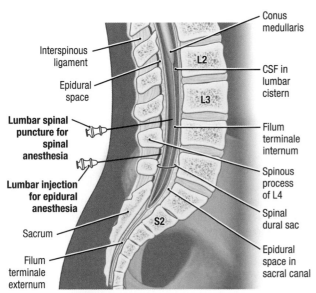

Conus medullaris

Interspinous ligament

L2

CSF in lumbar cistern

L3

Epidural space

Lumbar spinal puncture for spinal anesthesia

Filum terminale internum

Lumbar injection for epidural anesthesia

Spinous process of L4

Sacrum

S2

Spinal dural sac

Filum terminale externum

Epidural space in sacral canal

C. Sagittal Section

Inferior End of Dural Sac (II)

1.40

A. Inferior dural sac and lumbar cistern of subarachnoid space (opened). **B.** Myelogram of lumbar region of vertebral column (contrast injected into subarachnoid space). **C.** Lumbar spinal puncture and epidural anesthesia.

- The conus medullaris continues as a glistening thread, the filum terminale internum, which descends with the nerve roots, constituting the cauda equina.
- In the adult, the spinal cord usually ends at the level of the disc between vertebrae L1 and L2. Variations: 95% of cords end within the limits of the bodies of L1 and L2, whereas 3% end posterior to the inferior half of T12, and 2% posterior to L3.

To obtain a **sample of cerebrospinal fluid (CSF) from the lumbar cistern**, a lumbar puncture needle, fitted with a stylet, is inserted into the subarachnoid space. Flexion of the vertebral column facilitates insertion of the needle by stretching the ligamenta flava and spreading the laminae and spinous processes apart. The needle is inserted in the midline between the spinous processes of the L3 and L4 (or the L4 and L5) vertebrae. At these levels in adults, there is little danger of damaging the spinal cord.

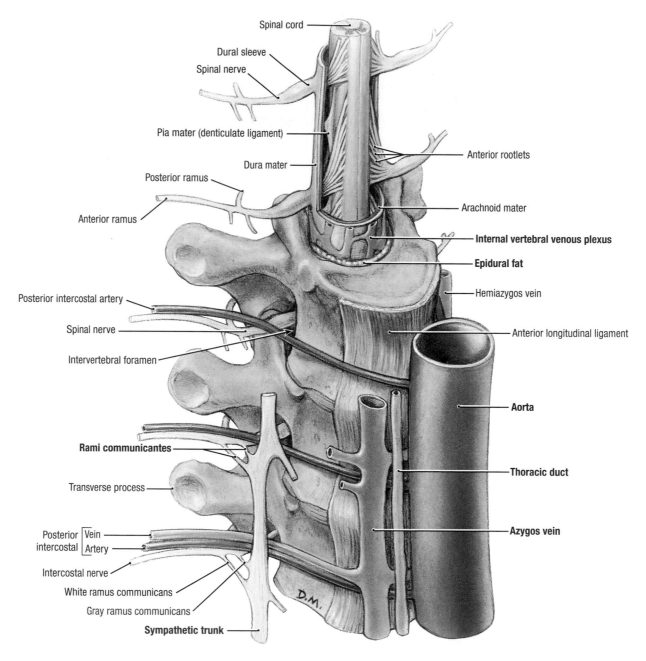

Spinal cord

Dural sleeve

Spinal nerve

Pia mater (denticulate ligament)

Dura mater

Posterior ramus

Anterior ramus

Posterior intercostal artery

Spinal nerve

Intervertebral foramen

Rami communicantes

Transverse process

Posterior Vein
intercostal Artery

Intercostal nerve

White ramus communicans

Gray ramus communicans

Sympathetic trunk

Anterior rootlets

Arachnoid mater

Internal vertebral venous plexus

Epidural fat

Hemiazygos vein

Anterior longitudinal ligament

Aorta

Thoracic duct

Azygos vein

D.M.

Right Anterolateral View

1.41 | **Spinal Cord and Prevertebral Structures**

The vertebrae have been removed superiorly to expose the spinal cord and meninges.

- The aorta descends to the left of the midline, with the thoracic duct and azygos vein to its right.
- Typically, the azygos vein is on the right side of the vertebral bodies, and the hemiazygos vein is on the left.

- The thoracic sympathetic trunk and ganglia lie lateral to the thoracic vertebrae; the rami communicantes connect the sympathetic ganglia with the spinal nerve.
- A sleeve of dura mater surrounds the spinal nerves and blends with the sheath (epineurium) of the spinal nerve.
- The dura mater is separated from the walls of the vertebral canal by epidural fat and the internal vertebral venous plexus.

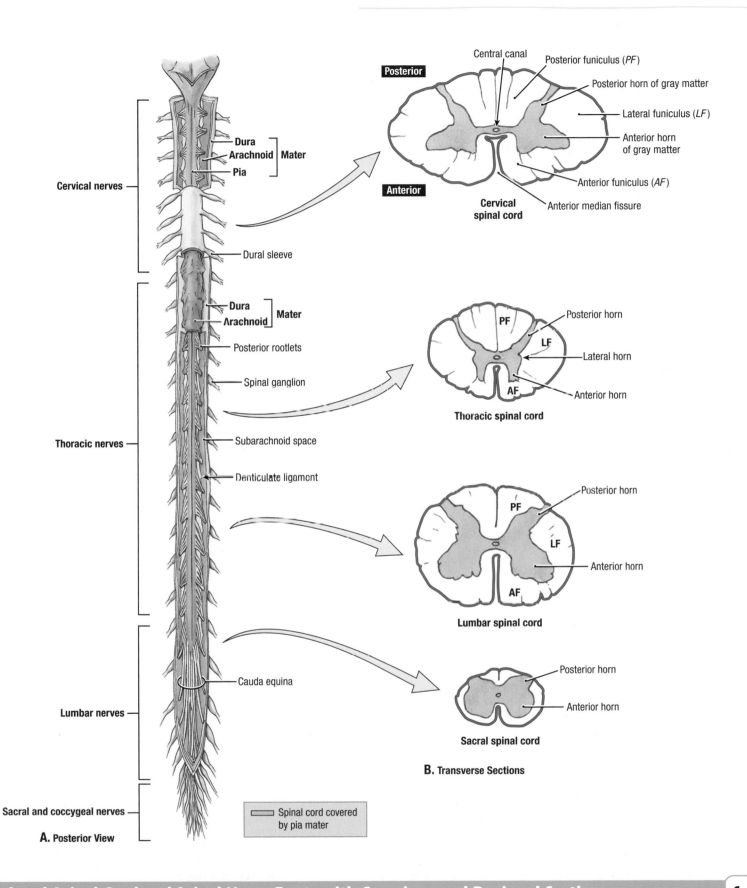

Central canal
Posterior funiculus (*PF*)
Posterior
Posterior horn of gray matter
Lateral funiculus (*LF*)
Dura
Arachnoid | **Mater**
Pia
Anterior horn of gray matter
Anterior
Anterior funiculus (*AF*)
Cervical spinal cord
Anterior median fissure

Cervical nerves

Dural sleeve

Dura] **Mater**
Arachnoid
Posterior rootlets
Spinal ganglion

Posterior horn
PF
LF
Lateral horn
AF
Anterior horn
Thoracic spinal cord

Subarachnoid space

Denticulate ligament

Thoracic nerves

Posterior horn
PF
LF
Anterior horn
AF
Lumbar spinal cord

Cauda equina

Posterior horn
Anterior horn
Sacral spinal cord

B. Transverse Sections

Lumbar nerves

Sacral and coccygeal nerves

A. Posterior View

Spinal cord covered by pia mater

Isolated Spinal Cord and Spinal Nerve Roots with Coverings and Regional Sections   **1.42**

A. Spinal cord and dural sac. The sac has been opened to reveal arachnoid and pia mater as well as spinal cord and posterior nerve rootlets.
B. Cervical, thoracic, lumbar, and sacral spinal cord.

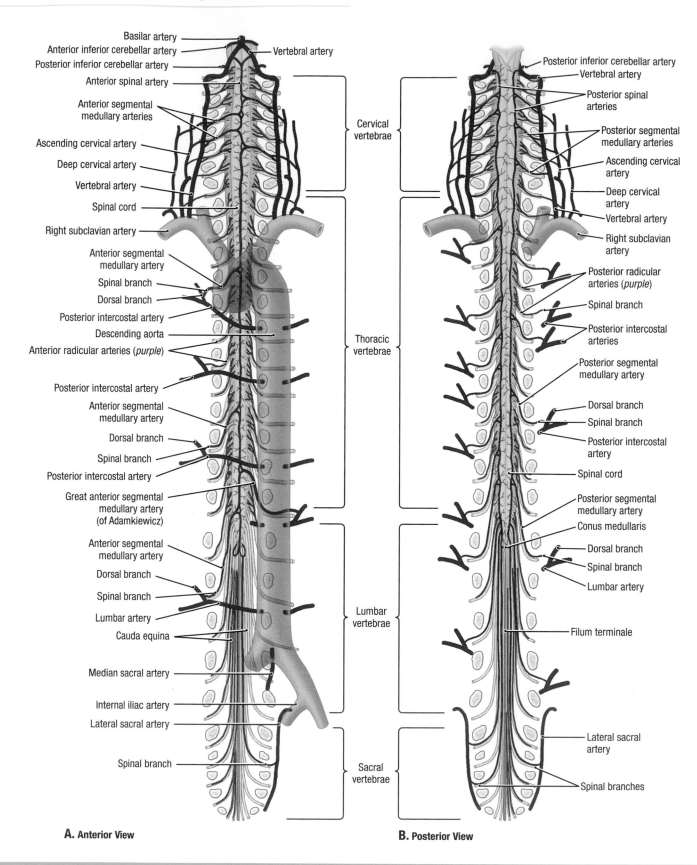

Basilar artery
Anterior inferior cerebellar artery
Posterior inferior cerebellar artery
Anterior spinal artery
Anterior segmental medullary arteries
Ascending cervical artery
Deep cervical artery
Vertebral artery
Spinal cord
Right subclavian artery
Anterior segmental medullary artery
Spinal branch
Dorsal branch
Posterior intercostal artery
Descending aorta
Anterior radicular arteries (*purple*)
Posterior intercostal artery
Anterior segmental medullary artery
Dorsal branch
Spinal branch
Posterior intercostal artery
Great anterior segmental medullary artery (of Adamkiewicz)
Anterior segmental medullary artery
Dorsal branch
Spinal branch
Lumbar artery
Cauda equina
Median sacral artery
Internal iliac artery
Lateral sacral artery
Spinal branch

Vertebral artery

Cervical vertebrae
Thoracic vertebrae
Lumbar vertebrae
Sacral vertebrae

Posterior inferior cerebellar artery
Vertebral artery
Posterior spinal arteries
Posterior segmental medullary arteries
Ascending cervical artery
Deep cervical artery
Vertebral artery
Right subclavian artery
Posterior radicular arteries (*purple*)
Spinal branch
Posterior intercostal arteries
Posterior segmental medullary artery
Dorsal branch
Spinal branch
Posterior intercostal artery
Spinal cord
Posterior segmental medullary artery
Conus medullaris
Dorsal branch
Spinal branch
Lumbar artery
Filum terminale
Lateral sacral artery
Spinal branches

A. Anterior View

B. Posterior View

1.43 Blood Supply of Spinal Cord

A. and **B.** **Arteries of spinal cord.** The segmental reinforcements of blood supply from the segmental medullary arteries are important in supplying blood to the anterior and posterior spinal arteries.

Back injuries. Fractures, dislocations, and fracture-dislocations may interfere with the blood supply to the spinal cord from the spinal and medullary arteries.

POSTERIOR

Posterior spinal veins

Posterior internal vertebral venous plexus

Pial venous plexus

Spinal nerve

Intervertebral vein

**Anterior internal
vertebral venous plexus**

Anterior spinal veins

Basivertebral vein

Posterior spinal artery

Spinal cord

Posterior radicular artery

Pial arterial plexus

Spinal nerve

Spinal branch

**Anterior segmental
medullary artery**

Anterior spinal artery

C. Transverse Section

ANTERIOR

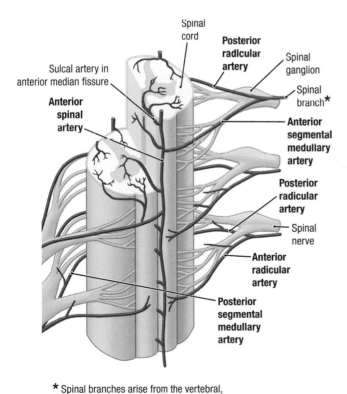

Spinal cord

Posterior radicular artery

Spinal ganglion

Spinal branch*

Anterior segmental medullary artery

Posterior radicular artery

Spinal nerve

Anterior radicular artery

Posterior segmental medullary artery

Sulcal artery in anterior median fissure

Anterior spinal artery

*Spinal branches arise from the vertebral, intercostal, lumbar, or sacral artery, depending on level of spinal cord.

D. Anterolateral View

Blood Supply of Spinal Cord (continued) 1.43

C. Arterial supply and venous drainage. **D.** Segmental medullary and radicular arteries.

- The spinal arteries run longitudinally from the brainstem to the conus medullaris of the spinal cord. By themselves, the anterior and posterior spinal arteries supply only the short superior part of the spinal cord.
- The anterior and posterior segmental medullary arteries enter the IV foramen to unite with the spinal arteries to supply blood to the spinal cord. The great anterior segmental medullary artery (Adamkiewicz artery) occurs on the left side in 65% of people. It reinforces the circulation to two thirds of the spinal cord.
- Posterior and anterior roots of the spinal nerves and their coverings are supplied by posterior and anterior radicular arteries, which run along the nerve roots. These vessels do not reach the posterior or anterior spinal arteries.
- The anterior and posterior spinal veins are arranged longitudinally; they communicate freely with each other and are drained by anterior and posterior medullary and radicular veins. The veins draining the spinal cord join the internal vertebral plexus in the epidural space.

Ischemia. Deficiency of blood supply (ischemia) of the spinal cord can lead to muscle weakness and paralysis. The spinal cord may also suffer circulatory impairment if the segmental medullary arteries, particularly the great anterior segmental medullary artery (of Adamkiewicz), are narrowed by obstructive arterial disease or aortic clamping during surgery.

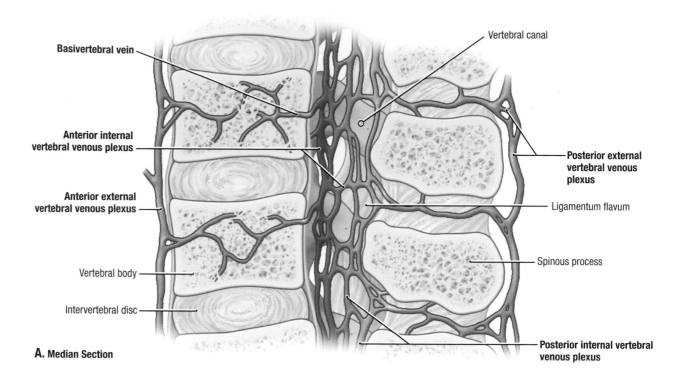

Basivertebral vein

Vertebral canal

Anterior internal
vertebral venous plexus

Anterior external
vertebral venous plexus

Posterior external
vertebral venous
plexus

Ligamentum flavum

Vertebral body

Spinous process

Intervertebral disc

Posterior internal vertebral
venous plexus

A. Median Section

1.44 Vertebral Venous Plexuses

A. Lumbar spine. **B.** Lumbar vertebra with vertebral body
sectioned transversely.

- There are internal and external vertebral venous plexuses, communicating with each other and with both
  systemic veins and the portal system. **Infection and
  tumors can spread** from the areas drained by the
  systemic and portal veins to the vertebral venous system
  and lodge in the vertebrae, spinal cord, brain, or skull.
- The internal vertebral venous plexus, located in the vertebral canal, consists of a plexus of thin-walled, valveless
  veins that surround the dura mater. Cranially, the internal venous plexus communicates through the foramen
  magnum with the occipital and basilar sinuses; at each
  spinal segment, the plexus receives veins from the spinal
  cord and a basivertebral vein from the vertebral body.
  The plexus is drained by IV veins that pass through the
  intervertebral and sacral foramina to the vertebral, intercostal, lumbar, and lateral sacral veins.
- The anterior external vertebral venous plexus is formed
  by veins that course through the body of each vertebra.
  Veins that pass through the ligamenta flava form the
  posterior external vertebral venous plexus. In the cervical
  region, these plexuses communicate with the occipital
  and deep cervical veins. In the thoracic, lumbar, and
  pelvic regions, the azygos (or hemiazygos), ascending
  lumbar, and lateral sacral veins, respectively, further link
  segment to segment.

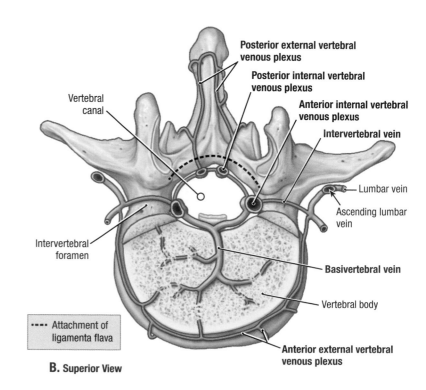

Posterior external vertebral
venous plexus

Posterior internal vertebral
venous plexus

Vertebral
canal

Anterior internal vertebral
venous plexus

Intervertebral vein

Lumbar vein

Ascending lumbar
vein

Intervertebral
foramen

Basivertebral vein

Vertebral body

- - - - Attachment of
ligamenta flava

Anterior external vertebral
venous plexus

B. Superior View

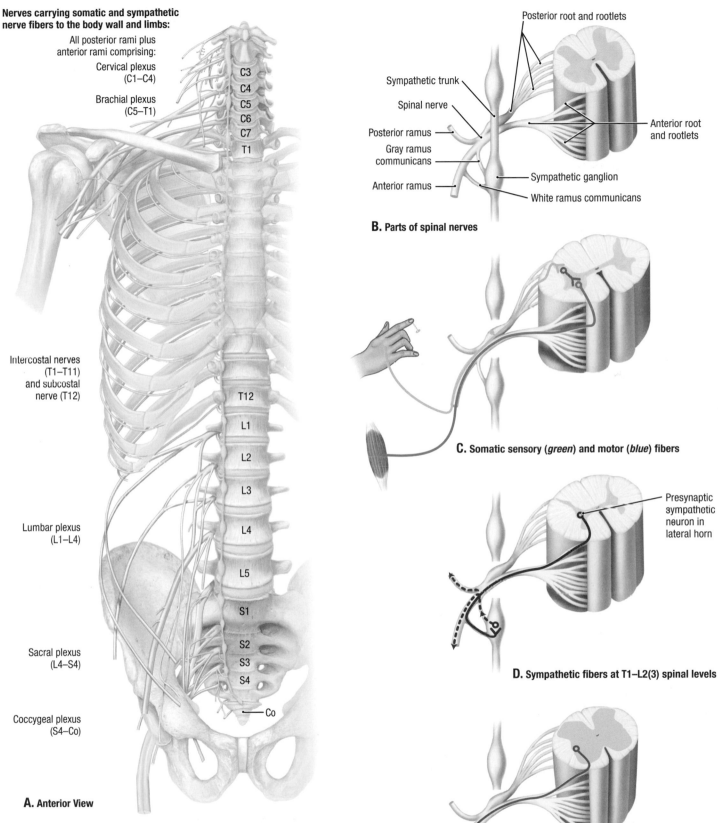

Nerves carrying somatic and sympathetic nerve fibers to the body wall and limbs:

All posterior rami plus anterior rami comprising:

Cervical plexus (C1–C4)

Brachial plexus (C5–T1)

C3
C4
C5
C6
C7
T1

Intercostal nerves (T1–T11) and subcostal nerve (T12)

T12
L1
L2
L3
L4
L5

Lumbar plexus (L1–L4)

S1

Sacral plexus (L4–S4)

S2
S3
S4

Co

Coccygeal plexus (S4–Co)

A. Anterior View

Posterior root and rootlets

Sympathetic trunk

Spinal nerve

Posterior ramus

Gray ramus communicans

Anterior ramus

Anterior root and rootlets

Sympathetic ganglion

White ramus communicans

B. Parts of spinal nerves

C. Somatic sensory (*green*) and motor (*blue*) fibers

Presynaptic sympathetic neuron in lateral horn

D. Sympathetic fibers at T1–L2(3) spinal levels

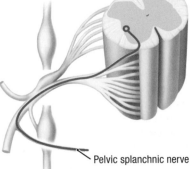

Pelvic splanchnic nerve

E. Parasympathetic fibers at S2–S4 spinal cord levels

B–E. Superoanterolateral Views

Overview of Innervation of Limbs and Body Wall **1.45**

A. Overview. **B.** Parts of spinal nerve. **C.** Somatic sensory and motor fibers. **D.** Pathway for presynaptic sympathetic fibers exiting central nervous system (CNS). **E.** Pathway for presynaptic parasympathetic fibers exiting sacral spinal cord.

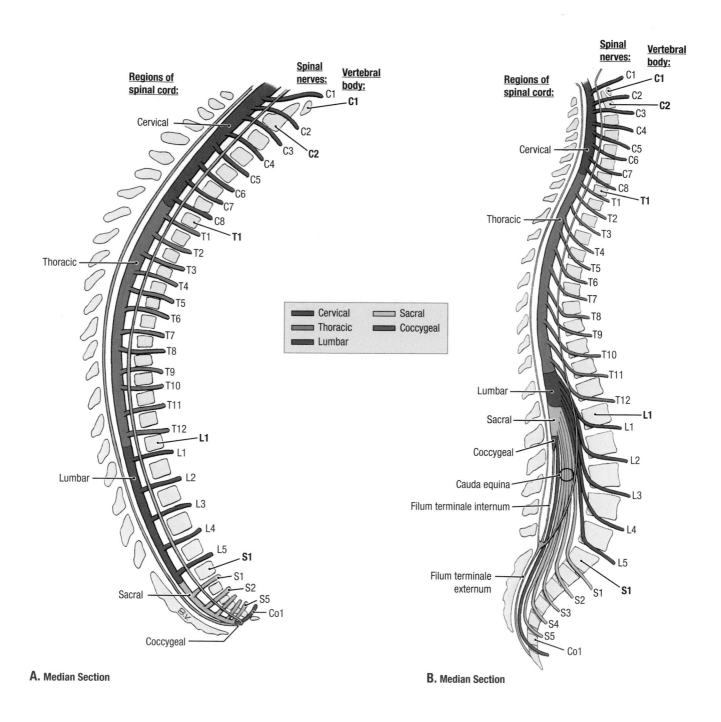

Regions of spinal cord:
Cervical
Thoracic
Lumbar
Sacral
Coccygeal

Spinal nerves:
C1
C2
C3
C4
C5
C6
C7
C8
T1
T2
T3
T4
T5
T6
T7
T8
T9
T10
T11
T12
L1
L2
L3
L4
L5
S1
S2
S5
Co1

Vertebral body:
C1
C2
T1
L1
S1

B.V.

Cervical	Sacral
Thoracic	Coccygeal
Lumbar	

A. Median Section

Regions of spinal cord:
Cervical
Thoracic
Lumbar
Sacral
Coccygeal
Cauda equina
Filum terminale internum
Filum terminale externum

Spinal nerves:
C1
C2
C3
C4
C5
C6
C7
C8
T1
T2
T3
T4
T5
T6
T7
T8
T9
T10
T11
T12
L1
L2
L3
L4
L5
S1
S2
S3
S4
S5
Co1

Vertebral body:
C1
C2
T1
L1
S1

B. Median Section

1.46 **Spinal Cord and Spinal Nerves**

A. Spinal cord at 12 weeks of gestation. **B.** Spinal cord of an adult.

- Early in development, the spinal cord and vertebral (spinal) canal are nearly equal in length. The canal grows longer, so spinal nerves have an increasingly longer course to reach the IV foramen at the correct level for their exit. The spinal cord of adults terminates between vertebral bodies L1–L2. The remaining spinal nerves, seeking their IV foramen of exit, form the cauda equina.

- All 31 pairs of spinal nerves—8 cervical (C), 12 thoracic (T), 5 lumbar (L), 5 sacral (S), and 1 coccygeal (Co)—arise from the spinal cord and exit through the IV foramina in the vertebral column.

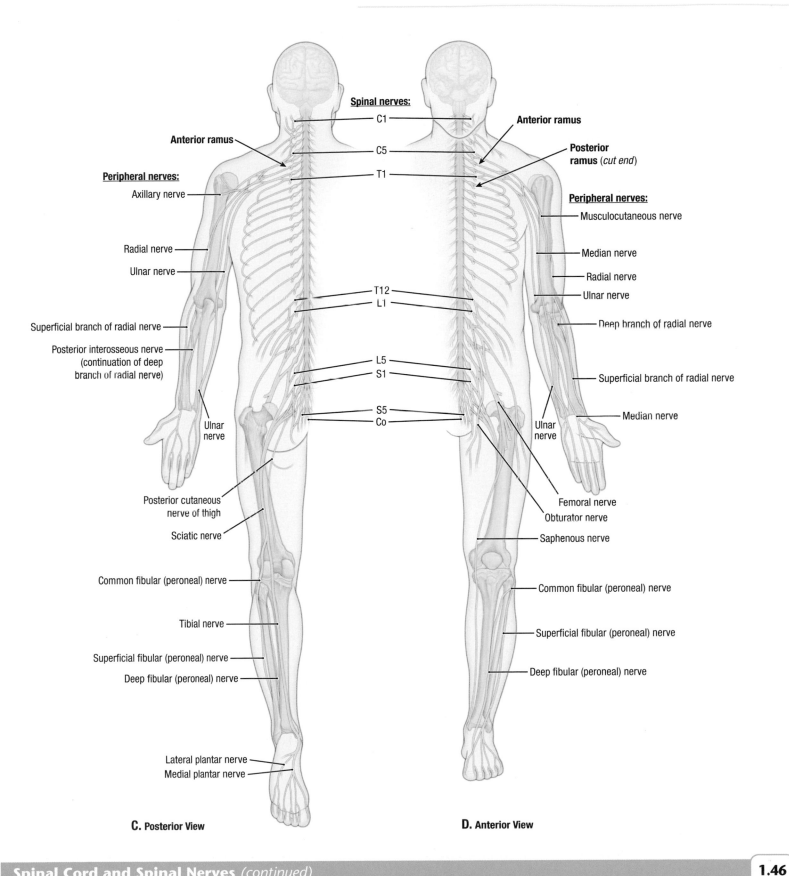

Spinal nerves:
- C1
- C5
- T1
- T12
- L1
- L5
- S1
- S5
- Co

Anterior ramus

Peripheral nerves:
- Axillary nerve
- Radial nerve
- Ulnar nerve
- Superficial branch of radial nerve
- Posterior interosseous nerve (continuation of deep branch of radial nerve)
- Ulnar nerve
- Posterior cutaneous nerve of thigh
- Sciatic nerve
- Common fibular (peroneal) nerve
- Tibial nerve
- Superficial fibular (peroneal) nerve
- Deep fibular (peroneal) nerve
- Lateral plantar nerve
- Medial plantar nerve

Anterior ramus

Posterior ramus (*cut end*)

Peripheral nerves:
- Musculocutaneous nerve
- Median nerve
- Radial nerve
- Ulnar nerve
- Deep branch of radial nerve
- Superficial branch of radial nerve
- Median nerve
- Ulnar nerve
- Femoral nerve
- Obturator nerve
- Saphenous nerve
- Common fibular (peroneal) nerve
- Superficial fibular (peroneal) nerve
- Deep fibular (peroneal) nerve

C. Posterior View   **D. Anterior View**

Spinal Cord and Spinal Nerves (continued)   **1.46**

C. and **D.** Peripheral nerves.
- The anterior rami supply nerve fibers to the anterior and lateral regions of the trunk and upper and lower limbs.
- The posterior rami supply nerve fibers to synovial joints of the vertebral column, deep muscles of the back, and overlying skin.

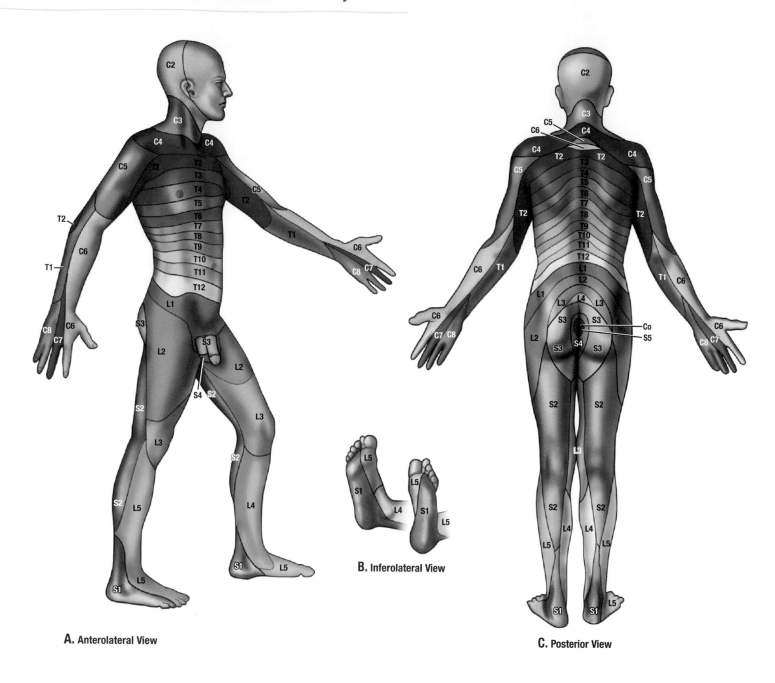

A. Anterolateral View

B. Inferolateral View

C. Posterior View

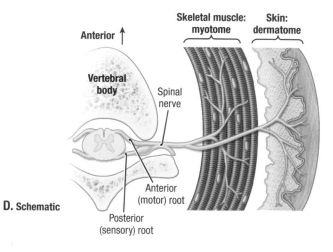

D. Schematic

1.47   **Dermatomes**

A–C. Dermatome map. From clinical studies of lesions in the posterior roots or spinal nerves, dermatome maps have been devised that indicate the typical patterns of innervation of the skin by specific spinal nerves. **D. Schematic of dermatome and myotome.** The unilateral area of skin innervated by the general sensory fibers of a single spinal nerve is called a dermatome.

A. Anterior View

Lateral rotation (shoulder) C5

Medial rotation (shoulder) C6, C7, C8

Finger flexion C7, **C8**

Abduction (shoulder)

Adduction (shoulder) C6, C7, **C8**

C5

Lateral external rotation (hip) L5, **S1**

Medial internal rotation (hip) L4, L5

Finger extension **C7**, C8

40°

0°

50°

Adduction (hip) L2, L3, L4

Abduction (hip) L5, S1

B. Lateral View

Flexion (elbow) C5, **C6**

Extension (elbow) C6, **C7**

Extension (wrist) **C6**, C7

Flexion (wrist) C6, **C7**

C. Anterior View

Supination (forearm) C6

Pronation (forearm) C7, C8

D. Anterior View

Abduction T1

Abduction **T1**

T1 Adduction

Abduction and Adduction of Digits (Metacarpophalangeal Joints)

E. Lateral View

Extension (shoulder) C6, C7, C8

Flexion (shoulder) C5

Extension (hip) L4, L5

Flexion (hip) **L2**, L3

Flexion (knee) L5, S1

Extension (knee) **L3**, L4

Dorsiflexion (ankle) **L4**, L5

Plantarflexion (ankle) **S1**, S2

Movements, mostly shown in antagonistic pairs

The movements associated with each **bolded** segment are most commonly tested to determine the neurologic level of a lesion.

Myotomes

Somatic motor (general somatic efferent) fibers transmit impulses to skeletal (voluntary) muscles. The unilateral muscle mass receiving innervation from the somatic motor fibers conveyed by a single spinal nerve is a myotome. Each skeletal muscle is innervated by the somatic motor fibers of several spinal nerves; therefore, the muscle myotome will consist of several segments. The muscle myotomes have been grouped by joint movement to facilitate clinical testing. The intrinsic muscles of the hand constitute a single myotome: T1.

1.48

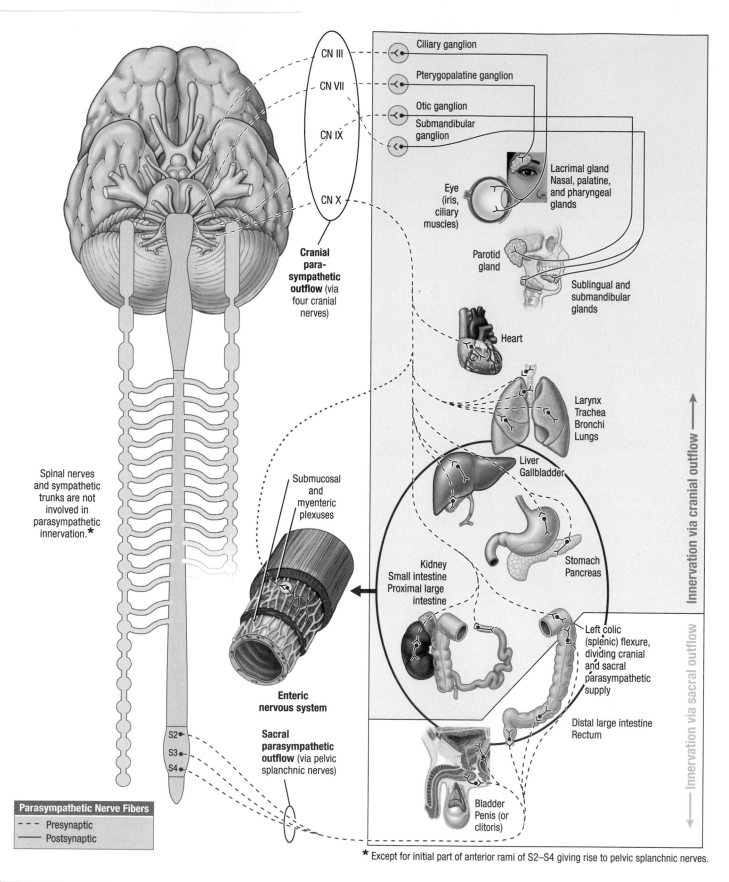

Ciliary ganglion

Pterygopalatine ganglion

Otic ganglion

Submandibular ganglion

CN III

CN VII

CN IX

CN X

Cranial parasympathetic outflow (via four cranial nerves)

Lacrimal gland Nasal, palatine, and pharyngeal glands

Eye (iris, ciliary muscles)

Parotid gland

Sublingual and submandibular glands

Heart

Larynx Trachea Bronchi Lungs

Liver Gallbladder

Stomach Pancreas

Kidney Small intestine Proximal large intestine

Left colic (splenic) flexure, dividing cranial and sacral parasympathetic supply

Distal large intestine Rectum

Bladder Penis (or clitoris)

Spinal nerves and sympathetic trunks are not involved in parasympathetic innervation.*

Submucosal and myenteric plexuses

Enteric nervous system

Sacral parasympathetic outflow (via pelvic splanchnic nerves)

S2
S3
S4

Innervation via cranial outflow

Innervation via sacral outflow

Parasympathetic Nerve Fibers

– – –   Presynaptic
———   Postsynaptic

*Except for initial part of anterior rami of S2–S4 giving rise to pelvic splanchnic nerves.

1.49   **Distribution of Parasympathetic Nerve Fibers**

The presynaptic nerve cell bodies of the parasympathetic system are located in two sites: in the gray matter of the brainstem (cranial parasympathetic outflow) and in the gray matter of the sacral segments of the spinal cord (sacral parasympathetic outflow).

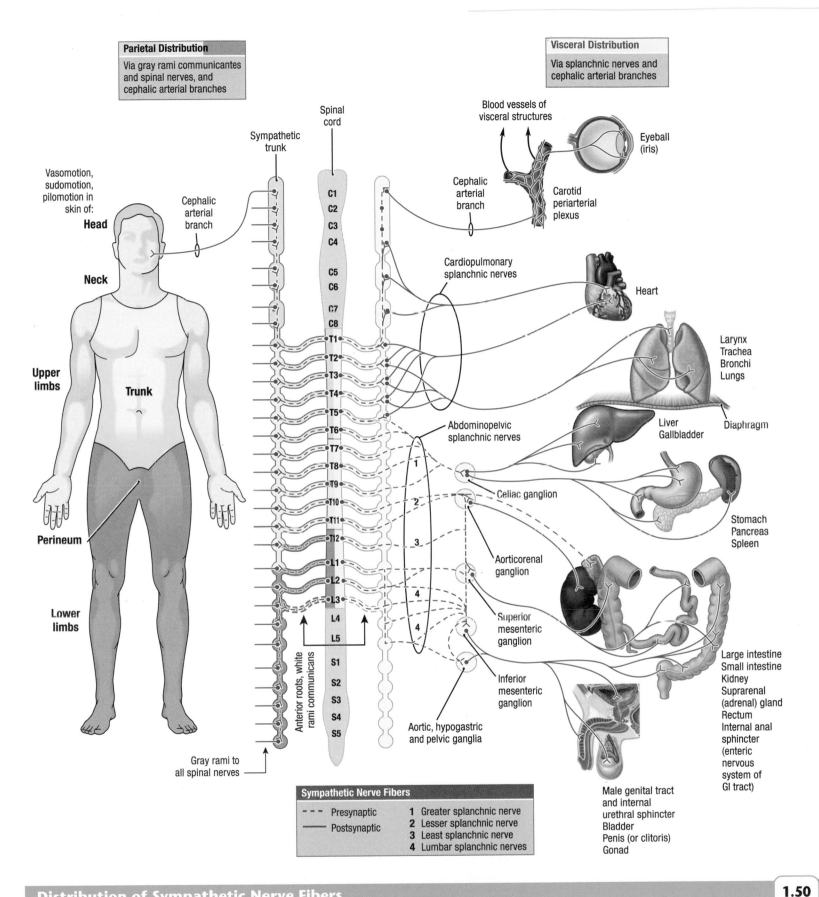

Blood vessels of visceral structures

Spinal cord

Eyeball (iris)

Sympathetic trunk

Vasomotion, sudomotion, pilomotion in skin of:

Head

Cephalic arterial branch

Cephalic arterial branch

Carotid periarterial plexus

Neck

C1
C2
C3
C4
C5
C6
C7
C8

Cardiopulmonary splanchnic nerves

Heart

Upper limbs

Trunk

T1
T2
T3
T4
T5
T6
T7
T8
T9
T10
T11
T12

Larynx
Trachea
Bronchi
Lungs

Diaphragm

Liver
Gallbladder

Abdominopelvic splanchnic nerves

1

Celiac ganglion

Stomach
Pancreas
Spleen

Perineum

L1
L2
L3
L4
L5

2

3

4

4

Aorticorenal ganglion

Superior mesenteric ganglion

Lower limbs

S1
S2
S3
S4
S5

Anterior roots, white rami communicans

Inferior mesenteric ganglion

Aortic, hypogastric and pelvic ganglia

Large intestine
Small intestine
Kidney
Suprarenal (adrenal) gland
Rectum
Internal anal sphincter (enteric nervous system of GI tract)

Gray rami to all spinal nerves

Male genital tract and internal urethral sphincter
Bladder
Penis (or clitoris)
Gonad

Sympathetic Nerve Fibers

- - -	Presynaptic	**1** Greater splanchnic nerve
———	Postsynaptic	**2** Lesser splanchnic nerve
		3 Least splanchnic nerve
		4 Lumbar splanchnic nerves

Distribution of Sympathetic Nerve Fibers

1.50

The cell bodies of presynaptic neurons of the sympathetic system are located in the intermediolateral cell column and extend between the first thoracic and the second lumbar segments of the spinal cord.

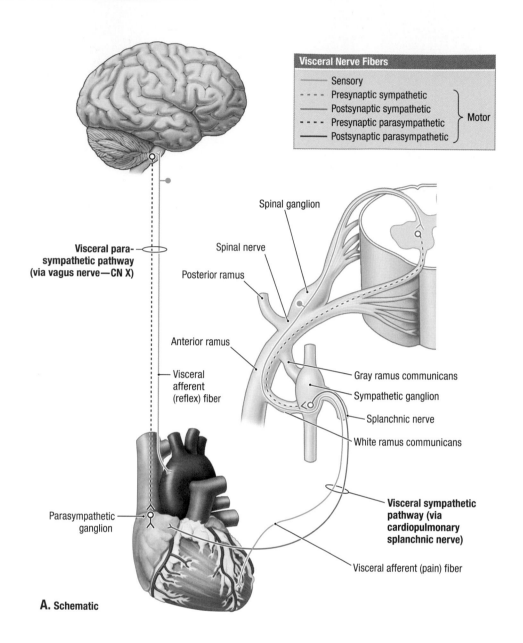

Visceral Nerve Fibers

———	Sensory
- - - -	Presynaptic sympathetic
———	Postsynaptic sympathetic
- - - -	Presynaptic parasympathetic
———	Postsynaptic parasympathetic

Motor

Spinal ganglion

Spinal nerve

Posterior ramus

Anterior ramus

Visceral afferent (reflex) fiber

Visceral para-sympathetic pathway (via vagus nerve—CN X)

Gray ramus communicans

Sympathetic ganglion

Splanchnic nerve

White ramus communicans

Parasympathetic ganglion

Visceral sympathetic pathway (via cardiopulmonary splanchnic nerve)

Visceral afferent (pain) fiber

A. Schematic

1.51   **Visceral Afferent and Visceral Efferent (Motor) Innervation**

A. Overview. Visceral afferent fibers have important relationships to the central nervous system (CNS), both anatomically and functionally. We are usually unaware of the sensory input of these fibers, which provides information about the condition of the body's internal environment. This information is integrated in the CNS, often triggering visceral or somatic reflexes or both. Visceral reflexes regulate blood pressure and chemistry by altering such functions as heart and respiratory rates and vascular resistance. Visceral sensation that reaches a conscious level is generally categorized as pain that is usually poorly localized and may be perceived as hunger or nausea. However, adequate stimulation may elicit true pain. Most visceral/reflex (unconscious) sensation and some pain travel in visceral afferent fibers that accompany the parasympathetic fibers retrograde. Most visceral pain impulses (from the heart and most organs of the peritoneal cavity) travel along visceral afferent fibers accompanying sympathetic fibers.

Visceral efferent (motor) innervation. The efferent nerve fibers and ganglia of the autonomic nervous system (ANS) are organized into two systems or divisions.
1. **Sympathetic (thoracolumbar) division.** In general, the effects of sympathetic stimulation are catabolic (preparing the body for "flight or fight").
2. **Parasympathetic (craniosacral) division.** In general, the effects of parasympathetic stimulation are anabolic (promoting normal function and conserving energy).

Conduction of impulses from the CNS to the effector organ involves a series of two neurons in both sympathetic and parasympathetic systems. The cell body of the presynaptic (preganglionic) neuron (first neuron) is located in the gray matter of the CNS. Its fiber (axon) synapses on the cell body of a postsynaptic (postganglionic) neuron, the second neuron in the series. The cell bodies of such second neurons are located in autonomic ganglia outside the CNS, and the postsynaptic fibers terminate on the effector organ (smooth muscle, modified cardiac muscle, or glands).

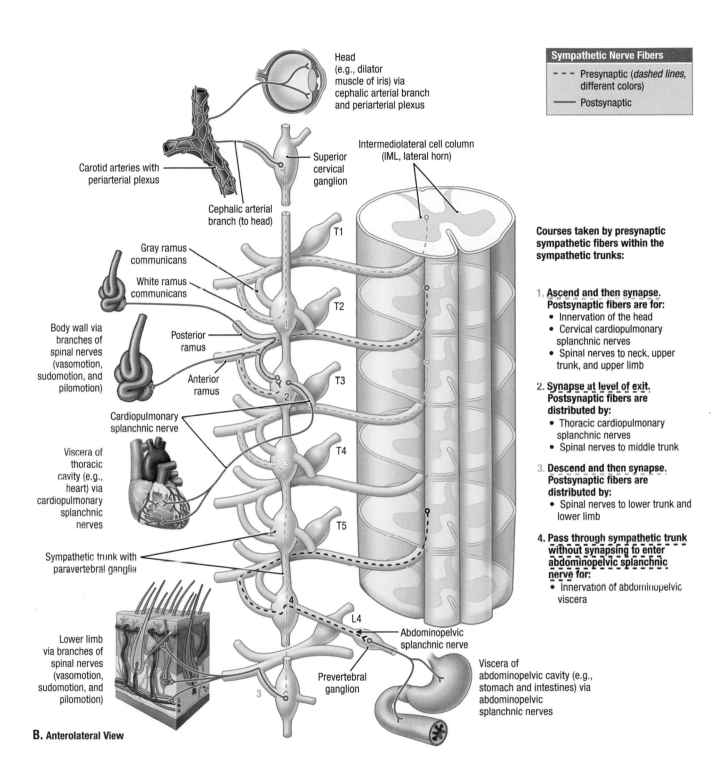

Head
(e.g., dilator
muscle of iris) via
cephalic arterial branch
and periarterial plexus

Carotid arteries with
periarterial plexus

Cephalic arterial
branch (to head)

Gray ramus
communicans

White ramus
communicans

Body wall via
branches of
spinal nerves
(vasomotion,
sudomotion, and
pilomotion)

Posterior
ramus

Anterior
ramus

Cardiopulmonary
splanchnic nerve

Viscera of
thoracic
cavity (e.g.,
heart) via
cardiopulmonary
splanchnic
nerves

Sympathetic trunk with
paravertebral ganglia

Lower limb
via branches of
spinal nerves
(vasomotion,
sudomotion, and
pilomotion)

Prevertebral
ganglion

Superior
cervical
ganglion

Intermediolateral cell column
(IML, lateral horn)

T1
T2
T3
T4
T5
L4

Abdominopelvic
splanchnic nerve

Viscera of
abdominopelvic
cavity (e.g.,
stomach and intestines) via
abdominopelvic
splanchnic nerves

Sympathetic Nerve Fibers

- - - Presynaptic (*dashed lines*,
different colors)

—— Postsynaptic

**Courses taken by presynaptic
sympathetic fibers within the
sympathetic trunks:**

1. **Ascend and then synapse.**
Postsynaptic fibers are for:
   - Innervation of the head
   - Cervical cardiopulmonary
splanchnic nerves
   - Spinal nerves to neck, upper
trunk, and upper limb

2. **Synapse at level of exit.**
Postsynaptic fibers are
distributed by:
   - Thoracic cardiopulmonary
splanchnic nerves
   - Spinal nerves to middle trunk

3. **Descend and then synapse.**
Postsynaptic fibers are
distributed by:
   - Spinal nerves to lower trunk and
lower limb

4. **Pass through sympathetic trunk
without synapsing to enter
abdominopelvic splanchnic
nerve for:**
   - Innervation of abdominopelvic
viscera

B. Anterolateral View

Visceral Afferent and Visceral Efferent (Motor) Innervation (continued)   1.51

B. Courses taken by sympathetic motor fibers. Presynaptic fibers all follow the same course until they reach the sympathetic trunks. In the sympathetic trunks, they follow one of four possible courses. Fibers involved in providing sympathetic innervation to the body wall and limbs or viscera above the level of the diaphragm follow paths 1 to 3. They synapse in the paravertebral ganglia of the sympathetic trunks. Fibers involved in innervating abdominopelvic viscera follow path 4 to prevertebral ganglion via abdominopelvic splanchnic nerves. Postsynaptic fibers usually do not ascend or descend within the sympathetic trunks, exiting at the level of synapse.

ANTERIOR

RIGHT

LEFT

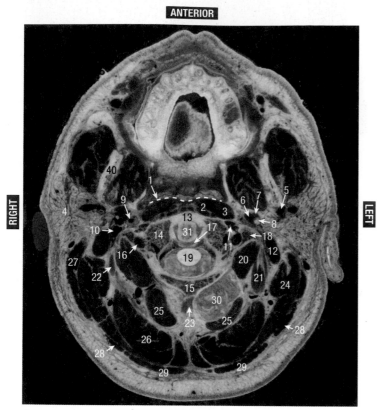

**A. Inferior View,
Anatomic Section**

POSTERIOR

ANTERIOR

RIGHT

LEFT

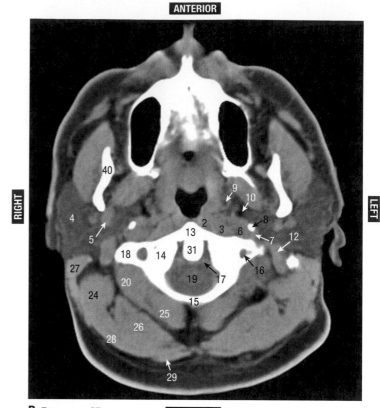

B. Transverse CT

POSTERIOR

1	Site of retropharyngeal space	21	Obliquus capitis inferior
2	Longus colli	22	Obliquus capitis superior
3	Longus capitis	23	Spinous process of atlas (C1)
4	Parotid gland	24	Longissimus capitis
5	Retromandibular vein	25	Rectus capitis posterior minor
6	Stylopharyngeus	26	Semispinalis capitis
7	Styloglossus	27	Sternocleidomastoid
8	Stylohyoid muscle and ligament/process	28	Splenius capitis
9	Internal carotid artery	29	Trapezius
10	Internal jugular vein	30	Fatty mass
11	Rectus capitis lateralis	31	Dens of axis (C2 vertebra)
12	Posterior belly of digastric	32	Anterior tubercle of atlas (C1)
13	Anterior arch of atlas (C1 vertebra)	33	Inferior articular facet of atlas (C1)
14	Lateral mass of atlas (C1)	34	Foramen magnum
15	Posterior arch of atlas (C1)	35	Foramen transversarium
16	Vertebral artery	36	Posterior tubercle of atlas (C1)
17	Transverse ligament of atlas (C1)	37	Mastoid process
18	Transverse process of atlas (C1)	38	Occipital bone of skull
19	Spinal cord	39	External occipital protuberance
20	Rectus capitis posterior major	40	Ramus of mandible

ANTERIOR

RIGHT

LEFT

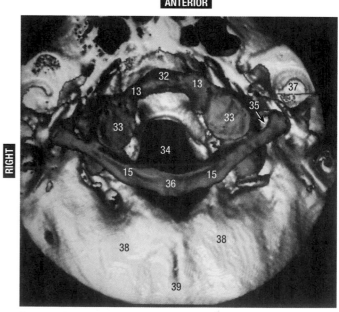

**C. 3D CT Reconstruction,
Inferior View**

POSTERIOR

1.52   **Imaging of Superior Nuchal Region at Level of Atlas**

A. Transverse section of specimen. **B.** Transverse CT image. **C.** Three-dimensional CT image of base of skull and atlas.

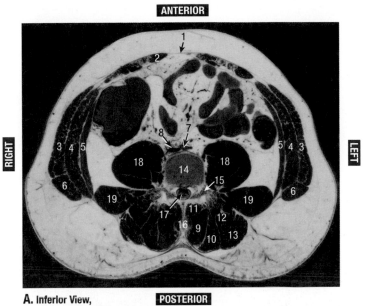

A. Inferior View, Anatomic Section

B. Transverse CT

1 Linea alba	6 Latissimus dorsi	11 Multifidus	16 Spinous process
2 Rectus abdominis	7 Descending aorta	12 Rotatores	17 Cauda equina
3 External oblique	8 Inferior vena cava	13 Iliocostalis	18 Psoas major
4 Internal oblique	9 Spinalis	14 4th lumbar vertebra	19 Quadratus lumborum
5 Transversus abdominis	10 Longissimus	15 Transverse process	

Imaging of Lumbar Spine at L4 — 1.53

A. Transverse section of specimen. **B.** Transverse CT image.

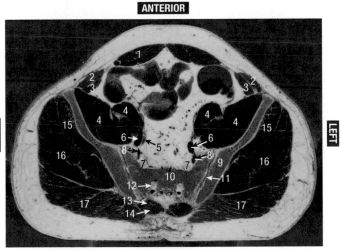

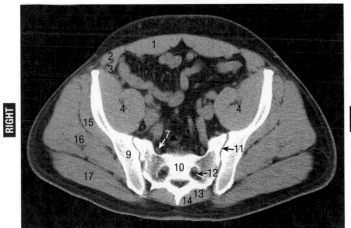

A. Inferior View, Anatomic Section

B. Transverse CT

1 Rectus abdominis	6 Internal iliac vein	10 2nd sacral vertebra	14 Erector spinae
2 External oblique	7 Anterior rami	11 Sacroiliac joint	15 Gluteus minimus
3 Internal oblique	8 Superior gluteal vessels	12 Sacral nerve root	16 Gluteus medius
4 Iliopsoas	9 Body of ilium	13 Multifidus	17 Gluteus maximus
5 Internal iliac artery			

Imaging of Sacroiliac Joint — 1.54

A. Transverse section of specimen. **B.** Transverse CT image.

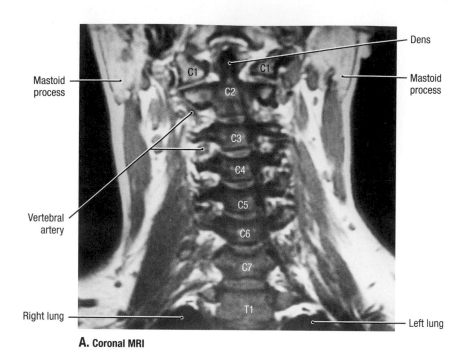

Dens

Mastoid process

C1 C1

C2

Mastoid process

C3

Vertebral artery

C4

C5

C6

C7

Right lung

T1

Left lung

A. Coronal MRI

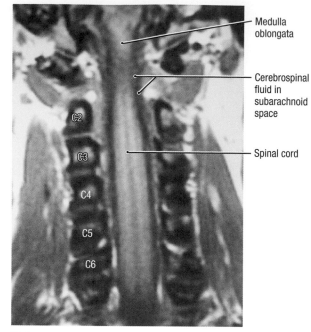

Medulla oblongata

Cerebrospinal fluid in subarachnoid space

C2

C3

Spinal cord

C4

C5

C6

B. Coronal MRI

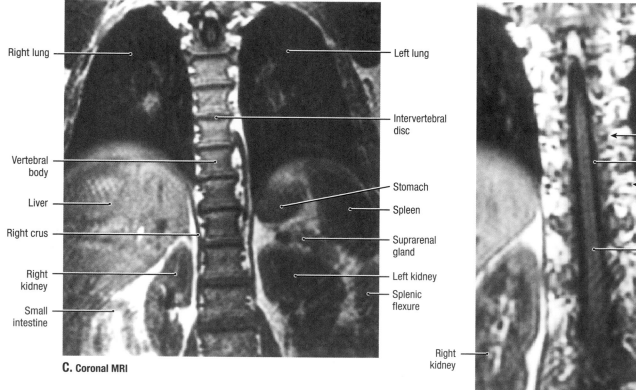

Right lung

Left lung

Intervertebral disc

Vertebral body

Liver

Stomach

Spleen

Right crus

Suprarenal gland

Right kidney

Left kidney

Small intestine

Splenic flexure

C. Coronal MRI

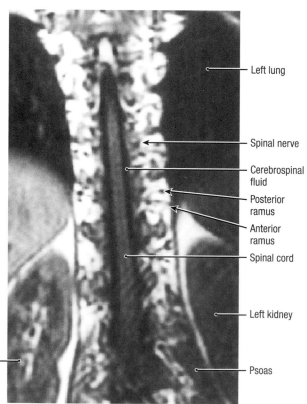

Left lung

Spinal nerve

Cerebrospinal fluid

Posterior ramus

Anterior ramus

Spinal cord

Left kidney

Right kidney

Psoas

D. Coronal MRI

1.55 **Coronal MRIs of Cervical and Thoracic Spine**

A. and **B.** Cervical spine. **C.** and **D.** Thoracic spine.

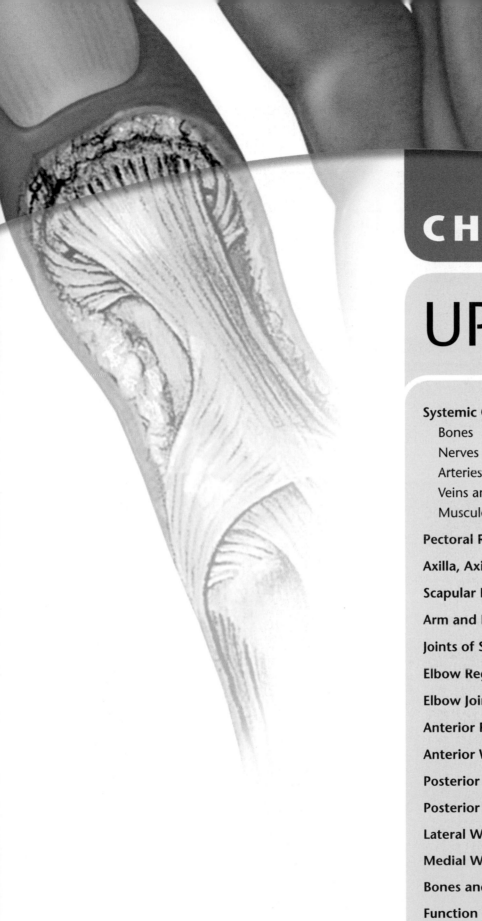

CHAPTER 2

UPPER LIMB

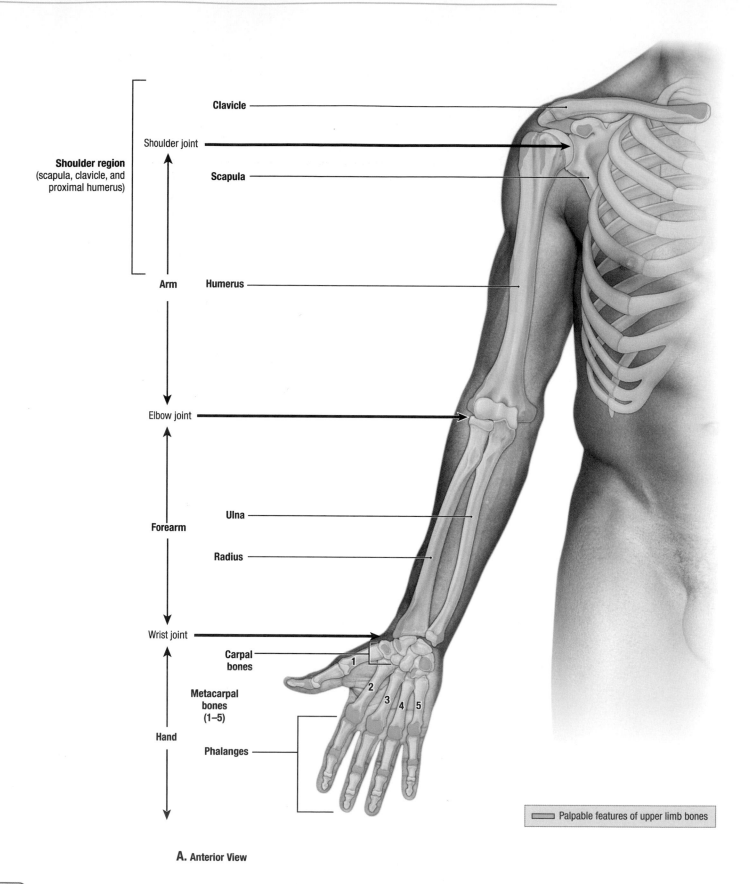

Clavicle

Shoulder joint

Shoulder region
(scapula, clavicle, and
proximal humerus)

Scapula

Arm   **Humerus**

Elbow joint

Forearm

Ulna

Radius

Wrist joint

Carpal
bones

Metacarpal
bones
(1–5)

Hand

Phalanges

Palpable features of upper limb bones

A. Anterior View

2.1   **Regions, Bones, and Major Joints of Upper Limb**

Joints divide the upper limb into four main regions: the shoulder, arm, forearm, and hand.

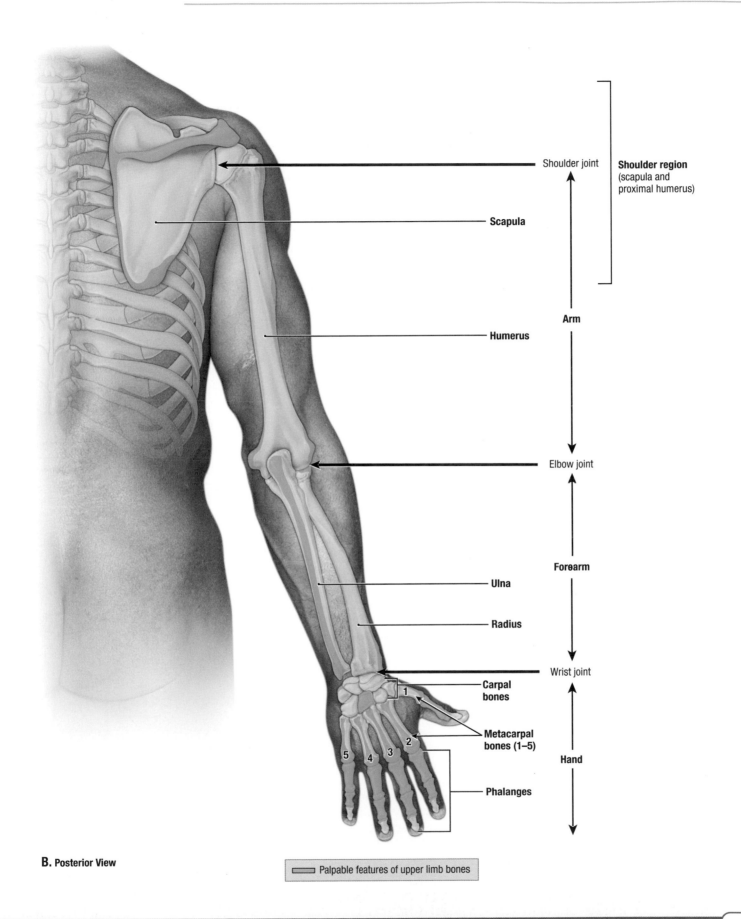

Shoulder joint

Shoulder region
(scapula and
proximal humerus)

Scapula

Arm

Humerus

Elbow joint

Forearm

Ulna

Radius

Wrist joint

Carpal
bones

Metacarpal
bones (1–5)

Hand

Phalanges

B. **Posterior View**

Palpable features of upper limb bones

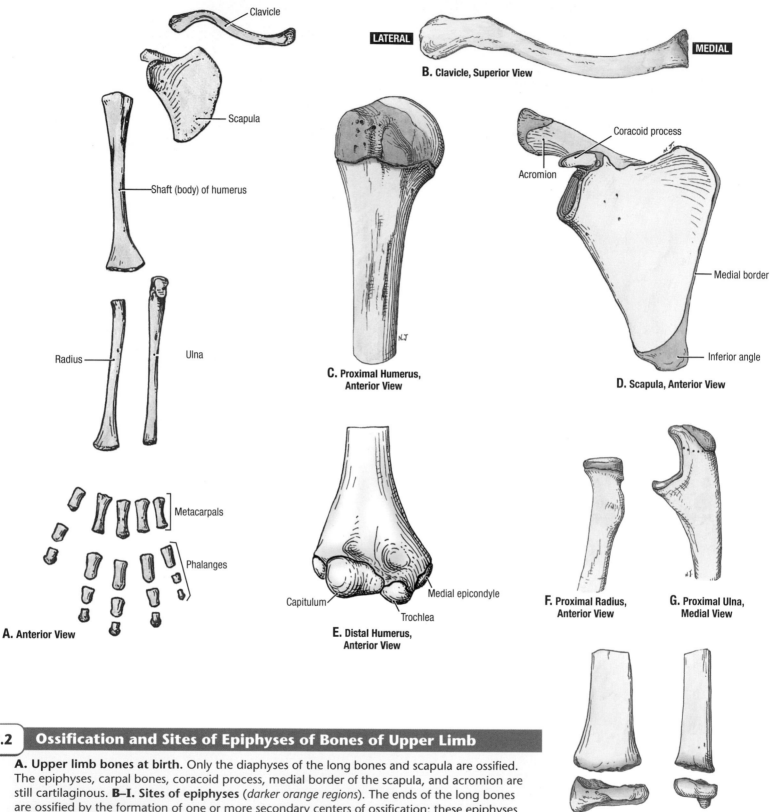

Clavicle

B. Clavicle, Superior View

LATERAL MEDIAL

Scapula

Shaft (body) of humerus

Coracoid process

Acromion

Medial border

Inferior angle

C. Proximal Humerus, Anterior View

D. Scapula, Anterior View

Radius Ulna

Metacarpals

Phalanges

Capitulum

Medial epicondyle

Trochlea

F. Proximal Radius, Anterior View

G. Proximal Ulna, Medial View

A. Anterior View

E. Distal Humerus, Anterior View

H. Distal Radius, Anterior View

I. Distal Ulna, Anterior View

2.2 **Ossification and Sites of Epiphyses of Bones of Upper Limb**

A. Upper limb bones at birth. Only the diaphyses of the long bones and scapula are ossified. The epiphyses, carpal bones, coracoid process, medial border of the scapula, and acromion are still cartilaginous. **B–I. Sites of epiphyses** (*darker orange regions*). The ends of the long bones are ossified by the formation of one or more secondary centers of ossification; these epiphyses develop from birth to approximately 20 years of age in the clavicle, humerus, radius, ulna, metacarpals, and phalanges.

Epiphyses. Without knowledge of bone growth and the appearance of bones in radiographic and other diagnostic images at various ages, a displaced epiphysial plate could be mistaken for a fracture, and separation of an epiphysis could be interpreted as a displaced piece of fractured bone. Knowledge of the patient's age and the location of epiphyses can prevent these errors.

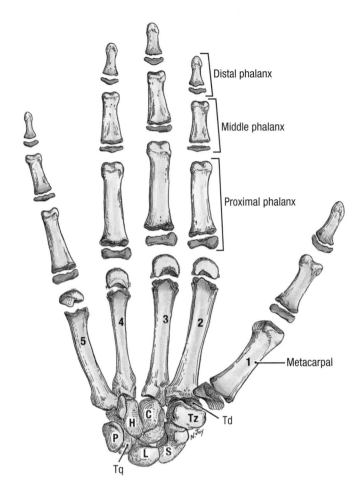

Distal phalanx

Middle phalanx

Proximal phalanx

Metacarpal

J. Anterior View

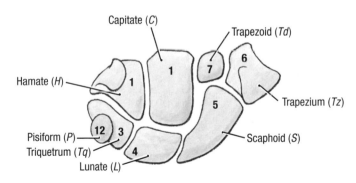

Capitate (*C*)

Trapezoid (*Td*)

Hamate (*H*)

Trapezium (*Tz*)

Scaphoid (*S*)

Pisiform (*P*)

Triquetrum (*Tq*)

Lunate (*L*)

Numbers: approximate age of ossification of carpal bones in years

K. Anterior View

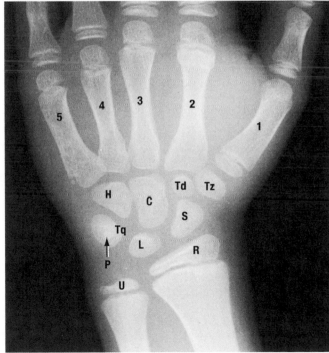

Note epiphyses in radiographs appear as radiolucent lines.

L. Anteroposterior Radiographs

Ossification and Sites of Epiphyses of Bones of Upper Limb (continued)   **2.2**

J. Ossification of bones of hand. Note the phalanges have a single proximal epiphysis and metacarpals 2, 3, 4, and 5 have single distal epiphyses. The 1st metacarpal behaves as a phalanx by having proximal epiphysis. Short-lived epiphyses may appear at the other ends of metacarpals 1 and/or 2. There are individual and gender differences in sequence and timing of ossification. **K. Sequence of ossification of carpal bones. L. Radiographs of stages of ossification of wrist and hand.** A 2½-year-old child (*top*): The lunate is ossifying, and the distal radial epiphysis (*R*) is present. An 11-year-old child (*bottom*): All carpal bones are ossified, and the distal epiphysis of the ulna (*U*) has ossified.

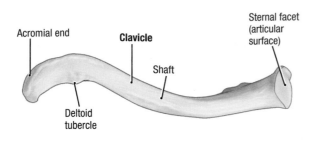

Acromial end — Clavicle — Shaft — Sternal facet (articular surface)

Deltoid tubercle

A. Superior Surface

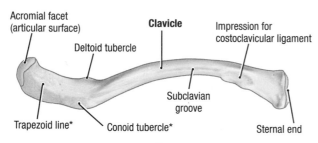

Acromial facet (articular surface) — Clavicle — Impression for costoclavicular ligament

Deltoid tubercle

Trapezoid line* — Conoid tubercle* — Subclavian groove — Sternal end

B. Inferior Surface   * Tuberosity for coracoclavicular ligament (conoid and trapezoid parts)

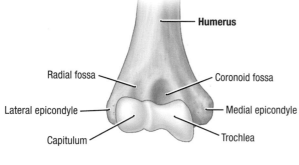

Humerus

Radial fossa — Coronoid fossa

Lateral epicondyle — Medial epicondyle

Capitulum — Trochlea

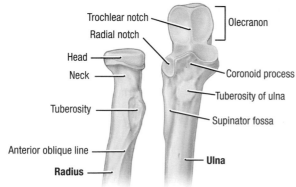

Trochlear notch — Olecranon
Radial notch
Head — Coronoid process
Neck
Tuberosity of ulna
Tuberosity — Supinator fossa

Anterior oblique line — Ulna

Radius

C. Anterior Views

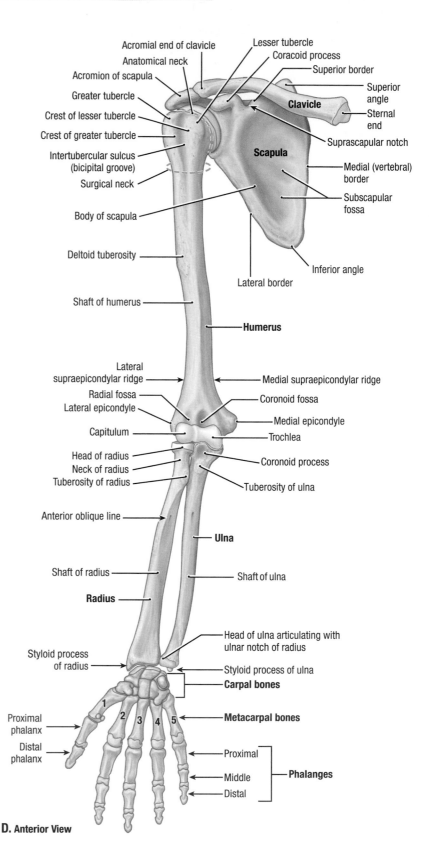

Acromial end of clavicle — Lesser tubercle — Coracoid process
Anatomical neck — Superior border
Acromion of scapula — Superior angle
Greater tubercle — Clavicle — Sternal end
Crest of lesser tubercle
Crest of greater tubercle — Suprascapular notch
Intertubercular sulcus (bicipital groove) — Scapula — Medial (vertebral) border
Surgical neck — Subscapular fossa
Body of scapula
Deltoid tuberosity — Inferior angle
Lateral border
Shaft of humerus
Humerus
Lateral supraepicondylar ridge — Medial supraepicondylar ridge
Radial fossa — Coronoid fossa
Lateral epicondyle — Medial epicondyle
Capitulum — Trochlea
Head of radius — Coronoid process
Neck of radius
Tuberosity of radius — Tuberosity of ulna
Anterior oblique line
Ulna
Shaft of radius — Shaft of ulna
Radius
Head of ulna articulating with ulnar notch of radius
Styloid process of radius — Styloid process of ulna
Carpal bones
Metacarpal bones
Proximal phalanx — Proximal
Distal phalanx — Middle — Phalanges
Distal

D. Anterior View

2.3   Features of Bones of Upper Limb

A. and **B.** Clavicle. **C.** Anterior aspect of disarticulated distal end of humerus and proximal end of radius and ulna. **D.** Anterior aspect of articulated upper limb.

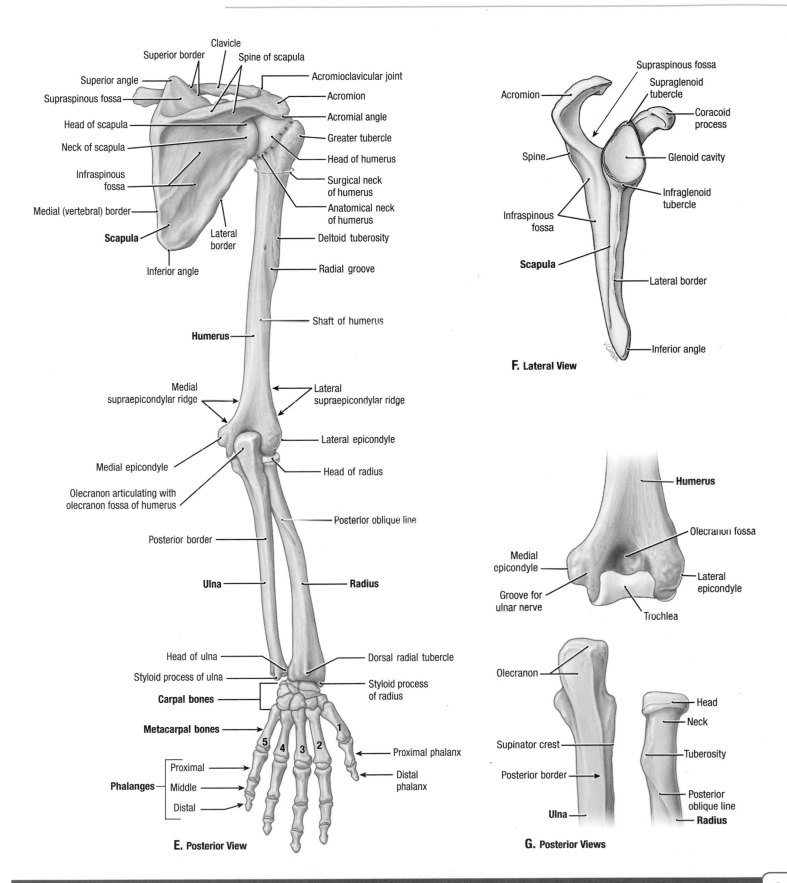

Clavicle
Superior border
Spine of scapula
Superior angle
Supraspinous fossa
Head of scapula
Neck of scapula
Infraspinous fossa
Medial (vertebral) border
Scapula
Lateral border
Inferior angle

Acromioclavicular joint
Acromion
Acromial angle
Greater tubercle
Head of humerus
Surgical neck of humerus
Anatomical neck of humerus
Deltoid tuberosity
Radial groove

Shaft of humerus
Humerus

Medial supraepicondylar ridge
Lateral supraepicondylar ridge

Medial epicondyle
Olecranon articulating with olecranon fossa of humerus
Lateral epicondyle
Head of radius

Posterior border
Posterior oblique line

Ulna
Radius

Head of ulna
Styloid process of ulna
Carpal bones
Metacarpal bones
Dorsal radial tubercle
Styloid process of radius

5 4 3 2 1
Proximal phalanx
Distal phalanx

Proximal
Phalanges Middle
Distal

E. Posterior View

Supraspinous fossa
Supraglenoid tubercle
Acromion
Coracoid process
Spine
Glenoid cavity
Infraglenoid tubercle
Infraspinous fossa
Scapula
Lateral border
Inferior angle

F. Lateral View

Humerus
Olecranon fossa
Medial epicondyle
Lateral epicondyle
Groove for ulnar nerve
Trochlea

Olecranon
Head
Neck
Supinator crest
Tuberosity
Posterior border
Posterior oblique line
Ulna
Radius

G. Posterior Views

Features of Bones of Upper Limb (continued)

2.3

E. Posterior aspect of articulated upper limb bones. **F.** Lateral aspect of scapula. **G.** Posterior aspect of disarticulated distal end of humerus and proximal ends of radius and ulna.

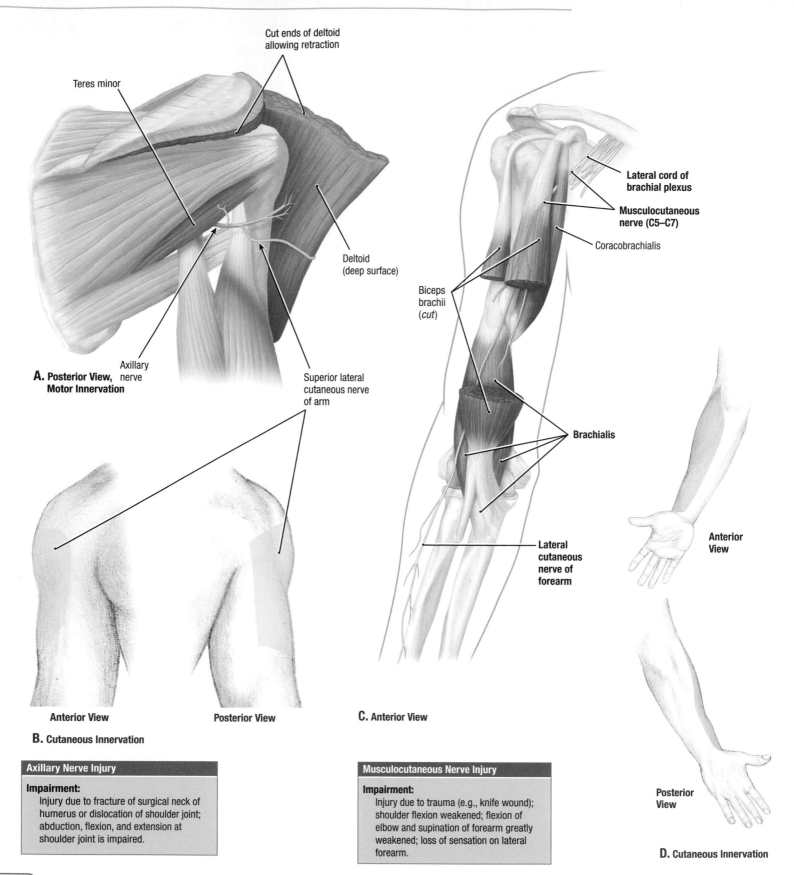

Cut ends of deltoid
allowing retraction

Teres minor

Deltoid
(deep surface)

Axillary
nerve

**A. Posterior View,
Motor Innervation**

Superior lateral
cutaneous nerve
of arm

Lateral cord of
brachial plexus

**Musculocutaneous
nerve (C5–C7)**

Coracobrachialis

Biceps
brachii
(*cut*)

Brachialis

Lateral
cutaneous
nerve of
forearm

Anterior
View

Anterior View   Posterior View

B. Cutaneous Innervation

C. Anterior View

Posterior
View

D. Cutaneous Innervation

Axillary Nerve Injury

Impairment:
Injury due to fracture of surgical neck of
humerus or dislocation of shoulder joint;
abduction, flexion, and extension at
shoulder joint is impaired.

Musculocutaneous Nerve Injury

Impairment:
Injury due to trauma (e.g., knife wound);
shoulder flexion weakened; flexion of
elbow and supination of forearm greatly
weakened; loss of sensation on lateral
forearm.

2.4 **Overview of Innervation of Upper Limb: Axillary and Musculocutaneous Nerves**

A. Motor innervation of axillary nerve. **B.** Cutaneous innervation of axillary nerve (*green area*). **C.** Overview of innervation of musculocutaneous nerve. **D.** Cutaneous innervation of musculocutaneous nerve.

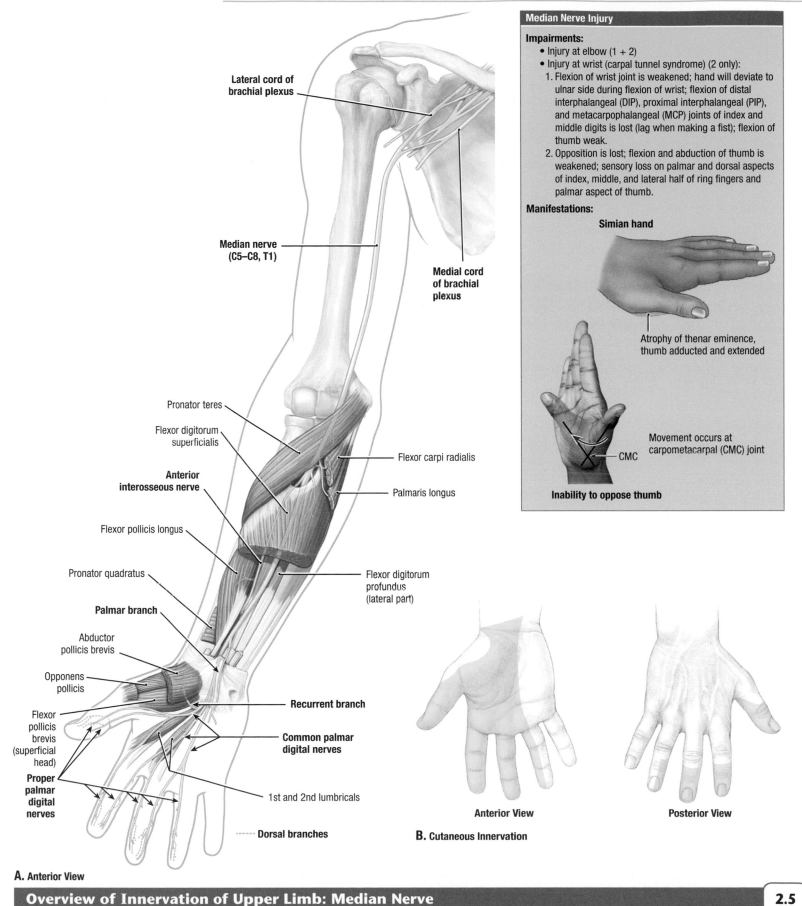

Lateral cord of brachial plexus

Median nerve (C5–C8, T1)

Medial cord of brachial plexus

Pronator teres

Flexor digitorum superficialis

Anterior interosseous nerve

Flexor pollicis longus

Pronator quadratus

Palmar branch

Abductor pollicis brevis

Opponens pollicis

Flexor pollicis brevis (superficial head)

Proper palmar digital nerves

Flexor carpi radialis

Palmaris longus

Flexor digitorum profundus (lateral part)

Recurrent branch

Common palmar digital nerves

1st and 2nd lumbricals

- - - - - **Dorsal branches**

A. Anterior View

Median Nerve Injury

Impairments:
- Injury at elbow (1 + 2)
- Injury at wrist (carpal tunnel syndrome) (2 only):
  1. Flexion of wrist joint is weakened; hand will deviate to ulnar side during flexion of wrist; flexion of distal interphalangeal (DIP), proximal interphalangeal (PIP), and metacarpophalangeal (MCP) joints of index and middle digits is lost (lag when making a fist); flexion of thumb weak.
  2. Opposition is lost; flexion and abduction of thumb is weakened; sensory loss on palmar and dorsal aspects of index, middle, and lateral half of ring fingers and palmar aspect of thumb.

Manifestations:

Simian hand

Atrophy of thenar eminence, thumb adducted and extended

Movement occurs at carpometacarpal (CMC) joint

CMC

Inability to oppose thumb

Anterior View

Posterior View

B. Cutaneous Innervation

Overview of Innervation of Upper Limb: Median Nerve **2.5**

A. Overview. **B.** Cutaneous innervation (*green area*).

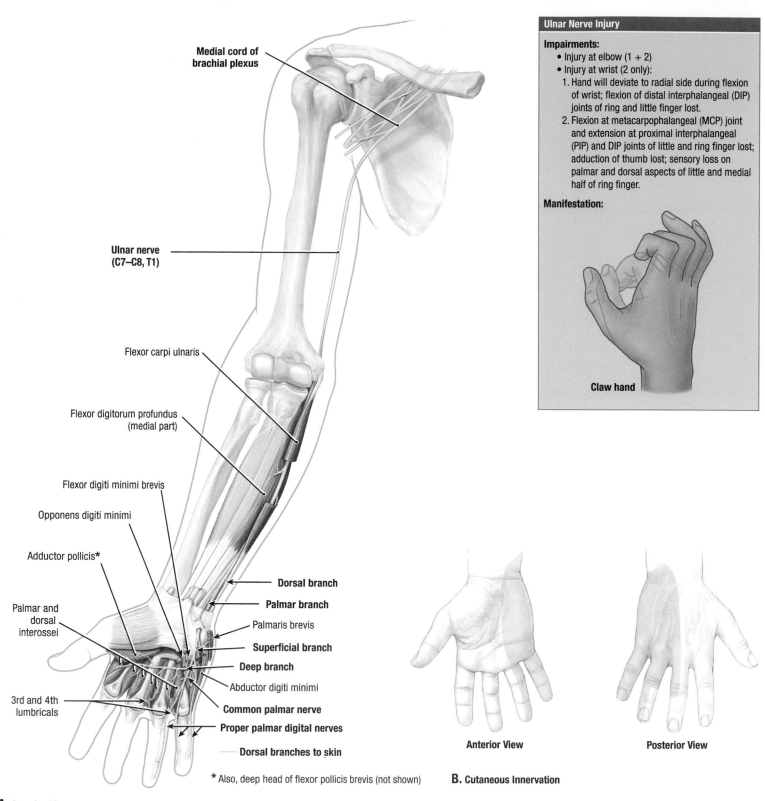

Medial cord of
brachial plexus

Ulnar nerve
(C7–C8, T1)

Flexor carpi ulnaris

Flexor digitorum profundus
(medial part)

Flexor digiti minimi brevis

Opponens digiti minimi

Adductor pollicis*

Palmar and
dorsal
interossei

3rd and 4th
lumbricals

Dorsal branch

Palmar branch

Palmaris brevis

Superficial branch

Deep branch

Abductor digiti minimi

Common palmar nerve

Proper palmar digital nerves

----- **Dorsal branches to skin**

* Also, deep head of flexor pollicis brevis (not shown)

A. Anterior View

Ulnar Nerve Injury

Impairments:
- Injury at elbow (1 + 2)
- Injury at wrist (2 only):
  1. Hand will deviate to radial side during flexion of wrist; flexion of distal interphalangeal (DIP) joints of ring and little finger lost.
  2. Flexion at metacarpophalangeal (MCP) joint and extension at proximal interphalangeal (PIP) and DIP joints of little and ring finger lost; adduction of thumb lost; sensory loss on palmar and dorsal aspects of little and medial half of ring finger.

Manifestation:

Claw hand

Anterior View

Posterior View

B. Cutaneous Innervation

A. Overview. **B.** Cutaneous innervation (*green area*).

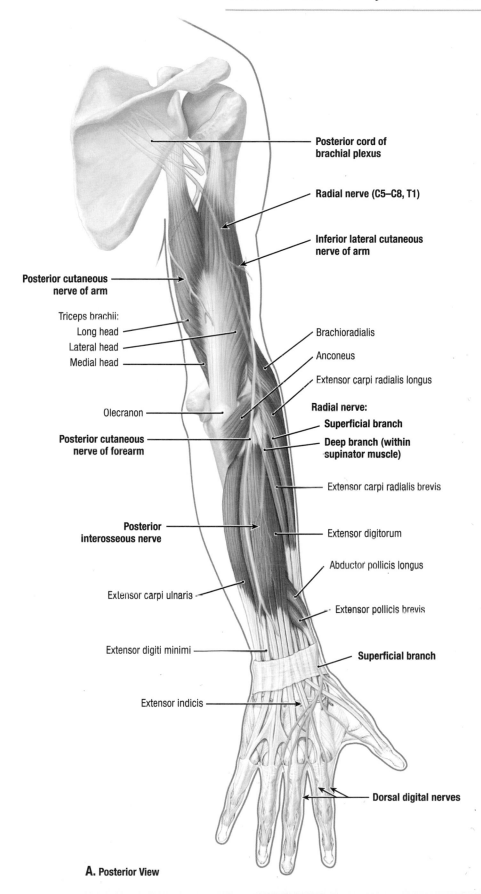

Posterior cord of
brachial plexus

Radial nerve (C5–C8, T1)

Inferior lateral cutaneous
nerve of arm

**Posterior cutaneous
nerve of arm**

Triceps brachii:
Long head
Lateral head
Medial head

Brachioradialis

Anconeus

Extensor carpi radialis longus

Olecranon

Radial nerve:

Superficial branch

**Deep branch (within
supinator muscle)**

**Posterior cutaneous
nerve of forearm**

Extensor carpi radialis brevis

Extensor digitorum

**Posterior
interosseous nerve**

Abductor pollicis longus

Extensor carpi ulnaris

Extensor pollicis brevis

Extensor digiti minimi

Superficial branch

Extensor indicis

Dorsal digital nerves

A. Posterior View

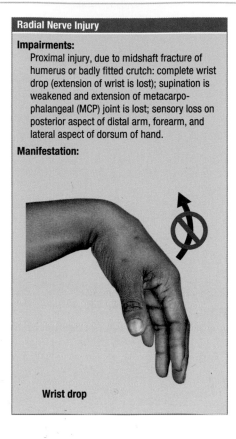

Radial Nerve Injury

Impairments:
Proximal injury, due to midshaft fracture of
humerus or badly fitted crutch: complete wrist
drop (extension of wrist is lost); supination is
weakened and extension of metacarpophalangeal (MCP) joint is lost; sensory loss on
posterior aspect of distal arm, forearm, and
lateral aspect of dorsum of hand.

Manifestation:

Wrist drop

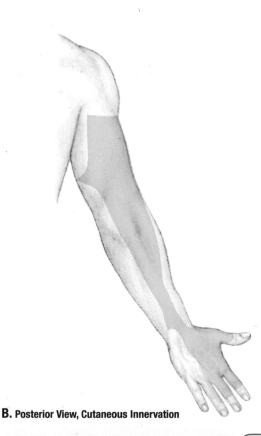

B. Posterior View, Cutaneous Innervation

Overview of Innervation of Upper Limb: Radial Nerve   **2.7**

A. Overview. **B.** Cutaneous innervation (*green area*).

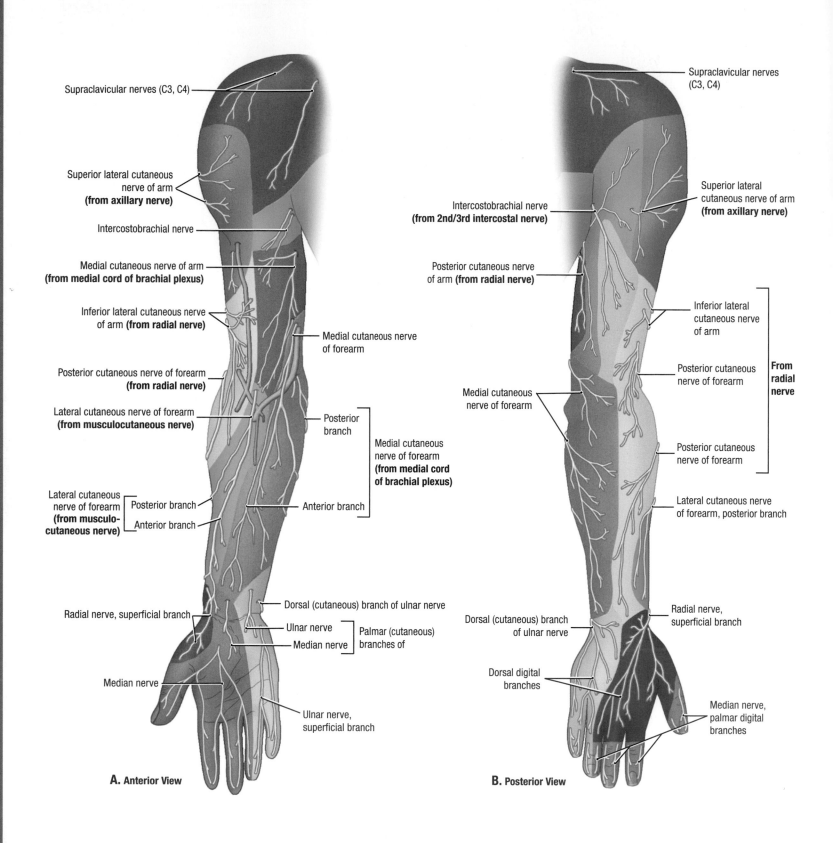

Supraclavicular nerves (C3, C4)

Superior lateral cutaneous nerve of arm **(from axillary nerve)**

Intercostobrachial nerve

Medial cutaneous nerve of arm **(from medial cord of brachial plexus)**

Inferior lateral cutaneous nerve of arm **(from radial nerve)**

Posterior cutaneous nerve of forearm **(from radial nerve)**

Lateral cutaneous nerve of forearm **(from musculocutaneous nerve)**

Lateral cutaneous nerve of forearm **(from musculo-cutaneous nerve)** — Posterior branch — Anterior branch

Radial nerve, superficial branch

Median nerve

Medial cutaneous nerve of forearm

Posterior branch

Medial cutaneous nerve of forearm **(from medial cord of brachial plexus)**

Anterior branch

Dorsal (cutaneous) branch of ulnar nerve

Ulnar nerve
Median nerve } Palmar (cutaneous) branches of

Ulnar nerve, superficial branch

A. Anterior View

Supraclavicular nerves (C3, C4)

Intercostobrachial nerve **(from 2nd/3rd intercostal nerve)**

Superior lateral cutaneous nerve of arm **(from axillary nerve)**

Posterior cutaneous nerve of arm **(from radial nerve)**

Inferior lateral cutaneous nerve of arm

Posterior cutaneous nerve of forearm

Medial cutaneous nerve of forearm

Posterior cutaneous nerve of forearm

From radial nerve

Lateral cutaneous nerve of forearm, posterior branch

Radial nerve, superficial branch

Dorsal (cutaneous) branch of ulnar nerve

Dorsal digital branches

Median nerve, palmar digital branches

B. Posterior View

2.8 **Cutaneous Nerves of Upper Limb**

Summary of distribution of the peripheral (named) cutaneous nerves in upper limb. Most nerves are branches of nerve plexuses and therefore contain fibers from more than one spinal nerve.

TABLE 2.1 Cutaneous Nerves of Upper Limb

Nerve	Spinal Nerve Components	Source	Course/Distribution
Supraclavicular nerves	C3–C4	Cervical plexus	Pass anterior to clavicle, immediately deep to platysma, and supply the skin over the clavicle and superolateral aspect of the pectoralis major muscle
Superior lateral cutaneous nerve of arm	C5–C6	Axillary nerve (posterior cord of brachial plexus)	Emerges from posterior margin of deltoid to supply skin over lower part of this muscle and the lateral side of the midarm
Inferior lateral cutaneous nerve of arm		Radial nerve (posterior cord of brachial plexus)	Arises with the posterior cutaneous nerve of forearm; pierces lateral head of triceps brachii to supply skin over the inferolateral aspect of the arm
Posterior cutaneous nerve of arm	C5–C8		Arises in axilla and supplies skin on posterior surface of the arm to olecranon
Posterior cutaneous nerve of forearm			Arises with the inferior lateral cutaneous nerve of the arm; pierces lateral head of triceps brachii to supply skin over the posterior aspect of the arm
Superficial branch of radial nerve			Arises in cubital fossa; supplies lateral (radial) half of the dorsal aspect of hand and thumb, the proximal portion of the dorsal aspects of digits 2 and 3, and the lateral (radial) half of dorsal aspect of digit 4
Lateral cutaneous nerve of forearm	C6–C7	Musculocutaneous nerve (lateral cord of brachial plexus)	Arises between biceps brachii and brachialis muscle as continuation of musculocutaneous nerve distal to branch to brachialis; emerges in cubital fossa lateral to biceps tendon and median cubital vein; supplies skin along radial (lateral) border of forearm to base of thenar eminence
Median nerve	C6–C7 (via lateral root); C8–T1 (via medial root)	Lateral and medial cords of brachial plexus	Courses with brachial artery in arm and deep to flexor digitorum superficialis in forearm; distal to origin of palmar cutaneous branch, traverses carpal tunnel to supply skin of palmar aspect of radial 3½ digits and adjacent palm, plus distal dorsal aspects of same, including nail beds
Ulnar nerve	(C7), C8–T1		Courses with brachial, superior ulnar collateral, and ulnar arteries; supplies skin of palmar and dorsal aspects of medial (ulnar) 1½ digits and palm and dorsum of hand proximal to those digits
Medial cutaneous nerve of forearm	C8–T1	Medial cord of brachial plexus	Pierces deep fascia with basilic vein in midarm; divides into anterior and posterior branches supplying skin over anterior and medial surfaces of forearm to wrist
Medial cutaneous nerve of arm	C8–T2		Smallest and most medial branch of brachial plexus; communicates with intercostobrachial nerve and then descends medial to brachial artery and basilic vein to innervate skin of distal medial arm
Intercostobrachial nerve	T2	Lateral cutaneous branch of 2nd intercostal nerve	Arises distal to angle of 2nd rib; supplies skin of axilla and proximal medial arm

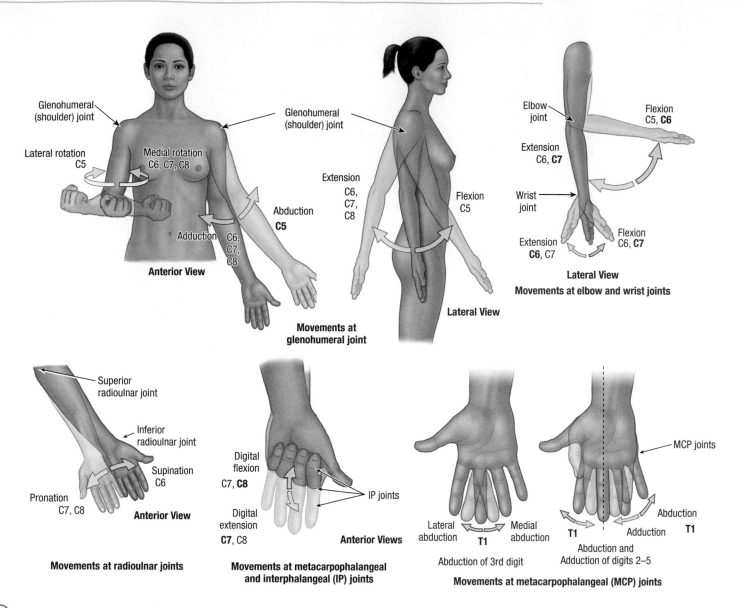

Movements at glenohumeral joint (Anterior View / Lateral View)

Lateral View — Movements at elbow and wrist joints

Movements at radioulnar joints (Anterior View)

Movements at metacarpophalangeal and interphalangeal (IP) joints (Anterior Views)

Movements at metacarpophalangeal (MCP) joints

2.9   Myotomes and Myotatic (Deep Tendon Stretch) Reflexes

Myotomes. Somatic motor (general somatic efferent) fibers transmit impulses to skeletal (voluntary) muscles. The unilateral muscle mass receiving information from the somatic motor fibers conveyed by a single spinal nerve is a myotome. The movements associated with each bolded segment in Figure 2.9 are most commonly tested to determine the neurologic level of a lesion. **Myotatic reflexes.** A myotatic reflex (deep tendon or stretch reflex) is an involuntary contraction of a muscle in response to sudden stretching. Myotatic reflexes are elicited by briskly tapping the tendon with a reflex hammer. Each tendon reflex is mediated by specific spinal nerves.

TABLE 2.2 | Clinical Manifestations of Nerve Root Compression: Upper Limb

Herniated Disc Between	Compressed Nerve Root	Dermatome Affected	Muscles Affected	Movement Weakness	Nerve and Myotatic Reflex Involved
C4 and C5	C5	C5 Shoulder Lateral surface UL	Deltoid	Abduction of shoulder	Axillary nerve ↓ Biceps jerk
C5 and C6	C6	C6 Thumb	Biceps Brachialis Brachioradialis	Flexion of elbow Supination/pronation of forearm	Musculocutaneous nerve ↓ Biceps jerk ↓ Brachioradialis jerk
C6 and C7	C7	C7 Posterior surface UL Middle and index fingers	Triceps Wrist extensors	Extension of elbow Extension of wrist	↓ Triceps reflex

UL, upper limb.

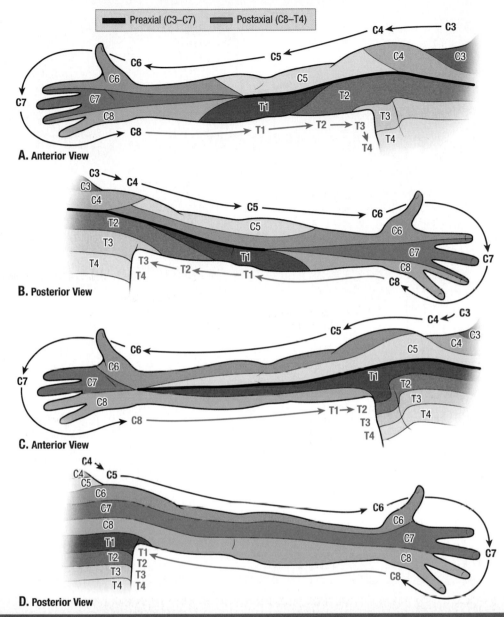

A. Anterior View

B. Posterior View

C. Anterior View

D. Posterior View

Preaxial (C3–C7)   Postaxial (C8–T4)

Dermatomes of Upper Limb

2.10

Two different dermatome maps are commonly used. **A.** and **B. Dermatome pattern according to Foerster** (1933). This map is preferred by many because of its correlation with clinical findings. In the Foerster schema, dermatomes C6–T1 are displaced from the trunk to limbs. **C.** and **D. Dermatome pattern according to Keegan and Garrett** (1948). This map is preferred by others for its correlation with development. Although depicted as distinct zones, adjacent dermatomes overlap considerably except along the axial line.

TABLE 2.3	Dermatomes of Upper Limb
Spinal Segment/Nerve(s)	**Description of Dermatome(s)**
C3, C4	Region at base of neck extending laterally over shoulder
C5	Lateral aspect of arm (i.e., superior aspect of abducted arm)
C6	Lateral forearm and thumb
C7	Middle and ring fingers (or middle three fingers) and center of posterior aspect of forearm
C8	Little finger, medial side of hand and forearm (i.e., inferior aspect of abducted arm)
T1	Medial aspect of forearm and inferior arm
T2	Medial aspect of superior arm and skin of axilla[a]

[a]Not indicated on the Keegan and Garrett map. However, pain experienced during a heart attack, considered to be mediated by T1 and T2, is commonly described as "radiating down the medial side of the left arm."

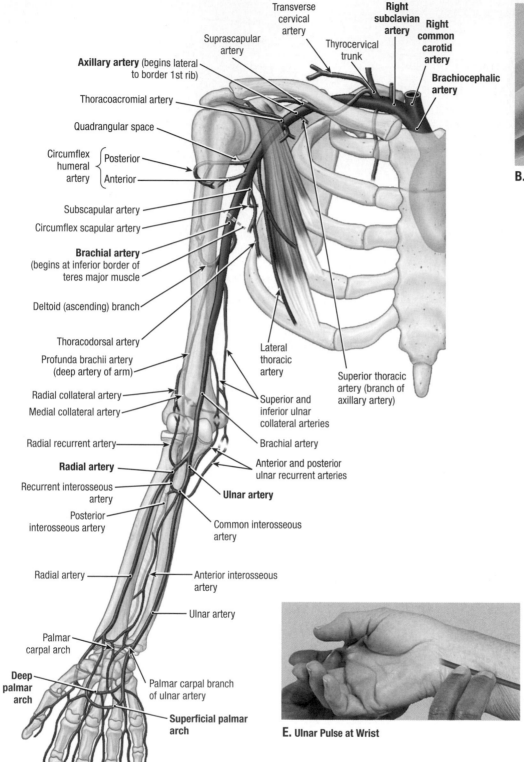

Transverse cervical artery

Suprascapular artery

Axillary artery (begins lateral to border 1st rib)

Thoracoacromial artery

Quadrangular space

Circumflex humeral artery { Posterior / Anterior }

Subscapular artery

Circumflex scapular artery

Brachial artery (begins at inferior border of teres major muscle)

Deltoid (ascending) branch

Thoracodorsal artery

Profunda brachii artery (deep artery of arm)

Radial collateral artery

Medial collateral artery

Radial recurrent artery

Radial artery

Recurrent interosseous artery

Posterior interosseous artery

Radial artery

Ulnar artery

Palmar carpal arch

Deep palmar arch

Thyrocervical trunk

Right subclavian artery

Right common carotid artery

Brachiocephalic artery

Lateral thoracic artery

Superior thoracic artery (branch of axillary artery)

Superior and inferior ulnar collateral arteries

Brachial artery

Anterior and posterior ulnar recurrent arteries

Ulnar artery

Common interosseous artery

Anterior interosseous artery

Ulnar artery

Palmar carpal branch of ulnar artery

Superficial palmar arch

A. Anterior View

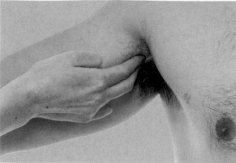

B. Axillary Pulse in Axilla

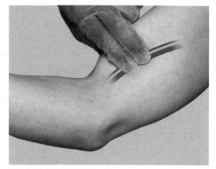

C. Brachial Pulse in Bicipital Groove

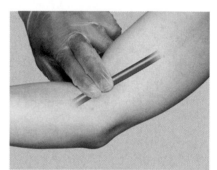

D. Brachial Pulse in Cubital Fossa

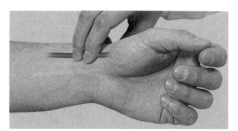

E. Ulnar Pulse at Wrist

F. Radial Pulse at Wrist

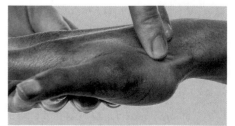

G. Radial Pulse in Anatomical Snuff Box

2.11   Arteries, Arterial Anastomoses, and Palpation Sites of Pulses of Upper Limb

A. Overview. **B–G.** Sites for palpation of arteries of upper limb.

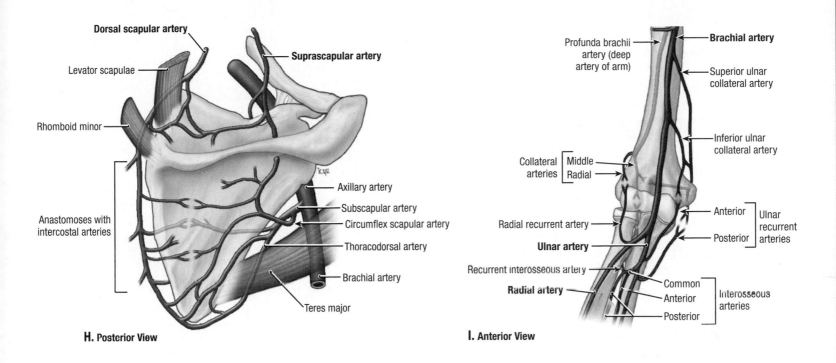

Dorsal scapular artery

Levator scapulae

Rhomboid minor

Anastomoses with intercostal arteries

Suprascapular artery

Axillary artery
Subscapular artery
Circumflex scapular artery
Thoracodorsal artery
Brachial artery
Teres major

H. Posterior View

Profunda brachii artery (deep artery of arm)

Brachial artery

Superior ulnar collateral artery

Inferior ulnar collateral artery

Collateral arteries { Middle / Radial }

Radial recurrent artery

Ulnar artery

Recurrent interosseous artery

Radial artery

Anterior } Ulnar recurrent arteries
Posterior

Common
Anterior } Interosseous arteries
Posterior

I. Anterior View

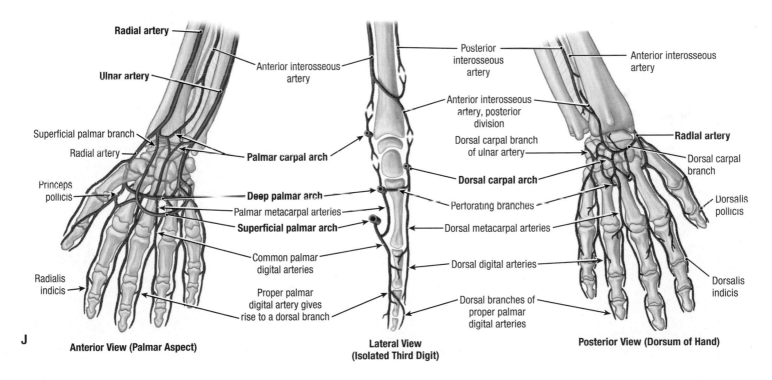

Radial artery

Anterior interosseous artery

Ulnar artery

Superficial palmar branch
Radial artery

Princeps pollicis

Radialis indicis

Palmar carpal arch

Deep palmar arch
Palmar metacarpal arteries
Superficial palmar arch

Common palmar digital arteries

Proper palmar digital artery gives rise to a dorsal branch

J   Anterior View (Palmar Aspect)

Posterior interosseous artery

Anterior interosseous artery, posterior division

Dorsal carpal branch of ulnar artery

Dorsal carpal arch

Perforating branches

Dorsal metacarpal arteries

Dorsal digital arteries

Dorsal branches of proper palmar digital arteries

Lateral View (Isolated Third Digit)

Anterior interosseous artery

Radial artery

Dorsal carpal branch

Dorsalis pollicis

Dorsalis indicis

Posterior View (Dorsum of Hand)

Arteries, Arterial Anastomoses, and Palpation Sites of Pulses of Upper Limb (continued)   **2.11**

H. Scapular anastomoses. **I.** Anastomoses of elbow. **J.** Anastomoses of hand.

Joints receive blood from articular arteries that arise from vessels around joints. The arteries often anastomose or communicate to form networks to ensure blood supply distal to the joint throughout the range of movement.

Arterial occlusion. If a main channel is occluded, the smaller alternate channels can usually increase in size, providing a collateral circulation that ensures the blood supply to structures distal to the blockage. However, collateral pathways require time to develop; they are usually insufficient to compensate for sudden occlusions.

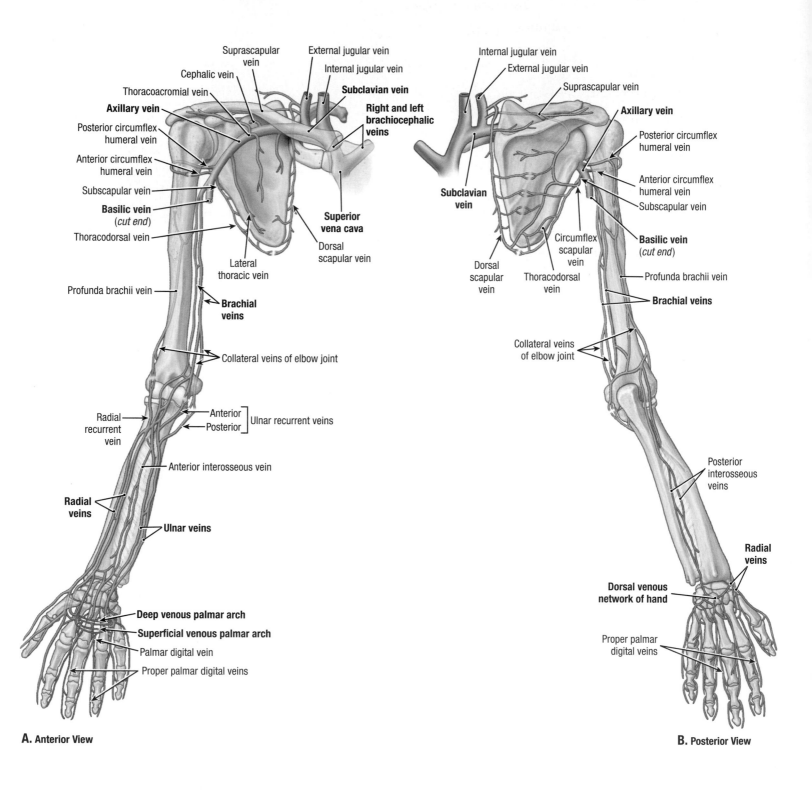

Suprascapular vein

Cephalic vein

Thoracoacromial vein

Axillary vein

Posterior circumflex humeral vein

Anterior circumflex humeral vein

Subscapular vein

Basilic vein (*cut end*)

Thoracodorsal vein

Profunda brachii vein

Brachial veins

Collateral veins of elbow joint

Radial recurrent vein

Anterior interosseous vein

Radial veins

Ulnar veins

External jugular vein

Internal jugular vein

Subclavian vein

Right and left brachiocephalic veins

Superior vena cava

Dorsal scapular vein

Lateral thoracic vein

Anterior / Posterior] Ulnar recurrent veins

Deep venous palmar arch

Superficial venous palmar arch

Palmar digital vein

Proper palmar digital veins

A. Anterior View

Internal jugular vein

External jugular vein

Suprascapular vein

Axillary vein

Posterior circumflex humeral vein

Anterior circumflex humeral vein

Subscapular vein

Basilic vein (*cut end*)

Profunda brachii vein

Brachial veins

Subclavian vein

Dorsal scapular vein

Circumflex scapular vein

Thoracodorsal vein

Collateral veins of elbow joint

Posterior interosseous veins

Radial veins

Dorsal venous network of hand

Proper palmar digital veins

B. Posterior View

2.12   **Overview of Deep Veins of Upper Limb**

Deep veins lie internal to the deep fascia and occur as paired, continually interanastomosing accompanying veins (e.g., venae comitantes) surrounding and sharing the name of the artery they accompany.

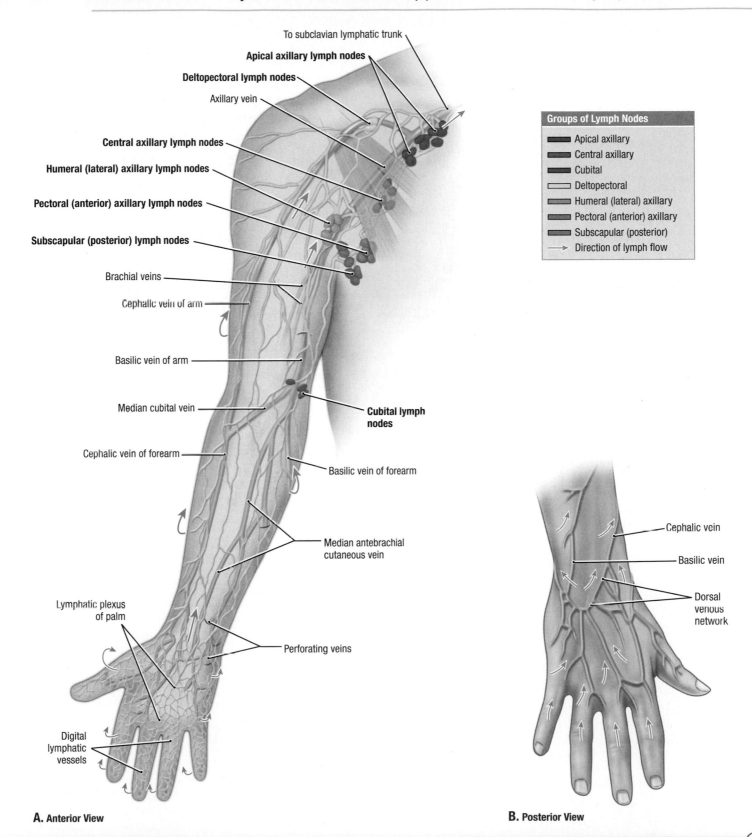

To subclavian lymphatic trunk

Apical axillary lymph nodes

Deltopectoral lymph nodes

Axillary vein

Central axillary lymph nodes

Humeral (lateral) axillary lymph nodes

Pectoral (anterior) axillary lymph nodes

Subscapular (posterior) lymph nodes

Brachial veins

Cephalic vein of arm

Basilic vein of arm

Median cubital vein

Cubital lymph nodes

Cephalic vein of forearm

Basilic vein of forearm

Median antebrachial cutaneous vein

Lymphatic plexus of palm

Perforating veins

Digital lymphatic vessels

A. Anterior View

Groups of Lymph Nodes

- Apical axillary
- Central axillary
- Cubital
- Deltopectoral
- Humeral (lateral) axillary
- Pectoral (anterior) axillary
- Subscapular (posterior)
- → Direction of lymph flow

Cephalic vein

Basilic vein

Dorsal venous network

B. Posterior View

Superficial Venous and Lymphatic Drainage of Upper Limb

2.13

A. Upper extremity. **B.** Dorsum of hand.

Superficial lymphatic vessels arise from lymphatic plexuses in the digits, and the hand and ascend with the superficial veins of the upper limb in the subcutaneous tissue. The superficial lymphatic vessels ascend through the forearm and arm, converging toward the cephalic and especially to the basilic vein to reach the axillary lymph nodes. Some lymph passes through the cubital nodes at the elbow. Deep lymphatic vessels accompany the neurovascular bundles internal to the deep fascia and end primarily in the humeral (lateral) and central axillary lymph nodes.

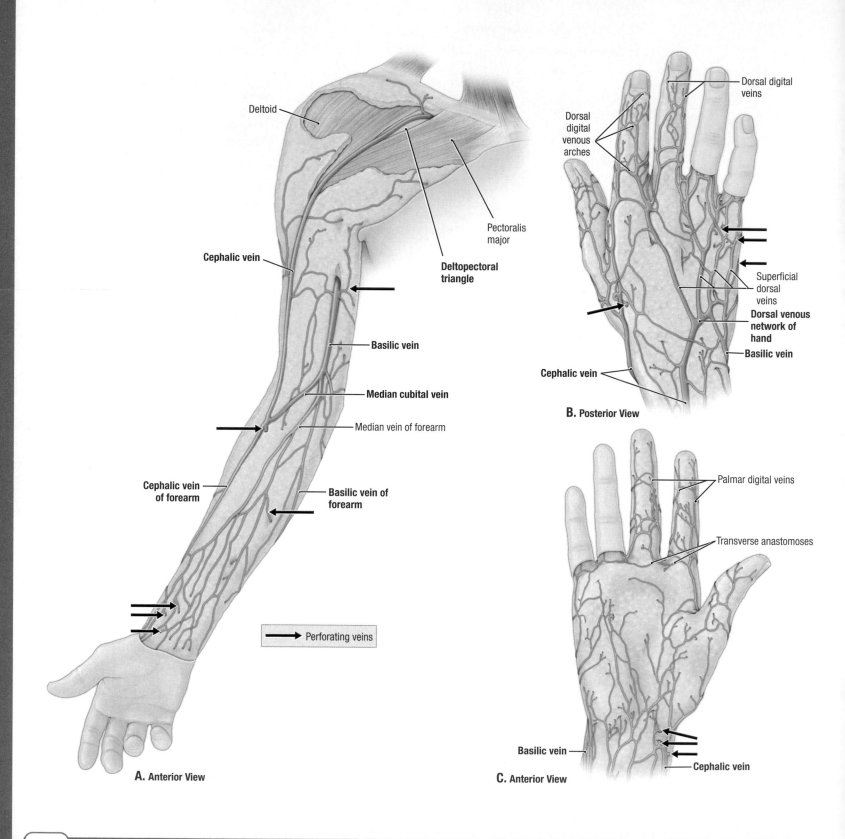

Deltoid

Pectoralis major

Cephalic vein

Deltopectoral triangle

Basilic vein

Median cubital vein

Median vein of forearm

Cephalic vein of forearm

Basilic vein of forearm

→ Perforating veins

A. Anterior View

Dorsal digital veins

Dorsal digital venous arches

Superficial dorsal veins

Dorsal venous network of hand

Basilic vein

Cephalic vein

B. Posterior View

Palmar digital veins

Transverse anastomoses

Basilic vein

C. Anterior View

Cephalic vein

2.14 **Superficial Venous Drainage of Upper Limb**

A. Forearm, arm, and pectoral region. B. Dorsal surface of hand. C. Palmar surface of hand. *Arrows* indicate where perforating veins penetrate the deep fascia. Blood is continuously shunted from these superficial veins in the subcutaneous tissue to deep veins via the perforating veins.

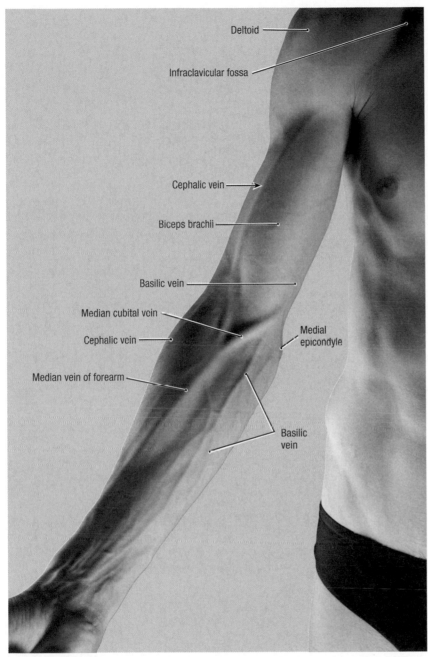

Deltoid

Infraclavicular fossa

Cephalic vein

Biceps brachii

Basilic vein

Median cubital vein

Cephalic vein

Median vein of forearm

Medial epicondyle

Basilic vein

D. Anterior View

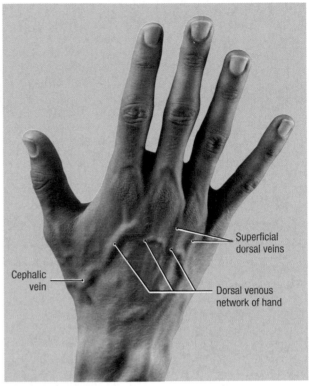

Superficial dorsal veins

Cephalic vein

Dorsal venous network of hand

E. Posterior View

Superficial Venous Drainage of Upper Limb *(continued)*   **2.14**

D. Surface anatomy of veins of forearm and arm. **E.** Surface anatomy of veins of dorsal surface of hand.

Because of the prominence and accessibility of the superficial veins, they are commonly used for **venipuncture** (puncture of a vein to draw blood or inject a solution). By applying a tourniquet to the arm, the venous return is occluded, and the veins distend and usually are visible and/or palpable. Once a vein is punctured, the tourniquet is removed so that when the needle is removed, the vein will not bleed extensively. The median cubital vein is commonly used for venipuncture. The veins forming the dorsal venous network of the hand and the cephalic and basilic veins arising from it are commonly used for long-term introduction of fluids (**intravenous feeding**). The cubital veins are also a site for the **introduction of cardiac catheters** to secure blood samples from the great vessels and chambers of the heart.

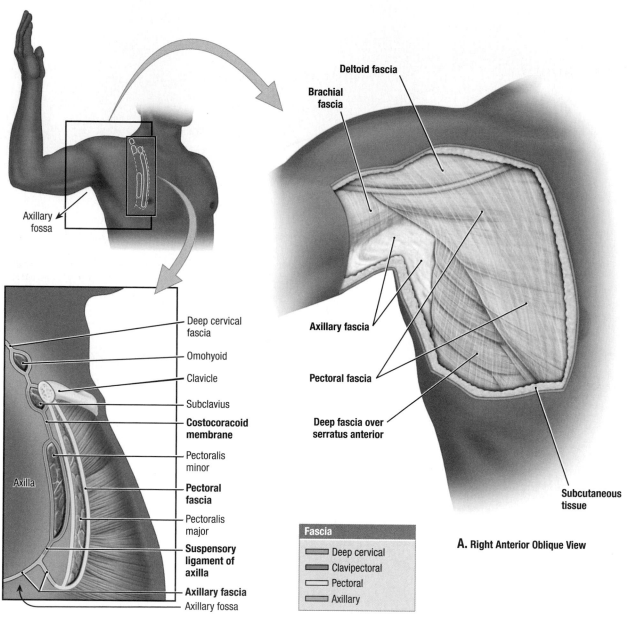

Deltoid fascia

Brachial fascia

Axillary fascia

Pectoral fascia

Deep fascia over serratus anterior

Subcutaneous tissue

A. Right Anterior Oblique View

Deep cervical fascia

Omohyoid

Clavicle

Subclavius

Costocoracoid membrane

Pectoralis minor

Pectoral fascia

Axilla

Pectoralis major

Suspensory ligament of axilla

Axillary fascia

Axillary fossa

B. Lateral View of Sagittal Section of Anterior Axillary Wall

Axillary fossa

Fascia	
▭	Deep cervical
▭	Clavipectoral
▭	Pectoral
▭	Axillary

2.15 Deep Fascia of Upper Limb, Axillary and Clavipectoral Fascia

A. Axillary fascia. The axillary fascia forms the floor of the axillary fossa and is continuous with the pectoral fascia covering the pectoralis major muscle and the brachial fascia of the arm. **B. Clavipectoral fascia.** The clavipectoral fascia extends from the axillary fascia to enclose the pectoralis minor and subclavius muscles and then attaches to the clavicle. The part of the clavipectoral fascia superior to the pectoralis minor is the costocoracoid membrane, and the part of the clavipectoral fascia inferior to the pectoralis minor is the suspensory ligament of the axilla. The suspensory ligament of the axilla, an extension of the axillary fascia, supports the axillary fascia and pulls the axillary fascia and the skin inferior to it superiorly when the arm is abducted, forming the axillary fossa or "armpit."

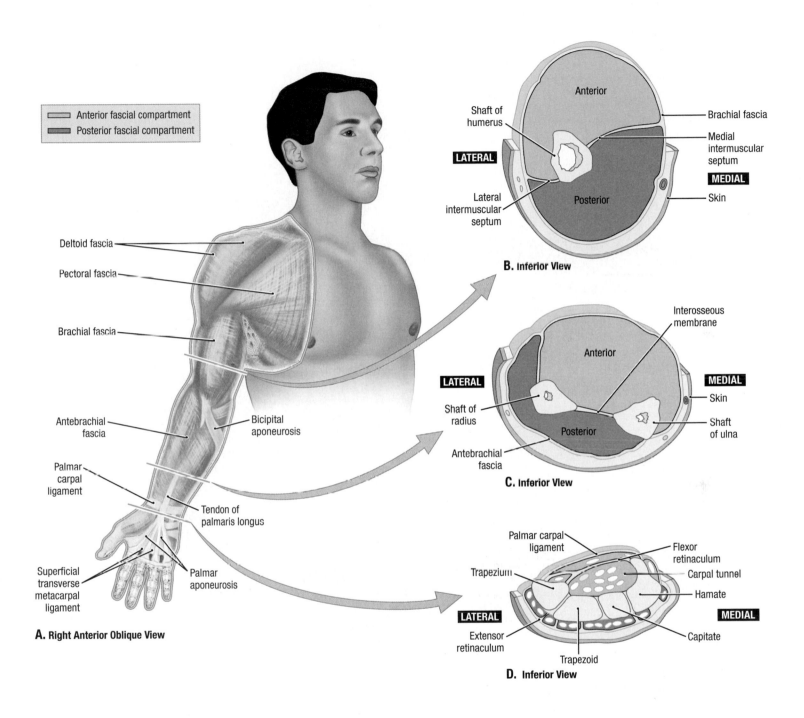

Anterior fascial compartment
Posterior fascial compartment

Deltoid fascia
Pectoral fascia
Brachial fascia
Antebrachial fascia
Bicipital aponeurosis
Palmar carpal ligament
Tendon of palmaris longus
Superficial transverse metacarpal ligament
Palmar aponeurosis

A. Right Anterior Oblique View

Anterior
Shaft of humerus
Brachial fascia
Medial intermuscular septum
LATERAL
MEDIAL
Lateral intermuscular septum
Posterior
Skin

B. Inferior View

Interosseous membrane
Anterior
LATERAL
MEDIAL
Shaft of radius
Skin
Antebrachial fascia
Posterior
Shaft of ulna

C. Inferior View

Palmar carpal ligament
Flexor retinaculum
Trapezium
Carpal tunnel
Hamate
LATERAL
MEDIAL
Extensor retinaculum
Capitate
Trapezoid

D. Inferior View

Deep Fascia of Upper Limb, Brachial and Antebrachial Fascia   2.16

A. Overview of upper limb. B. Brachial fascia. The brachial fascia is the deep fascia of the arm and is continuous superiorly with the pectoral and axillary layers of fascia. Medial and lateral intermuscular septa extend from the deep aspect of the brachial fascia to the humerus, dividing the arm into anterior and posterior musculofascial compartments. **C. Antebrachial fascia.** The antebrachial fascia surrounds the forearm and is continuous with the brachial fascia and deep fascia of the hand. The interosseous membrane separates the forearm into anterior and posterior musculofascial compartments. Distally, the fascia thickens to form the palmar carpal ligament, which is continuous with the flexor retinaculum and dorsally with the extensor expansion. The deep fascia of the hand is continuous with the antebrachial fascia, and on the palmar surface of the hand, it thickens to form the palmar aponeurosis. **D. Flexor retinaculum** (transverse carpal ligament). The flexor retinaculum extends between the medial and lateral carpal bones to form the carpal tunnel.

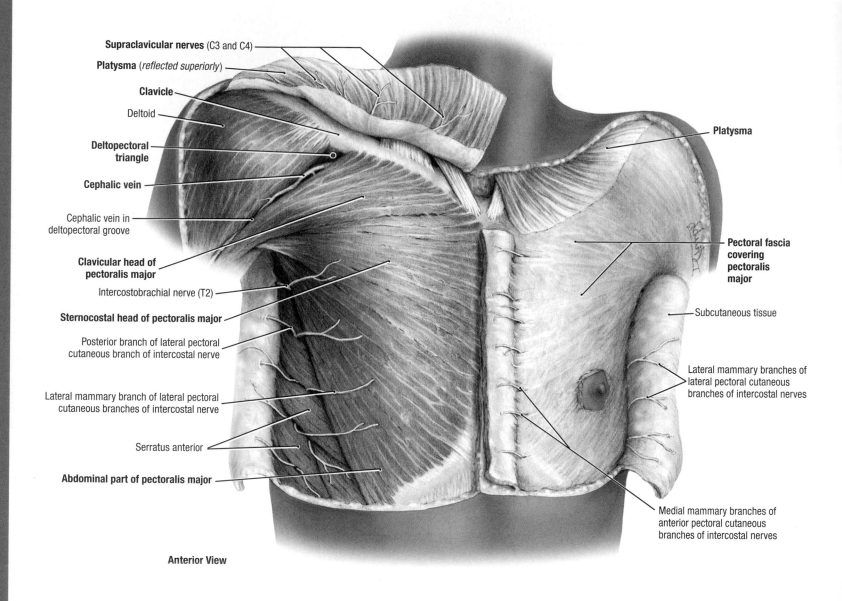

Supraclavicular nerves (C3 and C4)

Platysma (reflected superiorly)

Clavicle

Deltoid

Deltopectoral triangle

Cephalic vein

Cephalic vein in deltopectoral groove

Clavicular head of pectoralis major

Intercostobrachial nerve (T2)

Sternocostal head of pectoralis major

Posterior branch of lateral pectoral cutaneous branch of intercostal nerve

Lateral mammary branch of lateral pectoral cutaneous branches of intercostal nerve

Serratus anterior

Abdominal part of pectoralis major

Platysma

Pectoral fascia covering pectoralis major

Subcutaneous tissue

Lateral mammary branches of lateral pectoral cutaneous branches of intercostal nerves

Medial mammary branches of anterior pectoral cutaneous branches of intercostal nerves

Anterior View

2.17 **Superficial Dissection, Male Pectoral Region**

- The platysma muscle, which usually descends to the 2nd or 3rd rib, is cut short on the right side and, together with the supraclavicular nerves, is reflected on the left side.
- The exposed intermuscular bony strip of the clavicle is subcutaneous and subplatysmal.
- The cephalic vein passes deeply to join the axillary vein in the deltopectoral triangle.

- The cutaneous innervation of the pectoral region is by the supraclavicular nerves (C3 and C4) and upper thoracic nerves (T2–T6); the brachial plexus (C5–T1) does not supply cutaneous branches to the pectoral region.

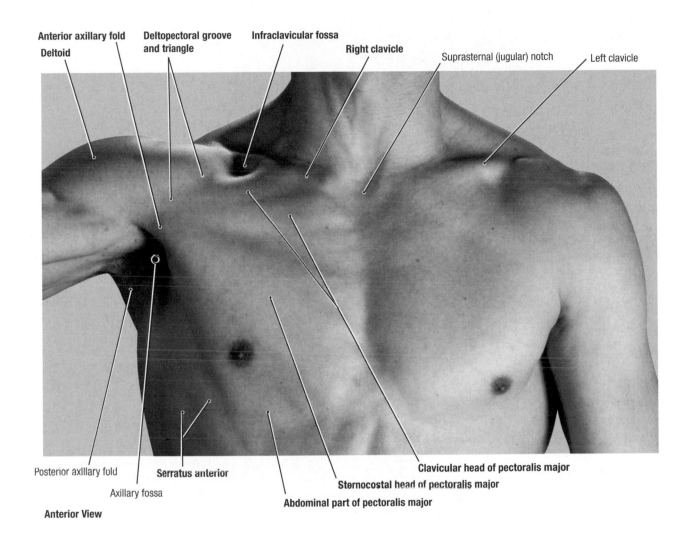

Anterior axillary fold

Deltoid

Deltopectoral groove and triangle

Infraclavicular fossa

Right clavicle

Suprasternal (jugular) notch

Left clavicle

Posterior axillary fold

Axillary fossa

Serratus anterior

Abdominal part of pectoralis major

Sternocostal head of pectoralis major

Clavicular head of pectoralis major

Anterior View

Surface Anatomy, Male Pectoral Region

2.18

The deltopectoral triangle is the depressed area just inferior to the lateral part of the clavicle, bounded by the clavicle superiorly, the deltoid laterally, and the clavicular head of pectoralis major medially. The infraclavicular fossa and the intermuscular deltopectoral groove extending from its inferior apex demarcate an "internervous plane" (plane not crossed by motor nerves) for an **anterior or deltopectoral surgical incision** to approach the axilla, shoulder joint, or proximal humerus.

When the arm is abducted and then adducted against resistance, the two heads of the pectoralis major are visible and palpable. As this muscle extends from the thoracic wall to the arm, it forms the anterior axillary fold. Digitations of the serratus anterior appear inferolateral to the pectoralis major. The coracoid process of the scapula is covered by the anterior part of deltoid; however, the tip of the process can be felt on deep palpation in the clavipectoral triangle. The deltoid forms the contour of the shoulder.

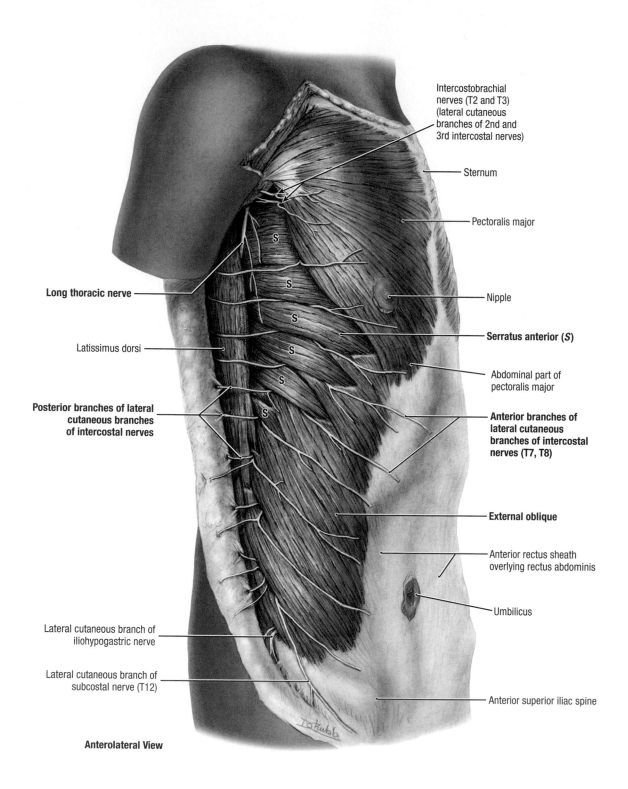

Intercostobrachial nerves (T2 and T3) (lateral cutaneous branches of 2nd and 3rd intercostal nerves)

Sternum

Pectoralis major

Long thoracic nerve

Nipple

Serratus anterior (*S*)

Latissimus dorsi

Abdominal part of pectoralis major

Posterior branches of lateral cutaneous branches of intercostal nerves

Anterior branches of lateral cutaneous branches of intercostal nerves (T7, T8)

External oblique

Anterior rectus sheath overlying rectus abdominis

Umbilicus

Lateral cutaneous branch of iliohypogastric nerve

Lateral cutaneous branch of subcostal nerve (T12)

Anterior superior iliac spine

Anterolateral View

| 2.19 | **Superficial Dissection of Trunk** |

- The slips of the serratus anterior interdigitate with the external oblique.
- The long thoracic nerve (nerve to serratus anterior) lies on the lateral (superficial) aspect of the serratus anterior; this nerve is vulnerable to damage from stab wounds and during surgery (e.g., radical mastectomy).
- The anterior and posterior branches of the lateral cutaneous branches of intercostal and thoracoabdominal nerves are dissected.

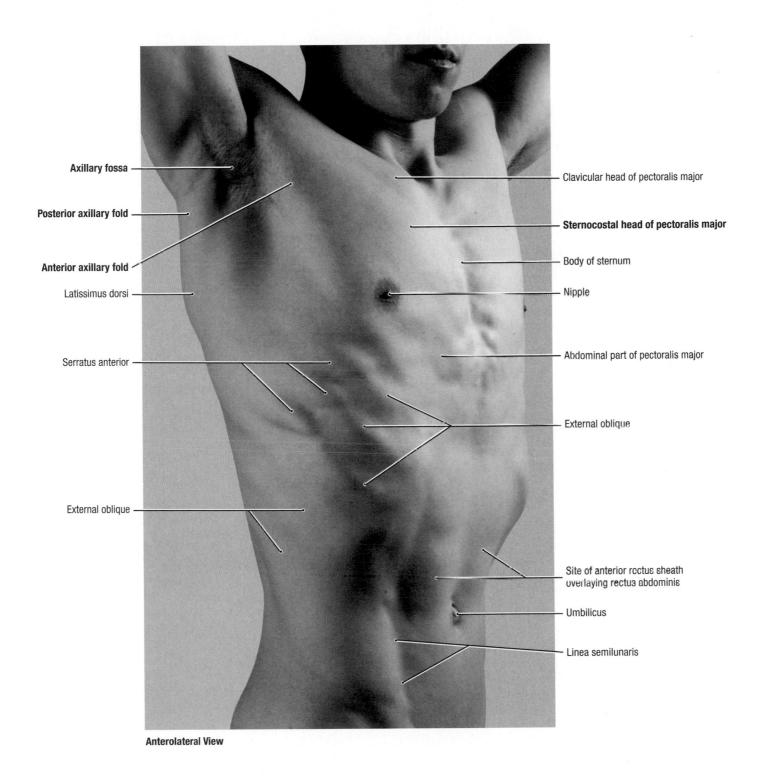

Axillary fossa

Posterior axillary fold

Anterior axillary fold

Latissimus dorsi

Serratus anterior

External oblique

Clavicular head of pectoralis major

Sternocostal head of pectoralis major

Body of sternum

Nipple

Abdominal part of pectoralis major

External oblique

Site of anterior rectus sheath
overlaying rectus abdominis

Umbilicus

Linea semilunaris

Anterolateral View

Surface Anatomy of Anterolateral Aspect of Trunk

2.20

When the arm is abducted and then adducted against resistance, the sternocostal part of the pectoralis major can be seen and palpated. If the anterior axillary fold bounding the axilla is grasped between the fingers and thumb, the inferior border of the sternocostal head of the pectoralis major can be felt. Several digitations of the serratus anterior are visible inferior to the anterior axillary fold. The posterior axillary fold is composed of skin and muscular tissue (latissimus dorsi and teres major) bounding the axilla posteriorly.

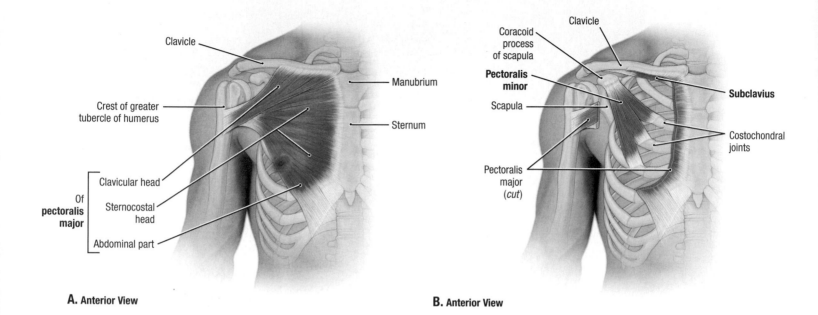

Clavicle

Manubrium

Crest of greater tubercle of humerus

Sternum

Clavicular head

Of **pectoralis major**

Sternocostal head

Abdominal part

A. Anterior View

Coracoid process of scapula

Clavicle

Pectoralis minor

Subclavius

Scapula

Pectoralis major (*cut*)

Costochondral joints

B. Anterior View

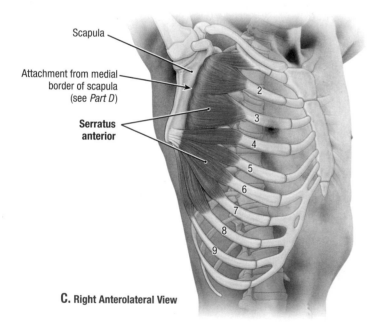

Scapula

Attachment from medial border of scapula (see *Part D*)

Serratus anterior

2
3
4
5
6
7
8
9

C. Right Anterolateral View

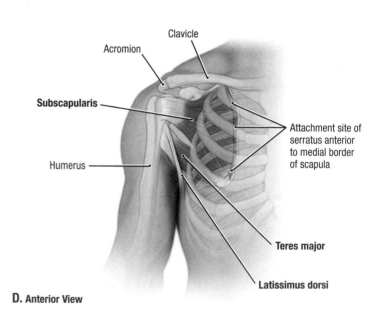

Acromion

Clavicle

Subscapularis

Humerus

Attachment site of serratus anterior to medial border of scapula

Teres major

Latissimus dorsi

D. Anterior View

2.21   **Muscles of Axillary Walls**

A. and **B.** Anterior axillary wall muscles: pectoralis major (*Part A*), pectoralis minor, and subclavius (*Part B*). **C.** Medial axillary wall muscle: serratus anterior. **D.** Posterior axillary wall muscles: subscapularis, teres major, and latissimus dorsi.

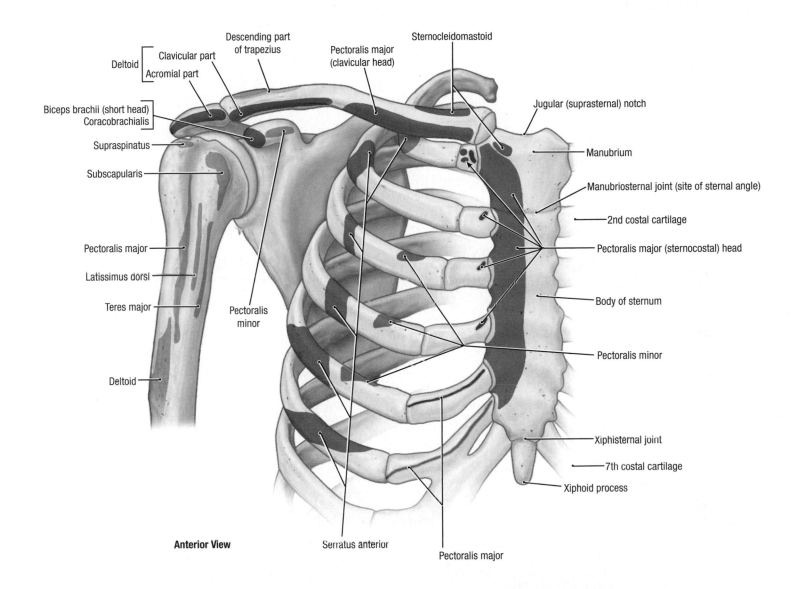

Anterior View

Anterior Attachments of Anterior and Posterior Axioappendicular and Scapulohumeral Muscles   2.22

TABLE 2.4	Anterior Axioappendicular Muscles			
Muscle	**Proximal Attachment (*red*)**	**Distal Attachment (*blue*)**	**Innervation*ᵃ***	**Main Actions**
Pectoralis major	*Clavicular head:* anterior surface of medial half of clavicle *Sternocostal head:* anterior surface of sternum, superior six costal cartilages *Abdominal part:* aponeurosis of external oblique muscle	Crest of greater tubercle of intertubercular sulcus (lateral lip of bicipital groove)	Lateral and medial pectoral nerves; clavicular head (C5 and C6), sternocostal head (**C7**, **C8**, and T1)	Adducts and medially rotates humerus at shoulder joint Acting alone: clavicular head flexes shoulder joint, and sternocostal head extends it from the flexed position
Pectoralis minor	3rd–5th ribs in midclavicular line near their costal cartilages	Medial border and superior surface of coracoid process of scapula	Medial and lateral pectoral nerves (C6–T1)	Stabilizes scapula by drawing it inferiorly and anteriorly against thoracic wall
Subclavius	Junction of 1st rib and its costal cartilage	Inferior surface of middle third of clavicle	Nerve to subclavius (C5 and C6)	Anchors and depresses clavicle at sternoclavicular joint
Serratus anterior	External surfaces of lateral parts of 1st to 8th–9th ribs	Anterior surface of medial border of scapula	Long thoracic nerve (C5, **C6**, and **C7**)	Protracts scapula and holds it against thoracic wall; rotates scapula

*ᵃ*Numbers indicate spinal cord segmental innervation (e.g., C5 and C6 indicate that nerves supplying the clavicular head of pectoralis major are derived from 5th and 6th cervical segments of spinal cord). Boldface numbers indicate the main segmental innervation. Damage to these segments or to motor nerve roots arising from them results in paralysis of the muscles concerned.

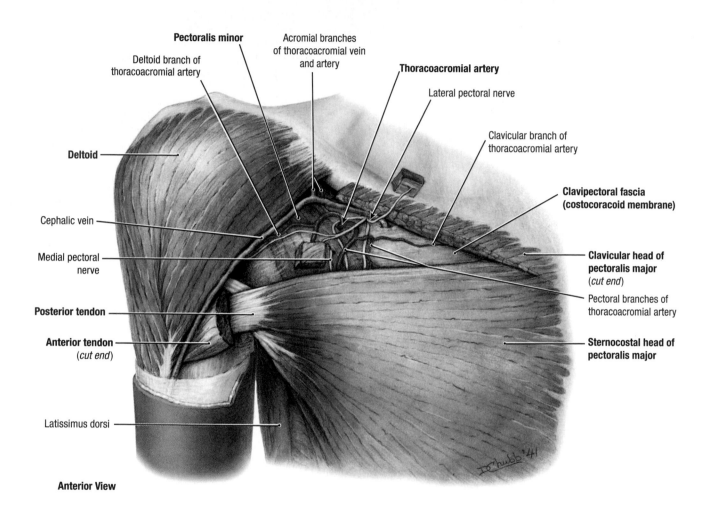

Pectoralis minor

Deltoid branch of
thoracoacromial artery

Acromial branches
of thoracoacromial vein
and artery

Thoracoacromial artery

Lateral pectoral nerve

Clavicular branch of
thoracoacromial artery

Deltoid

Cephalic vein

Medial pectoral
nerve

Posterior tendon

Anterior tendon
(cut end)

Latissimus dorsi

Anterior View

**Clavipectoral fascia
(costocoracoid membrane)**

**Clavicular head of
pectoralis major**
(cut end)

Pectoral branches of
thoracoacromial artery

**Sternocostal head of
pectoralis major**

2.23   **Anterior Wall of Axilla and Clavipectoral Fascia**

Anterior wall of axilla. The clavicular head of the pectoralis major is excised, except for two cubes of muscle that remain to identify the branches of the lateral pectoral nerve.

- The clavipectoral fascia (costocoracoid membrane) superior to the pectoralis minor is pierced by the cephalic vein, the lateral pectoral nerve, and the thoracoacromial vessels.

- The pectoralis minor and clavipectoral fascia are pierced by the medial pectoral nerve.
- Observe the insertion of the pectoralis major from deep to superficial: inferior part of the sternocostal head, superior part of the sternocostal head (posterior tendon), and clavicular head (anterior tendon).

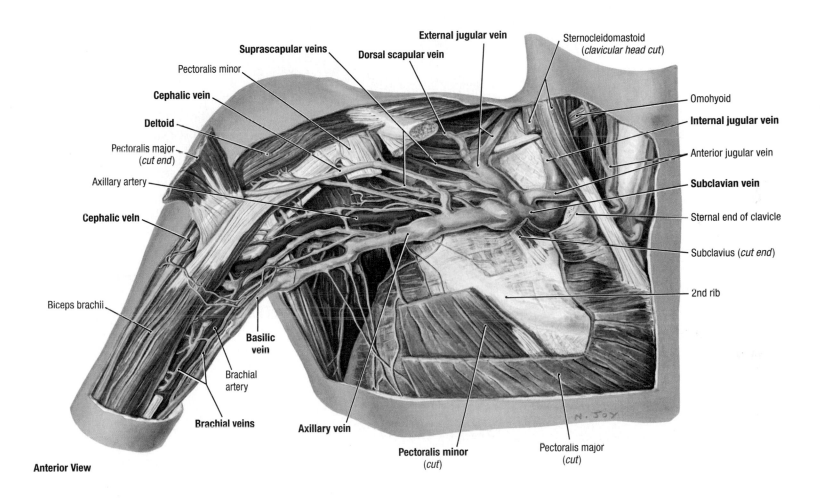

Suprascapular veins

External jugular vein

Dorsal scapular vein

Sternocleidomastoid
(*clavicular head cut*)

Pectoralis minor

Cephalic vein

Omohyoid

Deltoid

Internal jugular vein

Pectoralis major
(*cut end*)

Anterior jugular vein

Axillary artery

Subclavian vein

Cephalic vein

Sternal end of clavicle

Subclavius (*cut end*)

2nd rib

Biceps brachii

**Basilic
vein**

Brachial
artery

Brachial veins

Axillary vein

Pectoralis minor
(*cut*)

Pectoralis major
(*cut*)

N. JOY

Anterior View

Veins of Axilla

2.24

- The basilic vein joins the brachial veins to become the axillary vein near the inferior border of teres major, the axillary vein becomes the subclavian vein at the lateral border of the 1st rib, and the subclavian joins the internal jugular to become the brachiocephalic vein posterior to the sternal end of the clavicle.

- Numerous valves, enlargements in the vein, are shown.
- The cephalic vein in this specimen bifurcates to end in the axillary and external jugular veins.

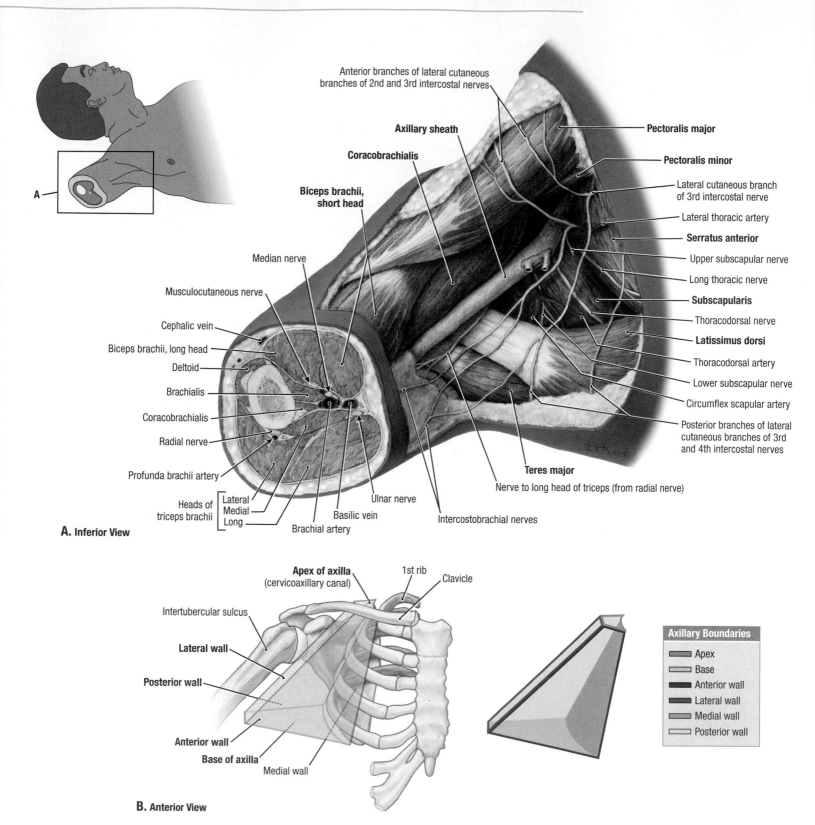

Anterior branches of lateral cutaneous branches of 2nd and 3rd intercostal nerves

Axillary sheath

Coracobrachialis

Biceps brachii, short head

Median nerve

Musculocutaneous nerve

Cephalic vein

Biceps brachii, long head

Deltoid

Brachialis

Coracobrachialis

Radial nerve

Profunda brachii artery

Heads of triceps brachii { Lateral / Medial / Long }

Brachial artery

Basilic vein

Ulnar nerve

Intercostobrachial nerves

Nerve to long head of triceps (from radial nerve)

Teres major

Posterior branches of lateral cutaneous branches of 3rd and 4th intercostal nerves

Circumflex scapular artery

Lower subscapular nerve

Thoracodorsal artery

Latissimus dorsi

Thoracodorsal nerve

Thoracodorsal nerve

Subscapularis

Long thoracic nerve

Upper subscapular nerve

Serratus anterior

Lateral thoracic artery

Lateral cutaneous branch of 3rd intercostal nerve

Pectoralis minor

Pectoralis major

A. Inferior View

Apex of axilla (cervicoaxillary canal)

1st rib

Clavicle

Intertubercular sulcus

Lateral wall

Posterior wall

Anterior wall

Base of axilla

Medial wall

B. Anterior View

Axillary Boundaries
Apex
Base
Anterior wall
Lateral wall
Medial wall
Posterior wall

2.25   Walls and Contents of Axilla

A. Dissection. **B.** Location and walls of axilla.

- The four axillary walls are (1) anterior, formed by the pectoralis major and minor and subclavius; (2) posterior, formed by the subscapularis, latissimus dorsi and teres major; (3) medial, formed by serratus anterior; and (4) lateral, formed by the

intertubercular sulcus of the humerus, occupied by the biceps and coracobrachialis tendons and muscles.

- The axillary sheath surrounds the nerves and vessels (neurovascular bundle) of the upper limb.

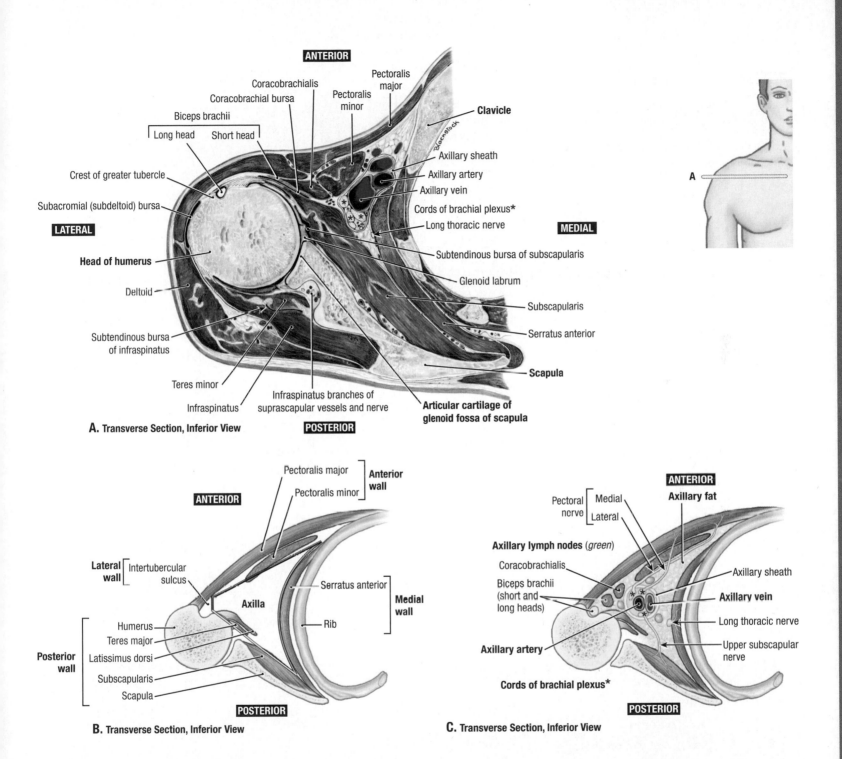

A. Transverse Section, Inferior View

ANTERIOR
Coracobrachialis
Coracobrachial bursa
Pectoralis minor
Pectoralis major
Biceps brachii
Long head Short head
Clavicle
Crest of greater tubercle
Axillary sheath
Axillary artery
Subacromial (subdeltoid) bursa
Axillary vein
Cords of brachial plexus*
LATERAL
Long thoracic nerve
MEDIAL
Head of humerus
Subtendinous bursa of subscapularis
Deltoid
Glenoid labrum
Subscapularis
Serratus anterior
Subtendinous bursa of infraspinatus
Teres minor
Infraspinatus
Infraspinatus branches of suprascapular vessels and nerve
Scapula
Articular cartilage of glenoid fossa of scapula
POSTERIOR

B. Transverse Section, Inferior View

Pectoralis major
Pectoralis minor
Anterior wall
ANTERIOR
Lateral wall Intertubercular sulcus
Serratus anterior
Axilla
Medial wall
Humerus
Rib
Teres major
Latissimus dorsi
Posterior wall
Subscapularis
Scapula
POSTERIOR

C. Transverse Section, Inferior View

ANTERIOR
Pectoral nerve Medial
Lateral
Axillary fat
Axillary lymph nodes (*green*)
Coracobrachialis
Axillary sheath
Biceps brachii (short and long heads)
Axillary vein
Axillary artery
Long thoracic nerve
Upper subscapular nerve
Cords of brachial plexus*
POSTERIOR

Transverse Sections through Shoulder Joint and Axilla

2.26

A. Anatomical section. **B.** Walls of axilla. **C.** Walls and contents of axilla.

- The intertubercular sulcus containing the tendon of the long head of the biceps brachii muscle is directed anteriorly; the short head of the biceps muscle and the coracobrachialis and pectoralis minor muscles are sectioned just inferior to their attachments to the coracoid process.
- The small glenoid cavity is deepened by the glenoid labrum.

- Bursae include the subdeltoid (subacromial) bursa, between the deltoid and greater tubercle; the subtendinous bursa of subscapularis, between the subscapularis tendon and scapula; and coracobrachial bursa, between the coracobrachialis and subscapularis.
- The axillary sheath encloses the axillary artery and vein and the three cords of the brachial plexus to form a neurovascular bundle, surrounded by axillary fat.

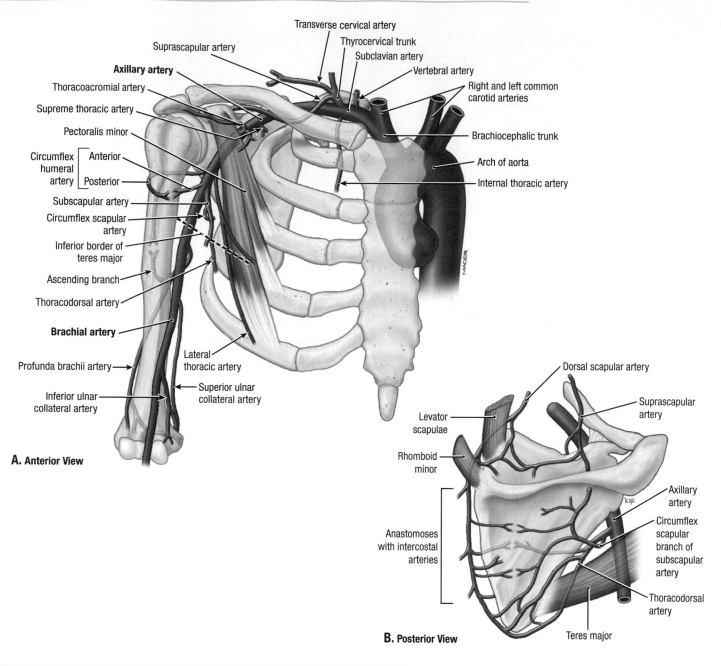

2.27 **Arteries of Proximal Upper Limb**

A. and **B.** Schematics.

TABLE 2.5	Arteries of Proximal Upper Limb (Shoulder Region and Arm)	
Artery	**Origin**	**Course**
Thyrocervical trunk	Subclavian artery	Ascends as a short, wide trunk, often giving rise to the suprascapular artery and/or cervicodorsal trunk and terminating by bifurcating into the ascending cervical and inferior thyroid arteries
Suprascapular	Subclavian artery Thyrocervical trunk/subclavian artery	Passes inferolaterally over anterior scalene muscle and phrenic nerve, subclavian artery and brachial plexus running laterally posterior and parallel to clavicle; next passes over transverse scapular ligament to supraspinous fossa and then lateral to scapular spine (deep to acromion) to infraspinous fossa
Dorsal scapular	Independently, directly from the third (or, less often, the second) part of the subclavian artery	When it is a branch of the subclavian, the dorsal scapular artery passes laterally through the trunks of the brachial plexus, anterior to the middle scalene. Regardless of its origin, its distal portion runs deep to the levator scapulae and rhomboid muscles, supplying both and participating in the arterial anastomoses around the scapula.

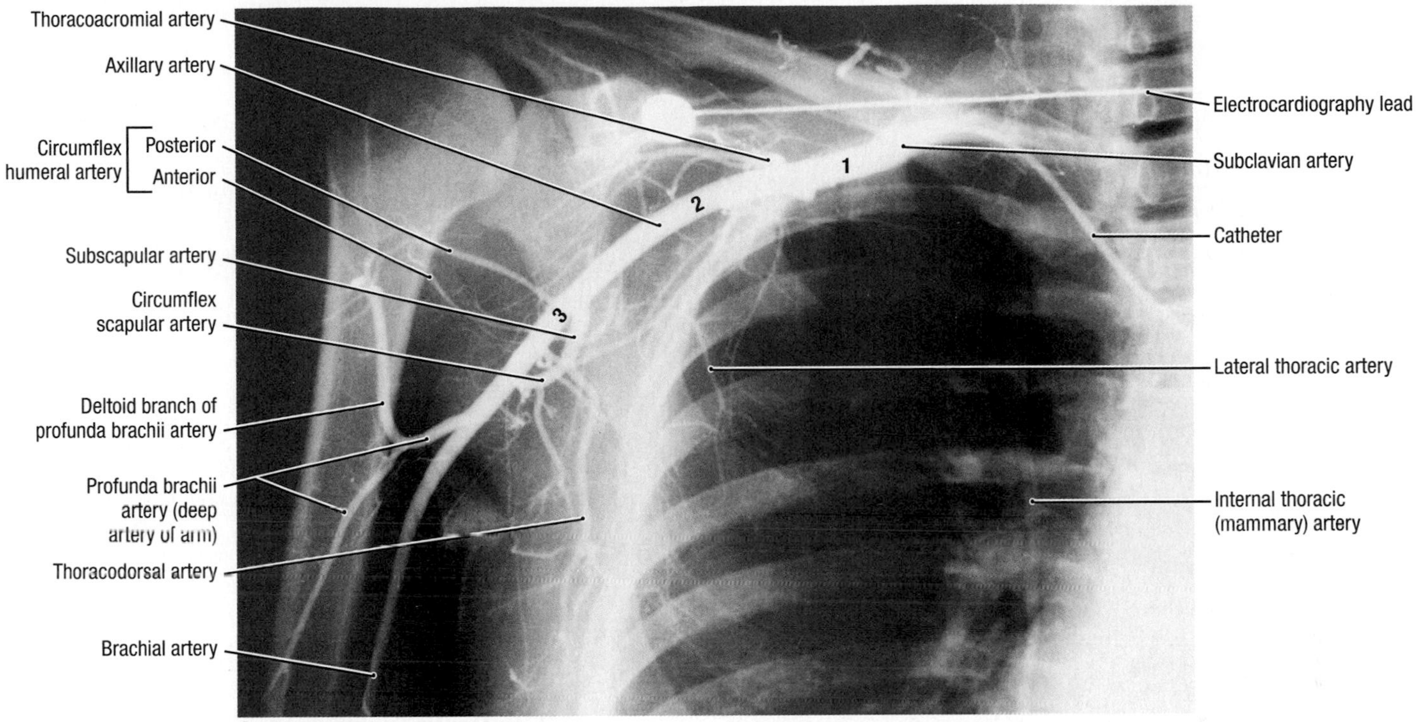
Thoracoacromial artery
Axillary artery
Circumflex humeral artery
Posterior
Anterior
Subscapular artery
Circumflex scapular artery
Deltoid branch of profunda brachii artery
Profunda brachii artery (deep artery of arm)
Thoracodorsal artery
Brachial artery
1
2
3
Electrocardiography lead
Subclavian artery
Catheter
Lateral thoracic artery
Internal thoracic (mammary) artery

C. Anteroposterior Axillary Arteriogram

1 First part of the axillary artery between lateral border of 1st rib and medial border of pectoralis minor
2 Second part of the axillary artery posterior to pectoralis minor
3 Third part of the axillary artery from lateral border of pectoralis minor to inferior border of teres major, where it becomes brachial artery

Arteries of Proximal Upper Limb *(continued)* 2.27

C. Radiographic image of axillary artery and its branches.

TABLE 2.5 Arteries of Proximal Upper Limb (Shoulder Region and Arm) *(continued)*

Artery	Origin		Course
Supreme thoracic	1st part (as only branch)	Of axillary artery	Runs anteromedially along superior border of pectoralis minor; then passes between it and pectoralis major to thoracic wall; helps supply 1st and 2nd intercostal spaces and superior part of serratus anterior
Thoracoacromial	2nd part (medial branch)	Of axillary artery	Curls around superomedial border of pectoralis minor, pierces costocoracoid membrane (clavipectoral fascia), and divides into four branches: pectoral, deltoid, acromial, and clavicular
Lateral thoracic	2nd part (lateral branch)	Of axillary artery	Descends along axillary border of pectoralis minor; follows it onto thoracic wall, supplying lateral aspect of breast
Circumflex humeral (anterior and posterior)	3rd part (sometimes via a common trunk)	Of axillary artery	Encircle surgical neck of humerus, anastomosing with each other laterally; larger posterior branch traverses quadrangular space
Subscapular	3rd part (largest branch)	Of axillary artery	Descends from level of inferior border of subscapularis along lateral border of scapula, dividing within 2–3 cm into terminal branches, the circumflex scapular and thoracodorsal arteries
Circumflex scapular	Subscapular artery	Of axillary artery	Curves around lateral border of scapula to enter infraspinous fossa, anastomosing with suprascapular and dorsal scapular arteries
Thoracodorsal	Subscapular artery	Of axillary artery	Continuation of subscapular artery; accompanies thoracodorsal nerve to enter latissimus dorsi
Profunda brachii (deep brachial) artery	Near middle of arm	Brachial artery	Accompanies radial nerve through radial groove of humerus, supplying posterior compartment of arm and participating in periarticular arterial anastomosis around elbow joint
Superior ulnar collateral	Inferior to teres major	Brachial artery	Accompanies ulnar nerve to posterior aspect of elbow; anastomoses with posterior ulnar recurrent artery
Inferior ulnar collateral	Superior to medial epicondyle of humerus	Brachial artery	Passes anterior to medial epicondyle of humerus to anastomose with anterior ulnar collateral artery around elbow joint

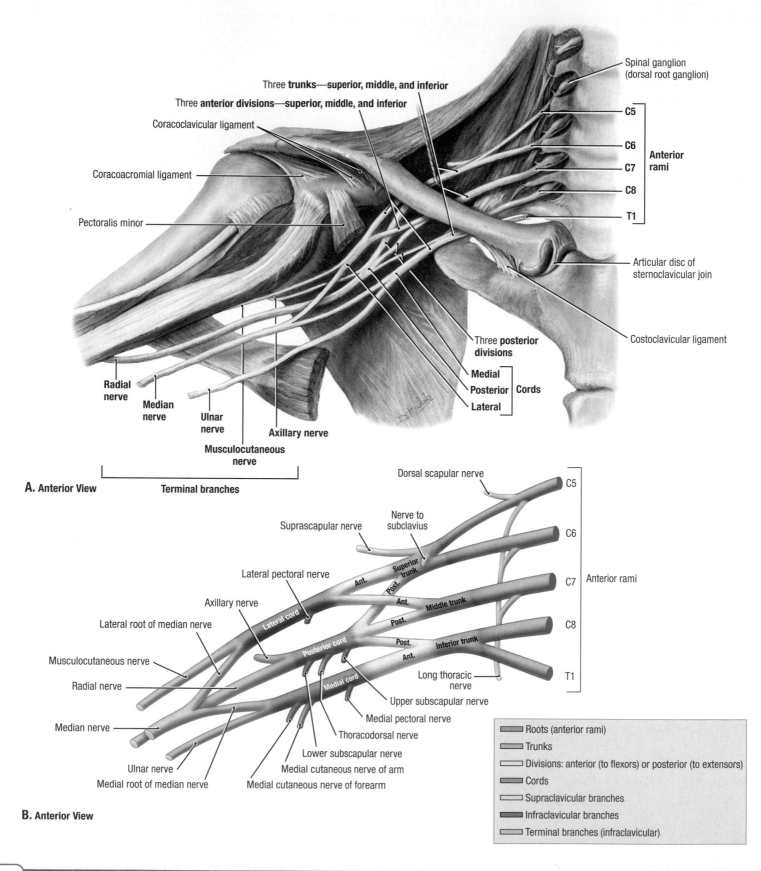

Three **trunks—superior, middle, and inferior**

Three **anterior divisions—superior, middle, and inferior**

Coracoclavicular ligament

Coracoacromial ligament

Pectoralis minor

Spinal ganglion (dorsal root ganglion)

C5

C6

C7 **Anterior rami**

C8

T1

Articular disc of sternoclavicular join

Costoclavicular ligament

Three **posterior divisions**

Medial

Posterior **Cords**

Lateral

Radial nerve

Median nerve

Ulnar nerve

Axillary nerve

Musculocutaneous nerve

A. Anterior View **Terminal branches**

Dorsal scapular nerve

Suprascapular nerve

Nerve to subclavius

Lateral pectoral nerve

Axillary nerve

Lateral root of median nerve

Musculocutaneous nerve

Radial nerve

Median nerve

Ulnar nerve

Medial root of median nerve

Medial cutaneous nerve of forearm

Medial cutaneous nerve of arm

Lower subscapular nerve

Thoracodorsal nerve

Medial pectoral nerve

Upper subscapular nerve

Long thoracic nerve

Lateral cord

Posterior cord

Medial cord

Superior trunk

Ant.

Post.

Ant.

Middle trunk

Post.

Post.

Inferior trunk

Ant.

C5

C6

C7 Anterior rami

C8

T1

B. Anterior View

Roots (anterior rami)

Trunks

Divisions: anterior (to flexors) or posterior (to extensors)

Cords

Supraclavicular branches

Infraclavicular branches

Terminal branches (infraclavicular)

2.28 **Brachial Plexus**

A. Dissection. **B.** Schematic.

TABLE 2.6	Brachial Plexus		
Nerve	**Origin**	**Course**	**Distribution/Structure(s) Supplied**
Supraclavicular branches			
Dorsal scapular	Anterior ramus of C5 with a frequent contribution from C4	Pierces scalenus medius, descends on deep surface of rhomboids	Rhomboids and occasionally supplies levator scapulae
Long thoracic	Anterior rami of C5–C7	Descends posterior to C8 and T1 rami and passes distally on external surface of serratus anterior	Serratus anterior
Nerve to subclavius	Superior trunk receiving fibers from C5 and C6 and often C4	Descends posterior to clavicle and anterior to brachial plexus and subclavian artery	Subclavius and sternoclavicular joint
Suprascapular		Passes laterally across posterior triangle of neck, through suprascapular notch deep to superior transverse scapular ligament	Supraspinatus, infraspinatus, and glenohumeral (shoulder) joint
Infraclavicular branches			
Lateral pectoral	Lateral cord receiving fibers from C5–C7	Pierces clavipectoral fascia to reach deep surface of pectoral muscles	Primarily pectoralis major but sends a loop to medial pectoral nerve that innervates pectoralis minor
Musculocutaneous		Pierces coracobrachialis and descends between biceps brachii and brachialis	Coracobrachialis, biceps brachii, and brachialis; continues as lateral cutaneous nerve of forearm
Median	Lateral root of median nerve is a terminal branch of lateral cord (C6–C7); medial root of median nerve is a terminal branch of medial cord (C8–T1)	Lateral and medial roots merge to form median nerve lateral to axillary artery; crosses anterior to brachial artery to lie medial to artery in cubital fossa	Flexor muscles in forearm (except flexor carpi ulnaris, ulnar half of flexor digitorum profundus), 3½ thumb muscles (except adductor pollicis and deep head of flexor pollicis brevis), and 2 lateral lumbricals and skin of palm and 3½ digits lateral to a line bisecting 4th digit and the dorsum of the distal halves of these digits
Medial pectoral	Medial cord receiving fibers from C8–T1	Passes between axillary artery and vein and enters deep surface of pectoralis minor	Pectoralis minor and part of pectoralis major
Medial cutaneous nerve of arm		Runs along the medial side of axillary vein and communicates with intercostobrachial nerve	Skin on medial side of arm
Medial cutaneous nerve of forearm		Runs between axillary artery and vein	Skin over medial side of forearm
Ulnar	Terminal branch of medial cord receiving fibers from C8, T1, and often C7	Passes down medial view of arm and runs posterior to medial epicondyle to enter forearm	Innervates flexor carpi ulnaris and ulnar half of flexor digitorum profundus in forearm, deep head of flexor pollicis brevis and adductor pollicis, and skin of hand medial to a line bisecting 4th digit (ring finger) anteriorly and posteriorly
Upper subscapular	Branch of posterior cord receiving fibers from C5	Passes posteriorly and enters subscapularis	Superior portion of subscapularis
Thoracodorsal	Branch of posterior cord receiving fibers from C6–C8	Arises between upper and lower subscapular nerves and runs inferolaterally to latissimus dorsi	Latissimus dorsi
Lower subscapular	Branch of posterior cord receiving fibers from C6	Passes inferolaterally, deep to subscapular artery and vein, to subscapularis and teres major	Inferior portion of subscapularis and teres major
Axillary	Terminal branch of posterior cord receiving fibers from C5 and C6	Passes to posterior aspect of arm through quadrangular space[a] with posterior circumflex humeral artery and then winds around surgical neck of humerus; gives rise to lateral cutaneous nerve of arm	Teres minor and deltoid, glenohumeral (shoulder) joint, and skin of superolateral arm
Radial	Terminal branch of posterior cord receiving fibers from C5–T1	Descends posterior to axillary artery; passes between long and medial heads of triceps to course along radial groove between medial and lateral heads of triceps brachii	Triceps brachii, anconeus, brachioradialis, and extensor muscles of forearm; supplies skin on posterior and inferolateral aspect of arm and forearm and dorsum of hand lateral to axial line of digit 4

[a]Quadrangular space is bounded superiorly by subscapularis and teres minor, inferiorly by teres major, medially by long head of triceps brachii, and laterally by humerus.

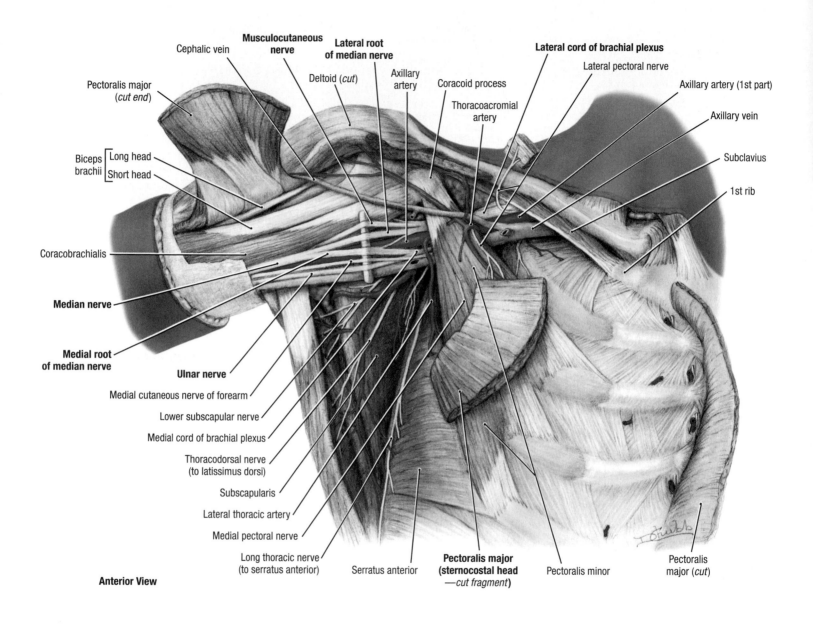

Cephalic vein

Musculocutaneous nerve

Lateral root of median nerve

Lateral cord of brachial plexus

Pectoralis major (*cut end*)

Deltoid (*cut*)

Axillary artery

Coracoid process

Lateral pectoral nerve

Thoracoacromial artery

Axillary artery (1st part)

Axillary vein

Biceps brachii [Long head / Short head]

Subclavius

1st rib

Coracobrachialis

Median nerve

Medial root of median nerve

Ulnar nerve

Medial cutaneous nerve of forearm

Lower subscapular nerve

Medial cord of brachial plexus

Thoracodorsal nerve (to latissimus dorsi)

Subscapularis

Lateral thoracic artery

Medial pectoral nerve

Long thoracic nerve (to serratus anterior)

Serratus anterior

Pectoralis major (sternocostal head —*cut fragment*)

Pectoralis minor

Pectoralis major (*cut*)

Anterior View

2.29   **Structures of Axilla: Deep Dissection (I)**

- The pectoralis major muscle is cut with attachments reflected, the anterior deltoid is cut, and the clavipectoral fascia is removed; the cube of muscle superior to the clavicle is cut from the clavicular head of the pectoralis major muscle.
- The subclavius and pectoralis minor are the two deep muscles of the anterior wall.
- The second part of the axillary artery passes posterior to the pectoralis minor muscle, a fingerbreadth from the tip of the coracoid process; the axillary vein lies anterior and then medial to the axillary artery.

- The median nerve, followed proximally, leads by its lateral root to the lateral cord and musculocutaneous nerve and by its medial root to the medial cord and ulnar nerve. These four nerves and the medial cutaneous nerve of the forearm are derived from the anterior divisions of the brachial plexus and are raised on a stick. The lateral root of the median nerve may occur as several strands.
- The musculocutaneous nerve enters the flexor compartment of the arm by piercing the coracobrachialis muscle.

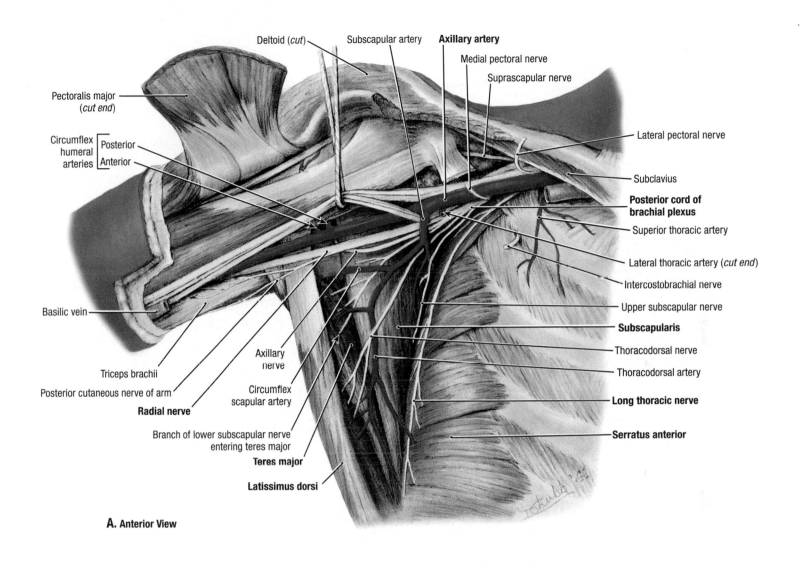

Deltoid (*cut*)
Subscapular artery
Axillary artery
Medial pectoral nerve
Suprascapular nerve

Pectoralis major
(*cut end*)

Circumflex humeral arteries — Posterior / Anterior

Lateral pectoral nerve

Subclavius

Posterior cord of brachial plexus

Superior thoracic artery

Lateral thoracic artery (*cut end*)

Intercostobrachial nerve

Basilic vein

Upper subscapular nerve

Subscapularis

Triceps brachii

Axillary nerve

Thoracodorsal nerve

Thoracodorsal artery

Posterior cutaneous nerve of arm

Circumflex scapular artery

Long thoracic nerve

Radial nerve

Branch of lower subscapular nerve entering teres major

Serratus anterior

Teres major

Latissimus dorsi

A. Anterior View

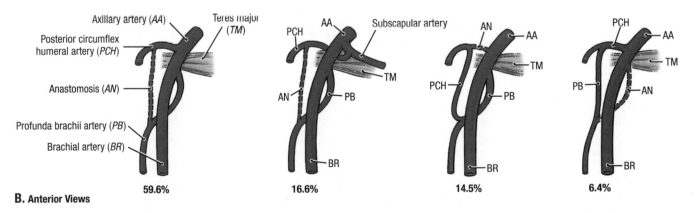

Axillary artery (*AA*)
Teres major (*TM*)
Posterior circumflex humeral artery (*PCH*)
Anastomosis (*AN*)
Profunda brachii artery (*PB*)
Brachial artery (*BR*)

Subscapular artery

PCH   AA
AN   PB   TM
BR

AN   AA
PCH   PB   TM
BR

PCH   AA
PB   AN   TM
BR

59.6%   **16.6%**   **14.5%**   **6.4%**

B. Anterior Views

Posterior and Medial Walls of Axilla: Deep Dissection (II)

2.30

A. Dissection. The pectoralis minor muscle is excised, the terminal branches of lateral and medial cords of the brachial plexus are retracted, and the axillary vein is removed. **B. Variations of posterior** **circumflex humeral artery and profunda brachii artery.** Frequency of occurrences is based on 235 specimens dissected in Dr. Grant's laboratory.

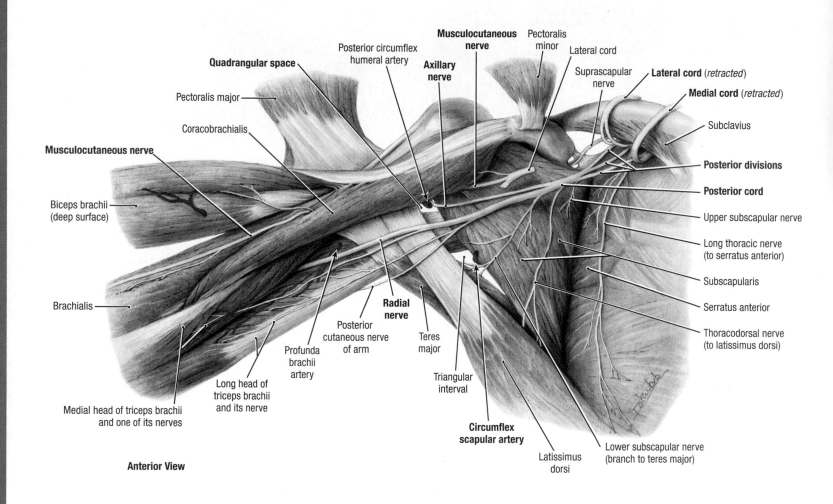

Musculocutaneous nerve
Posterior circumflex humeral artery
Quadrangular space
Axillary nerve
Pectoralis major
Coracobrachialis
Musculocutaneous nerve
Biceps brachii (deep surface)
Brachialis
Medial head of triceps brachii and one of its nerves
Long head of triceps brachii and its nerve
Profunda brachii artery
Posterior cutaneous nerve of arm
Radial nerve
Teres major
Triangular interval
Circumflex scapular artery
Latissimus dorsi
Lower subscapular nerve (branch to teres major)
Anterior View

Musculocutaneous nerve
Pectoralis minor
Lateral cord
Suprascapular nerve
Lateral cord (*retracted*)
Medial cord (*retracted*)
Subclavius
Posterior divisions
Posterior cord
Upper subscapular nerve
Long thoracic nerve (to serratus anterior)
Subscapularis
Serratus anterior
Thoracodorsal nerve (to latissimus dorsi)

2.31 Posterior Wall of Axilla, Musculocutaneous Nerve, and Posterior Cord: Deep Dissection (III)

- The pectoralis major and minor muscles are reflected laterally; the lateral and medial cords of the brachial plexus are reflected superiorly; and the arteries, veins, and median and ulnar nerves are removed.
- Coracobrachialis arises with the short head of the biceps brachii muscle from the tip of the coracoid process and attaches halfway down the medial aspect of the humerus.
- The musculocutaneous nerve pierces the coracobrachialis muscle and supplies it, the biceps, and the brachialis before becoming the lateral cutaneous nerve of the forearm.
- The posterior cord of the plexus is formed by the union of the three posterior divisions; it supplies the three muscles of the posterior wall of the axilla and then bifurcates into the radial and axillary nerves.

- In the axilla, the radial nerve gives off the nerve to the long head of the triceps brachii muscle and a cutaneous branch; in this specimen, it also gives off a branch to the medial head of the triceps. It then enters the radial groove of the humerus with the profunda brachii (deep brachial) artery.
- The axillary nerve passes through the quadrangular space along with the posterior circumflex humeral artery. The borders of the quadrangular space are superiorly, the lateral border of the scapula; inferiorly, the teres major; laterally, the humerus (surgical neck); and medially, the long head of triceps brachii. The circumflex scapular artery traverses the triangular interval.

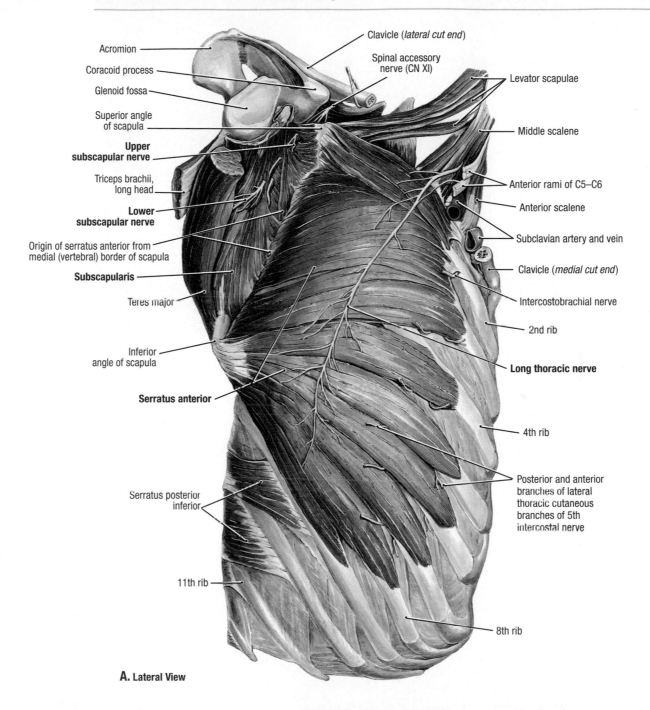

Clavicle (*lateral cut end*)

Acromion

Spinal accessory
nerve (CN XI)

Coracoid process

Levator scapulae

Glenoid fossa

Superior angle
of scapula

Middle scalene

**Upper
subscapular nerve**

Anterior rami of C5–C6

Triceps brachii,
long head

Anterior scalene

**Lower
subscapular nerve**

Subclavian artery and vein

Origin of serratus anterior from
medial (vertebral) border of scapula

Clavicle (*medial cut end*)

Subscapularis

Intercostobrachial nerve

Teres major

2nd rib

Inferior
angle of scapula

Long thoracic nerve

Serratus anterior

4th rib

Serratus posterior
inferior

Posterior and anterior
branches of lateral
thoracic cutaneous
branches of 5th
intercostal nerve

11th rib

8th rib

A. Lateral View

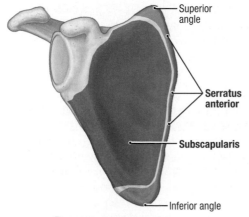

Superior
angle

**Serratus
anterior**

Subscapularis

Inferior angle

B. Anterior View

Serratus Anterior and Subscapularis   2.32

A. Serratus anterior. B. Sites of muscle attachment of serratus anterior and subscapularis to scapula. The serratus anterior muscle, which forms the medial wall of the axilla, has a fleshy belly extending from the superior 8 or 9 ribs in the midclavicular line to the medial border of the scapula.

Winged scapula. When the serratus anterior is paralyzed because of injury to the long thoracic nerve, the medial border of the scapula moves laterally and posteriorly, away from the thoracic wall. When the arm is abducted, the medial border and the inferior angle of the scapula pull away from the posterior thoracic wall, a deformation known as a winged scapula. In addition, the arm cannot be abducted above the horizontal position because the serratus anterior is unable to rotate the glenoid cavity superiorly.

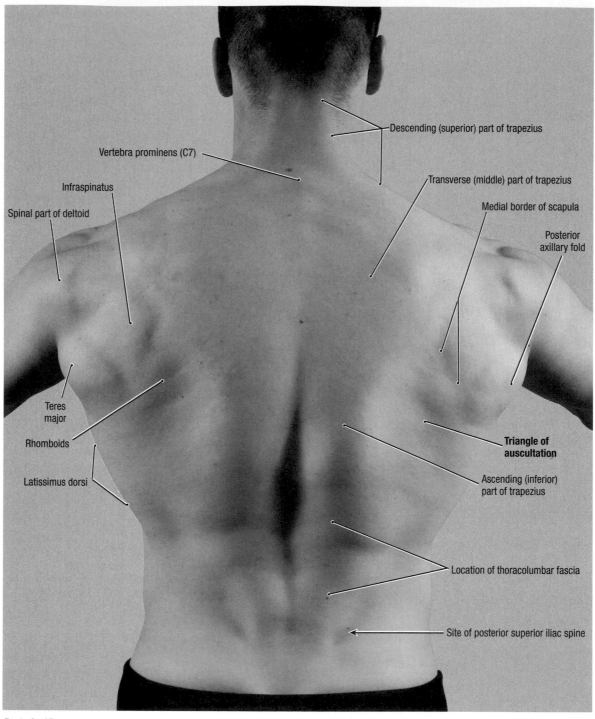

Descending (superior) part of trapezius

Vertebra prominens (C7)

Infraspinatus

Spinal part of deltoid

Transverse (middle) part of trapezius

Medial border of scapula

Posterior axillary fold

Teres major

Rhomboids

Latissimus dorsi

Triangle of auscultation

Ascending (inferior) part of trapezius

Location of thoracolumbar fascia

Site of posterior superior iliac spine

Posterior View

2.33 Surface Anatomy of Superficial Back

The superior border of the latissimus dorsi and a part of the rhomboid major are overlapped by the trapezius. The area formed by the superior border of latissimus dorsi, the medial border of the scapula, and the inferolateral border of the trapezius is called the **triangle of auscultation**. This gap in the thick back musculature is a good place to examine posterior segments of the lungs with a stethoscope. When the scapulae are drawn anteriorly by folding the arms across the thorax and the trunk is flexed, the auscultatory triangle enlarges. The teres major forms a raised oval area on the inferolateral third of the posterior aspect of the scapula when the arm is adducted against resistance. The posterior axillary fold is formed by the teres major and the tendon of the latissimus dorsi.

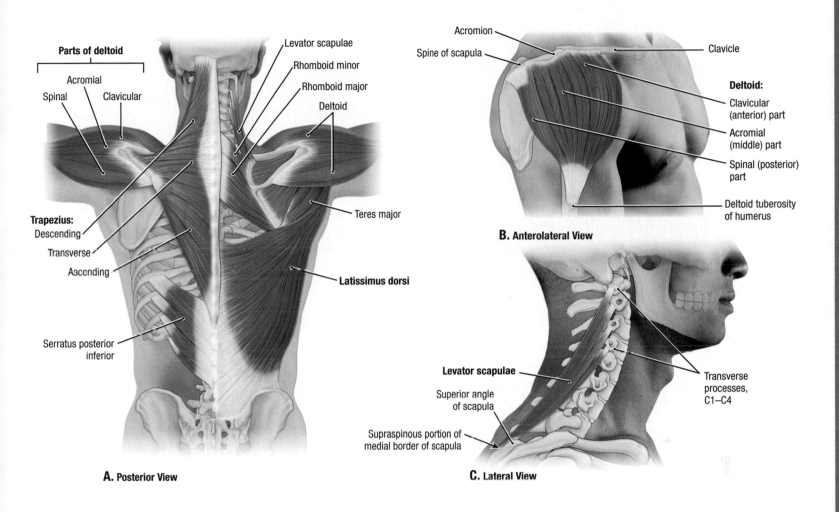

A. Posterior View

B. Anterolateral View

C. Lateral View

Superficial Back Muscles

2.34

A. Overview. **B.** Deltoid. **C.** Levator scapulae.

TABLE 2.7	Superficial Back (Posterior Axioappendicular) and Deltoid Muscles			
Muscle	**Proximal Attachment**	**Distal Attachment**	**Innervation**	**Main Actions**
Trapezius	Medial third of superior nuchal line; external occipital protuberance, nuchal ligament, and spinous processes of C7–T12 vertebrae	Lateral third of clavicle, acromion, and spine of scapula	Spinal accessory nerve (CN XI—motor) and cervical nerves (C3–C4—sensory)	Elevates, retracts, and rotates scapula; *descending part* elevates, *transverse part* retracts, and *ascending part* depresses scapula; descending and ascending parts act together in superior rotation of scapula
Latissimus dorsi	Spinous processes of inferior six thoracic vertebrae, thoracolumbar fascia, iliac crest, and inferior three or four ribs, inferior angle of scapula[a]	Intertubercular sulcus (bicipital groove) of humerus	Thoracodorsal nerve (**C6, C7,** and **C8**)	Extends, adducts, and medially rotates shoulder joint; elevates body toward arms during climbing
Levator scapulae	Posterior tubercles of transverse processes of C1–C4 vertebrae	Superior part of medial border of scapula	Dorsal scapular (C5) and cervical (C3–C4) nerves	Elevates scapula and tilts its glenoid cavity inferiorly by rotating scapula
Rhomboid minor and major	*Minor:* inferior part of nuchal ligament and spinous processes of C7 and T1 vertebrae *Major:* spinous processes of T2–T5 vertebrae	Medial border of scapula from level of spine to inferior angle	Dorsal scapular nerve (C4 and **C5**)	Retract scapula and rotate it to depress glenoid cavity; fix scapula to thoracic wall

[a]Intermediate attachment.

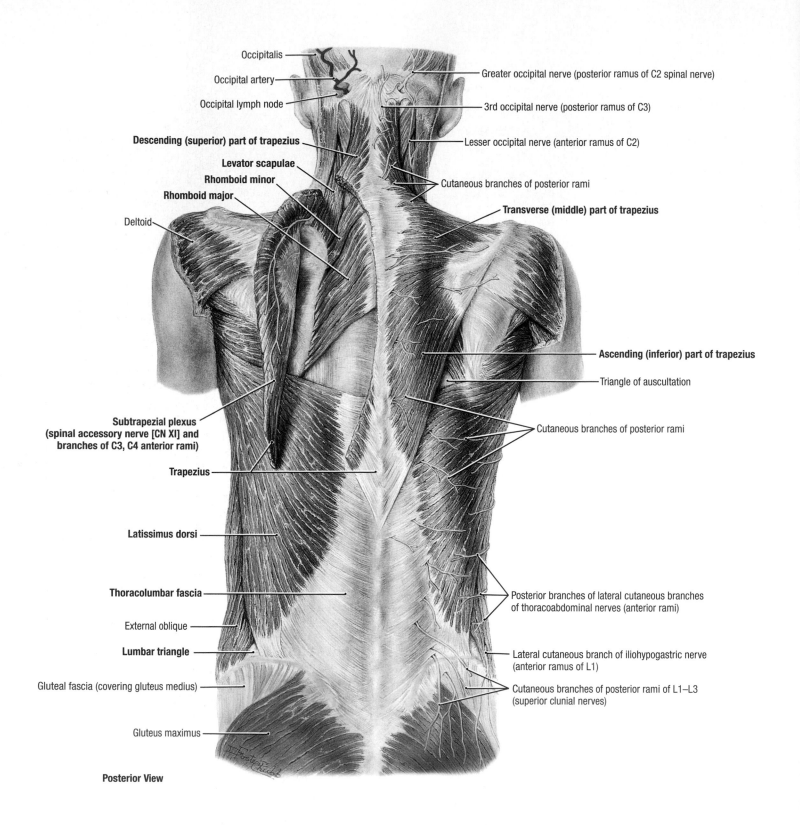

Occipitalis

Occipital artery

Occipital lymph node

Descending (superior) part of trapezius

Levator scapulae

Rhomboid minor

Rhomboid major

Deltoid

Subtrapezial plexus (spinal accessory nerve [CN XI] and branches of C3, C4 anterior rami)

Trapezius

Latissimus dorsi

Thoracolumbar fascia

External oblique

Lumbar triangle

Gluteal fascia (covering gluteus medius)

Gluteus maximus

Posterior View

Greater occipital nerve (posterior ramus of C2 spinal nerve)

3rd occipital nerve (posterior ramus of C3)

Lesser occipital nerve (anterior ramus of C2)

Cutaneous branches of posterior rami

Transverse (middle) part of trapezius

Ascending (inferior) part of trapezius

Triangle of auscultation

Cutaneous branches of posterior rami

Posterior branches of lateral cutaneous branches of thoracoabdominal nerves (anterior rami)

Lateral cutaneous branch of iliohypogastric nerve (anterior ramus of L1)

Cutaneous branches of posterior rami of L1–L3 (superior clunial nerves)

2.35 **Posterior Axioappendicular Muscles**

The trapezius muscle is cut and reflected on the left side. A superficial or first muscle layer consists of the trapezius and latissimus dorsi muscles, and a second layer of the levator scapulae and rhomboids.

Cutaneous branches of posterior rami penetrate but do not supply the superficial back muscles.

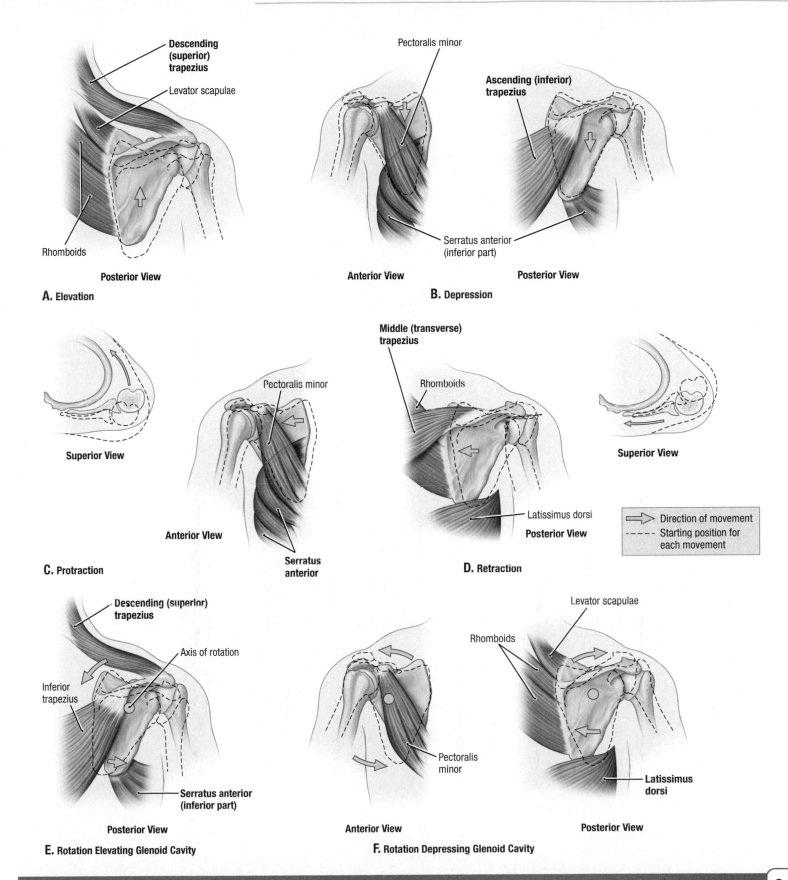

A. Elevation

Descending (superior) trapezius
Levator scapulae
Rhomboids
Posterior View

B. Depression

Pectoralis minor
Ascending (inferior) trapezius
Serratus anterior (inferior part)
Anterior View   Posterior View

C. Protraction

Pectoralis minor
Superior View
Anterior View
Serratus anterior

D. Retraction

Middle (transverse) trapezius
Rhomboids
Latissimus dorsi
Posterior View
Superior View

Direction of movement
Starting position for each movement

E. Rotation Elevating Glenoid Cavity

Descending (superior) trapezius
Axis of rotation
Inferior trapezius
Serratus anterior (inferior part)
Posterior View

F. Rotation Depressing Glenoid Cavity

Pectoralis minor
Anterior View

Levator scapulae
Rhomboids
Latissimus dorsi
Posterior View

Scapular Movements   **2.36**

A–F. Overview of muscles producing scapular movements. The scapula moves on the thoracic wall at the conceptual "scapulothoracic joint." Boldface refers to the prime movers.

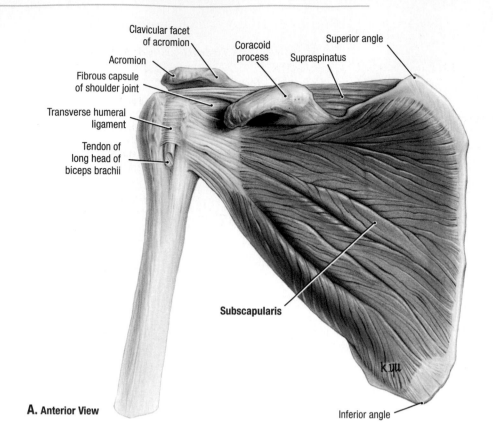

Clavicular facet
of acromion

Acromion

Coracoid
process

Superior angle

Supraspinatus

Fibrous capsule
of shoulder joint

Transverse humeral
ligament

Tendon of
long head of
biceps brachii

Subscapularis

A. Anterior View

Inferior angle

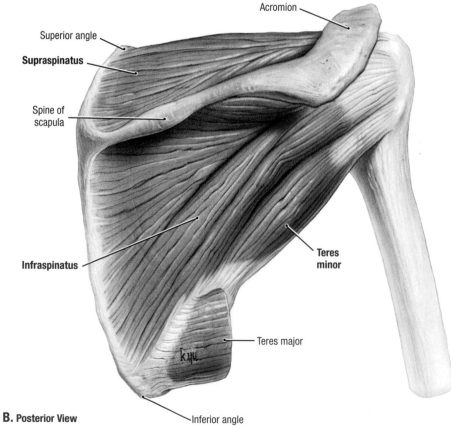

Acromion

Superior angle

Supraspinatus

Spine of
scapula

Infraspinatus

**Teres
minor**

Teres major

Inferior angle

B. Posterior View

2.37 **Rotator Cuff**

A. Subscapularis. **B.** Supraspinatus, infraspinatus, and teres minor.

Four of the scapulohumeral muscles (supraspinatus, infraspinatus, teres minor, and subscapularis) are called rotator cuff muscles because they form a musculotendinous rotator cuff around the glenohumeral (shoulder) joint. All except the supraspinatus are rotators of the humerus.

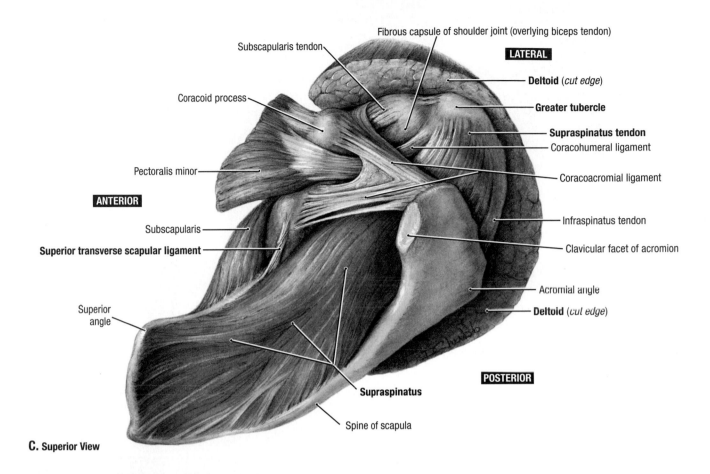

Fibrous capsule of shoulder joint (overlying biceps tendon)

Subscapularis tendon

Coracoid process

LATERAL

Deltoid (*cut edge*)

Greater tubercle

Supraspinatus tendon

Coracohumeral ligament

Pectoralis minor

Coracoacromial ligament

ANTERIOR

Subscapularis

Infraspinatus tendon

Superior transverse scapular ligament

Clavicular facet of acromion

Acromial angle

Deltoid (*cut edge*)

Superior angle

POSTERIOR

Supraspinatus

Spine of scapula

C. Superior View

Rotator Cuff (*continued*)

2.37

C. Supraspinatus. The supraspinatus, also part of the rotator cuff, initiates and assists the deltoid in abducting the shoulder joint. The tendons of the rotator cuff muscles blend with and reinforce the joint capsule of the glenohumeral joint, protecting the joint and giving it stability.

Injury or disease may damage the rotator cuff, producing instability of the glenohumeral joint. **Rupture or tear of the supraspinatus tendon** is the most common injury of the rotator cuff. **Degenerative tendinitis of the rotator cuff** is common, especially in older people.

TABLE 2.8	**Scapulohumeral Muscles**			
Muscle	**Proximal Attachment**	**Distal Attachment**	**Innervation**	**Main Actions**
Deltoid	Lateral third of clavicle (*clavicular part*), acromion (*acromial part*), and spine (*spinal part*) of scapula	Deltoid tuberosity of humerus	Axillary nerve (**C5** and C6)	*Clavicular* (*anterior*) *part:* flexes and medially rotates shoulder joint *Acromial* (*middle*) *part:* abducts shoulder joint *Spinal* (*posterior*) *part:* extends and laterally rotates shoulder joint
Supraspinatus (S)	Supraspinous fossa of scapula	Superior facet on greater tubercle of humerus	Suprascapular nerve (C4, **C5**, and C6)	Initiates abduction at shoulder joint and acts with other rotator cuff muscles[a]
Infraspinatus (I)	Infraspinous fossa of scapula	Middle facet on greater tubercle of humerus	Suprascapular nerve (**C5** and C6)	Laterally rotates shoulder joint; helps to hold humeral head in glenoid cavity of scapula
Teres minor (T)	Middle part of lateral border of scapula	Inferior facet on greater tubercle of humerus	Axillary nerve (**C5** and C6)	
Subscapularis (S)	Subscapular fossa	Lesser tubercle of humerus	Upper and lower subscapular nerves (C5, **C6**, and C7)	Medially rotates shoulder joint and adducts it; helps to hold humeral head in glenoid cavity
Teres major[b]	Posterior surface of inferior angle of scapula	Crest of lesser tubercle (medial lip of bicipital groove) of humerus	Lower subscapular nerve (**C6** and C7)	Adducts and medially rotates shoulder joint

[a]Collectively, the supraspinatus, infraspinatus, teres minor, and subscapularis muscles are referred to as the rotator cuff muscles or "SITS" muscles. They function together during all movements of the shoulder joint to hold the head of the humerus in the glenoid cavity of scapula.
[b]Not a rotator cuff muscle.

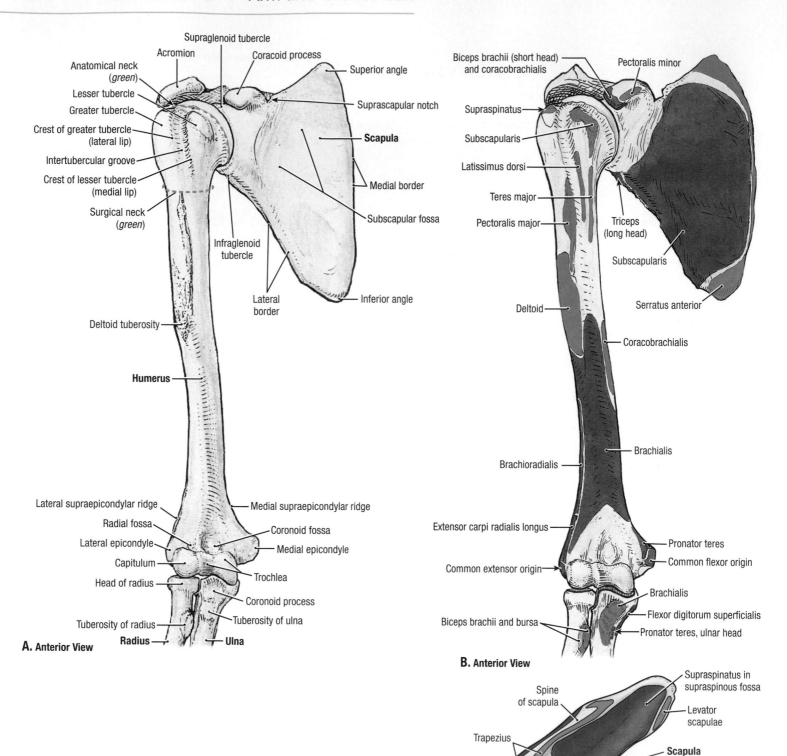

A. Anterior View

Supraglenoid tubercle
Acromion
Coracoid process
Anatomical neck (*green*)
Lesser tubercle
Greater tubercle
Crest of greater tubercle (lateral lip)
Intertubercular groove
Crest of lesser tubercle (medial lip)
Surgical neck (*green*)
Superior angle
Suprascapular notch
Scapula
Medial border
Subscapular fossa
Infraglenoid tubercle
Lateral border
Inferior angle
Deltoid tuberosity
Humerus
Lateral supraepicondylar ridge
Medial supraepicondylar ridge
Radial fossa
Coronoid fossa
Lateral epicondyle
Medial epicondyle
Capitulum
Trochlea
Head of radius
Coronoid process
Tuberosity of radius
Tuberosity of ulna
Radius
Ulna

B. Anterior View

Biceps brachii (short head) and coracobrachialis
Pectoralis minor
Supraspinatus
Subscapularis
Latissimus dorsi
Teres major
Pectoralis major
Triceps (long head)
Subscapularis
Serratus anterior
Deltoid
Coracobrachialis
Brachialis
Brachioradialis
Extensor carpi radialis longus
Pronator teres
Common flexor origin
Common extensor origin
Brachialis
Biceps brachii and bursa
Flexor digitorum superficialis
Pronator teres, ulnar head

C. Superior View

Supraspinatus in supraspinous fossa
Spine of scapula
Levator scapulae
Trapezius
Scapula
Acromion
Inferior belly of omohyoid
Long head of biceps brachii
Clavicle
Pectoralis minor
Deltoid
Coracobrachialis and short head of biceps brachii
Coracoid process
Pectoralis major
Sternocleidomastoid

2.38   **Bones of Proximal Upper Limb**

A. Bony features, anterior aspect. **B.** Muscle attachment sites, anterior aspect. **C.** Muscle attachment sites, clavicle and scapula.

Fractures of the clavicle are common, often caused by indirect force transmitted from an outstretched hand through the bones of the forearm and arm to the shoulder during a fall. A fracture may also result from a fall directly on the shoulder. The weakest part of the clavicle is at the junction of its middle and lateral thirds.

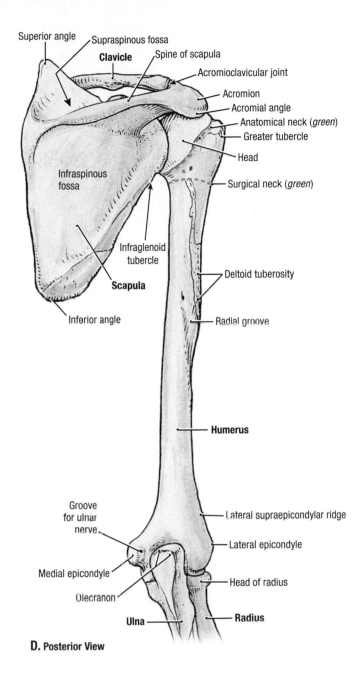

Superior angle
Supraspinous fossa
Clavicle
Spine of scapula
Acromioclavicular joint
Acromion
Acromial angle
Anatomical neck (*green*)
Greater tubercle
Head
Surgical neck (*green*)
Infraspinous fossa
Infraglenoid tubercle
Scapula
Inferior angle
Radial groove
Humerus
Groove for ulnar nerve
Lateral supraepicondylar ridge
Lateral epicondyle
Medial epicondyle
Olecranon
Head of radius
Ulna
Radius

D. Posterior View

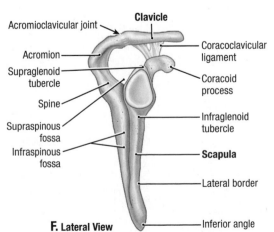

Acromioclavicular joint
Clavicle
Acromion
Coracoclavicular ligament
Supraglenoid tubercle
Coracoid process
Spine
Supraspinous fossa
Infraglenoid tubercle
Infraspinous fossa
Scapula
Lateral border
Inferior angle

F. Lateral View

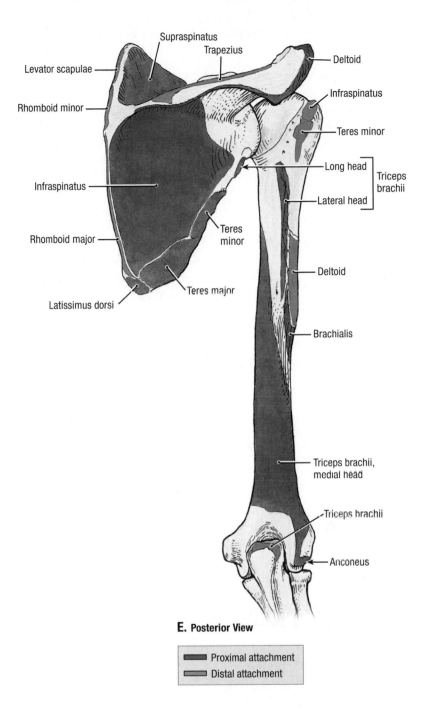

Supraspinatus
Trapezius
Levator scapulae
Deltoid
Rhomboid minor
Infraspinatus
Teres minor
Infraspinatus
Long head
Lateral head
Triceps brachii
Rhomboid major
Teres minor
Deltoid
Latissimus dorsi
Teres major
Brachialis
Triceps brachii, medial head
Triceps brachii
Anconeus

E. Posterior View

Proximal attachment
Distal attachment

Bones of Proximal Upper Limb (*continued*)   **2.38**

D. Bony features, posterior aspect. **E.** Muscle attachment sites, posterior aspect. **F.** Lateral aspect of scapula.

Fractures of the surgical neck of the humerus are especially common in elderly people with **osteoporosis** (degeneration of bone). Even a low energy fall on the hand, with the force being transmitted up the forearm bones of the extended limb, may result in a fracture. **Transverse fractures of the shaft of humerus** frequently result from a direct blow to the arm. Fracture of the distal part of the humerus, near the supraepicondylar ridges, is a **supraepicondylar (supracondylar) fracture**.

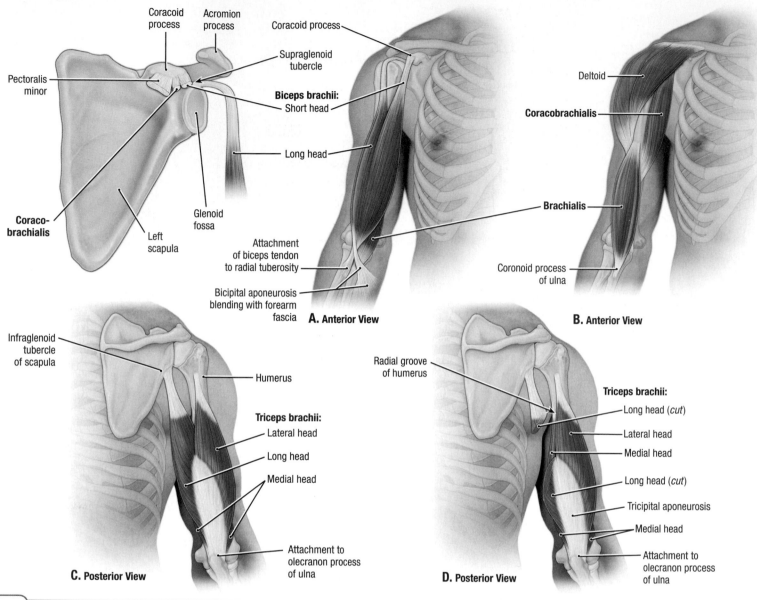

A. Anterior View

B. Anterior View

C. Posterior View

D. Posterior View

2.39 **Arm Muscles**

TABLE 2.9	Arm Muscles			
Muscle	**Proximal Attachment**	**Distal Attachment**	**Innervation**	**Main Actions**
Biceps brachii	*Short head:* tip of coracoid process of scapula *Long head:* supraglenoid tubercle of scapula and glenoid labrum	Tuberosity of radius and fascia of forearm through bicipital aponeurosis	Musculocutaneous nerve (C5, **C6**, and C7)	Supinates forearm and, when forearm is supine, flexes elbow joint; short head flexes shoulder joint; long head helps to stabilize shoulder joint during abduction.
Brachialis	Distal half of anterior surface of humerus	Coronoid process and tuberosity of ulna	Musculocutaneous nerve (C5–C7) and radial (C5–C7)	Flexes elbow joint in all positions
Coracobrachialis	Tip of coracoid process of scapula	Middle third of medial surface of humerus	Musculocutaneous nerve (C5, **C6**, and C7)	Assists with flexion and adduction of shoulder joint
Triceps brachii	*Long head:* infraglenoid tubercle of scapula *Lateral head:* posterior surface of humerus, superior to radial groove *Medial head:* posterior surface of humerus, inferior to radial groove	Proximal end of olecranon of ulna and fascia of forearm	Radial nerve (C6, **C7**, and **C8**)	Extends the elbow joint; long head steadies head of humerus when shoulder joint is abducted
Anconeus	Lateral epicondyle of humerus	Lateral surface of olecranon and superior part of posterior surface of ulna	Radial nerve (C7–T1)	Assists triceps in extending elbow joint; stabilizes elbow joint; abducts ulna during pronation

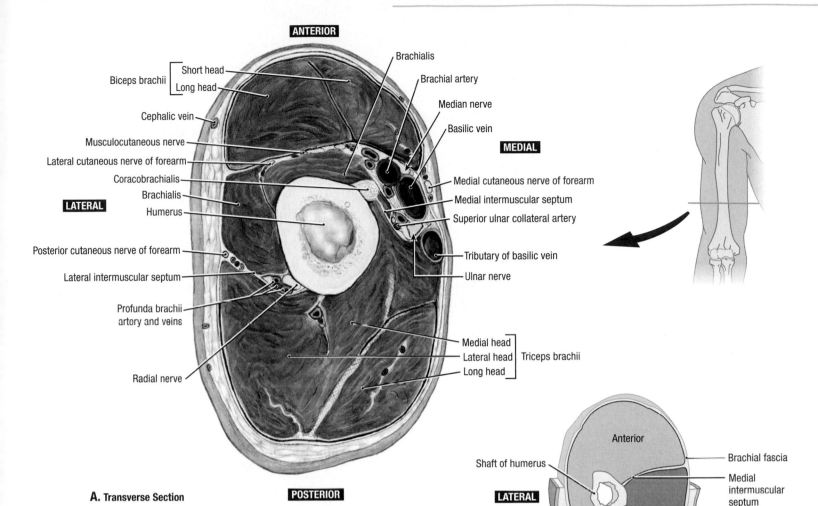

ANTERIOR

Biceps brachii — Short head
— Long head

Cephalic vein

Musculocutaneous nerve

Lateral cutaneous nerve of forearm

Coracobrachialis

Brachialis

Humerus

LATERAL

Posterior cutaneous nerve of forearm

Lateral intermuscular septum

Profunda brachii artery and veins

Radial nerve

Brachialis

Brachial artery

Median nerve

Basilic vein

MEDIAL

Medial cutaneous nerve of forearm

Medial intermuscular septum

Superior ulnar collateral artery

Tributary of basilic vein

Ulnar nerve

Medial head
Lateral head   Triceps brachii
Long head

A. Transverse Section

POSTERIOR

Shaft of humerus

Anterior

Brachial fascia

Medial intermuscular septum

LATERAL

Lateral intermuscular septum

Posterior

MEDIAL

Skin

C. Transverse Section

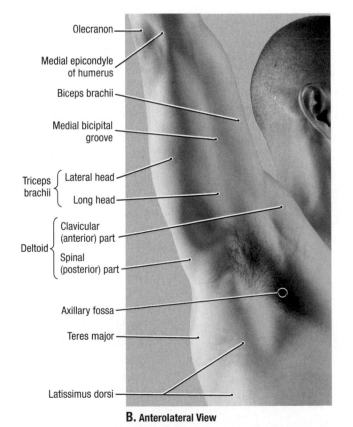

Olecranon

Medial epicondyle of humerus

Biceps brachii

Medial bicipital groove

Triceps brachii { Lateral head
Long head

Deltoid { Clavicular (anterior) part
Spinal (posterior) part

Axillary fossa

Teres major

Latissimus dorsi

B. Anterolateral View

Anterior and Posterior Compartments of Arm   2.40

A. Anatomical section. **B.** Surface anatomy. **C.** Compartments of arm.

- Three muscles, the biceps brachii, brachialis, and coracobrachialis, lie in the anterior compartment of the arm; the triceps brachii lies in the posterior compartment.
- The medial and lateral intermuscular septum separates these two muscle groups.
- The radial nerve and profunda brachii artery and veins serving the posterior compartment lie in contact with the radial groove of the humerus.
- The musculocutaneous nerve serving the anterior compartment lies in the plane between the biceps and the brachialis muscles.
- The median nerve crosses to the medial side of the brachial artery.
- The ulnar nerve passes posteriorly onto the medial side of the triceps muscle.

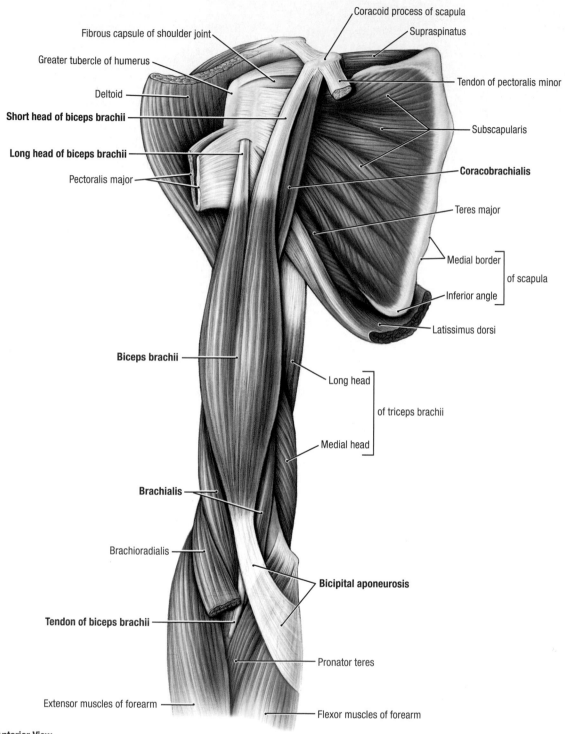

Coracoid process of scapula

Fibrous capsule of shoulder joint

Supraspinatus

Greater tubercle of humerus

Tendon of pectoralis minor

Deltoid

Short head of biceps brachii

Subscapularis

Long head of biceps brachii

Coracobrachialis

Pectoralis major

Teres major

Medial border

of scapula

Inferior angle

Latissimus dorsi

Biceps brachii

Long head

of triceps brachii

Medial head

Brachialis

Brachioradialis

Bicipital aponeurosis

Tendon of biceps brachii

Pronator teres

Extensor muscles of forearm

Flexor muscles of forearm

A. Anterior View

2.41 Muscles of Anterior Aspect of Arm (I)

- The biceps brachii has two heads: a long head and a short head.
- When the elbow joint is flexed approximately 90 degrees, the biceps is a flexor from the supinated position of the forearm but a very powerful supinator from the pronated position.

- A triangular membranous band, the bicipital aponeurosis, runs from the biceps tendon across the cubital fossa and merges with the antebrachial (deep) fascia covering the flexor muscles on the medial side of the forearm.

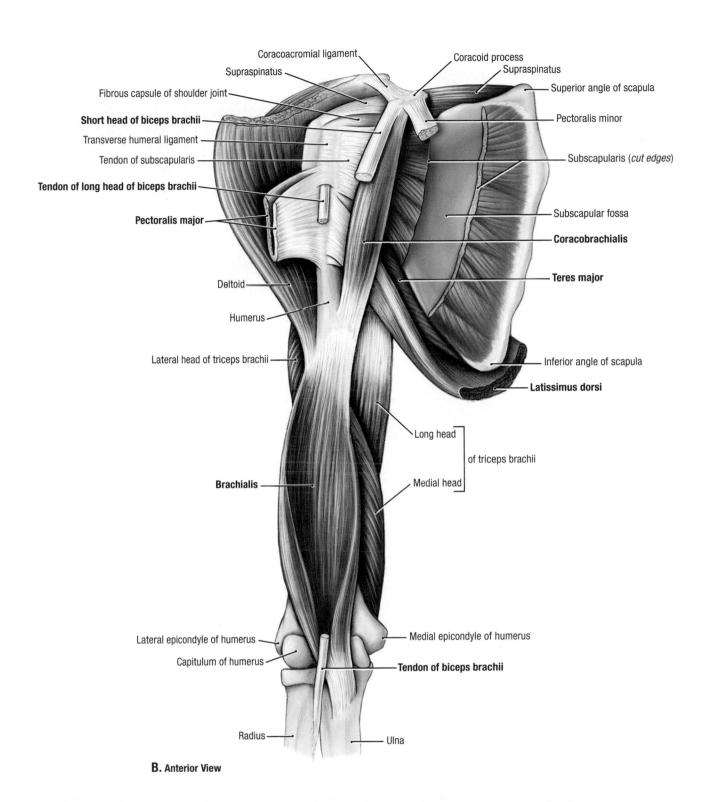

Coracoacromial ligament

Supraspinatus

Fibrous capsule of shoulder joint

Short head of biceps brachii

Transverse humeral ligament

Tendon of subscapularis

Tendon of long head of biceps brachii

Pectoralis major

Deltoid

Humerus

Lateral head of triceps brachii

Brachialis

Lateral epicondyle of humerus

Capitulum of humerus

Radius

Coracoid process
Supraspinatus

Superior angle of scapula

Pectoralis minor

Subscapularis (*cut edges*)

Subscapular fossa

Coracobrachialis

Teres major

Inferior angle of scapula

Latissimus dorsi

Long head
of triceps brachii
Medial head

Medial epicondyle of humerus

Tendon of biceps brachii

Ulna

B. Anterior View

Muscles of Anterior Aspect of Arm (II)　　　　　　　　　　　　　　　　　　　　　　　　**2.41**

- The brachialis, a flattened fusiform muscle, lies posterior (deep) to the biceps and produces the greatest amount of flexion force.
- The coracobrachialis, an elongated muscle in the superomedial part of the arm, is pierced by the musculocutaneous nerve. It helps flex and adduct the shoulder joint.

- **Rupture of the tendon of the long head of the biceps** usually results from wear and tear of an inflamed tendon (**biceps tendinitis**). Normally, the tendon is torn from its attachment to the supraglenoid tubercle of the scapula. The detached muscle belly forms a ball near the center of the distal part of the anterior aspect of the arm.

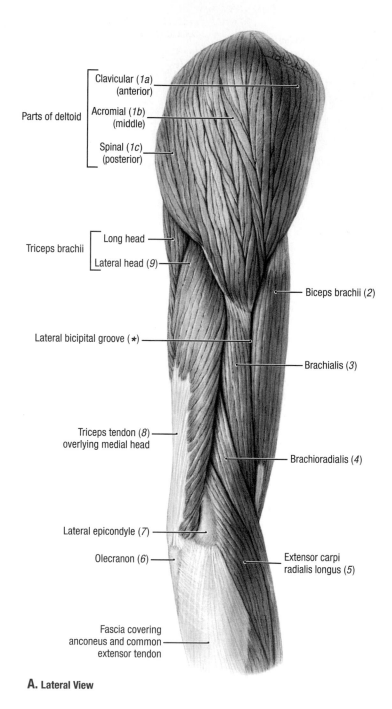

Parts of deltoid

Clavicular (*1a*)
(anterior)

Acromial (*1b*)
(middle)

Spinal (*1c*)
(posterior)

Triceps brachii

Long head

Lateral head (*9*)

Biceps brachii (*2*)

Lateral bicipital groove (✶)

Brachialis (*3*)

Triceps tendon (*8*)
overlying medial head

Brachioradialis (*4*)

Lateral epicondyle (*7*)

Olecranon (*6*)

Extensor carpi
radialis longus (*5*)

Fascia covering
anconeus and common
extensor tendon

A. Lateral View

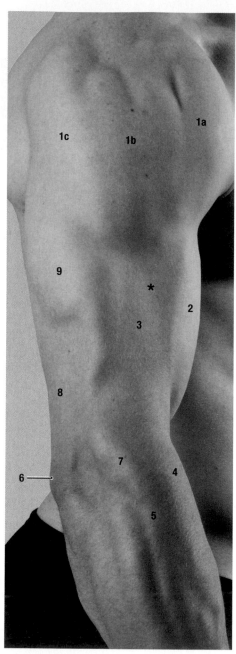

B. Lateral View

2.42   **Muscles of Lateral Aspect of Arm**

A. Dissection. Numbers in parentheses refer to structures in *Part B*.
B. Surface anatomy.

    Atrophy of the deltoid occurs when the axillary nerve (C5 and C6) is severely damaged (e.g., as might occur when the surgical neck of the humerus is fractured). As the deltoid atrophies, the rounded contour of the shoulder disappears. This gives the shoulder a flattened appearance and produces a slight hollow inferior to the acromion. A loss of sensation may occur over the lateral side of the proximal part of the arm, the area supplied by the superior lateral cutaneous nerve of the arm. To test the deltoid (or the function of the axillary nerve), the shoulder joint is abducted against resistance, starting from approximately 15 degrees. Supraspinatus initiates abduction at the shoulder joint.

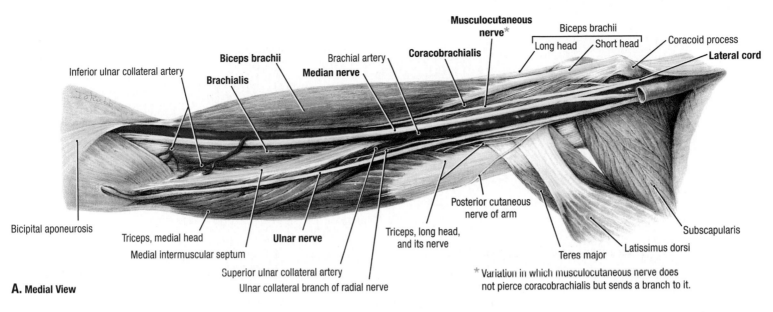

Musculocutaneous nerve*
Biceps brachii
Long head   Short head
Coracoid process
Lateral cord
Biceps brachii
Brachialis
Brachial artery
Median nerve
Coracobrachialis
Inferior ulnar collateral artery
Bicipital aponeurosis
Triceps, medial head
Medial intermuscular septum
Superior ulnar collateral artery
Ulnar collateral branch of radial nerve
Ulnar nerve
Triceps, long head, and its nerve
Posterior cutaneous nerve of arm
Teres major
Latissimus dorsi
Subscapularis

*Variation in which musculocutaneous nerve does not pierce coracobrachialis but sends a branch to it.

A. Medial View

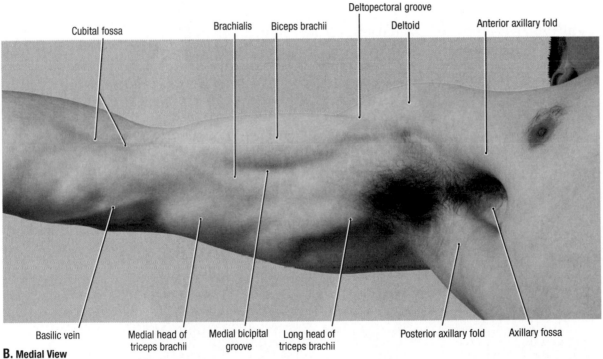

Cubital fossa
Brachialis
Biceps brachii
Deltopectoral groove
Deltoid
Anterior axillary fold
Basilic vein
Medial head of triceps brachii
Medial bicipital groove
Long head of triceps brachii
Posterior axillary fold
Axillary fossa

B. Medial View

Medial Aspect of Arm

2.43

A. Dissection. **B.** Surface anatomy.

- The axillary artery passes just inferior to the tip of the coracoid process and courses posterior to the coracobrachialis. At the inferior border of the teres major, the axillary artery changes names to become the brachial artery and continues distally on the anterior aspect of the brachialis.
- Although collateral pathways confer some protection against gradual temporary and partial occlusion, sudden complete **occlusion or laceration of the brachial artery** creates a surgical emergency because paralysis of muscles results from ischemia within a few hours.

- The median nerve lies adjacent to the axillary and brachial arteries and then crosses the artery from lateral to medial.
- Proximally, the ulnar nerve is adjacent to the medial side of the artery, passes posterior to the medial intermuscular septum, and descends on the medial head of triceps to pass posterior to the medial epicondyle; here, the ulnar nerve is palpable.
- The superior ulnar collateral artery and ulnar collateral branch of the radial nerve (to medial head of the triceps) accompany the ulnar nerve in the arm.

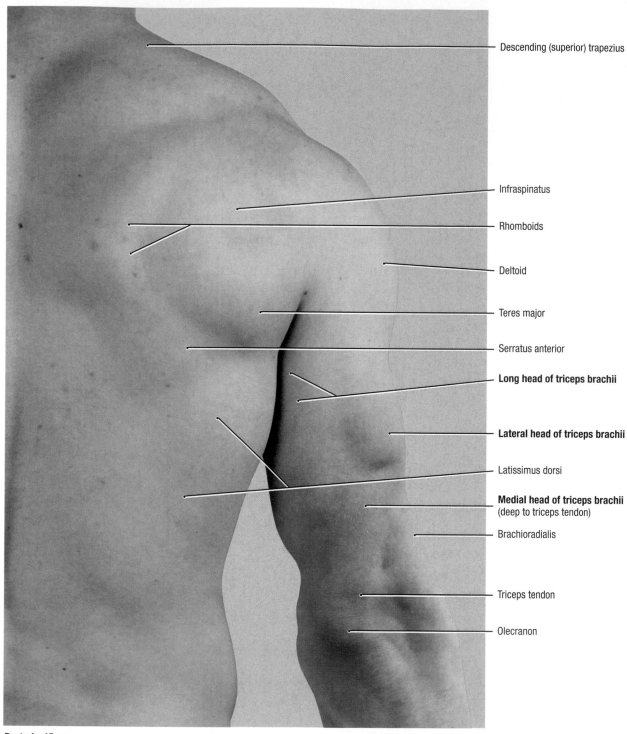

Descending (superior) trapezius

Infraspinatus

Rhomboids

Deltoid

Teres major

Serratus anterior

Long head of triceps brachii

Lateral head of triceps brachii

Latissimus dorsi

Medial head of triceps brachii
(deep to triceps tendon)

Brachioradialis

Triceps tendon

Olecranon

Posterior View

2.44 **Surface Anatomy of Scapular Region and Posterior Aspect of Arm**

The three heads of the triceps brachii form a bulge on the posterior aspect of the arm and are identifiable in a lean individual when the elbow joint is extended from the flexed position against resistance.

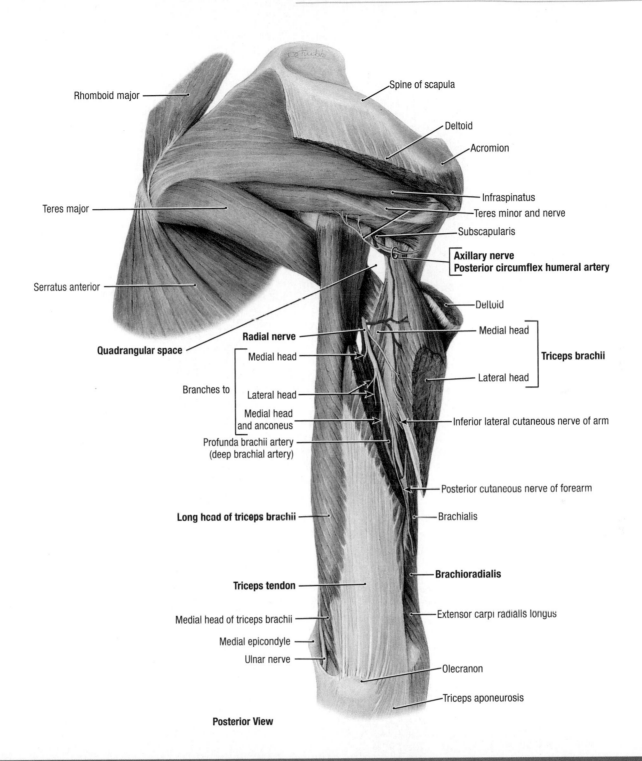

Rhomboid major

Teres major

Serratus anterior

Quadrangular space

Spine of scapula

Deltoid

Acromion

Infraspinatus

Teres minor and nerve

Subscapularis

Axillary nerve
Posterior circumflex humeral artery

Deltoid

Radial nerve

Medial head

Triceps brachii

Lateral head

Branches to

Medial head

Lateral head

Medial head
and anconeus

Profunda brachii artery
(deep brachial artery)

Inferior lateral cutaneous nerve of arm

Long head of triceps brachii

Posterior cutaneous nerve of forearm

Brachialis

Brachioradialis

Triceps tendon

Medial head of triceps brachii

Extensor carpi radialis longus

Medial epicondyle

Ulnar nerve

Olecranon

Triceps aponeurosis

Posterior View

Triceps Brachii and Related Nerves

2.45

- The lateral head is reflected laterally, and the medial head is attached to the deep surface of the triceps tendon, which attaches to the olecranon.
- The radial nerve and profunda brachii artery pass between the proximal attachments of the lateral and medial heads of the triceps brachii in the middle third of the arm, directly contacting the radial groove of the humerus.
- **Midarm fracture.** The middle third of the arm is a common site for fractures of the humerus, often with associated **radial nerve trauma**. When the radial nerve is injured in the radial groove,

the triceps brachii muscle typically is only weakened because only the medial head is affected. However, the muscles in the posterior compartment of the forearm, supplied by more distal branches of the radial nerve, are paralyzed. The characteristic clinical sign of radial nerve injury is **wrist drop** (inability to extend the wrist joint and fingers at the metacarpophalangeal joints).
- The axillary nerve passes through the quadrangular space along with the posterior circumflex humeral artery.
- The ulnar nerve follows the medial border of the triceps then passes posterior to the medial epicondyle.

Suprascapular artery

Suprascapular nerve

Supraspinatus

Infraspinatus
(*cut end reflected*)

Fibrous capsule of glenohumeral
(shoulder) joint

Teres minor

Acromial (central) — Parts of deltoid
Spinal (posterior) — (*cut and reflected*)

Infraspinatus
(*cut*)

Axillary nerve

**Posterior circumflex
humeral artery**

Teres major

Superior lateral cutaneous nerve of arm

Radial nerve

Profunda brachii artery (deep artery of arm)

Triangular interval

Triangular space

Lateral head of triceps brachii

Circumflex scapular artery

Quadrangular space

**Long head of
triceps brachii**

Tendon overlying medial
head of triceps brachii

Posterior View

2.46 **Dorsal Scapular and Subdeltoid Regions**

- The infraspinatus muscle, aided by the teres minor and spinal (posterior) part of the deltoid muscle, rotates the shoulder joint laterally.
- The long head of the triceps muscle passes between the teres minor and teres major and separates the quadrangular space from the triangular interval.
- Regarding the distribution of the suprascapular and axillary nerves, each comes from C5 and C6; each supplies two muscles—the suprascapular nerve innervates the supraspinatus

and infraspinatus, and the axillary nerve innervates the teres minor and deltoid muscles. Both nerves supply the shoulder joint, but only the axillary nerve has a cutaneous branch.

- **Axillary nerve injury** may occur when the glenohumeral (shoulder) joint dislocates because of its close relation to the inferior part of the joint capsule. Subglenoid displacement of the head of the humerus into the quadrangular space may damage the axillary nerve. Axillary nerve injury is indicated by paralysis of the deltoid and sensory loss over the lateral side of the proximal part of the arm.

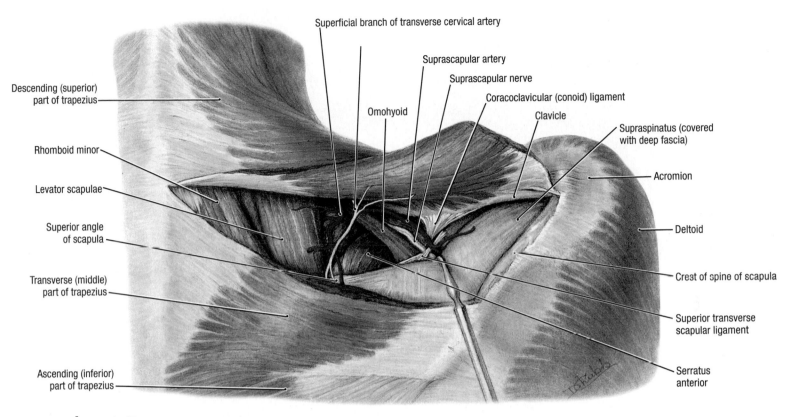

A. Posterior View

Labels (clockwise from top):
Superficial branch of transverse cervical artery
Suprascapular artery
Suprascapular nerve
Coracoclavicular (conoid) ligament
Clavicle
Supraspinatus (covered with deep fascia)
Acromion
Deltoid
Crest of spine of scapula
Superior transverse scapular ligament
Serratus anterior
Ascending (inferior) part of trapezius
Transverse (middle) part of trapezius
Superior angle of scapula
Levator scapulae
Rhomboid minor
Descending (superior) part of trapezius
Omohyoid

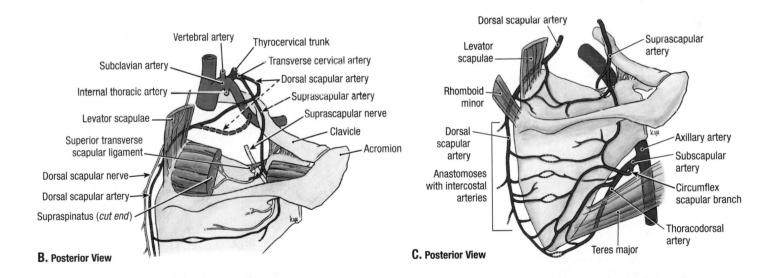

B. Posterior View

Labels:
Vertebral artery
Thyrocervical trunk
Subclavian artery
Transverse cervical artery
Internal thoracic artery
Dorsal scapular artery
Levator scapulae
Suprascapular artery
Suprascapular nerve
Superior transverse scapular ligament
Clavicle
Acromion
Dorsal scapular nerve
Dorsal scapular artery
Supraspinatus (*cut end*)

C. Posterior View

Labels:
Dorsal scapular artery
Levator scapulae
Suprascapular artery
Rhomboid minor
Dorsal scapular artery
Axillary artery
Subscapular artery
Anastomoses with intercostal arteries
Circumflex scapular branch
Thoracodorsal artery
Teres major

Suprascapular Region

2.47

A. Dissection. At the level of the superior angle of the scapula, the transverse part of the trapezius muscle is reflected. **B. Suprascapular and dorsal scapular arteries. C. Scapular anastomosis.**

Several arteries join to form anastomoses on the anterior and posterior surfaces of the scapula. The importance of the collateral circulation made possible by these anastomoses becomes apparent when **ligation of a lacerated subclavian or axillary artery** is necessary or there is occlusion of these vessels. The direction of blood flow in the subscapular artery is then reversed, enabling blood to reach the third part of the axillary artery. In contrast to a sudden occlusion, slow occlusion of an artery often enables sufficient lateral circulation to develop, preventing **ischemia** (deficiency of blood).

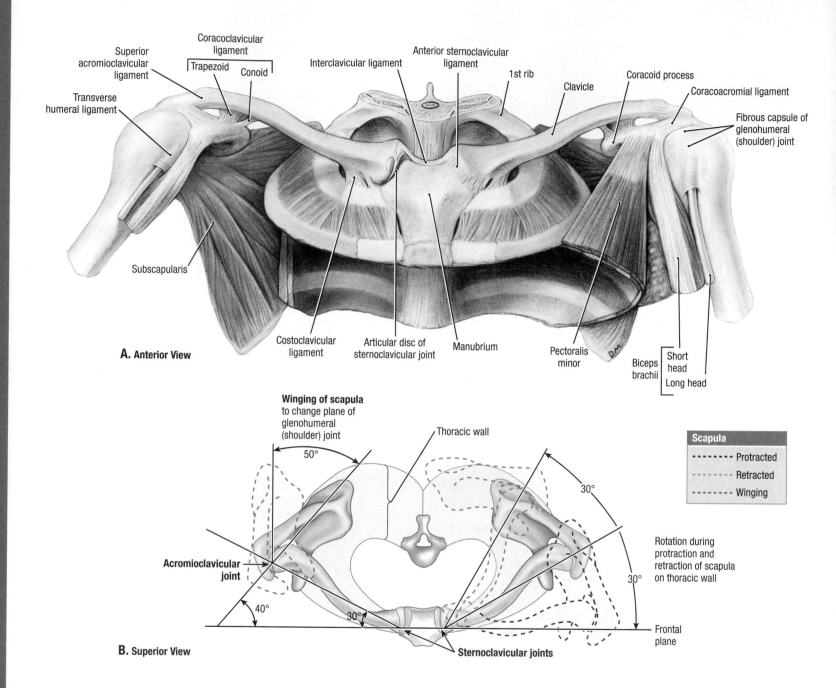

Superior acromioclavicular ligament

Coracoclavicular ligament
[Trapezoid   Conoid]

Transverse humeral ligament

Interclavicular ligament

Anterior sternoclavicular ligament

1st rib

Clavicle

Coracoid process

Coracoacromial ligament

Fibrous capsule of glenohumeral (shoulder) joint

Subscapularis

Costoclavicular ligament

Articular disc of sternoclavicular joint

Manubrium

Pectoralis minor

Biceps brachii
[Short head   Long head]

A. Anterior View

Winging of scapula to change plane of glenohumeral (shoulder) joint

Thoracic wall

50°

30°

Scapula
- - - - - Protracted
- - - - - Retracted
- - - - - Winging

Acromioclavicular joint

Rotation during protraction and retraction of scapula on thoracic wall

30°

30°

40°

Frontal plane

Sternoclavicular joints

B. Superior View

| 2.48 | **Pectoral Girdle** |

A. Ligaments of pectoral girdle. B. Clavicular and scapular movements at sternoclavicular and acromioclavicular joints. Movements demonstrated include rotation, protraction, and retraction of the scapula on the thoracic wall and winging of the scapula. Elevation and depression also involve these joints.

- The shoulder region includes the sternoclavicular, acromioclavicular, and shoulder (glenohumeral) joints; the mobility of the clavicle is essential to the movement of the upper limb.
- The sternoclavicular joint is the only joint connecting the upper limb (appendicular skeleton) to the trunk (axial skeleton).

- The articular disc of the sternoclavicular joint divides the joint cavity into two parts and attaches superiorly to the clavicle and inferiorly to the first costal cartilage; the disc resists superior and medial displacement of the clavicle.

Paralysis of serratus anterior. Note that when the serratus anterior is paralyzed because of injury to the long thoracic nerve (*Part B*), the medial border of the scapula moves laterally and posteriorly away from the thoracic wall, giving the scapula the appearance of a wing (**winged scapula**). (See Clinical Comment for Fig. 2.32.)

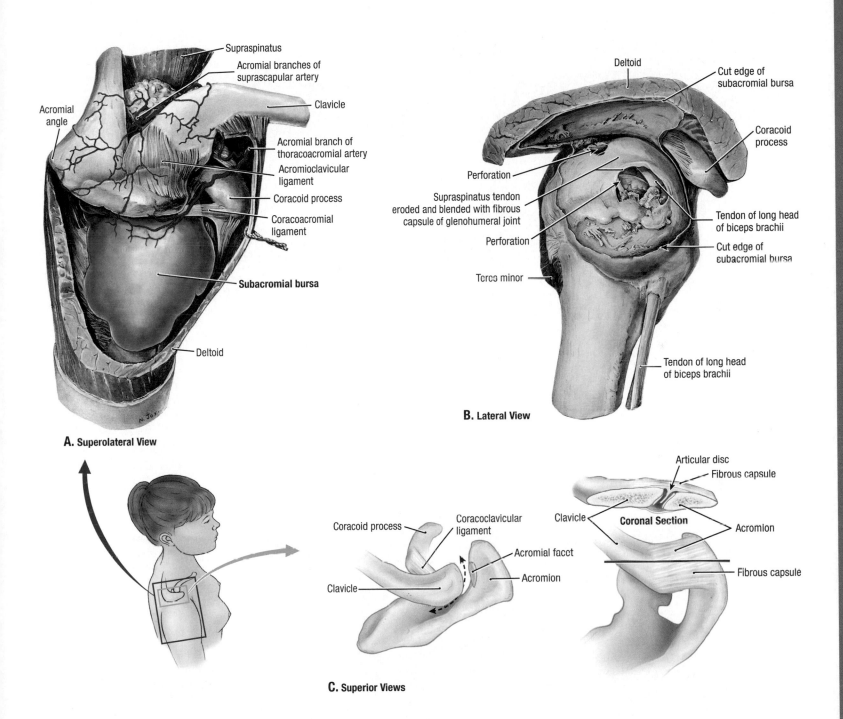

Supraspinatus

Acromial branches of
suprascapular artery

Acromial
angle

Clavicle

Acromial branch of
thoracoacromial artery

Acromioclavicular
ligament

Coracoid process

Coracoacromial
ligament

Subacromial bursa

Deltoid

A. **Superolateral View**

Deltoid

Cut edge of
subacromial bursa

Coracoid
process

Perforation

Supraspinatus tendon
eroded and blended with fibrous
capsule of glenohumeral joint

Perforation

Tendon of long head
of biceps brachii

Cut edge of
subacromial bursa

Teres minor

Tendon of long head
of biceps brachii

B. **Lateral View**

Coracoid process

Coracoclavicular
ligament

Acromial facet

Acromion

Clavicle

Articular disc

Fibrous capsule

Clavicle

Coronal Section

Acromion

Fibrous capsule

C. **Superior Views**

Subacromial Bursa and Acromioclavicular Joint

2.49

A. Subacromial bursa. The bursa has been injected with
purple latex. **B. Attrition of supraspinatus tendon.** As a result
of wearing away of the supraspinatus tendon and underlying
capsule, the subacromial bursa and shoulder joint come into
communication. The intracapsular part of the tendon of the long
head of biceps muscle becomes frayed, leaving it adherent to
the intertubercular groove. Of 95 dissecting room subjects in
Dr. Grant's lab, none of the 18 younger than 50 years of age had
a perforation, but 4 of the 19 who were 50 to 60 years and 23 of
the 57 older than 60 years had perforations. The perforation was
bilateral in 11 subjects and unilateral in 14. **C. Acromioclavicular
joint.**

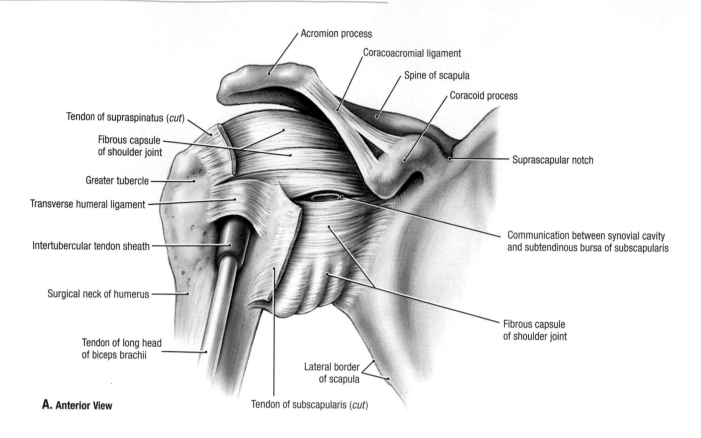

Acromion process

Coracoacromial ligament

Spine of scapula

Coracoid process

Tendon of supraspinatus (*cut*)

Fibrous capsule
of shoulder joint

Greater tubercle

Transverse humeral ligament

Intertubercular tendon sheath

Surgical neck of humerus

Tendon of long head
of biceps brachii

Suprascapular notch

Communication between synovial cavity
and subtendinous bursa of subscapularis

Fibrous capsule
of shoulder joint

Lateral border
of scapula

A. Anterior View

Tendon of subscapularis (*cut*)

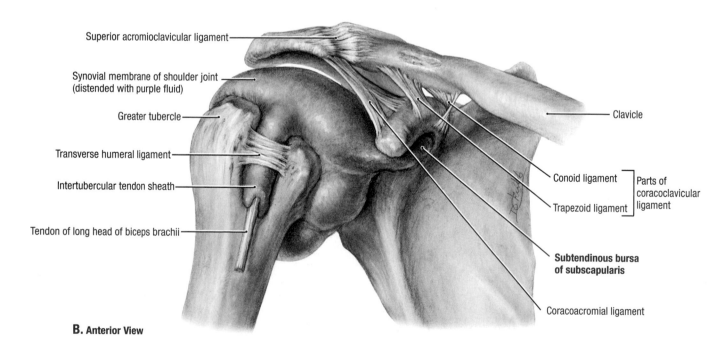

Superior acromioclavicular ligament

Synovial membrane of shoulder joint
(distended with purple fluid)

Greater tubercle

Transverse humeral ligament

Intertubercular tendon sheath

Tendon of long head of biceps brachii

Clavicle

Conoid ligament

Trapezoid ligament

Parts of
coracoclavicular
ligament

**Subtendinous bursa
of subscapularis**

Coracoacromial ligament

B. Anterior View

2.50 **Ligaments and Articular Capsule of Glenohumeral (Shoulder) Joint**

A. Fibrous capsule.
- The loose fibrous capsule is attached to the margin of the glenoid cavity and to the anatomical neck of the humerus.
- The strong coracoclavicular ligament provides stability to the acromioclavicular joint and prevents the scapula from being

driven medially and the acromion from being driven inferior to the clavicle.
- The coracoacromial ligament prevents superior displacement of the head of the humerus.

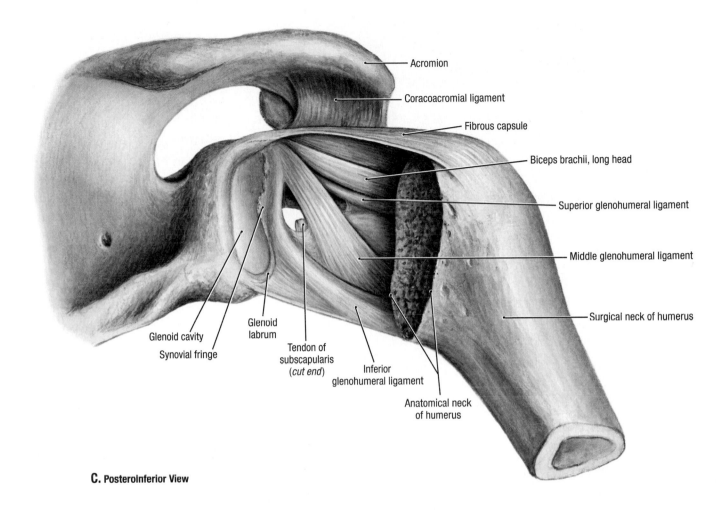

Acromion

Coracoacromial ligament

Fibrous capsule

Biceps brachii, long head

Superior glenohumeral ligament

Middle glenohumeral ligament

Surgical neck of humerus

Glenoid cavity

Synovial fringe

Glenoid labrum

Tendon of subscapularis (*cut end*)

Inferior glenohumeral ligament

Anatomical neck of humerus

C. Posteroinferior View

Ligaments and Articular Capsule of Glenohumeral (Shoulder) Joint *(continued)*   2.50

B. Synovial membrane of joint capsule. The synovial membrane lines the fibrous capsule and has two prolongations: (1) where it forms a synovial sheath for the tendon of the long head of the biceps muscle in its osseofibrous tunnel and (2) inferior to the coracoid process, where it forms a bursa between the subscapularis tendon and margin of the glenoid cavity—the subtendinous bursa of the subscapularis. **C. Glenohumeral ligaments viewed from interior of shoulder joint.**

- The joint is exposed from the posterior aspect by cutting away the thinner posteroinferior part of the capsule and sawing off the head of the humerus.
- The glenohumeral ligaments are visible from within the joint but are not easily seen externally.
- The glenohumeral ligaments and tendon of the long head of biceps brachii muscle converge on the supraglenoid tubercle.

- The slender superior glenohumeral ligament lies parallel to the tendon of the long head of biceps brachii. The middle ligament is free medially because the subtendinous bursa of subscapularis communicates with the joint cavity; usually, there is only a single site of communication. In this individual, there are openings on both sides of the ligament.

Because of its freedom of movement and instability, the glenohumeral joint is commonly dislocated by direct or indirect injury. Most **dislocations of the humeral head** occur in the downward (inferior) direction but are described clinically as anterior or (more rarely) posterior dislocations, indicating whether the humeral head has descended anterior or posterior to the infraglenoid tubercle and the long head of triceps. Anterior dislocation of the glenohumeral joint occurs most often in young adults, particularly athletes. It is usually caused by excessive extension and lateral rotation of the humerus.

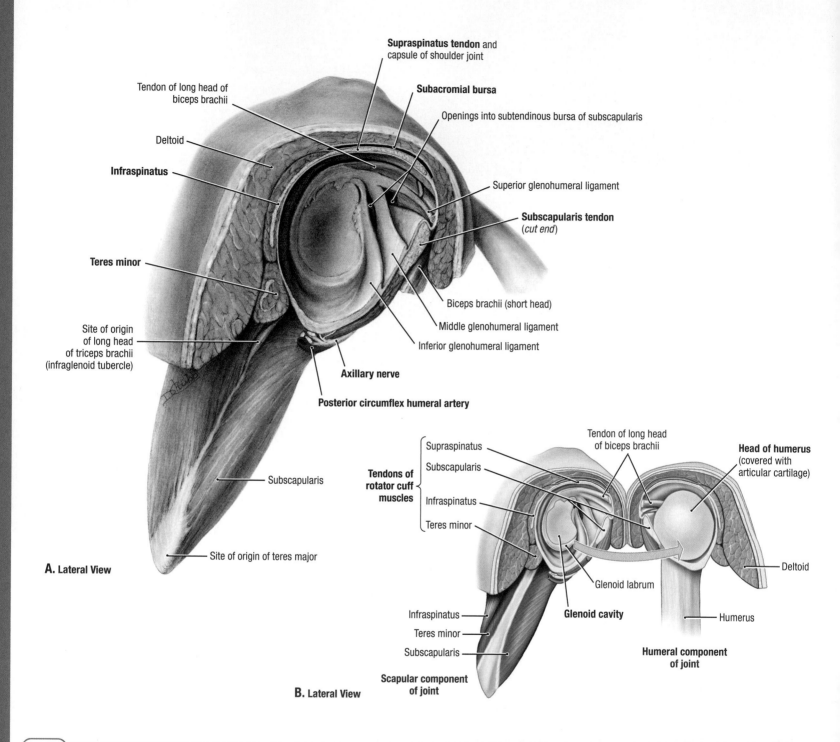

Tendon of long head of biceps brachii

Deltoid

Infraspinatus

Teres minor

Site of origin
of long head
of triceps brachii
(infraglenoid tubercle)

Supraspinatus tendon and
capsule of shoulder joint

Subacromial bursa

Openings into subtendinous bursa of subscapularis

Superior glenohumeral ligament

Subscapularis tendon
(*cut end*)

Biceps brachii (short head)

Middle glenohumeral ligament

Inferior glenohumeral ligament

Axillary nerve

Posterior circumflex humeral artery

Subscapularis

Site of origin of teres major

A. Lateral View

**Tendons of
rotator cuff
muscles**

Supraspinatus

Subscapularis

Infraspinatus

Teres minor

Tendon of long head
of biceps brachii

Head of humerus
(covered with
articular cartilage)

Deltoid

Glenoid labrum

Glenoid cavity

Humerus

Infraspinatus

Teres minor

Subscapularis

**Scapular component
of joint**

**Humeral component
of joint**

B. Lateral View

2.51 | **Interior of Glenohumeral (Shoulder) Joint and Relationship of Rotator Cuff**

A. Scapular component of joint and cuff. **B.** Overview of joint and cuff.

- The subacromial bursa is between the acromion and deltoid superiorly and the tendon of supraspinatus inferiorly.
- The four short rotator cuff muscles (supraspinatus, infraspinatus, teres minor, and subscapularis) cross the glenohumeral joint and blend with the capsule.
- The axillary nerve and posterior circumflex humeral artery are in contact with the capsule inferiorly and may be injured when the glenohumeral joint dislocates.

- Inflammation and calcification of the subacromial bursa result in pain, tenderness, and limitation of movement of the glenohumeral joint. This condition is also known as **calcific scapulohumeral bursitis**. Deposition of calcium in the supraspinatus tendon may irritate the overlying subacromial bursa, producing an inflammatory reaction, **subacromial bursitis**.

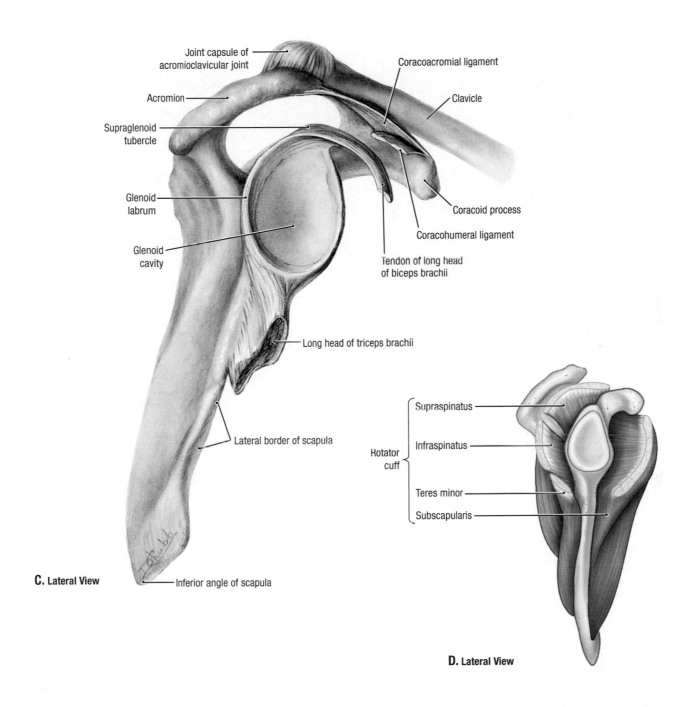

Joint capsule of acromioclavicular joint

Coracoacromial ligament

Acromion

Clavicle

Supraglenoid tubercle

Glenoid labrum

Coracoid process

Glenoid cavity

Coracohumeral ligament

Tendon of long head of biceps brachii

Long head of triceps brachii

Lateral border of scapula

Supraspinatus

Infraspinatus

Rotator cuff

Teres minor

Subscapularis

C. Lateral View

Inferior angle of scapula

D. Lateral View

Interior of Glenohumeral (Shoulder) Joint and Relationship of Rotator Cuff (continued)   2.51

C. Scapular elements. **D.** Muscles of rotator cuff and their relationship to glenoid cavity.

- The coracoacromial arch (coracoid process, coracoacromial ligament, and acromion) prevents superior displacement of the head of the humerus.
- The long head of the triceps brachii muscle arises just inferior to the glenoid cavity; the long head of biceps just superior to it.
- The main function of the musculotendinous rotator cuff is to hold the large head of the humerus in the smaller and shallow glenoid cavity of the scapula, both during the relaxed state (by tonic contraction) and during active abduction.

Tearing of the fibrocartilaginous glenoid labrum commonly occurs in the athletes who throw (e.g., a baseball) and in those who have shoulder instability and subluxation (partial dislocation) of the glenohumeral joint. The tear often results from sudden contraction of the biceps or forceful subluxation of the humeral head over the glenoid labrum. Usually, a tear occurs in the anterosuperior part of the labrum.

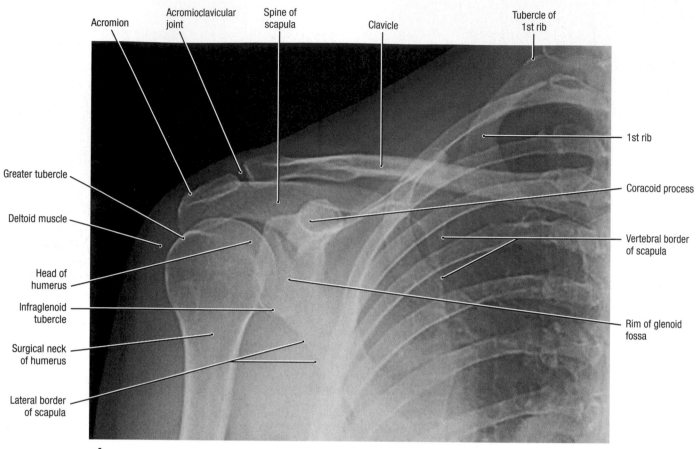

Acromion

Acromioclavicular joint

Spine of scapula

Clavicle

Tubercle of 1st rib

Greater tubercle

Deltoid muscle

Head of humerus

Infraglenoid tubercle

Surgical neck of humerus

Lateral border of scapula

1st rib

Coracoid process

Vertebral border of scapula

Rim of glenoid fossa

A. Anteroposterior Radiograph

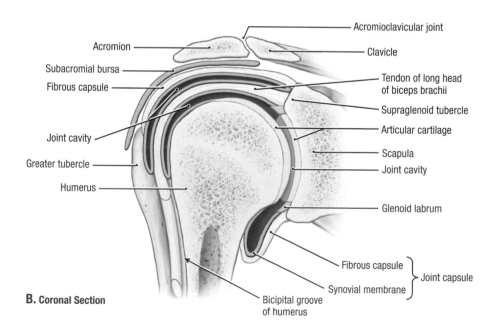

Acromion

Subacromial bursa

Fibrous capsule

Joint cavity

Greater tubercle

Humerus

Acromioclavicular joint

Clavicle

Tendon of long head of biceps brachii

Supraglenoid tubercle

Articular cartilage

Scapula

Joint cavity

Glenoid labrum

Fibrous capsule

Synovial membrane

} Joint capsule

Bicipital groove of humerus

B. Coronal Section

2.52 **Imaging of Glenohumeral (Shoulder) Joint**

A. Radiographic shoulder study. **B.** Anatomical section of joint to show location of subacromial bursa and joint cavity.

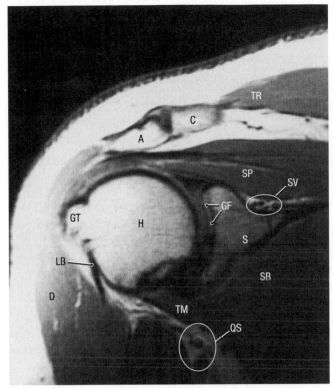

C. Coronal MRI

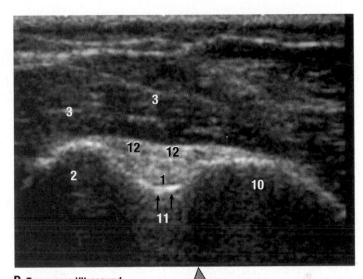

D. Transverse Ultrasound

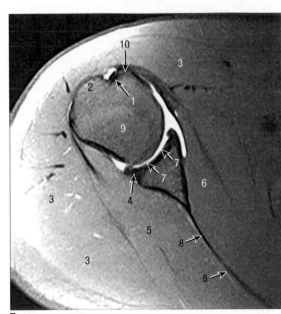

E. Transverse MRI

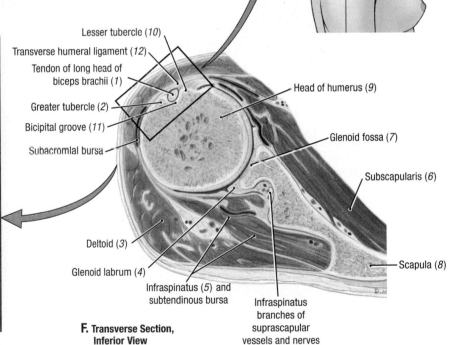

Lesser tubercle (*10*)
Transverse humeral ligament (*12*)
Tendon of long head of biceps brachii (*1*)
Greater tubercle (*2*)
Bicipital groove (*11*)
Subacromial bursa
Deltoid (*3*)
Glenoid labrum (*4*)
Infraspinatus (*5*) and subtendinous bursa
Head of humerus (*9*)
Glenoid fossa (*7*)
Subscapularis (*6*)
Scapula (*8*)
Infraspinatus branches of suprascapular vessels and nerves

F. Transverse Section, Inferior View

Imaging of Glenohumeral (Shoulder) Joint (*continued*)

2.52

C. MRI study including both shoulder and acromioclavicular joints. *A*, acromion; *C*, clavicle; *D*, deltoid; *GF*, glenoid cavity; *GT*, crest of greater tubercle; *H*, head of humerus; *LB*, long head of biceps brachii; *QS*, quadrangular space; *S*, scapula; *SB*, subscapularis; *SP*, supraspinatus; *SV*, suprascapular vessels and nerve; *TM*, teres minor; *TR*, trapezius. **D. Ultrasound scan of tendon of long head of biceps** (area indicated in *Part F*). **E. MRI with contrast agent in synovial cavity. F. Anatomical section.** Numbers in *Part F* refer to structures labeled in *Part D* and *Part E*.

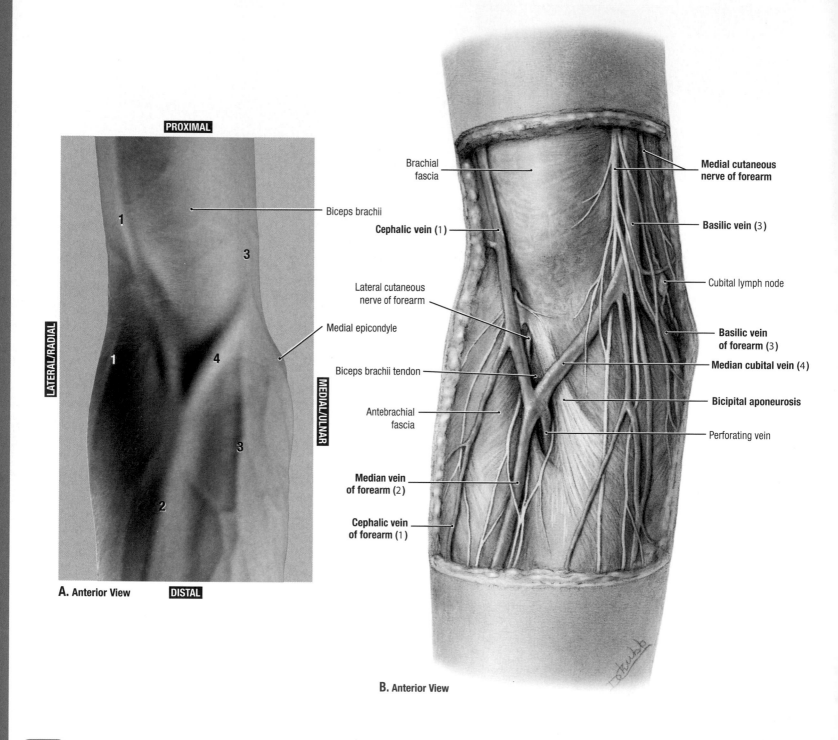

PROXIMAL

LATERAL/RADIAL

1

3

1   4

3

2

MEDIAL/ULNAR

A. Anterior View   DISTAL

Biceps brachii

Medial epicondyle

Brachial fascia

Medial cutaneous nerve of forearm

Cephalic vein (1)

Basilic vein (3)

Cubital lymph node

Lateral cutaneous nerve of forearm

Biceps brachii tendon

Antebrachial fascia

Median vein of forearm (2)

Cephalic vein of forearm (1)

Basilic vein of forearm (3)

Median cubital vein (4)

Bicipital aponeurosis

Perforating vein

B. Anterior View

2.53   **Cubital Fossa: Surface Anatomy and Superficial Dissection**

A. Surface anatomy. B. Cutaneous nerves and superficial veins. Numbers in parentheses refer to structures in *Part A*.

- The cubital fossa is a triangular space (compartment) inferior to the elbow crease, roofed by deep fascia.
- In the forearm, the superficial veins (cephalic, median, basilic, and their connecting veins) make a variable, M-shaped pattern.
- The cephalic and basilic veins occupy the bicipital grooves, one on each side of the biceps brachii. In the lateral bicipital groove,

the lateral cutaneous nerve of the forearm appears just superior to the elbow crease; in the medial bicipital groove, the medial cutaneous nerve of the forearm becomes cutaneous at approximately the midpoint of the arm.

- The cubital fossa is the common site for **sampling and transfusion of blood and intravenous injections** because of the prominence and accessibility of veins. Usually, the median cubital vein or basilic vein is selected.

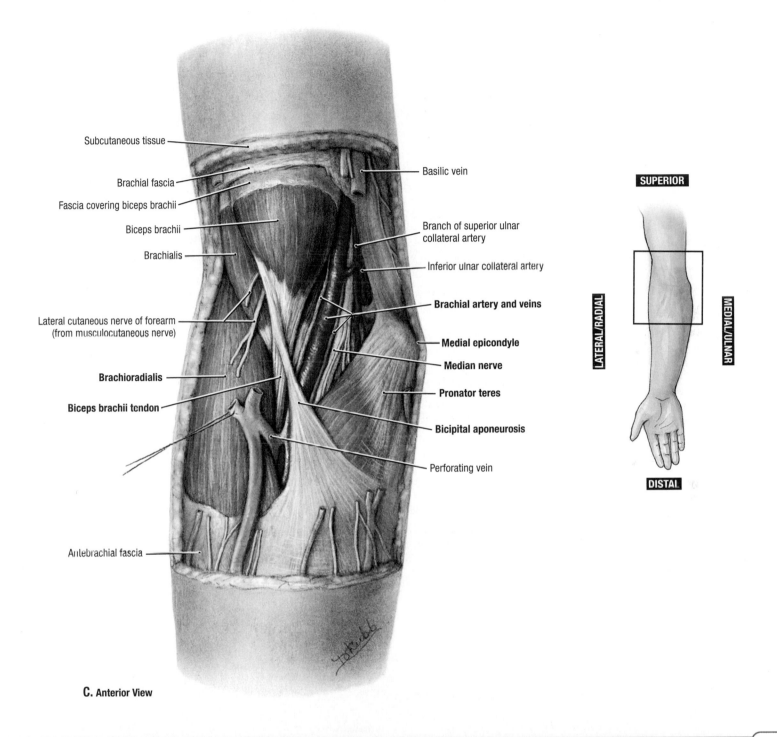

Subcutaneous tissue

Brachial fascia

Fascia covering biceps brachii

Biceps brachii

Brachialis

Lateral cutaneous nerve of forearm
(from musculocutaneous nerve)

Brachioradialis

Biceps brachii tendon

Antebrachial fascia

Basilic vein

Branch of superior ulnar
collateral artery

Inferior ulnar collateral artery

Brachial artery and veins

Medial epicondyle

Median nerve

Pronator teres

Bicipital aponeurosis

Perforating vein

SUPERIOR

LATERAL/RADIAL

MEDIAL/ULNAR

DISTAL

C. Anterior View

Cubital Fossa: Deep Dissection (I)

2.53

C. Bounding structures and contents of cubital fossa.
- The cubital fossa is bound laterally by the brachioradialis, medially by the pronator teres, and superiorly by a line joining the medial and lateral epicondyles.
- The three chief contents of the cubital fossa are the biceps brachii tendon, brachial artery, and median nerve.
- The biceps brachii tendon, on approaching its insertion, rotates through 90 degrees, and the bicipital aponeurosis extends medially from the proximal part of the tendon.

- A fracture of the distal part of the humerus, near the supraepicondylar ridges, is called a **supraepicondylar (supracondylar) fracture.** The distal bone fragment may be displaced anteriorly or posteriorly. Any of the nerves or branches of the brachial vessels related to the humerus may be injured by a displaced bone fragment.

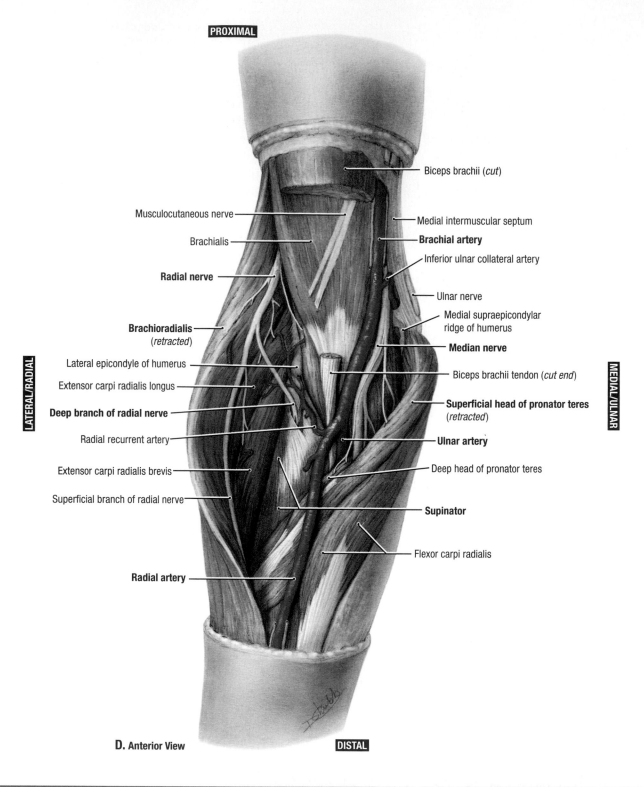

PROXIMAL

Biceps brachii (*cut*)

Musculocutaneous nerve

Brachialis

Medial intermuscular septum

Brachial artery

Inferior ulnar collateral artery

Radial nerve

Ulnar nerve

Medial supraepicondylar ridge of humerus

Brachioradialis
(*retracted*)

Median nerve

Lateral epicondyle of humerus

Extensor carpi radialis longus

Biceps brachii tendon (*cut end*)

Superficial head of pronator teres
(*retracted*)

Deep branch of radial nerve

Radial recurrent artery

Ulnar artery

Extensor carpi radialis brevis

Deep head of pronator teres

Superficial branch of radial nerve

Supinator

Flexor carpi radialis

Radial artery

LATERAL/RADIAL

MEDIAL/ULNAR

D. Anterior View

DISTAL

2.53 **Cubital Fossa: Deep Dissection (II)**

D. Floor of cubital fossa.
- Part of the biceps brachii muscle is excised, and the cubital fossa is opened widely, exposing the brachialis and supinator muscles in the floor of the fossa.
- The deep branch of the radial nerve pierces the supinator.
- The brachial artery lies between the biceps tendon and median nerve and divides into two branches, the ulnar and radial arteries.

- The median nerve supplies the flexor muscles. With the exception of the twig to the deep head of pronator teres, its motor branches arise from its medial side.
- The radial nerve supplies the extensor muscles. With the exception of the twig to brachioradialis, its motor branches arise from its lateral side. In this specimen, the radial nerve has been displaced laterally, so here, its lateral branches appear to run medially.

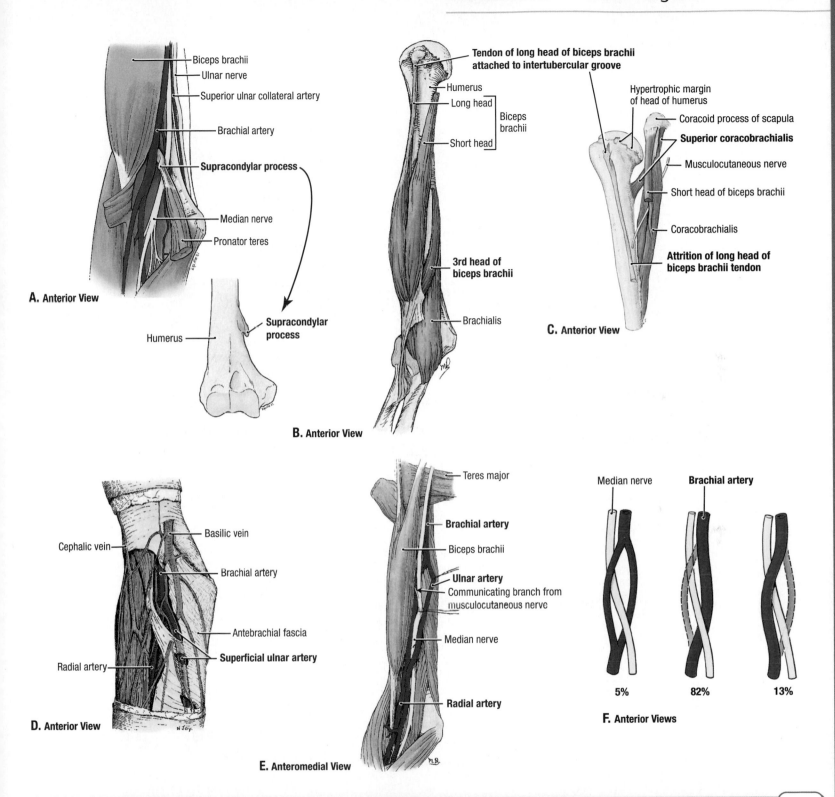

A. Anterior View
- Biceps brachii
- Ulnar nerve
- Superior ulnar collateral artery
- Brachial artery
- **Supracondylar process**
- Median nerve
- Pronator teres
- Humerus
- **Supracondylar process**

B. Anterior View
- Tendon of long head of biceps brachii attached to intertubercular groove
- Humerus
- Long head
- Short head
- Biceps brachii
- **3rd head of biceps brachii**
- Brachialis

C. Anterior View
- Hypertrophic margin of head of humerus
- Coracoid process of scapula
- **Superior coracobrachialis**
- Musculocutaneous nerve
- Short head of biceps brachii
- Coracobrachialis
- **Attrition of long head of biceps brachii tendon**

D. Anterior View
- Cephalic vein
- Basilic vein
- Brachial artery
- Antebrachial fascia
- **Superficial ulnar artery**
- Radial artery

E. Anteromedial View
- Teres major
- **Brachial artery**
- Biceps brachii
- **Ulnar artery**
- Communicating branch from musculocutaneous nerve
- Median nerve
- **Radial artery**

F. Anterior Views
- Median nerve
- **Brachial artery**
- 5%
- 82%
- 13%

Anomalies

2.54

A. Supracondylar process of humerus. A fibrous band, from which the pronator teres muscle arises, joins this supraepicondylar process to the medial epicondyle. The median nerve, often accompanied by the brachial artery, passes through the foramen formed by this band. This may be a cause of nerve entrapment. **B. Third head of biceps brachii.** In this case, there is also attrition of the biceps tendon. **C. Attrition of tendon of long head of biceps brachii and presence of a superior coracobrachialis** (variation).

D. Superficial ulnar artery. E. Anomalous division of brachial artery. In this case, the median nerve passes between the radial and ulnar arteries, which arise high in the arm. **F. Relationship of median nerve and brachial artery.** The variable relationship of these two structures can be explained developmentally. In a study of 307 limbs in Dr. Grant's lab, portions of both primitive brachial arteries persisted in 5%, the posterior in 82%, and the anterior in 13%.

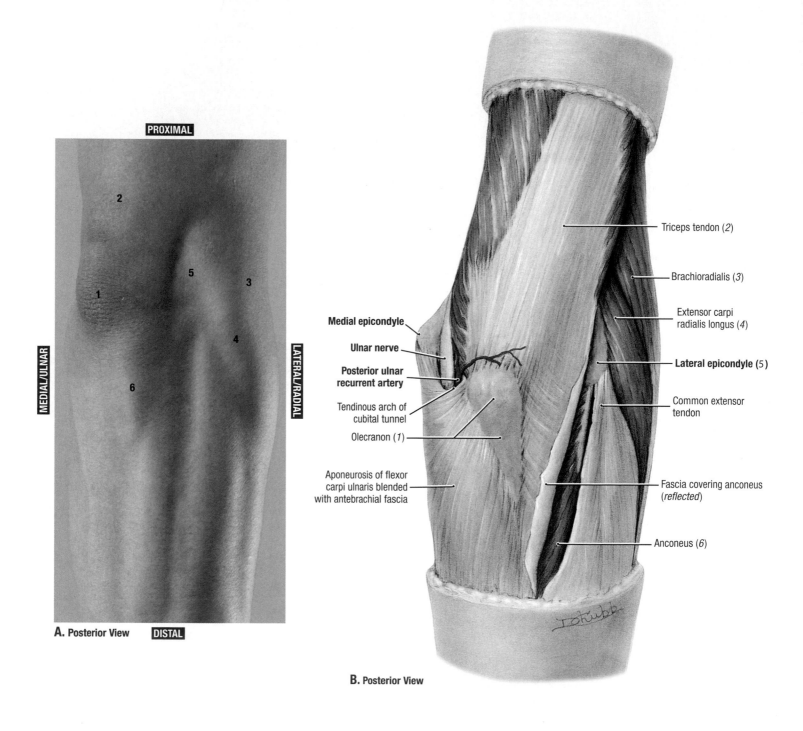

PROXIMAL

MEDIAL/ULNAR

LATERAL/RADIAL

2

5

1

3

4

6

A. Posterior View   **DISTAL**

Triceps tendon (*2*)

Brachioradialis (*3*)

Extensor carpi
radialis longus (*4*)

Medial epicondyle

Ulnar nerve

**Posterior ulnar
recurrent artery**

Tendinous arch of
cubital tunnel

Olecranon (*1*)

Aponeurosis of flexor
carpi ulnaris blended
with antebrachial fascia

Lateral epicondyle (5)

Common extensor
tendon

Fascia covering anconeus
(*reflected*)

Anconeus (*6*)

B. Posterior View

2.55   **Posterior Aspect of Elbow (I)**

A. Surface anatomy. B. Superficial dissection. Numbers in parentheses refer to structures in *Part A*.
- The triceps brachii is attached distally to the superior surface of the olecranon and, through the deep fascia covering the anconeus, into the lateral border of olecranon.

- The posterior surfaces of the medial epicondyle, lateral epicondyle, and olecranon are subcutaneous and palpable.
- The ulnar nerve, also palpable, runs subfascially posterior to the medial epicondyle; distal to this point, it disappears deep to the two heads of the flexor carpi ulnaris.

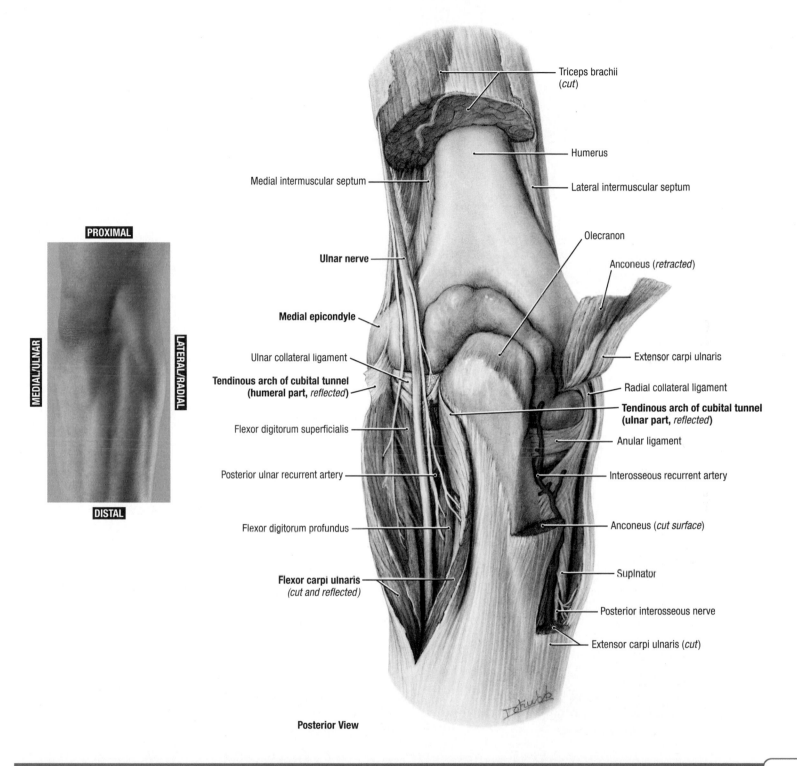

PROXIMAL

MEDIAL/ULNAR

LATERAL/RADIAL

DISTAL

Triceps brachii (*cut*)

Humerus

Medial intermuscular septum

Lateral intermuscular septum

Olecranon

Anconeus (*retracted*)

Ulnar nerve

Medial epicondyle

Ulnar collateral ligament

Extensor carpi ulnaris

Tendinous arch of cubital tunnel (humeral part, *reflected*)

Radial collateral ligament

Flexor digitorum superficialis

Tendinous arch of cubital tunnel (ulnar part, *reflected*)

Anular ligament

Posterior ulnar recurrent artery

Interosseous recurrent artery

Flexor digitorum profundus

Anconeus (*cut surface*)

Supinator

Flexor carpi ulnaris (*cut and reflected*)

Posterior interosseous nerve

Extensor carpi ulnaris (*cut*)

Posterior View

Posterior Aspect of Elbow (II)

2.56

Deep dissection. The distal portion of the triceps brachii muscle was removed. Note that the ulnar nerve descends subfascially within the posterior compartment of the arm, passing posterior to the medial epicondyle in the groove for the ulnar nerve. Next, it passes posterior to the ulnar collateral ligament of the elbow joint and then between the flexor carpi ulnaris and flexor digitorum profundus muscles.

Ulnar nerve injury occurs most commonly where the nerve passes posterior to the medial epicondyle of the humerus.

The injury results when the medial part of the elbow hits a hard surface, fracturing the medial epicondyle. The ulnar nerve may be compressed in the cubital tunnel, resulting in **cubital tunnel syndrome**. The cubital tunnel is formed by the tendinous arch joining the humeral and ulnar heads of attachment of the flexor carpi ulnaris muscle. Ulnar nerve injury can result in extensive motor and sensory loss to the hand.

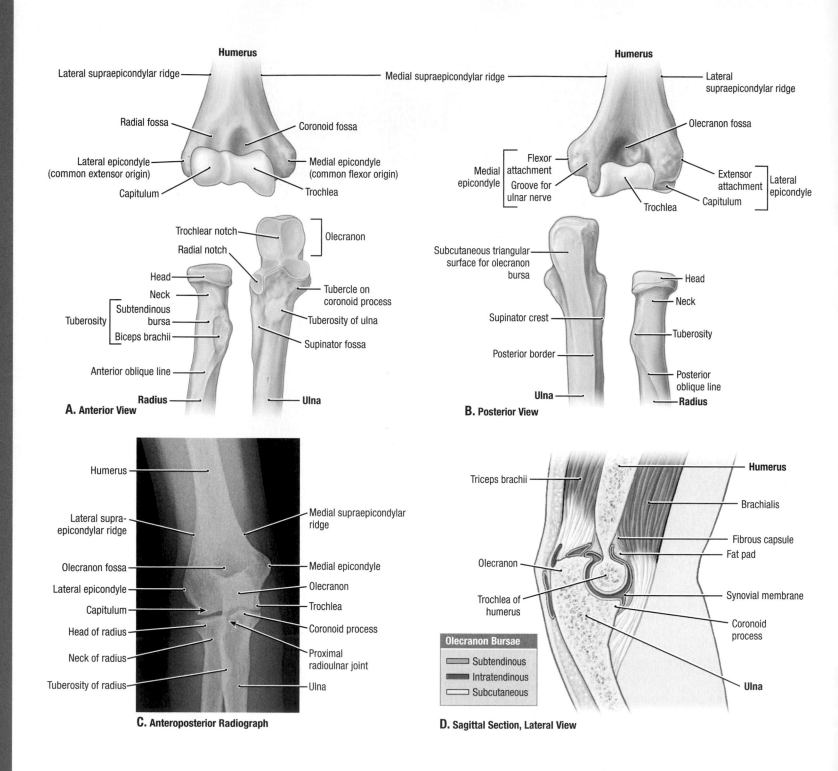

A. Anterior View

B. Posterior View

C. Anteroposterior Radiograph

D. Sagittal Section, Lateral View

Olecranon Bursae
- Subtendinous
- Intratendinous
- Subcutaneous

2.57   **Bones and Imaging of Elbow Region**

A. Anterior bony features. **B.** Posterior bony features. **C.** Radiographic study of bones of elbow joint. **D.** Bursae related to olecranon of ulna.

The subcutaneous olecranon bursa is exposed to injury during falls on the elbow and to infection from abrasions of the skin covering the olecranon. Repeated excessive pressure and friction produces a friction **subcutaneous olecranon bursitis** (e.g., "student's elbow").

Subtendinous olecranon bursitis results from excessive friction between the triceps tendon and the olecranon. For example, it may occur due to repeated flexion-extension of the forearm during certain assembly-line jobs. The pain is severe during flexion of the forearm because of pressure exerted on the inflamed subtendinous olecranon bursa by the triceps tendon.

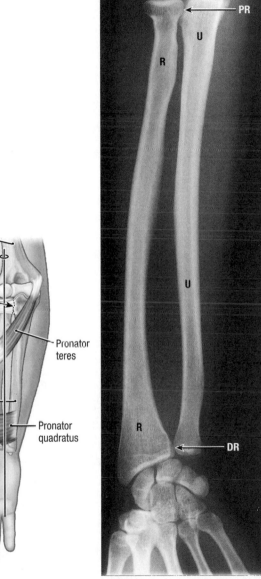

Humerus (*H*)

Axis of rotary movement of radius

Proximal radioulnar joint (*PR*)

Anular ligament of radius

Pronator teres

Radius (*R*)

Ulna (*U*)

Pronator quadratus

Distal radioulnar joint (*DR*)

A. Anterior View, Supination

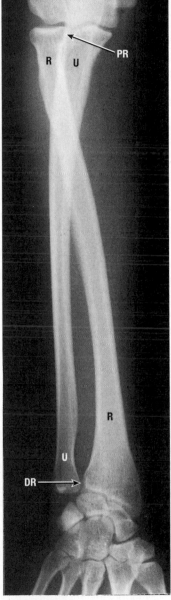

B. Anteroposterior Radiograph, Supination

C. Anteroposterior Radiograph, Pronation

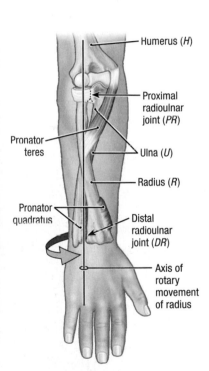

Humerus (*H*)

Proximal radioulnar joint (*PR*)

Pronator teres

Ulna (*U*)

Radius (*R*)

Pronator quadratus

Distal radioulnar joint (*DR*)

Axis of rotary movement of radius

D. Anterior View, Pronation

Supination and Pronation at Superior, Middle, and Inferior Radioulnar Joints   **2.58**

A. and **B.** Forearm in supination. **C.** and **D.** Forearm in pronation. The radius crosses the ulna when the forearm is pronated. The superior and inferior radioulnar joints are synovial joints; the middle radioulnar joint is a syndesmosis (fibrous joint) in which the interosseous membrane connects the forearm bones.

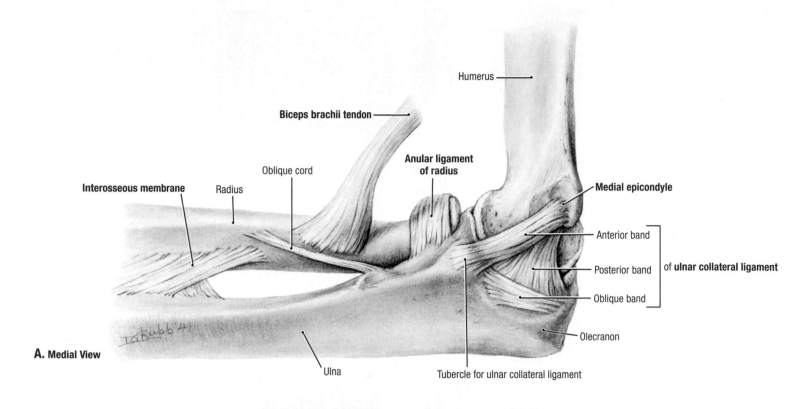

Humerus

Biceps brachii tendon

Oblique cord

Anular ligament of radius

Interosseous membrane   Radius

Medial epicondyle

Anterior band

Posterior band   of **ulnar collateral ligament**

Oblique band

Olecranon

A. Medial View

Ulna

Tubercle for ulnar collateral ligament

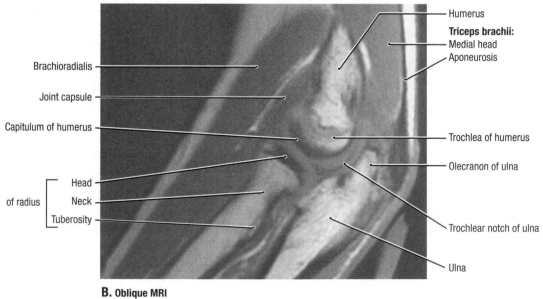

Humerus

Triceps brachii:
Medial head
Aponeurosis

Brachioradialis

Joint capsule

Capitulum of humerus

Trochlea of humerus

Olecranon of ulna

Head

Neck   of radius

Tuberosity

Trochlear notch of ulna

Ulna

B. Oblique MRI

2.59   **Medial Aspect of Bones and Ligaments of Elbow Region**

A. Ligaments. The anterior band of the ulnar (medial) collateral ligament is a strong, round cord that is taut when the elbow joint is extended. The posterior band is a weak fan that is taut in flexion of the joint. **B. Elbow joint in slight flexion.**

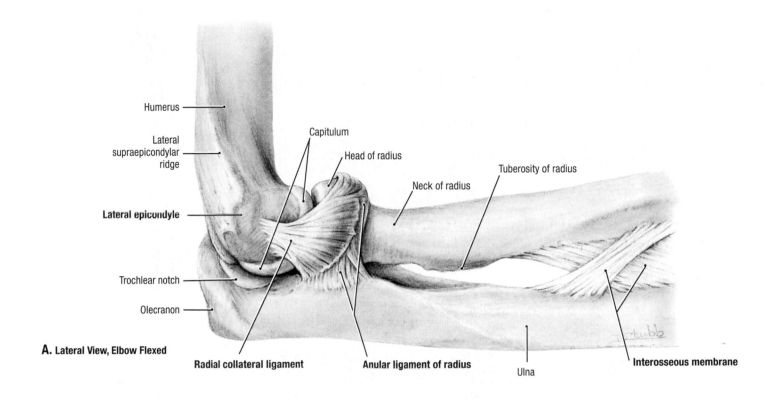

A. Lateral View, Elbow Flexed

Humerus

Capitulum

Head of radius

Lateral supraepicondylar ridge

Neck of radius

Tuberosity of radius

Lateral epicondyle

Trochlear notch

Olecranon

Radial collateral ligament

Anular ligament of radius

Ulna

Interosseous membrane

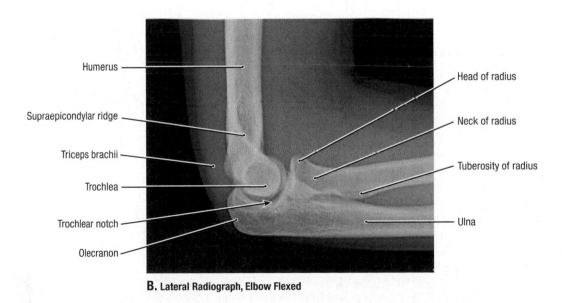

Humerus

Head of radius

Supraepicondylar ridge

Neck of radius

Triceps brachii

Tuberosity of radius

Trochlea

Trochlear notch

Ulna

Olecranon

B. Lateral Radiograph, Elbow Flexed

Lateral Aspect of Bones and Ligaments of Elbow Region   **2.60**

A. Ligaments. The fan-shaped radial (lateral) collateral ligament is primarily attached to the anular ligament of the radius; superficial fibers of the lateral ligament blend with the fibrous capsule and continue onto the radius. **B. Bony formations.**

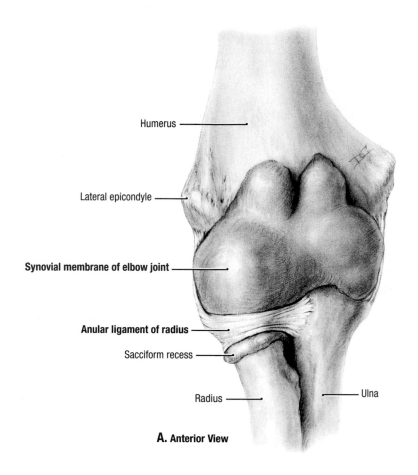

Humerus

Lateral epicondyle

Synovial membrane of elbow joint

Anular ligament of radius

Sacciform recess

Radius

Ulna

A. Anterior View

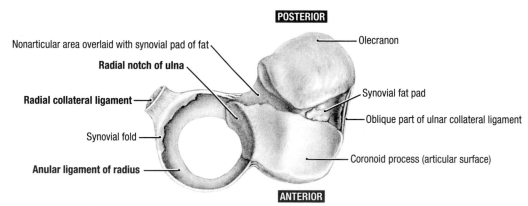

POSTERIOR

Olecranon

Nonarticular area overlaid with synovial pad of fat

Radial notch of ulna

Synovial fat pad

Radial collateral ligament

Oblique part of ulnar collateral ligament

Synovial fold

Coronoid process (articular surface)

Anular ligament of radius

ANTERIOR

B. Superior View of Ulna and Anular Ligament

| 2.61 | **Synovial Capsule of Elbow Joint and Anular Ligament** |

A. Synovial capsule of elbow and proximal radioulnar joints.
The cavity of the elbow was injected with purple fluid (wax). The
fibrous capsule was removed, and the synovial membrane remains.
B. Anular ligament.

- The anular ligament secures the head of the radius to the radial
  notch of the ulna and with it forms a tapering columnar socket
  (i.e., wide superiorly, narrow inferiorly).
- The anular ligament is bound to the humerus by the radial collateral ligament of the elbow.

A common childhood injury is **subluxation and dislocation of
the head of the radius** after traction on a pronated forearm (e.g.,
when lifting a child onto a bus). The sudden pulling of the upper
limb tears or stretches the distal attachment of the less tapering
anular ligament of a child. The radial head then moves distally,
partially out of the anular ligament. The proximal part of the torn
ligament may become trapped between the head of the radius and
the capitulum of the humerus. The source of pain is the pinched
anular ligament.

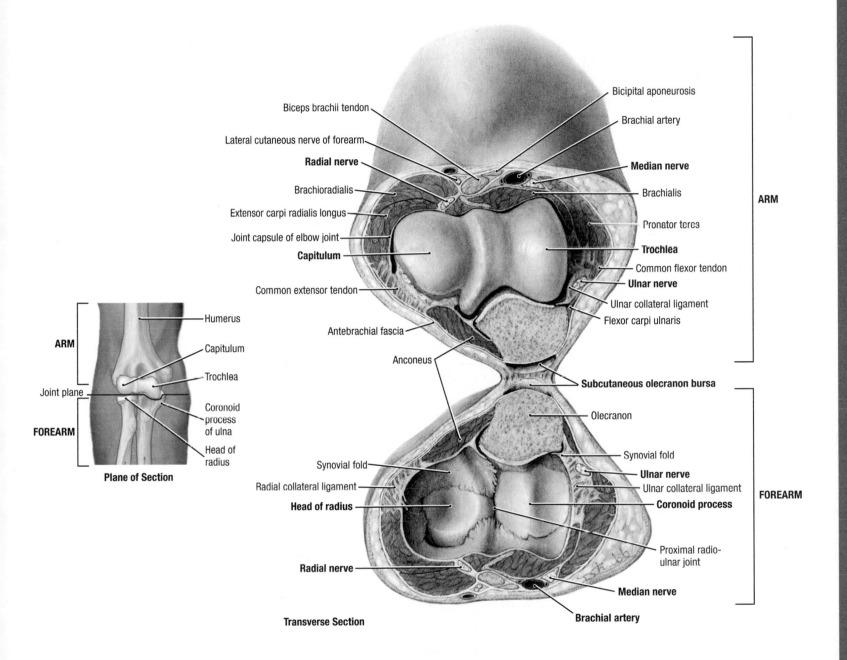

Biceps brachii tendon
Lateral cutaneous nerve of forearm
Radial nerve
Brachioradialis
Extensor carpi radialis longus
Joint capsule of elbow joint
Capitulum
Common extensor tendon
Antebrachial fascia
Anconeus
Synovial fold
Radial collateral ligament
Head of radius
Radial nerve

Bicipital aponeurosis
Brachial artery
Median nerve
Brachialis
Pronator teres
Trochlea
Common flexor tendon
Ulnar nerve
Ulnar collateral ligament
Flexor carpi ulnaris
Subcutaneous olecranon bursa
Olecranon
Synovial fold
Ulnar nerve
Ulnar collateral ligament
Coronoid process
Proximal radio-ulnar joint
Median nerve
Brachial artery

ARM

FOREARM

Transverse Section

Humerus
Capitulum
Trochlea
Coronoid process of ulna
Head of radius

ARM
Joint plane
FOREARM

Plane of Section

Articular Surfaces of Elbow Joint

2.62

The tissue surrounding the condyles of the humerus and the olecranon of the ulna have been sectioned in a transverse plane, followed by disarticulation and hyperextension of the elbow joint, revealing the articular surfaces. Compare the forearm (inferior) component with Figure 2.61B.

- Synovial folds containing fat overlie the periphery of the head of the radius and the nonarticular indentations on the trochlear notch of the ulna.

- The radial nerve is in contact with the joint capsule, the ulnar nerve is in contact with the ulnar collateral ligament, and the median nerve is separated from the joint capsule by the brachialis muscle.

TABLE 2.10 Arteries of Forearm

Radial Artery

Origin: In cubital fossa, as smaller terminal branch of brachial artery

Course/Distribution: Runs distally under brachioradialis, lateral to flexor carpi radialis, defining boundary between the flexor and extensor compartments and supplying the radial aspect of both. Gives rise to a superficial palmar branch near the radiocarpal joint; it then transverses the anatomical snuff box to pass between the heads of the first dorsal interosseous muscle joining the deep branch of the ulnar artery to form the deep palmar arch

Ulnar Artery

Origin: In cubital fossa, as larger terminal branch of brachial artery

Course/Distribution: Passes distally between second and third layers of forearm flexor muscles, supplying ulnar aspect of flexor compartment; passes superficial to flexor retinaculum at wrist, continuing as the superficial palmar arch (with superficial branch of radial) after its deep palmar branch joins the deep palmar arch

Radial Recurrent Artery

Origin: In cubital fossa, as first (lateral) branch of radial artery

Course/Distribution: Courses proximally, superficial to supinator, passing between brachioradialis and brachialis to anastomose with radial collateral artery

Anterior and Posterior Ulnar Recurrent Arteries

Origin: In and immediately distal to cubital fossa, as first and second medial branches of ulnar artery

Course/Distribution: Course proximally to anastomose with the inferior and superior ulnar collateral arteries, respectively, forming collateral pathways anterior and posterior to the medial epicondyle of the humerus

Common Interosseous Artery

Origin: Immediately distal to the cubital fossa, as first lateral branch of ulnar artery

Course/Distribution: Terminates almost immediately, dividing into anterior and posterior interosseous arteries

Anterior and Posterior Interosseous Arteries

Origin: Distal to radial tubercle, as terminal branches of common interosseous

Course/Distribution: Pass to opposite sides of interosseous membrane; anterior artery runs on interosseous membrane; posterior artery runs between superficial and deep layers of extensor muscles as primary artery of compartment

Interosseous Recurrent Artery

Origin: Initial part of posterior interosseous artery

Course/Distribution: Courses proximally between lateral epicondyle and olecranon, deep to anconeus, to anastomose with middle collateral artery

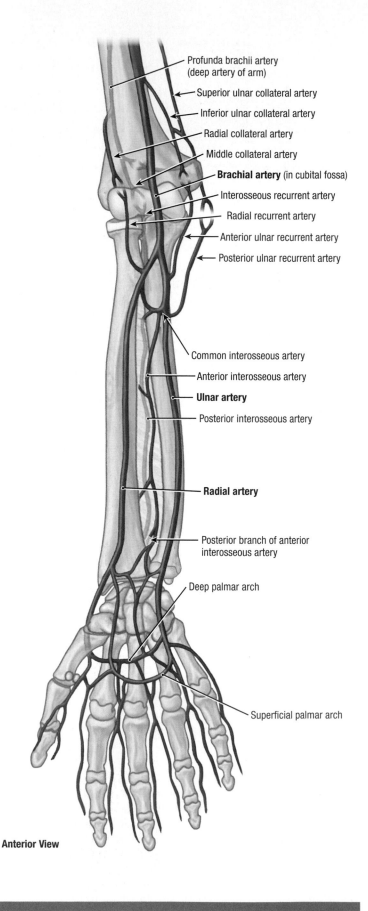

Profunda brachii artery (deep artery of arm)
Superior ulnar collateral artery
Inferior ulnar collateral artery
Radial collateral artery
Middle collateral artery
Brachial artery (in cubital fossa)
Interosseous recurrent artery
Radial recurrent artery
Anterior ulnar recurrent artery
Posterior ulnar recurrent artery
Common interosseous artery
Anterior interosseous artery
Ulnar artery
Posterior interosseous artery
Radial artery
Posterior branch of anterior interosseous artery
Deep palmar arch
Superficial palmar arch

Anterior View

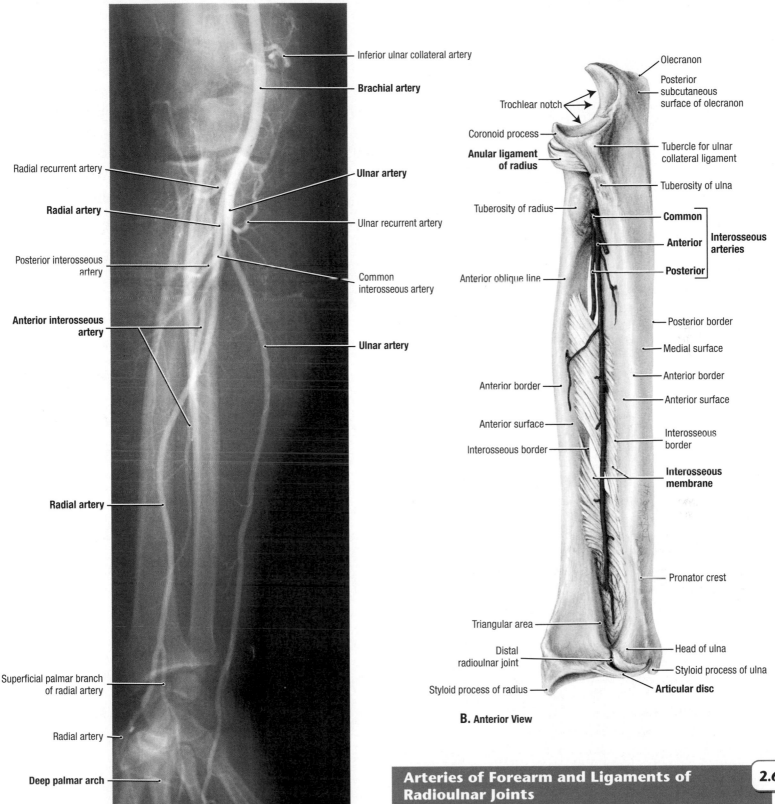

Inferior ulnar collateral artery

Brachial artery

Radial recurrent artery

Radial artery

Ulnar artery

Ulnar recurrent artery

Posterior interosseous artery

Common interosseous artery

Anterior interosseous artery

Ulnar artery

Radial artery

Superficial palmar branch of radial artery

Radial artery

Deep palmar arch

Superficial palmar arch

A. Anteroposterior Brachial Arteriogram

Olecranon

Posterior subcutaneous surface of olecranon

Trochlear notch

Coronoid process

Anular ligament of radius

Tubercle for ulnar collateral ligament

Tuberosity of ulna

Tuberosity of radius

Common

Anterior   Interosseous arteries

Posterior

Anterior oblique line

Posterior border

Medial surface

Anterior border

Anterior surface

Anterior border

Anterior surface

Interosseous border

Interosseous border

Interosseous membrane

Pronator crest

Triangular area

Distal radioulnar joint

Head of ulna

Styloid process of ulna

Styloid process of radius

Articular disc

B. Anterior View

Arteries of Forearm and Ligaments of Radioulnar Joints

2.64

A. Arteries and bones of forearm. B. Radioulnar ligaments and interosseous arteries. The ligament maintaining the proximal radioulnar joint is the anular ligament, that for the distal joint is the articular disc, and that for the middle joint is the interosseous membrane. The interosseous membrane is attached to the interosseous borders of the radius and ulna, but it also spreads onto their surfaces.

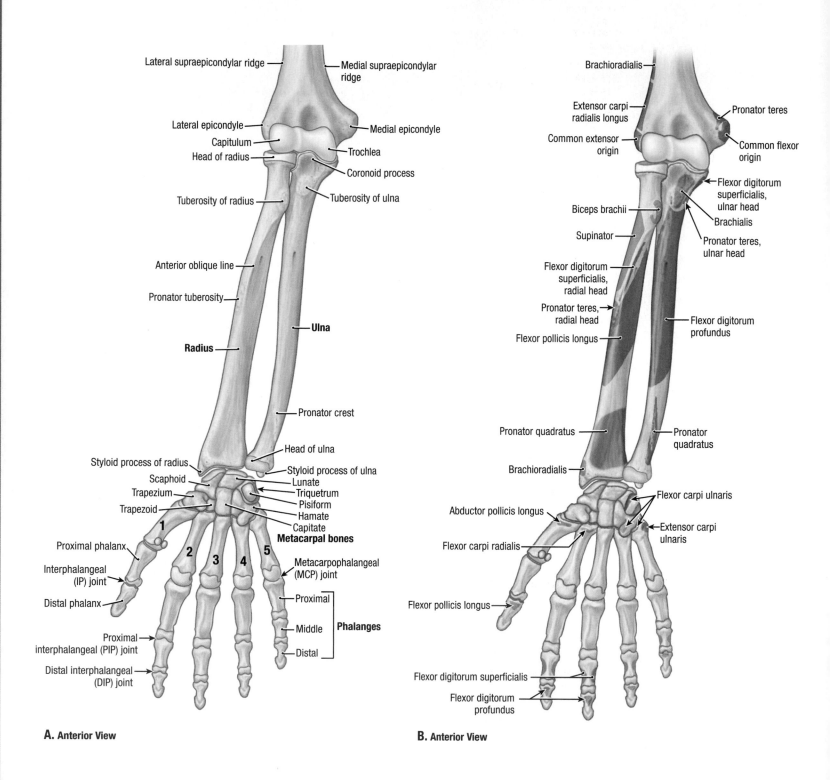

Lateral supraepicondylar ridge
Medial supraepicondylar ridge
Lateral epicondyle
Medial epicondyle
Capitulum
Head of radius
Trochlea
Coronoid process
Tuberosity of radius
Tuberosity of ulna
Anterior oblique line
Pronator tuberosity
Ulna
Radius
Pronator crest
Head of ulna
Styloid process of radius
Styloid process of ulna
Scaphoid
Lunate
Trapezium
Triquetrum
Trapezoid
Pisiform
Hamate
Capitate
Metacarpal bones
1
Proximal phalanx
2   3   4   5
Interphalangeal (IP) joint
Metacarpophalangeal (MCP) joint
Distal phalanx
Proximal
Proximal interphalangeal (PIP) joint
Middle
Phalanges
Distal interphalangeal (DIP) joint
Distal

A. Anterior View

Brachioradialis
Extensor carpi radialis longus
Pronator teres
Common extensor origin
Common flexor origin
Flexor digitorum superficialis, ulnar head
Biceps brachii
Brachialis
Supinator
Pronator teres, ulnar head
Flexor digitorum superficialis, radial head
Pronator teres, radial head
Flexor digitorum profundus
Flexor pollicis longus
Pronator quadratus
Pronator quadratus
Brachioradialis
Flexor carpi ulnaris
Abductor pollicis longus
Flexor carpi radialis
Extensor carpi ulnaris
Flexor pollicis longus
Flexor digitorum superficialis
Flexor digitorum profundus

B. Anterior View

2.65   Bones of Forearm and Hand and Attachments of Forearm Muscles

A. Bony features. **B.** Sites of muscle attachments.

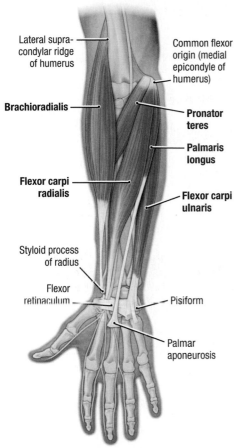

A. **Anterior View, 1st layer**

Lateral supra-condylar ridge of humerus

Common flexor origin (medial epicondyle of humerus)

Brachioradialis

Pronator teres

Palmaris longus

Flexor carpi radialis

Flexor carpi ulnaris

Styloid process of radius

Flexor retinaculum

Pisiform

Palmar aponeurosis

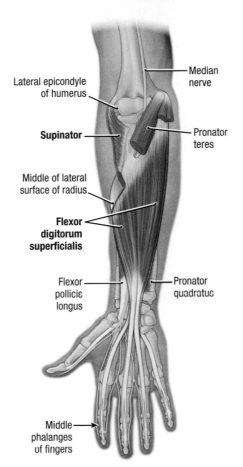

B. **Anterior View, 2nd layer**

Lateral epicondyle of humerus

Median nerve

Supinator

Pronator teres

Middle of lateral surface of radius

Flexor digitorum superficialis

Flexor pollicis longus

Pronator quadratus

Middle phalanges of fingers

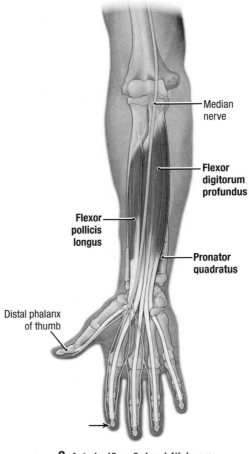

C. **Anterior View, 3rd and 4th layers**

Median nerve

Flexor digitorum profundus

Flexor pollicis longus

Pronator quadratus

Distal phalanx of thumb

Muscles of Anterior Forearm

2.66

The muscles of the anterior aspect of the forearm are arranged in three layers.

TABLE 2.11   Muscles of Anterior Forearm

Muscle	Proximal Attachment	Distal Attachment	Innervation	Main Actions
Pronator teres	Medial epicondyle of humerus and coronoid process of ulna	Middle of lateral surface of radius (pronator tuberosity)	Median nerve (C6–**C7**)	Pronates forearm and flexes elbow joint
Flexor carpi radialis	Medial epicondyle of humerus	Base of 2nd (and 3rd) metacarpals		Flexes and abducts wrist joint
Palmaris longus		Distal half of flexor retinaculum and palmar aponeurosis	Median nerve (C7–**C8**)	Flexes wrist joint and tightens palmar aponeurosis
Flexor carpi ulnaris	*Humeral head:* medial epicondyle of humerus *Ulnar head:* olecranon and posterior border of ulna	Pisiform, hook of hamate, and 5th metacarpal	Ulnar nerve (C7–**C8**)	Flexes and adducts wrist joint
Flexor digitorum superficialis	*Humeroulnar head:* medial epicondyle of humerus, ulnar collateral ligament, and coronoid process of ulna *Radial head:* superior half of anterior border of radius	Bodies of middle phalanges of medial four digits	Median nerve (C7, **C8**, and T1)	Flexes PIPs of medial four digits; acting more strongly, it flexes MCPs and wrist joint
Flexor digitorum profundus	Proximal three quarters of medial and anterior surfaces of ulna and interosseous membrane	Bases of distal phalanges of medial four digits	*Medial part:* ulnar nerve (**C8**–T1) *Lateral part:* median nerve (**C8**–T1)	Flexes DIPs of medial four digits; assists with flexion of wrist joint
Flexor pollicis longus	Anterior surface of radius and adjacent interosseous membrane	Base of distal phalanx of thumb	Anterior interosseous nerve from median (**C8**–T1)	Flexes IP joints of 1st digit (thumb) and assists flexion of wrist joint
Pronator quadratus	Distal fourth of anterior surface of ulna	Distal fourth of anterior surface of radius		Pronates forearm; deep fibers bind radius and ulna together

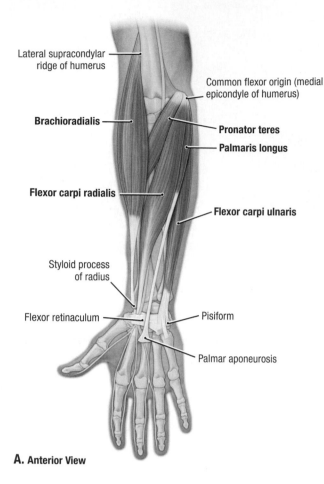

Lateral supracondylar
ridge of humerus

Common flexor origin (medial
epicondyle of humerus)

Brachioradialis

Pronator teres

Palmaris longus

Flexor carpi radialis

Flexor carpi ulnaris

Styloid process
of radius

Flexor retinaculum

Pisiform

Palmar aponeurosis

A. Anterior View

| 2.67 | **Superficial Muscles of Forearm and Palmar Aponeurosis** |

A. Muscles. **B.** Dissection.

- At the elbow, the brachial artery lies between the biceps tendon and median nerve. It then bifurcates into the radial and ulnar arteries.
- At the wrist, the radial artery is lateral to the flexor carpi radialis tendon, and the ulnar artery is lateral to flexor carpi ulnaris tendon.
- In the forearm, the radial artery lies between the flexor and extensor compartments. The muscles lateral to the artery are supplied by the radial nerve, and those medial to it by the median and ulnar nerves; thus, no motor nerve crosses the radial artery.
- The brachioradialis muscle slightly overlaps the radial artery, which is otherwise superficial.
- The four superficial muscles all attach proximally to the medial epicondyle of the humerus (common flexor origin).
- The palmaris longus muscle, in this specimen, has an anomalous distal belly; this muscle usually has a small belly at the common flexor origin and a long tendon that is continued into the palm as the palmar aponeurosis. The palmaris longus is absent unilaterally or bilaterally in approximately 14% of limbs.

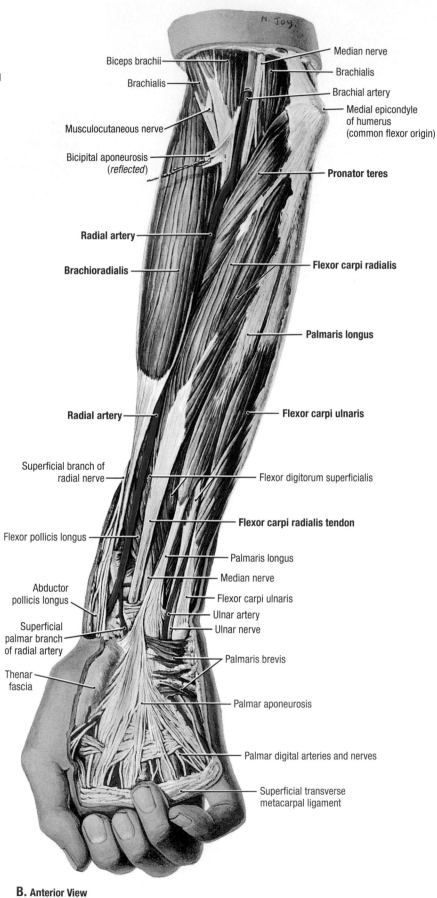

Biceps brachii

Brachialis

Musculocutaneous nerve

Bicipital aponeurosis
(reflected)

Radial artery

Brachioradialis

Radial artery

Superficial branch of
radial nerve

Flexor pollicis longus

Abductor
pollicis longus

Superficial
palmar branch
of radial artery

Thenar
fascia

Median nerve

Brachialis

Brachial artery

Medial epicondyle
of humerus
(common flexor origin)

Pronator teres

Flexor carpi radialis

Palmaris longus

Flexor carpi ulnaris

Flexor digitorum superficialis

Flexor carpi radialis tendon

Palmaris longus

Median nerve

Flexor carpi ulnaris

Ulnar artery

Ulnar nerve

Palmaris brevis

Palmar aponeurosis

Palmar digital arteries and nerves

Superficial transverse
metacarpal ligament

B. Anterior View

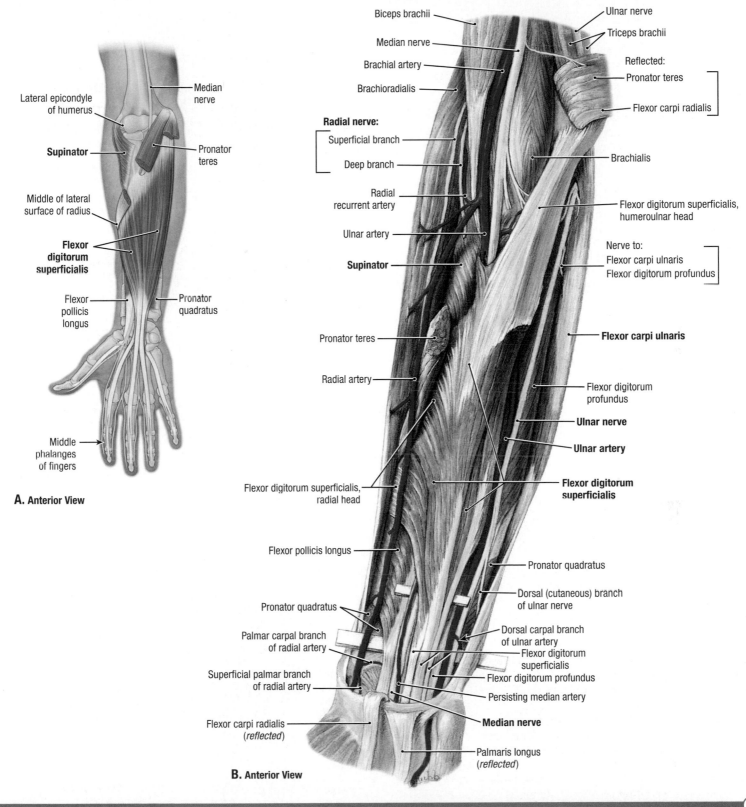

A. Anterior View

- Lateral epicondyle of humerus
- Median nerve
- **Supinator**
- Pronator teres
- Middle of lateral surface of radius
- **Flexor digitorum superficialis**
- Flexor pollicis longus
- Pronator quadratus
- Middle phalanges of fingers

B. Anterior View

- Biceps brachii
- Median nerve
- Brachial artery
- Brachioradialis
- **Radial nerve:**
  - Superficial branch
  - Deep branch
- Radial recurrent artery
- Ulnar artery
- **Supinator**
- Pronator teres
- Radial artery
- Flexor digitorum superficialis, radial head
- Flexor pollicis longus
- Pronator quadratus
- Palmar carpal branch of radial artery
- Superficial palmar branch of radial artery
- Flexor carpi radialis (*reflected*)
- Ulnar nerve
- Triceps brachii
- Reflected:
  - Pronator teres
  - Flexor carpi radialis
- Brachialis
- Flexor digitorum superficialis, humeroulnar head
- Nerve to:
  - Flexor carpi ulnaris
  - Flexor digitorum profundus
- **Flexor carpi ulnaris**
- Flexor digitorum profundus
- **Ulnar nerve**
- **Ulnar artery**
- **Flexor digitorum superficialis**
- Pronator quadratus
- Dorsal (cutaneous) branch of ulnar nerve
- Dorsal carpal branch of ulnar artery
- Flexor digitorum superficialis
- Flexor digitorum profundus
- Persisting median artery
- **Median nerve**
- Palmaris longus (*reflected*)

Flexor Digitorum Superficialis and Related Structures

2.68

A. Muscles. **B.** Dissection.
- The flexor digitorum superficialis muscle is attached proximally to the humerus, ulna, and radius.
- The ulnar artery passes obliquely posterior to the flexor digitorum superficialis; at the medial border of the muscle, the ulnar artery joins the ulnar nerve.
- The median nerve descends vertically posterior to the flexor digitorum superficialis and appears distally at its lateral border.
- The median artery of this specimen is a variation resulting from persistence of an embryologic vessel that usually disappears.

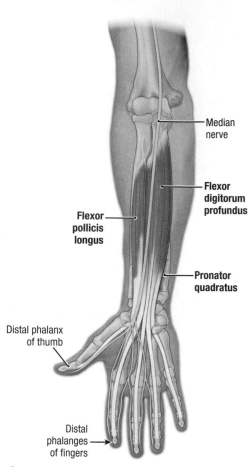

A. Anterior View

Labels (A): Median nerve; **Flexor digitorum profundus**; **Flexor pollicis longus**; **Pronator quadratus**; Distal phalanx of thumb; Distal phalanges of fingers

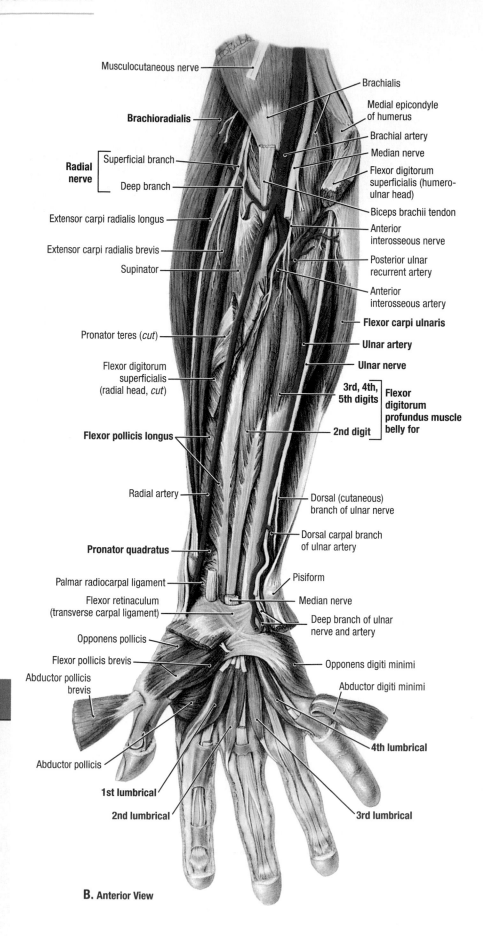

B. Anterior View

Labels (B): Musculocutaneous nerve; Brachialis; Medial epicondyle of humerus; Brachial artery; Median nerve; Flexor digitorum superficialis (humero-ulnar head); **Brachioradialis**; **Radial nerve** — Superficial branch, Deep branch; Biceps brachii tendon; Anterior interosseous nerve; Extensor carpi radialis longus; Extensor carpi radialis brevis; Posterior ulnar recurrent artery; Supinator; Anterior interosseous artery; **Flexor carpi ulnaris**; **Ulnar artery**; **Ulnar nerve**; Pronator teres (*cut*); 3rd, 4th, 5th digits / **Flexor digitorum profundus muscle belly for**; Flexor digitorum superficialis (radial head, *cut*); 2nd digit; **Flexor pollicis longus**; Radial artery; Dorsal (cutaneous) branch of ulnar nerve; Dorsal carpal branch of ulnar artery; **Pronator quadratus**; Pisiform; Palmar radiocarpal ligament; Median nerve; Flexor retinaculum (transverse carpal ligament); Deep branch of ulnar nerve and artery; Opponens pollicis; Flexor pollicis brevis; Opponens digiti minimi; Abductor pollicis brevis; Abductor digiti minimi; Abductor pollicis; **4th lumbrical**; **1st lumbrical**; **2nd lumbrical**; **3rd lumbrical**

2.69 **Deep Flexors of Digits and Related Structures**

A. Muscles. B. Dissection.

- The ulnar nerve enters the forearm posterior to the medial epicondyle, then descends between the flexor digitorum profundus and flexor carpi ulnaris, and is joined by the ulnar artery. At the wrist, the ulnar nerve and artery pass anterior to the flexor retinaculum and lateral to the pisiform to enter the palm.
- At the elbow, the ulnar nerve supplies the flexor carpi ulnaris and the medial half of the flexor digitorum profundus muscles; proximal to the wrist, it gives off the dorsal (cutaneous) branch.
- The four lumbricals arise from the flexor digitorum profundus tendons.

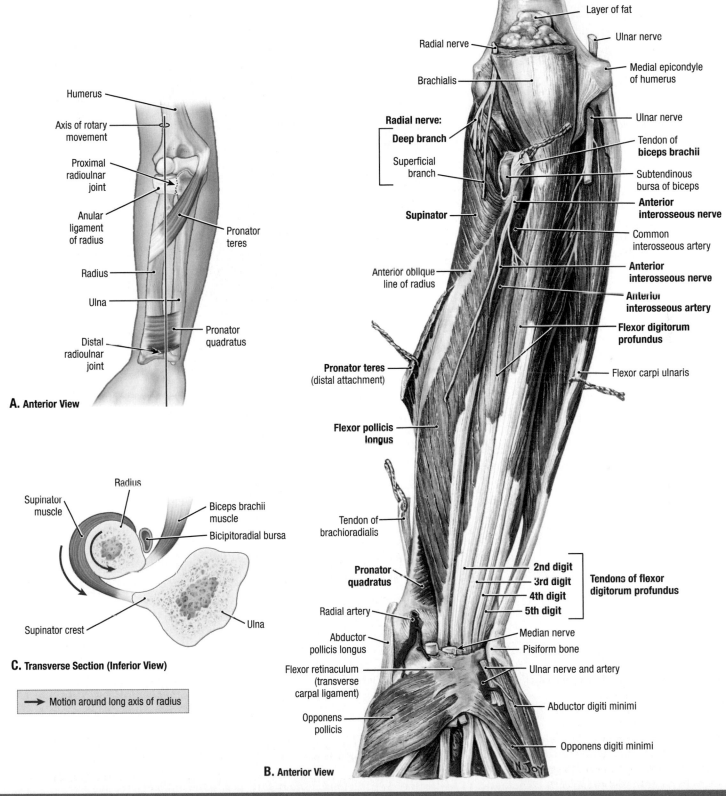

A. Anterior View

- Humerus
- Axis of rotary movement
- Proximal radioulnar joint
- Anular ligament of radius
- Radius
- Ulna
- Distal radioulnar joint
- Pronator teres
- Pronator quadratus

C. Transverse Section (Inferior View)

- Radius
- Supinator muscle
- Biceps brachii muscle
- Bicipitoradial bursa
- Ulna
- Supinator crest

→ Motion around long axis of radius

B. Anterior View

- Layer of fat
- Ulnar nerve
- Radial nerve
- Brachialis
- Medial epicondyle of humerus
- **Radial nerve:**
  - **Deep branch**
  - Superficial branch
- Ulnar nerve
- Tendon of **biceps brachii**
- Subtendinous bursa of biceps
- **Anterior interosseous nerve**
- **Supinator**
- Common interosseous artery
- Anterior oblique line of radius
- **Anterior interosseous nerve**
- **Anterior interosseous artery**
- **Flexor digitorum profundus**
- **Pronator teres** (distal attachment)
- Flexor carpi ulnaris
- **Flexor pollicis longus**
- Tendon of brachioradialis
- **Pronator quadratus**
- 2nd digit
- 3rd digit
- 4th digit
- 5th digit
- **Tendons of flexor digitorum profundus**
- Radial artery
- Median nerve
- Pisiform bone
- Abductor pollicis longus
- Ulnar nerve and artery
- Flexor retinaculum (transverse carpal ligament)
- Abductor digiti minimi
- Opponens pollicis
- Opponens digiti minimi

Deep Flexors of Digits and Supinator   2.70

A. Pronator quadratus. **B.** Dissection. **C.** Muscles producing supination of forearm.

- The anterior interosseous nerve and artery pass deeply between the flexor pollicis longus and flexor digitorum profundus muscles to lie on the interosseous membrane.

- The deep branch of the radial nerve pierces and innervates the supinator muscle.

Severance of the deep branch of the radial nerve results in an inability to extend the thumb and metacarpophalangeal (MCP) joints of the other digits. Loss of sensation does not occur because the deep branch is entirely muscular and articular in distribution.

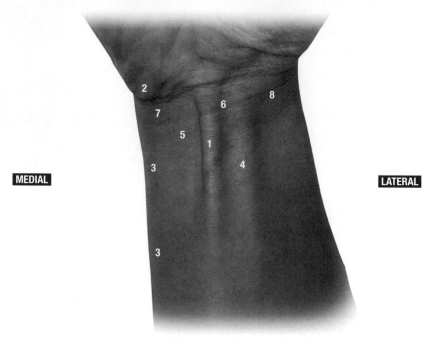

A. Anterior View of Right Hand and Wrist

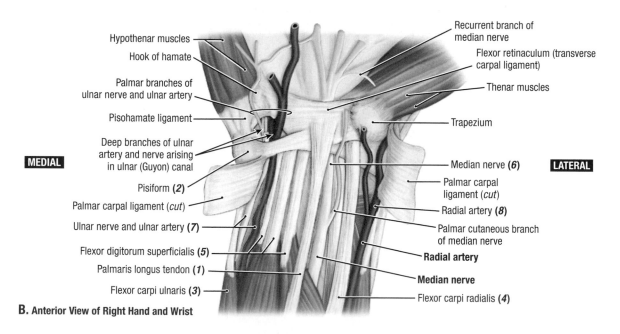

Hypothenar muscles

Hook of hamate

Palmar branches of
ulnar nerve and ulnar artery

Pisohamate ligament

Deep branches of ulnar
artery and nerve arising
in ulnar (Guyon) canal

Pisiform (*2*)

Palmar carpal ligament (*cut*)

Ulnar nerve and ulnar artery (*7*)

Flexor digitorum superficialis (*5*)

Palmaris longus tendon (*1*)

Flexor carpi ulnaris (*3*)

MEDIAL

Recurrent branch of
median nerve

Flexor retinaculum (transverse
carpal ligament)

Thenar muscles

Trapezium

Median nerve (*6*)

Palmar carpal
ligament (*cut*)

Radial artery (*8*)

Palmar cutaneous branch
of median nerve

Radial artery

Median nerve

Flexor carpi radialis (*4*)

LATERAL

B. Anterior View of Right Hand and Wrist

2.71   Structures of Anterior Wrist

A. Surface anatomy. Numbers refer to labels with corresponding numbers in parentheses in *Part B*. **B. Schematic. C. Dissection.**
- The distal skin incision follows the transverse skin crease at the wrist. The incision crosses the pisiform, to which the flexor carpi ulnaris muscle attaches, and the tubercle of the scaphoid, to which the tendon of flexor carpi radialis muscle is a guide.
- The palmaris longus tendon bisects the transverse skin crease; deep to the lateral margin of the tendon is the median nerve. The palmaris longus is absent in *Part A*—a variation in up to 20% of people.

- Note the ulnar (Guyon) canal through which the ulnar vessels and nerve pass medial to the pisiform.
- The radial artery passes deep to the tendon of the abductor pollicis longus muscle.
- The flexor digitorum superficialis tendons to the 3rd and 4th digits become anterior to those of the 2nd and 5th digits.
- The recurrent branch of the median nerve to the thenar muscles lies within a circle whose center is 2.5 to 4 cm distal to the tubercle of the scaphoid.

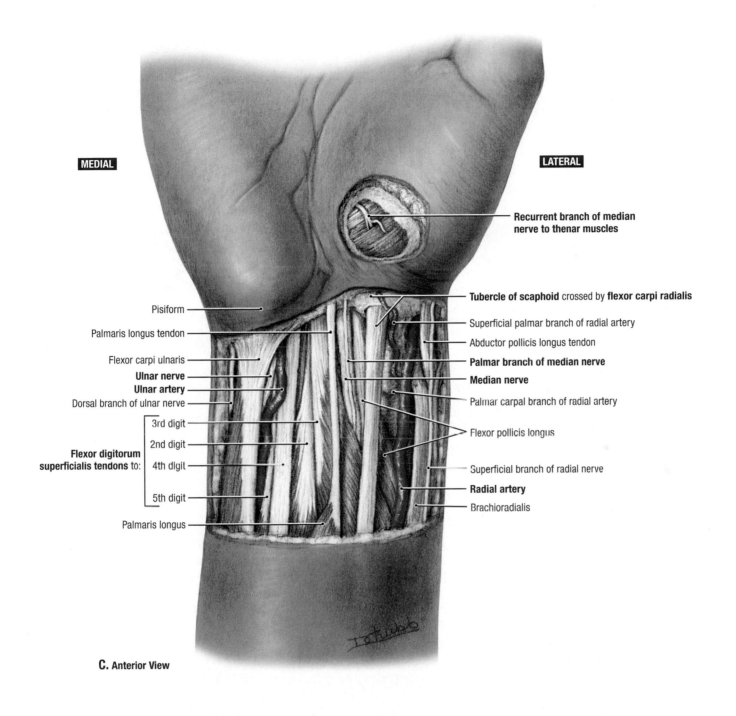

Recurrent branch of median nerve to thenar muscles

Tubercle of scaphoid crossed by **flexor carpi radialis**

Pisiform

Palmaris longus tendon

Flexor carpi ulnaris

Ulnar nerve

Ulnar artery

Dorsal branch of ulnar nerve

Superficial palmar branch of radial artery

Abductor pollicis longus tendon

Palmar branch of median nerve

Median nerve

Palmar carpal branch of radial artery

3rd digit

2nd digit

Flexor digitorum superficialis tendons to: 4th digit

5th digit

Palmaris longus

Flexor pollicis longus

Superficial branch of radial nerve

Radial artery

Brachioradialis

C. Anterior View

Structures of Anterior Wrist (*continued*)

2.71

Lesions of the median nerve usually occur in two places: the forearm and the wrist. The most common site is where the nerve passes though the carpal tunnel. Lacerations of the wrist often cause median nerve injury because this nerve is relatively close to the surface. This results in paralysis of the thenar muscles and the first two lumbricals. Hence, opposition of the thumb is not possible and fine control movements of the 2nd and 3rd digits are impaired. Sensation is also lost over the thumb and adjacent 2½ digits.

Median nerve injury resulting from a perforating wound in the elbow region results in loss of flexion of the proximal and distal interphalangeal (IP) joints of the 2nd and 3rd digits. The ability to flex the metacarpophalangeal joints of these digits is also affected because digital branches of the median nerve supply the 1st and 2nd lumbricals. The palmar cutaneous branch of the median nerve does not traverse the carpal tunnel. It supplies the skin of the central palm, which remains sensitive in carpal tunnel syndrome.

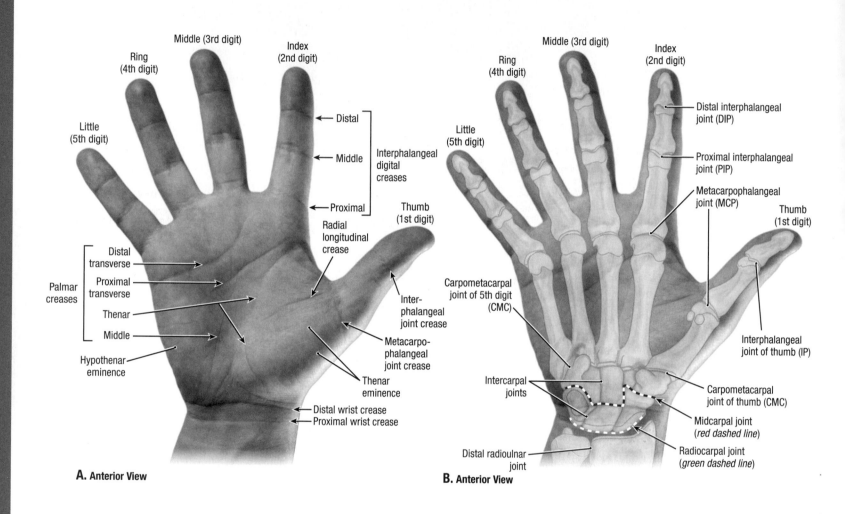

A. Anterior View

Ring (4th digit)
Middle (3rd digit)
Index (2nd digit)
Little (5th digit)
Distal
Middle
Proximal
Interphalangeal digital creases
Thumb (1st digit)
Radial longitudinal crease
Distal transverse
Proximal transverse
Thenar
Middle
Palmar creases
Hypothenar eminence
Inter-phalangeal joint crease
Metacarpo-phalangeal joint crease
Thenar eminence
Distal wrist crease
Proximal wrist crease

B. Anterior View

Middle (3rd digit)
Ring (4th digit)
Index (2nd digit)
Little (5th digit)
Distal interphalangeal joint (DIP)
Proximal interphalangeal joint (PIP)
Metacarpophalangeal joint (MCP)
Thumb (1st digit)
Carpometacarpal joint of 5th digit (CMC)
Interphalangeal joint of thumb (IP)
Intercarpal joints
Carpometacarpal joint of thumb (CMC)
Distal radioulnar joint
Midcarpal joint (*red dashed line*)
Radiocarpal joint (*green dashed line*)

| 2.72 | **Surface Anatomy of Hand and Wrist** |

A. Skin creases of wrist and hand. B. Surface projection of joints of wrist and hand. Note relationship of bones and joints to features of the hand.

The palmar skin presents several more or less constant *flexion creases* where the skin is firmly bound to the deep fascia:

- *Wrist creases*: **proximal, middle, distal**. The distal wrist crease indicates the proximal border of the flexor retinaculum.
- *Palmar creases*: **radial longitudinal crease** (the "life line" of palmistry), proximal and distal transverse palmar creases

- *Transverse digital flexion creases*: The **proximal digital crease** is located at the root of the digit, approximately 2 cm distal to the metacarpophalangeal joint. The proximal digital crease of the thumb crosses obliquely, proximal to the 1st metacarpophalangeal joint. The **middle digital crease** lies over the proximal interphalangeal joint, and the **distal digital crease** lies proximal to the distal interphalangeal joint. The thumb, having two phalanges, has only two flexion creases.

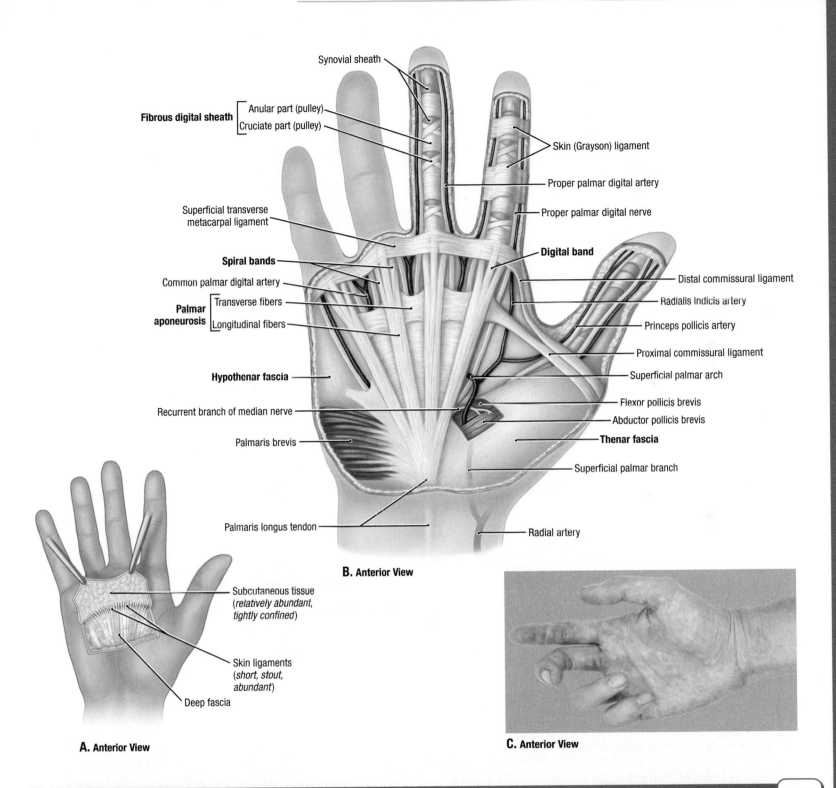

Synovial sheath

Fibrous digital sheath [Anular part (pulley)
Cruciate part (pulley)]

Skin (Grayson) ligament

Proper palmar digital artery

Proper palmar digital nerve

Superficial transverse metacarpal ligament

Spiral bands

Digital band

Common palmar digital artery

Distal commissural ligament

Palmar aponeurosis [Transverse fibers
Longitudinal fibers]

Radialis indicis artery

Princeps pollicis artery

Proximal commissural ligament

Hypothenar fascia

Superficial palmar arch

Recurrent branch of median nerve

Flexor pollicis brevis

Abductor pollicis brevis

Thenar fascia

Palmaris brevis

Superficial palmar branch

Palmaris longus tendon

Radial artery

B. Anterior View

Subcutaneous tissue (*relatively abundant, tightly confined*)

Skin ligaments (*short, stout, abundant*)

Deep fascia

A. Anterior View

C. Anterior View

Palmar (Deep) Fascia: Palmar Aponeurosis, Thenar and Hypothenar Fascia | **2.73**

A. Skin and subcutaneous tissue of palm. These layers are firmly attached to the deep fascia. **B. Superficial dissection.** The palmar fascia is thin over the thenar and hypothenar eminences but thick centrally, where it forms the palmar aponeurosis, and in the digits, where it forms the fibrous digital sheaths. At the distal end (base) of the palmar aponeurosis, four bundles of digital and spiral bands continue to the bases and fibrous digital sheaths of digits 2 to 5.

C. Dupuytren contracture is a disease of the palmar fascia resulting in progressive shortening, thickening, and fibrosis of the palmar fascia and palmar aponeurosis. The fibrous degeneration of the longitudinal digital bands of the aponeurosis on the medial side of the hand pulls the 4th and 5th fingers into partial flexion at the metacarpophalangeal and proximal interphalangeal joints. The contracture is frequently bilateral. Treatment of Dupuytren contracture usually involves surgical excision of all fibrotic parts of the palmar fascia to free the fingers.

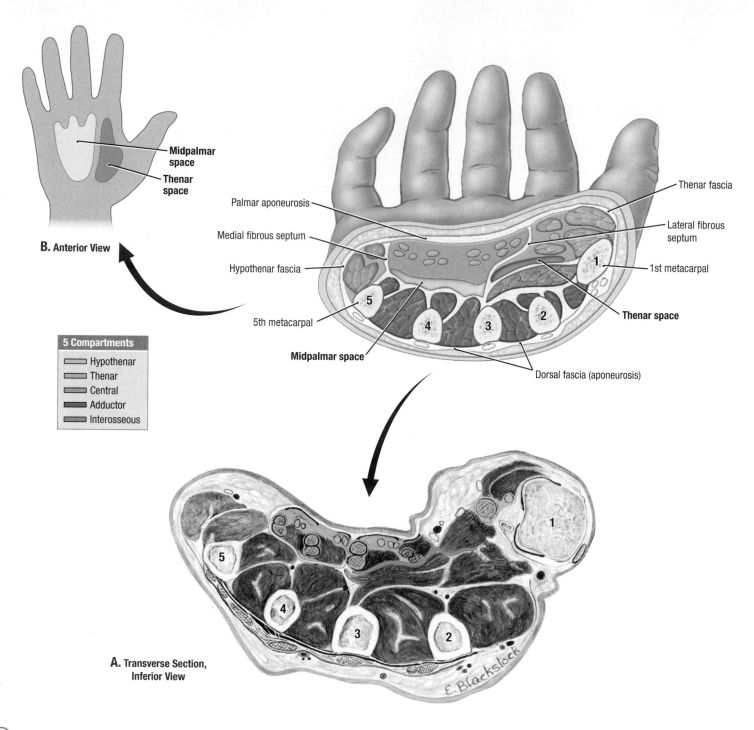

B. Anterior View

Midpalmar space

Thenar space

5 Compartments
	Hypothenar
	Thenar
	Central
	Adductor
	Interosseous

Palmar aponeurosis

Medial fibrous septum

Hypothenar fascia

5th metacarpal

Midpalmar space

Thenar fascia

Lateral fibrous septum

1st metacarpal

Thenar space

Dorsal fascia (aponeurosis)

A. Transverse Section, Inferior View

E. Blackstock

2.74   Spaces and Compartments of Palm of Hand

A. Fascial compartments of palm. Transverse section through middle of palm. **B. Potential fascial spaces of palm.**

- The potential midpalmar space lies posterior to the central compartment, is bounded medially by the hypothenar compartment, and is related distally to the synovial sheath of the 3rd, 4th, and 5th digits.
- The potential thenar space lies posterior to the thenar compartment and is related distally to the synovial sheath of the index finger.
- The potential midpalmar and thenar spaces are separated by a septum that passes from the palmar aponeurosis to the 3rd metacarpal.

Because the palmar fascia is thick and strong, **swellings resulting from hand infections** usually appear on the dorsum of the hand where the fascia is thinner. The potential fascial spaces of the palm are important because they may become infected. The fascial spaces determine the extent and direction of the spread of pus formed in the infected areas. Depending on the site of infection, pus will accumulate in the thenar, hypothenar, or adductor compartments. Antibiotic therapy has made infections that spread beyond one of these fascial compartments rare, but an untreated infection can spread proximally through the carpal tunnel into the forearm anterior to the pronator quadratus and its fascia.

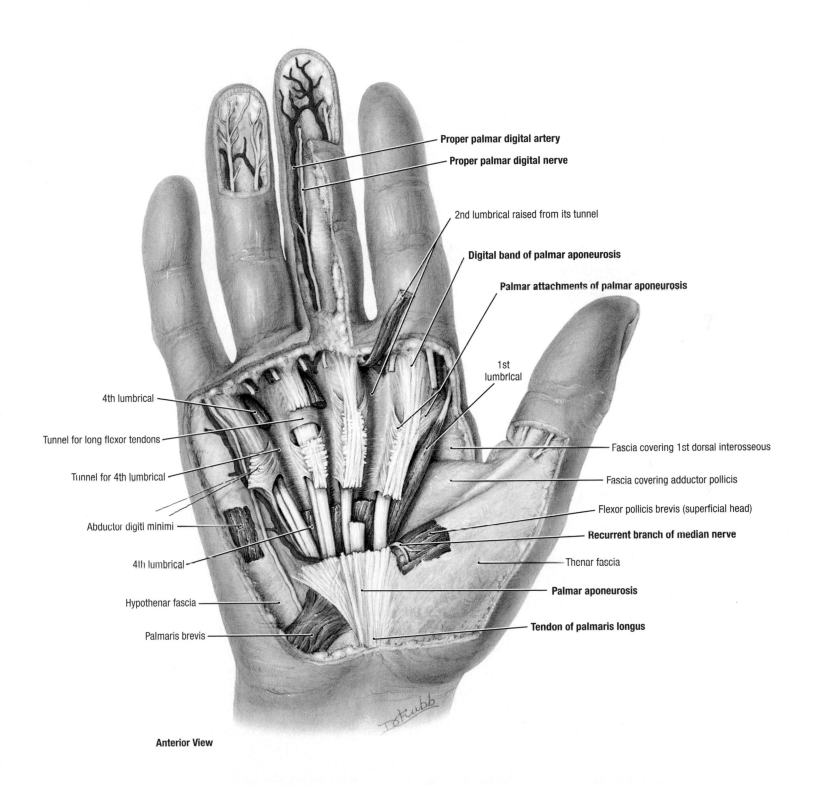

Proper palmar digital artery

Proper palmar digital nerve

2nd lumbrical raised from its tunnel

Digital band of palmar aponeurosis

Palmar attachments of palmar aponeurosis

1st lumbrical

4th lumbrical

Tunnel for long flexor tendons

Tunnel for 4th lumbrical

Abductor digiti minimi

4th lumbrical

Hypothenar fascia

Palmaris brevis

Fascia covering 1st dorsal interosseous

Fascia covering adductor pollicis

Flexor pollicis brevis (superficial head)

Recurrent branch of median nerve

Thenar fascia

Palmar aponeurosis

Tendon of palmaris longus

Anterior View

Palmar Aponeurosis

2.75

- From the palmar aponeurosis, four longitudinal digital bands enter the fingers; the other fibers form extensive fibroareolar septa that pass posteriorly to the palmar ligaments (see Fig. 2.82) and, more proximally, to the fascia covering the interossei. Thus, two sets of tunnels exist in the distal half of the palm: (1) tunnels for long flexor tendons and (2) tunnels for lumbricals, digital vessels, and digital nerves.
- In the dissected middle finger, note the absence of fat deep to the skin creases of the fingers.

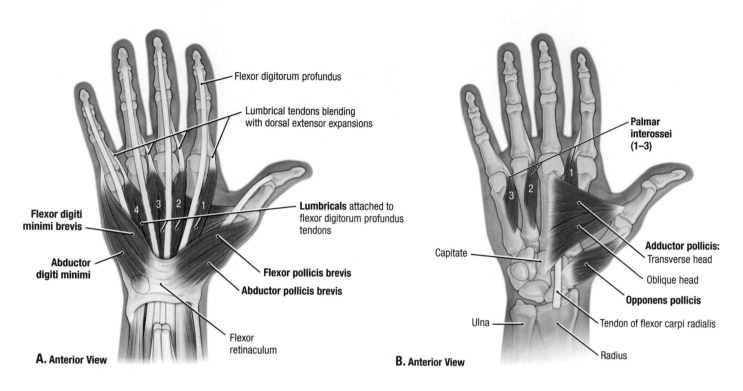

Flexor digitorum profundus

Lumbrical tendons blending
with dorsal extensor expansions

**Flexor digiti
minimi brevis**

Lumbricals attached to
flexor digitorum profundus
tendons

**Abductor
digiti minimi**

4 3 2 1

Flexor pollicis brevis

Abductor pollicis brevis

Flexor
retinaculum

A. Anterior View

**Palmar
interossei
(1–3)**

3 2 1

Capitate

Adductor pollicis:
Transverse head

Oblique head

Opponens pollicis

Ulna

Tendon of flexor carpi radialis

Radius

B. Anterior View

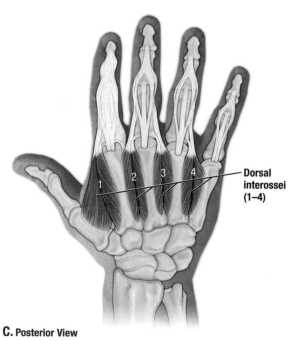

1 2 3 4

**Dorsal
interossei
(1–4)**

C. Posterior View

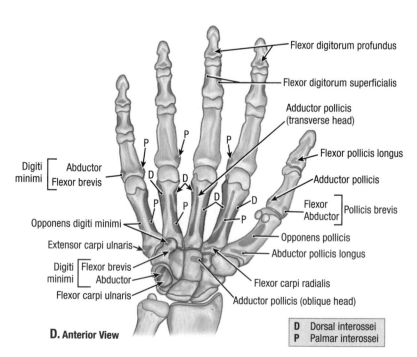

Flexor digitorum profundus

Flexor digitorum superficialis

Adductor pollicis
(transverse head)

Flexor pollicis longus

Adductor pollicis

P   P   P

Digiti
minimi ⌈ Abductor
       ⌊ Flexor brevis

D   D

Flexor ⌉
Abductor ⌋ Pollicis brevis

Opponens digiti minimi

D   D

Opponens pollicis

Extensor carpi ulnaris

P   P   P

Abductor pollicis longus

Digiti ⌈ Flexor brevis
minimi ⌊ Abductor

Flexor carpi radialis

Flexor carpi ulnaris

Adductor pollicis (oblique head)

| D | Dorsal interossei |
| P | Palmar interossei |

D. Anterior View

2.76   **Muscular Layers of Palm**

A. Lumbricals. **B.** Adductor pollicis and palmar interossei. **C.** Dorsal interossei. **D.** Bony attachments.

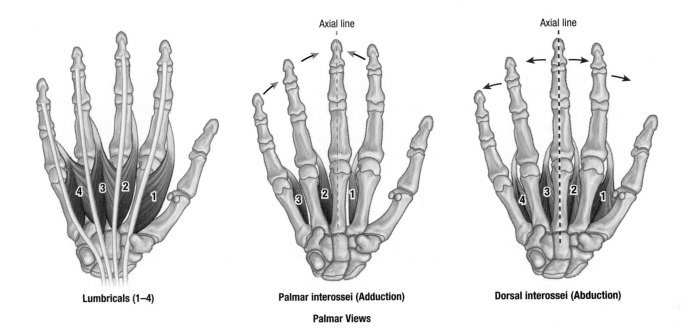

Lumbricals (1–4)   Palmar interossei (Adduction)   Dorsal interossei (Abduction)

Palmar Views

Lumbricals and Interossei

2.77

The lumbricals and interossei are intrinsic muscles of the hand. The actions of the palmar (adduction) and dorsal (abduction) interossei are shown with *arrows*.

TABLE 2.12   Muscles of Hand

Muscle	Proximal Attachment	Distal Attachment	Innervation	Main Actions
Abductor pollicis brevis	Flexor retinaculum and tubercles of scaphoid and trapezium	Lateral side of base of proximal phalanx of thumb	Recurrent branch of median nerve (**C8** and T1)	Abducts thumb and helps oppose it
Flexor pollicis brevis	Flexor retinaculum (transverse carpal ligament) and tubercle of trapezium			Flexes thumb
Opponens pollicis		Lateral side of 1st metacarpal		Opposes thumb toward center of palm and rotates it medially
Adductor pollicis	*Oblique head:* bases of 2nd and 3rd metacarpals, capitate, and adjacent carpal bones *Transverse head:* anterior surface of shaft of 3rd metacarpal	Medial side of base of proximal phalanx of thumb	Deep branch of ulnar nerve (C8 and **T1**)	Adducts thumb toward lateral border of palm
Abductor digiti minimi	Pisiform	Medial side of base of proximal phalanx of digit 5		Abducts digit 5; assists in flexion of its PIP joint
Flexor digiti minimi brevis	Hook of hamate and flexor retinaculum (transverse carpal ligament)			Flexes PIP joint of digit 5
Opponens digiti minimi		Medial border of 5th metacarpal		Draws 5th metacarpal anteriorly and rotates it, bringing digit 5 into opposition with thumb
Lumbricals 1 and 2	Lateral two tendons of flexor digitorum profundus	Lateral sides of extensor expansions of digits 2–5	Median nerve (C8 and **T1**)	Flex MCP joints and extend IP joints of digits 2–5
Lumbricals 3 and 4	Medial three tendons of flexor digitorum profundus			
Dorsal interossei 1–4	Adjacent sides of two metacarpals	Extensor expansions and bases of proximal phalanges of digits 2–4	Deep branch of ulnar nerve (C8 and **T1**)	Abduct 2nd–4th MCP joints; act with lumbricals to flex MCP and extend IP joints
Palmar interossei 1–3	Palmar surfaces of 2nd, 4th, and 5th metacarpals	Extensor expansions of digits and bases of proximal phalanges of digits 2, 4, and 5		Adduct 2nd, 4th, and 5th MCP joints; act with lumbricals to flex MCP and extend IP joints

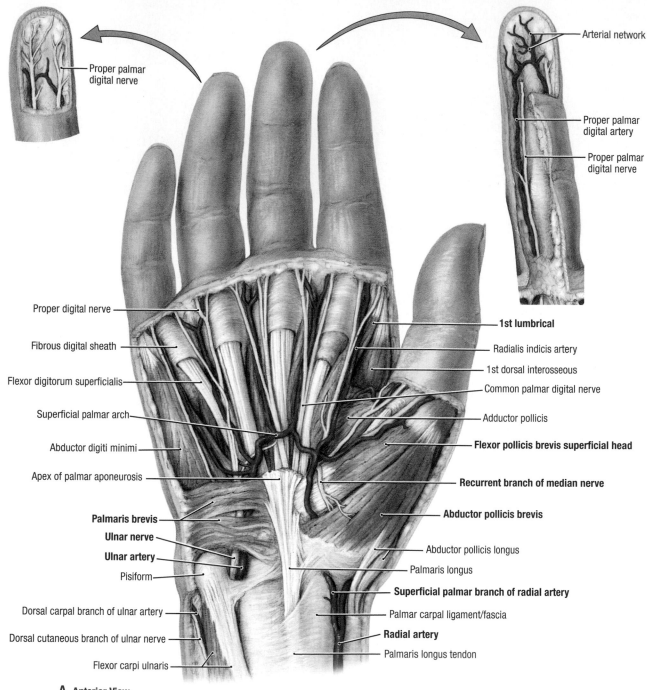

Proper palmar digital nerve

Arterial network

Proper palmar digital artery

Proper palmar digital nerve

Proper digital nerve

Fibrous digital sheath

Flexor digitorum superficialis

Superficial palmar arch

Abductor digiti minimi

Apex of palmar aponeurosis

Palmaris brevis

Ulnar nerve

Ulnar artery

Pisiform

Dorsal carpal branch of ulnar artery

Dorsal cutaneous branch of ulnar nerve

Flexor carpi ulnaris

1st lumbrical

Radialis indicis artery

1st dorsal interosseous

Common palmar digital nerve

Adductor pollicis

Flexor pollicis brevis superficial head

Recurrent branch of median nerve

Abductor pollicis brevis

Abductor pollicis longus

Palmaris longus

Superficial palmar branch of radial artery

Palmar carpal ligament/fascia

Radial artery

Palmaris longus tendon

A. Anterior View

2.78 | Superficial Dissection of Palm, Ulnar, and Median Nerves

A. Superficial palmar arch and digital nerves and vessels.
- The skin, superficial fascia, palmar aponeurosis, and thenar and hypothenar fasciae have been removed.
- The superficial palmar arch is formed by the ulnar artery and completed by the superficial palmar branch of the radial artery.
- The four lumbricals lie posterior to the digital vessels and nerves. The lumbricals arise from the lateral sides of the flexor digitorum profundus tendons and are inserted into the lateral sides of the dorsal expansions of the corresponding digits. The medial two lumbricals are bipennate and also arise from the medial sides of adjacent flexor digitorum profundus tendons.

- In the digits, a proper palmar digital artery and nerve lie on each side of the fibrous digital sheath.
- Note the canal (Guyon) through which the ulnar vessels and nerve pass lateral to the pisiform.

Laceration of palmar (arterial) arches. Bleeding is usually profuse when the palmar (arterial) arches are lacerated. It may not be sufficient to ligate (tie off) only one forearm artery when the arches are lacerated because these vessels usually have numerous communications in the forearm and hand and thus bleed from both ends.

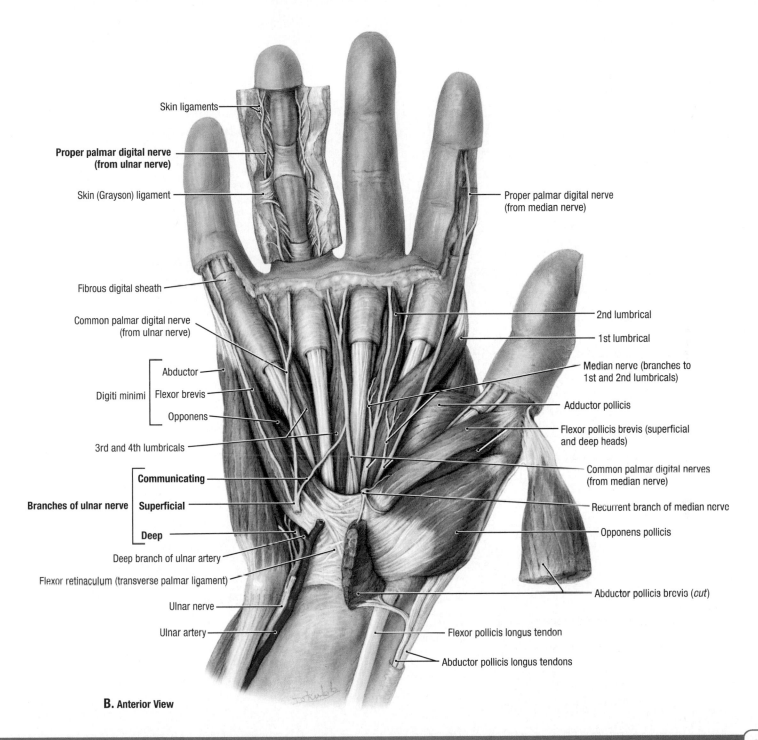

Skin ligaments

Proper palmar digital nerve (from ulnar nerve)

Skin (Grayson) ligament

Fibrous digital sheath

Common palmar digital nerve (from ulnar nerve)

Abductor

Digiti minimi — Flexor brevis

Opponens

3rd and 4th lumbricals

Communicating

Branches of ulnar nerve — **Superficial**

Deep

Deep branch of ulnar artery

Flexor retinaculum (transverse palmar ligament)

Ulnar nerve

Ulnar artery

Proper palmar digital nerve (from median nerve)

2nd lumbrical

1st lumbrical

Median nerve (branches to 1st and 2nd lumbricals)

Adductor pollicis

Flexor pollicis brevis (superficial and deep heads)

Common palmar digital nerves (from median nerve)

Recurrent branch of median nerve

Opponens pollicis

Abductor pollicis brevis (cut)

Flexor pollicis longus tendon

Abductor pollicis longus tendons

B. Anterior View

Superficial Dissection of Palm, Ulnar, and Median Nerves (continued)

2.78

B. Ulnar and median nerves.

Carpal tunnel syndrome results from any lesion that significantly reduces the size of the carpal tunnel or, more commonly, increases the size of some of the structures (or their coverings) that pass through it (e.g., inflammation of the synovial sheaths). The median nerve is the most vulnerable structure in the carpal tunnel. The median nerve has two terminal sensory branches that supply the skin of the hand; hence, paresthesia (tingling), hypoesthesia (diminished sensation), or anesthesia (absence of tactile sensation) may occur in the lateral 3½ digits. However, recall that the palmar cutaneous branch of the median nerve arises proximal

to and does not pass through the carpal tunnel; thus, sensation in the central palm remains unaffected. This nerve also has one terminal motor branch, the recurrent branch, which innervates the three thenar muscles. Wasting of the thenar eminence and progressive loss of coordination and strength in the thumb may occur. To relieve the compression, partial or complete surgical division of the flexor retinaculum, a procedure called **carpal tunnel release,** may be necessary. The incision is made toward the medial side of the wrist and flexor retinaculum to avoid possible injury to the recurrent branch of the median nerve. This procedure is also done laparoscopically.

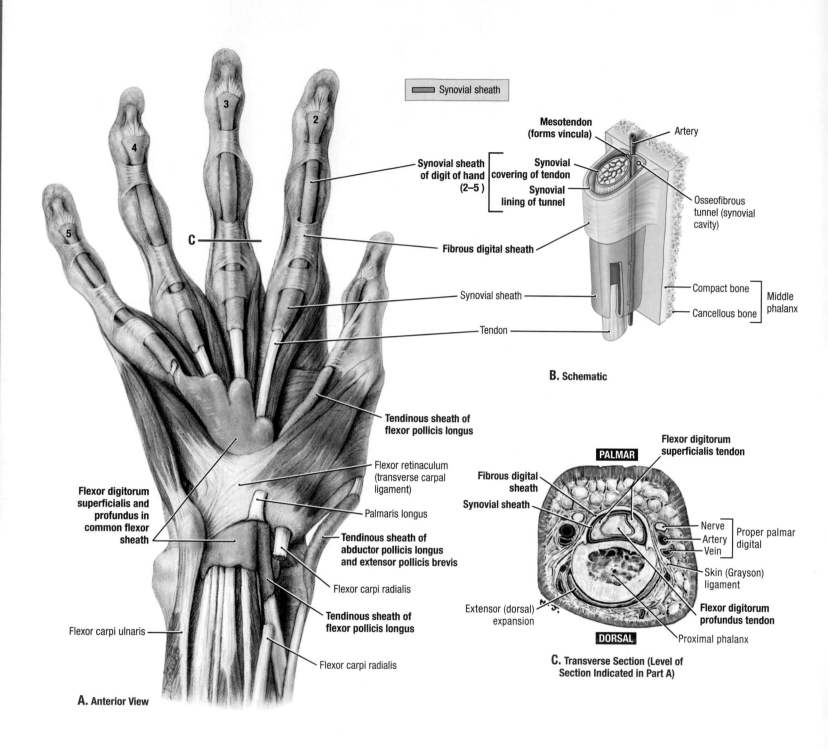

Synovial sheath

Mesotendon (forms vincula)
Artery

Synovial sheath of digit of hand (2–5)
Synovial covering of tendon
Synovial lining of tunnel

Osseofibrous tunnel (synovial cavity)

Fibrous digital sheath

Compact bone
Cancellous bone
Middle phalanx

Synovial sheath

Tendon

B. Schematic

Tendinous sheath of flexor pollicis longus

Flexor retinaculum (transverse carpal ligament)

Palmaris longus

Flexor digitorum superficialis and profundus in common flexor sheath

Tendinous sheath of abductor pollicis longus and extensor pollicis brevis

Flexor carpi radialis

Tendinous sheath of flexor pollicis longus

Flexor carpi ulnaris

Flexor carpi radialis

A. Anterior View

Flexor digitorum superficialis tendon

PALMAR

Fibrous digital sheath

Synovial sheath

Nerve
Artery
Vein
Proper palmar digital

Skin (Grayson) ligament

Extensor (dorsal) expansion

Flexor digitorum profundus tendon

DORSAL

Proximal phalanx

C. Transverse Section (Level of Section Indicated in Part A)

2.79 Synovial Sheaths of Palm of Hand

A. Tendinous (synovial) sheaths of long flexor tendons of digits.
B. Osseofibrous tunnel and tendinous (synovial) sheath.
C. Transverse section through proximal phalanx.

Injuries such as puncture of a finger by a rusty nail can cause **infection of the digital synovial sheaths**. When inflammation of the tendon and synovial sheath (**tenosynovitis**) occurs, the digit swells and movement becomes painful. Because the tendons of the 2nd to 4th digits nearly always have separate synovial sheaths, the infection usually is confined to the infected digits. If the infection is untreated, the proximal ends of these sheaths may rupture, allowing the infection to spread to the midpalmar space. Because the synovial sheath of the little finger is usually continuous with the common flexor sheath, tenosynovitis in this finger may spread to the common flexor sheath and through the palm and carpal tunnel to the anterior forearm. Likewise, tenosynovitis in the thumb may spread through the continuous tendinous sheath of flexor pollicis longus.

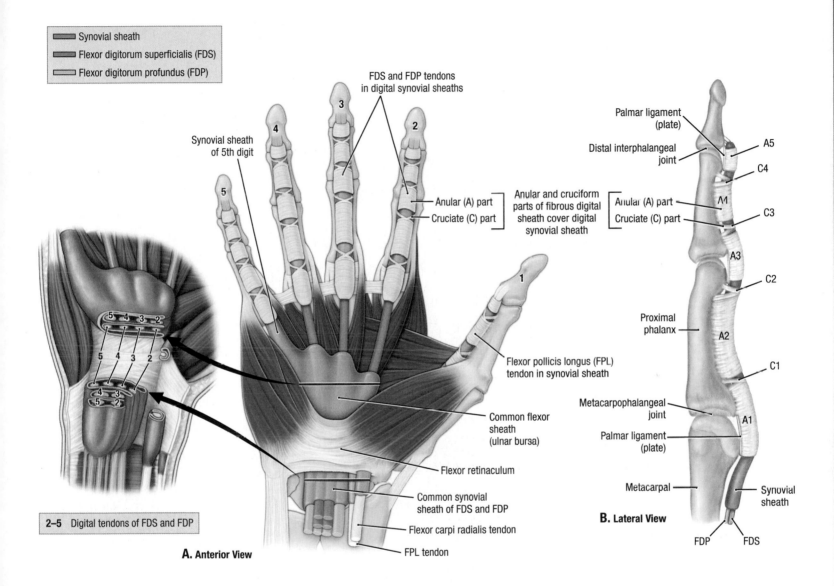

Synovial sheath
Flexor digitorum superficialis (FDS)
Flexor digitorum profundus (FDP)

FDS and FDP tendons
in digital synovial sheaths

Synovial sheath
of 5th digit

Anular (A) part
Cruciate (C) part

Anular and cruciform
parts of fibrous digital
sheath cover digital
synovial sheath

Flexor pollicis longus (FPL)
tendon in synovial sheath

Common flexor
sheath
(ulnar bursa)

Flexor retinaculum

Common synovial
sheath of FDS and FDP

Flexor carpi radialis tendon

FPL tendon

2–5 Digital tendons of FDS and FDP

A. Anterior View

Palmar ligament
(plate)

Distal interphalangeal
joint

A5

C4

Anular (A) part
Cruciate (C) part

M

C3

A3

C2

Proximal
phalanx

A2

C1

Metacarpophalangeal
joint

Palmar ligament
(plate)

A1

Metacarpal

Synovial
sheath

B. Lateral View

FDP   FDS

Fibrous Digital Sheaths   **2.80**

A. Fibrous digital and synovial sheaths. **B.** Anular and cruciate parts
(pulleys) of fibrous digital sheath.

Fibrous digital sheaths are the strong ligamentous tunnels
containing the flexor tendons and their synovial sheaths. The
sheaths extend from the heads of the metacarpals to the bases
of the distal phalanges. These sheaths prevent the tendons from
pulling away from the digits (bowstringing). The fibrous digital
sheaths combine with the bones to form osseofibrous tunnels
through which the tendons pass to reach the digits. The anular and cruciform (cruciate) parts, often referred to clinically as
"pulleys," are thickened reinforcements of the fibrous digital
sheaths.

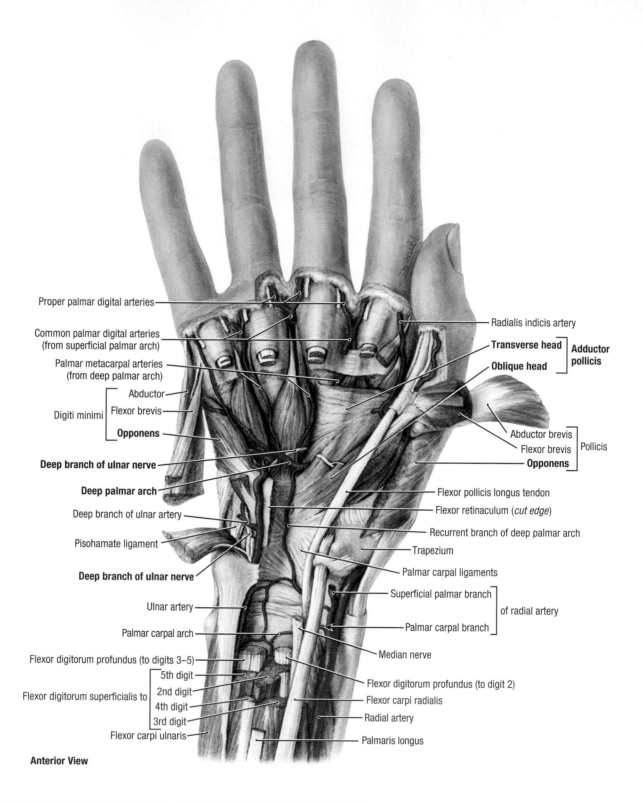

Proper palmar digital arteries

Common palmar digital arteries (from superficial palmar arch)

Palmar metacarpal arteries (from deep palmar arch)

Abductor

Digiti minimi | Flexor brevis

Opponens

Deep branch of ulnar nerve

Deep palmar arch

Deep branch of ulnar artery

Pisohamate ligament

Deep branch of ulnar nerve

Ulnar artery

Palmar carpal arch

Flexor digitorum profundus (to digits 3–5)

Flexor digitorum superficialis to | 5th digit | 2nd digit | 4th digit | 3rd digit

Flexor carpi ulnaris

Radialis indicis artery

Transverse head } **Adductor pollicis**

Oblique head

Abductor brevis } Pollicis
Flexor brevis
Opponens

Flexor pollicis longus tendon

Flexor retinaculum (*cut edge*)

Recurrent branch of deep palmar arch

Trapezium

Palmar carpal ligaments

Superficial palmar branch } of radial artery

Palmar carpal branch

Median nerve

Flexor digitorum profundus (to digit 2)

Flexor carpi radialis

Radial artery

Palmaris longus

Anterior View

2.81 Deep Dissection of Palm

- The deep branch of the ulnar artery joins the radial artery to form the deep palmar arch.
- The pisohamate ligament is often considered a continuation of the tendon of flexor carpi ulnaris, making the pisiform a sesamoid bone.

Compression of the ulnar nerve may occur at the wrist where it passes between the pisiform and the hook of hamate.

The depression between these bones is converted by the piso-hamate ligament into an osseofibrous ulnar canal. **Ulnar canal syndrome** is manifested by hypoesthesia in the medial one and one half digits and weakness of the intrinsic hand muscles. Clawing of the 4th and 5th digits may occur, but in contrast to proximal nerve injury, their ability to flex the wrist joint is unaffected.

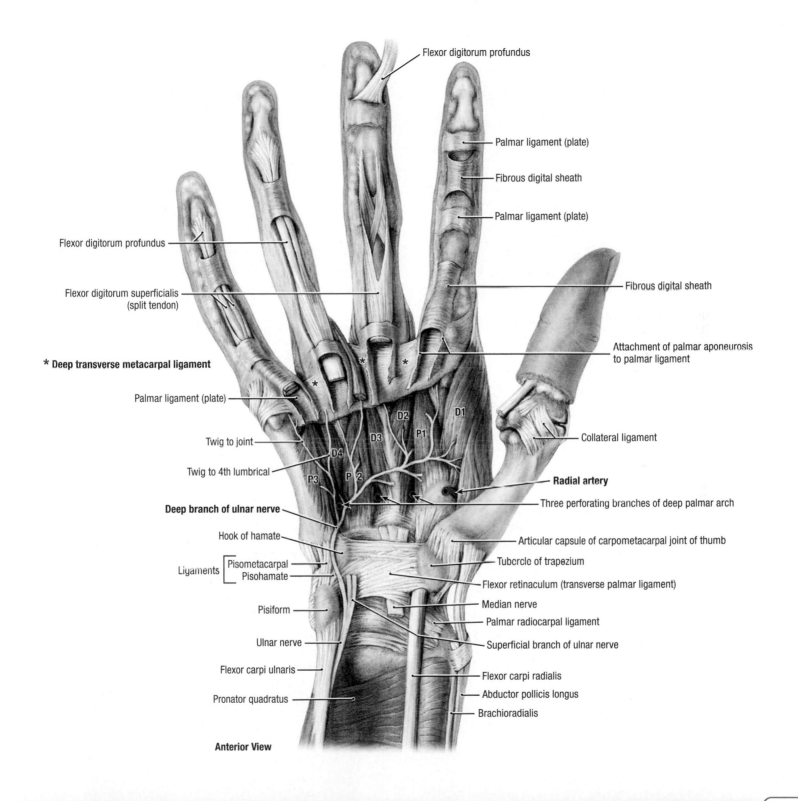

Flexor digitorum profundus

Palmar ligament (plate)

Fibrous digital sheath

Palmar ligament (plate)

Flexor digitorum profundus

Flexor digitorum superficialis
(split tendon)

Fibrous digital sheath

Attachment of palmar aponeurosis
to palmar ligament

* **Deep transverse metacarpal ligament**

Palmar ligament (plate)

D2   D1

D3   P1

Twig to joint

D4

Collateral ligament

Twig to 4th lumbrical

P3   P 2

Radial artery

Deep branch of ulnar nerve

Three perforating branches of deep palmar arch

Hook of hamate

Articular capsule of carpometacarpal joint of thumb

Ligaments [Pisometacarpal
              Pisohamate

Tubercle of trapezium

Flexor retinaculum (transverse palmar ligament)

Pisiform

Median nerve

Palmar radiocarpal ligament

Ulnar nerve

Superficial branch of ulnar nerve

Flexor carpi ulnaris

Flexor carpi radialis

Pronator quadratus

Abductor pollicis longus

Brachioradialis

Anterior View

Deep Dissection of Palm and Digits with Deep Branch of Ulnar Nerve   2.82

- Three unipennate palmar (*P1–P3*) and four bipennate dorsal (*D1–D4*) interosseous muscles are illustrated; the palmar interossei adduct the fingers, and the dorsal interossei abduct the fingers in relation to the axial line, an imaginary line through the long axis of the 3rd digit (see Table 2.12).
- The deep transverse metacarpal ligaments unite the palmar ligaments; the lumbricals pass anterior to the deep transverse metacarpal ligament, and the interossei pass posterior to the ligament.
- The pisohamate and pisometacarpal ligaments form the distal attachment of flexor carpi ulnaris.

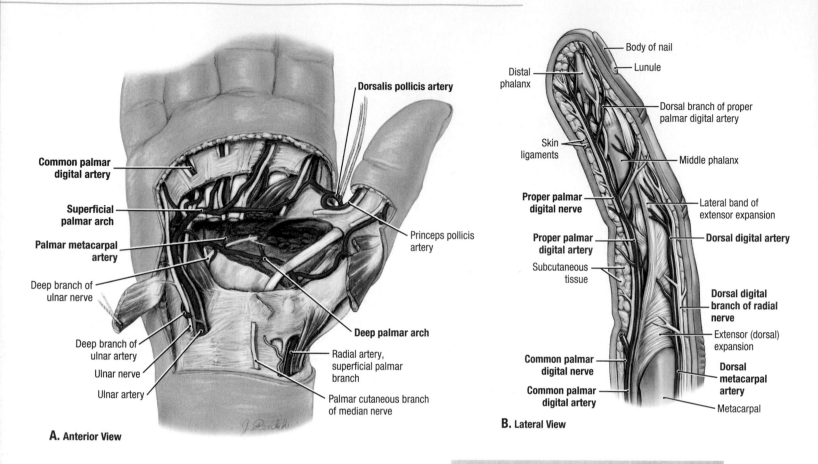

Common palmar digital artery

Superficial palmar arch

Palmar metacarpal artery

Deep branch of ulnar nerve

Deep branch of ulnar artery

Ulnar nerve

Ulnar artery

Dorsalis pollicis artery

Princeps pollicis artery

Deep palmar arch

Radial artery, superficial palmar branch

Palmar cutaneous branch of median nerve

A. Anterior View

Body of nail

Lunule

Distal phalanx

Dorsal branch of proper palmar digital artery

Skin ligaments

Middle phalanx

Proper palmar digital nerve

Lateral band of extensor expansion

Proper palmar digital artery

Dorsal digital artery

Subcutaneous tissue

Dorsal digital branch of radial nerve

Common palmar digital nerve

Extensor (dorsal) expansion

Common palmar digital artery

Dorsal metacarpal artery

Metacarpal

B. Lateral View

2.83   Arterial Supply of Hand (I)

A. Dissection of palmar arterial arches. **B.** Digital vessels and nerves. **C.** Arteriogram of hand.

Note that the superficial palmar arch is usually completed by the superficial palmar branch of the radial artery, but in this specimen, the dorsalis pollicis artery completes the arch.

The **superficial and deep palmar (arterial) arches** are not palpable, but their surface markings are visible. The superficial palmar arch occurs at the level of the distal border of the fully extended thumb. The deep palmar arch lies approximately 1 cm proximal to the superficial palmar arch. The location of these arches should be borne in mind in wounds of the palm and when palmar incisions are made.

Intermittent bilateral attacks of **ischemia of the digits**, marked by cyanosis and often accompanied by paresthesia and pain, are characteristically brought on by cold and emotional stimuli. The condition may result from an anatomical abnormality or an underlying disease. When the cause of the condition is idiopathic (unknown) or primary, it is called **Raynaud syndrome** (disease). Since arteries receive innervation from postsynaptic fibers from the sympathetic ganglia, it may be necessary to perform a cervicodorsal presynaptic sympathectomy to dilate the digital arteries.

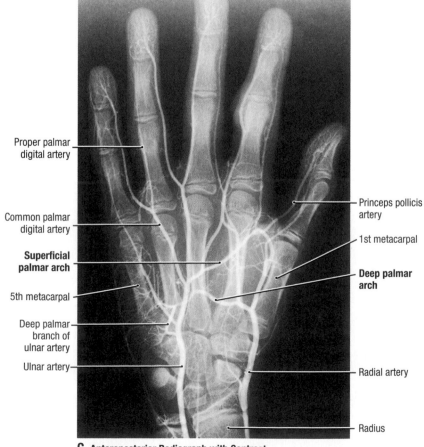

Proper palmar digital artery

Common palmar digital artery

Superficial palmar arch

5th metacarpal

Deep palmar branch of ulnar artery

Ulnar artery

Princeps pollicis artery

1st metacarpal

Deep palmar arch

Radial artery

Radius

C. Anteroposterior Radiograph with Contrast

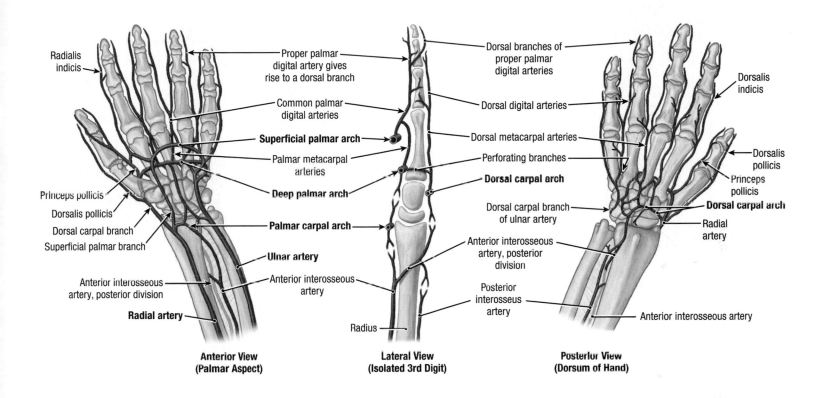

Radialis indicis

Proper palmar digital artery gives rise to a dorsal branch

Common palmar digital arteries

Superficial palmar arch

Palmar metacarpal arteries

Deep palmar arch

Princeps pollicis

Dorsalis pollicis

Dorsal carpal branch

Superficial palmar branch

Palmar carpal arch

Ulnar artery

Anterior interosseous artery, posterior division

Anterior interosseous artery

Radial artery

Anterior View (Palmar Aspect)

Dorsal branches of proper palmar digital arteries

Dorsal digital arteries

Dorsal metacarpal arteries

Perforating branches

Dorsal carpal arch

Dorsal carpal branch of ulnar artery

Anterior interosseous artery, posterior division

Posterior interosseus artery

Radius

Lateral View (Isolated 3rd Digit)

Dorsalis indicis

Dorsalis pollicis

Princeps pollicis

Dorsal carpal arch

Radial artery

Anterior interosseous artery

Posterior View (Dorsum of Hand)

Arterial Supply of Hand (II)	**2.84**

Since hand is placed and held in many different positions, it requires an abundance of highly branched and anastomosing arteries so that oxygenated blood is available in all positions.

TABLE 2.13   Arteries of Hand

Artery	Origin	Course
Superficial palmar arch	Direct continuation of ulnar artery; arch is completed on lateral side by superficial branch of radial artery or another of its branches	Curves laterally deep to palmar aponeurosis and superficial to long flexor tendons; curve of arch lies across palm at level of distal border of extended thumb
Deep palmar arch	Direct continuation of radial artery; arch is completed on medial side by deep branch of ulnar artery	Curves medially, deep to long flexor tendons and is in contact with bases of metacarpals
Common palmar digital	Superficial palmar arch	Pass directly on lumbricals to webbings of digits
Proper palmar digital	Common palmar digital arteries	Run along sides of digits 2–5
Princeps pollicis	Radial artery as it turns into palm	Descends on palmar aspect of 1st metacarpal and divides at the base of proximal phalanx into two branches that run along sides of thumb
Radialis indicis	Radial artery but may arise from princeps pollicis artery	Passes along lateral side of index finger to its distal end
Dorsal carpal arch	Radial and ulnar arteries	Arches within fascia on dorsum of hand

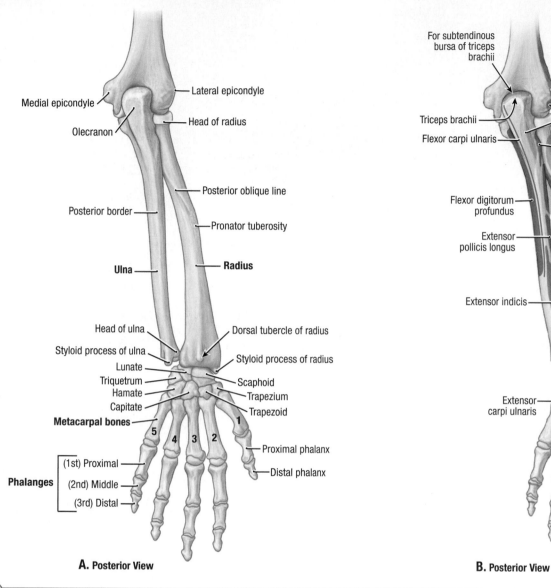

Medial epicondyle

Lateral epicondyle

Olecranon

Head of radius

Posterior oblique line

Posterior border

Pronator tuberosity

Ulna

Radius

Head of ulna

Dorsal tubercle of radius

Styloid process of ulna

Styloid process of radius

Lunate

Triquetrum

Scaphoid

Hamate

Trapezium

Capitate

Trapezoid

Metacarpal bones

5   4   3   2   1

Proximal phalanx

Distal phalanx

Phalanges

(1st) Proximal

(2nd) Middle

(3rd) Distal

A. Posterior View

For subtendinous bursa of triceps brachii

Common extensor origin

Triceps brachii

Anconeus

Flexor carpi ulnaris

Supinator

Flexor digitorum profundus

Extensor pollicis longus

Pronator teres

Abductor pollicis longus

Extensor indicis

Extensor pollicis brevis

Brachioradialis

Extensor carpi radialis brevis

Extensor carpi ulnaris

Extensor carpi radialis longus

Extensor pollicis brevis

Extensor pollicis longus

Extensor (dorsal) expansion

B. Posterior View

2.85   Bones and Muscle Attachments on Posterior Forearm and Hand

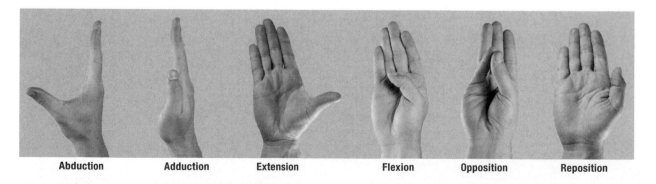

Abduction   Adduction   Extension   Flexion   Opposition   Reposition

2.86   Movements of Thumb

The thumb is rotated 90 degrees compared to the other digits. Abduction and adduction at the MCP joint occur in a sagittal plane; flexion and extension at the MCP and IP joints occur in frontal planes, opposite to these movements at other joints.

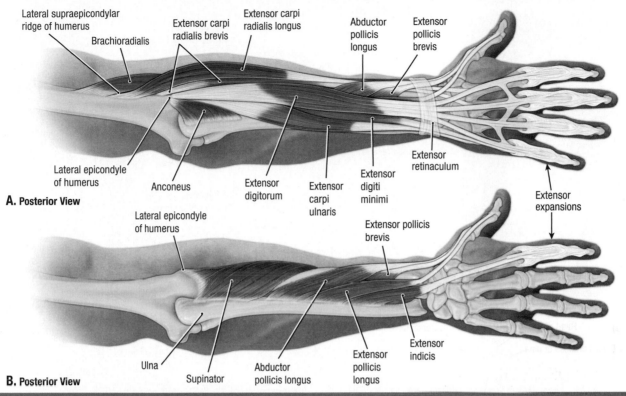

A. Posterior View

B. Posterior View

Muscles of Posterior Forearm

2.87

A. Superficial dissection. **B.** Deep dissection.

TABLE 2.14	Muscles of Posterior Surface of Forearm			
Muscle	**Proximal Attachment**	**Distal Attachment**	**Innervation**	**Main Actions**
Brachioradialis	Proximal two thirds of lateral supraepicondylar ridge of humerus	Lateral surface of distal end of radius	Radial nerve (C5, **C6**, and C7)	Flexes elbow joint
Extensor carpi radialis longus	Lateral supraepicondylar ridge of humerus	Base of 2nd metacarpal bone	Radial nerve (C6–C7)	Extend and abduct wrist joint
Extensor carpi radialis brevis		Base of 3rd metacarpal bone	Deep branch of radial nerve (**C7** and C8)	
Extensor digitorum	Lateral epicondyle of humerus	Extensor expansions of medial four digits	Posterior interosseous nerve (C7–C8), a branch of the radial nerve	Extends medial four metacarpophalangeal joints; extends wrist joint
Extensor digiti minimi		Extensor expansion of 5th digit		Extends MCP and IP joints of 5th digit; extends wrist joint
Extensor carpi ulnaris	Lateral epicondyle of humerus and posterior border of ulna	Base of 5th metacarpal bone		Extends and adducts wrist joint
Anconeus	Lateral epicondyle of humerus	Lateral surface of olecranon and superior part of posterior surface of ulna	Radial nerve (C7–C8 and T1)	Assists triceps brachii in extending elbow joint; stabilizes elbow joint; abducts ulna during pronation
Supinator	Lateral epicondyle of humerus, radial collateral and anular ligaments, supinator fossa, and crest of ulna	Lateral, posterior, and anterior surfaces of proximal third of radius	Deep branch of radial nerve (C6 and **C7**)	Supinates forearm
Abductor pollicis longus	Posterior surface of ulna, radius, and interosseous membrane	Base of 1st metacarpal bone	Posterior interosseous nerve (C7 and **C8**)	Abducts and extends carpometacarpal joint of thumb
Extensor pollicis brevis	Posterior surface of radius and interosseous membrane	Base of proximal phalanx of thumb		Extends MCP joint of thumb; extends wrist joint
Extensor pollicis longus	Posterior surface of middle third of ulna and interosseous membrane	Base of distal phalanx of thumb		Extends MCP and IP joints of thumb; extends wrist joint
Extensor indicis	Posterior surface of ulna and interosseous membrane	Extensor expansion of 2nd digit		Extends MCP and IP joints of 2nd digit; extends wrist joint

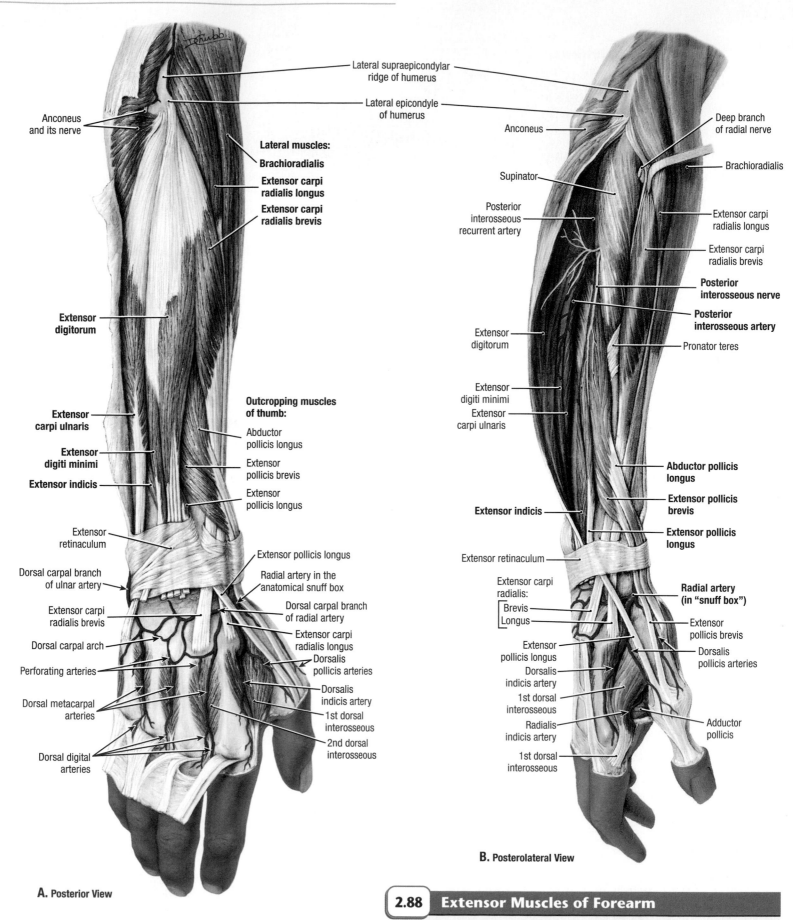

Lateral supraepicondylar ridge of humerus

Lateral epicondyle of humerus

Anconeus and its nerve

Lateral muscles:

Brachioradialis

Extensor carpi radialis longus

Extensor carpi radialis brevis

Extensor digitorum

Outcropping muscles of thumb:

Abductor pollicis longus

Extensor carpi ulnaris

Extensor pollicis brevis

Extensor digiti minimi

Extensor indicis

Extensor pollicis longus

Extensor retinaculum

Dorsal carpal branch of ulnar artery

Extensor pollicis longus

Radial artery in the anatomical snuff box

Dorsal carpal branch of radial artery

Extensor carpi radialis brevis

Extensor carpi radialis longus

Dorsal carpal arch

Dorsalis pollicis arteries

Perforating arteries

Dorsalis indicis artery

Dorsal metacarpal arteries

1st dorsal interosseous

2nd dorsal interosseous

Dorsal digital arteries

A. Posterior View

Anconeus

Deep branch of radial nerve

Supinator

Brachioradialis

Posterior interosseous recurrent artery

Extensor carpi radialis longus

Extensor carpi radialis brevis

Posterior interosseous nerve

Posterior interosseous artery

Extensor digitorum

Pronator teres

Extensor digiti minimi

Extensor carpi ulnaris

Abductor pollicis longus

Extensor pollicis brevis

Extensor indicis

Extensor pollicis longus

Extensor retinaculum

Extensor carpi radialis:
  Brevis
  Longus

Radial artery (in "snuff box")

Extensor pollicis longus

Extensor pollicis brevis

Dorsalis pollicis arteries

Dorsalis indicis artery

1st dorsal interosseous

Radialis indicis artery

Adductor pollicis

1st dorsal interosseous

B. Posterolateral View

2.88 **Extensor Muscles of Forearm**

A. Superficial dissection. **B.** Deep dissection.

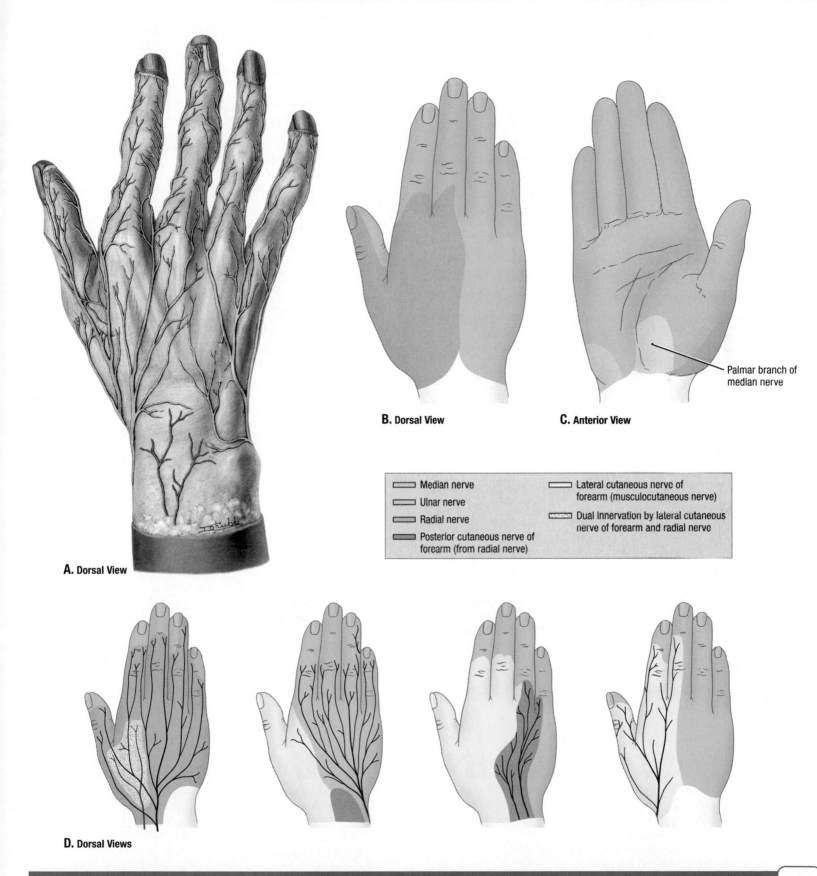

A. Dorsal View

B. Dorsal View

C. Anterior View

Palmar branch of median nerve

☐ Median nerve

☐ Ulnar nerve

☐ Radial nerve

☐ Posterior cutaneous nerve of forearm (from radial nerve)

☐ Lateral cutaneous nerve of forearm (musculocutaneous nerve)

☐ Dual innervation by lateral cutaneous nerve of forearm and radial nerve

D. Dorsal Views

Cutaneous Innervation of Hand   **2.89**

A. Dissection of nerves of dorsum of hand. **B.** and **C.** Distribution of cutaneous nerves to palm and dorsum of hand. **D.** Variations in pattern of cutaneous nerves in dorsum of hand.

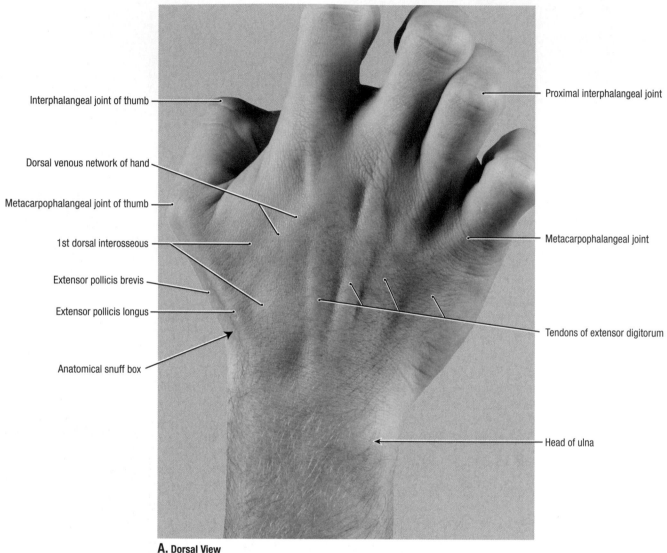

Interphalangeal joint of thumb

Dorsal venous network of hand

Metacarpophalangeal joint of thumb

1st dorsal interosseous

Extensor pollicis brevis

Extensor pollicis longus

Anatomical snuff box

Proximal interphalangeal joint

Metacarpophalangeal joint

Tendons of extensor digitorum

Head of ulna

A. Dorsal View

| 2.90 | **Dorsum of Hand** |

A. Surface anatomy. The interphalangeal joints are flexed, and the metacarpophalangeal joints are hyperextended to demonstrate the extensor digitorum tendons. **B. Tendinous (synovial) sheaths distended with blue fluid. C. Transverse section of distal forearm.** Numbers refer to structures in *Part B*. **D. Sites of bony attachments.**

- Six tendinous sheaths occupy the six osseofibrous tunnels deep to the extensor retinaculum. They contain nine tendons: tendons for the thumb in sheaths 1 and 3, tendons for the extensors of the wrist in sheaths 2 and 6, and tendons for the extensors of the wrist and fingers in sheaths 4 and 5.

- The tendon of the extensor pollicis longus hooks around the dorsal tubercle of radius to pass obliquely across the tendons of the extensor carpi radialis longus and brevis to the thumb.

The tendons of the abductor pollicis longus and extensor pollicis brevis are in the same tendinous sheath on the dorsum of the wrist. Excessive friction of these tendons results in fibrous thickening of the sheath and stenosis of the osseofibrous tunnel, **Quervain tenovaginitis stenosans**. This condition causes pain in the wrist that radiates proximally to the forearm and distally to the thumb.

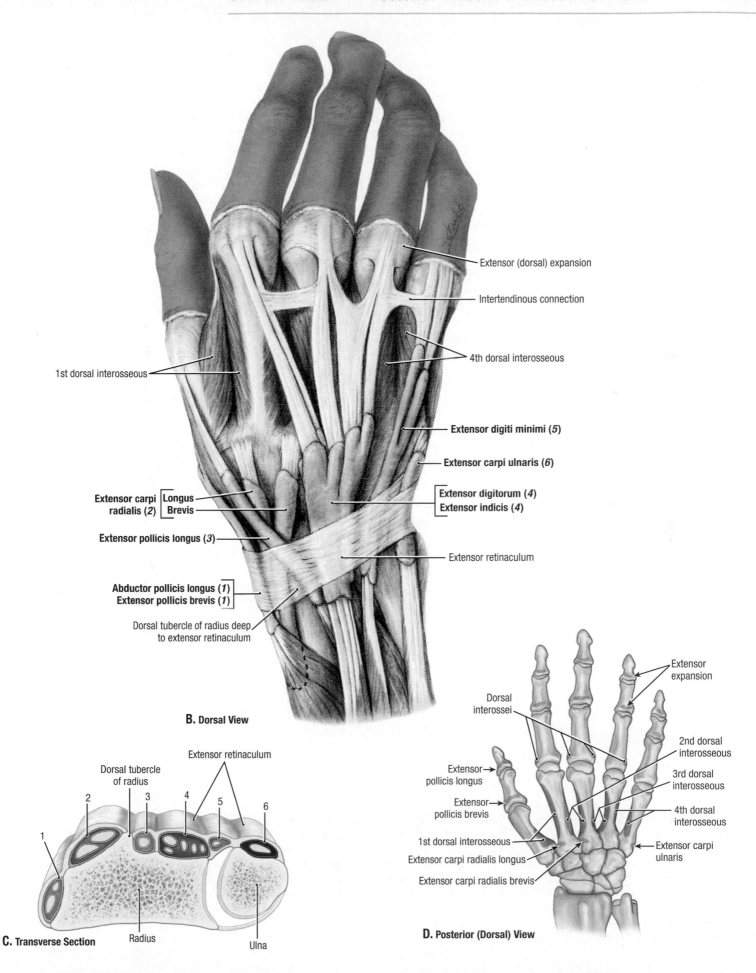

Extensor (dorsal) expansion

Intertendinous connection

4th dorsal interosseous

1st dorsal interosseous

Extensor digiti minimi (5)

Extensor carpi ulnaris (6)

Extensor carpi [Longus
radialis (2)] [Brevis]

Extensor digitorum (4)
Extensor indicis (4)

Extensor pollicis longus (3)

Extensor retinaculum

Abductor pollicis longus (1)
Extensor pollicis brevis (1)

Dorsal tubercle of radius deep
to extensor retinaculum

B. Dorsal View

Extensor retinaculum

Dorsal tubercle
of radius

2   3   4   5   6

1

C. Transverse Section   Radius   Ulna

Extensor
expansion

Dorsal
interossei

2nd dorsal
interosseous

Extensor→
pollicis longus

3rd dorsal
interosseous

Extensor→
pollicis brevis

4th dorsal
interosseous

1st dorsal interosseous

Extensor carpi radialis longus

Extensor carpi radialis brevis

Extensor carpi
ulnaris

D. Posterior (Dorsal) View

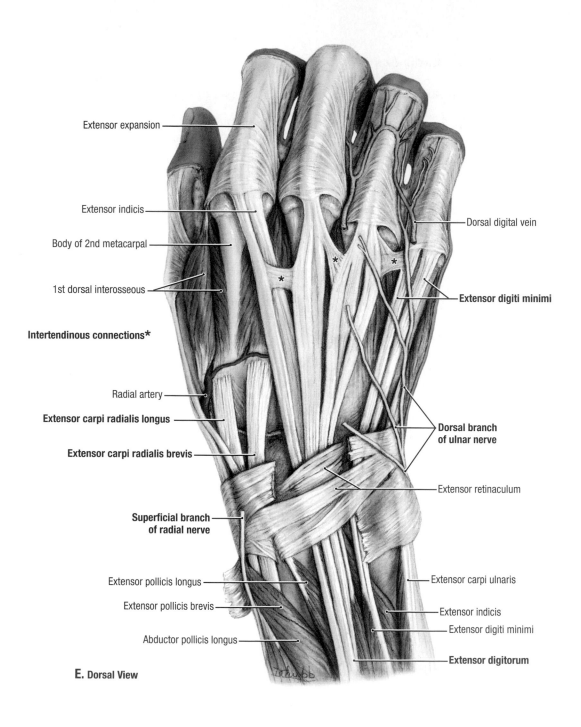

Extensor expansion

Extensor indicis

Body of 2nd metacarpal

1st dorsal interosseous

Intertendinous connections*

Radial artery

Extensor carpi radialis longus

Extensor carpi radialis brevis

Superficial branch of radial nerve

Extensor pollicis longus

Extensor pollicis brevis

Abductor pollicis longus

Dorsal digital vein

Extensor digiti minimi

Dorsal branch of ulnar nerve

Extensor retinaculum

Extensor carpi ulnaris

Extensor indicis

Extensor digiti minimi

Extensor digitorum

E. Dorsal View

2.90 **Dorsum of Hand** (continued)

E. Tendons on dorsum of hand and extensor retinaculum.
- The deep fascia is thickened to form the extensor retinaculum.
- Proximal to the knuckles, intertendinous connections extend between the tendons of the digital extensors and, thereby, restrict the independent action of the fingers.

Ganglion cyst. Sometimes a nontender cystic swelling appears on the hand, most commonly on the dorsum of the wrist.

The thin-walled cyst contains clear mucinous fluid. Clinically, this type of swelling is called a ganglion (a swelling or knot). These synovial cysts are close to and often communicate with the synovial sheaths. The distal attachment of the extensor carpi radialis brevis tendon is a common site for such a cyst.

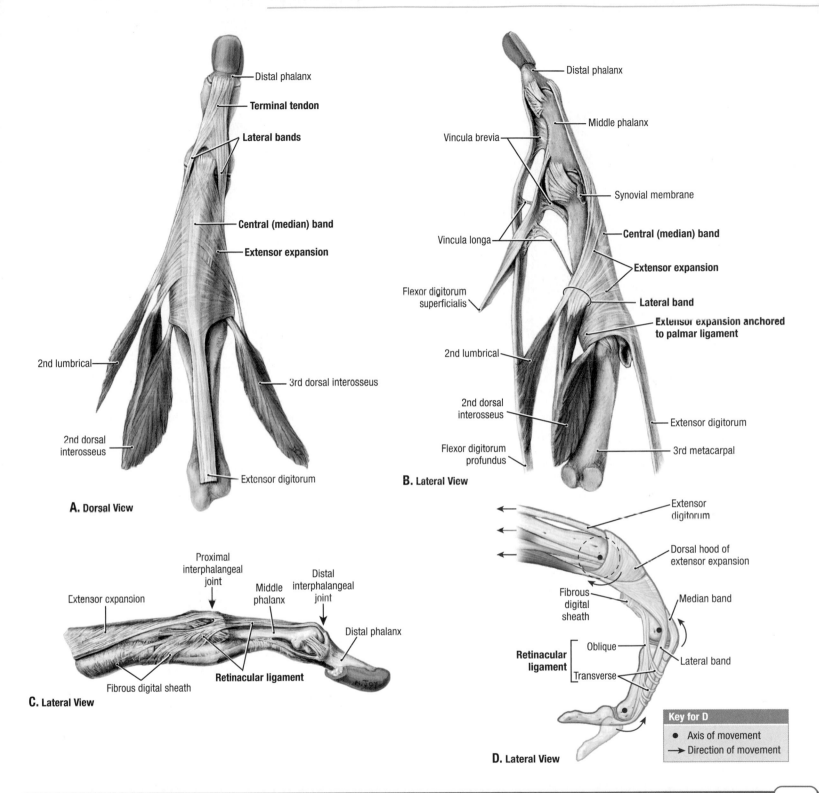

Distal phalanx

Terminal tendon

Lateral bands

Central (median) band

Extensor expansion

2nd lumbrical

3rd dorsal interosseus

2nd dorsal interosseus

Extensor digitorum

A. Dorsal View

Distal phalanx

Middle phalanx

Vincula brevia

Synovial membrane

Central (median) band

Vincula longa

Extensor expansion

Flexor digitorum superficialis

Lateral band

Extensor expansion anchored to palmar ligament

2nd lumbrical

2nd dorsal interosseus

Flexor digitorum profundus

Extensor digitorum

3rd metacarpal

B. Lateral View

Proximal interphalangeal joint

Distal interphalangeal joint

Middle phalanx

Extensor expansion

Distal phalanx

Retinacular ligament

Fibrous digital sheath

C. Lateral View

Extensor digitorum

Dorsal hood of extensor expansion

Fibrous digital sheath

Median band

Retinacular ligament Oblique

Lateral band

Transverse

Key for D
● Axis of movement
→ Direction of movement

D. Lateral View

Extensor (Dorsal) Expansion of Third Digit

2.91

A. Dorsal aspect of digit. **B.** Lateral aspect of digit. **C.** Retinacular ligaments of extended digit. **D.** Retinacular ligaments of flexed digit.

- The hood covering the head of the metacarpal is attached to the palmar ligament.
- Contraction of the muscles attaching to the lateral band will produce flexion of the metacarpophalangeal joint and extension of the interphalangeal joints.

- The retinacular ligament is a fibrous band that runs from the proximal phalanx and fibrous digital sheath obliquely across the middle phalanx and two interphalangeal joints to join the extensor (dorsal) expansion and then to the distal phalanx.
- On flexion of the distal interphalangeal joint, the retinacular ligament becomes taut and pulls the proximal joint into flexion; on extension of the proximal joint, the distal joint is pulled by the ligament into nearly complete extension.

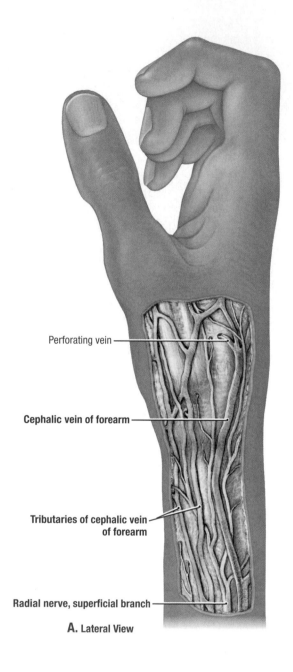

Perforating vein

Cephalic vein of forearm

Tributaries of cephalic vein of forearm

Radial nerve, superficial branch

A. Lateral View

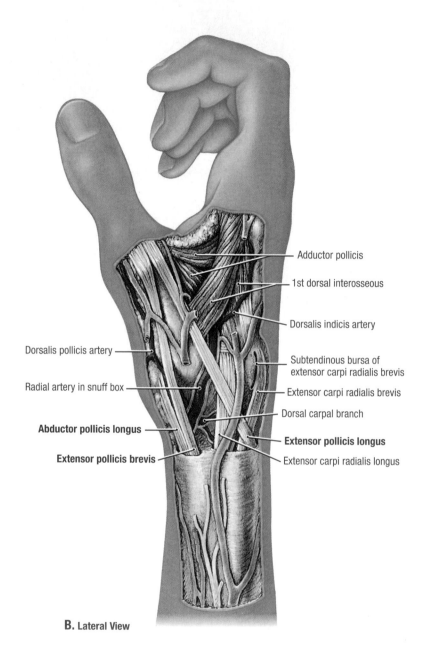

Adductor pollicis

1st dorsal interosseous

Dorsalis indicis artery

Dorsalis pollicis artery

Subtendinous bursa of extensor carpi radialis brevis

Extensor carpi radialis brevis

Radial artery in snuff box

Dorsal carpal branch

Abductor pollicis longus

Extensor pollicis longus

Extensor pollicis brevis

Extensor carpi radialis longus

B. Lateral View

2.92   **Lateral Wrist and Hand**

A. Anatomical snuff box (I).
- The depression at the base of the thumb, the "anatomical snuff box," retains its name from an archaic habit.
- Note the superficial veins, including the cephalic vein of forearm and/or its tributaries, and cutaneous nerves crossing the snuff box.

B. Anatomical snuff box (II).
- Three long tendons of the thumb form the boundaries of the snuff box; the extensor pollicis longus forms the medial boundary and the abductor pollicis longus and extensor pollicis brevis the lateral boundary.
- The radial artery crosses the floor of the snuff box and travels between the two heads of the 1st dorsal interosseous.

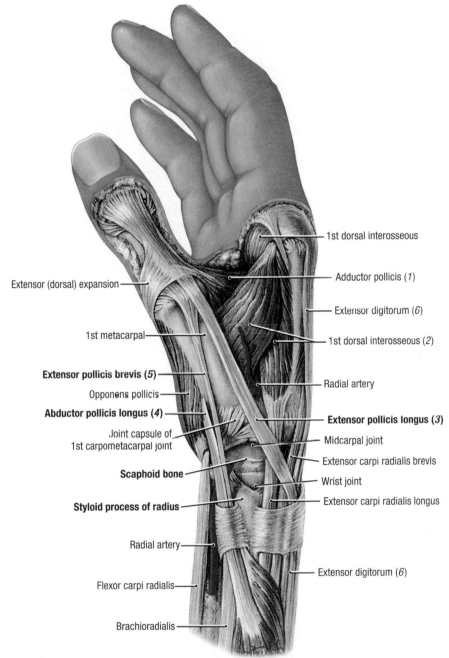

1st dorsal interosseous

Extensor (dorsal) expansion

Adductor pollicis (*1*)

Extensor digitorum (*6*)

1st metacarpal

1st dorsal interosseous (*2*)

Extensor pollicis brevis (*5*)

Opponens pollicis

Radial artery

Abductor pollicis longus (*4*)

Extensor pollicis longus (*3*)

Joint capsule of
1st carpometacarpal joint

Midcarpal joint

Extensor carpi radialis brevis

Scaphoid bone

Wrist joint

Styloid process of radius

Extensor carpi radialis longus

Radial artery

Flexor carpi radialis

Extensor digitorum (*6*)

Brachioradialis

C. Lateral View

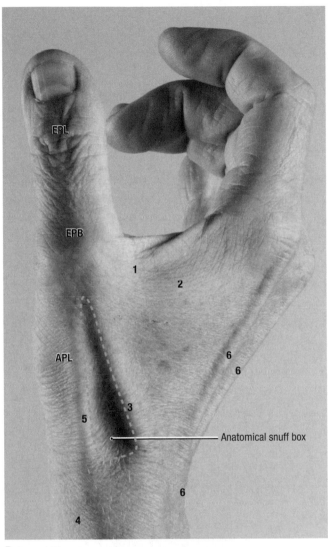

D. Lateral View

Distal Extent of	
APL	Abductor pollicis longus
EPB	Extensor pollicis brevis
EPL	Extensor pollicis longus

Lateral Wrist and Hand (*continued*)

C. Anatomical snuff box (III). Note the scaphoid bone, the wrist joint proximal to the scaphoid, and the midcarpal joint distal to it.
D. Surface anatomy.
   Fracture of the scaphoid often results from a fall on the palm with the hand abducted. The fracture occurs across the narrow part ("waist") of the scaphoid. Pain occurs primarily on the lateral side of the wrist, especially during dorsiflexion and abduction of the hand.

Initial radiographs of the wrist may not reveal a fracture, but radiographs taken 10 to 14 days later reveal a fracture because bone resorption has occurred. Owing to the poor blood supply to the proximal part of the scaphoid, union of the fractured parts may take several months. **Avascular necrosis of the proximal fragment of the scaphoid** (pathological death of bone resulting from poor blood supply) may occur and produce degenerative joint disease of the wrist.

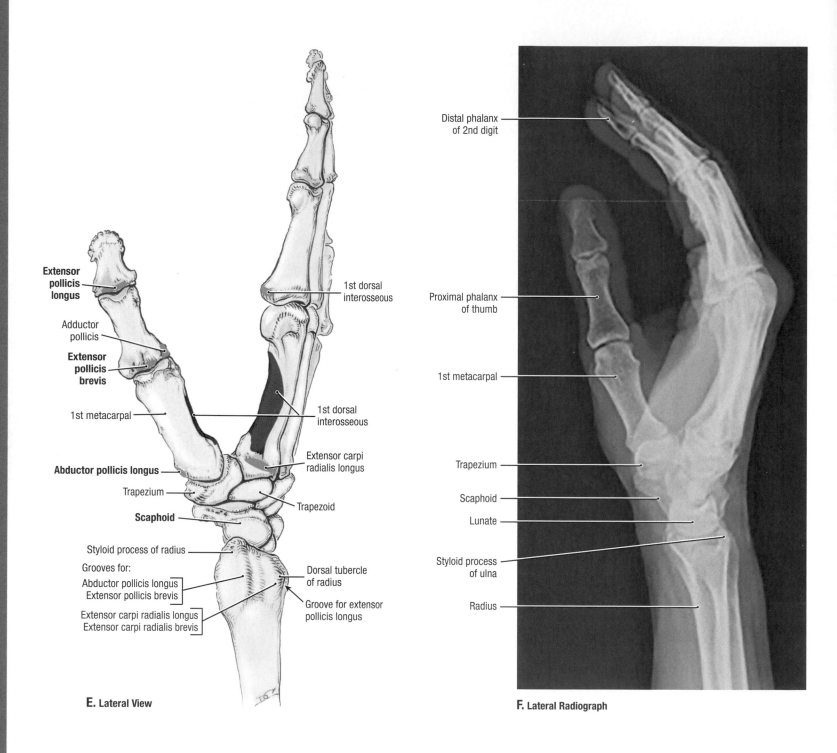

Extensor pollicis longus

Adductor pollicis

Extensor pollicis brevis

1st metacarpal

Abductor pollicis longus

Trapezium

Scaphoid

Styloid process of radius

Grooves for:
Abductor pollicis longus
Extensor pollicis brevis

Extensor carpi radialis longus
Extensor carpi radialis brevis

1st dorsal interosseous

1st dorsal interosseous

Extensor carpi radialis longus

Trapezoid

Dorsal tubercle of radius

Groove for extensor pollicis longus

E. Lateral View

Distal phalanx of 2nd digit

Proximal phalanx of thumb

1st metacarpal

Trapezium

Scaphoid

Lunate

Styloid process of ulna

Radius

F. Lateral Radiograph

2.92   Lateral Wrist and Hand (continued)

E. Bony hand showing muscle attachments. **F.** Bones of hand and wrist.

Note that the anatomical snuff box is limited proximally by the styloid process of the radius and distally by the base of the 1st metacarpal; parts of the two lateral bones of the carpus (scaphoid and trapezium) form the floor of the snuff box.

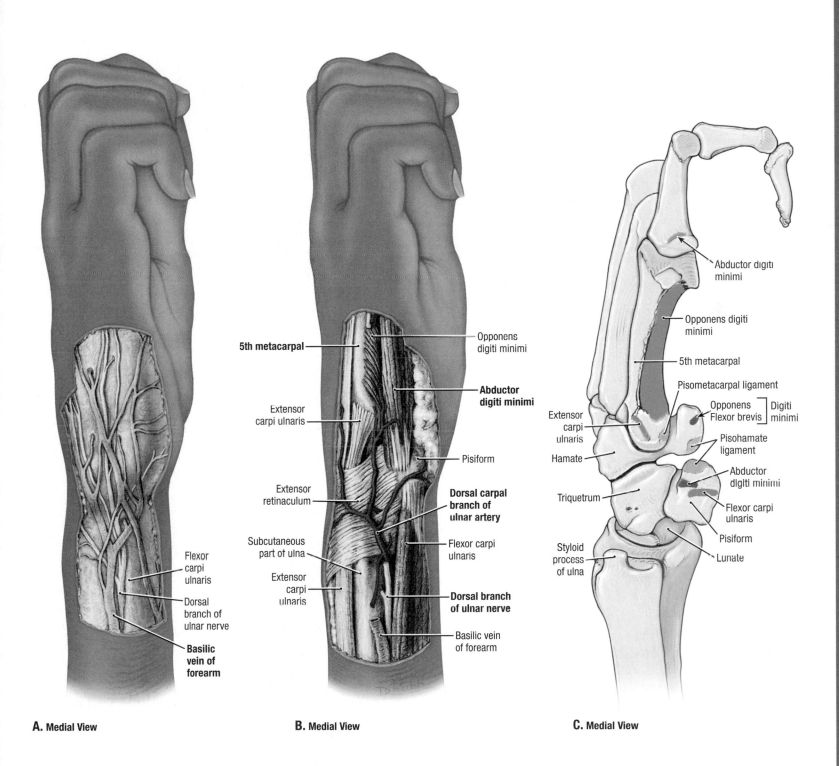

A. Medial View

B. Medial View

C. Medial View

A. Medial View labels:
- Flexor carpi ulnaris
- Dorsal branch of ulnar nerve
- **Basilic vein of forearm**

B. Medial View labels:
- **5th metacarpal**
- Extensor carpi ulnaris
- Extensor retinaculum
- Subcutaneous part of ulna
- Extensor carpi ulnaris
- Opponens digiti minimi
- **Abductor digiti minimi**
- Pisiform
- **Dorsal carpal branch of ulnar artery**
- Flexor carpi ulnaris
- **Dorsal branch of ulnar nerve**
- Basilic vein of forearm

C. Medial View labels:
- Abductor digiti minimi
- Opponens digiti minimi
- 5th metacarpal
- Pisometacarpal ligament
- Opponens / Flexor brevis } Digiti minimi
- Extensor carpi ulnaris
- Pisohamate ligament
- Hamate
- Abductor digiti minimi
- Triquetrum
- Flexor carpi ulnaris
- Pisiform
- Styloid process of ulna
- Lunate

Medial Wrist and Hand

2.93

A. Superficial dissection. **B.** Deep dissection. **C.** Bony hand showing sites of muscular and ligamentous attachments.

The extensor carpi ulnaris is inserted directly into the base of the 5th metacarpal, but the flexor carpi ulnaris inserts indirectly to the base of the 5th metacarpal via the pisiform and pisohamate and pisometacarpal ligaments. These ligaments are often considered to be a part of the distal attachment of flexor carpi ulnaris.

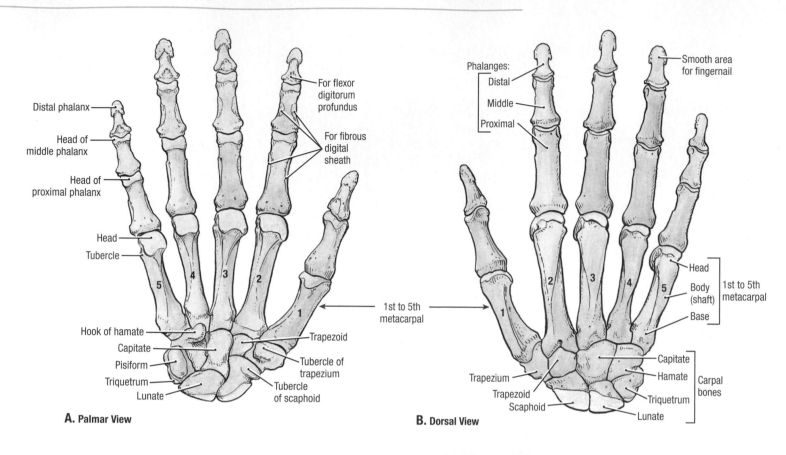

A. Palmar View

Distal phalanx

Head of middle phalanx

Head of proximal phalanx

Head

Tubercle

Hook of hamate

Capitate

Pisiform

Triquetrum

Lunate

For flexor digitorum profundus

For fibrous digital sheath

Trapezoid

Tubercle of trapezium

Tubercle of scaphoid

B. Dorsal View

Phalanges:
Distal
Middle
Proximal

Smooth area for fingernail

Head

Body (shaft)

Base

1st to 5th metacarpal

Capitate

Hamate

Triquetrum

Lunate

Carpal bones

Trapezium

Trapezoid

Scaphoid

1st to 5th metacarpal

2.94 Bones and Imaging of Wrist and Hand

A. Palmar view. **B.** Dorsal view. **C.** Three-dimensional computer-generated image of wrist and hand. Letters refer to structures in *Part D*.

The eight carpal bones form two rows: in the distal row, the hamate, capitate, trapezoid, and trapezium, the trapezium forming a saddle-shaped joint with the 1st metacarpal; and in the proximal row, the scaphoid, lunate, and pisiform, the pisiform being superimposed on the triquetrum.

Severe **crushing injuries of the hand** may produce multiple metacarpal fractures, resulting in instability of the hand. Similar injuries of the distal phalanges are common (e.g., when a finger is caught in a car door). A **fracture of a distal phalanx** is usually comminuted, and a painful **hematoma** (collection of blood) develops. **Fractures of the proximal and middle phalanges** are usually the result of crushing or hypertension injuries.

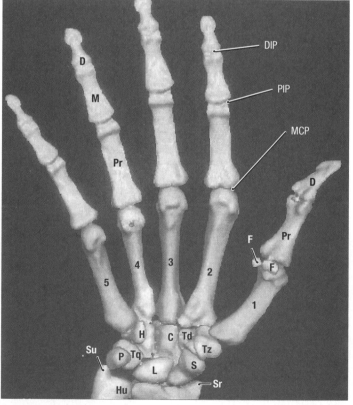

C. Anterior 3D CT Reconstruction

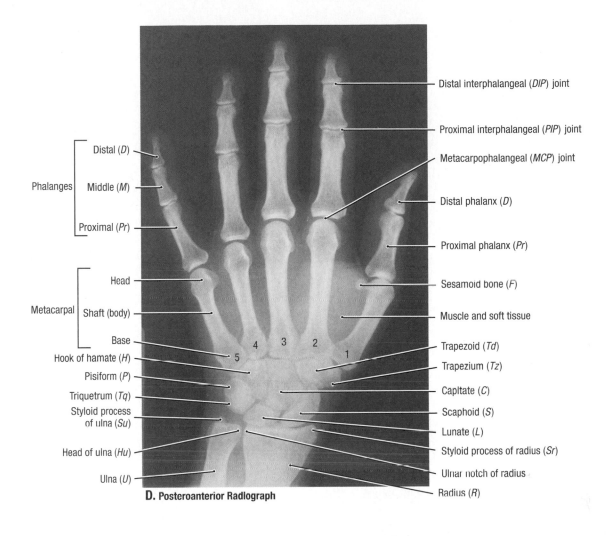

Phalanges
- Distal (*D*)
- Middle (*M*)
- Proximal (*Pr*)

Metacarpal
- Head
- Shaft (body)
- Base

Hook of hamate (*H*)
Pisiform (*P*)
Triquetrum (*Tq*)
Styloid process of ulna (*Su*)
Head of ulna (*Hu*)
Ulna (*U*)

Distal interphalangeal (*DIP*) joint
Proximal interphalangeal (*PIP*) joint
Metacarpophalangeal (*MCP*) joint
Distal phalanx (*D*)
Proximal phalanx (*Pr*)
Sesamoid bone (*F*)
Muscle and soft tissue
Trapezoid (*Td*)
Trapezium (*Tz*)
Capitate (*C*)
Scaphoid (*S*)
Lunate (*L*)
Styloid process of radius (*Sr*)
Ulnar notch of radius
Radius (*R*)

D. Posteroanterior Radiograph

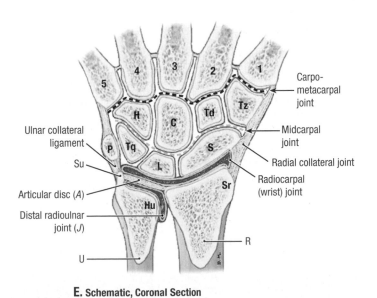

Ulnar collateral ligament
Su
Articular disc (*A*)
Distal radioulnar joint (*J*)
U

Carpo-metacarpal joint
Midcarpal joint
Radial collateral joint
Radiocarpal (wrist) joint

E. Schematic, Coronal Section

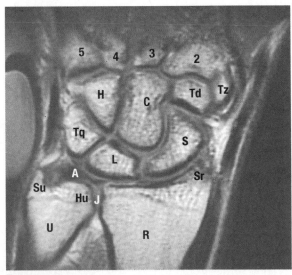

F. Coronal MRI

Bones and Imaging of Wrist and Hand *(continued)*   **2.94**

D. Bones and joints of hand and wrist. **E.** and **F.** Sectional studies of bones and joints of wrist. Letters refer to structures in *Parts D and E.*

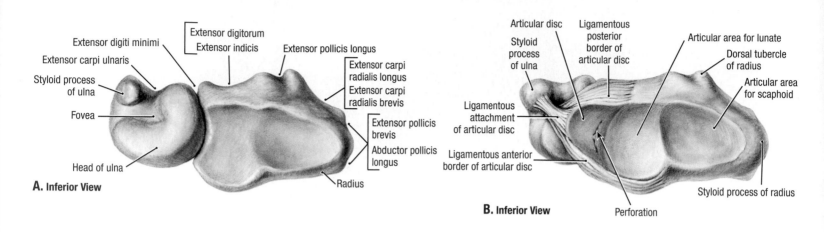

A. Inferior View

Extensor digiti minimi
Extensor carpi ulnaris
Styloid process of ulna
Fovea
Head of ulna
Extensor digitorum
Extensor indicis
Extensor pollicis longus
Extensor carpi radialis longus
Extensor carpi radialis brevis
Extensor pollicis brevis
Abductor pollicis longus
Radius

B. Inferior View

Articular disc
Styloid process of ulna
Ligamentous posterior border of articular disc
Articular area for lunate
Dorsal tubercle of radius
Articular area for scaphoid
Ligamentous attachment of articular disc
Ligamentous anterior border of articular disc
Perforation
Styloid process of radius

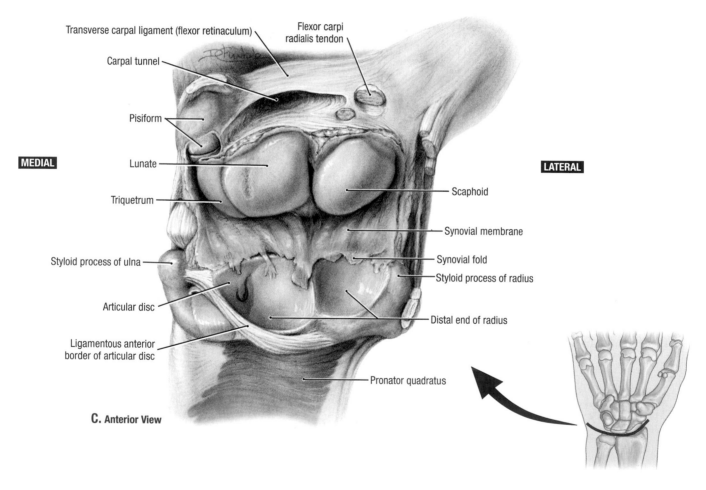

Transverse carpal ligament (flexor retinaculum)
Flexor carpi radialis tendon
Carpal tunnel
Pisiform
Lunate
Triquetrum
Styloid process of ulna
Articular disc
Ligamentous anterior border of articular disc
Scaphoid
Synovial membrane
Synovial fold
Styloid process of radius
Distal end of radius
Pronator quadratus

MEDIAL LATERAL

C. Anterior View

2.95 **Radiocarpal (Wrist) Joint**

A. Distal ends of radius and ulna showing grooves for tendons on posterior aspects. B. Articular disc. The articular disc unites the distal ends of the radius and ulna; it is fibrocartilaginous at the triangular area between the head of the ulna and the lunate bone but ligamentous and pliable elsewhere. The cartilaginous part of the articular disc commonly has a fissure or perforation, as shown here, associated with a roughened surface of the lunate. **C. Articular surface of radiocarpal joint.** The joint is opened anteriorly. The lunate articulates with the radius and articular disc; only during adduction of the wrist does the triquetrum come into articulation with the disc.

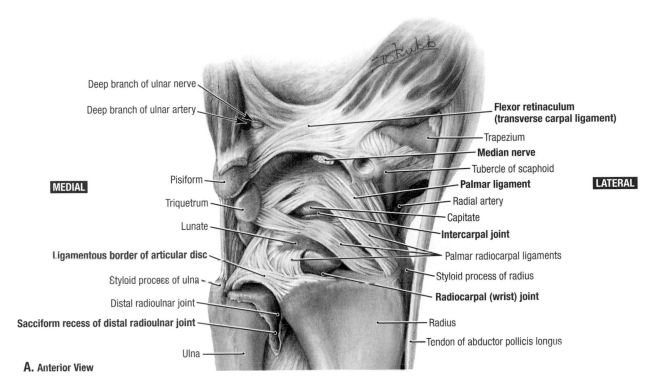

Deep branch of ulnar nerve
Deep branch of ulnar artery
Flexor retinaculum (transverse carpal ligament)
Trapezium
Median nerve
Tubercle of scaphoid
MEDIAL
Pisiform
Palmar ligament
LATERAL
Triquetrum
Radial artery
Lunate
Capitate
Intercarpal joint
Ligamentous border of articular disc
Palmar radiocarpal ligaments
Styloid process of ulna
Styloid process of radius
Distal radioulnar joint
Radiocarpal (wrist) joint
Sacciform recess of distal radioulnar joint
Radius
Tendon of abductor pollicis longus
Ulna

A. Anterior View

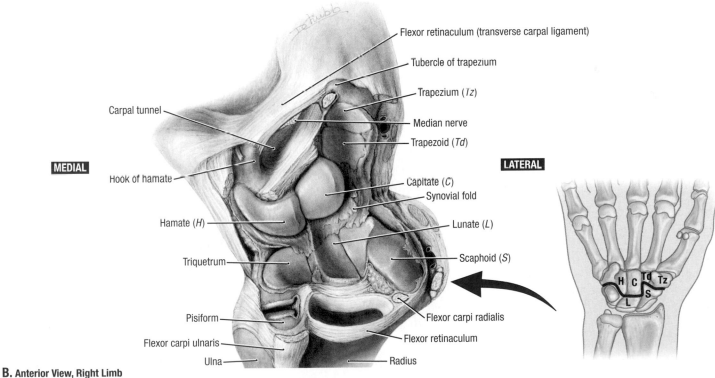

Flexor retinaculum (transverse carpal ligament)
Tubercle of trapezium
Trapezium (*Tz*)
Carpal tunnel
Median nerve
Trapezoid (*Td*)
MEDIAL
LATERAL
Hook of hamate
Capitate (*C*)
Synovial fold
Hamate (*H*)
Lunate (*L*)
Triquetrum
Scaphoid (*S*)
Pisiform
Flexor carpi radialis
Flexor carpi ulnaris
Flexor retinaculum
Ulna
Radius

B. Anterior View, Right Limb

Radiocarpal (Wrist) and Midcarpal (Transverse Carpal) Joint

2.96

A. Ligaments. The hand is forcibly extended. The palmar radiocarpal ligaments pass from the radius to the two rows of carpal bones; they are strong and directed so that the hand moves with the radius during supination. **B. Articular surfaces of midcarpal (transverse carpal) joint, opened anteriorly.**

Note that the flexor retinaculum (transverse carpal ligament) is cut. The proximal part of the ligament, which spans from the pisiform to the scaphoid, is relatively weak; the distal part, which passes from the hook of the hamate to the tubercle of the trapezium, is strong.

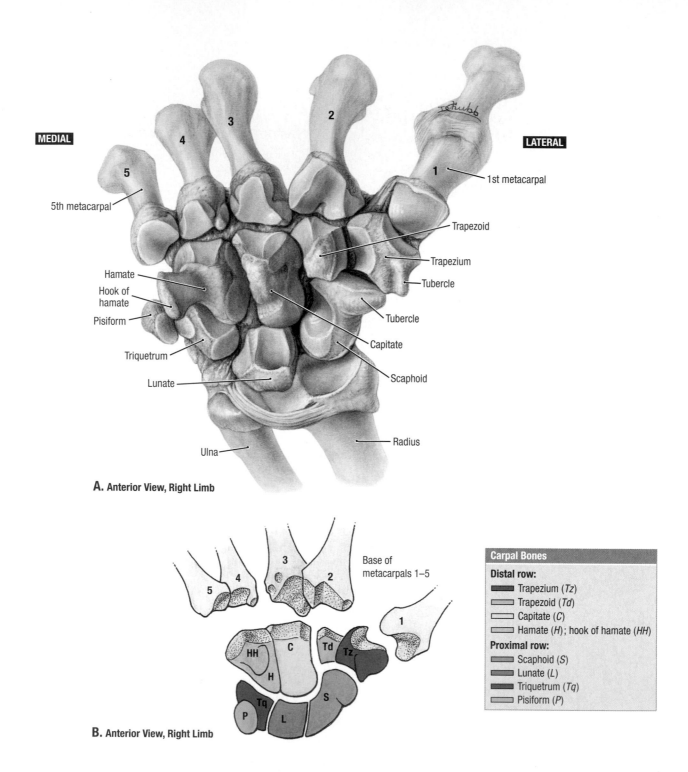

MEDIAL

LATERAL

3

2

4

5

1st metacarpal

5th metacarpal

Trapezoid

Trapezium

Hamate

Tubercle

Hook of hamate

Pisiform

Tubercle

Triquetrum

Capitate

Lunate

Scaphoid

Ulna

Radius

A. Anterior View, Right Limb

3

2

Base of metacarpals 1–5

4

5

1

HH   C   Td   Tz

H

Tq   S

P   L

B. Anterior View, Right Limb

Carpal Bones	
Distal row:	
	Trapezium (*Tz*)
	Trapezoid (*Td*)
	Capitate (*C*)
	Hamate (*H*); hook of hamate (*HH*)
Proximal row:	
	Scaphoid (*S*)
	Lunate (*L*)
	Triquetrum (*Tq*)
	Pisiform (*P*)

2.97   **Carpal Bones and Bases of Metacarpals**

A. Open intercarpal and carpometacarpal (CMC) joints. The dorsal ligaments remain intact and all the joints have been hyperextended. **B. Articular surfaces of CMC joints.**

Note that the 1st CMC joint is saddle-shaped and especially mobile, allowing opposition of the thumb; the 2nd and 3rd CMC joints have interlocking surfaces and are practically immobile; and the 4th and 5th are hinge-shaped synovial joints with limited movement.

Anterior dislocation of the lunate is a serious injury that usually results from a fall on the extended wrist. The lunate is pushed to the palmar surface of the wrist and may compress the median nerve and lead to carpal tunnel syndrome. Because of poor blood supply, **avascular necrosis of the lunate** may occur.

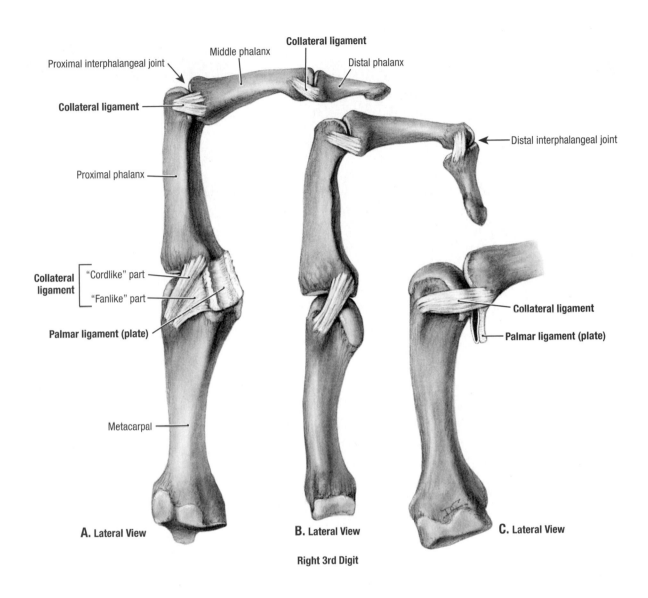

Proximal interphalangeal joint

Middle phalanx

Collateral ligament

Distal phalanx

Collateral ligament

Distal interphalangeal joint

Proximal phalanx

Collateral ligament

"Cordlike" part

"Fanlike" part

Palmar ligament (plate)

Collateral ligament

Palmar ligament (plate)

Metacarpal

A. Lateral View

B. Lateral View

C. Lateral View

Right 3rd Digit

| **Collateral Ligaments of Metacarpophalangeal and Interphalangeal Joints of Third Digit** | **2.98** |

A. Extended metacarpophalangeal (MCP) and distal interphalangeal (IP) joints. **B.** Flexed interphalangeal joints. **C.** Flexed MCP joint.

- A fibrocartilaginous plate, the palmar ligament, hangs from the base of the proximal phalanx; is fixed to the head of the metacarpal by the weaker, fanlike part of the collateral ligament (*Part A*); and moves like a visor across the metacarpal head (*Part C*). The IP joints have similar palmar ligaments.
- The extremely strong, cordlike parts of the collateral ligaments of this joint (*Part A* and *Part B*) are eccentrically attached to the metacarpal heads; they are slack during extension and taut during flexion (*Part C*), so the fingers cannot be spread (abducted) unless the hand is open; the IP joints have similar collateral ligaments.

Skier's thumb refers to the rupture or chronic laxity of the collateral ligament of the 1st metacarpophalangeal joint. The injury results from hyperextension of the joint, which occurs when the thumb is held by the ski pole while the rest of the hand hits the ground or enters the snow.

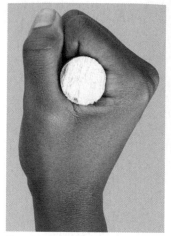

A. Lateral View

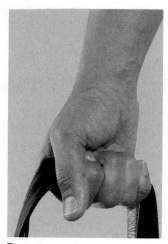

B. Anterior View

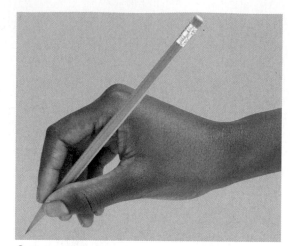

C. Medial View

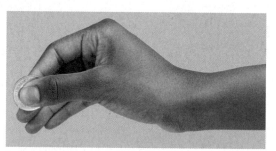

D. Medial View

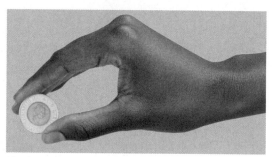

E. Medial View

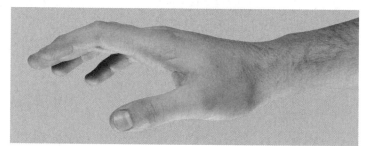

F. Medial View

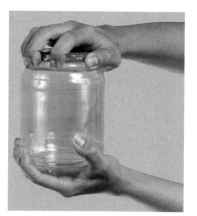

I. Lateral View

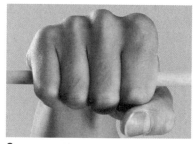

G. Anterior View

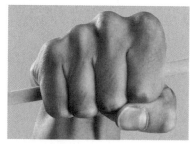

H. Anterior View

2.99 **Functional Positions of Hand**

A. Cylindrical (power) grasp. When grasping an object, the metacarpophalangeal and interphalangeal joints are flexed, but the radiocarpal joints are extended. Without wrist extension, the grip is weak and insecure. **B. Hook grasp.** This grasp involves primarily the long flexors of the fingers, which are flexed to a varying degree depending on the size of the object. **C.** and **D. Tripod (three-jaw chuck) pinch. E. Fingertip pinch. F. Rest position of hand.** Casts for fractures are applied most often with the hand in this position. **G. Loose cylindrical grasp. H. Firm cylindrical (power) grasp. I. Disc (power) grasp.**

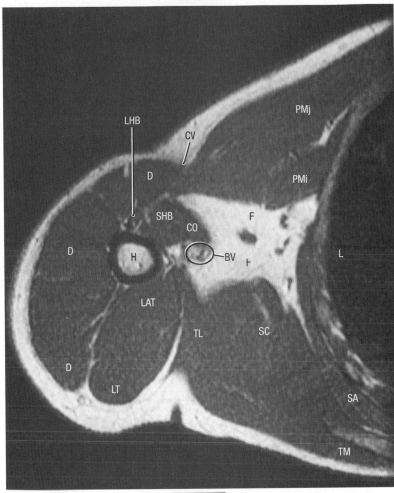

A. Transverse MRI

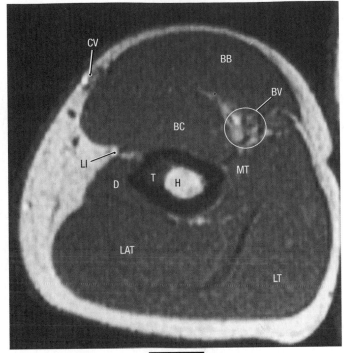

B. Transverse MRI

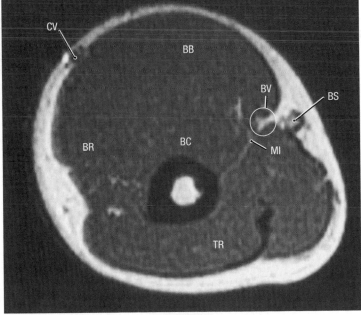

C. Transverse MRI

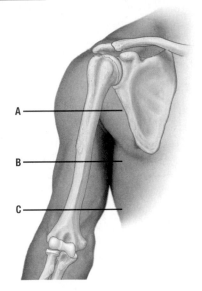

BB	Biceps brachii
BC	Brachialis
BR	Brachioradialis
BS	Basilic vein
BV	Brachial vessels and nerves
CO	Coracobrachialis
CV	Cephalic vein
D	Deltoid
F	Fat in axilla
H	Humerus
L	Lung
LAT	Lateral head of triceps brachii
LHB	Long head of biceps brachii
LI	Lateral intermuscular septum
LT	Long head of triceps brachii
MI	Medial intermuscular septum
MT	Medial head of triceps brachii
PMi	Pectoralis minor
PMj	Pectoralis major
SA	Serratus anterior
SC	Subscapularis
SHB	Short head of biceps brachii
T	Deltoid tuberosity
TL	Teres major and latissimus dorsi
TM	Teres minor
TR	Triceps brachii

Transverse (Axial) MRIs of Arm | 2.100

A. Transverse MRI through proximal arm. **B.** Transverse MRI through middle of arm. **C.** Transverse MRI through distal arm.

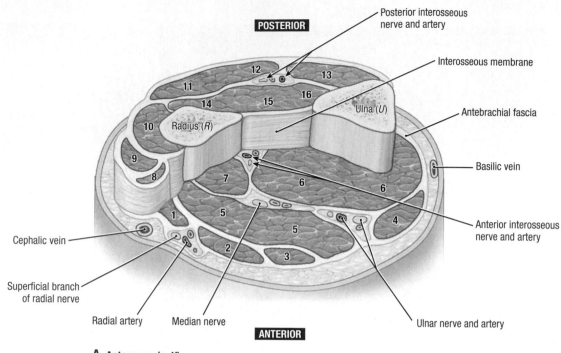

POSTERIOR

Posterior interosseous nerve and artery

Interosseous membrane

Antebrachial fascia

Basilic vein

Anterior interosseous nerve and artery

Ulnar nerve and artery

Ulnar nerve and artery

Cephalic vein

Superficial branch of radial nerve

Radial artery

Median nerve

ANTERIOR

A. Anterosuperior View

Ulna (U)

Radius (R)

A. Anterosuperior View

Muscle Compartments of Forearm

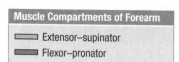

☐ Extensor–supinator
▬ Flexor–pronator

Flexors

1	Pronator teres
2	Flexor carpi radialis
3	Palmaris longus
4	Flexor carpi ulnaris
5	Flexor digitorum superficialis
6	Flexor digitorum profundus
7	Flexor pollicis longus

Extensors

8	Brachioradialis
9	Extensor carpi radialis longus
10	Extensor carpi radialis brevis
11	Extensor digitorum
12	Extensor digiti minimi
13	Extensor carpi ulnaris
14	Abductor pollicis longus
15	Extensor pollicis brevis
16	Extensor pollicis longus (extensor indicis)

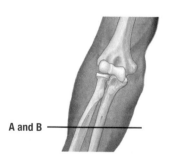

A and B

ANTERIOR

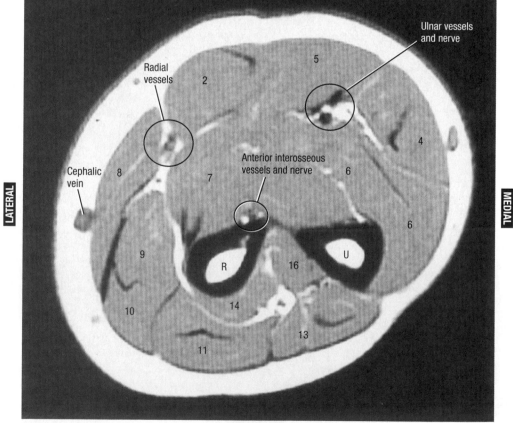

Ulnar vessels and nerve

Radial vessels

Cephalic vein

Anterior interosseous vessels and nerve

LATERAL

MEDIAL

B. Transverse MRI

POSTERIOR

Transverse Sections and Transverse (Axial) MRIs of Forearm

A. Stepped transverse sections of anterior and posterior compartments. **B.** Transverse MRI through proximal forearm.

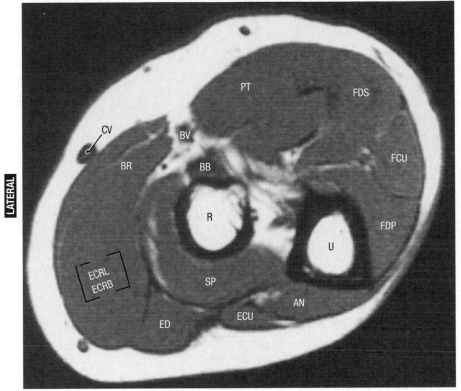

C. Transverse MRI

AN	Anconeus
APL	Abductor pollicis longus
BB	Biceps brachii
BR	Brachioradialis
BV	Brachial vessels
CV	Cephalic vein
ECRB	Extensor carpi radialis brevis
ECRL	Extensor carpi radialis longus
ECU	Extensor carpi ulnaris
ED	Extensor digitorum
EPB	Extensor pollicis brevis
EPL	Extensor pollicis longus
FCR	Flexor carpi radialis
FCU	Flexor carpi ulnaris
FDP	Flexor digitorum profundus
FDS	Flexor digitorum superficialis
FPL	Flexor pollicis longus
PQ	Pronator quadratus
PT	Pronator teres
R	Radius
SP	Supinator
U	Ulna
UV	Ulnar vessels and nerve

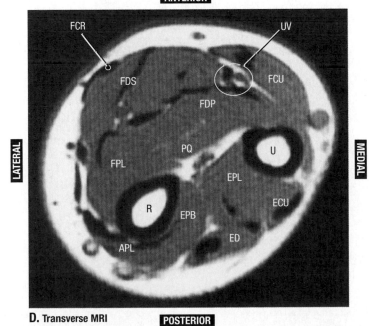

D. Transverse MRI

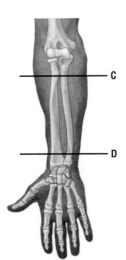

Transverse Sections and Transverse (Axial) MRIs of Forearm *(continued)* **2.101**

C. Transverse MRI through middle forearm. **D.** Transverse MRI through distal forearm.

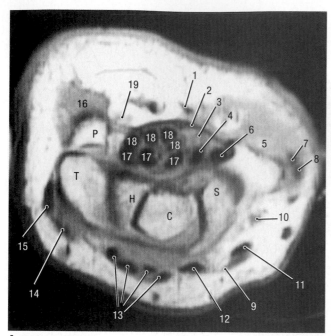

A. Transverse MRI

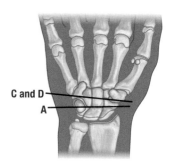

Pisiform (*P*)
Triquetrum (*T*)
Flexor retinaculum
Carpal tunnel
Lunate
Scaphoid (*S*)

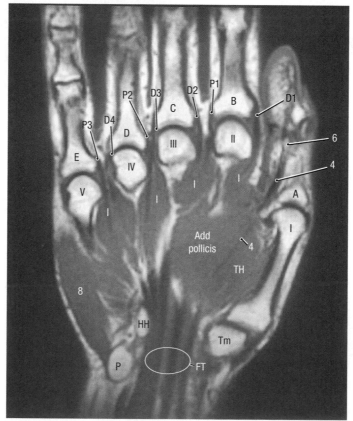

B. Coronal MRI

2.102 **Transverse (Axial) Section and MRIs through Carpal Tunnel**

A. Transverse MRI through proximal carpal tunnel. Numbers and letters in MRI refer to structures in *Part D*. **B. Coronal MRI of wrist and hand showing course of long flexor tendons in carpal tunnel.** Numbers and letters in MRI refer to structures in *Part D*.

A–E, proximal phalanges; *FT*, long flexor tendons; *HH*, hook of hamate; *I*, interossei; *P*, pisiform; *TH*, thenar muscles; *Tm*, trapezium; *I–V*, heads of metacarpals.

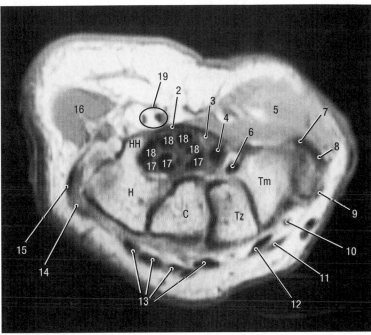

C. Transverse MRI

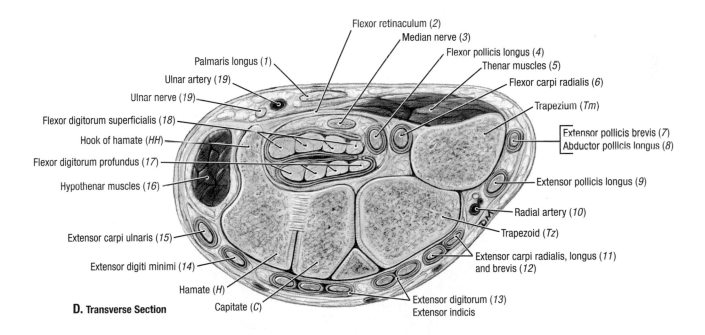

Flexor retinaculum (*2*)
Median nerve (*3*)
Flexor pollicis longus (*4*)
Thenar muscles (*5*)
Flexor carpi radialis (*6*)
Trapezium (*Tm*)
Extensor pollicis brevis (*7*)
Abductor pollicis longus (*8*)
Extensor pollicis longus (*9*)
Radial artery (*10*)
Trapezoid (*Tz*)
Extensor carpi radialis, longus (*11*)
and brevis (*12*)
Extensor digitorum (*13*)
Extensor indicis

Palmaris longus (*1*)
Ulnar artery (*19*)
Ulnar nerve (*19*)
Flexor digitorum superficialis (*18*)
Hook of hamate (*HH*)
Flexor digitorum profundus (*17*)
Hypothenar muscles (*16*)
Extensor carpi ulnaris (*15*)
Extensor digiti minimi (*14*)
Hamate (*H*)
Capitate (*C*)

D. Transverse Section

Transverse (Axial) Section and MRIs through Carpal Tunnel (*continued*)   2.102

C. Transverse MRI through distal carpal tunnel. Numbers and letters in MRI refer to structures in *Part D*. **D.** Transverse section of carpal tunnel through distal row of carpal bones.

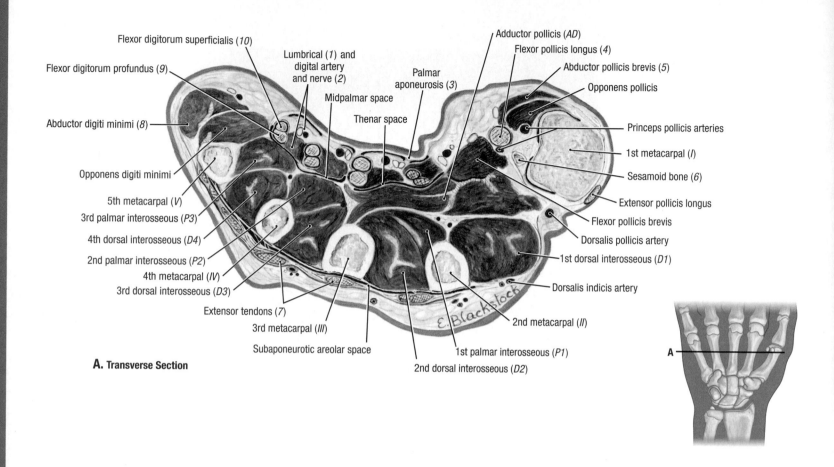

Flexor digitorum superficialis (*10*)
Flexor digitorum profundus (*9*)
Abductor digiti minimi (*8*)
Opponens digiti minimi
5th metacarpal (*V*)
3rd palmar interosseous (*P3*)
4th dorsal interosseous (*D4*)
2nd palmar interosseous (*P2*)
4th metacarpal (*IV*)
3rd dorsal interosseous (*D3*)
Extensor tendons (*7*)
3rd metacarpal (*III*)
Subaponeurotic areolar space

Lumbrical (*1*) and digital artery and nerve (*2*)
Midpalmar space
Thenar space
Palmar aponeurosis (*3*)

Adductor pollicis (*AD*)
Flexor pollicis longus (*4*)
Abductor pollicis brevis (*5*)
Opponens pollicis
Princeps pollicis arteries
1st metacarpal (*I*)
Sesamoid bone (*6*)
Extensor pollicis longus
Flexor pollicis brevis
Dorsalis pollicis artery
1st dorsal interosseous (*D1*)
Dorsalis indicis artery

2nd metacarpal (*II*)
1st palmar interosseous (*P1*)
2nd dorsal interosseous (*D2*)

A. Transverse Section

A

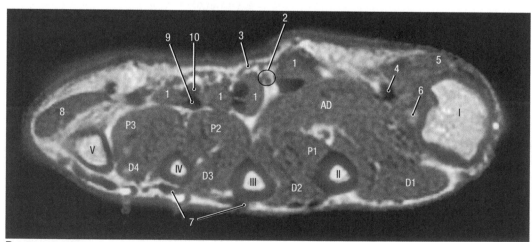

B. Transverse MRI

2.103 **Transverse Section and MRI through Palm (Metacarpals) at Level of Adductor Pollicis**

A. Anatomical section. (See Fig. 2.74 for demonstration of compartment of palm.) **B.** MRI.

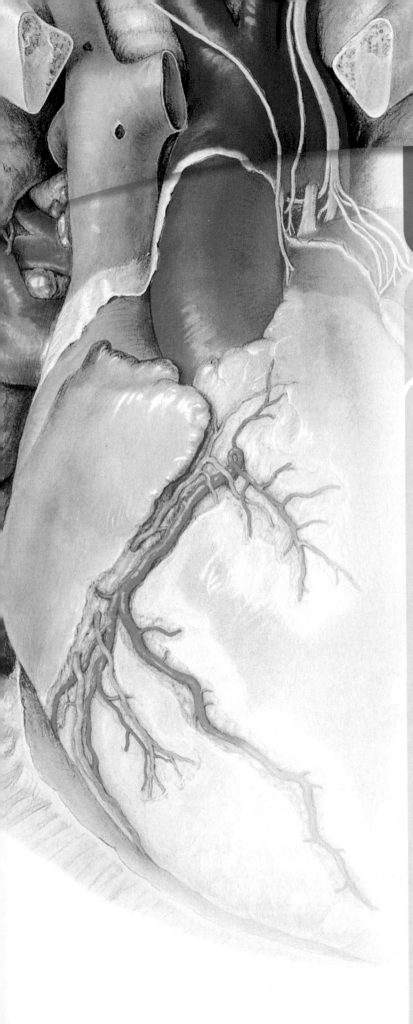

CHAPTER 3

THORAX

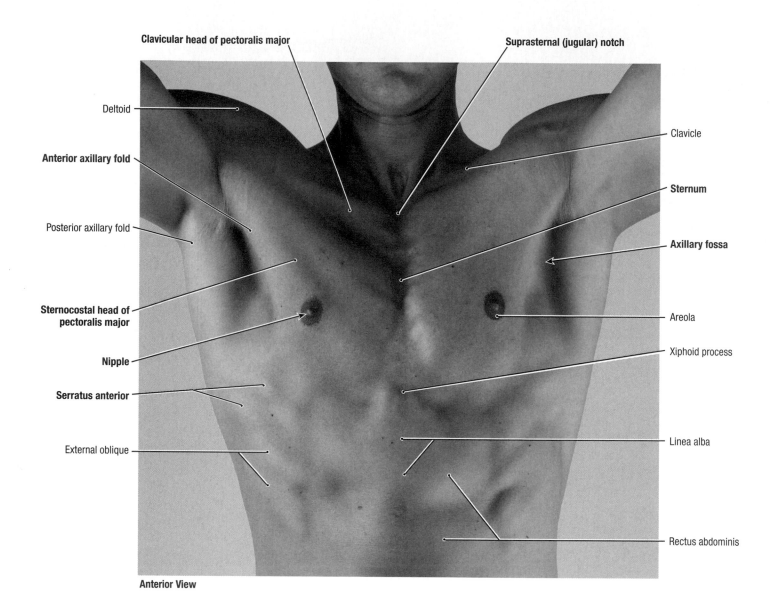

Clavicular head of pectoralis major

Suprasternal (jugular) notch

Deltoid

Clavicle

Anterior axillary fold

Sternum

Posterior axillary fold

Axillary fossa

Sternocostal head of pectoralis major

Areola

Nipple

Xiphoid process

Serratus anterior

Linea alba

External oblique

Rectus abdominis

Anterior View

| 3.1 | **Surface Anatomy of Male Pectoral Region** |

- The subject is adducting the shoulders against resistance to demonstrate the pectoralis major muscle.
- The sternum (breastbone) lies subcutaneously in the anterior median line and is palpable throughout its length.
- The suprasternal notch can be palpated between the prominent medial ends of the clavicles.
- The pectoralis major muscle has two parts: the sternocostal and clavicular heads.
- The inferior border of the sternocostal head of the pectoralis major muscle forms the anterior axillary fold. The axillary fossa ("armpit") is a surface feature overlying a fat-filled space, the axilla, posterior to the anterior fold.
- The male nipple overlies the 4th intercostal space.

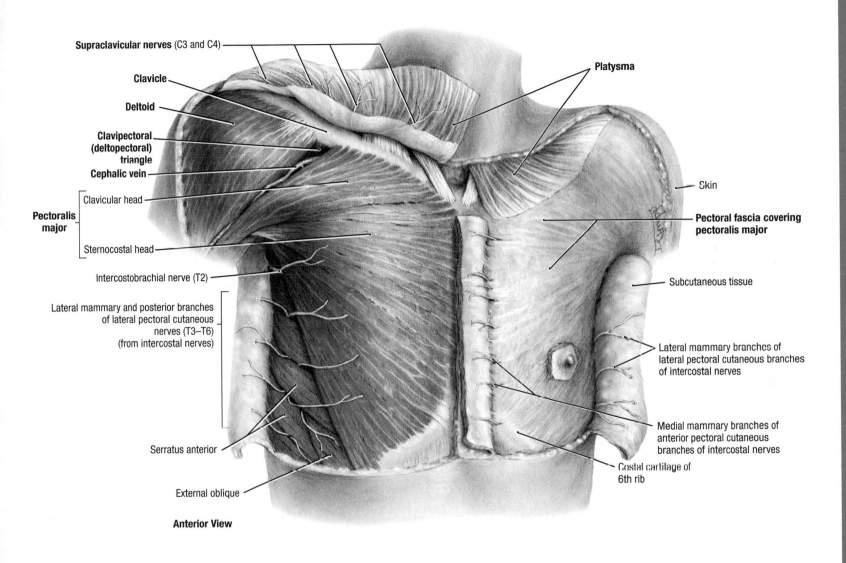

Supraclavicular nerves (C3 and C4)

Platysma

Clavicle

Deltoid

Clavipectoral (deltopectoral) triangle

Cephalic vein

Skin

Clavicular head

Pectoral fascia covering pectoralis major

Pectoralis major

Sternocostal head

Intercostobrachial nerve (T2)

Subcutaneous tissue

Lateral mammary and posterior branches of lateral pectoral cutaneous nerves (T3–T6) (from intercostal nerves)

Lateral mammary branches of lateral pectoral cutaneous branches of intercostal nerves

Medial mammary branches of anterior pectoral cutaneous branches of intercostal nerves

Serratus anterior

Costal cartilage of 6th rib

External oblique

Anterior View

Superficial Dissection, Male Pectoral Region

3.2

- The platysma muscle, which descends to the 2nd or 3rd rib, is cut short on both sides of the specimen; together with the supraclavicular nerves, it is reflected superiorly on the right side.
- The pectoral fascia covers the pectoralis major.
- The clavicle lies deep to the subcutaneous tissue and the platysma muscle.
- The cephalic vein passes deeply in the clavipectoral (deltopectoral) triangle to join the axillary vein.

- Supraclavicular (C3–C4) and upper thoracic nerves (T2–T6) supply cutaneous innervation to the pectoral region.
- The clavipectoral (deltopectoral) triangle, bounded by the clavicle superiorly, the deltoid muscle laterally, and the clavicular head of the pectoralis major muscle medially, underlies a surface depression called the infraclavicular fossa (see Fig. 3.3A).

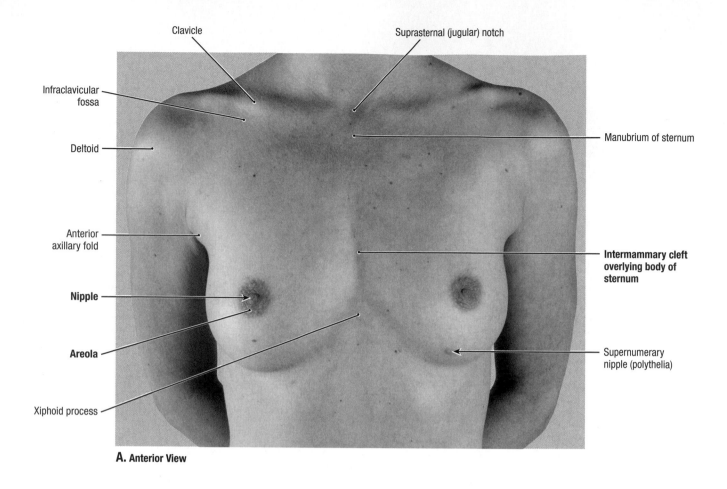

Clavicle

Suprasternal (jugular) notch

Infraclavicular fossa

Deltoid

Manubrium of sternum

Anterior axillary fold

Intermammary cleft overlying body of sternum

Nipple

Areola

Supernumerary nipple (polythelia)

Xiphoid process

A. Anterior View

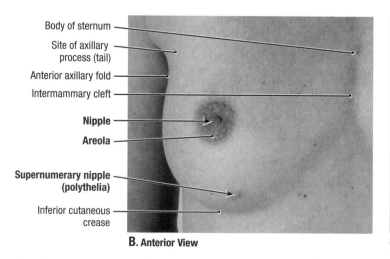

Body of sternum

Site of axillary process (tail)

Anterior axillary fold

Intermammary cleft

Nipple

Areola

Supernumerary nipple (polythelia)

Inferior cutaneous crease

B. Anterior View

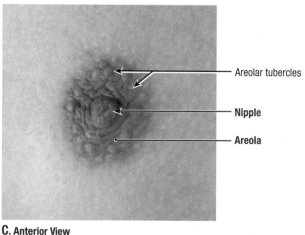

Areolar tubercles

Nipple

Areola

C. Anterior View

3.3 | **Surface Anatomy of Female Pectoral Region**

A. Overview. B. Breast. The roughly circular base of the female breast extends transversely from the lateral border of the sternum to the midaxillary line and vertically from the 2nd to 6th ribs. A small part of the breast may extend along the inferolateral edge of the pectoralis major muscle toward the axillary fossa, forming an axillary process or tail (of Spence) (see Figs. 3.4A & B). **C. Areola and nipple.** The pigmented areola surrounds the nipple.

Polymastia (supernumerary breasts) or **polythelia** (accessory nipples) may occur superior or inferior to the normal pair, occasionally developing in the axillary fossa or anterior abdominal wall. Supernumerary breasts usually consist of only a rudimentary nipple and areola, which may be mistaken for a mole (nevus) until they change pigmentation with the normal nipples during pregnancy.

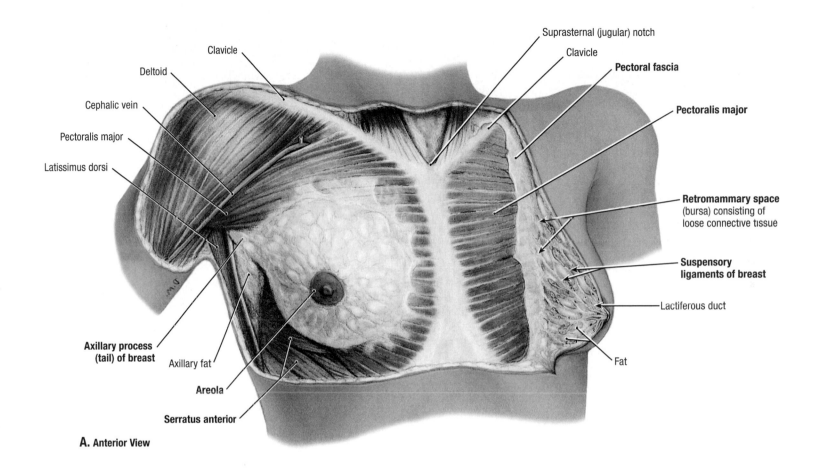

Suprasternal (jugular) notch

Clavicle

Clavicle

Deltoid

Pectoral fascia

Cephalic vein

Pectoralis major

Pectoralis major

Latissimus dorsi

Retromammary space
(bursa) consisting of
loose connective tissue

**Suspensory
ligaments of breast**

Lactiferous duct

**Axillary process
(tail) of breast**

Axillary fat

Fat

Areola

Serratus anterior

A. Anterior View

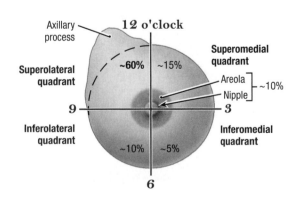

Axillary
process

12 o'clock

**Superomedial
quadrant**

**Superolateral
quadrant**

~60%

~15%

Areola

Nipple

~10%

9

3

**Inferolateral
quadrant**

~10%

~5%

**Inferomedial
quadrant**

6

B. Right Breast, Anterior View

Superficial Dissection, Female   **3.4**

A. Dissection.
- On the specimen's right side, the skin is removed; on the left side, the breast is sagittally sectioned.
- Two thirds of the breast rests on the pectoral fascia covering the pectoralis major; the other third rests on the fascia covering the serratus anterior muscle.
- The region of loose connective tissue between the pectoral fascia and the deep surface of the breast, the retromammary space (bursa), permits the breast to move on the deep fascia.

Cancer can spread by contiguity (invasion of adjacent tissue). When breast cancer cells invade the retromammary space, attach to or invade the pectoral fascia overlying the pectoralis major, or metastasize to the interpectoral nodes (see Fig. 3.7), the breast elevates when the muscle contracts. This movement is a clinical sign of **advanced cancer of the breast.**

    B. Breast quadrants: percentage of malignant tumors. For the anatomical location and description of tumors and cysts, the surface of the breast is divided into four quadrants. For example, "A hard irregular mass was felt in the superomedial quadrant of the breast at the 2 o'clock position, approximately 2.5 cm from the margin of the areola."

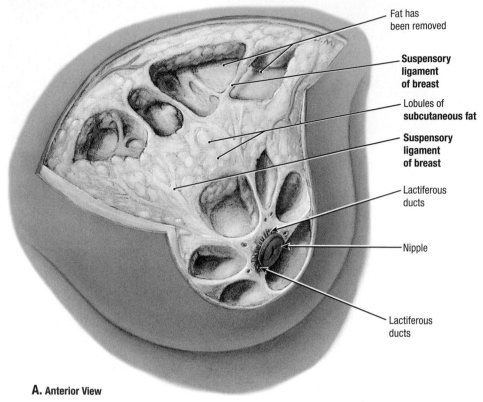

Fat has
been removed

**Suspensory
ligament
of breast**

Lobules of
subcutaneous fat

**Suspensory
ligament
of breast**

Lactiferous
ducts

Nipple

Lactiferous
ducts

A. Anterior View

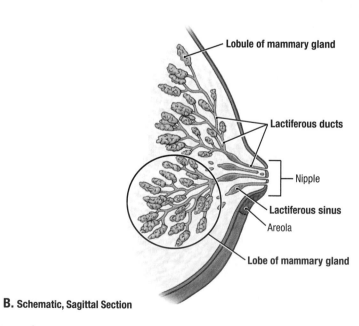

Lobule of mammary gland

Lactiferous ducts

Nipple

Lactiferous sinus

Areola

Lobe of mammary gland

B. Schematic, Sagittal Section

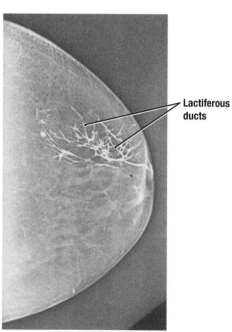

**Lactiferous
ducts**

C. Galactogram

3.5   Female Mammary Gland

A. Dissection. Areas of subcutaneous fat were removed to show the suspensory ligaments of the breast. **B. Sagittal section.** The glandular tissue consists of 15 to 20 lobes, each composed of lobules. Each lobe has a lactiferous duct that widens to form the lactiferous sinus before opening on the nipple. **C. Galactogram.** This is used to image the duct system of the breast. Contrast material is injected into the ducts, and mammograms are then taken.

Interference with the lymphatic drainage by cancer may cause **lymphedema** (edema, excess fluid in the subcutaneous tissue), which in turn may result in deviation of the nipple and a leathery, thickened appearance of the breast skin. Prominent (puffy) skin between dimpled pores may develop, which gives the skin an orange-peel appearance (*peau d'orange* sign). Larger dimples may form if pulled by cancerous invasion of the suspensory ligaments of the breast.

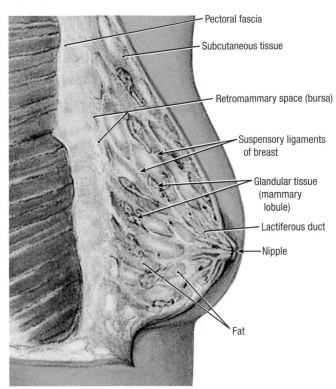

Pectoral fascia

Subcutaneous tissue

Retromammary space (bursa)

Suspensory ligaments of breast

Glandular tissue (mammary lobule)

Lactiferous duct

Nipple

Fat

A. Sagittal Breast Section

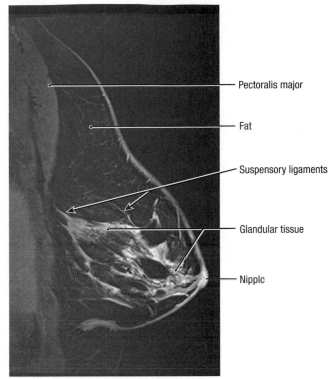

Pectoralis major

Fat

Suspensory ligaments

Glandular tissue

Nipplc

B. Sagittal Breast MRI

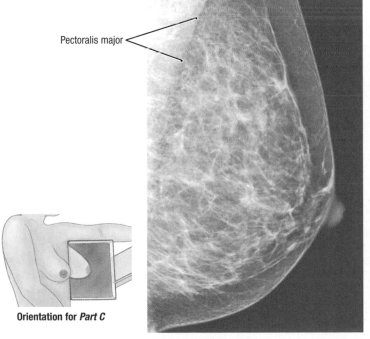

Pectoralis major

Orientation for *Part C*

C. Sagittal Mammogram

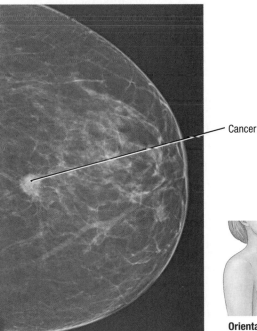

Cancer

D. Transverse Mammogram

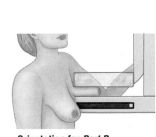

Orientation for *Part D*

Imaging of Breast   **3.6**

A. Illustration. B. Sagittal MRI of breast. The scan shows many of the features visible in *Part A*. In this MRI, fat appears very dark, whereas glandular tissue is brighter and the linear suspensory ligaments clearly visible. The pectoralis major is also apparent as is the pectoralis minor posterior to it.

C. and **D. Scanning mammograms.** Mammograms, which use x-rays, are done with a sagittal *mediolateral oblique* (*MLO*) and a transverse *craniocaudal* (*CC*) orientation. These two orientations allow the entire breast to be imaged. A speculated mass (cancer) is identified in *Part D*.

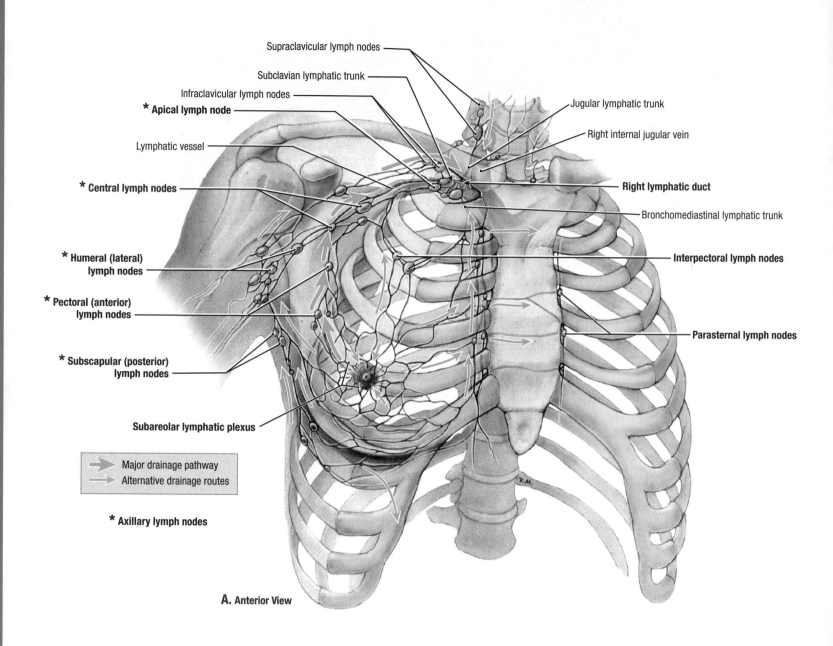

Supraclavicular lymph nodes

Subclavian lymphatic trunk

Infraclavicular lymph nodes

* **Apical lymph node**

Lymphatic vessel

* **Central lymph nodes**

* **Humeral (lateral) lymph nodes**

* **Pectoral (anterior) lymph nodes**

* **Subscapular (posterior) lymph nodes**

Subareolar lymphatic plexus

Jugular lymphatic trunk

Right internal jugular vein

Right lymphatic duct

Bronchomediastinal lymphatic trunk

Interpectoral lymph nodes

Parasternal lymph nodes

Major drainage pathway
Alternative drainage routes

* **Axillary lymph nodes**

A. Anterior View

3.7 | **Lymphatic Drainage of Breast**

A. Overview. Lymph drained from the upper limb and breast passes through nodes arranged irregularly in groups of axillary lymph nodes: (1) pectoral, along the inferior border of the pectoralis minor muscle; (2) subscapular, along the subscapular artery and veins; (3) humeral, along the distal part of the axillary vein; (4) central, at the base of the axilla, embedded in axillary fat; and (5) apical, along the axillary vein between the clavicle and the pectoralis minor muscle. Most of the breast drains via the pectoral, central, and apical axillary nodes to the subclavian lymph trunk, which joins the venous system at the venous angle (the junction of the subclavian and internal jugular veins). The medial part of the breast drains to the parasternal nodes, which are located along the internal thoracic vessels.

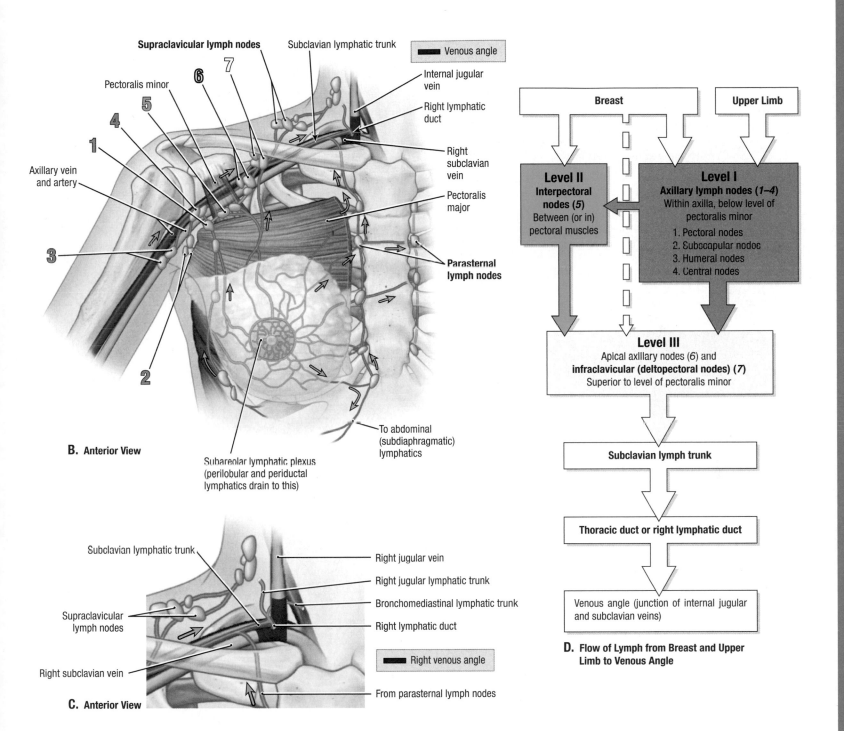

Supraclavicular lymph nodes

Subclavian lymphatic trunk

Pectoralis minor

⑥ ⑦

⑤

④

① Internal jugular vein

Right lymphatic duct

Axillary vein and artery

Right subclavian vein

③

Pectoralis major

② Parasternal lymph nodes

B. Anterior View

Subareolar lymphatic plexus (perilobular and periductal lymphatics drain to this)

To abdominal (subdiaphragmatic) lymphatics

Venous angle

Subclavian lymphatic trunk

Right jugular vein

Right jugular lymphatic trunk

Supraclavicular lymph nodes

Bronchomediastinal lymphatic trunk

Right lymphatic duct

Right subclavian vein

From parasternal lymph nodes

Right venous angle

C. Anterior View

Breast | Upper Limb

Level II
Interpectoral nodes (5)
Between (or in) pectoral muscles

Level I
Axillary lymph nodes (1–4)
Within axilla, below level of pectoralis minor
1. Pectoral nodes
2. Subscapular nodes
3. Humeral nodes
4. Central nodes

Level III
Apical axillary nodes (6) and
infraclavicular (deltopectoral nodes) (7)
Superior to level of pectoralis minor

Subclavian lymph trunk

Thoracic duct or right lymphatic duct

Venous angle (junction of internal jugular and subclavian veins)

D. Flow of Lymph from Breast and Upper Limb to Venous Angle

Lymphatic Drainage of Breast *(continued)* **3.7**

B. Pattern of lymphatic drainage. Breast cancer typically spreads by means of lymphatic vessels (lymphogenic metastasis), which carry cancer cells from the breast to the lymph nodes, chiefly those in the axilla. The cells lodge in the nodes, producing nests of tumor cells (metastases). Abundant communications among lymphatic pathways and among axillary, cervical, and parasternal nodes may also cause metastases from the breast to develop in the supraclavicular lymph nodes, the opposite breast, or the abdomen. The prognosis of breast cancer has been correlated with the level of metastasis (Level I, II, or III in *Part D*) and to the number of involved axillary lymph nodes. **C. Venous angle. D. Flow of lymph from breast and upper limb.**

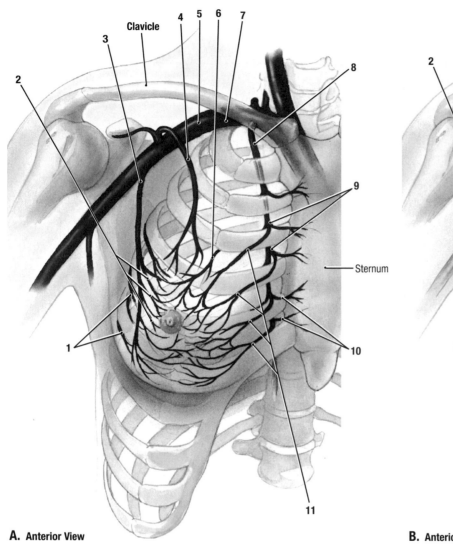

A. Anterior View

B. Anterior View

Arteries of Breast
1   Lateral mammary branches of lateral cutaneous branches of posterior intercostal arteries
2   Lateral mammary branches of lateral thoracic artery
3   Lateral thoracic artery
4   Pectoral branch of thoracoacromial artery
5   Axillary artery
6   Mammary branch of anterior intercostal artery
7   Subclavian artery
8   Internal thoracic artery
9   Perforating branches
10   Sternal branches
11   Medial mammary branches

Veins of Breast
1   Lateral mammary branches of lateral cutaneous branches of posterior intercostal veins
2   Lateral mammary branches of lateral thoracic vein
3   Lateral thoracic vein
4   Pectoral branch of thoracoacromial vein
5   Axillary vein
6   Mammary branch of anterior intercostal vein
7   Subclavian vein
8   Internal thoracic vein
9   Perforating branches
10   Sternal branches
11   Medial mammary veins

3.8   Arterial Supply and Venous Drainage of Breast

Arteries (*Part A*) enter and veins (*Part B*) drain the breast from its superomedial and superolateral aspects; vessels also penetrate the deep surface of the breast. The vessels branch profusely and anastomose with each other.

Breast incisions are placed in the inferior breast quadrants when possible because these quadrants are less vascular than the superior ones.

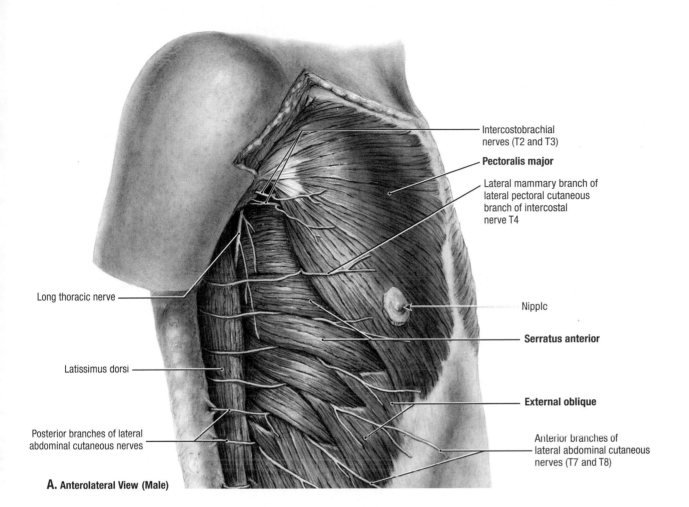

Intercostobrachial nerves (T2 and T3)

Pectoralis major

Lateral mammary branch of lateral pectoral cutaneous branch of intercostal nerve T4

Long thoracic nerve

Nipple

Serratus anterior

Latissimus dorsi

External oblique

Posterior branches of lateral abdominal cutaneous nerves

Anterior branches of lateral abdominal cutaneous nerves (T7 and T8)

A. Anterolateral View (Male)

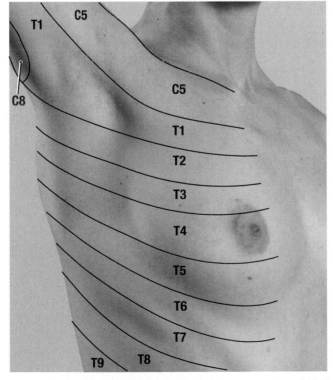

C5
T1
C8
C5
T1
T2
T3
T4
T5
T6
T7
T8
T9

B. Anterolateral View (Female)

Muscles and Nerves of Bed of Breast 3.9

A. Muscles comprising bed and cutaneous nerves. **B.** Dermatomes.

Local anesthesia of an intercostal space (intercostal nerve block) is produced by injecting a local anesthetic agent around the intercostal nerves between the paravertebral line and the area of required anesthesia. Because any particular area of skin usually receives innervation from two adjacent nerves, considerable overlapping of contiguous dermatomes occurs. Therefore, complete loss of sensation usually does not occur unless two or more intercostal nerves are anesthetized.

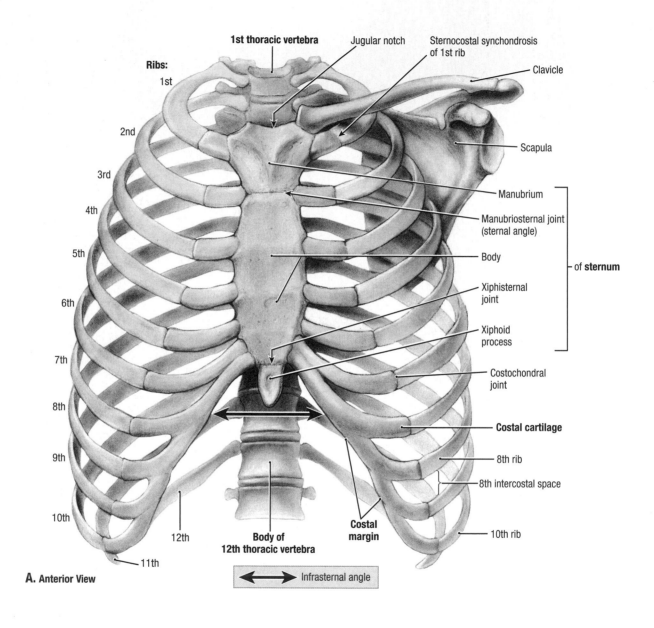

1st thoracic vertebra

Jugular notch

Sternocostal synchondrosis of 1st rib

Clavicle

Ribs:

1st

2nd

Scapula

3rd

Manubrium

4th

Manubriosternal joint (sternal angle)

5th

Body

— of **sternum**

Xiphisternal joint

6th

Xiphoid process

7th

Costochondral joint

8th

Costal cartilage

9th

8th rib

8th intercostal space

10th

12th

Body of 12th thoracic vertebra

Costal margin

10th rib

11th

A. Anterior View

Infrasternal angle

3.10 Bony Thorax

- The thoracic cage consists of 12 thoracic vertebrae, 12 pairs of ribs and costal cartilages, and the sternum.
- Anteriorly, the superior seven costal cartilages articulate with the sternum; the 8th, 9th, and 10th cartilages articulate with the cartilage above forming the costal margin; the 11th and 12th are "floating" ribs, that is, their cartilages do not articulate anteriorly.
- The clavicle lies over the 1st rib, making it difficult to palpate. The 2nd rib is easily palpable because its costal cartilage

- articulates with the sternum at the sternal angle, located at the junction of the manubrium and body of the sternum.
- The 3rd to 10th ribs can be palpated in sequence inferolaterally from the 2nd rib; the fused costal cartilages of the 7th to 10th ribs form the costal arch (margin), and the tips of the 11th and 12th ribs can be palpated posterolaterally.
- A rib dislocation is the displacement of a costal cartilage from the sternum; a rib separation refers to dislocation of the costochondral joint.

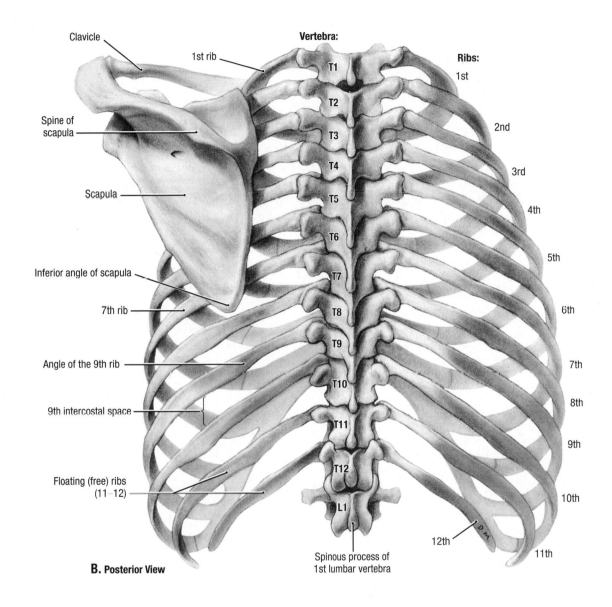

Clavicle

1st rib

Spine of scapula

Scapula

Inferior angle of scapula

7th rib

Angle of the 9th rib

9th intercostal space

Floating (free) ribs (11–12)

Vertebra:

T1
T2
T3
T4
T5
T6
T7
T8
T9
T10
T11
T12
L1

Ribs:

1st
2nd
3rd
4th
5th
6th
7th
8th
9th
10th
11th
12th

Spinous process of 1st lumbar vertebra

B. Posterior View

Bony Thorax *(continued)*

3.10

- The superior thoracic aperture (thoracic inlet) is the doorway between the thoracic cavity and the neck region; it is bounded by the 1st thoracic vertebra, the 1st ribs and their cartilages, and the manubrium of the sternum.
- Each rib articulates posteriorly with the vertebral column.
- Posteriorly, all ribs angle inferiorly; anteriorly, the 3rd to 10th costal cartilages angle superiorly.
- The scapula is suspended from the clavicle and extends across the 2nd to 7th ribs posteriorly.

- The spinous process of vertebra T6 overlaps vertebra T7 (the palpable tip of the T6 spinous process actually indicates the T7 vertebral level).
- When clinicians refer to the superior thoracic aperture as the thoracic "outlet," they are emphasizing the important nerves and arteries that pass through this aperture into the lower neck and upper limb. Hence, various types of thoracic outlet syndromes exist, such as the costoclavicular syndrome—pallor and coldness of the skin of the upper limb and diminished radial pulse—resulting from compression of the subclavian artery between the clavicle and the 1st rib.

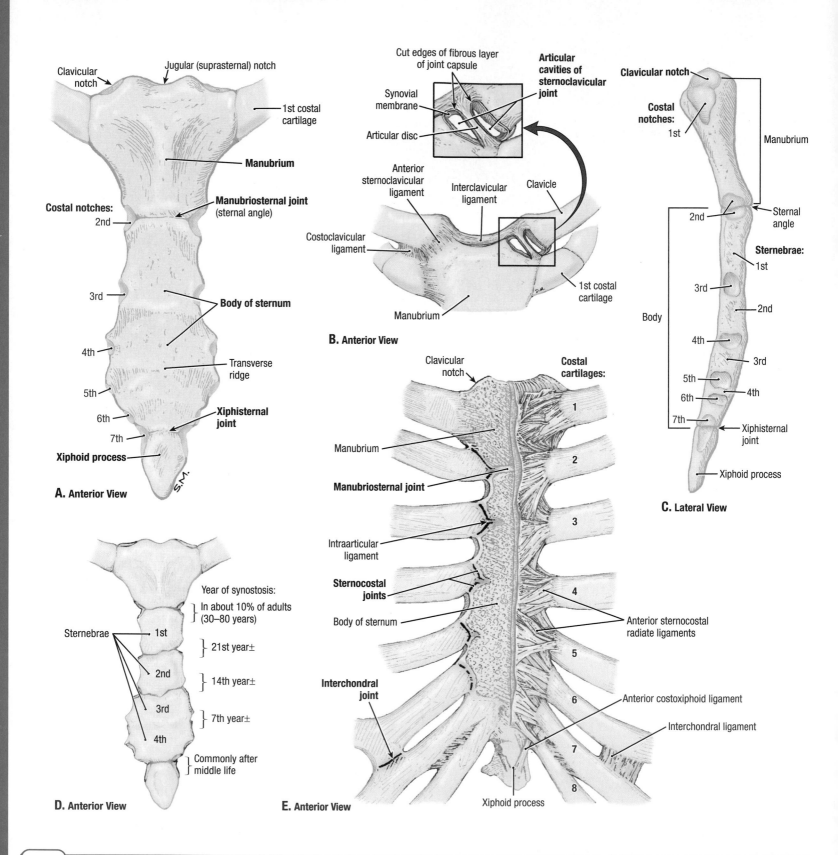

A. Anterior View

Clavicular notch

Jugular (suprasternal) notch

1st costal cartilage

Manubrium

Manubriosternal joint (sternal angle)

Costal notches:
2nd
3rd
Body of sternum
4th
5th
6th
7th

Transverse ridge

Xiphisternal joint

Xiphoid process

B. Anterior View

Cut edges of fibrous layer of joint capsule

Synovial membrane

Articular disc

Articular cavities of sternoclavicular joint

Anterior sternoclavicular ligament

Interclavicular ligament

Clavicle

Costoclavicular ligament

Manubrium

1st costal cartilage

C. Lateral View

Clavicular notch

Costal notches:
1st
2nd

Manubrium

Sternal angle

Sternebrae:
1st
3rd
2nd
4th
3rd
5th
6th
4th
7th

Body

Xiphisternal joint

Xiphoid process

D. Anterior View

Sternebrae
1st
2nd
3rd
4th

Year of synostosis:

In about 10% of adults (30–80 years)

21st year±

14th year±

7th year±

Commonly after middle life

E. Anterior View

Clavicular notch

Costal cartilages:
1
2
3
4
5
6
7
8

Manubrium

Manubriosternal joint

Intraarticular ligament

Sternocostal joints

Body of sternum

Interchondral joint

Anterior sternocostal radiate ligaments

Anterior costoxiphoid ligament

Interchondral ligament

Xiphoid process

A. Parts of sternum. **B.** Sternoclavicular joint. **C.** Features of lateral aspect of sternum. **D.** Ages of ossification of sternum. **E.** Sternocostal, manubriosternal, and interchondral joints.

On the right side of the specimen, the cortex of the sternum and the external surface of the costal cartilages have been shaved away.

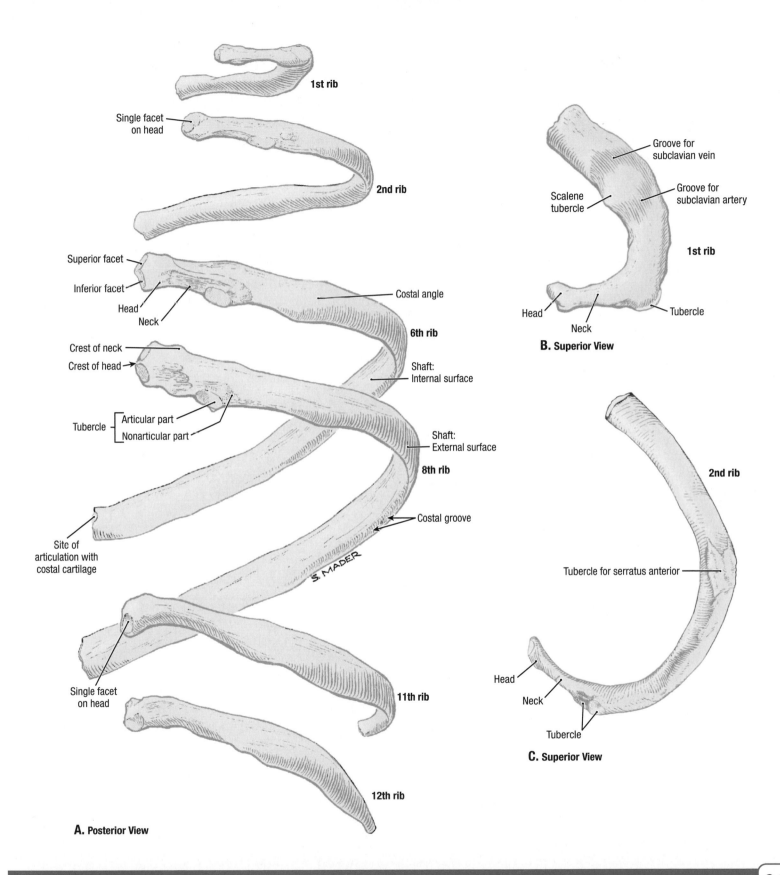

1st rib

Single facet on head

2nd rib

Superior facet

Inferior facet

Head

Neck

Costal angle

6th rib

Crest of neck

Crest of head

Shaft: Internal surface

Articular part

Nonarticular part

Tubercle

Shaft: External surface

8th rib

Site of articulation with costal cartilage

Costal groove

S. MADER

11th rib

Single facet on head

12th rib

A. Posterior View

Groove for subclavian vein

Scalene tubercle

Groove for subclavian artery

1st rib

Head

Neck

Tubercle

B. Superior View

2nd rib

Tubercle for serratus anterior

Head

Neck

Tubercle

C. Superior View

Ribs **3.12**

A. "Typical" (6th and 8th) and "atypical" (1st and 2nd and 11th and 12th) ribs. **B.** First rib. **C.** Second rib.

Rib fractures. The weakest part of a rib is immediately anterior to its angle. The middle ribs are most commonly fractured.

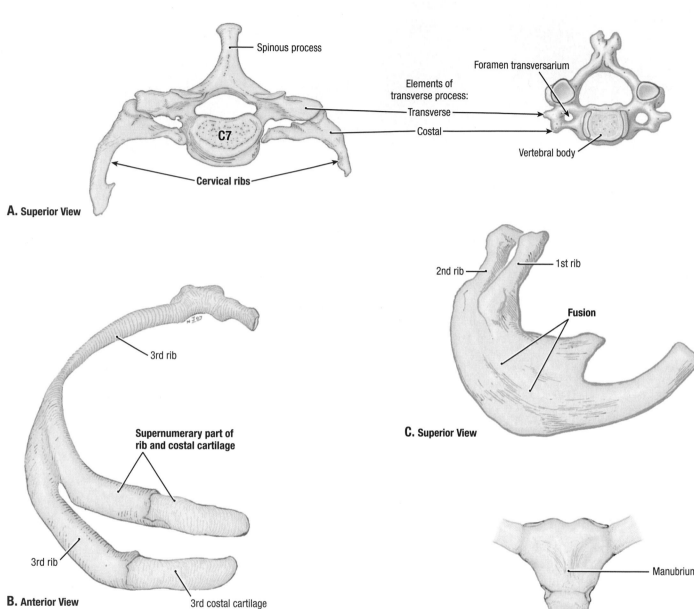

Spinous process

Foramen transversarium

Elements of transverse process:

Transverse

Costal

Vertebral body

C7

Cervical ribs

A. **Superior View**

3rd rib

2nd rib

1st rib

Fusion

Supernumerary part of rib and costal cartilage

C. **Superior View**

3rd rib

B. **Anterior View**   3rd costal cartilage

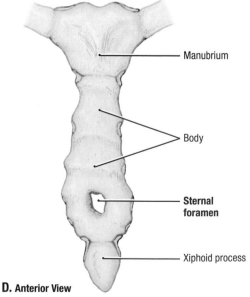

Manubrium

Body

Sternal foramen

Xiphoid process

D. **Anterior View**

3.13   Rib and Sternum Anomalies

A. Cervical ribs. People usually have 12 ribs on each side, but the number may be increased by the presence of cervical and/or lumbar ribs (supernumerary ribs) or decreased by a failure of the 12th pair to form. **Cervical ribs** (present in up to 1% of people) articulate with the C7 vertebra and are clinically significant because they may compress spinal nerves C8 and T1 or the inferior trunk of the brachial plexus supplying the upper limb. Tingling and numbness may occur along the medial border of the forearm. They may also compress the subclavian artery, resulting in **ischemic muscle pain** (caused by poor blood supply) in the upper limb. **Lumbar ribs** are less common than cervical ribs but have clinical significance in that they may confuse the identity of vertebral levels in diagnostic images. **B. Bifid rib.** The superior component of this 3rd rib is supernumerary and articulated with the lateral aspect of the 1st sternebra. The inferior component articulated at the junction of the 1st and 2nd sternebrae. **C. Bicipital rib.** In this specimen, there has been partial fusion of the first two thoracic ribs. **D. Sternal foramen.**

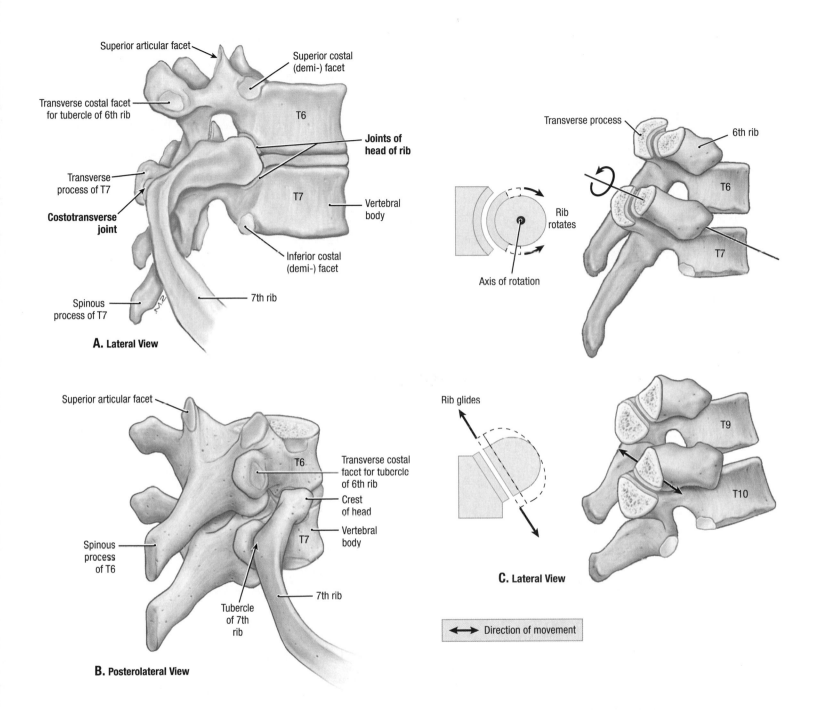

A. Lateral View

B. Posterolateral View

C. Lateral View

Direction of movement

Costovertebral Articulations

3.14

A. and **B. Articulating structures.**

- There are two articular facets on the head of the rib: a larger, inferior costal facet for articulation with the vertebral body of its own number and a smaller, superior costal facet for articulation with the vertebral body of the vertebra superior to the rib.
- The crest of the head of the rib separates the superior and inferior costal facets.

- The smooth articular part of the tubercle of the rib, the transverse costal facet, articulates with the transverse process of the same numbered vertebra at the costotransverse joint.

C. Movements at costotransverse joints. At the 1st to 7th costotransverse joints, the ribs rotate, increasing the anteroposterior diameter of the thorax; at the 8th, 9th, and 10th, they glide, increasing the transverse diameter of the upper abdomen.

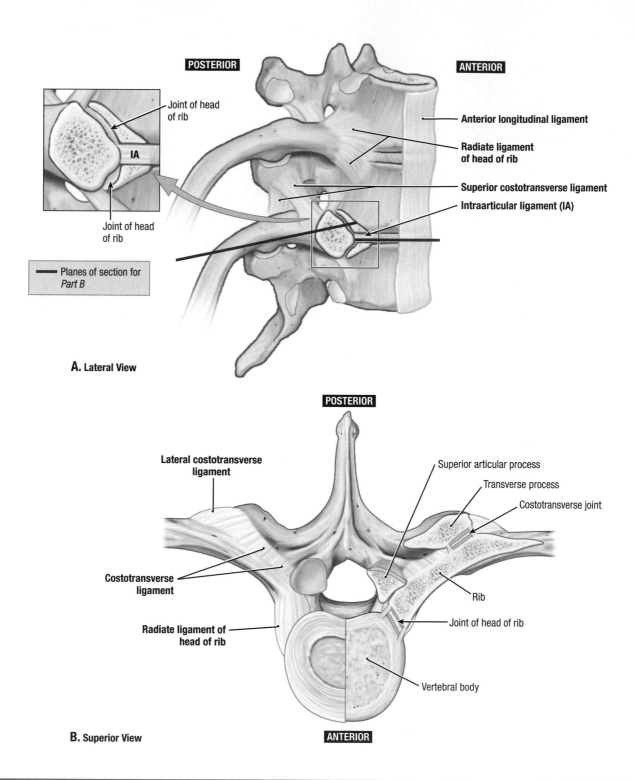

POSTERIOR   ANTERIOR

Joint of head
of rib

IA

Joint of head
of rib

Anterior longitudinal ligament

Radiate ligament
of head of rib

Superior costotransverse ligament

Intraarticular ligament (IA)

Planes of section for
Part B

A. Lateral View

POSTERIOR

Lateral costotransverse
ligament

Superior articular process

Transverse process

Costotransverse joint

Costotransverse
ligament

Radiate ligament of
head of rib

Rib

Joint of head of rib

Vertebral body

B. Superior View   ANTERIOR

3.15   Ligaments of Costovertebral Articulations

A. External and internal costovertebral ligaments.
- The radiate ligament joins the head of the rib to two vertebral bodies and the interposed intervertebral disc.
- The superior costotransverse ligament joins the crest of the neck of the rib to the transverse process above.
- The intraarticular ligament joins the crest of the head of the rib to the intervertebral disc.

B. Transverse section of costovertebral joints.
- The vertebral body, transverse processes, superior articulating processes, and posterior elements of the articulating ribs have been transversely sectioned to visualize the joint surfaces and ligaments.
- The costotransverse ligament joins the posterior aspect of the neck of the rib to the adjacent transverse process.
- The lateral costotransverse ligament joins the nonarticulating part of the tubercle of the rib to the tip (apex) of the transverse process.

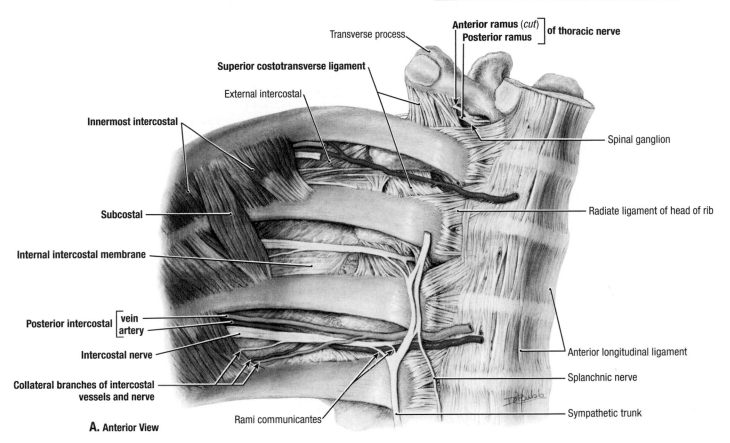

Transverse process

Anterior ramus (*cut*) } of thoracic nerve
Posterior ramus

Superior costotransverse ligament

External intercostal

Innermost intercostal

Spinal ganglion

Subcostal

Radiate ligament of head of rib

Internal intercostal membrane

Posterior intercostal [vein
                          artery

Intercostal nerve

Anterior longitudinal ligament

**Collateral branches of intercostal
vessels and nerve**

Splanchnic nerve

Rami communicantes

Sympathetic trunk

A. Anterior View

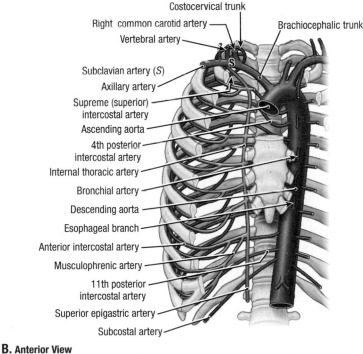

Costocervical trunk

Right common carotid artery

Brachiocephalic trunk

Vertebral artery

Subclavian artery (*S*)

Axillary artery

Supreme (superior)
intercostal artery

Ascending aorta

4th posterior
intercostal artery

Internal thoracic artery

Bronchial artery

Descending aorta

Esophageal branch

Anterior intercostal artery

Musculophrenic artery

11th posterior
intercostal artery

Superior epigastric artery

Subcostal artery

B. Anterior View

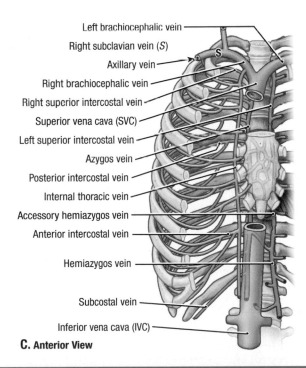

Left brachiocephalic vein

Right subclavian vein (*S*)

Axillary vein

Right brachiocephalic vein

Right superior intercostal vein

Superior vena cava (SVC)

Left superior intercostal vein

Azygos vein

Posterior intercostal vein

Internal thoracic vein

Accessory hemiazygos vein

Anterior intercostal vein

Hemiazygos vein

Subcostal vein

Inferior vena cava (IVC)

C. Anterior View

Neurovasculature of Intercostal Spaces

3.16

A. Vertebral ends of intercostal spaces. **B.** Arteries. **C.** Veins.
- Portions of the innermost intercostal muscle that bridge two intercostal spaces are called subcostales muscles.
- Note the order of the structures in the most inferior space: posterior intercostal vein and artery and intercostal nerve; note also their collateral branches.

- The intercostal nerves attach to the sympathetic trunk by rami communicantes; the splanchnic nerves are visceral branches.
- While the arterial and venous systems of the trunk and limbs run similar, generally parallel courses, that pattern does not apply to the aorta and azygos system of veins.

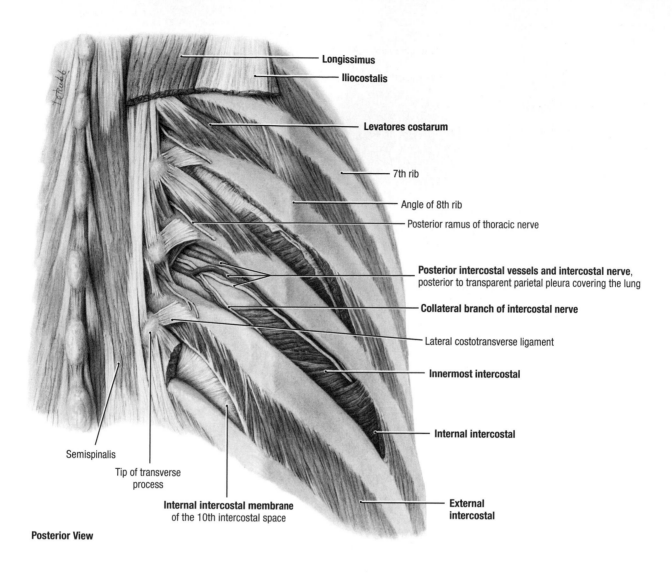

Longissimus

Iliocostalis

Levatores costarum

7th rib

Angle of 8th rib

Posterior ramus of thoracic nerve

Posterior intercostal vessels and intercostal nerve,
posterior to transparent parietal pleura covering the lung

Collateral branch of intercostal nerve

Lateral costotransverse ligament

Innermost intercostal

Internal intercostal

**External
intercostal**

Semispinalis

Tip of transverse
process

Internal intercostal membrane
of the 10th intercostal space

Posterior View

| **3.17** | **Vertebral Ends of External Aspect of Inferior Intercostal Spaces** |

- Most of the iliocostalis and longissimus muscles have been removed, exposing the levatores costarum muscle. Of the five intercostal spaces shown, the superior two (6th and 7th) are intact. In the 8th and 10th spaces, varying portions of the external intercostal muscle have been removed to reveal the underlying internal intercostal membrane, which is continuous with the internal intercostal muscle. In the 9th space, the levatores costarum muscle has been removed to show the posterior intercostal vessels and intercostal nerve.
- The intercostal vessels and nerve disappear laterally between the internal and innermost intercostal muscles.
- The intercostal nerve is the most inferior of the neurovascular trio (posterior intercostal vein and artery and intercostal nerve) and the least sheltered in the intercostal groove; a collateral branch arises near the angle of the rib.
- **Thoracocentesis.** Sometimes it is necessary to insert a hypodermic needle through an intercostal space into the pleural cavity (see Fig. 3.27) to obtain a sample of pleural fluid or to remove blood or pus. To avoid damage to the intercostal nerve and vessels, the needle is inserted superior to the rib, high enough to avoid the collateral branches.

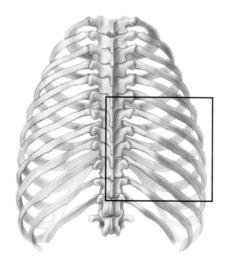

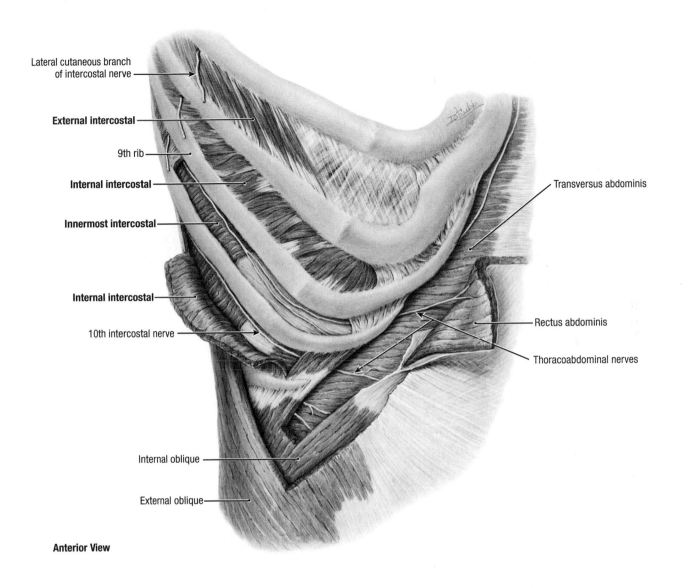

Lateral cutaneous branch of intercostal nerve

External intercostal

9th rib

Internal intercostal

Innermost intercostal

Internal intercostal

10th intercostal nerve

Internal oblique

External oblique

Transversus abdominis

Rectus abdominis

Thoracoabdominal nerves

Anterior View

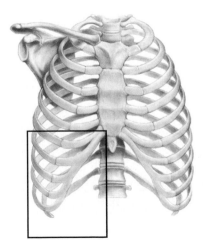

| **Anterior Ends of Inferior Intercostal Spaces** | **3.18** |

- The fibers of the external intercostal and external oblique muscles run inferomedially.
- The internal intercostal and internal oblique muscles are in continuity at the ends of the 9th, 10th, and 11th intercostal spaces.
- The intercostal nerves lie deep to the internal intercostal muscle but superficial to the innermost intercostal muscle; anteriorly, these nerves lie superficial to the transversus thoracis or become thoracoabdominal nerves, distal to the costal margin and anterior to the transversus abdominis muscles.
- Intercostal nerves run parallel to the ribs and costal cartilages; on reaching the abdominal wall, nerves T7 and T8 continue superiorly, T9 continues nearly horizontally, and T10 continues inferomedially toward the umbilicus. The intercostal/thoracoabdominal nerves provide cutaneous innervation in overlapping segmental bands.

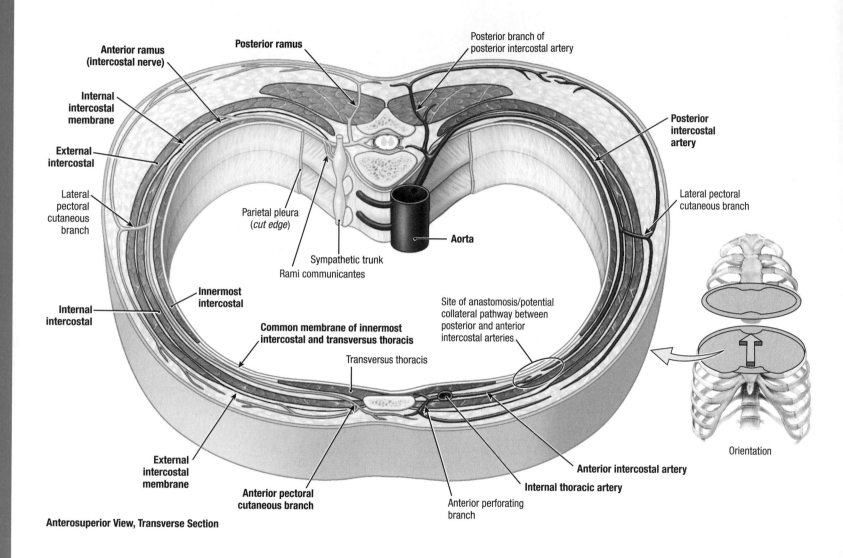

Anterosuperior View, Transverse Section

3.19 | Contents of Intercostal Space, Transverse Section

- The diagram is simplified by showing nerves on the right and arteries on the left.
- The layers from superficial to deep are the external intercostal muscle and membrane, internal intercostal muscle and membrane, innermost intercostal muscle, and transversus thoracis muscle and associated membrane.
- The intercostal nerves are the anterior rami of spinal nerves T1–T11; the anterior ramus of T12 is the subcostal nerve.

- Posterior intercostal arteries are branches of the aorta (the superior two spaces are supplied from the superior intercostal branch of the costocervical trunk); the anterior intercostal arteries are branches of the internal thoracic artery or its branch, the musculophrenic artery.
- The posterior rami innervate the deep back muscles and skin adjacent to the vertebral column.

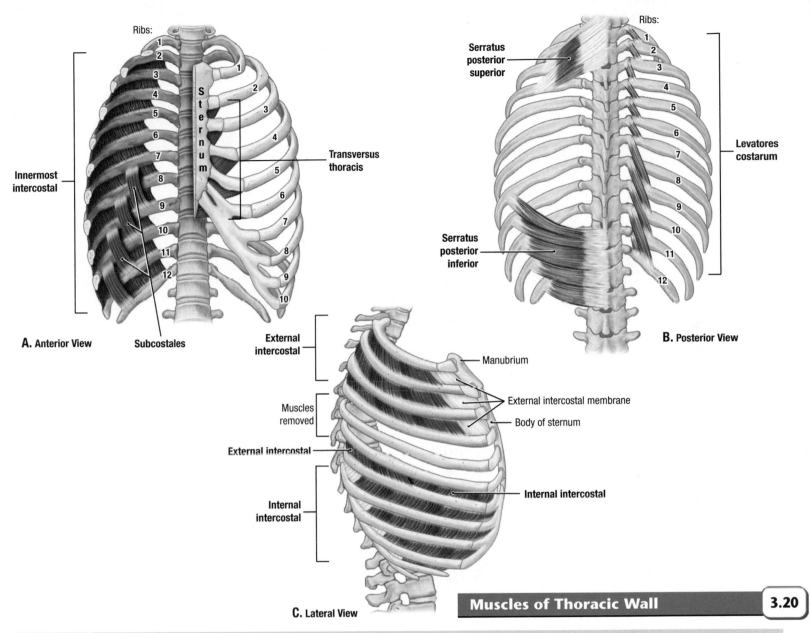

Ribs:
1 2 3 4 5 6 7 8 9 10 11 12

Innermost intercostal

S t e r n u m

1 2 3 4 5 6 7 8 9 10

Transversus thoracis

A. Anterior View   **Subcostales**

Serratus posterior superior

Ribs:
1 2 3 4 5 6 7 8 9 10 11 12

Levatores costarum

Serratus posterior inferior

B. Posterior View

External intercostal

Muscles removed

External intercostal

Internal intercostal

Manubrium

External intercostal membrane

Body of sternum

Internal intercostal

C. Lateral View

Muscles of Thoracic Wall   **3.20**

TABLE 3.1	Muscles of Thoracic Wall			
Muscles	**Superior Attachment**	**Inferior Attachment**	**Innervation**	**Main Action**[a]
External intercostal				During forced inspiration: elevate ribs[a]
Internal intercostal[b]	Inferior border of ribs	Superior border of ribs below		During forced respiration: interosseous part depresses ribs; interchondral part elevates ribs[a]
Innermost intercostal[b]			Intercostal nerve	
Transversus thoracis	Posterior surface of lower sternum	Internal surface of costal cartilages 2–6		Weakly depress ribs
Subcostales	Internal surface of lower ribs near their angles	Superior borders of 2nd or 3rd rib below		Probably act in same manner as internal intercostal muscles
Levatores costarum	Transverse processes of C7–T11	Subjacent ribs between tubercle and angle	Posterior rami of C8–T11 nerves	Elevate ribs
Serratus posterior superior	Nuchal ligament, spinous processes of C7–T3 vertebrae	2nd–4th ribs near their angles	2nd–5th intercostal nerves	Elevate ribs[c]
Serratus posterior inferior	Spinous processes of T11–L2 vertebrae	Inferior borders of 8th–12th ribs near their angles	9th–11th intercostal nerves, subcostal (T12) nerve	Depress ribs[c]

[a]The tonus of the intercostal muscles keep intercostal spaces rigid, thereby preventing them from billowing (bulging) out during expiration and from being drawn in during inspiration. The role of individual intercostal muscles and accessory muscles of respiration in moving the ribs is difficult to interpret despite many electromyographic studies.
[b]Internal and innermost intercostal muscles are essentially the same muscle: Muscle fibers passing superficial to the intercostal neurovasculature are "internal" and those passing deep to the neurovasculature are "innermost."
[c]Action traditionally assigned on the basis of attachments; these muscles appear to be largely proprioceptive in function.

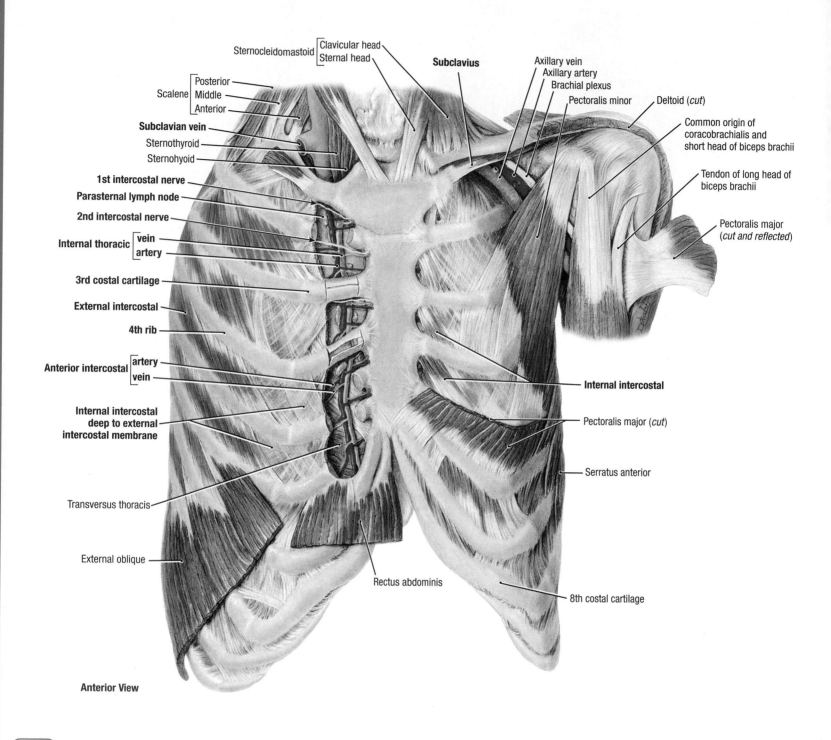

Sternocleidomastoid — Clavicular head / Sternal head

Subclavius

Axillary vein / Axillary artery / Brachial plexus

Pectoralis minor — Deltoid (*cut*)

Scalene — Posterior / Middle / Anterior

Common origin of coracobrachialis and short head of biceps brachii

Subclavian vein

Sternothyroid

Sternohyoid

Tendon of long head of biceps brachii

1st intercostal nerve

Parasternal lymph node

2nd intercostal nerve

Pectoralis major (*cut and reflected*)

Internal thoracic — vein / artery

3rd costal cartilage

External intercostal

4th rib

Anterior intercostal — artery / vein

Internal intercostal

Internal intercostal deep to external intercostal membrane

Pectoralis major (*cut*)

Serratus anterior

Transversus thoracis

External oblique

Rectus abdominis

8th costal cartilage

Anterior View

| **3.21** | **External Aspect of Thoracic Wall** |

- H-shaped cuts were made through the perichondrium of the 3rd and 4th costal cartilages to shell out segments of cartilage.
- During surgery, **retaining perichondrium** promotes regrowth of removed cartilages.
- The internal thoracic (internal mammary) vessels run inferiorly deep to the costal cartilages and just lateral to the edge of the sternum, providing anterior intercostal branches.

- The parasternal lymph nodes (*green*) receive lymphatic vessels from the anterior parts of intercostal spaces, the costal pleura and diaphragm, and the medial part of the breast.
- The subclavian vessels are "sandwiched" between the 1st rib and clavicle and are "padded" by the subclavius.
- **Surgical access to thorax.** To gain access to the thoracic cavity for surgical procedures, the sternum is divided in the median plane (median sternotomy) and retracted (spread apart). After surgery, the halves of the sternum are held together with wire sutures.

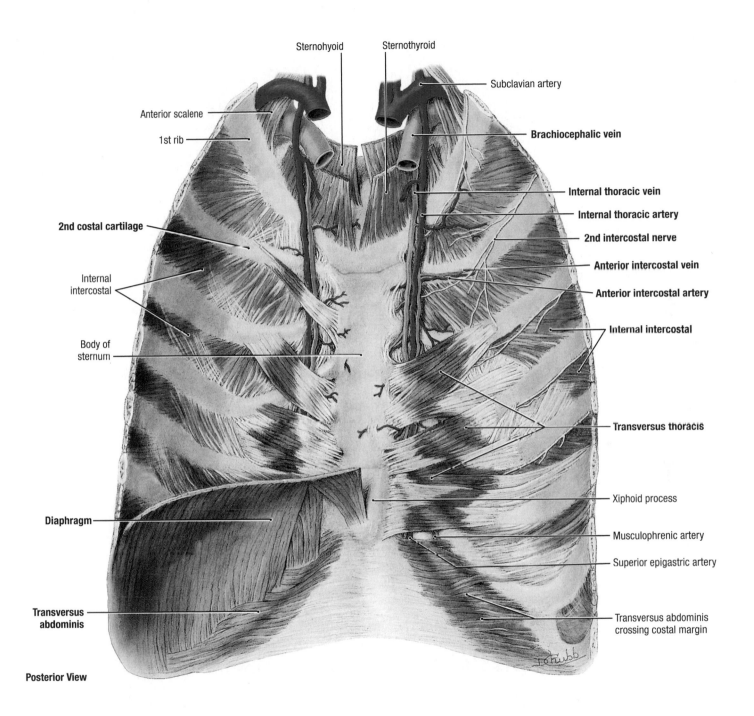

Sternohyoid

Sternothyroid

Subclavian artery

Anterior scalene

Brachiocephalic vein

1st rib

Internal thoracic vein

Internal thoracic artery

2nd costal cartilage

2nd intercostal nerve

Anterior intercostal vein

Internal intercostal

Anterior intercostal artery

Internal intercostal

Body of sternum

Transversus thoracis

Xiphoid process

Diaphragm

Musculophrenic artery

Superior epigastric artery

Transversus abdominis

Transversus abdominis crossing costal margin

Posterior View

Internal Aspect of Anterior Thoracic Wall

3.22

- The inferior portions of the internal thoracic vessels are covered posteriorly by the transversus thoracis muscle; the superior portions are in contact with the parietal pleura (removed).
- The transversus thoracis muscle (superior to diaphragm) is continuous with the transversus abdominis muscle (inferior to diaphragm); these form the innermost layer of the three flat muscles of the thoracoabdominal wall.

- The internal thoracic (internal mammary) artery arises from the subclavian artery and is accompanied by two venae comitantes up to the 2nd costal cartilage in this specimen and, superior to this, by the single internal thoracic vein, which drains into the brachiocephalic vein.

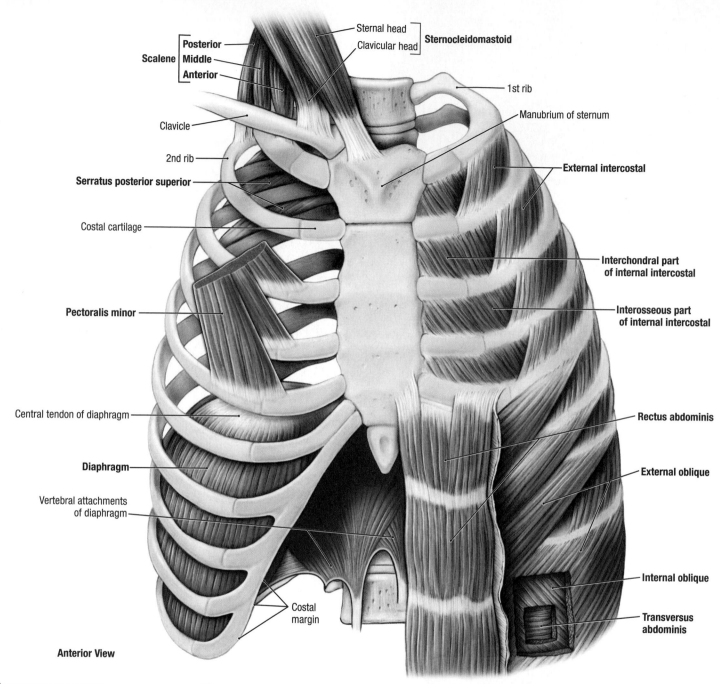

Anterior View

3.23　**Muscles of Respiration**

TABLE 3.2		**Muscles of Respiration**	
Inspiration			**Expiration**
Normal (Quiet)	Major	Diaphragm (active contraction)	Passive (elastic) recoil of lungs and thoracic cage
	Minor	*Tonic contraction* of external intercostals and interchondral portion of internal intercostals to resist negative pressure	*Tonic contraction* of muscles of anterolateral abdominal walls (rectus abdominis, external and internal obliques, transversus abdominis) to antagonize diaphragm by maintaining intraabdominal pressure
Active (Forced)		In addition to the above, *active contraction* of sternocleidomastoid, descending (superior) trapezius, pectoralis minor, and scalenes to elevate and fix upper rib cage	In addition to the above, *active contraction* of muscles of anterolateral abdominal wall (antagonizing diaphragm by increasing intraabdominal pressure and by pulling inferiorly and fixing inferior costal margin): rectus abdominis, external and internal obliques, and transversus abdominis
		External intercostals, interchondral portion of internal intercostals, subcostales, levatores costarum, and serratus posterior superior[a] to elevate ribs	Internal intercostal (interosseous part) and serratus posterior inferior[a] to depress ribs

[a]Recent studies indicate that the serratus posterior superior and inferior muscles may serve primarily as organs of proprioception rather than motion.

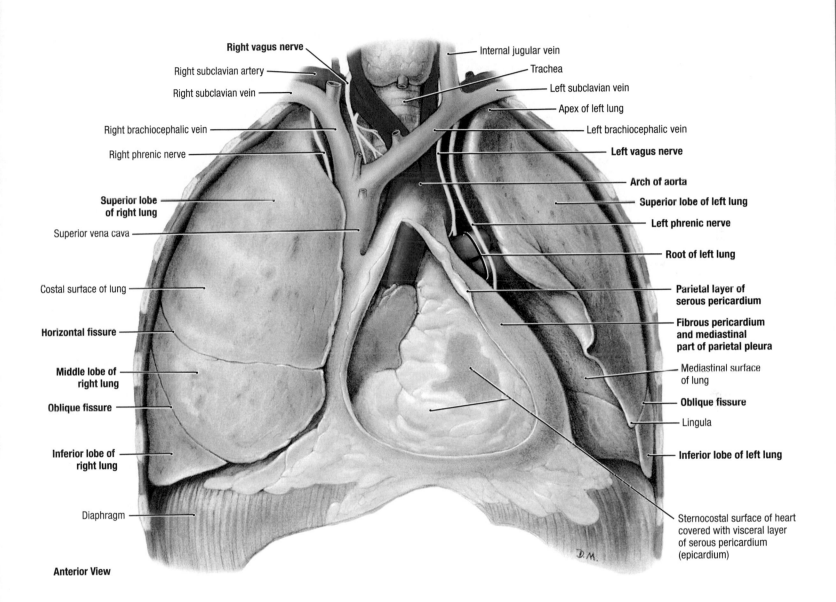

Right vagus nerve

Right subclavian artery

Right subclavian vein

Right brachiocephalic vein

Right phrenic nerve

Superior lobe of right lung

Superior vena cava

Costal surface of lung

Horizontal fissure

Middle lobe of right lung

Oblique fissure

Inferior lobe of right lung

Diaphragm

Anterior View

Internal jugular vein

Trachea

Left subclavian vein

Apex of left lung

Left brachiocephalic vein

Left vagus nerve

Arch of aorta

Superior lobe of left lung

Left phrenic nerve

Root of left lung

Parietal layer of serous pericardium

Fibrous pericardium and mediastinal part of parietal pleura

Mediastinal surface of lung

Oblique fissure

Lingula

Inferior lobe of left lung

Sternocostal surface of heart covered with visceral layer of serous pericardium (epicardium)

D. M.

Thoracic Contents *In Situ*

3.24

- The fibrous pericardium, lined by the parietal layer of serous pericardium, is removed anteriorly to expose the heart and great vessels.
- The right lung has three lobes; the superior lobe is separated from the middle lobe by the horizontal fissure, and the middle lobe is separated from the inferior lobe by the oblique fissure.

The left lung has two lobes, superior and inferior, separated by the oblique fissure.
- The anterior border of the left lung is reflected laterally to visualize the phrenic nerve passing anterior to the root of the lung and the vagus nerve lying anterior to the arch of the aorta and then passing posterior to the root of the lung.

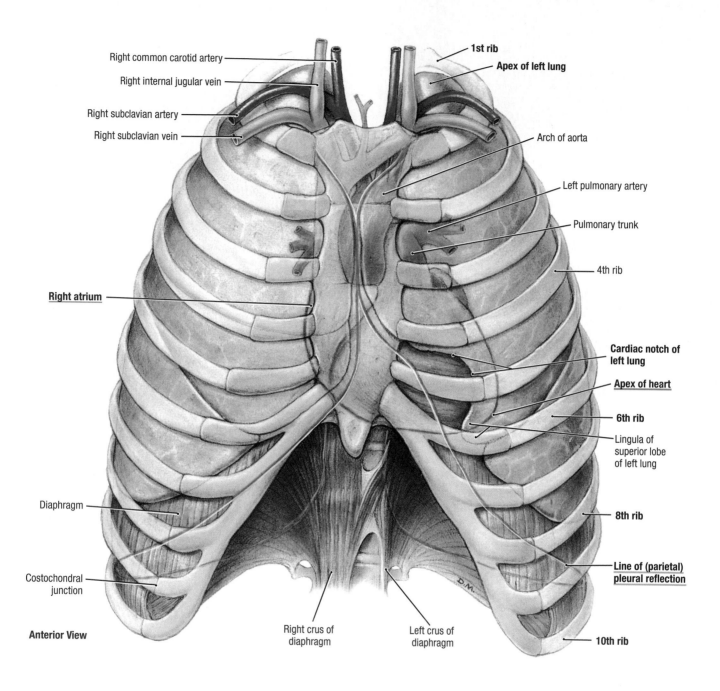

Right common carotid artery

Right internal jugular vein

Right subclavian artery

Right subclavian vein

Right atrium

Diaphragm

Costochondral
junction

Anterior View

1st rib

Apex of left lung

Arch of aorta

Left pulmonary artery

Pulmonary trunk

4th rib

**Cardiac notch of
left lung**

Apex of heart

6th rib

Lingula of
superior lobe
of left lung

8th rib

**Line of (parietal)
pleural reflection**

10th rib

Right crus of
diaphragm

Left crus of
diaphragm

3.25   Topography of Lungs and Mediastinum

- The mediastinum is located between the pleural cavities and is occupied by the heart and the tissues anterior, posterior, and superior to the heart.
- The apex of the lungs is at the level of the neck of the 1st rib, and the inferior border of the lungs is at the 6th rib in the left midclavicular line and the 8th rib at the lateral aspect of the bony thorax at the midaxillary line.
- The cardiac notch of the left lung and the corresponding deviation of the parietal pleura are away from the median plane toward the left side.

- The inferior line of reflection of parietal pleura is at the 8th costochondral junction in the midclavicular line and at the 10th rib in the midaxillary line.
- The apex of the heart is in the 5th intercostal space at the left midclavicular line.
- The right atrium forms the right border of the heart and extends just beyond the lateral margin of the sternum.
- The branches of the great vessels pass through the superior thoracic aperture.

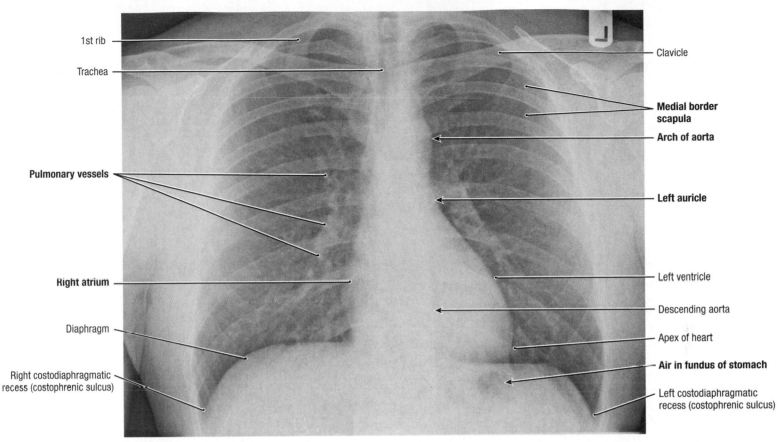

1st rib
Trachea
Pulmonary vessels
Right atrium
Diaphragm
Right costodiaphragmatic recess (costophrenic sulcus)

Clavicle
Medial border scapula
Arch of aorta
Left auricle
Left ventricle
Descending aorta
Apex of heart
Air in fundus of stomach
Left costodiaphragmatic recess (costophrenic sulcus)

A. Posteroanterior Radiograph

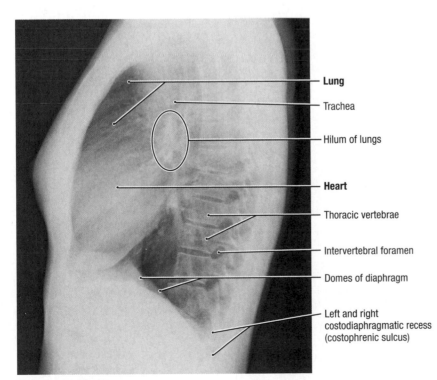

Lung
Trachea
Hilum of lungs
Heart
Thoracic vertebrae
Intervertebral foramen
Domes of diaphragm
Left and right costodiaphragmatic recess (costophrenic sulcus)

B. Lateral Radiograph

Radiograph of Chest   3.26

A. Standard chest x-ray (chest film).

- Unless a patient is bedridden, a chest radiograph is done with the x-ray beam traversing the patient from posterior to anterior (PA) because this minimizes distortion. The scapula is protracted and not in the main field of view.
- Right atrium is the primary discernible structure along the right border of the heart.
- Within the dark gray (radiolucent) regions of both sides that show air in the lung, most of the linear denser (whiter) elements are pulmonary veins.
- Along the upper left mediastinal border, the arch of aorta is visible, and the aorta can be followed inferiorly.
- Left auricle is often visible along the left border of the heart; inferiorly is the border of the left ventricle.
- In a standing PA radiograph, air is often seen in the fundus of the stomach.

B. Standard lateral chest x-ray (lateral chest film).

- Note that the left and right are not precisely superimposed on one another.
- Notice how well the heart is shown relative to the aerated lungs, which are radiopaque because they do not block many photons. A loss of this clear differentiation is known as the silhouette sign and suggests lung disease.
- Any structure in the mediastinum may contribute to **pathological widening of the mediastinal silhouette** (e.g., after trauma that produces hemorrhage into the mediastinum), malignant lymphoma (cancer of lymphatic tissue) that produces massive enlargement of mediastinal lymph nodes, or enlargement (hypertrophy) of the heart occurring with congestive heart failure.

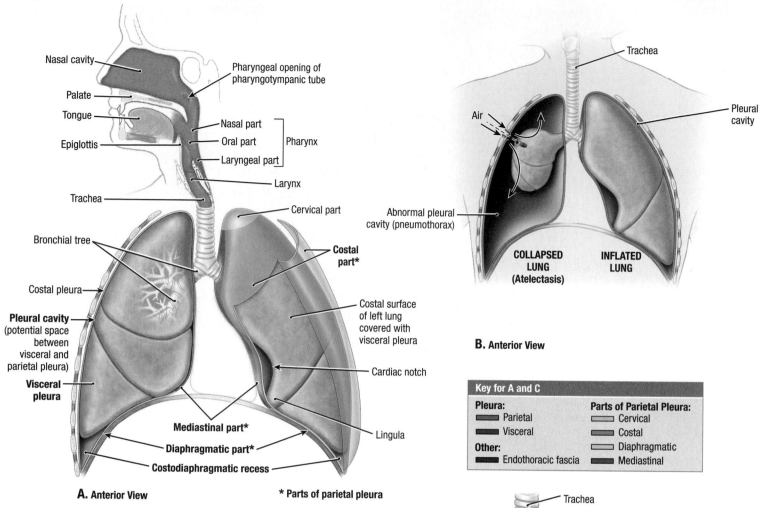

A. Anterior View

* Parts of parietal pleura

Labels (A. Anterior View):
Nasal cavity; Pharyngeal opening of pharyngotympanic tube; Palate; Tongue; Nasal part; Oral part; Pharynx; Epiglottis; Laryngeal part; Larynx; Trachea; Cervical part; Bronchial tree; Costal part*; Costal pleura; Costal surface of left lung covered with visceral pleura; Pleural cavity (potential space between visceral and parietal pleura); Visceral pleura; Cardiac notch; Mediastinal part*; Diaphragmatic part*; Costodiaphragmatic recess; Lingula

B. Anterior View

Labels (B): Trachea; Pleural cavity; Air; Abnormal pleural cavity (pneumothorax); COLLAPSED LUNG (Atelectasis); INFLATED LUNG

Key for A and C

Pleura:	Parts of Parietal Pleura:
Parietal	Cervical
Visceral	Costal
Other:	Diaphragmatic
Endothoracic fascia	Mediastinal

3.27 Respiratory System and Pleura

A. Overview. **B.** Pleural cavity and pleura.
C. Diagrammatic section through lungs with pulmonary vessels and tracheobronchial tree.

- The lungs invaginate a continuous membranous pleural sac; the visceral (pulmonary) pleura covers the lungs, and the parietal pleura lines the thoracic cavity; the visceral and parietal pleurae are continuous around the root of the lung.
- The parietal pleura can be divided regionally into the costal, diaphragmatic, mediastinal, and cervical parts; note the costodiaphragmatic recess.
- The pleural cavity is a potential space between the visceral and parietal pleurae that contains a thin layer of fluid. If a sufficient amount of air enters the pleural cavity, the surface tension adhering visceral to parietal pleura (lung to thoracic wall) is broken, and the lung collapses (**atelectasis**) because of its inherent elasticity (elastic recoil). When a lung collapses, the pleural cavity becomes a real space (as in *Part B*) and may contain air (**pneumothorax**), blood (**hemothorax**), etc.

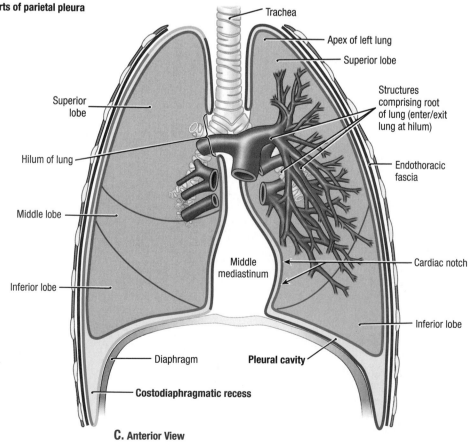

C. Anterior View

Labels (C): Trachea; Apex of left lung; Superior lobe; Structures comprising root of lung (enter/exit lung at hilum); Superior lobe; Hilum of lung; Endothoracic fascia; Middle lobe; Middle mediastinum; Cardiac notch; Inferior lobe; Inferior lobe; Diaphragm; Pleural cavity; Costodiaphragmatic recess

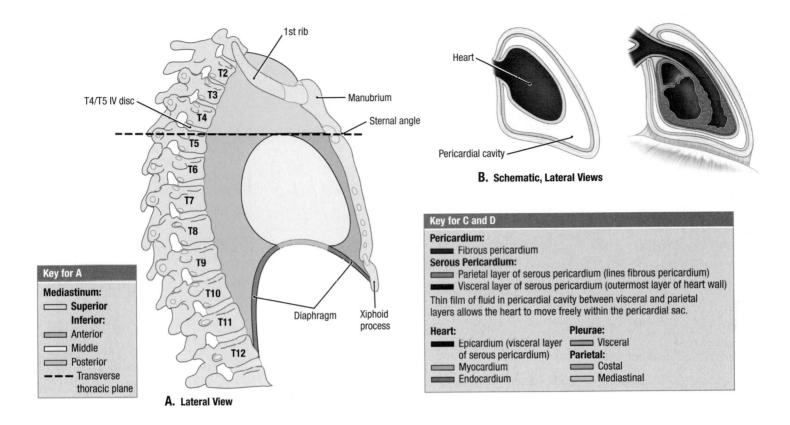

A. Lateral View

- 1st rib
- T2
- T3
- T4/T5 IV disc
- T4
- Manubrium
- Sternal angle
- T5
- T6
- T7
- T8
- T9
- T10
- T11
- Diaphragm
- Xiphoid process
- T12

Key for A

Mediastinum:
- **Superior**
- **Inferior:**
  - Anterior
  - Middle
  - Posterior
- - - Transverse thoracic plane

B. Schematic, Lateral Views

- Heart
- Pericardial cavity

Key for C and D

Pericardium:
- Fibrous pericardium

Serous Pericardium:
- Parietal layer of serous pericardium (lines fibrous pericardium)
- Visceral layer of serous pericardium (outermost layer of heart wall)

Thin film of fluid in pericardial cavity between visceral and parietal layers allows the heart to move freely within the pericardial sac.

Heart:
- Epicardium (visceral layer of serous pericardium)
- Myocardium
- Endocardium

Pleurae:
- Visceral

Parietal:
- Costal
- Mediastinal

C. Median Section

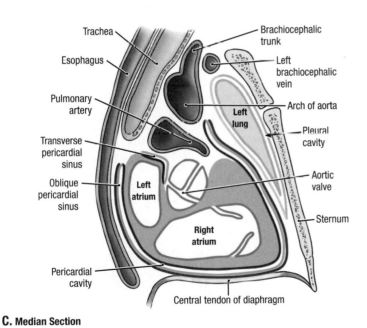

- Trachea
- Esophagus
- Pulmonary artery
- Transverse pericardial sinus
- Oblique pericardial sinus
- Left atrium
- Right atrium
- Pericardial cavity
- Central tendon of diaphragm
- Brachiocephalic trunk
- Left brachiocephalic vein
- Arch of aorta
- Left lung
- Pleural cavity
- Aortic valve
- Sternum

D. Transverse Section

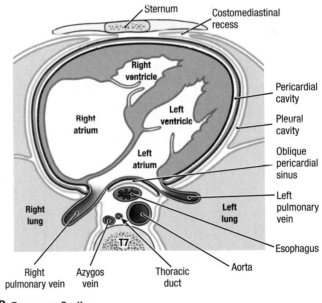

- Sternum
- Costomediastinal recess
- Right ventricle
- Right atrium
- Left ventricle
- Left atrium
- Pericardial cavity
- Pleural cavity
- Oblique pericardial sinus
- Left pulmonary vein
- Right lung
- Left lung
- Esophagus
- Right pulmonary vein
- Azygos vein
- Thoracic duct
- Aorta
- T7

Mediastinum and Pericardium

3.28

A. Subdivisions of mediastinum. B. Development of pericardial cavity. The embryonic heart invaginates the wall of the serous sac (*left*) and soon practically obliterates the pericardial cavity, leaving only a potential space between the layers of serous pericardium (*right*). **C.** and **D. Layers of pericardium and heart in sectional views.**

Cardiac tamponade (heart compression) is a potentially lethal condition because heart volume is increasingly compromised by the fluid outside the heart but inside the pericardial cavity. The heart is increasingly compressed and circulation fails. Blood in the pericardial cavity, **hemopericardium**, produces cardiac tamponade.

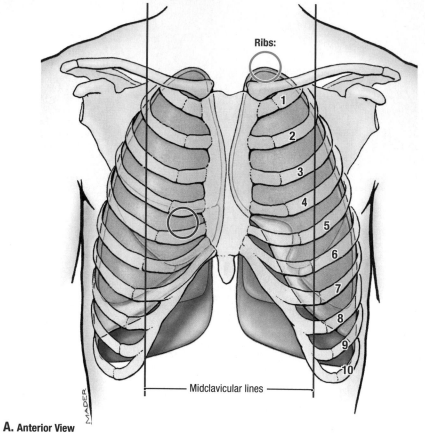

Ribs:

Midclavicular lines

A. Anterior View

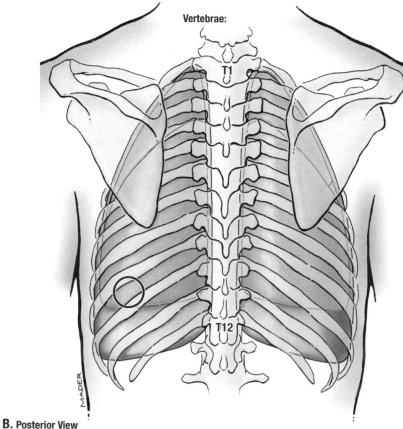

Vertebrae:

T1

T12

B. Posterior View

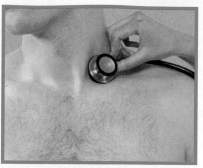

Anterior View

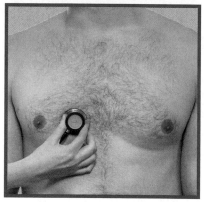

Anterior View

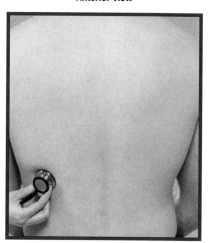

Posterior View

C. Auscultation

3.29 Pleura and Auscultation of Lungs

A. Extent of pleura, anterior aspect. **B.** Extent of pleura, posterior aspect. **C.** Auscultation of lungs.

Auscultation of lungs. Note the position of the fissures in relation to overlying ribs. To auscultate the upper lobes, place the stethoscope on the anterior thoracic wall superior to the 4th rib on the right and 6th rib on the left; for the middle lobe, place it medial to the right nipple; for the inferior lobes, place it on the posterior thoracic wall below the 3rd rib.

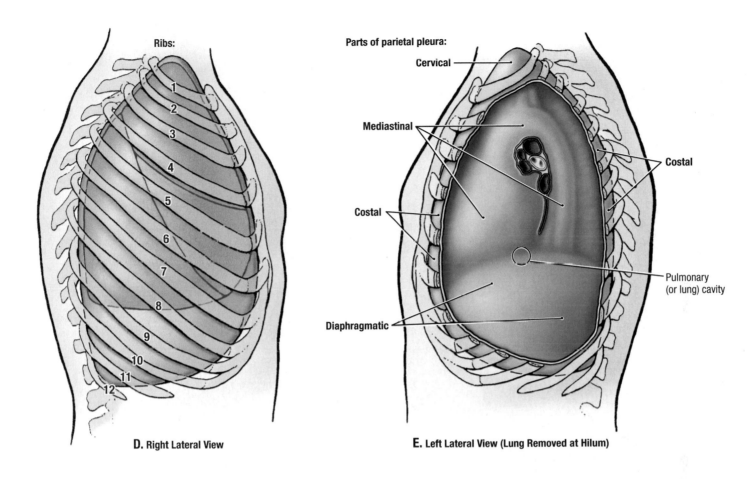

D. Right Lateral View

E. Left Lateral View (Lung Removed at Hilum)

Pleura and Auscultation of Lungs *(continued)* 3.29

TABLE 3.3	Surface Markings of Lines of Reflection of Parietal Pleura and Borders of Lungs	
Level	**Left Pleura**	**Right Pleura**
Apex	About 4 cm superior to middle of clavicle	About 4 cm superior to middle of clavicle
4th costal cartilage	Midline (anteriorly)	Midline (anteriorly)
6th costal cartilage	Lateral margin of sternum	Midline (anteriorly)
8th costal cartilage	Midclavicular line	Midclavicular line
10th rib	Midaxillary line	Midaxillary line
11th rib	Scapular line (vertical line passing through inferior angle of scapula)	Scapular line (vertical line passing through inferior angle of scapula)
12th rib	Lateral border of erector spinae to T12 spinous process (slightly lower level than right pleura)	Lateral border of erector spinae to T12 spinous process

Level	**Left Lung**	**Right Lung**
Apex	About 4 cm superior to middle of clavicle	About 4 cm superior to middle of clavicle
2nd costal cartilage	Midline (anteriorly)	Midline (anteriorly)
4th costal cartilage	Leaves lateral margin of sternum, follows 4th costal cartilage	Lateral margin of sternum
6th costal cartilage	Turns inferiorly to 6th costal cartilage in the midclavicular line (cardiac notch)	Follows 6th costal cartilage to midclavicular line
8th rib	Midaxillary line	Midaxillary line
10th rib	Scapular line (vertical line passing through inferior angle of scapula)	Scapular line (vertical line passing through inferior angle of scapula)

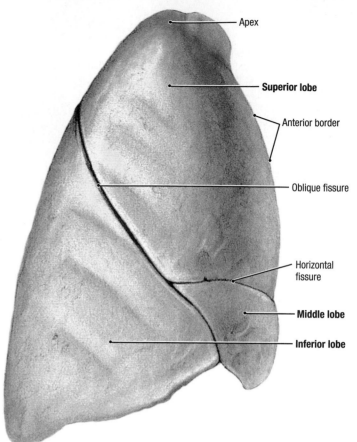

Apex

Superior lobe

Anterior border

Oblique fissure

Horizontal fissure

Middle lobe

Inferior lobe

B. Lateral View

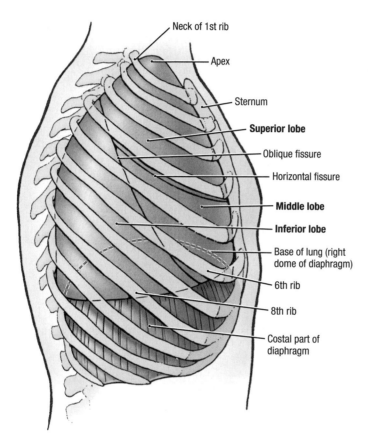

Neck of 1st rib

Apex

Sternum

Superior lobe

Oblique fissure

Horizontal fissure

Middle lobe

Inferior lobe

Base of lung (right dome of diaphragm)

6th rib

8th rib

Costal part of diaphragm

A. Lateral View

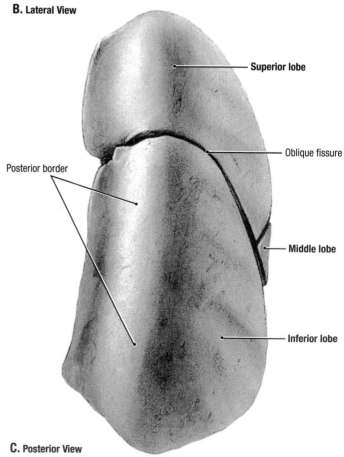

Superior lobe

Posterior border

Oblique fissure

Middle lobe

Inferior lobe

C. Posterior View

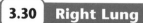

3.30 **Right Lung**

- The oblique and horizontal fissures divide the right lung into three lobes: superior, middle, and inferior.
- The right lung is larger and heavier than the left but is shorter and wider because the right dome of the diaphragm is higher and the heart bulges more to the left.
- Cadaveric lungs may be shrunken, firm, and discolored, whereas healthy lungs in living people are normally soft, light, and spongy.
- Each lung has an apex and base, three surfaces (costal, mediastinal, and diaphragmatic), and three borders (anterior, inferior, and posterior).

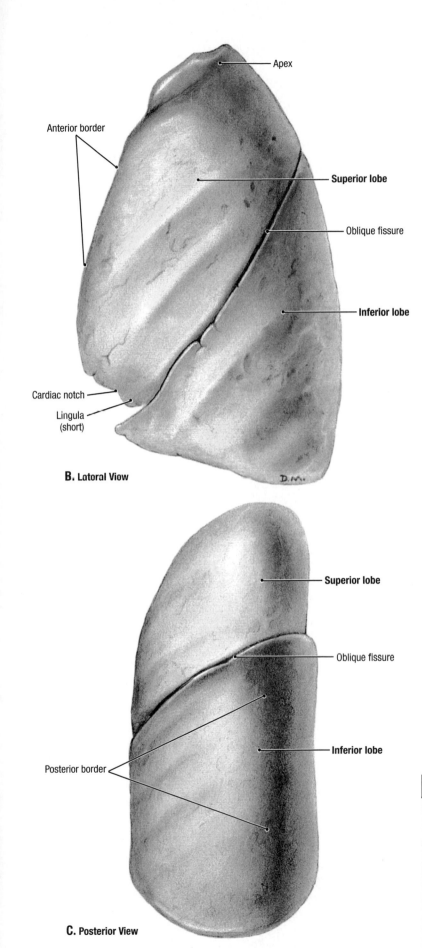

B. Lateral View

- Apex
- Anterior border
- **Superior lobe**
- Oblique fissure
- **Inferior lobe**
- Cardiac notch
- Lingula (short)

C. Posterior View

- **Superior lobe**
- Oblique fissure
- **Inferior lobe**
- Posterior border

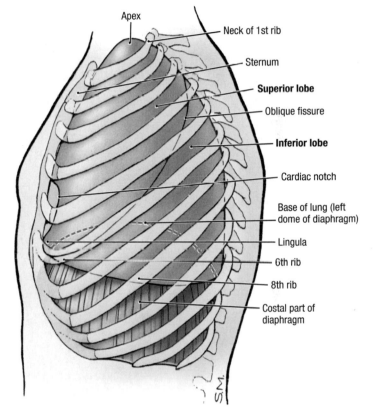

A. Lateral View

- Apex
- Neck of 1st rib
- Sternum
- **Superior lobe**
- Oblique fissure
- **Inferior lobe**
- Cardiac notch
- Base of lung (left dome of diaphragm)
- Lingula
- 6th rib
- 8th rib
- Costal part of diaphragm

Left Lung
3.31

- The left lung has two lobes (superior and inferior) separated by the oblique fissure.
- The anterior border has a deep cardiac notch that indents the anteroinferior aspect of the superior lobe.
- The lingula, a tongue-like process of the superior lobe, extends below the cardiac notch and slides in and out of the costomediastinal recess during inspiration and expiration.
- The lungs of an embalmed cadaver usually retain impressions of structures that lie adjacent to them, such as the ribs and heart.

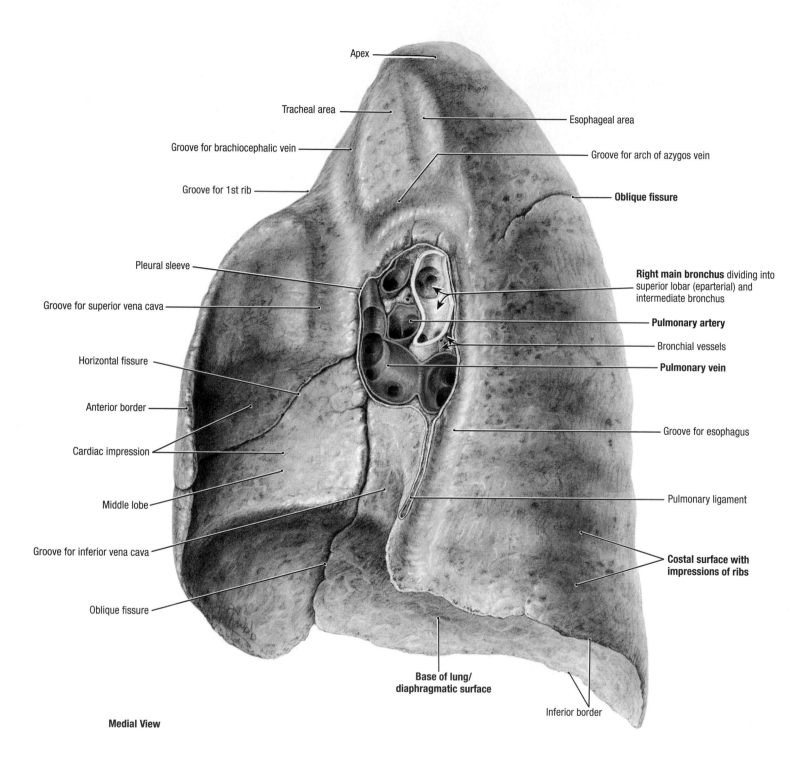

Apex

Tracheal area

Esophageal area

Groove for brachiocephalic vein

Groove for arch of azygos vein

Groove for 1st rib

Oblique fissure

Pleural sleeve

Right main bronchus dividing into superior lobar (eparterial) and intermediate bronchus

Groove for superior vena cava

Pulmonary artery

Bronchial vessels

Horizontal fissure

Pulmonary vein

Anterior border

Cardiac impression

Groove for esophagus

Middle lobe

Pulmonary ligament

Groove for inferior vena cava

Costal surface with impressions of ribs

Oblique fissure

Base of lung/ diaphragmatic surface

Inferior border

Medial View

3.32 **Mediastinal (Medial) Surface and Hilum of Right Lung**

The embalmed lung shows impressions of the structures with which it comes into contact, clearly demarcated as surface features; the base is contoured by the domes of the diaphragm; the costal surface bears the impressions of the ribs; distended vessels leave their mark, but nerves do not. The oblique fissure is incomplete superiorly and medially here.

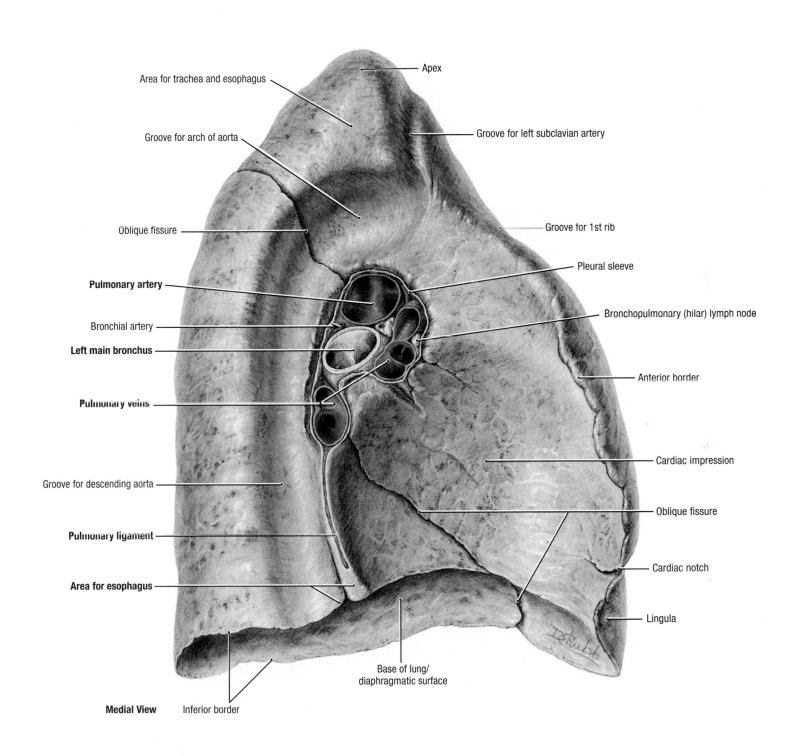

Apex

Area for trachea and esophagus

Groove for arch of aorta

Groove for left subclavian artery

Oblique fissure

Groove for 1st rib

Pleural sleeve

Pulmonary artery

Bronchopulmonary (hilar) lymph node

Bronchial artery

Left main bronchus

Pulmonary veins

Anterior border

Groove for descending aorta

Cardiac impression

Pulmonary ligament

Oblique fissure

Area for esophagus

Cardiac notch

Lingula

Base of lung/
diaphragmatic surface

Medial View   Inferior border

Mediastinal (Medial) Surface and Hilum of Left Lung

Note the site of contact with esophagus, between the descending aorta and the inferior end of the pulmonary ligament. At the right and left hila, the artery is superior, the bronchus is posterior, one vein is anterior, and the other is inferior; at the right hilum, the superior lobar bronchus (eparterial bronchus) is the most superior structure.

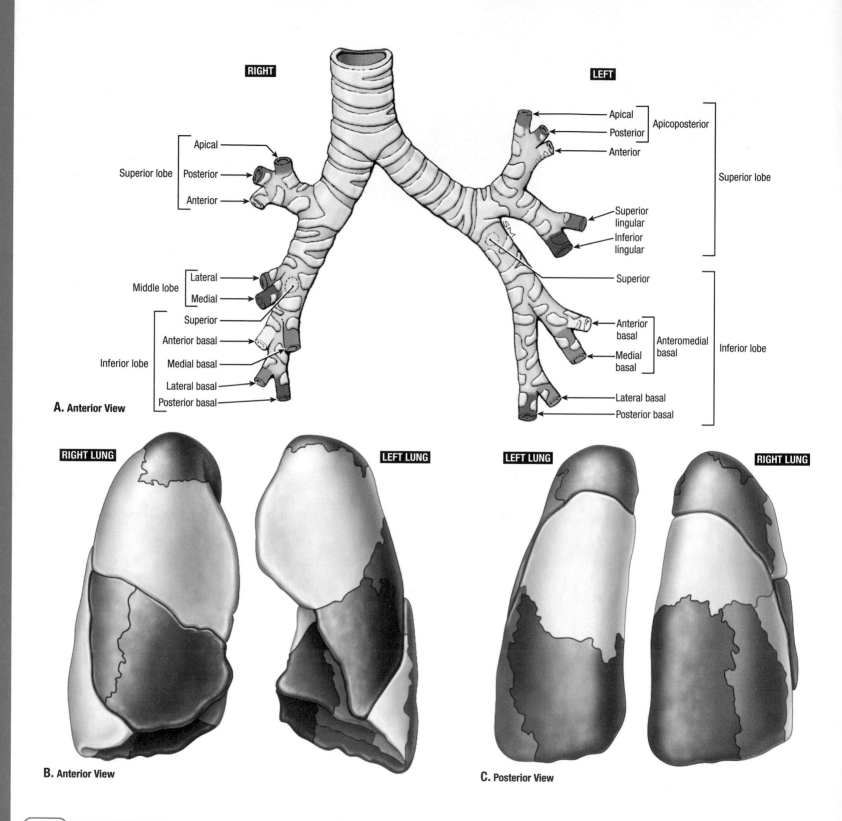

A. Anterior View

RIGHT

Superior lobe
- Apical
- Posterior
- Anterior

Middle lobe
- Lateral
- Medial

Inferior lobe
- Superior
- Anterior basal
- Medial basal
- Lateral basal
- Posterior basal

LEFT

Superior lobe
- Apical } Apicoposterior
- Posterior
- Anterior
- Superior lingular
- Inferior lingular

Inferior lobe
- Superior
- Anterior basal } Anteromedial basal
- Medial basal
- Lateral basal
- Posterior basal

RIGHT LUNG   LEFT LUNG

B. Anterior View

LEFT LUNG   RIGHT LUNG

C. Posterior View

3.34 Segmental Bronchi and Bronchopulmonary Segments

A. Tertiary or segmental bronchi (10 right and 8 left). Note that in the left lung, the apical and posterior bronchi arise from a single stem, as do the anterior basal and medial basal. **B–F. Bronchopulmonary segments.** Each consists of a tertiary bronchus, pulmonary artery, and the portion of lung they serve. These structures are surgically separable to allow segmental resection of the lung. To prepare these specimens, the tertiary bronchi of fresh lungs were isolated within the hilum and injected with latex of various colors. Minor variations in the branching of the bronchi result in variations in the surface patterns.

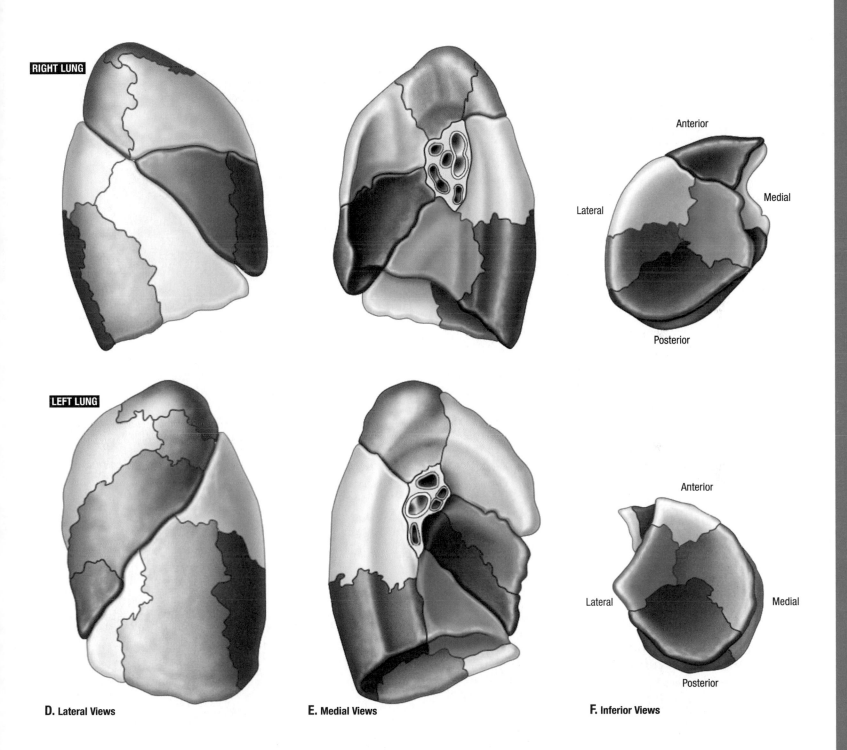

RIGHT LUNG

LEFT LUNG

Anterior

Lateral

Medial

Posterior

Anterior

Lateral

Medial

Posterior

D. Lateral Views

E. Medial Views

F. Inferior Views

Segmental Bronchi and Bronchopulmonary Segments (*continued*) **3.34**

Knowledge of the anatomy of the bronchopulmonary segments is essential for precise interpretations of diagnostic images of the lungs and for surgical resection (removal) of diseased segments. During the treatment of lung cancer, the surgeon may remove a whole lung (**pneumonectomy**), a lobe (**lobectomy**), or one or more bronchopulmonary segments

(**segmentectomy**). Knowledge and understanding of the bronchopulmonary segments and their relationship to the bronchial tree are also essential for planning drainage and clearance techniques used in physical therapy for enhancing drainage from specific areas (e.g., in patients with pneumonia or cystic fibrosis).

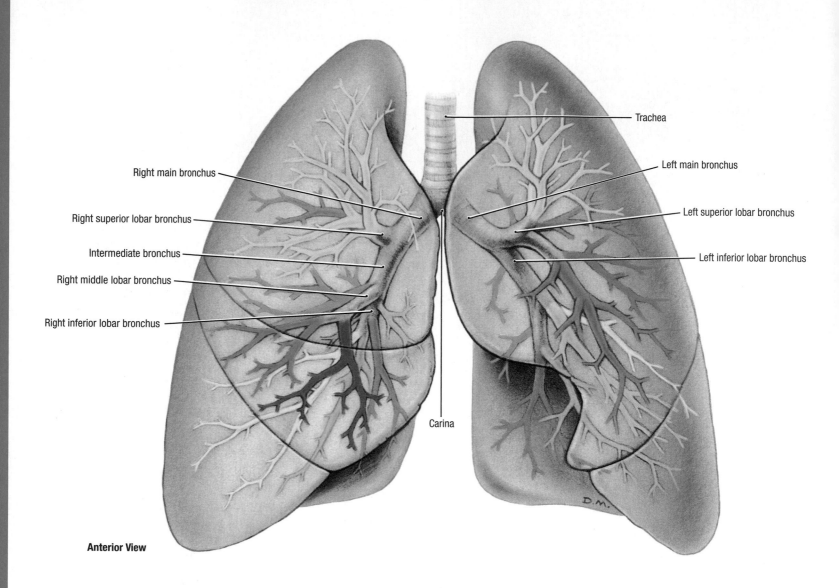

Trachea

Right main bronchus

Right superior lobar bronchus

Intermediate bronchus

Right middle lobar bronchus

Right inferior lobar bronchus

Left main bronchus

Left superior lobar bronchus

Left inferior lobar bronchus

Carina

D.M.

Anterior View

3.35 **Trachea and Bronchi** *In Situ*

- The segmental (tertiary) bronchi are color coded.
- The trachea bifurcates into right and left main (primary) bronchi; the right main bronchus is shorter, wider, and more vertical than the left.
- Therefore, it is more likely that **aspirated foreign bodies** will enter and lodge in the right main bronchus or one of its descending branches.
- The right main bronchus gives off the right superior lobe bronchus (eparterial bronchus) before entering the hilum (hilus) of the lung; after entering the hilum, the continuing intermediate bronchus divides into the right middle and inferior lobar bronchi.
- The left main bronchus divides at the hilum into the left superior and left inferior lobar bronchi; the lobar bronchi further divide into segmental (tertiary) bronchi.

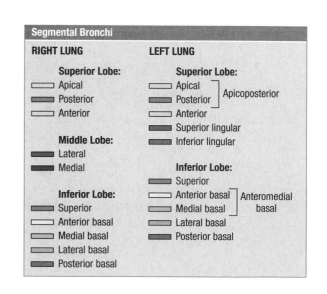

Segmental Bronchi

RIGHT LUNG	LEFT LUNG
Superior Lobe:	**Superior Lobe:**
Apical	Apical ⎤ Apicoposterior
Posterior	Posterior ⎦
Anterior	Anterior
	Superior lingular
Middle Lobe:	Inferior lingular
Lateral	
Medial	**Inferior Lobe:**
	Superior
Inferior Lobe:	Anterior basal ⎤ Anteromedial
Superior	Medial basal ⎦ basal
Anterior basal	Lateral basal
Medial basal	Posterior basal
Lateral basal	
Posterior basal	

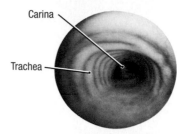

Trachea and carina

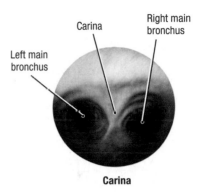

Carina

Trachea

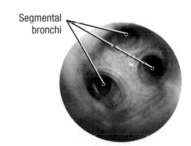

Carina

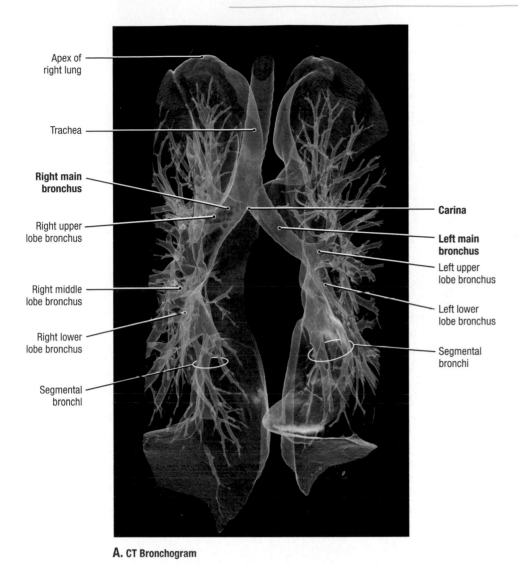

Apex of
right lung

Trachea

**Right main
bronchus**

Right upper
lobe bronchus

Right middle
lobe bronchus

Right lower
lobe bronchus

Segmental
bronchl

Carina

**Left main
bronchus**

Left upper
lobe bronchus

Left lower
lobe bronchus

Segmental
bronchi

Carina

Right main
bronchus

Left main
bronchus

Segmental
bronchi

Right upper lobe bronchus

B. Bronchoscopic Views

A. CT Bronchogram

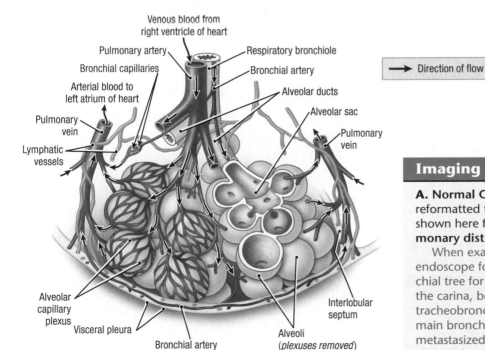

Venous blood from
right ventricle of heart

Pulmonary artery

Bronchial capillaries

Arterial blood to
left atrium of heart

Pulmonary
vein

Lymphatic
vessels

Alveolar
capillary
plexus

Visceral pleura

Bronchial artery

Respiratory bronchiole

Bronchial artery

Alveolar ducts

Alveolar sac

Pulmonary
vein

Interlobular
septum

Alveoli
(*plexuses removed*)

→ Direction of flow

C. Schematic

Imaging of Lungs   3.36

A. Normal CT 3D airway study. CT imaging data can be
reformatted to demonstrate specific anatomical structures as
shown here for the bronchi. **B. Bronchoscopy. C. Intrapulmonary distribution of vasculature.**

When examining the bronchi with a **bronchoscope**—an
endoscope for inspecting the interior of the tracheobronchial tree for diagnostic purposes—one can observe a ridge,
the carina, between the orifices of the main bronchi. If the
tracheobronchial lymph nodes in the angle between the
main bronchi are enlarged (e.g., because cancer cells have
metastasized from a **bronchogenic carcinoma**), the carina is
distorted, widened posteriorly, and immobile.

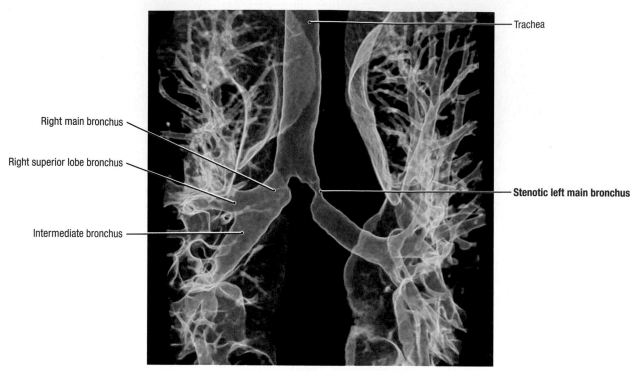

Trachea

Right main bronchus

Right superior lobe bronchus

Stenotic left main bronchus

Intermediate bronchus

D. CT Bronchogram, Airway Stenosis

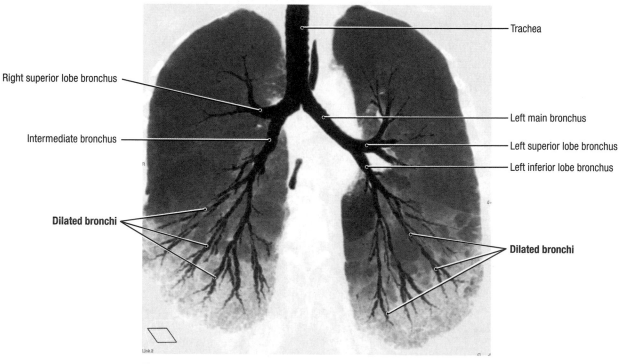

Trachea

Right superior lobe bronchus

Left main bronchus

Intermediate bronchus

Left superior lobe bronchus

Left inferior lobe bronchus

Dilated bronchi

Dilated bronchi

E. CT Minimum Intensity Projection (MinIP), Bronchiectasis

3.36   **Imaging of Lungs** (continued)

D. Stenotic main bronchi. This patient complained of difficulty breathing. A stent was inserted into the bronchus to widen it.
E. CT MinIP. Minimum intensity projection (MinIP) is used to visualize low-density structures within a given volume. This technique is used to reveal abnormally dilated bronchi, a condition called **bronchiectasis**. The abnormal dilation of these bronchi interferes with mucus removal and is associated with repeated pulmonary infections.

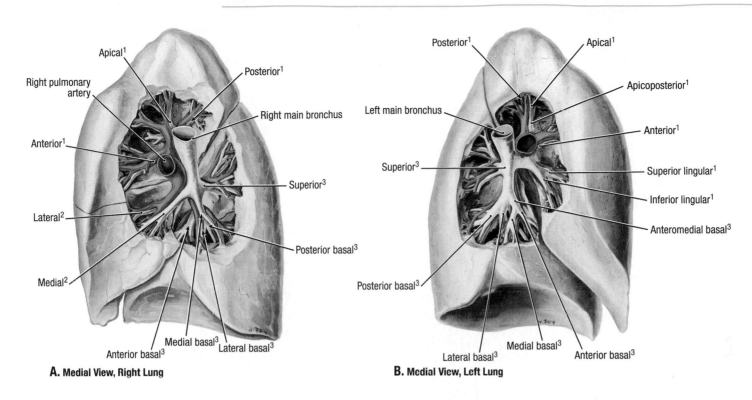

Apical¹

Posterior¹

Right pulmonary artery

Right main bronchus

Anterior¹

Superior³

Lateral²

Posterior basal³

Medial²

Anterior basal³   Medial basal³   Lateral basal³

A. **Medial View, Right Lung**

Posterior¹

Apical¹

Apicoposterior¹

Left main bronchus

Anterior¹

Superior³

Superior lingular¹

Inferior lingular¹

Anteromedial basal³

Posterior basal³

Lateral basal³   Medial basal³   Anterior basal³

B. **Medial View, Left Lung**

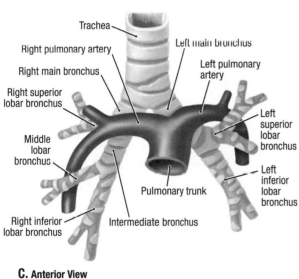

Trachea

Right pulmonary artery

Left main bronchus

Right main bronchus

Left pulmonary artery

Right superior lobar bronchus

Left superior lobar bronchus

Middle lobe bronchus

Left inferior lobar bronchus

Right inferior lobar bronchus

Pulmonary trunk

Intermediate bronchus

C. **Anterior View**

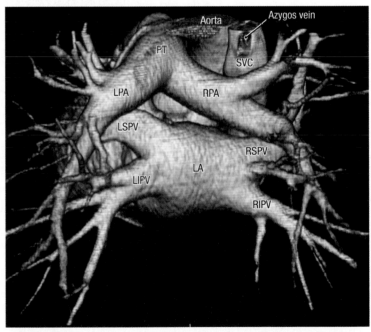

Aorta   Azygos vein

PT

SVC

LPA   RPA

LSPV

RSPV

LIPV   LA

RIPV

Posterior 3DVR

Relationship of Bronchi and Pulmonary Arteries

3.37

A. Right lung. B. Left lung. C. Pulmonary arteries and main and lobar bronchi. Superscripts in *Parts A* and *B* indicate segmental bronchi to the superior lobe (¹), middle lobe (²), and inferior lobe (³). The pulmonary arteries of fresh lungs were filled with latex; the bronchi were inflated with air. The tissues surrounding the bronchi and vessels were removed.

Obstruction of a pulmonary artery by a blood clot (**pulmonary embolism**) results in partial or complete obstruction of blood flow to the lung.

3D Volume Reconstruction (3DVR) of Pulmonary Arteries and Veins and Left Atrium

3.38

The pulmonary trunk (*PT*) divides into a longer right pulmonary artery (*RPA*) and shorter left pulmonary artery (*LPA*); the left superior (*LSPV*) and inferior (*LIPV*) and the right superior (*RSPV*) and inferior (*RIPV*) pulmonary veins drain into the left atrium (*LA*). *SVC*, superior vena cava.

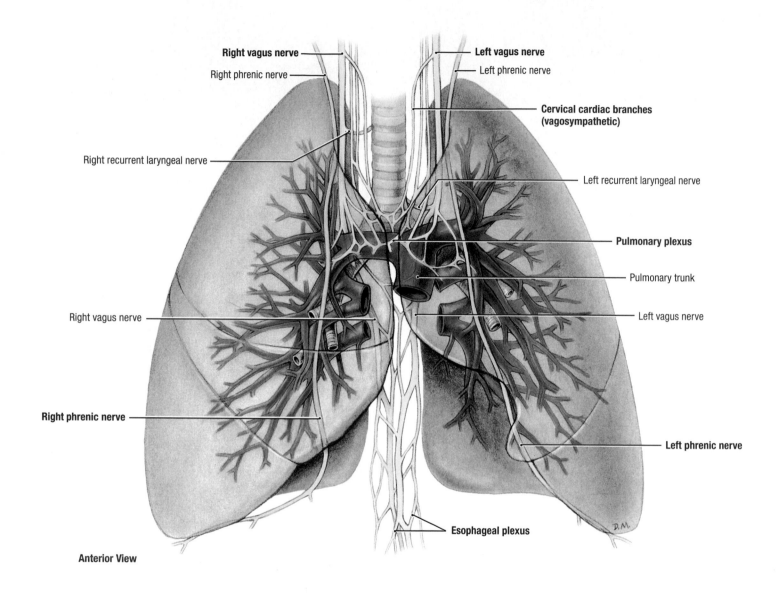

Right vagus nerve

Right phrenic nerve

Right recurrent laryngeal nerve

Right vagus nerve

Right phrenic nerve

Left vagus nerve

Left phrenic nerve

Cervical cardiac branches (vagosympathetic)

Left recurrent laryngeal nerve

Pulmonary plexus

Pulmonary trunk

Left vagus nerve

Left phrenic nerve

Esophageal plexus

Anterior View

| 3.39 | **Innervation of Lungs** |

- The pulmonary plexuses, located anterior and posterior to the roots of the lungs, receive sympathetic contributions from the right and left sympathetic trunks (2nd to 5th thoracic ganglia, not shown) and parasympathetic contributions from the right and left vagus nerves; cell bodies of postsynaptic parasympathetic neurons are in the pulmonary plexuses and along the branches of the pulmonary tree.
- The right and left vagus nerves continue inferiorly from the posterior pulmonary plexus to contribute fibers to the esophageal plexus.

- The phrenic nerves pass anterior to the root of the lung on their way to the diaphragm.
- Visceral pleura is insensitive to pain. The autonomic nerves reach the visceral pleura in company with the bronchial vessels. The visceral pleura receives no nerves of general sensation.
- Parietal pleura is richly supplied by branches of the somatic intercostal and phrenic nerves. Irritation of the parietal pleura **pleuritis** produces local pain **pleurisy** and referred pain to the areas sharing innervation by the same segments of the spinal cord.

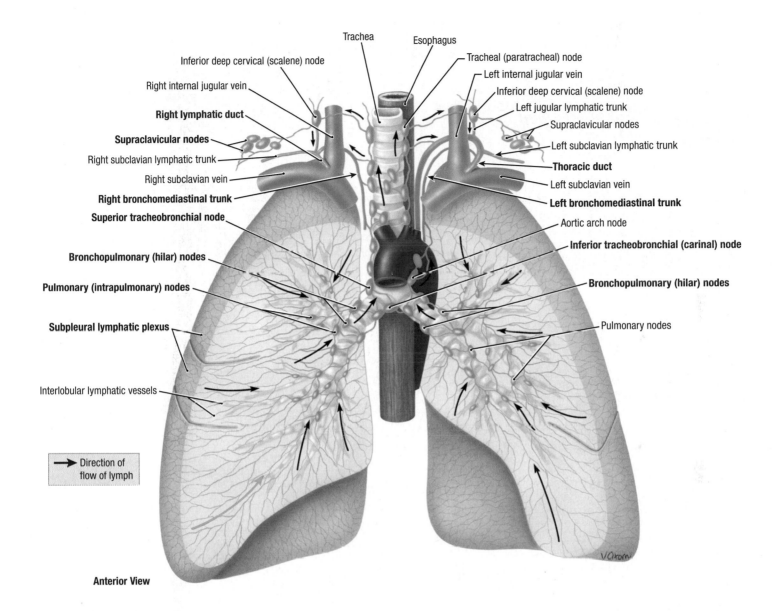

Trachea

Esophagus

Inferior deep cervical (scalene) node

Tracheal (paratracheal) node

Right internal jugular vein

Left internal jugular vein

Inferior deep cervical (scalene) node

Right lymphatic duct

Left jugular lymphatic trunk

Supraclavicular nodes

Supraclavicular nodes

Right subclavian lymphatic trunk

Left subclavian lymphatic trunk

Right subclavian vein

Thoracic duct

Right bronchomediastinal trunk

Left subclavian vein

Superior tracheobronchial node

Left bronchomediastinal trunk

Aortic arch node

Bronchopulmonary (hilar) nodes

Inferior tracheobronchial (carinal) node

Pulmonary (intrapulmonary) nodes

Bronchopulmonary (hilar) nodes

Subpleural lymphatic plexus

Pulmonary nodes

Interlobular lymphatic vessels

→ Direction of
flow of lymph

Anterior View

V Chron

Lymphatic Drainage of Lungs

3.40

- Lymphatic vessels originate in the subpleural (superficial) and deep lymphatic plexuses.
- The subpleural lymphatic plexus is superficial, lying deep to the visceral pleura, and drains lymph from the surface of the lung to the bronchopulmonary (hilar) nodes.
- The deep lymphatic plexus is in the lung and follows the bronchi and pulmonary vessels to the pulmonary, and then bronchopulmonary, nodes located at the root of the lung.
- All lymph from the lungs enters the inferior (carinal) and superior tracheobronchial nodes and then continues to the right and left bronchomediastinal trunks to drain into the venous system via the right lymphatic and thoracic ducts; lymph from the left inferior lobe passes largely to the right side.
- Lymph from the parietal pleura drains into lymph nodes of the thoracic wall (see Fig. 3.71).

Lung cancer (carcinoma) metastasizes early to the bronchopulmonary lymph nodes and subsequently to the other thoracic lymph nodes. Common sites of **hematogenous metastases** (spreading through the blood) of cancer cells from a bronchogenic carcinoma are the brain, bones, lungs, and suprarenal glands. Often the lymph nodes superior to the clavicle—the supraclavicular lymph nodes—are enlarged when lung (bronchogenic) carcinoma develops owing to metastasis of cancer cells from the tumor. Consequently, the supraclavicular nodes were once referred to as sentinel lymph nodes. More recently, the term *sentinel lymph node* has been applied to a node or nodes that first receive lymph drainage from a cancer-containing area, regardless of location, following injection of blue dye containing radioactive tracer (technetium-99).

Intercostal spaces:

Ribs:

	Tricuspid valve (T)
	Mitral valve (M)
	Pulmonary valve (P)
	Aortic valve (A)

A. Anterior View

3.41 **Surface Projections of Heart, Heart Valves, and Auscultation Areas**

A. Overview of surface anatomy of heart and areas of auscultation.
- The location of each heart valve *in situ* is indicated by a colored oval and the area of auscultation of the valve is indicated as a circle of the same color containing the first letter of the valve name.

- The **auscultation areas** are sites where the sounds of each of the heart's valves can be heard most distinctly through a stethoscope (**cardiac auscultation**).

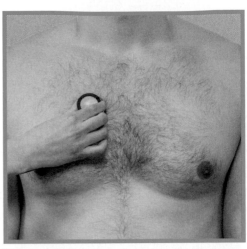

C. Anterior View

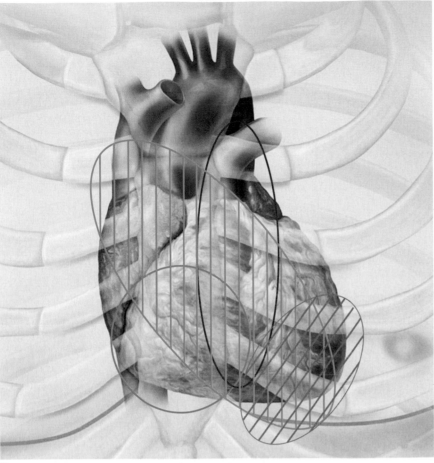

B. Anterior View

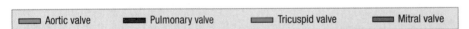

| Aortic valve | Pulmonary valve | Tricuspid valve | Mitral valve |

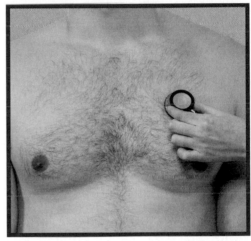

D. Anterior View

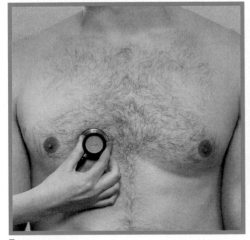

E. Anterior View

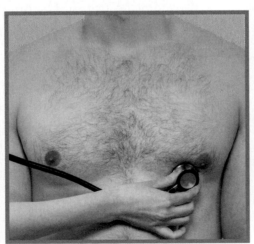

F. Anterior View

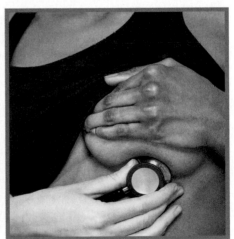

G. Anterior View

Surface Projections of Heart, Heart Valves, and Auscultation Areas (continued)   **3.41**

B. Overlapping of areas of auscultation. Each area, although overlapping, is located superficial to the chamber or vessel into which the blood has passed and in a direct line with the valve orifice. **C–G. Stethoscope placement for auscultation of:** Aortic valve (Part C), pulmonary valve (Part D), tricuspid valve (Part E), mitral valve in male (Part F), and mitral valve in female (Part G).

The aortic (A) and pulmonary (P) auscultation areas are in the 2nd intercostal space to the right and left of the sternal border; the tricuspid area (T) is near the left sternal border in the 5th or 6th intercostal space; the mitral valve (M) is heard best near the apex of the heart in the 5th intercostal space in the midclavicular line.

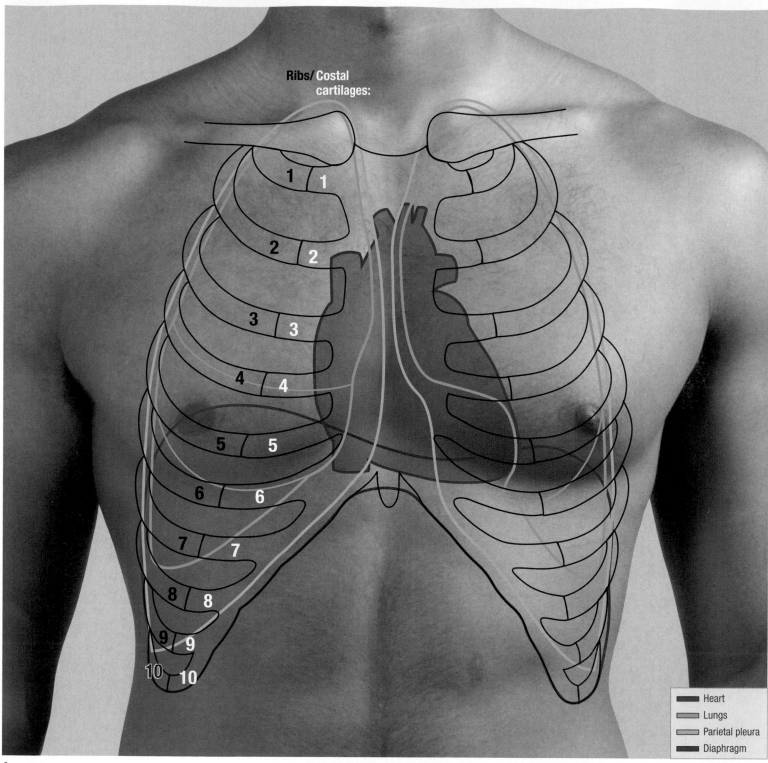

Ribs/ Costal
cartilages:

	Heart
	Lungs
	Parietal pleura
	Diaphragm

A. Anterior View

3.42 **Surface Markings of Heart and Lungs, Areas of Auscultation and Percussion**

A. Overview.

- The superior border of the heart is represented by a slightly oblique line joining the 3rd costal cartilages; the convex right side of the heart projects lateral to the sternum and inferiorly, lying at the 6th or 7th costochondral junction; the inferior border of the heart is lying superior to the central tendon of the diaphragm and sloping slightly inferiorly to the apex at the 5th interspace at the midclavicular line.

- The right dome of the diaphragm is higher than the left because of the large size of the liver inferior to the dome; during expiration, the right dome reaches as high as the 5th rib and the left dome ascends to the 5th intercostal space.
- The left pleural cavity is smaller than the right because of the projection of the heart to the left side.

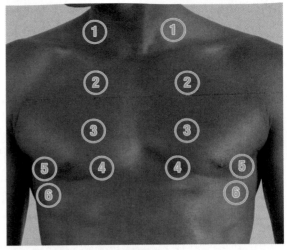

D. Anterior View

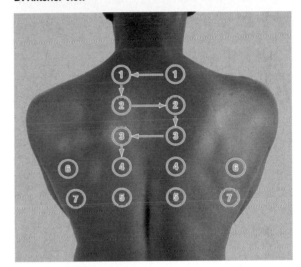

E. Posterior View

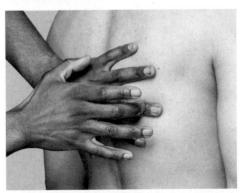

F. Posterolateral View, 3rd Digits in Contact for Percussion

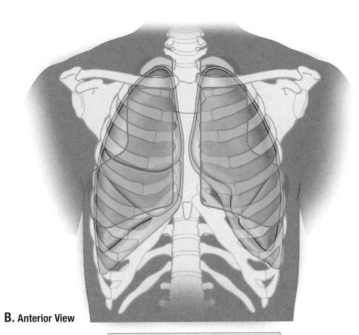

B. Anterior View

Normal area for resonant sound

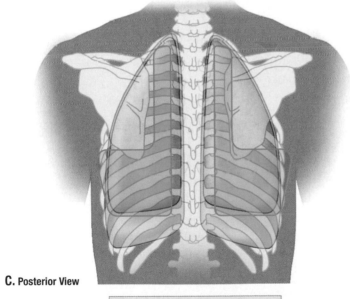

C. Posterior View

Normal area for resonant sound

Surface Markings of Heart and Lungs, Areas of Auscultation and Percussion (continued)   3.42

B. and **C.** Areas of resonant sound. These are areas where the lungs are not overlapped by bone (e.g., scapula and sternum).
D. and **E.** Areas of auscultation of lungs. **F.** Percussion of lungs.
   Auscultation of the lungs (listening to their sounds with a stethoscope) and **percussion of the thorax** (tapping on fingers pressed firmly on the thoracic wall over the lungs to detect sounds in the lungs) are important techniques used during physical examination. Auscultation assesses airflow through the tracheobronchial tree into the lobes of the lung. The patterns of breath sounds can be characterized by their intensity, pitch, and relative duration throughout inspiration and expiration. Percussion helps establish whether the underlying tissues are air filled (*resonant* sound), fluid filled (*dull* sound), or solid (*flat* sound). An awareness of normal anatomy, particularly the projection of the lungs and the portions that are overlapped by bone, enables the examiner to know where flat and resonant sounds should be expected.

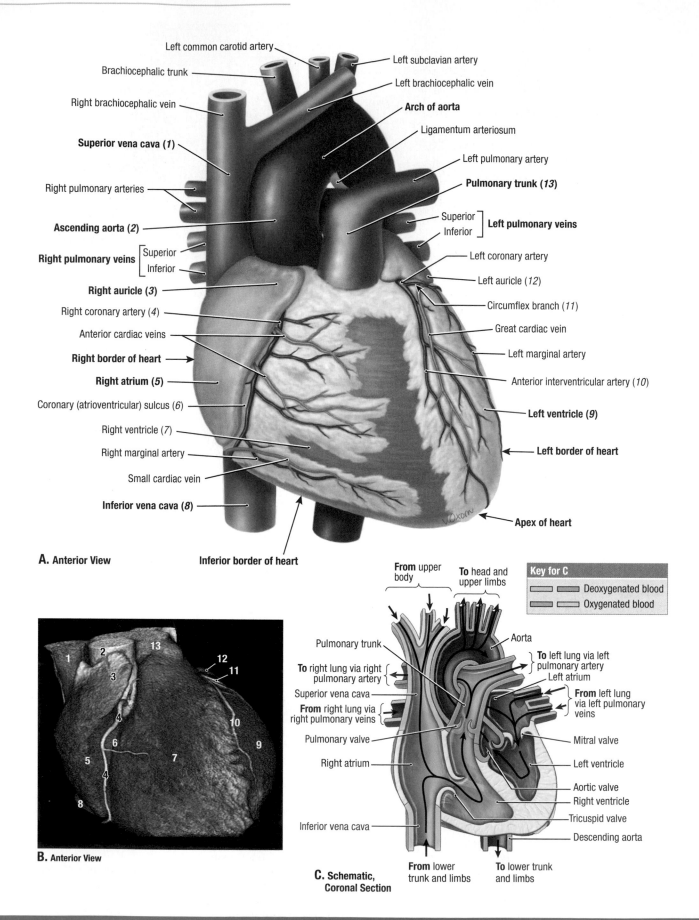

Left common carotid artery

Brachiocephalic trunk

Right brachiocephalic vein

Superior vena cava (1)

Right pulmonary arteries

Ascending aorta (2)

Right pulmonary veins — Superior / Inferior

Right auricle (3)

Right coronary artery (4)

Anterior cardiac veins

Right border of heart

Right atrium (5)

Coronary (atrioventricular) sulcus (6)

Right ventricle (7)

Right marginal artery

Small cardiac vein

Inferior vena cava (8)

Left subclavian artery

Left brachiocephalic vein

Arch of aorta

Ligamentum arteriosum

Left pulmonary artery

Pulmonary trunk (13)

Superior / Inferior **Left pulmonary veins**

Left coronary artery

Left auricle (12)

Circumflex branch (11)

Great cardiac vein

Left marginal artery

Anterior interventricular artery (10)

Left ventricle (9)

Left border of heart

Apex of heart

A. Anterior View

Inferior border of heart

B. Anterior View

From upper body

To head and upper limbs

Pulmonary trunk

To right lung via right pulmonary artery

Superior vena cava

From right lung via right pulmonary veins

Pulmonary valve

Right atrium

Inferior vena cava

Aorta

To left lung via left pulmonary artery

Left atrium

From left lung via left pulmonary veins

Mitral valve

Left ventricle

Aortic valve

Right ventricle

Tricuspid valve

Descending aorta

From lower trunk and limbs

To lower trunk and limbs

Key for C

Deoxygenated blood

Oxygenated blood

C. Schematic, Coronal Section

Left common carotid artery

Left subclavian artery

Brachiocephalic trunk

Right brachiocephalic vein

Arch of aorta

Ligamentum arteriosum

Superior vena cava

Arch of azygos vein

Left pulmonary artery (1)

Right pulmonary artery (15)

Left pulmonary veins Superior (2) / Inferior (3)

Superior (14) / Inferior (13) **Right pulmonary veins**

Left auricle (4)

Left atrium (5)

Great cardiac vein

Right atrium (12)

Circumflex branch (6)

Coronary sinus (11)

Oblique vein of left atrium

Inferior vena cava

Small cardiac vein

Left posterior ventricular vein

Right coronary artery (10)

Middle cardiac vein (9)

Posterior interventricular artery (8)

Left ventricle (7)

Right ventricle

Anterior interventricular artery

D. Posteroinferior View

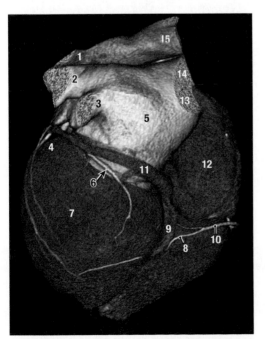

E. 3D Volume Reconstruction from MRI, Posteroinferior View

Heart and Great Vessels (continued)   3.43

A. Anatomical specimen.
- The right border of the heart, formed by the right atrium, is slightly convex and almost in line with the superior vena cava.
- The inferior border is formed primarily by the right ventricle and part of the left ventricle.
- The left border is formed primarily by the left ventricle and part of the left auricle.

B. 3D volume reconstruction from MRI of heart and coronary vessels (living patient). Numbers refer to structures in *Part A*.
C. Circulation of blood through heart. D. Anatomical specimen, posterior view.
- Most of the left atrium and left ventricle are visible in this posteroinferior view.
- The right and left pulmonary veins open into the left atrium.
- The arch of the aorta extends superiorly, posteriorly, and to the left, in a nearly sagittal plane.

E. Heart and coronary vessels (living patient). Numbers refer to structures in *Part D*.

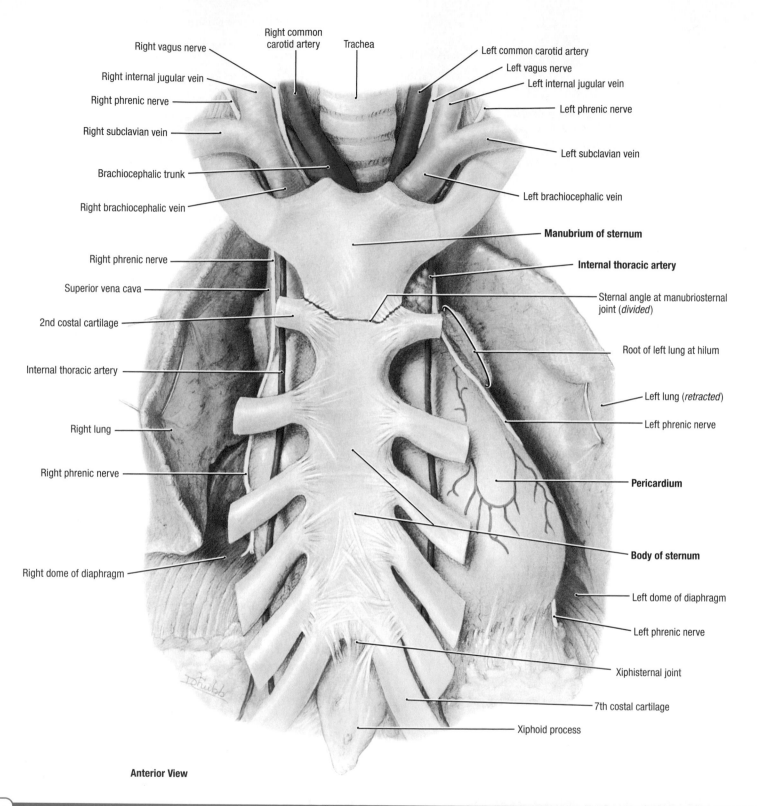

Right vagus nerve

Right common carotid artery

Trachea

Left common carotid artery

Right internal jugular vein

Left vagus nerve

Right phrenic nerve

Left internal jugular vein

Left phrenic nerve

Right subclavian vein

Left subclavian vein

Brachiocephalic trunk

Left brachiocephalic vein

Right brachiocephalic vein

Manubrium of sternum

Right phrenic nerve

Internal thoracic artery

Superior vena cava

Sternal angle at manubriosternal joint (*divided*)

2nd costal cartilage

Root of left lung at hilum

Internal thoracic artery

Left lung (*retracted*)

Right lung

Left phrenic nerve

Right phrenic nerve

Pericardium

Body of sternum

Right dome of diaphragm

Left dome of diaphragm

Left phrenic nerve

Xiphisternal joint

7th costal cartilage

Xiphoid process

Anterior View

3.44 Pericardium in Relation to Sternum

- The pericardium lies posterior to the body of the sternum, extending from just superior to the sternal angle to the level of the xiphisternal joint; approximately two thirds lies to the left of the median plane.
- The heart lies between the body of the sternum and the anterior mediastinum anteriorly and the T5–T9 vertebrae and the posterior mediastinum posteriorly (see Fig. 3.28A).

- In **cardiac compression**, the sternum is depressed 4 to 5 cm, forcing blood out of the heart and into the great vessels.
- Internal thoracic arteries arise from the subclavian arteries and descend posterior to the costal cartilages, running lateral to the sternum and anterior to the pleura.

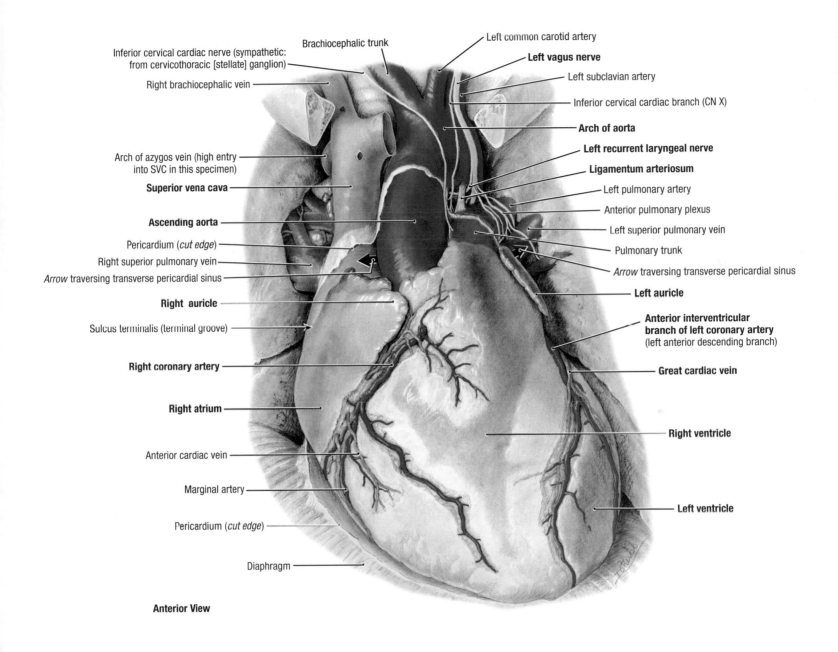

Inferior cervical cardiac nerve (sympathetic: from cervicothoracic [stellate] ganglion)

Brachiocephalic trunk

Left common carotid artery

Left vagus nerve

Right brachiocephalic vein

Left subclavian artery

Inferior cervical cardiac branch (CN X)

Arch of aorta

Arch of azygos vein (high entry into SVC in this specimen)

Left recurrent laryngeal nerve

Ligamentum arteriosum

Superior vena cava

Left pulmonary artery

Anterior pulmonary plexus

Ascending aorta

Left superior pulmonary vein

Pericardium (*cut edge*)

Right superior pulmonary vein

Pulmonary trunk

Arrow traversing transverse pericardial sinus

Arrow traversing transverse pericardial sinus

Right auricle

Left auricle

Sulcus terminalis (terminal groove)

Anterior interventricular branch of left coronary artery (left anterior descending branch)

Right coronary artery

Great cardiac vein

Right atrium

Right ventricle

Anterior cardiac vein

Marginal artery

Left ventricle

Pericardium (*cut edge*)

Diaphragm

Anterior View

Sternocostal (Anterior) Surface of Heart and Great Vessels *In Situ*   **3.45**

- The right ventricle forms most of the sternocostal surface.
- The entire right auricle and much of the right atrium are visible anteriorly, but only a small portion of the left auricle is visible; the auricles, like a closing claw, grasp the origins of the pulmonary trunk and ascending aorta from a posterior approach.
- The ligamentum arteriosum passes from the origin of the left pulmonary artery to the arch of the aorta.
- The right coronary artery courses in the anterior atrioventricular groove, and the anterior interventricular branch of the left coronary artery (anterior descending branch) courses in or parallel to the anterior interventricular groove (see Fig. 3.43B).
- The left vagus nerve passes lateral to the arch of the aorta and then posterior to the root of the lung; the left recurrent laryngeal nerve passes inferior to the arch of the aorta posterior to the ligamentum arteriosum.
- The great cardiac vein ascends beside the anterior interventricular branch of the left coronary artery to drain into the coronary sinus posteriorly.

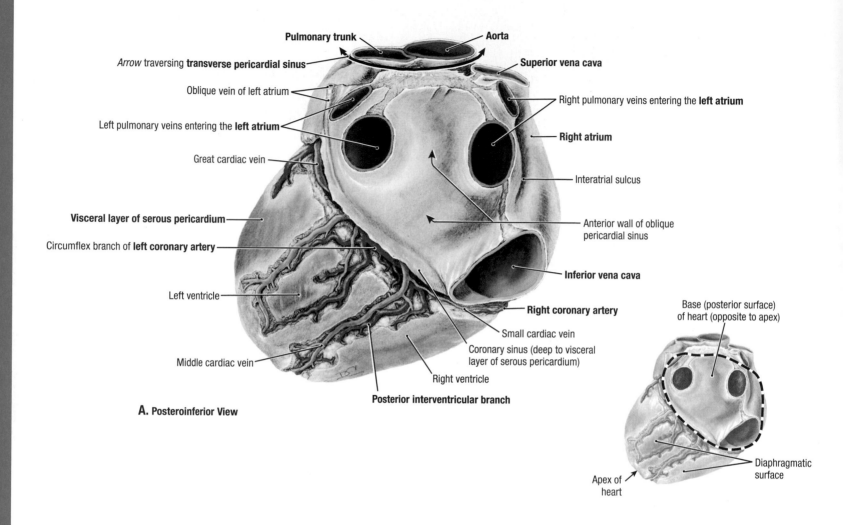

Pulmonary trunk · Aorta

Arrow traversing **transverse pericardial sinus** · Superior vena cava

Oblique vein of left atrium · Right pulmonary veins entering the **left atrium**

Left pulmonary veins entering the **left atrium** · **Right atrium**

Great cardiac vein · Interatrial sulcus

Visceral layer of serous pericardium · Anterior wall of oblique pericardial sinus

Circumflex branch of **left coronary artery**

Left ventricle · **Inferior vena cava**

· **Right coronary artery**

Middle cardiac vein · Small cardiac vein

· Coronary sinus (deep to visceral layer of serous pericardium)

Right ventricle

Posterior interventricular branch

A. Posteroinferior View

Base (posterior surface) of heart (opposite to apex)

Diaphragmatic surface

Apex of heart

3.46 **Heart and Pericardium**

A. Heart removed from interior of pericardial sac (*Part B*).
- The entire base, or posterior surface, and part of the diaphragmatic or inferior surface of the heart are in view (*dashed line*).
- The superior vena cava and larger inferior vena cava join the superior and inferior aspects of the right atrium.
- The left atrium forms the greater part of the base (posterior surface) of the heart (*inset*).
- The left coronary artery in this specimen is dominant, since it supplies the posterior interventricular branch.
- Most branches of cardiac veins cross branches of the coronary arteries superficially.
- The visceral layer of serous pericardium (epicardium) covers the surface of the heart and reflects onto the great vessels; from around the great vessels, the serous pericardium reflects to line the internal aspect of the fibrous pericardium as the parietal layer

of serous pericardium. The fibrous pericardium and the parietal layer of serous pericardium form the pericardial sac that encases the heart.
- Note the cut edges of the reflections of serous pericardia around the arterial vessels (the pulmonary trunk and aorta) and venous vessels (the superior and inferior venae cavae and the pulmonary veins).
- **Surgical isolation of cardiac outflow.** The transverse pericardial sinus is especially important to cardiac surgeons. After the pericardial sac has been opened anteriorly, a finger can be passed through the transverse pericardial sinus posterior to the aorta and pulmonary trunk. By passing a surgical clamp or placing a ligature around these vessels, inserting the tubes of a coronary bypass machine, and then tightening the ligature, surgeons can stop or divert the circulation of blood in these large arteries while performing cardiac surgery.

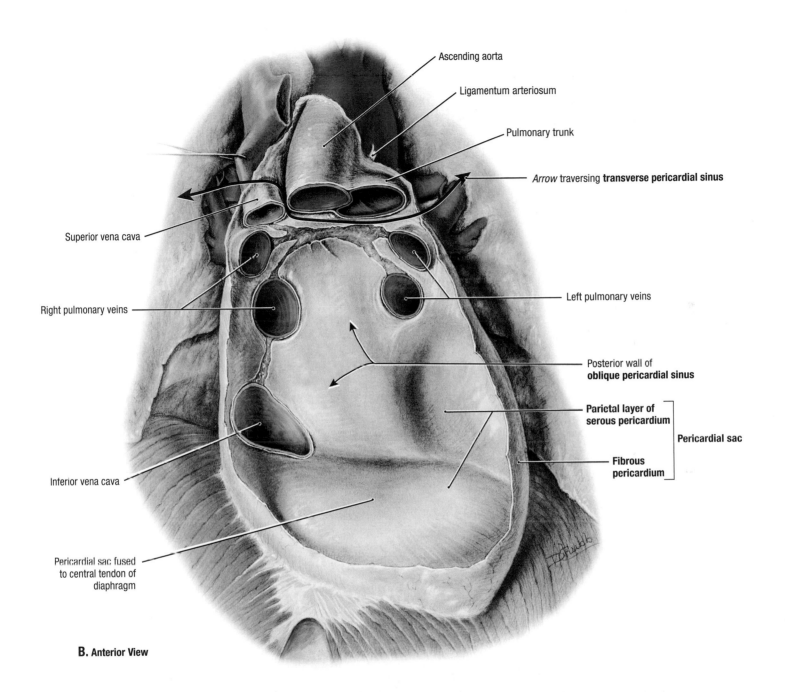

Ascending aorta

Ligamentum arteriosum

Pulmonary trunk

Arrow traversing **transverse pericardial sinus**

Superior vena cava

Left pulmonary veins

Right pulmonary veins

Posterior wall of **oblique pericardial sinus**

Parietal layer of serous pericardium

Pericardial sac

Inferior vena cava

Fibrous pericardium

Pericardial sac fused to central tendon of diaphragm

B. Anterior View

Heart and Pericardium (*continued*)

3.46

B. Interior of pericardial sac.
- Eight vessels were severed to excise the heart: superior and inferior venae cavae, four pulmonary veins, and two pulmonary arteries.
- The oblique sinus is bounded anteriorly by the visceral layer of serous pericardium covering the left atrium (*Part A*), posteriorly by the parietal layer of serous pericardium lining the fibrous pericardium, and superiorly and laterally by the reflection of serous pericardium around the four pulmonary veins and the superior and inferior venae cavae (*Part B*).
- The transverse sinus is bounded anteriorly by the serous pericardium covering the posterior aspect of the pulmonary trunk and

aorta and posteriorly by the visceral pericardium reflecting from the atria (*Part A*) inferiorly and the superior vena cava superiorly on the right.
- Blood in the pericardial cavity, **hemopericardium**, produces **cardiac tamponade**. Hemopericardium may result from perforation of a weakened area of the heart muscle owing to a previous **myocardial infarction (MI)** or heart attack, from bleeding into the pericardial cavity after cardiac operations, or from stab wounds. Heart volume is increasingly compromised and circulation fails.

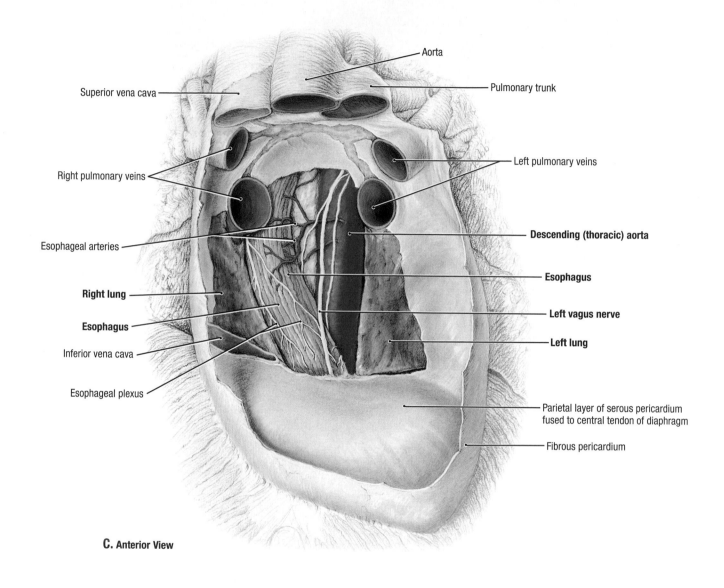

Aorta

Superior vena cava

Pulmonary trunk

Right pulmonary veins

Left pulmonary veins

Esophageal arteries

Descending (thoracic) aorta

Esophagus

Right lung

Left vagus nerve

Esophagus

Left lung

Inferior vena cava

Esophageal plexus

Parietal layer of serous pericardium fused to central tendon of diaphragm

Fibrous pericardium

C. Anterior View

3.46 **Heart and Pericardium** *(continued)*

C. Posterior relationships, dissection. The fibrous and parietal layers of serous pericardium have been removed from posterior and lateral to the oblique sinus. The esophagus in this specimen is deflected to the right; it usually lies in contact with the aorta, forming primary posterior relationships of the heart.

Surgical exposure of venae cavae. After ascending through the diaphragm, the entire thoracic part of the inferior vena cava (IVC)

(approximately 2 cm) is enclosed by the pericardium. Consequently, the pericardial sac must be opened to expose the terminal part of the IVC. The same is true for the terminal part of the superior vena cava (SVC), which is partly inside and partly outside the pericardial sac.

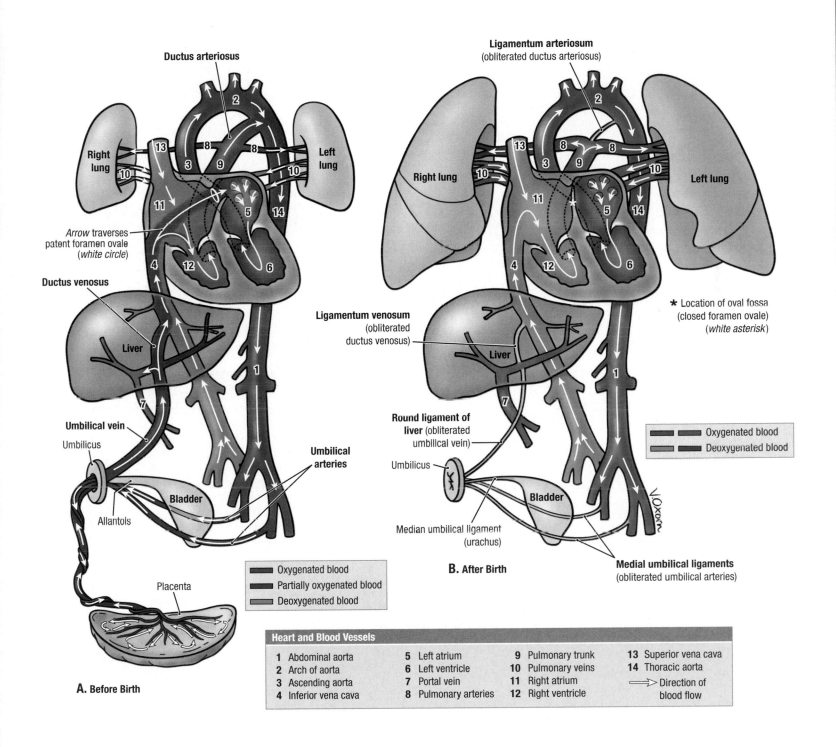

Ductus arteriosus

Ligamentum arteriosum
(obliterated ductus arteriosus)

Right lung

Left lung

Right lung

Left lung

Arrow traverses
patent foramen ovale
(*white circle*)

Ductus venosus

Liver

Ligamentum venosum
(obliterated
ductus venosus)

Liver

* Location of oval fossa
(closed foramen ovale)
(*white asterisk*)

Umbilical vein

Umbilicus

Allantois

Bladder

Umbilical
arteries

Round ligament of
liver (obliterated
umbilical vein)

Umbilicus

Bladder

Median umbilical ligament
(urachus)

Medial umbilical ligaments
(obliterated umbilical arteries)

B. After Birth

▬▬▬	Oxygenated blood
▬▬▬	Deoxygenated blood

Placenta

A. Before Birth

▬▬▬	Oxygenated blood
▬▬▬	Partially oxygenated blood
▬▬▬	Deoxygenated blood

Heart and Blood Vessels

1	Abdominal aorta	5	Left atrium	9	Pulmonary trunk	13	Superior vena cava
2	Arch of aorta	6	Left ventricle	10	Pulmonary veins	14	Thoracic aorta
3	Ascending aorta	7	Portal vein	11	Right atrium	⟹	Direction of
4	Inferior vena cava	8	Pulmonary arteries	12	Right ventricle		blood flow

A. Before birth. B. After birth. At birth, two major changes take place: (1) pulmonary respiration starts, and (2) after the umbilical cord is ligated, the umbilical arteries (except the most proximal part), umbilical vein, and ductus venosus are occluded and become the medial umbilical ligament, round ligament of liver, and the ligamentum venosum, respectively.

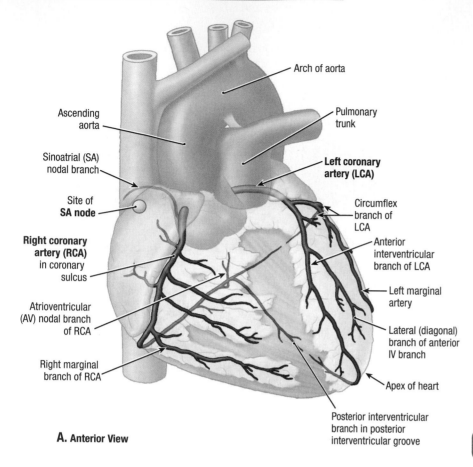

Arch of aorta

Ascending aorta

Pulmonary trunk

Sinoatrial (SA) nodal branch

Left coronary artery (LCA)

Site of **SA node**

Circumflex branch of LCA

Right coronary artery (RCA) in coronary sulcus

Anterior interventricular branch of LCA

Atrioventricular (AV) nodal branch of RCA

Left marginal artery

Lateral (diagonal) branch of anterior IV branch

Right marginal branch of RCA

Apex of heart

Posterior interventricular branch in posterior interventricular groove

A. Anterior View

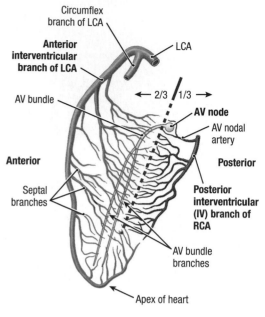

Circumflex branch of LCA

LCA

Anterior interventricular branch of LCA

AV bundle

← 2/3 | 1/3 →

AV node

AV nodal artery

Anterior

Posterior

Septal branches

Posterior interventricular (IV) branch of RCA

AV bundle branches

Apex of heart

C. Left Lateral View

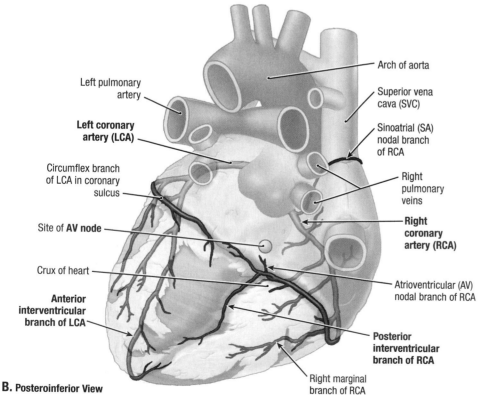

Left pulmonary artery

Arch of aorta

Superior vena cava (SVC)

Left coronary artery (LCA)

Sinoatrial (SA) nodal branch of RCA

Circumflex branch of LCA in coronary sulcus

Right pulmonary veins

Site of **AV node**

Right coronary artery (RCA)

Crux of heart

Atrioventricular (AV) nodal branch of RCA

Anterior interventricular branch of LCA

Posterior interventricular branch of RCA

Right marginal branch of RCA

B. Posteroinferior View

3.48 **Coronary Arteries**

A. Anterior view. **B.** Posteroinferior view.
C. Arteries of isolated interventricular septum.

- In the most common pattern, the right coronary artery travels in the coronary sulcus to reach the posterior surface of the heart, where it anastomoses with the circumflex branch of the left coronary artery. Early in its course, it gives off the right atrial branch, which supplies the sinoatrial (SA) node via its sinoatrial nodal branch. Major branches are a marginal branch supplying much of the anterior wall of the right ventricle, an atrioventricular (AV) nodal branch given off near the posterior border of the interventricular septum, and a posterior interventricular branch in the interventricular groove that anastomoses with the anterior interventricular branch of the left coronary artery.

- The left coronary artery divides into a circumflex branch that passes posteriorly to anastomose with the right coronary artery on the posterior aspect of the heart and an anterior interventricular branch in the interventricular groove; the origin of the SA nodal branch is variable and may be a branch of the left coronary artery.

- The interventricular septum receives its blood supply from septal branches of the two interventricular (descending) branches: typically the anterior two thirds from the left coronary and the posterior one third from the right (as in *Part C*).

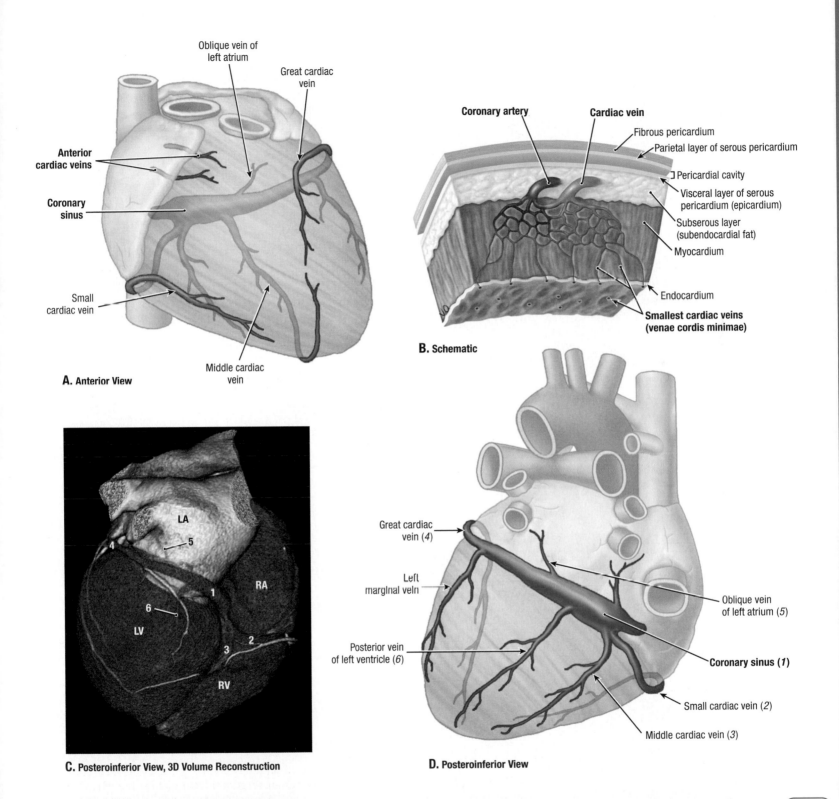

Oblique vein of left atrium

Great cardiac vein

Anterior cardiac veins

Coronary sinus

Small cardiac vein

Middle cardiac vein

A. Anterior View

Coronary artery

Cardiac vein

Fibrous pericardium

Parietal layer of serous pericardium

Pericardial cavity

Visceral layer of serous pericardium (epicardium)

Subserous layer (subendocardial fat)

Myocardium

Endocardium

Smallest cardiac veins (venae cordis minimae)

B. Schematic

LA
5
4
1
RA
6
LV
3
2
RV

C. Posteroinferior View, 3D Volume Reconstruction

Great cardiac vein (4)

Left marginal vein

Posterior vein of left ventricle (6)

Oblique vein of left atrium (5)

Coronary sinus (1)

Small cardiac vein (2)

Middle cardiac vein (3)

D. Posteroinferior View

Cardiac Veins

3.49

A. Anterior aspect. B. Smallest cardiac veins. C. Heart and cardiac veins (living patient). Numbers refer to veins in *Part D. LA*, left atrium; *LV*, left ventricle; *RA*, right atrium; *RV*, right ventricle. **D. Posteroinferior aspect.**

The coronary sinus is the major venous drainage vessel of the heart; it is located posteriorly in the atrioventricular (coronary) groove and drains into the right atrium. The coronary sinus begins at the merger of the great cardiac vein and the oblique vein of the left atrium. The anterior cardiac veins drain directly into the right atrium. The smallest cardiac veins (venae cordis minimae) drain the myocardium directly into the atria and ventricles as in *Part B*. Most cardiac veins accompany the coronary arteries and their branches.

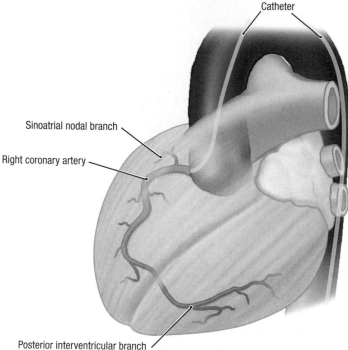

Catheter

Sinoatrial nodal branch

Right coronary artery

Posterior interventricular branch
(posterior descending artery)

A. Schematic

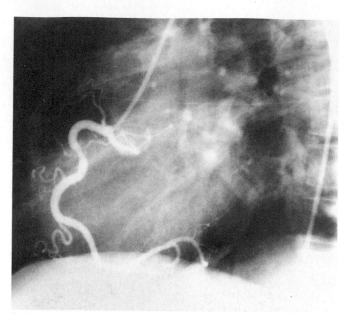

B. Left Anterior Oblique Right Coronary Arteriogram

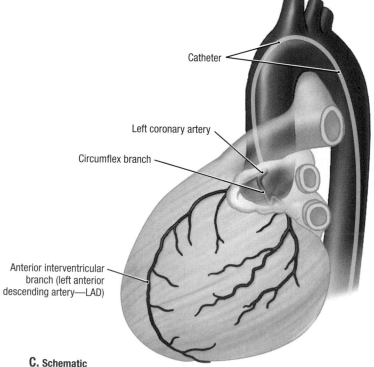

Catheter

Left coronary artery

Circumflex branch

Anterior interventricular
branch (left anterior
descending artery—LAD)

C. Schematic

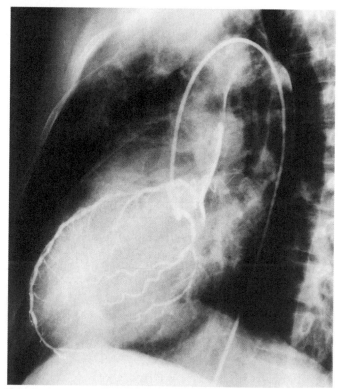

D. Left Anterior Oblique Left Coronary Arteriogram

3.50 Coronary Arteriograms with Orientation Drawings

Right (*Part A* and *Part B*) and left (*Part C* and *Part D*) coronary arteriograms.

Coronary artery disease (CAD), one of the leading causes of death, results in a reduced blood supply to the vital myocardial tissue. The three most common sites of coronary artery occlusion and the approximate percentage of occlusions involving each artery are the (1) anterior interventricular (clinically referred to as LAD) branch of the left coronary artery (LCA) (40% to 50%), (2) right coronary artery (RCA) (30% to 40%), and (3) circumflex branch of the LCA (15% to 20%).

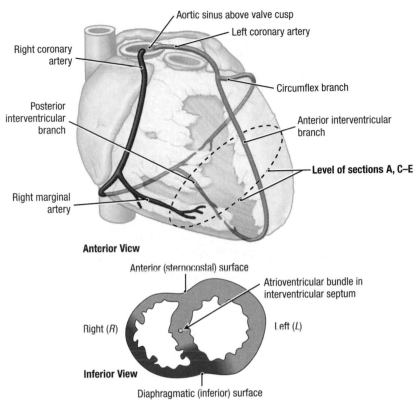

Aortic sinus above valve cusp

Left coronary artery

Right coronary artery

Circumflex branch

Posterior interventricular branch

Anterior interventricular branch

Level of sections A, C–E

Right marginal artery

Anterior View

Anterior (sternocostal) surface

Atrioventricular bundle in interventricular septum

Right (*R*)

Left (*L*)

Inferior View

Diaphragmatic (inferior) surface

A. Most Common Pattern (67%)

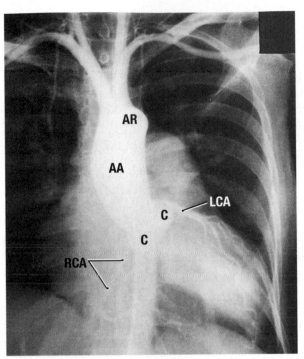

AR

AA

LCA

C

C

RCA

B. Anteroposterior Coronary Angiogram

Key for B		
AA Ascending aorta	**LCA**	Left coronary artery
AR Arch of aorta	**RCA**	Right coronary artery
C Cusp of aortic valve		

Key for A and C–E	
▬▬	Myocardium supplied by RCA
▬▬	Myocardium supplied by LCA

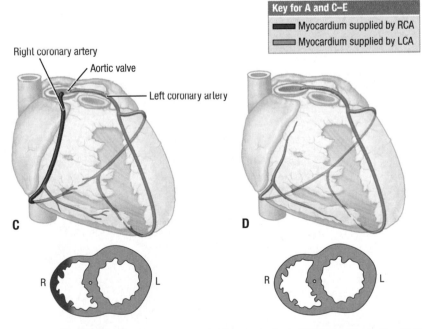

Right coronary artery

Aortic valve

Left coronary artery

C

D

E

R L

R L

R L

C. and D. Left Coronary Artery Gives Rise to the Posterior Interventricular Branch (15%)

E. Circumflex Branch Emerging from Right Coronary Sinus

Variations in Distribution of Coronary Arteries

3.51

A. Most common pattern. Right coronary artery is dominant, giving rise to the posterior interventricular branch (67%). **B.** Coronary angiogram of most common pattern. **C–E.** Less common patterns.

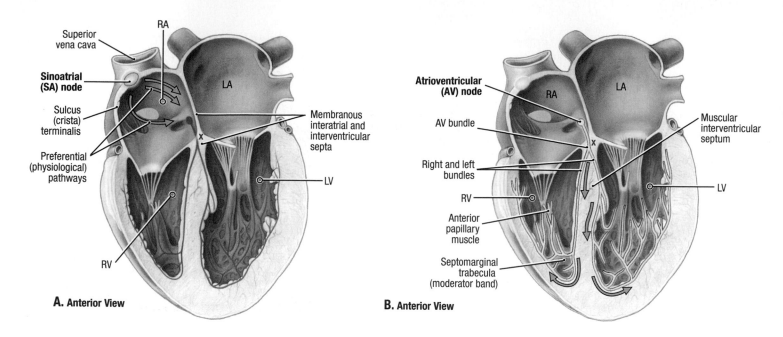

A. Anterior View

B. Anterior View

3.52   Conduction System of Heart, Coronal Section

A. Impulses (*arrows*) initiated at sinoatrial (SA) node. **B.** Atrioventricular (AV) node, AV bundle, and bundle branches. **C.** Echocardiogram, apical four-chamber view.

- The SA node is in the wall of the right atrium near the superior end of the sulcus terminalis (internally crista terminalis) at the opening of the superior vena cava. The SA node is the "pacemaker" of the heart because it initiates muscle contraction and determines the heart rate. It is supplied by the sinoatrial nodal artery, usually a branch of the right atrial branch of the right coronary artery, but it may arise from the left coronary artery.
- Contraction spreads through the atrial wall (myogenic induction) until it reaches the AV node in the interatrial septum, superomedial to the opening of the coronary sinus. The AV node is supplied by the AV nodal artery, usually arising from the right coronary artery posteriorly at the inferior margin of the interatrial septum.
- The AV bundle, usually supplied by the right coronary artery, passes from the AV node in the membranous part of the interventricular septum, dividing into right and left bundle branches on either side of the muscular part of the interventricular septum.
- The right bundle branch travels inferiorly in the interventricular septum to the anterior wall of the ventricle, with part passing via the septomarginal trabecula to the anterior papillary muscle; excitation spreads throughout the right ventricular wall through a network of subendocardial branches (Purkinje fibers) from the right bundle.
- The left bundle branch lies beneath the endocardium on the left side of the interventricular septum and branches to enter the anterior and posterior papillary muscles and the wall of the left ventricle; further branching into a plexus of subendocardial branches allows the impulses to be conveyed throughout the left ventricular wall. The bundle branches are mostly supplied by the left coronary artery except the posterior limb of the left bundle branch, which is supplied by both coronary arteries.
- **Damage to the cardiac conduction system** (often by compromised blood supply as in coronary artery disease) leads to disturbances of muscle contraction. Damage to the AV node results in "heart block" because the atrial excitation wave does not reach the ventricles, which begin to contract independently at their own slower rate. Damage to one of the bundle branches results in "bundle branch block," in which excitation goes down the unaffected branch to cause systole of that ventricle; the impulse then spreads to the other ventricle, producing later asynchronous contraction.

Key for A and B

LA	Left atrium
LV	Left ventricle
RA	Right atrium
RV	Right ventricle
x	Crux (cross) of heart
⇒	Direction of impulses

C. Apical Four-Chamber Echocardiogram. For this ultrasound image, the transducer is usually placed on the chest wall in the left 5th intercostal space and aimed so that the beam obliquely transects the heart and penetrates all four chambers.

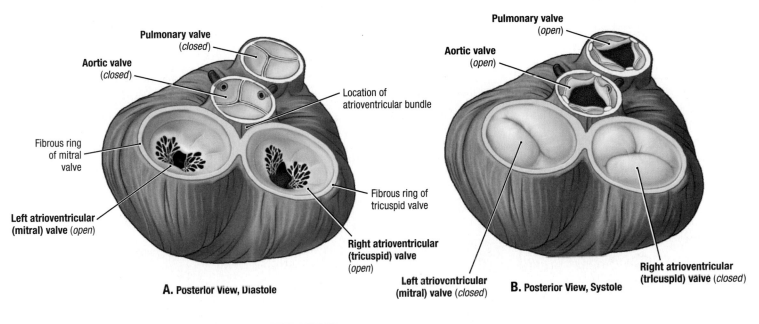

Pulmonary valve
(*closed*)

Aortic valve
(*closed*)

**Fibrous ring
of mitral
valve**

Location of
atrioventricular bundle

**Left atrioventricular
(mitral) valve** (*open*)

Fibrous ring of
tricuspid valve

**Right atrioventricular
(tricuspid) valve**
(*open*)

A. Posterior View, Diastole

Pulmonary valve
(*open*)

Aortic valve
(*open*)

**Left atrioventricular
(mitral) valve** (*closed*)

**Right atrioventricular
(tricuspid) valve** (*closed*)

B. Posterior View, Systole

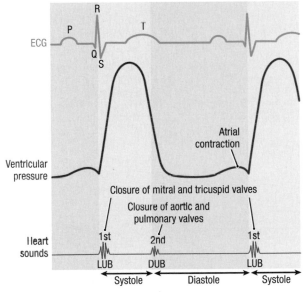

ECG

P
R
Q S
T

Ventricular
pressure

Atrial
contraction

Closure of mitral and tricuspid valves

Closure of aortic and
pulmonary valves

Heart
sounds

1st   2nd   1st
LUB   DUB   LUB

Systole   Diastole   Systole

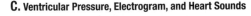

C. Ventricular Pressure, Electrogram, and Heart Sounds

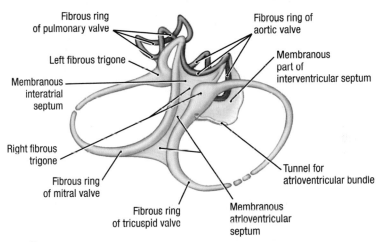

Fibrous ring
of pulmonary valve

Fibrous ring of
aortic valve

Left fibrous trigone

Membranous
part of
interventricular septum

Membranous
interatrial
septum

Right fibrous
trigone

Tunnel for
atrioventricular bundle

Fibrous ring
of mitral valve

Fibrous ring
of tricuspid valve

Membranous
atrioventricular
septum

D. Posteroinferior View

Cardiac Cycle and Cardiac Skeleton

3.53

A. Ventricular diastole. B. Ventricular systole. C. Correlation of ventricular pressure, electrocardiogram (ECG), and heart sounds. The cardiac cycle describes the complete movement of the heart or heartbeat and includes the period from the beginning of one heartbeat to the beginning of the next one. The cycle consists of diastole (ventricular relaxation and filling) and systole (ventricular contraction and emptying). The right heart is the pump for the pulmonary circuit; the left heart is the pump for the systemic circuit (see Fig. 3.43C). **D. Cardiac skeleton.** The fibrous framework of dense collagen forms four fibrous rings, which provide attachment for the leaflets and cusps of the valves, and two fibrous trigones that connect the rings and the membranous parts of the interatrial and interventricular septa. The fibrous skeleton keeps the orifices of the valves patent and separates the myenterically conducted impulses of the atria.

Disorders involving the valves of the heart disturb the pumping efficiency of the heart. **Valvular heart disease** produces either stenosis (narrowing) or insufficiency. **Valvular stenosis** is the failure of a valve to open fully, slowing blood flow from a chamber. **Valvular insufficiency**, or regurgitation, is the failure of the valve to close completely, usually owing to nodule formation on (or scarring and contraction of) the cusps so that the edges do not meet or align. This allows a variable amount of blood (depending on the severity) to flow back into the chamber it was just ejected from. Both stenosis and insufficiency result in an increased workload for the heart. Because valvular diseases are mechanical problems, damaged or defective cardiac valves are often replaced surgically in a procedure called **valvuloplasty.**

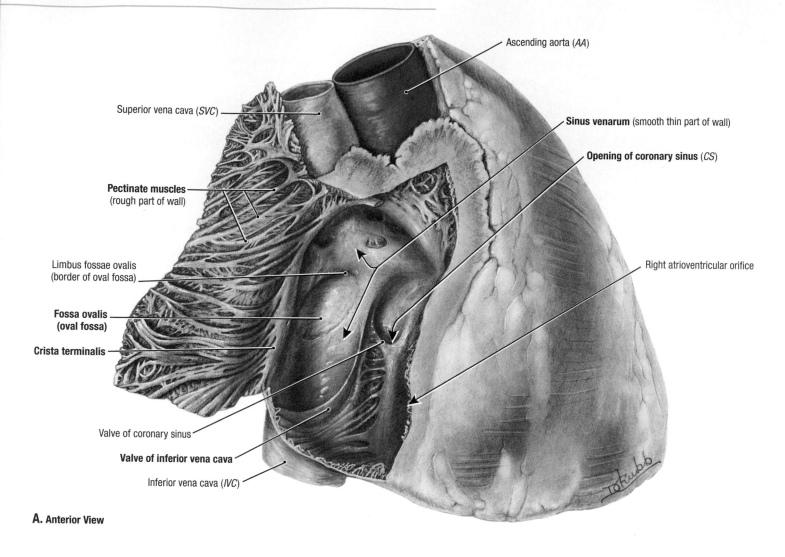

Ascending aorta (*AA*)

Superior vena cava (*SVC*)

Sinus venarum (smooth thin part of wall)

Opening of coronary sinus (*CS*)

Pectinate muscles
(rough part of wall)

Limbus fossae ovalis
(border of oval fossa)

Right atrioventricular orifice

Fossa ovalis
(oval fossa)

Crista terminalis

Valve of coronary sinus

Valve of inferior vena cava

Inferior vena cava (*IVC*)

A. Anterior View

3.54 Right Atrium

A. Interior of right atrium. The anterior wall of the right atrium is reflected. **B. Blood flow into right atrium.**

- The smooth part of the atrial wall is formed by the absorption of the right horn of the sinus venosus, and the rough part is formed from the primitive atrium.
- The floor of the fossa ovalis is the remnant of the fetal septum primum; the crescent-shaped ridge (limbus fossae ovalis) partially surrounding the fossa is the remnant of the septum secundum.
- Inflow from the superior vena cava is directed toward the tricuspid orifice, whereas blood from the inferior vena cava is directed toward the fossa ovalis, as in *Part B*.
- Congenital anomalies of the interatrial septum, most often incomplete closure of the oval foramen (patent foramen ovale), are **atrial septal defects (ASDs)** with an incidence of 6.4/10,000 births (Sadler, 2024). A probe-size patency is present in the superior part of the oval fossa in 15% to 25% of adults (Moore et al., 2016). These small openings, by themselves, cause no hemodynamic abnormalities. Large ASDs allow oxygenated blood from the lungs to be shunted from the left atrium through the ASD into the right atrium, causing enlargement of the right atrium and ventricle and dilation of the pulmonary trunk.

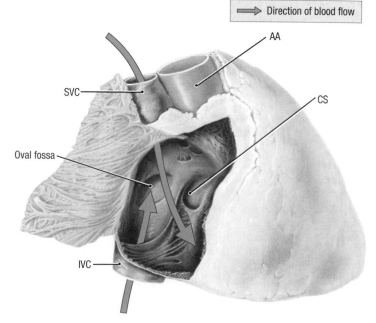

Direction of blood flow

AA

SVC

CS

Oval fossa

IVC

B. Anterior View

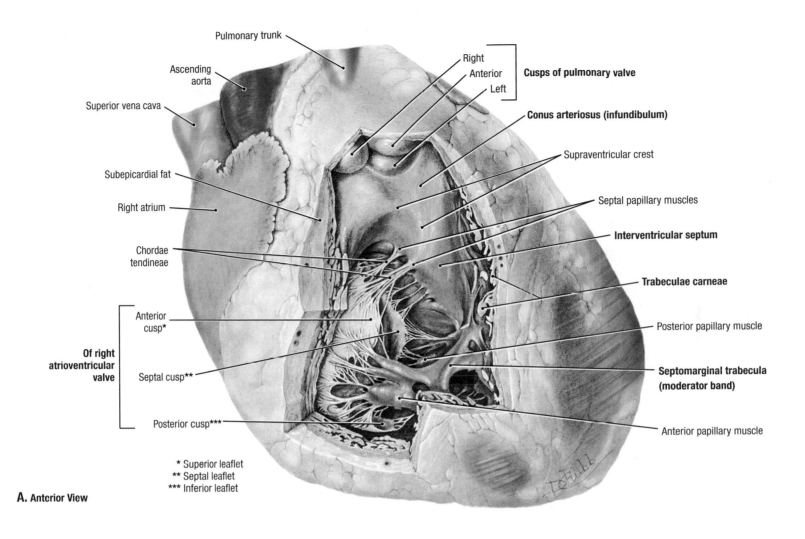

Pulmonary trunk

Ascending aorta

Superior vena cava

Subepicardial fat

Right atrium

Chordae tendineae

Anterior cusp*

Of right atrioventricular valve

Septal cusp**

Posterior cusp***

Right
Anterior
Left
} **Cusps of pulmonary valve**

Conus arteriosus (infundibulum)

Supraventricular crest

Septal papillary muscles

Interventricular septum

Trabeculae carneae

Posterior papillary muscle

Septomarginal trabecula (moderator band)

Anterior papillary muscle

* Superior leaflet
** Septal leaflet
*** Inferior leaflet

A. Anterior View

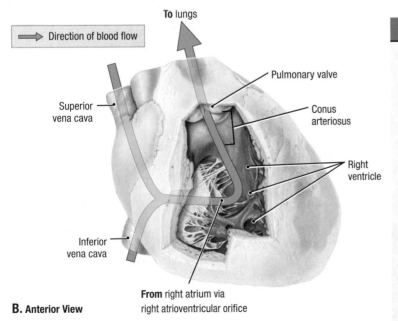

To lungs

→ Direction of blood flow

Pulmonary valve

Superior vena cava

Conus arteriosus

Right ventricle

Inferior vena cava

From right atrium via right atrioventricular orifice

B. Anterior View

Right Ventricle 3.55

A. Interior of right ventricle. **B.** Blood flow through right heart.

- The entrance to this chamber, the right atrioventricular or tricuspid orifice, is situated posteriorly; the exit, the orifice of the pulmonary trunk, is superior.
- The outflow portion of the chamber inferior to the pulmonary orifice (conus arteriosus or infundibulum) has a smooth, funnel-shaped wall; the remainder of the ventricle is rough with fleshy trabeculae.
- The septomarginal trabecula, here thick, extends from the septum to the base of the anterior papillary muscle.
- The membranous part of the interventricular septum develops separately from the muscular part and has a complex embryological origin. Consequently, this part is the common site of **ventricular septal defects (VSDs)**, although defects also occur in the muscular part. VSDs rank first on all lists of cardiac defects. The size of the defect varies from 1 to 25 mm. A VSD causes a left-to-right shunt of blood through the defect. A large shunt increases pulmonary blood flow, which causes severe pulmonary disease (**pulmonary hypertension**, or increased blood pressure) and may cause **cardiac failure**.

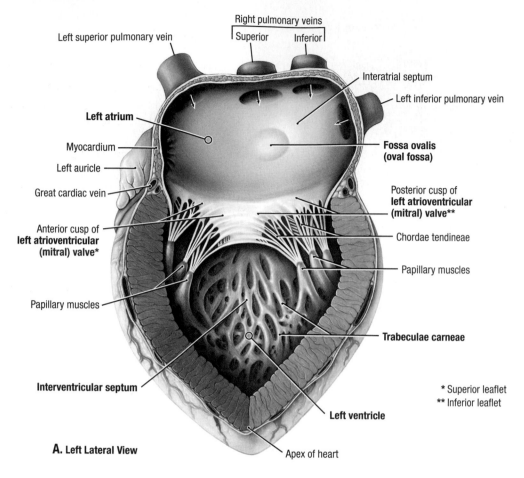

Right pulmonary veins
Superior   Inferior

Left superior pulmonary vein

Interatrial septum

Left inferior pulmonary vein

Left atrium

Myocardium

**Fossa ovalis
(oval fossa)**

Left auricle

Great cardiac vein

Posterior cusp of
**left atrioventricular
(mitral) valve****

Anterior cusp of
**left atrioventricular
(mitral) valve***

Chordae tendineae

Papillary muscles

Papillary muscles

Trabeculae carneae

Interventricular septum

* Superior leaflet
** Inferior leaflet

Left ventricle

A. Left Lateral View

Apex of heart

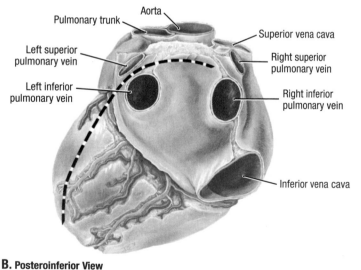

Aorta

Pulmonary trunk

Superior vena cava

Left superior
pulmonary vein

Right superior
pulmonary vein

Left inferior
pulmonary vein

Right inferior
pulmonary vein

Inferior vena cava

B. Posteroinferior View

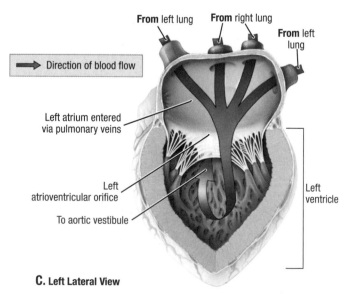

From left lung   **From** right lung

From left
lung

→ Direction of blood flow

Left atrium entered
via pulmonary veins

Left
ventricle

Left
atrioventricular orifice

To aortic vestibule

C. Left Lateral View

3.56   **Left Atrium and Left Ventricle**

A. Interior of left heart. **B.** Line of incision (*black dashed line*) for
Part A and *Part C*. **C.** Blood flow through left heart.
- A diagonal cut was made from the base of the heart to the apex,
  passing between the superior and inferior pulmonary veins and
  through the posterior cusp of the mitral valve, followed by retraction (spreading) of the left heart wall on each side of the incision.

- The entrances (pulmonary veins) to the left atrium are posterior,
  and the exit (left atrioventricular or mitral orifice) is anterior.
- The left side of the fossa ovalis is also seen on the left side of the
  interatrial septum, although the left side is not usually as distinct
  as the right side is within the right atrium.
- Except for that of the auricle, the atrial wall is smooth.

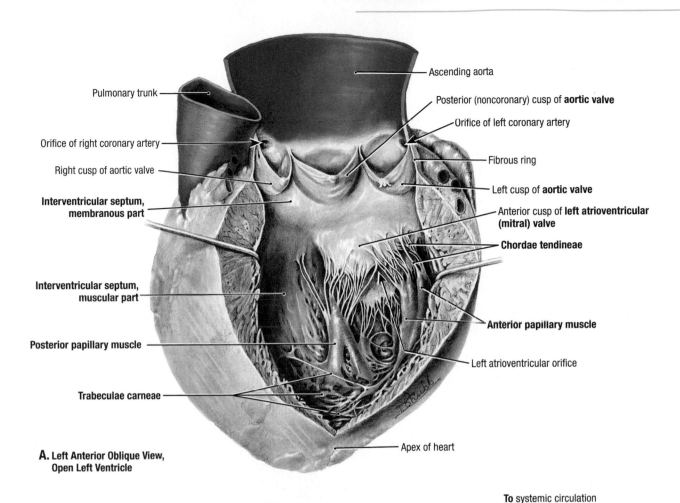

Pulmonary trunk

Orifice of right coronary artery

Right cusp of aortic valve

**Interventricular septum,
membranous part**

**Interventricular septum,
muscular part**

Posterior papillary muscle

Trabeculae carneae

Ascending aorta

Posterior (noncoronary) cusp of **aortic valve**

Orifice of left coronary artery

Fibrous ring

Left cusp of **aortic valve**

Anterior cusp of **left atrioventricular
(mitral) valve**

Chordae tendineae

Anterior papillary muscle

Left atrioventricular orifice

Apex of heart

**A. Left Anterior Oblique View,
Open Left Ventricle**

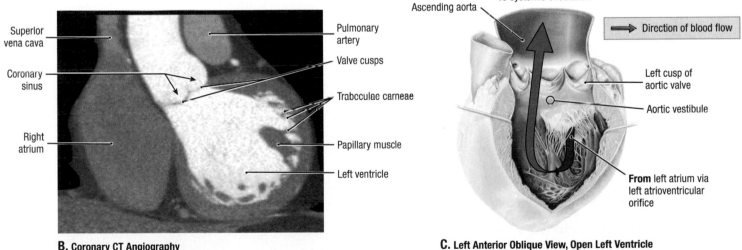

B. Coronary CT Angiography

Superior
vena cava

Coronary
sinus

Right
atrium

Pulmonary
artery

Valve cusps

Trabeculae carneae

Papillary muscle

Left ventricle

To systemic circulation

Ascending aorta

Direction of blood flow

Left cusp of
aortic valve

Aortic vestibule

From left atrium via
left atrioventricular
orifice

C. Left Anterior Oblique View, Open Left Ventricle

Left Ventricle

3.57

**A. Interior of left ventricle. B. CT with an intravenous (IV)
contrast agent.** A series of CT images was taken as the contrast
material traveled through the heart. For this image, the material
has mainly passed through the right side of the heart and is primarily now in the left ventricle and aorta. **C. Blood flow through left
ventricle.**

- A cut was made from the apex along the left margin of the
  heart, passing posterior to the pulmonary trunk, to open the
  aortic vestibule and ascending aorta.

- The entrance (left atrioventricular, bicuspid, or mitral orifice) is
  situated posteriorly, and the exit (aortic orifice) is superior.
- The left ventricular wall is thin and muscular near the apex, thick
  and muscular superiorly, and thin and fibrous (nonelastic) at the
  aortic orifice.
- Two large papillary muscles, the anterior from the anterior
  wall and the posterior from the posterior wall, control the
  adjacent halves of two cusps of the mitral valve with chordae
  tendineae.

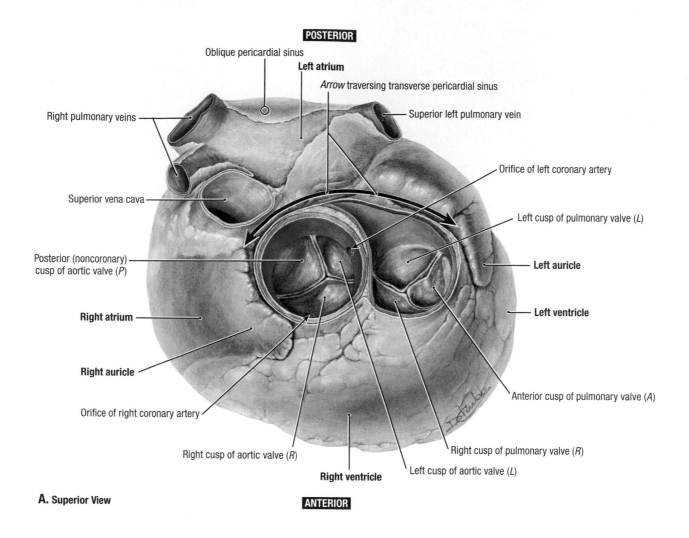

POSTERIOR

Oblique pericardial sinus

Left atrium

Arrow traversing transverse pericardial sinus

Right pulmonary veins

Superior left pulmonary vein

Superior vena cava

Orifice of left coronary artery

Left cusp of pulmonary valve (*L*)

Posterior (noncoronary) cusp of aortic valve (*P*)

Left auricle

Right atrium

Left ventricle

Right auricle

Anterior cusp of pulmonary valve (*A*)

Orifice of right coronary artery

Right cusp of pulmonary valve (*R*)

Right cusp of aortic valve (*R*)

Left cusp of aortic valve (*L*)

A. Superior View

Right ventricle

ANTERIOR

3.58 Valves of Heart (I)

A. Excised heart.
- The ventricles are positioned anteriorly and to the left, and the atria posteriorly and to the right.
- The roots of the aorta and pulmonary artery, which conduct blood from the ventricles, are placed anterior to the atria.
- The aorta and pulmonary artery are enclosed within a common tube of serous pericardium and partly embraced by the auricles of the atria.
- The transverse pericardial sinus curves posterior to the enclosed stems of the aorta and pulmonary trunk and anterior to the superior vena cava and upper limits of the atria.

B. Developmental basis for naming of pulmonary and aortic valve cusps. The truncus arteriosus with four cusps (I) splits to form two valves, each with three cusps (II). The heart undergoes partial rotation to the left on its axis, resulting in the arrangement of cusps shown in (III).

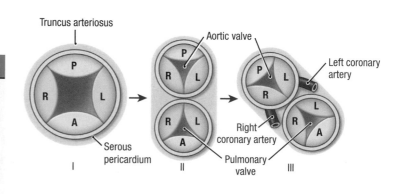

Truncus arteriosus

Aortic valve

Left coronary artery

Serous pericardium

Right coronary artery

Pulmonary valve

I

II

III

B. Schematic

Semilunar Valves/Cusps	
R Right	**A** Anterior
L Left	**P** Posterior

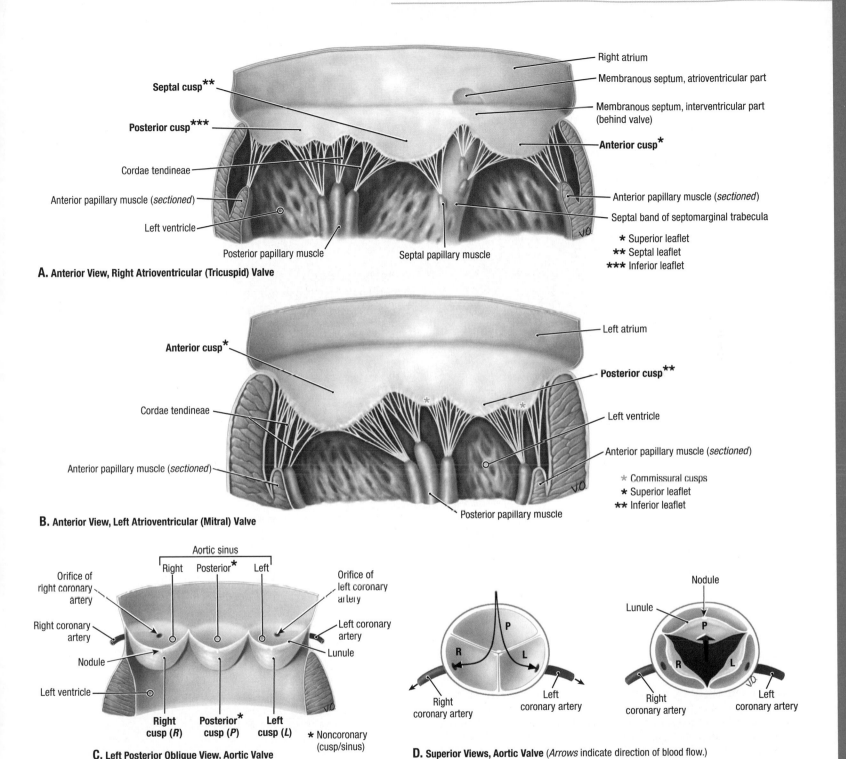

A. Anterior View, Right Atrioventricular (Tricuspid) Valve

Septal cusp**
Posterior cusp***
Cordae tendineae
Anterior papillary muscle (*sectioned*)
Left ventricle
Posterior papillary muscle
Septal papillary muscle

Right atrium
Membranous septum, atrioventricular part
Membranous septum, interventricular part (behind valve)
Anterior cusp*
Anterior papillary muscle (*sectioned*)
Septal band of septomarginal trabecula

★ Superior leaflet
★★ Septal leaflet
★★★ Inferior leaflet

B. Anterior View, Left Atrioventricular (Mitral) Valve

Anterior cusp*
Cordae tendineae
Anterior papillary muscle (*sectioned*)
Posterior papillary muscle

Left atrium
Posterior cusp**
Left ventricle
Anterior papillary muscle (*sectioned*)

＊ Commissural cusps
★ Superior leaflet
★★ Inferior leaflet

C. Left Posterior Oblique View, Aortic Valve

Aortic sinus
Right Posterior* Left
Orifice of right coronary artery
Right coronary artery
Nodule
Left ventricle
Right cusp (R) Posterior* cusp (P) Left cusp (L)
Orifice of left coronary artery
Left coronary artery
Lunule
★ Noncoronary (cusp/sinus)

D. Superior Views, Aortic Valve (*Arrows* indicate direction of blood flow.)

Nodule
Lunule
P
R L
Right coronary artery Left coronary artery
Right coronary artery Left coronary artery

Valves of Heart (II)

3.59

A. and **B.** Atrioventricular valves. **C.** and **D.** Semilunar valves.
Tendinous cords pass from the tips of the papillary muscles to the free margins and ventricular surfaces of the cusps of the tricuspid (*Part A*) and mitral (*Part B*) valves. Each papillary muscle or muscle group controls the adjacent sides of two cusps, resisting valve prolapse during systole. In *Part C*, the anulus of the aortic valve has been incised between the right and left cusps and spread open. Each cusp of the semilunar valves bears a nodule in the midpoint of its free edge, flanked by thin connective tissue areas (lunules). When the ventricles relax to fill (diastole), backflow of blood from aortic recoil or pulmonary resistance fills the sinus (space between cusp and dilated part of the aortic or pulmonary wall), causing the nodules and lunules to meet centrally, closing the valve (*Part D, left*). Filling of the coronary arteries occurs during diastole (when ventricular walls are relaxed) as backflow "inflates" the cusps to close the valve.

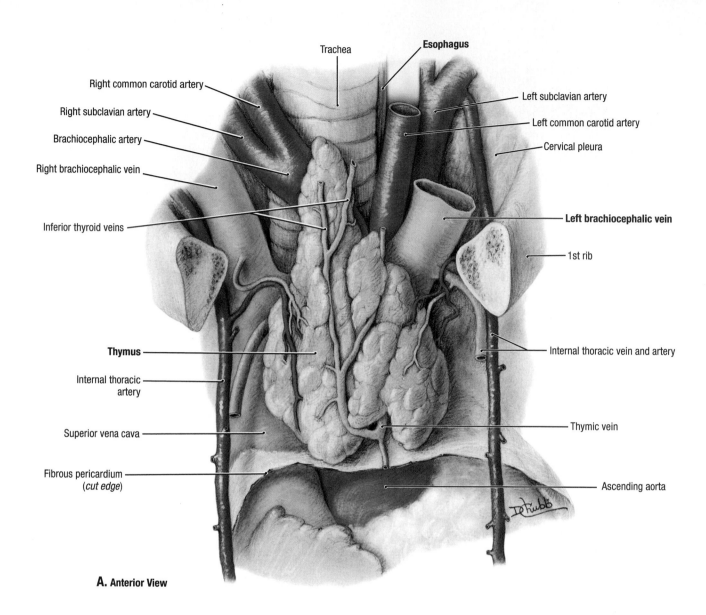

Trachea

Esophagus

Right common carotid artery

Right subclavian artery

Brachiocephalic artery

Right brachiocephalic vein

Inferior thyroid veins

Left subclavian artery

Left common carotid artery

Cervical pleura

Left brachiocephalic vein

1st rib

Thymus

Internal thoracic artery

Superior vena cava

Fibrous pericardium (*cut edge*)

Internal thoracic vein and artery

Thymic vein

Ascending aorta

A. Anterior View

3.60   **Superior Mediastinum (I and II): Superficial Dissections**

A. Dissection (I): thymus *in situ*. The sternum and ribs have been excised and the pleurae removed. It is unusual in an adult to see such a discrete thymus, which is large during puberty but subsequently regresses and is for the most part replaced by fat and fibrous tissue. **B. Dissection (II): thymus removed. C. Relationship of nerves and vessels.** The right vagus nerve (CN X) crosses anterior to the right subclavian artery and gives off the right recurrent laryngeal nerve, which passes medially to reach the trachea and esophagus. The left recurrent laryngeal nerve passes inferior and then posterior to the arch of the aorta and ascends between the trachea and esophagus to the larynx.

The distal part of the ascending aorta receives a strong thrust of blood when the left ventricle contracts. Because its wall is not reinforced by fibrous pericardium (the fibrous pericardium blends with the aortic adventitia at the beginning of the arch), an aneurysm may develop. An **aortic aneurysm** is evident on chest film (radiograph of the thorax) or a magnetic resonance angiogram as an enlarged area

of the ascending aorta silhouette. Individuals with an aneurysm usually complain of chest pain that radiates to the back. The aneurysm may exert pressure on the trachea, esophagus, and recurrent laryngeal nerve, causing difficulty in breathing and swallowing.

Mediastinal compression. The recurrent laryngeal nerves supply all the intrinsic muscles of the larynx, except the cricothyroid. Consequently, any investigative procedure or disease process in the superior mediastinum may involve these nerves and affect the voice. Because the left recurrent laryngeal nerve hooks around the arch of the aorta and ascends between the trachea and the esophagus, it may be involved when there is a bronchial or esophageal carcinoma, enlargement of mediastinal lymph nodes, or an aneurysm of the arch of the aorta.

The thymus is a prominent feature during infancy and childhood. In some infants, the thymus may compress the trachea. The thymus plays an important role in the development and maintenance of the immune system.

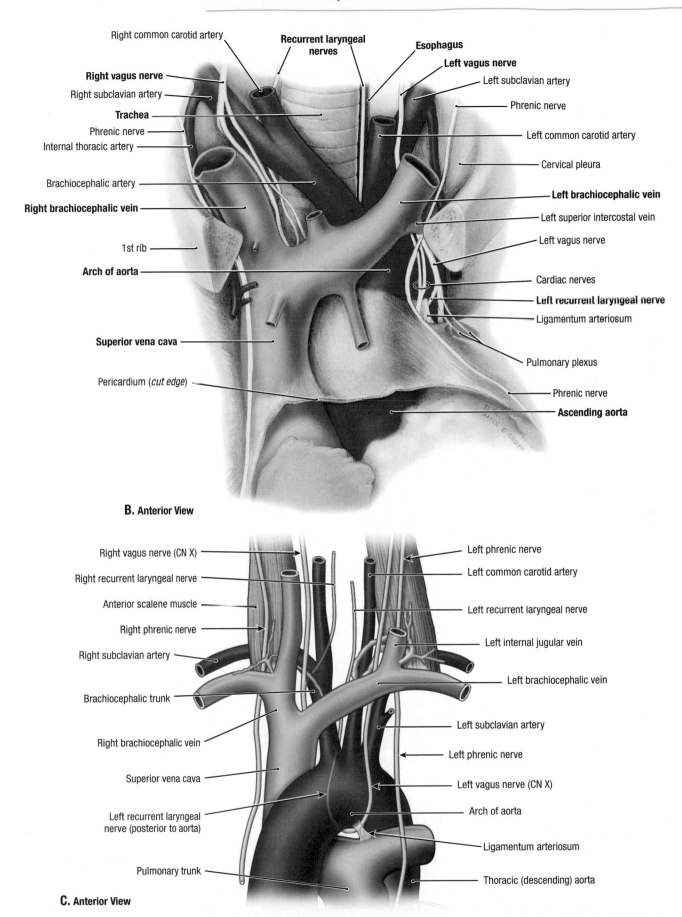

Right common carotid artery

Recurrent laryngeal nerves

Esophagus

Right vagus nerve

Left vagus nerve

Right subclavian artery

Left subclavian artery

Phrenic nerve

Trachea

Phrenic nerve

Left common carotid artery

Internal thoracic artery

Brachiocephalic artery

Cervical pleura

Right brachiocephalic vein

Left brachiocephalic vein

Left superior intercostal vein

1st rib

Left vagus nerve

Arch of aorta

Cardiac nerves

Left recurrent laryngeal nerve

Ligamentum arteriosum

Superior vena cava

Pulmonary plexus

Pericardium (*cut edge*)

Phrenic nerve

Ascending aorta

B. Anterior View

Right vagus nerve (CN X)

Left phrenic nerve

Right recurrent laryngeal nerve

Left common carotid artery

Anterior scalene muscle

Left recurrent laryngeal nerve

Right phrenic nerve

Left internal jugular vein

Right subclavian artery

Brachiocephalic trunk

Left brachiocephalic vein

Right brachiocephalic vein

Left subclavian artery

Left phrenic nerve

Superior vena cava

Left vagus nerve (CN X)

Left recurrent laryngeal nerve (posterior to aorta)

Arch of aorta

Ligamentum arteriosum

Pulmonary trunk

Thoracic (descending) aorta

C. Anterior View

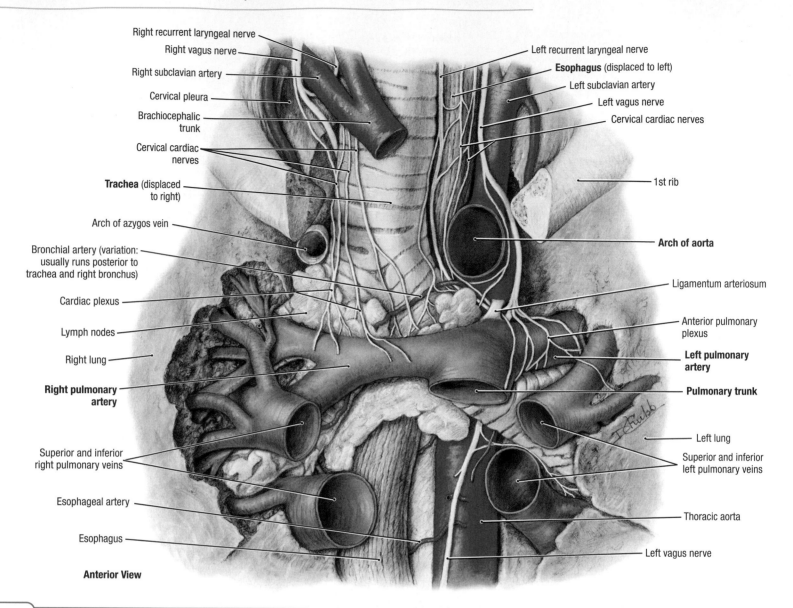

Right recurrent laryngeal nerve
Right vagus nerve
Right subclavian artery
Cervical pleura
Brachiocephalic trunk
Cervical cardiac nerves
Trachea (displaced to right)
Arch of azygos vein
Bronchial artery (variation: usually runs posterior to trachea and right bronchus)
Cardiac plexus
Lymph nodes
Right lung
Right pulmonary artery
Superior and inferior right pulmonary veins
Esophageal artery
Esophagus

Left recurrent laryngeal nerve
Esophagus (displaced to left)
Left subclavian artery
Left vagus nerve
Cervical cardiac nerves
1st rib
Arch of aorta
Ligamentum arteriosum
Anterior pulmonary plexus
Left pulmonary artery
Pulmonary trunk
Left lung
Superior and inferior left pulmonary veins
Thoracic aorta
Left vagus nerve

Anterior View

| 3.61 | **Superior Mediastinum (III): Cardiac Plexus and Pulmonary Arteries** |

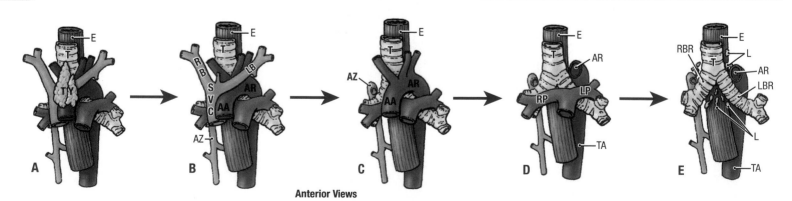

Anterior Views

| 3.62 | **Relations of Great Vessels and Trachea from Superficial to Deep** |

A. Thymus (*TY*). **B.** Right (*RB*) and left (*LB*) brachiocephalic veins form superior vena cava (*SVC*), which receives the arch of the azygos vein (*AZ*) posteriorly. **C.** Ascending aorta (*AA*) and arch of aorta (*AR*) arch over right pulmonary artery and left main bronchus. **D.** Right and left pulmonary arteries (*RP* and *LP*). **E.** Tracheobronchial lymph nodes (*L*) at tracheal bifurcation (*T*). *E*, esophagus; *LBR*, left main bronchus; *RBR*, right main bronchus; *TA*, thoracic aorta.

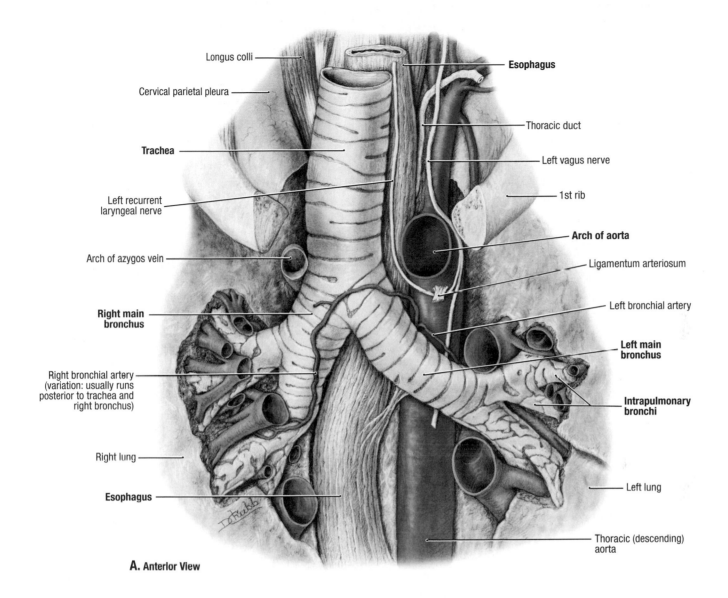

Longus colli
Cervical parietal pleura
Trachea
Left recurrent laryngeal nerve
Arch of azygos vein
Right main bronchus
Right bronchial artery (variation: usually runs posterior to trachea and right bronchus)
Right lung
Esophagus

Esophagus
Thoracic duct
Left vagus nerve
1st rib
Arch of aorta
Ligamentum arteriosum
Left bronchial artery
Left main bronchus
Intrapulmonary bronchi
Left lung
Thoracic (descending) aorta

A. Anterior View

Right vagus nerve
Right recurrent laryngeal nerve
Right 4th aortic arch
Right 5th aortic arch (degenerated)
Right 6th aortic arch (distal half degenerates)
Foregut

Left vagus nerve
Left 4th aortic arch
Left recurrent laryngeal nerve
Left 6th aortic arch
Dorsal aorta

B. Embryonic (6 Weeks), Anterior View

Right vagus nerve
Right recurrent laryngeal nerve
Right subclavian artery (from right 4th aortic arch)
Trachea
Esophagus

Left vagus nerve
Left recurrent laryngeal nerve
Arch of aorta (from left 4th aortic arch)
Ligamentum arteriosum (from left 6th aortic arch)
Left pulmonary artery
Thoracic aorta

C. Child, Anterior View

Superior Mediastinum (IV): Tracheal Bifurcation and Bronchi

3.63

A. Dissection. B. and C. Asymmetrical course of right and left recurrent laryngeal nerves. Arch VI disappears on the right, leaving the right recurrent laryngeal nerve (*green circle*) to pass under arch IV, which becomes the right subclavian artery. Arch VI becomes part of the ductus arteriosus on the left side, and arch IV "descends" to become the arch of the aorta; thus, the left recurrent laryngeal nerve (*blue circle*) is pulled into the thorax.

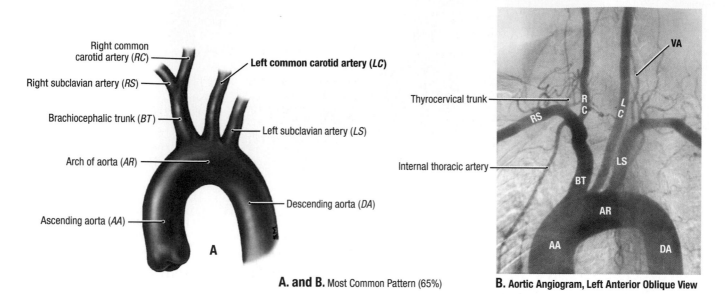

Right common carotid artery (*RC*)

Right subclavian artery (*RS*)

Brachiocephalic trunk (*BT*)

Arch of aorta (*AR*)

Ascending aorta (*AA*)

Left common carotid artery (*LC*)

Left subclavian artery (*LS*)

Descending aorta (*DA*)

A

A. and B. Most Common Pattern (65%)

VA

Thyrocervical trunk

Internal thoracic artery

RC
RS
LC
LS
BT
AR
AA
DA

B. Aortic Angiogram, Left Anterior Oblique View

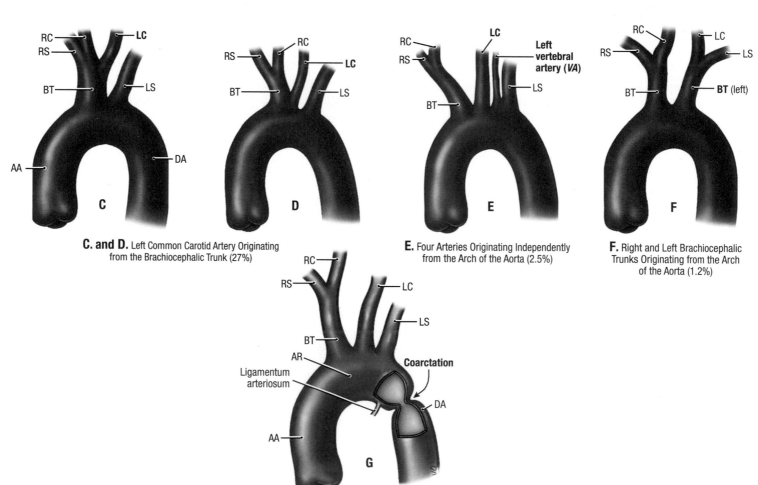

RC — LC
RS
BT — LS
AA — DA

C

RS — RC
BT — LC
— LS

D

RC — LC
RS — Left vertebral artery (*VA*)
BT — LS

E

RC — LC
RS — LS
BT — **BT** (left)

F

C. and D. Left Common Carotid Artery Originating from the Brachiocephalic Trunk (27%)

E. Four Arteries Originating Independently from the Arch of the Aorta (2.5%)

F. Right and Left Brachiocephalic Trunks Originating from the Arch of the Aorta (1.2%)

RC
RS — LC
BT — LS
AR — **Coarctation**
Ligamentum arteriosum — DA
AA

G

3.64   **Branches of Aortic Arch**

A. and **B.** Most common pattern (65%). **C–F.** Variations. **G.** In **coarctation of the aorta**, the arch or descending aorta has an abnormal narrowing (stenosis) that diminishes the caliber of the aortic lumen, producing an obstruction to blood flow. The most common site is near the ligamentum arteriosum. When the coarctation is inferior to this site (**postductal coarctation**), a good collateral circulation usually develops between the proximal and distal parts of the aorta through the intercostal and internal thoracic arteries.

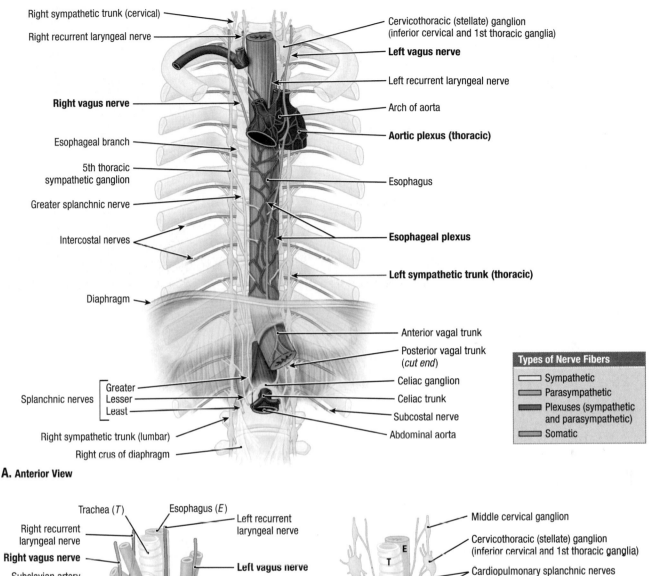

Right sympathetic trunk (cervical)
Right recurrent laryngeal nerve
Right vagus nerve
Esophageal branch
5th thoracic sympathetic ganglion
Greater splanchnic nerve
Intercostal nerves
Diaphragm
Splanchnic nerves — Greater / Lesser / Least
Right sympathetic trunk (lumbar)
Right crus of diaphragm

Cervicothoracic (stellate) ganglion (inferior cervical and 1st thoracic ganglia)
Left vagus nerve
Left recurrent laryngeal nerve
Arch of aorta
Aortic plexus (thoracic)
Esophagus
Esophageal plexus
Left sympathetic trunk (thoracic)
Anterior vagal trunk
Posterior vagal trunk (*cut end*)
Celiac ganglion
Celiac trunk
Subcostal nerve
Abdominal aorta

Types of Nerve Fibers
- Sympathetic
- Parasympathetic
- Plexuses (sympathetic and parasympathetic)
- Somatic

A. Anterior View

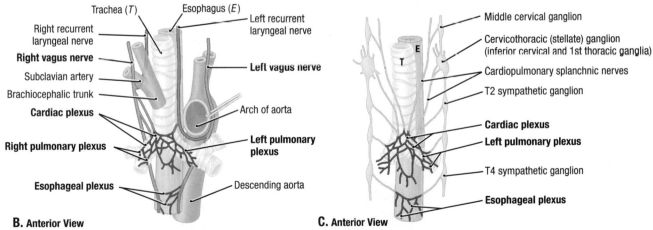

Trachea (*T*) Esophagus (*E*)
Right recurrent laryngeal nerve
Right vagus nerve
Subclavian artery
Brachiocephalic trunk
Cardiac plexus
Right pulmonary plexus
Esophageal plexus

Left recurrent laryngeal nerve
Left vagus nerve
Arch of aorta
Left pulmonary plexus
Descending aorta

B. Anterior View

Middle cervical ganglion
Cervicothoracic (stellate) ganglion (inferior cervical and 1st thoracic ganglia)
Cardiopulmonary splanchnic nerves
T2 sympathetic ganglion
Cardiac plexus
Left pulmonary plexus
T4 sympathetic ganglion
Esophageal plexus

C. Anterior View

Cardiac and Pulmonary Plexuses

3.65

A. Overview. **B.** Parasympathetic contribution. **C.** Sympathetic contribution.

Heart. Sympathetic stimulation increases the heart's rate and the force of its contractions. Parasympathetic stimulation slows the heart rate, reduces the force of contraction, and constricts the coronary arteries, saving energy between periods of increased demand. While the cardiac plexus is shown in relation to the bifurcation of the trachea, note that it lies directly posterior to the superior margin of the heart (see Fig. 3.28C) and in close proximity to the nodal tissue and origins of the coronary arteries.

Lungs. Sympathetic fibers are inhibitory to the bronchial muscle (bronchodilator), motor to pulmonary vessels (vasoconstrictor), and inhibitory to the alveolar glands of the bronchial tree. Parasympathetic fibers from CN X are bronchoconstrictors, secretory to the glands of the bronchial tree (secretomotor).

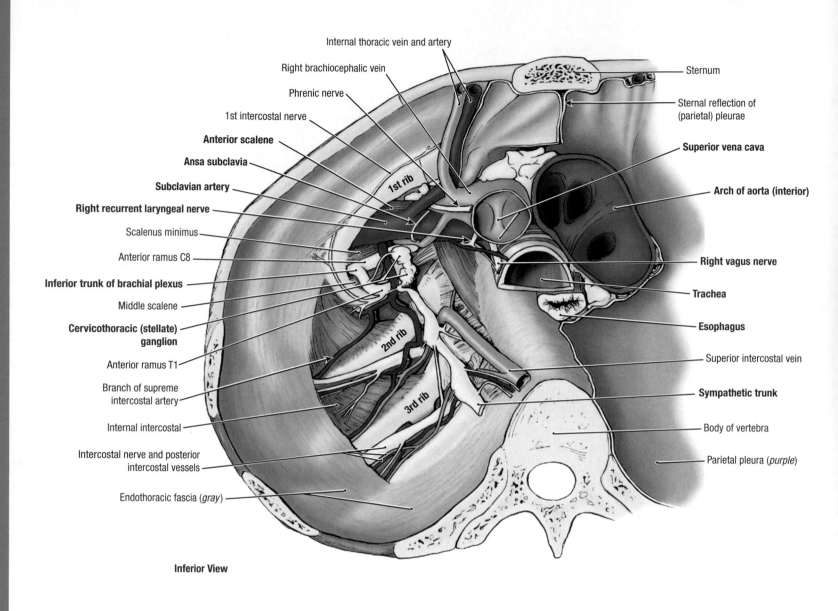

Internal thoracic vein and artery

Right brachiocephalic vein

Phrenic nerve

1st intercostal nerve

Anterior scalene

Ansa subclavia

Subclavian artery

Right recurrent laryngeal nerve

Scalenus minimus

Anterior ramus C8

Inferior trunk of brachial plexus

Middle scalene

Cervicothoracic (stellate) ganglion

Anterior ramus T1

Branch of supreme intercostal artery

Internal intercostal

Intercostal nerve and posterior intercostal vessels

Endothoracic fascia (*gray*)

1st rib

2nd rib

3rd rib

Sternum

Sternal reflection of (parietal) pleurae

Superior vena cava

Arch of aorta (interior)

Right vagus nerve

Trachea

Esophagus

Superior intercostal vein

Sympathetic trunk

Body of vertebra

Parietal pleura (*purple*)

Inferior View

| 3.66 | **Superior Mediastinum and Roof of Pleural Cavity** |

- The cervical, costal, and mediastinal parietal pleura (*purple*) and portions of the endothoracic fascia (*gray*) have been removed from the right side of the specimen to demonstrate structures traversing the superior thoracic aperture.
- The first part of the subclavian artery disappears as it crosses the 1st rib anterior to the anterior scalene muscle.
- The ansa subclavia from the sympathetic trunk and right recurrent laryngeal nerve from the vagus are seen looping inferior to the subclavian artery.
- The anterior rami of C8 and T1 merge to form the inferior trunk of the brachial plexus, which crosses the 1st rib posterior to the anterior scalene muscle.

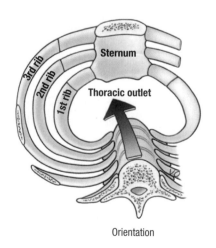

Orientation

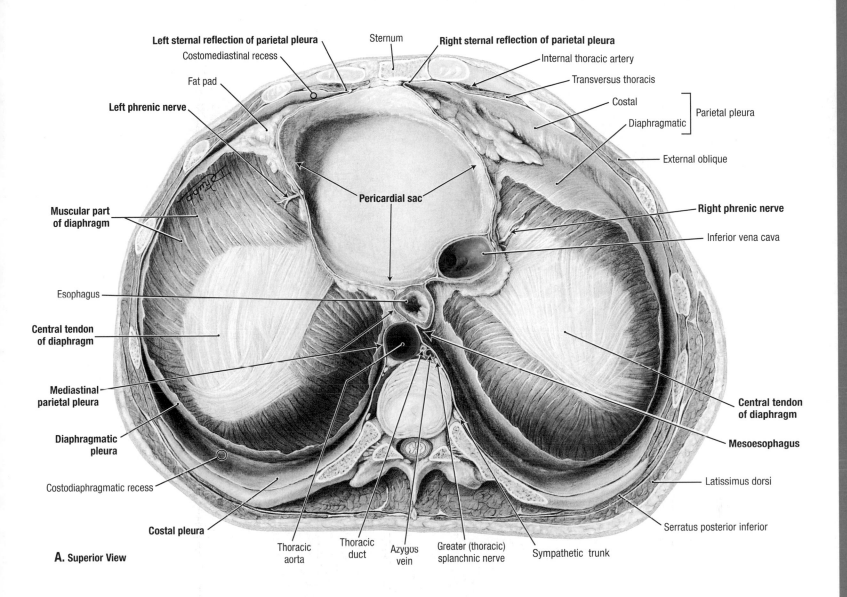

Left sternal reflection of parietal pleura
Costomediastinal recess
Fat pad
Left phrenic nerve
Sternum
Right sternal reflection of parietal pleura
Internal thoracic artery
Transversus thoracis
Costal
Diaphragmatic
Parietal pleura
External oblique
Pericardial sac
Muscular part of diaphragm
Right phrenic nerve
Inferior vena cava
Esophagus
Central tendon of diaphragm
Central tendon of diaphragm
Mediastinal parietal pleura
Mesoesophagus
Diaphragmatic pleura
Latissimus dorsi
Costodiaphragmatic recess
Costal pleura
Serratus posterior inferior
Thoracic aorta
Thoracic duct
Azygos vein
Greater (thoracic) splanchnic nerve
Sympathetic trunk

A. Superior View

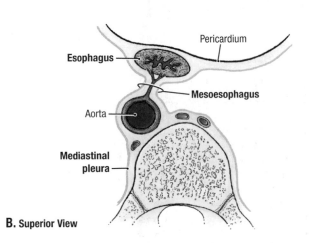

Pericardium
Esophagus
Mesoesophagus
Aorta
Mediastinal pleura

B. Superior View

Diaphragm, Pericardial Sac, and Pleura   3.67

A. Dissection. The diaphragmatic pleura is mostly removed. The pericardial sac is situated on the anterior half of the diaphragm; one third is to the right of the median plane and two thirds is to the left. Note also that anterior to the pericardium, the sternal reflection of the left pleural sac approaches but fails to meet that of the right sac in the median plane; and on reaching the vertebral column, the costal pleura becomes the mediastinal pleura.

Irritation of the parietal pleura produces local pain and referred pain to the areas sharing innervation by the same segments of the spinal cord. **Irritation of the costal and peripheral parts of the diaphragmatic pleura** results in local pain and referred pain along the intercostal nerves to the thoracic and abdominal walls. **Irritation of the mediastinal and central diaphragmatic parts of the parietal pleura** results in pain that is referred to the root of the neck and over the shoulder (C3–C5 dermatomes). **B. Mesoesophagus.** The inferior part of the esophagus and the aorta, the right and left layers of mediastinal pleura form a dorsal mesoesophagus, especially when the body is in the prone position.

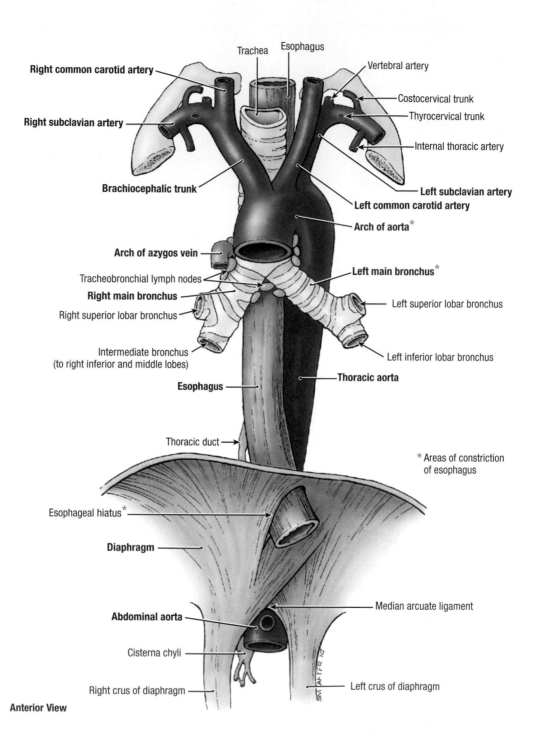

Trachea

Esophagus

Right common carotid artery

Vertebral artery

Costocervical trunk

Thyrocervical trunk

Right subclavian artery

Internal thoracic artery

Brachiocephalic trunk

Left subclavian artery

Left common carotid artery

Arch of aorta*

Arch of azygos vein

Left main bronchus*

Tracheobronchial lymph nodes

Right main bronchus

Left superior lobar bronchus

Right superior lobar bronchus

Intermediate bronchus
(to right inferior and middle lobes)

Left inferior lobar bronchus

Thoracic aorta

Esophagus

Thoracic duct

* Areas of constriction
of esophagus

Esophageal hiatus*

Diaphragm

Median arcuate ligament

Abdominal aorta

Cisterna chyli

Right crus of diaphragm

Left crus of diaphragm

Anterior View

3.68 **Esophagus, Trachea, and Aorta**

- The anterior relations of the thoracic part of the esophagus from superior to inferior are the trachea (from origin at cricoid cartilage to bifurcation), right and left bronchi, inferior tracheobronchial lymph nodes, pericardium (not shown), and, finally, the diaphragm.
- The arch of the aorta passes posterior to the left of these four structures as it arches over the left main bronchus; the arch of the azygos vein passes anterior to their right as it arches over the right main bronchus.

- **Esophageal impressions.** The impressions produced in the esophagus by adjacent structures (aorta, left main bronchus, and esophageal hiatus) are of clinical interest because of the slower passage of substances at these sites. The impressions indicate where swallowed foreign bodies are most likely to lodge and where a stricture may develop after the accidental drinking of a caustic liquid such as lye.

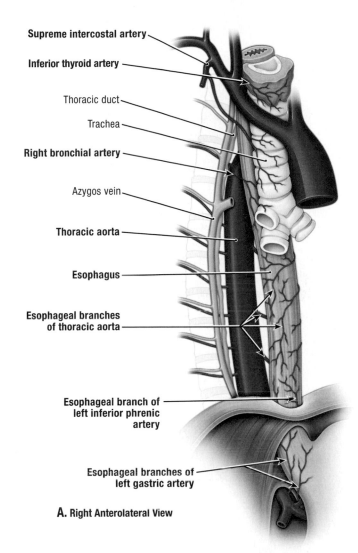

Supreme intercostal artery

Inferior thyroid artery

Thoracic duct

Trachea

Right bronchial artery

Azygos vein

Thoracic aorta

Esophagus

Esophageal branches of thoracic aorta

Esophageal branch of left inferior phrenic artery

Esophageal branches of left gastric artery

A. Right Anterolateral View

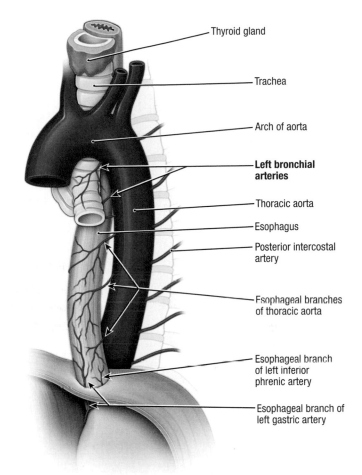

Thyroid gland

Trachea

Arch of aorta

Left bronchial arteries

Thoracic aorta

Esophagus

Posterior intercostal artery

Esophageal branches of thoracic aorta

Esophageal branch of left inferior phrenic artery

Esophageal branch of left gastric artery

B. Left Anterolateral View

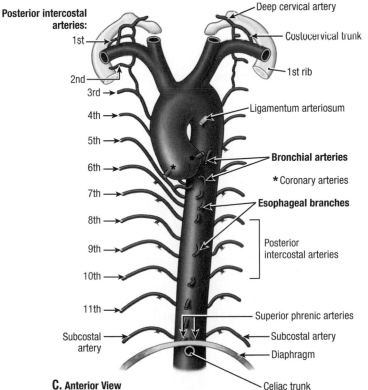

Posterior intercostal arteries:

1st

2nd

3rd

4th

5th

6th

7th

8th

9th

10th

11th

Subcostal artery

Deep cervical artery

Costocervical trunk

1st rib

Ligamentum arteriosum

Bronchial arteries

* Coronary arteries

Esophageal branches

Posterior intercostal arteries

Superior phrenic arteries

Subcostal artery

Diaphragm

Celiac trunk

C. Anterior View

Arterial Supply to Trachea and Esophagus 3.69

A. and **B. Arteries of trachea and esophagus.** The continuous anastomotic chain of arteries on the esophagus is formed (1) by branches of the right and left inferior thyroid and right supreme intercostal arteries superiorly, (2) by the unpaired median aortic (bronchial and esophageal) branches, and (3) by branches of the left gastric and left inferior phrenic arteries inferiorly. The right bronchial artery usually arises from the superior left bronchial or 3rd right posterior intercostal artery (here the 5th) or from the aorta directly. The unpaired median aortic branches also supply the trachea and bronchi. **C. Branches of thoracic aorta.**

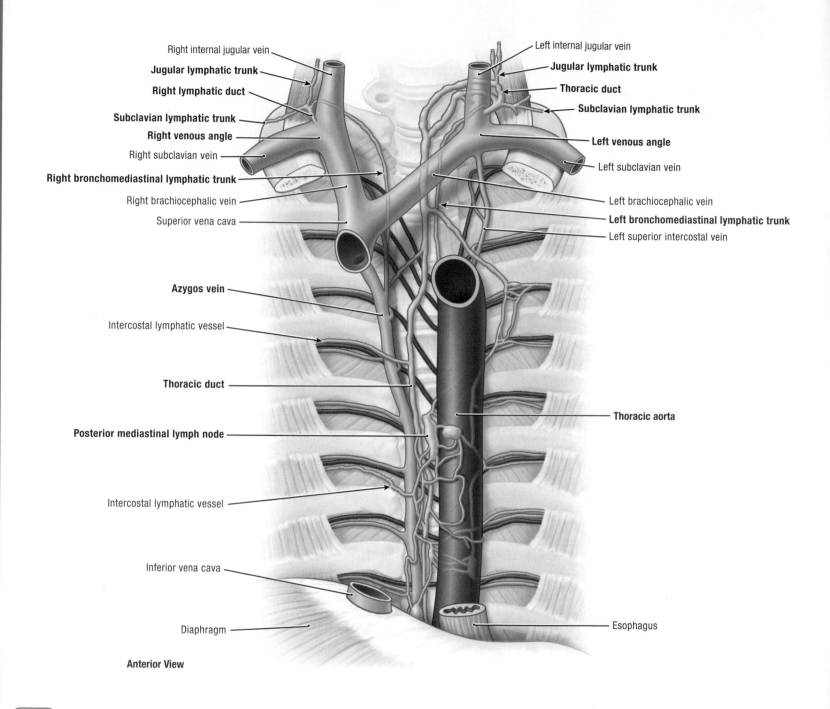

Right internal jugular vein

Jugular lymphatic trunk

Right lymphatic duct

Subclavian lymphatic trunk

Right venous angle

Right subclavian vein

Right bronchomediastinal lymphatic trunk

Right brachiocephalic vein

Superior vena cava

Azygos vein

Intercostal lymphatic vessel

Thoracic duct

Posterior mediastinal lymph node

Intercostal lymphatic vessel

Inferior vena cava

Diaphragm

Left internal jugular vein

Jugular lymphatic trunk

Thoracic duct

Subclavian lymphatic trunk

Left venous angle

Left subclavian vein

Left brachiocephalic vein

Left bronchomediastinal lymphatic trunk

Left superior intercostal vein

Thoracic aorta

Esophagus

Anterior View

3.70 | **Thoracic Duct**

- The thoracic aorta is located to the left and the azygos vein slightly to the right of the midline.
- The thoracic duct (1) originates from the cisterna chyli at the T12 vertebral level, (2) ascends on the vertebral column between the azygos vein and the thoracic aorta, (3) passes to the left at the junction of the posterior and superior mediastina, and continues its ascent to the neck, where (4) it arches laterally to enter the venous system near or at the angle of union of the left internal jugular and subclavian veins (left venous angle).
- The thoracic duct is commonly plexiform (resembling a network) in the posterior mediastinum.

- The termination of the thoracic duct typically receives the left jugular, subclavian, and bronchomediastinal trunks.
- The right lymph duct is short and formed by the union of the right jugular, subclavian, and bronchomediastinal trunks.
- Because the thoracic duct is thin walled and may be colorless, it may not be easily identified. Consequently, it is vulnerable to inadvertent injury during investigative and/or surgical procedures in the posterior mediastinum. **Laceration of the thoracic duct** results in chyle escaping into the thoracic cavity. Chyle may also enter the pleural cavity, producing chylothorax.

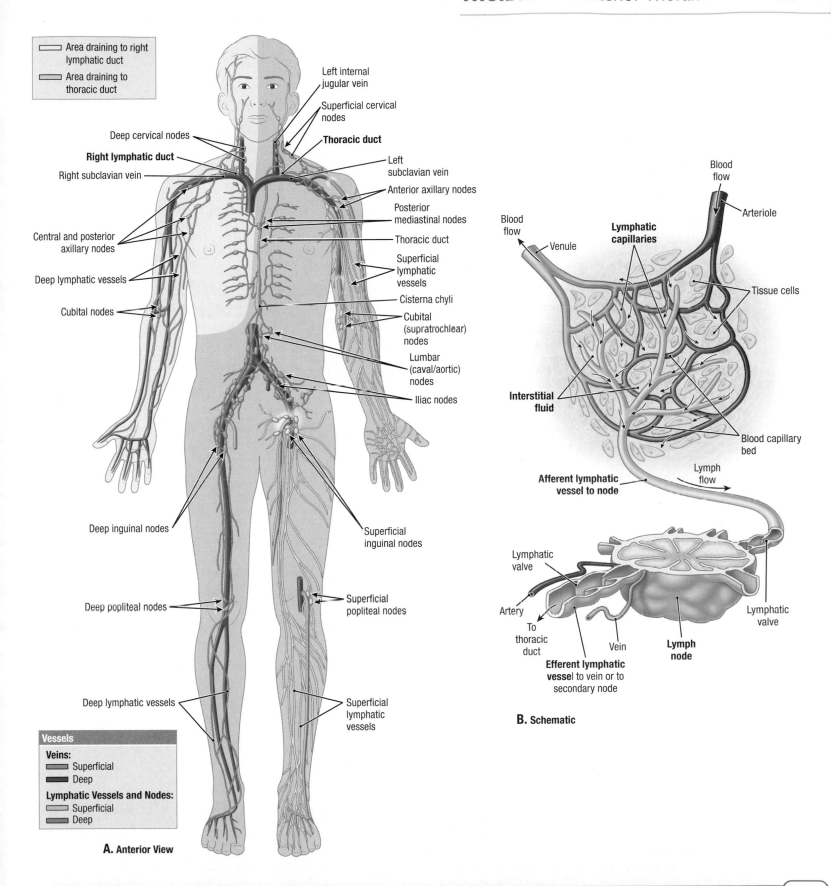

Area draining to right lymphatic duct

Area draining to thoracic duct

Left internal jugular vein

Superficial cervical nodes

Thoracic duct

Deep cervical nodes

Right lymphatic duct

Right subclavian vein

Left subclavian vein

Anterior axillary nodes

Posterior mediastinal nodes

Thoracic duct

Central and posterior axillary nodes

Superficial lymphatic vessels

Deep lymphatic vessels

Cisterna chyli

Cubital (supratrochlear) nodes

Cubital nodes

Lumbar (caval/aortic) nodes

Iliac nodes

Deep inguinal nodes

Superficial inguinal nodes

Deep popliteal nodes

Superficial popliteal nodes

Deep lymphatic vessels

Superficial lymphatic vessels

Vessels

Veins:
Superficial
Deep

Lymphatic Vessels and Nodes:
Superficial
Deep

A. Anterior View

Blood flow

Arteriole

Blood flow

Lymphatic capillaries

Venule

Tissue cells

Interstitial fluid

Blood capillary bed

Lymph flow

Afferent lymphatic vessel to node

Lymphatic valve

Artery

Lymphatic valve

To thoracic duct

Vein

Lymph node

Efferent lymphatic vessel to vein or to secondary node

B. Schematic

Lymphatic System

3.71

A. Overview of superficial and deep lymphatics. B. Lymphatic capillaries, vessels, and nodes. *Black arrows* indicate the flow (leaking of interstitial fluid out of blood vessels and absorption) into the lymphatic capillaries.

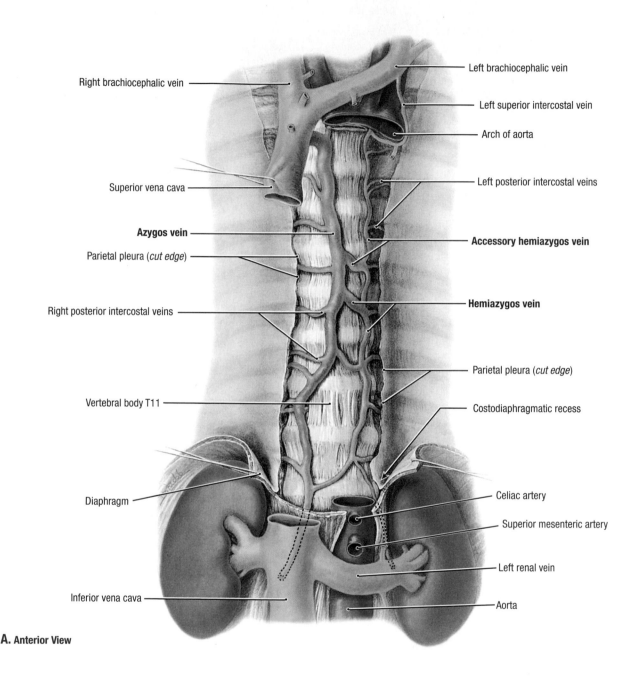

A. Anterior View

3.72   **Azygos System of Veins**

A. Dissection. B. Schematic. The ascending lumbar veins connect the common iliac veins to the lumbar veins and join the subcostal veins to become the lateral roots of the azygos and hemiazygos veins; the medial roots of the azygos and hemiazygos veins are usually from the inferior vena cava and left renal vein, if present. Typically, the upper four left posterior intercostal veins drain into the left brachiocephalic vein, directly and via the left superior intercostal veins.

The hemiazygos, accessory hemiazygos, and left superior intercostals veins are continuous (*Part A*), but most commonly, they are discontinuous (*Part B*). The hemiazygos vein crosses the vertebral column at approximately T9, and the accessory hemiazygos vein crosses at T8, to enter the azygos vein (*Part B*). In contrast, there are four cross-connecting channels between the azygos and hemiazygos systems (*Part A*). The azygos vein arches superior to the root of the right lung at T4 to drain into the superior vena cava.

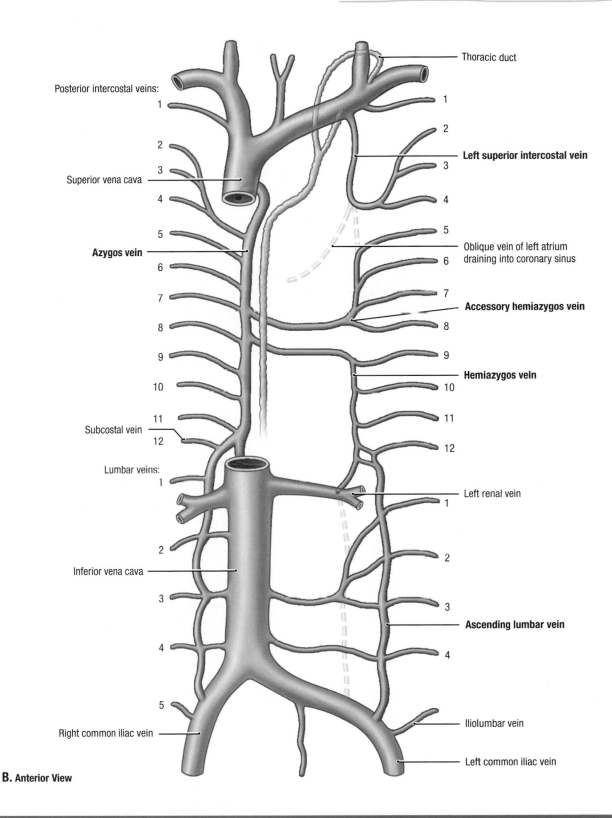

Thoracic duct

Posterior intercostal veins:
1
2
3
Superior vena cava
4
5
Azygos vein
6
7
8
9
10
11
Subcostal vein
12

Lumbar veins:
1

2
Inferior vena cava
3

4

5
Right common iliac vein

B. Anterior View

1
2
3 — **Left superior intercostal vein**
4
5 — Oblique vein of left atrium
6   draining into coronary sinus
7 — **Accessory hemiazygos vein**
8
9
10 — **Hemiazygos vein**
11
12

1 — Left renal vein

2

3 — **Ascending lumbar vein**

4

Iliolumbar vein

Left common iliac vein

Azygos System of Veins (continued)   **3.72**

The azygos, hemiazygos, and accessory hemiazygos veins offer alternate means of venous drainage from the thoracic, abdominal, and back regions when **obstruction of the IVC** occurs. In some people, an accessory azygos vein parallels the main azygos vein on the right side. Other people have no hemiazygos system of veins. A clinically important variation, although uncommon, is when the azygos system receives all the blood from the IVC, except that from the liver. In these people, the azygos system drains nearly all the blood inferior to the diaphragm, except that from the digestive tract. When **obstruction of the SVC** occurs superior to the entrance of the azygos vein, blood can drain inferiorly into the veins of the abdominal wall and return to the right atrium through the IVC and azygos system of veins.

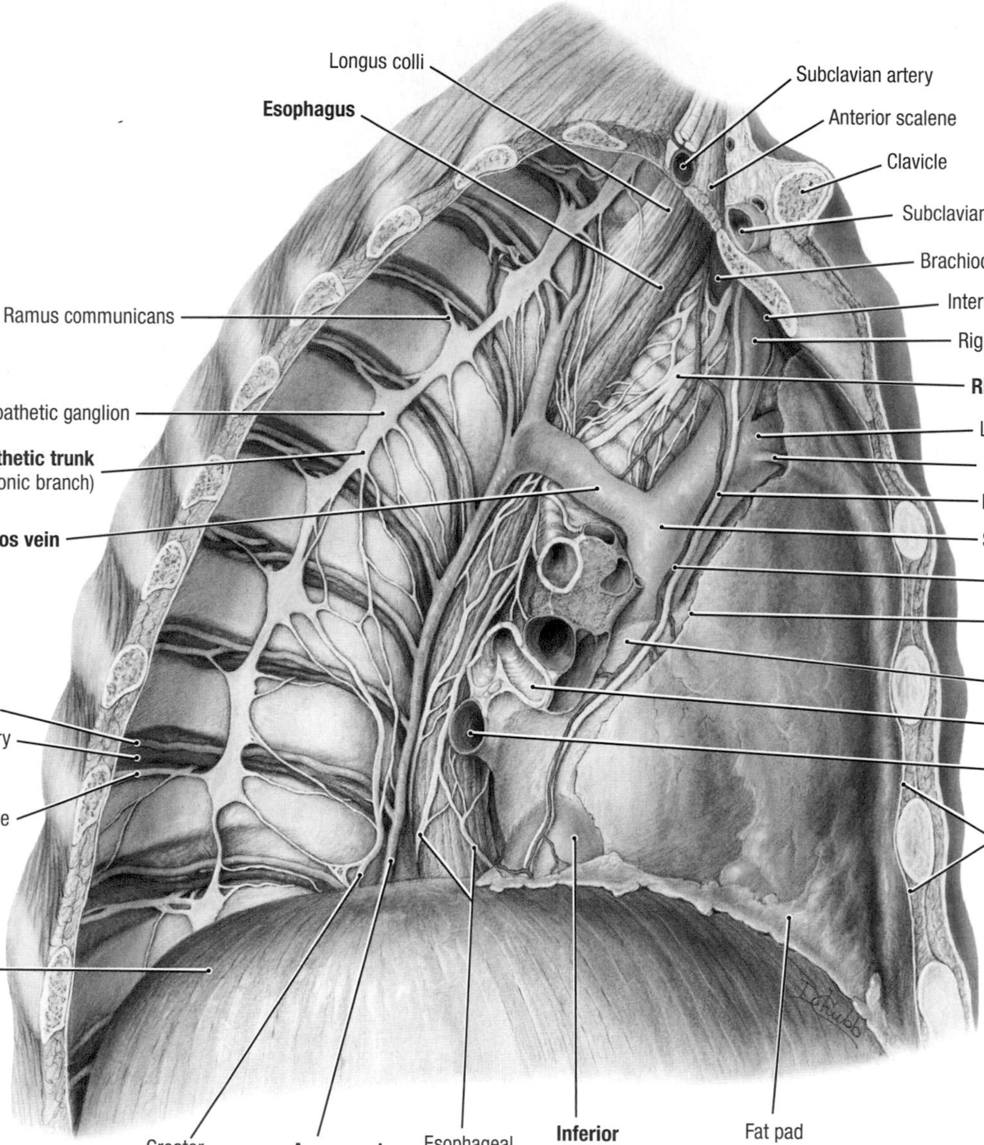

Longus colli

Esophagus

Subclavian artery

Anterior scalene

Clavicle

Subclavian vein

Brachiocephalic trunk

Ramus communicans

Internal thoracic artery

Right brachiocephalic vein

Right vagus nerve on trachea

Sympathetic ganglion

Left brachiocephalic vein

Internal thoracic vein

Sympathetic trunk
(interganglionic branch)

Phrenic nerve

Superior vena cava

Arch of azygos vein

Pericardiacophrenic artery

Mediastinal part of parietal pleura
(*cut edge*)

Pericardial sac

Posterior [vein
intercostal [artery

Bronchus

Inferior pulmonary vein

Intercostal nerve

Costal part of parietal pleura
(*cut edge*)

Diaphragm

Right Lateral View

Greater
splanchnic nerve

Azygos vein

Esophageal
plexus

**Inferior
vena cava**

Fat pad

| 3.73 | **Mediastinum, Right Side** |

- The costal and mediastinal pleurae have mostly been removed, exposing the underlying structures. Compare with the mediastinal surface of the right lung in Figure 3.32.
- The right side of the mediastinum is the "blue side," dominated by the arch of the azygos vein and the superior vena cava.
- Both the trachea and the esophagus are visible from the right side.

- The right vagus nerve descends on the medial surface of the trachea, passes medial to the arch of the azygos vein, posterior to the root of the lung, and then enters the esophageal plexus.
- The right phrenic nerve passes anterior to the root of the lung lateral to both venae cavae.

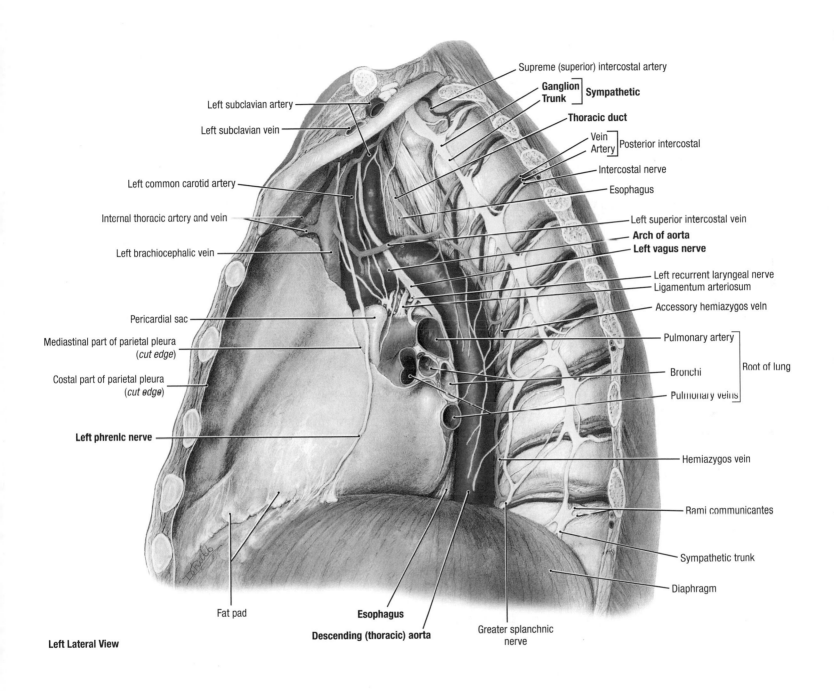

Left subclavian artery

Left subclavian vein

Left common carotid artery

Internal thoracic artery and vein

Left brachiocephalic vein

Pericardial sac

Mediastinal part of parietal pleura
(*cut edge*)

Costal part of parietal pleura
(*cut edge*)

Left phrenic nerve

Fat pad

Esophagus

Descending (thoracic) aorta

Greater splanchnic
nerve

Supreme (superior) intercostal artery

Ganglion
Trunk   Sympathetic

Thoracic duct

Vein
Artery   Posterior intercostal

Intercostal nerve

Esophagus

Left superior intercostal vein

Arch of aorta

Left vagus nerve

Left recurrent laryngeal nerve

Ligamentum arteriosum

Accessory hemiazygos vein

Pulmonary artery

Bronchi   Root of lung

Pulmonary veins

Hemiazygos vein

Rami communicantes

Sympathetic trunk

Diaphragm

Left Lateral View

Mediastinum, Left Side

- Compare with the mediastinal surface of the left lung in Figure 3.33.
- The left side of the mediastinum is the "red side," dominated by the arch and descending portion of the aorta, the left common carotid and subclavian arteries; the latter obscure the trachea from view.
- The thoracic duct can be seen on the left side of the esophagus.

- The left vagus nerve passes posterior to the root of the lung, sending its recurrent laryngeal branch around the ligamentum arteriosum inferior and then medial to the aortic arch.
- The phrenic nerve passes anterior to the root of the lung and penetrates the diaphragm more anteriorly than on the right side.

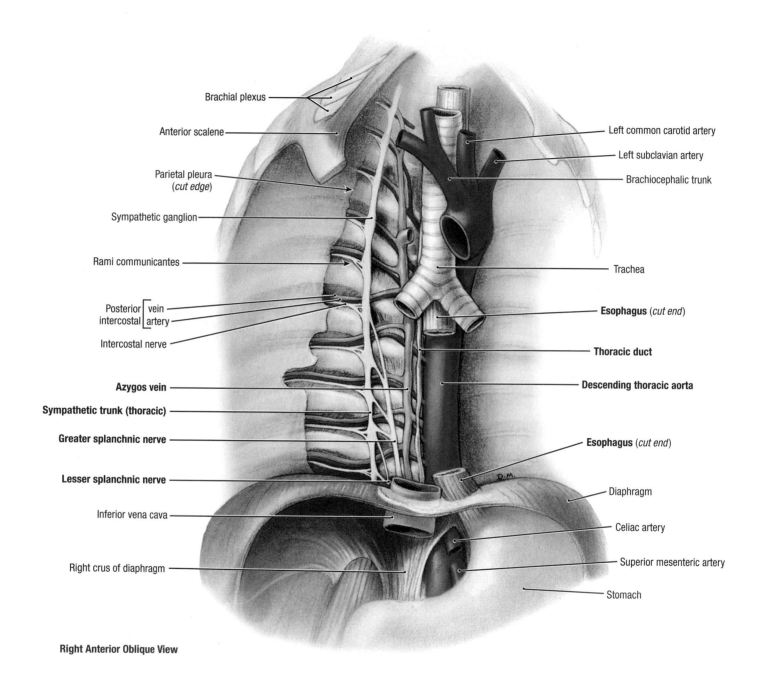

Brachial plexus

Anterior scalene

Parietal pleura
(*cut edge*)

Sympathetic ganglion

Rami communicantes

Posterior [vein
intercostal [artery

Intercostal nerve

Azygos vein

Sympathetic trunk (thoracic)

Greater splanchnic nerve

Lesser splanchnic nerve

Inferior vena cava

Right crus of diaphragm

Left common carotid artery

Left subclavian artery

Brachiocephalic trunk

Trachea

Esophagus (*cut end*)

Thoracic duct

Descending thoracic aorta

Esophagus (*cut end*)

Diaphragm

Celiac artery

Superior mesenteric artery

Stomach

Right Anterior Oblique View

| 3.75 | **Structures of Posterior Mediastinum (I)** |

- In this specimen, the parietal pleura is intact on the left side and partially removed on the right side. A portion of the esophagus, between the bifurcation of the trachea and the diaphragm, is also removed.
- The thoracic sympathetic trunk is connected to each intercostal nerve by rami communicantes.
- The greater splanchnic nerve is formed by fibers from the 5th to 10th thoracic sympathetic ganglia, and the lesser splanchnic nerve receives fibers from the 10th and 11th thoracic ganglia. Both nerves contain presynaptic and visceral afferent fibers.
- The azygos vein ascends anterior to the intercostal vessels and to the right of the thoracic duct and aorta and drains into the superior vena cava.

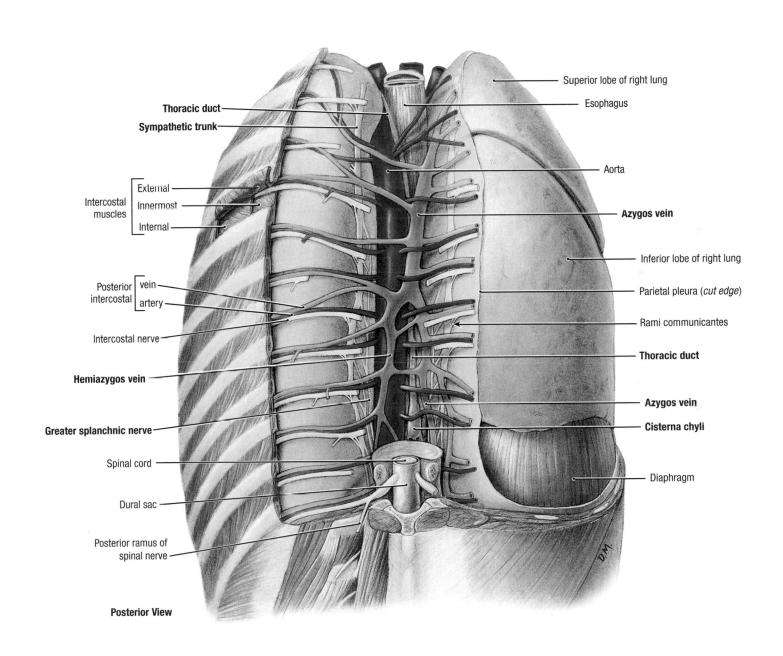

Superior lobe of right lung

Esophagus

Thoracic duct

Sympathetic trunk

Aorta

Intercostal muscles
- External
- Innermost
- Internal

Azygos vein

Inferior lobe of right lung

Posterior intercostal
- vein
- artery

Parietal pleura (*cut edge*)

Rami communicantes

Intercostal nerve

Thoracic duct

Hemiazygos vein

Azygos vein

Greater splanchnic nerve

Cisterna chyli

Spinal cord

Dural sac

Diaphragm

Posterior ramus of spinal nerve

Posterior View

Structures of Posterior Mediastinum (II)

- The thoracic vertebral column and thoracic cage are removed on the right. On the left, the ribs and intercostal musculature are removed posteriorly as far laterally as the angles of the ribs. The parietal pleura is intact on the left side but partially removed on the right to reveal the visceral pleura covering the right lung.

- The azygos vein is on the right side, and the hemiazygos vein is on the left, crossing the midline (usually at T9 but higher in this specimen) to join the azygos vein. The accessory hemiazygos vein is absent in this specimen; instead, three most superior posterior intercostal veins drain directly into the azygos vein.

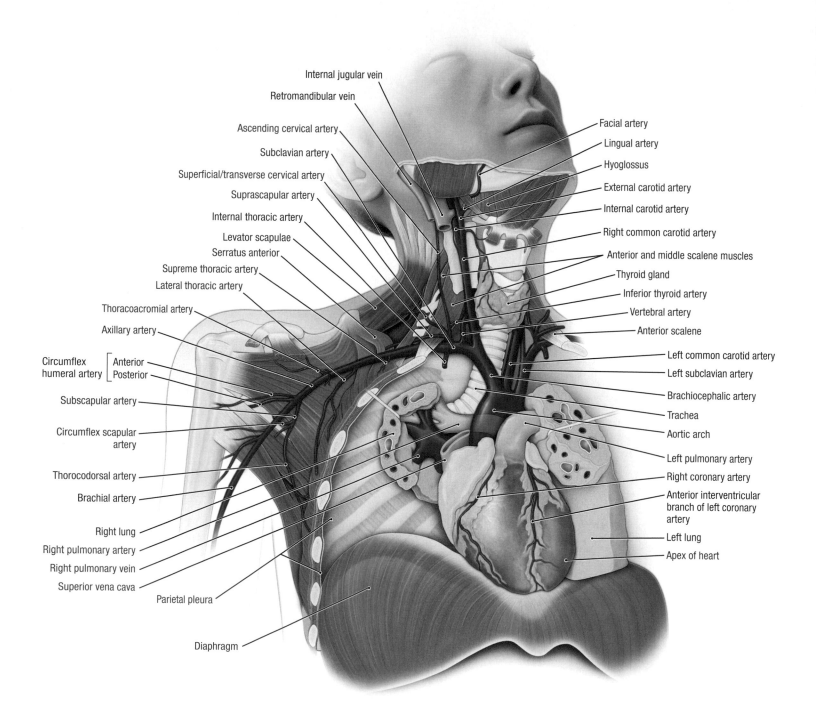

Internal jugular vein

Retromandibular vein

Ascending cervical artery

Subclavian artery

Superficial/transverse cervical artery

Suprascapular artery

Internal thoracic artery

Levator scapulae

Serratus anterior

Supreme thoracic artery

Lateral thoracic artery

Thoracoacromial artery

Axillary artery

Circumflex humeral artery [Anterior / Posterior]

Subscapular artery

Circumflex scapular artery

Thorocodorsal artery

Brachial artery

Right lung

Right pulmonary artery

Right pulmonary vein

Superior vena cava

Parietal pleura

Diaphragm

Facial artery

Lingual artery

Hyoglossus

External carotid artery

Internal carotid artery

Right common carotid artery

Anterior and middle scalene muscles

Thyroid gland

Inferior thyroid artery

Vertebral artery

Anterior scalene

Left common carotid artery

Left subclavian artery

Brachiocephalic artery

Trachea

Aortic arch

Left pulmonary artery

Right coronary artery

Anterior interventricular branch of left coronary artery

Left lung

Apex of heart

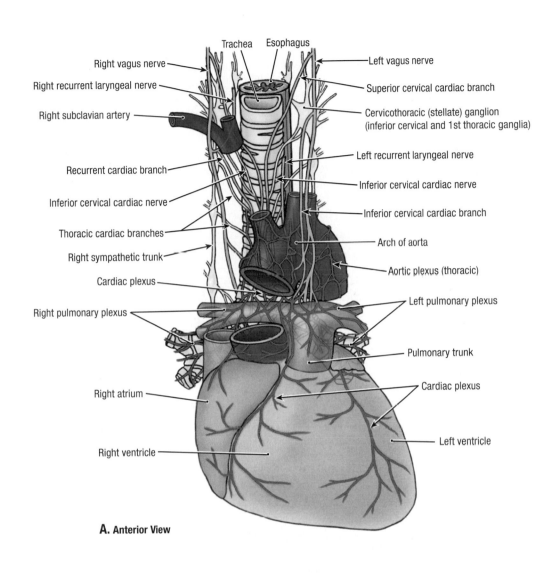

Trachea   Esophagus

Right vagus nerve
Right recurrent laryngeal nerve
Right subclavian artery

Recurrent cardiac branch

Inferior cervical cardiac nerve

Thoracic cardiac branches
Right sympathetic trunk
Cardiac plexus
Right pulmonary plexus

Right atrium

Right ventricle

Left vagus nerve
Superior cervical cardiac branch
Cervicothoracic (stellate) ganglion
(inferior cervical and 1st thoracic ganglia)

Left recurrent laryngeal nerve
Inferior cervical cardiac nerve
Inferior cervical cardiac branch

Arch of aorta
Aortic plexus (thoracic)

Left pulmonary plexus

Pulmonary trunk

Cardiac plexus

Left ventricle

A. Anterior View

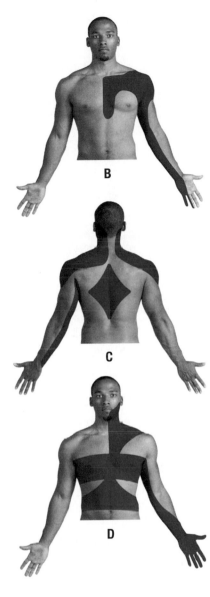

B

C

D

Overview of Autonomic and Visceral Afferent Innervation of Thorax

3.78

A. Innervation of heart. **B–D.** Areas of cardiac referred pain (*red*). **E.** Innervation of posterior and superior mediastina.

The heart is insensitive to touch, cutting, cold, and heat; however, ischemia and the accumulation of metabolic products stimulate pain endings in the myocardium. The afferent pain fibers run centrally in the middle and inferior cervical branches and especially in the thoracic cardiac branches of the sympathetic trunk. The axons of these primary sensory neurons enter spinal cord segments T1 through T4 or T5, especially on the left side.

Cardiac referred pain is a phenomenon whereby noxious stimuli originating in the heart are perceived by a person as pain arising from a superficial part of the body—the skin on the left upper limb, for example. Visceral referred pain is transmitted by visceral afferent fibers accompanying sympathetic fibers and is typically referred to somatic structures or areas such as a limb having afferent fibers with cell bodies in the same spinal ganglion

and central processes that enter the spinal cord through the same posterior roots.

Anginal pain is commonly felt as radiating from the substernal and left pectoral regions to the left shoulder and the medial aspect of the left upper limb (*Part B*). This part of the limb is supplied by the medial cutaneous nerve of the arm. Often, the lateral cutaneous branches of the 2nd and 3rd intercostal nerves (the intercostobrachial nerves) join or overlap in their distribution with the medial cutaneous nerve of the arm. Consequently, cardiac pain is referred to the upper limb because the spinal cord segments of these cutaneous nerves (T1–T3) are also common to the visceral afferent terminations for the coronary arteries. Synaptic contacts may also be made with commissural (connector) neurons, which conduct impulses to neurons on the right side of comparable areas of the spinal cord. This occurrence explains why pain of cardiac origin, although usually referred to the left side, may be referred to the right side, both sides, or the back (*Parts C and D*).

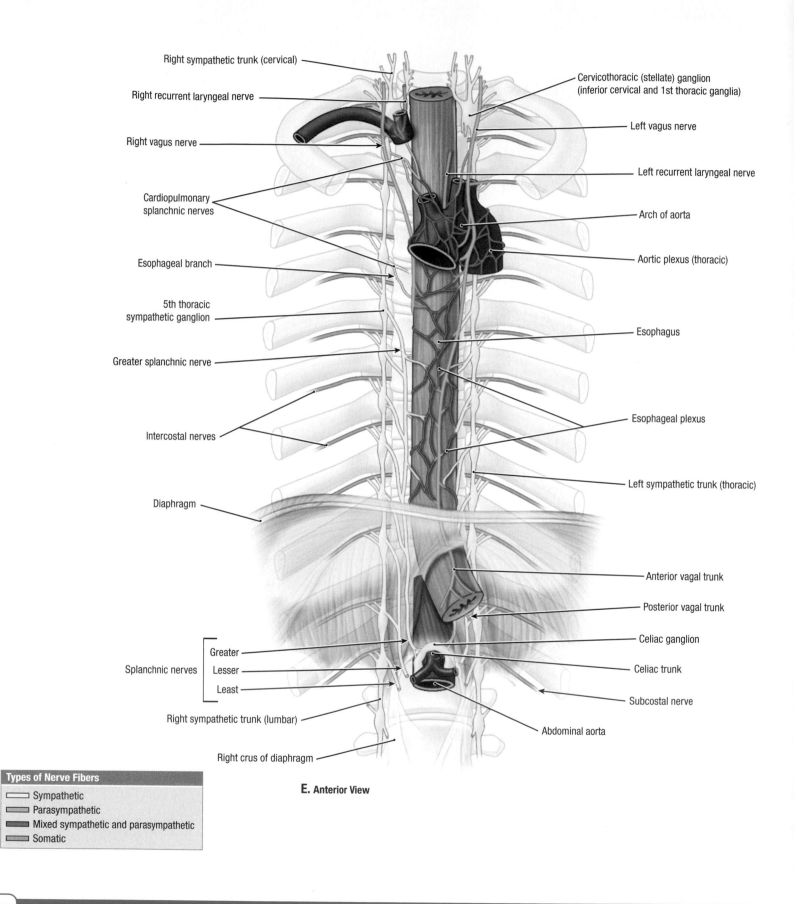

Right sympathetic trunk (cervical)

Right recurrent laryngeal nerve

Right vagus nerve

Cardiopulmonary splanchnic nerves

Esophageal branch

5th thoracic sympathetic ganglion

Greater splanchnic nerve

Intercostal nerves

Diaphragm

Splanchnic nerves
Greater
Lesser
Least

Right sympathetic trunk (lumbar)

Right crus of diaphragm

Cervicothoracic (stellate) ganglion (inferior cervical and 1st thoracic ganglia)

Left vagus nerve

Left recurrent laryngeal nerve

Arch of aorta

Aortic plexus (thoracic)

Esophagus

Esophageal plexus

Left sympathetic trunk (thoracic)

Anterior vagal trunk

Posterior vagal trunk

Celiac ganglion

Celiac trunk

Subcostal nerve

Abdominal aorta

E. Anterior View

Types of Nerve Fibers
- Sympathetic
- Parasympathetic
- Mixed sympathetic and parasympathetic
- Somatic

3.78 **Overview of Autonomic and Visceral Afferent Innervation of Thorax** *(continued)*

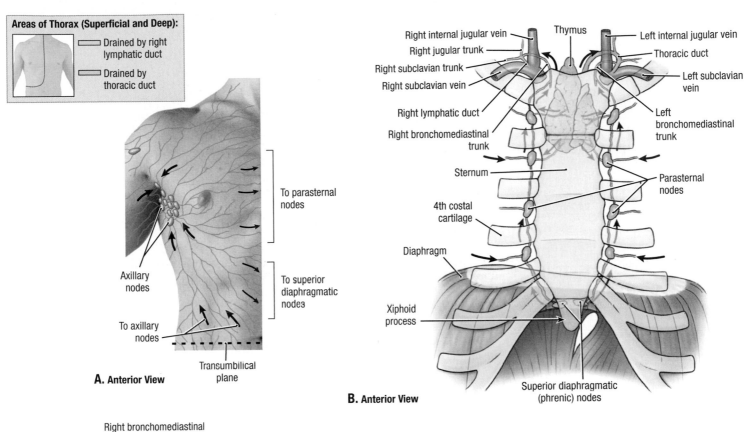

Areas of Thorax (Superficial and Deep):
☐ Drained by right lymphatic duct
☐ Drained by thoracic duct

To parasternal nodes

To superior diaphragmatic nodes

Axillary nodes

To axillary nodes

Transumbilical plane

A. Anterior View

Right internal jugular vein — Thymus — Left internal jugular vein
Right jugular trunk — Thoracic duct
Right subclavian trunk — Left subclavian vein
Right subclavian vein
Right lymphatic duct — Left bronchomediastinal trunk
Right bronchomediastinal trunk
Sternum — Parasternal nodes
4th costal cartilage
Diaphragm
Xiphoid process
Superior diaphragmatic (phrenic) nodes

B. Anterior View

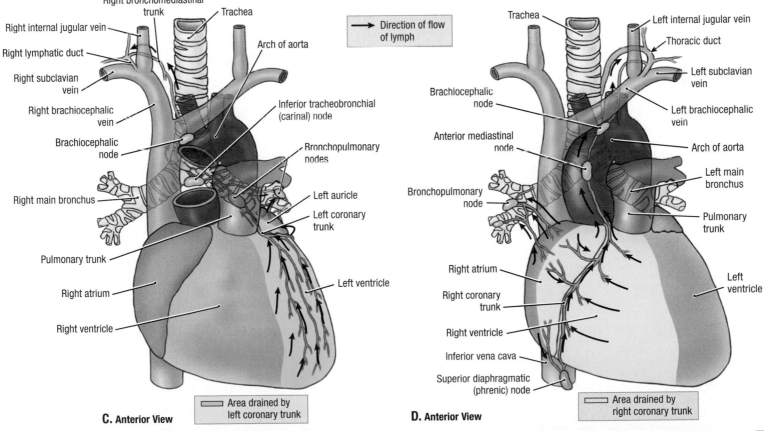

Right bronchomediastinal trunk — Trachea
Right internal jugular vein — Arch of aorta
Right lymphatic duct
Right subclavian vein — Inferior tracheobronchial (carinal) node
Right brachiocephalic vein
Brachiocephalic node — Bronchopulmonary nodes
Right main bronchus — Left auricle
Left coronary trunk
Pulmonary trunk
Right atrium — Left ventricle
Right ventricle

→ Direction of flow of lymph

Area drained by left coronary trunk

C. Anterior View

Trachea — Left internal jugular vein
Thoracic duct
Brachiocephalic node — Left subclavian vein
Left brachiocephalic vein
Anterior mediastinal node — Arch of aorta
Bronchopulmonary node — Left main bronchus
Pulmonary trunk
Right atrium
Right coronary trunk — Left ventricle
Right ventricle
Inferior vena cava
Superior diaphragmatic (phrenic) node

Area drained by right coronary trunk

D. Anterior View

Overview of Lymphatic Drainage of Thorax

A. Superficial lymphatic drainage. **B.** Deep lymphatic drainage of parasternal nodes. **C.** Lymphatic drainage of left side of heart.
D. Lymphatic drainage of right side of heart.

3.79

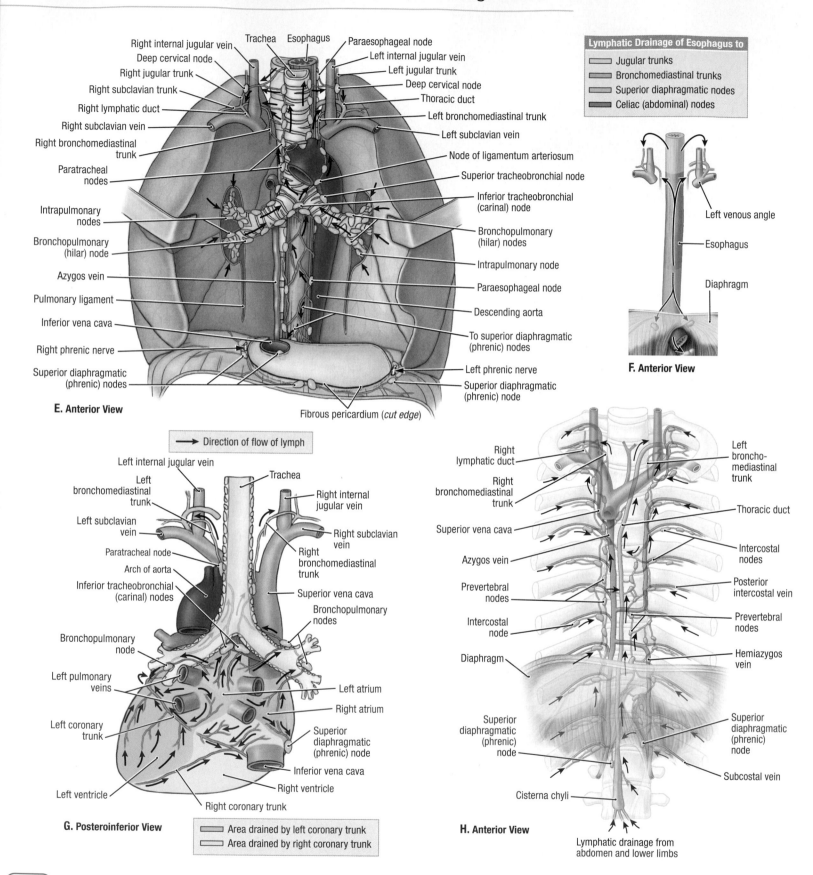

Lymphatic Drainage of Esophagus to
- Jugular trunks
- Bronchomediastinal trunks
- Superior diaphragmatic nodes
- Celiac (abdominal) nodes

E. Anterior View

Right internal jugular vein — Trachea — Esophagus — Paraesophageal node
Deep cervical node — Left internal jugular vein
Right jugular trunk — Left jugular trunk
Right subclavian trunk — Deep cervical node
Right lymphatic duct — Thoracic duct
Right subclavian vein — Left bronchomediastinal trunk
Right bronchomediastinal trunk — Left subclavian vein
Paratracheal nodes — Node of ligamentum arteriosum
Intrapulmonary nodes — Superior tracheobronchial node
Bronchopulmonary (hilar) node — Inferior tracheobronchial (carinal) node
Azygos vein — Bronchopulmonary (hilar) nodes
Pulmonary ligament — Intrapulmonary node
Inferior vena cava — Paraesophageal node
Right phrenic nerve — Descending aorta
Superior diaphragmatic (phrenic) nodes — To superior diaphragmatic (phrenic) nodes
Fibrous pericardium (cut edge) — Left phrenic nerve
Superior diaphragmatic (phrenic) node

F. Anterior View

Left venous angle
Esophagus
Diaphragm

→ Direction of flow of lymph

G. Posteroinferior View

Left internal jugular vein — Trachea
Left bronchomediastinal trunk — Right internal jugular vein
Left subclavian vein — Right subclavian vein
Paratracheal node — Right bronchomediastinal trunk
Arch of aorta — Superior vena cava
Inferior tracheobronchial (carinal) nodes — Bronchopulmonary nodes
Bronchopulmonary node — Left atrium
Left pulmonary veins — Right atrium
Left coronary trunk — Superior diaphragmatic (phrenic) node
Left ventricle — Inferior vena cava
Right coronary trunk — Right ventricle

- Area drained by left coronary trunk
- Area drained by right coronary trunk

H. Anterior View

Right lymphatic duct — Left bronchomediastinal trunk
Right bronchomediastinal trunk — Thoracic duct
Superior vena cava — Intercostal nodes
Azygos vein — Posterior intercostal vein
Prevertebral nodes — Prevertebral nodes
Intercostal node — Hemiazygos vein
Diaphragm — Superior diaphragmatic (phrenic) node
Superior diaphragmatic (phrenic) node — Subcostal vein
Cisterna chyli
Lymphatic drainage from abdomen and lower limbs

3.79 **Overview of Lymphatic Drainage of Thorax** (continued)

E. Lymphatic drainage of lungs, esophagus, and superior surface of diaphragm. **F.** Lymphatic drainage of esophagus. **G.** Lymphatic drainage of posterior and inferior surfaces of heart. **H.** Lymphatic drainage of posterior mediastinum.

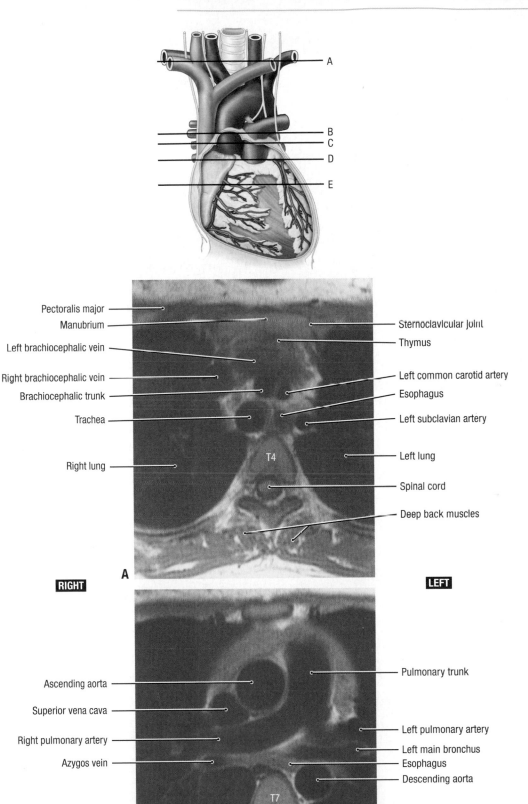

A

B

Pectoralis major

Manubrium

Left brachiocephalic vein

Right brachiocephalic vein

Brachiocephalic trunk

Trachea

Right lung

T4

Sternoclavicular joint

Thymus

Left common carotid artery

Esophagus

Left subclavian artery

Left lung

Spinal cord

Deep back muscles

Ascending aorta

Superior vena cava

Right pulmonary artery

Azygos vein

Right lung

T7

Pulmonary trunk

Left pulmonary artery

Left main bronchus

Esophagus

Descending aorta

Spinal cord

Deep back muscles

RIGHT   **LEFT**

Transverse (Axial) MRIs of Thorax (A–E)   **3.80**

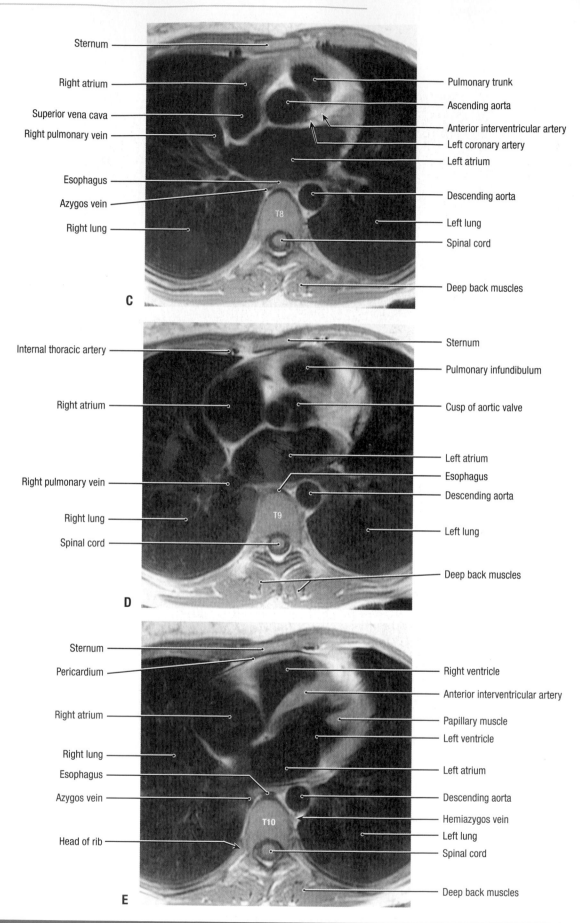

Sternum

Right atrium

Superior vena cava

Right pulmonary vein

Esophagus

Azygos vein

Right lung

Pulmonary trunk

Ascending aorta

Anterior interventricular artery

Left coronary artery

Left atrium

Descending aorta

Left lung

Spinal cord

Deep back muscles

T8

C

Internal thoracic artery

Right atrium

Right pulmonary vein

Right lung

Spinal cord

Sternum

Pulmonary infundibulum

Cusp of aortic valve

Left atrium

Esophagus

Descending aorta

Left lung

Deep back muscles

T9

D

Sternum

Pericardium

Right atrium

Right lung

Esophagus

Azygos vein

Head of rib

Right ventricle

Anterior interventricular artery

Papillary muscle

Left ventricle

Left atrium

Descending aorta

Hemiazygos vein

Left lung

Spinal cord

Deep back muscles

T10

E

3.80 **Transverse (Axial) MRIs of Thorax (A–E)** (continued)

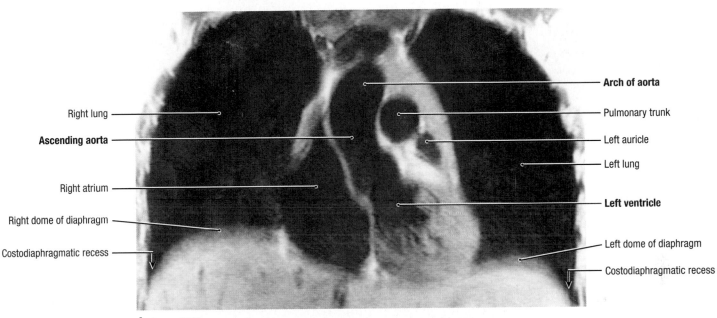

Arch of aorta

Right lung

Ascending aorta

Pulmonary trunk

Left auricle

Left lung

Right atrium

Left ventricle

Right dome of diaphragm

Costodiaphragmatic recess

Left dome of diaphragm

Costodiaphragmatic recess

A. Coronal MRI

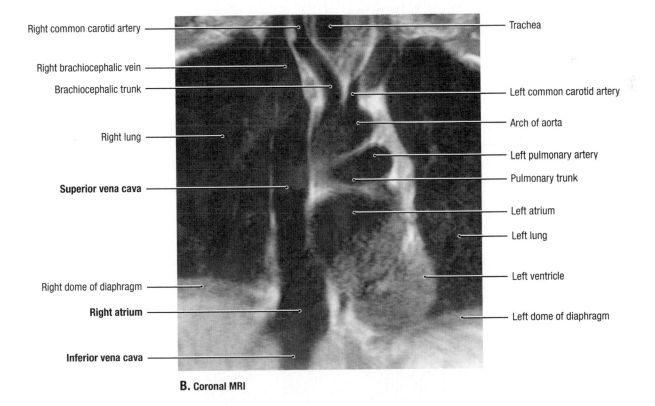

Right common carotid artery

Trachea

Right brachiocephalic vein

Brachiocephalic trunk

Left common carotid artery

Arch of aorta

Right lung

Left pulmonary artery

Pulmonary trunk

Superior vena cava

Left atrium

Left lung

Right dome of diaphragm

Left ventricle

Right atrium

Left dome of diaphragm

Inferior vena cava

B. Coronal MRI

Coronal MRIs of Thorax

A. In plane of ascending and arch of aorta. **B.** In plane of superior and inferior vena cava.

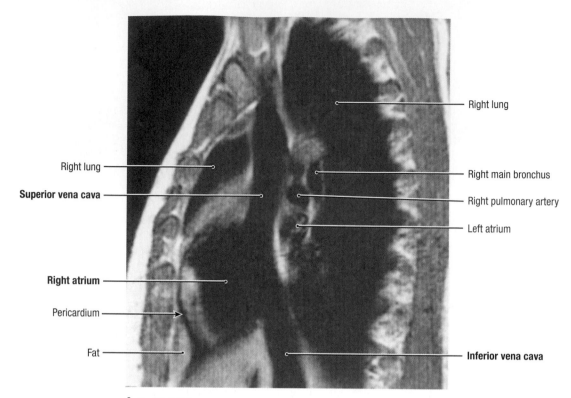

Right lung

Right lung

Superior vena cava

Right main bronchus

Right pulmonary artery

Left atrium

Right atrium

Pericardium

Fat

Inferior vena cava

A. Sagittal MRI

ANTERIOR

POSTERIOR

Left common carotid artery

Left brachiocephalic vein

Left lung

Left subclavian artery

Arch of aorta

Right pulmonary artery

Left lung

Ascending aorta

Left main bronchus

Left atrium

Right ventricle

Left ventricle

Descending (thoracic) aorta

B. Sagittal MRI

3.82 **Sagittal MRIs of Thorax**

A. In plane of superior and inferior vena cava. **B.** In plane of arch of aorta.

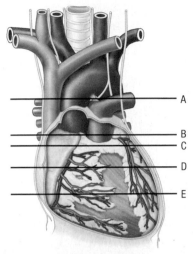

Level of Scans in A–E

3D Volume Reconstructions:

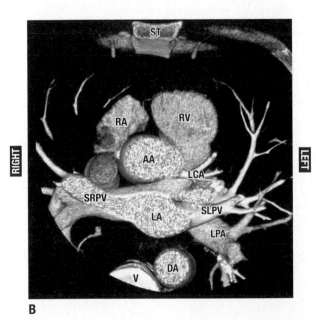

RIGHT | LEFT

SRPV
SVC
AA
PT
RPA
SLPV
LPA

A

Transverse MRIs:

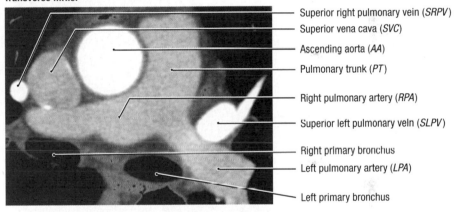

Superior right pulmonary vein (*SRPV*)
Superior vena cava (*SVC*)
Ascending aorta (*AA*)
Pulmonary trunk (*PT*)
Right pulmonary artery (*RPA*)
Superior left pulmonary vein (*SLPV*)
Right primary bronchus
Left pulmonary artery (*LPA*)
Left primary bronchus

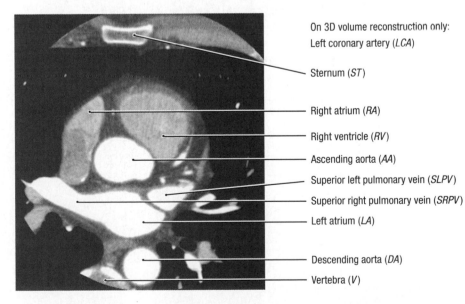

RIGHT | LEFT

ST
RA
RV
AA
LCA
SRPV
LA
SLPV
LPA
DA
V

B

On 3D volume reconstruction only:
Left coronary artery (*LCA*)

Sternum (*ST*)

Right atrium (*RA*)

Right ventricle (*RV*)

Ascending aorta (*AA*)

Superior left pulmonary vein (*SLPV*)

Superior right pulmonary vein (*SRPV*)

Left atrium (*LA*)

Descending aorta (*DA*)

Vertebra (*V*)

Transverse (Axial) 3D Volume Reconstructions (*Left Side of Page*) and CT Angiograms of Thorax (A–E)

3.83

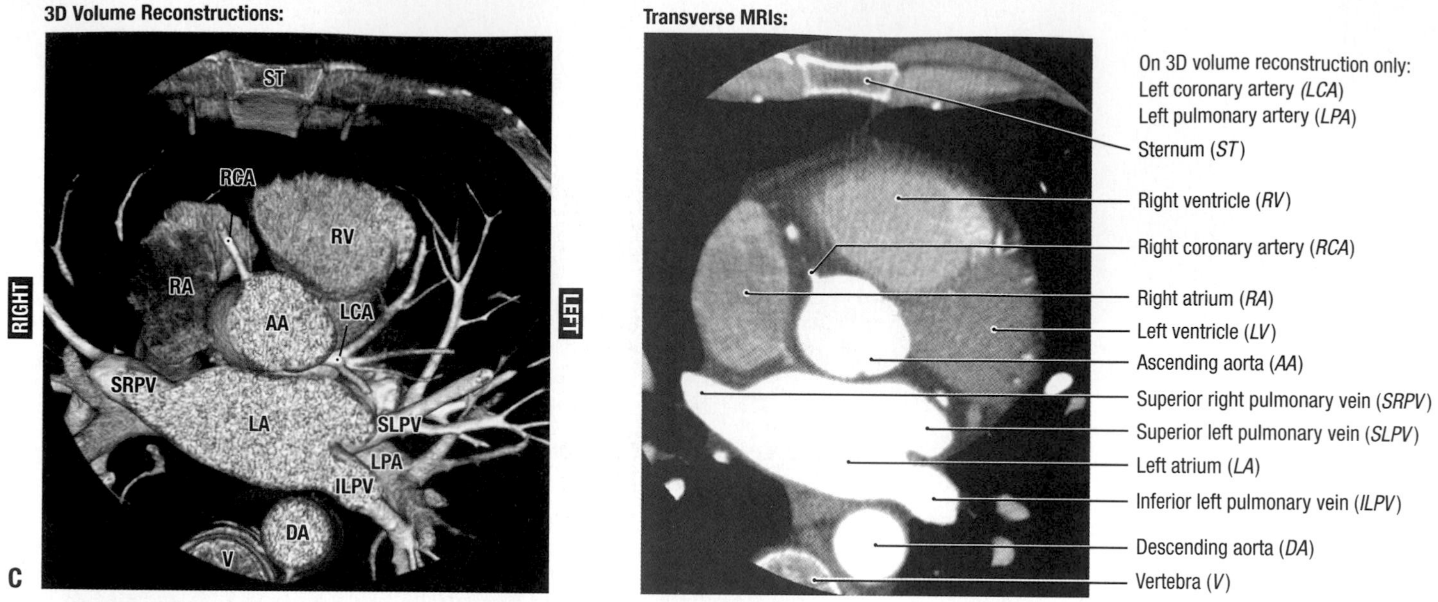

3D Volume Reconstructions:
Transverse MRIs:
ST
RCA
RV
RA
AA
LCA
SRPV
LA
SLPV
LPA
ILPV
DA
V
RIGHT
LEFT
On 3D volume reconstruction only:
Left coronary artery (LCA)
Left pulmonary artery (LPA)
Sternum (ST)
Right ventricle (RV)
Right coronary artery (RCA)
Right atrium (RA)
Left ventricle (LV)
Ascending aorta (AA)
Superior right pulmonary vein (SRPV)
Superior left pulmonary vein (SLPV)
Left atrium (LA)
Inferior left pulmonary vein (ILPV)
Descending aorta (DA)
Vertebra (V)

C

ST
RV
IVS
RA
LV
MV
LA
IRPV
ILPV
DA
V
RIGHT
LEFT
On 3D volume reconstruction only:
Inferior left pulmonary vein (ILPV)
Sternum (ST)
Right ventricle (RV)
Right atrium (RA)
Interventricular septum (IVS)
Left ventricle (LV)
Mitral valve (MV)
Left atrium (LA)
Inferior right pulmonary vein (IRPV)
Descending aorta (DA)
Vertebra (V)

D

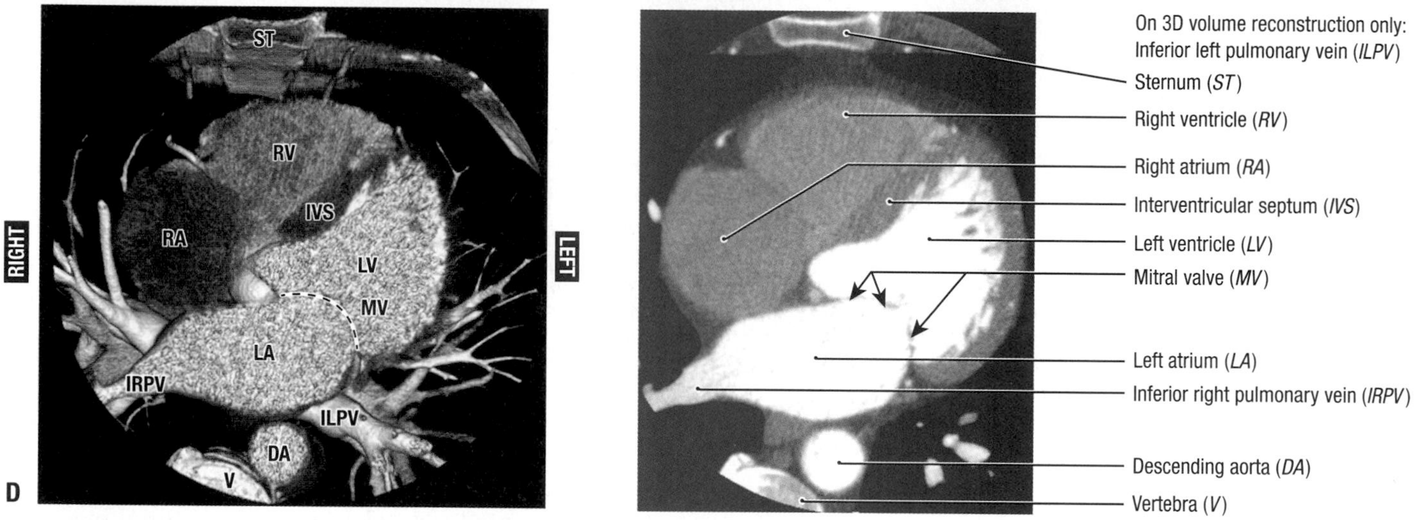

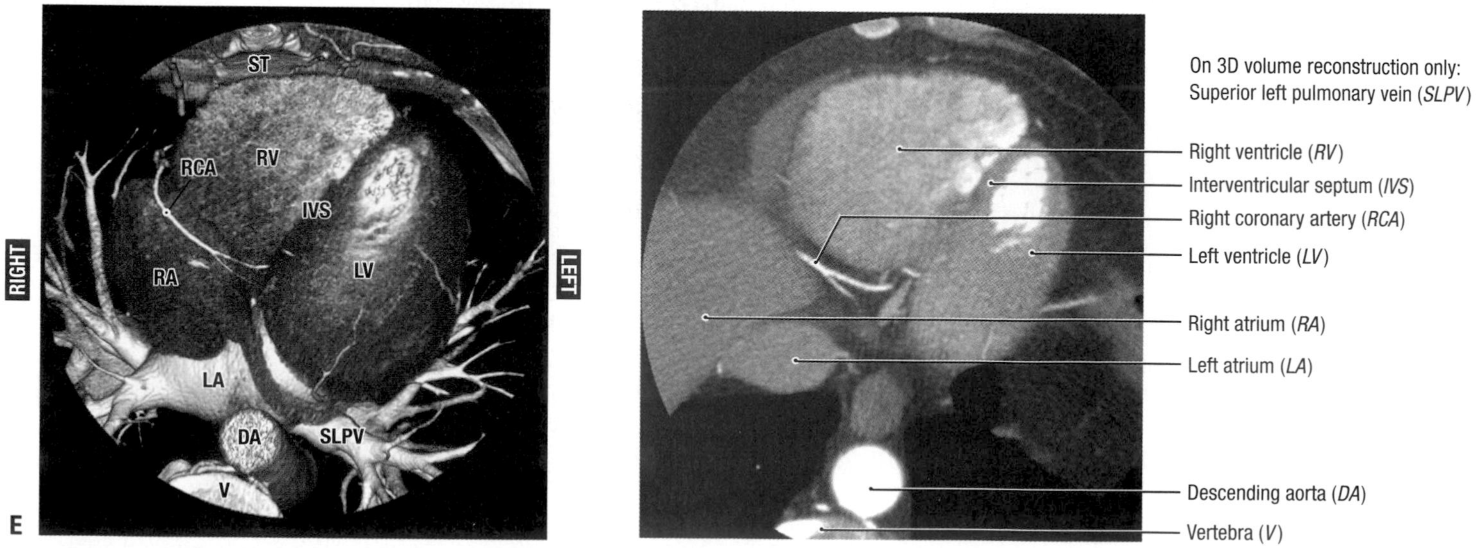

ST
RCA
RV
IVS
RA
LV
LA
DA
SLPV
V
RIGHT
LEFT
On 3D volume reconstruction only:
Superior left pulmonary vein (SLPV)
Right ventricle (RV)
Interventricular septum (IVS)
Right coronary artery (RCA)
Left ventricle (LV)
Right atrium (RA)
Left atrium (LA)
Descending aorta (DA)
Vertebra (V)

E

3.83 Transverse (Axial) 3D Volume Reconstructions (*Left Side of Page*) and CT Angiograms of Thorax (A–E) *(continued)*

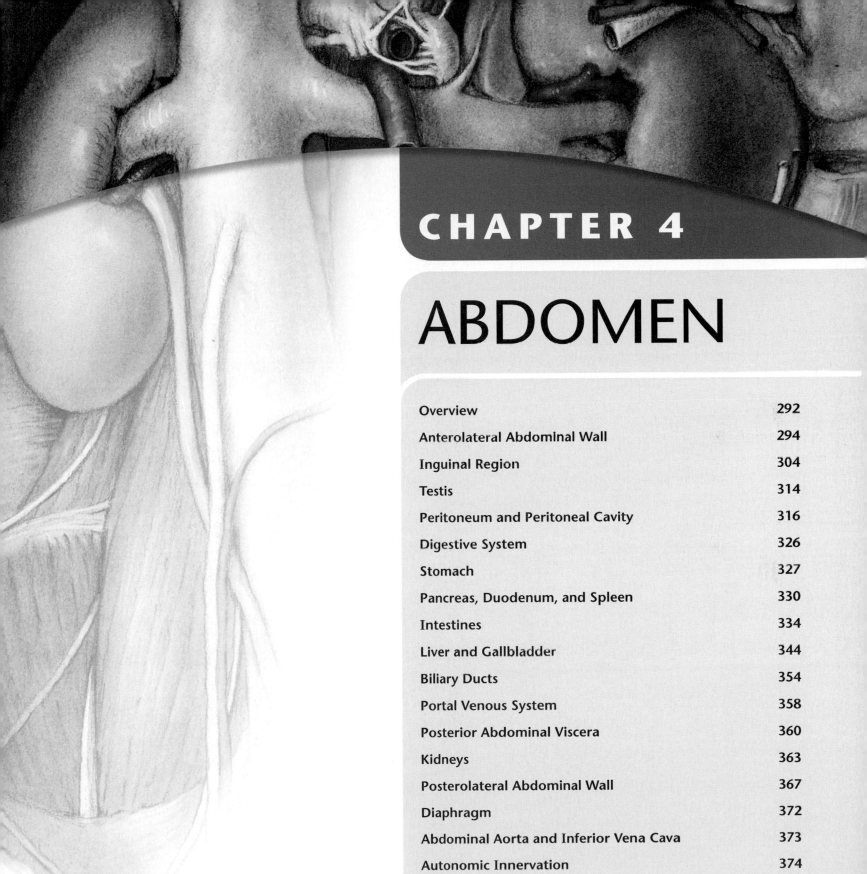

ABDOMEN

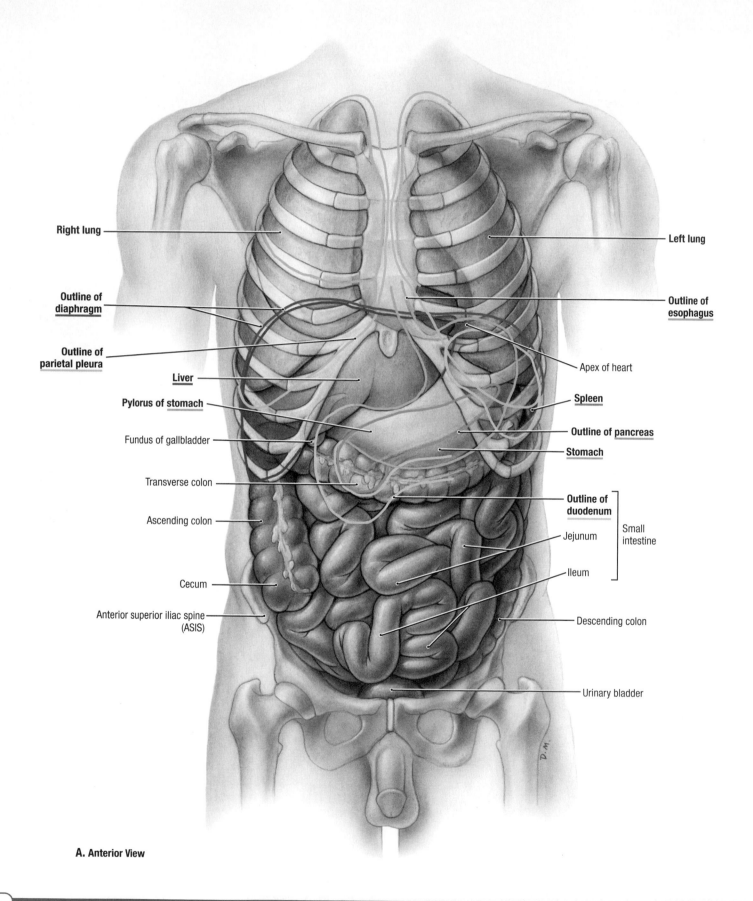

Right lung

Outline of diaphragm

Outline of parietal pleura

Liver

Pylorus of stomach

Fundus of gallbladder

Transverse colon

Ascending colon

Cecum

Anterior superior iliac spine (ASIS)

Left lung

Outline of esophagus

Apex of heart

Spleen

Outline of pancreas

Stomach

Outline of duodenum

Jejunum

Ileum

Small intestine

Descending colon

Urinary bladder

A. Anterior View

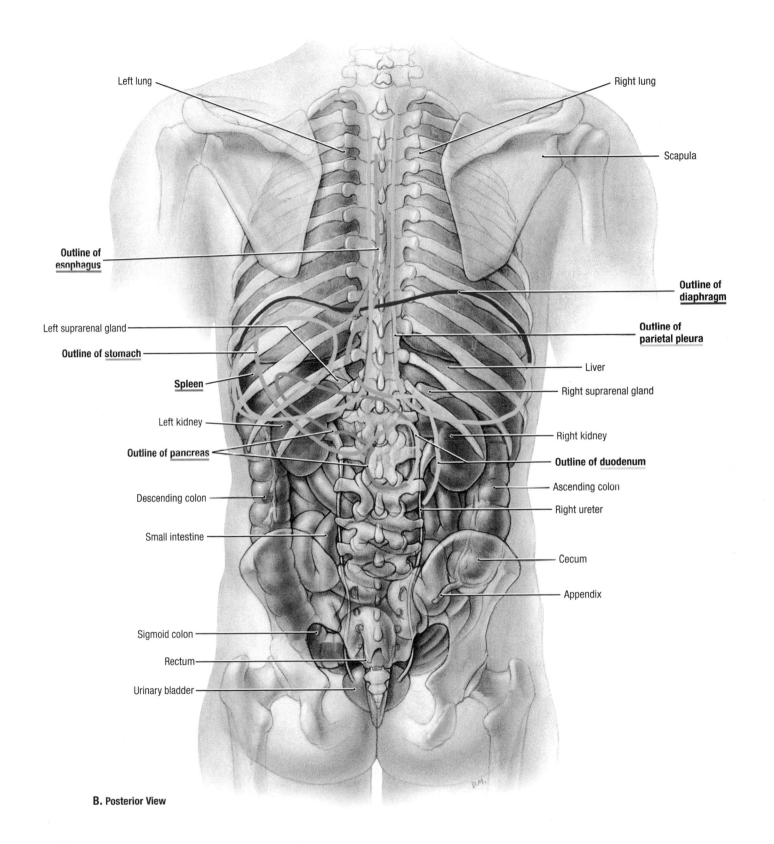

Left lung

Right lung

Scapula

Outline of esophagus

Outline of diaphragm

Left suprarenal gland

Outline of parietal pleura

Outline of stomach

Liver

Spleen

Right suprarenal gland

Left kidney

Right kidney

Outline of pancreas

Outline of duodenum

Descending colon

Ascending colon

Right ureter

Small intestine

Cecum

Appendix

Sigmoid colon

Rectum

Urinary bladder

B. Posterior View

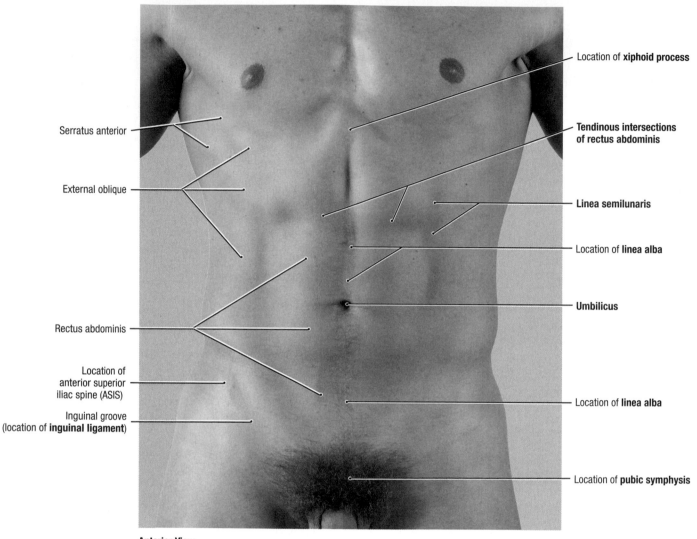

Serratus anterior

External oblique

Rectus abdominis

Location of
anterior superior
iliac spine (ASIS)

Inguinal groove
(location of **inguinal ligament**)

Location of **xiphoid process**

**Tendinous intersections
of rectus abdominis**

Linea semilunaris

Location of **linea alba**

Umbilicus

Location of **linea alba**

Location of **pubic symphysis**

Anterior View

<hr/>

4.2 | **Surface Anatomy**

- The umbilicus is where the umbilical cord entered the fetus and indicates the anterior level of the T10 dermatome. Typically, the umbilicus lies at the level of the intervertebral disc between the L3 and L4 vertebrae.
- The linea alba is a fibrous band formed by the fusion of the right and left abdominal aponeuroses between the xiphoid process and the pubic symphysis demarcated superficially by a midline vertical skin groove.
- A curved skin groove, the linea semilunaris, demarcates the lateral border of the right and left rectus abdominis muscles and rectus sheath.

- In lean individuals with good muscle development, three to four transverse skin grooves overlie the tendinous intersections of the rectus abdominis muscle.
- The site of the inguinal ligament is indicated by a skin crease, the inguinal groove, just inferior and parallel to the ligament, marking the division between the anterolateral abdominal wall and the thigh.

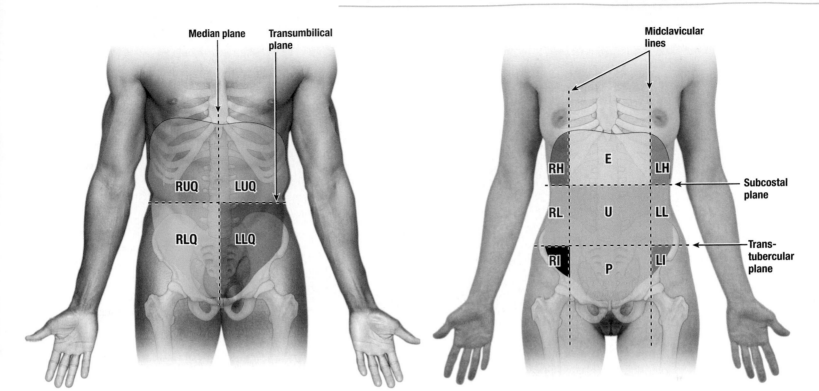

Median plane · Transumbilical plane

Midclavicular lines

RUQ · LUQ · RLQ · LLQ

RH · E · LH · Subcostal plane
RL · U · LL
RI · P · LI · Trans-tubercular plane

A. Anterior View

B. Anterior View

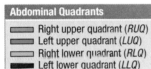

Abdominal Quadrants

- Right upper quadrant (*RUQ*)
- Left upper quadrant (*LUQ*)
- Right lower quadrant (*RLQ*)
- Left lower quadrant (*LLQ*)

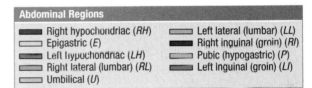

Abdominal Regions

- Right hypochondriac (*RH*)
- Epigastric (*E*)
- Left hypochondriac (*LH*)
- Right lateral (lumbar) (*RL*)
- Umbilical (*U*)
- Left lateral (lumbar) (*LL*)
- Right inguinal (groin) (*RI*)
- Pubic (hypogastric) (*P*)
- Left inguinal (groin) (*LI*)

Right upper quadrant (RUQ)

Liver: right lobe
Gallbladder
Stomach: pylorus
Duodenum: parts 1–3
Pancreas: head
Right suprarenal gland
Right kidney
Right colic (hepatic) flexure
Ascending colon: superior part
Transverse colon: right half

Left upper quadrant (LUQ)

Liver: left lobe
Spleen
Stomach
Jejunum and proximal ileum
Pancreas: body and tail
Left kidney
Left suprarenal gland
Left colic (splenic) flexure
Transverse colon: left half
Descending colon: superior part

Right lower quadrant (RLQ)

Cecum
Appendix
Most of ileum
Ascending colon: inferior part
Right ovary
Right uterine tube
Right ureter: abdominal part
Right spermatic cord:
   abdominal part
Uterus (if enlarged)
Urinary bladder (if very full)

Left lower quadrant (LLQ)

Sigmoid colon
Descending colon: inferior part
Left ovary
Left uterine tube
Left ureter: abdominal part
Left spermatic cord:
   abdominal part
Uterus (if enlarged)
Urinary bladder (if very full)

Abdominal Regions and Quadrants

4.3

A. Quadrants. B. Regions. It is important to know what organs are located in each abdominal region or quadrant so that one knows where to auscultate, percuss, and palpate them and to record the locations of findings during a physical exam.

The six common causes of **abdominal protrusion** begin with the letter F: food, fluid, fat, feces, flatus, and fetus. Eversion of the umbilicus may be a sign of increased intraabdominal pressure, usually resulting from ascites (abdominal accumulation of serous fluid in the peritoneal cavity), or a large mass (e.g., a tumor, fetus, or enlarged organ such as the liver [hepatomegaly]).

Warm hands are important when palpating the abdominal wall because cold hands make the anterolateral abdominal muscles tense, producing involuntary muscle spasms known as guarding. Intense guarding, boardlike reflexive muscular rigidity that cannot be willfully suppressed, occurs during palpation when an organ (such as the appendix) is inflamed and in itself constitutes a clinically significant sign of **acute abdomen**. The involuntary muscular spasms attempt to protect the viscera from pressure, which is painful when an abdominal infection is present. The common nerve supply of the skin and muscles of the wall explains why these spasms occur.

Lateral View

4.4 Dermatomes

The thoracoabdominal (T7–T11) nerves run between the internal oblique and transversus abdominis muscles giving rise to branches that supply sensory innervation to the overlying skin. The T10 nerve supplies the region of the umbilicus. The subcostal nerve (T12) runs along the inferior border of the 12th rib to supply the skin over the anterior superior iliac spine and hip. The iliohypogastric nerve (also L1) innervates the skin over the iliac crest and lower pubic region, and the ilioinguinal nerve (also L1) innervates the skin of the mons pubis, anterior scrotum or labium majus, and superomedial aspect of thigh.

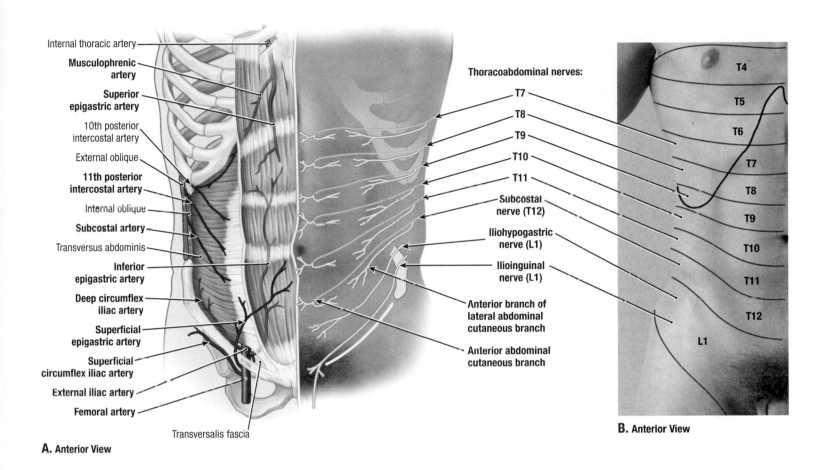

A. Anterior View

Internal thoracic artery
Musculophrenic artery
Superior epigastric artery
10th posterior intercostal artery
External oblique
11th posterior intercostal artery
Internal oblique
Subcostal artery
Transversus abdominis
Inferior epigastric artery
Deep circumflex iliac artery
Superficial epigastric artery
Superficial circumflex iliac artery
External iliac artery
Femoral artery
Transversalis fascia

Thoracoabdominal nerves:
T7
T8
T9
T10
T11
Subcostal nerve (T12)
Iliohypogastric nerve (L1)
Ilioinguinal nerve (L1)
Anterior branch of lateral abdominal cutaneous branch
Anterior abdominal cutaneous branch

T4
T5
T6
T7
T8
T9
T10
T11
T12
L1

B. Anterior View

Arteries and Nerves of Anterolateral Abdominal Wall

4.5

The skin and muscles of the anterolateral abdominal wall are supplied mainly by the:
- Thoracoabdominal nerves: distal, abdominal parts of the anterior rami of the inferior six thoracic spinal nerves (T7–T11), which have muscular branches and anterior and lateral abdominal cutaneous branches. The anterior abdominal cutaneous branches pierce the rectus sheath a short distance from the median plane, after the rectus abdominis muscle has been supplied. Spinal nerves T7–T9 supply the skin superior to the umbilicus; T10 innervates the skin around the umbilicus.
- Spinal nerve T11, plus the cutaneous branches of the subcostal (T12) and iliohypogastric and ilioinguinal (L1) nerves: supply the skin inferior to the umbilicus.
- Subcostal nerve: large anterior ramus of spinal nerve T12.

The blood vessels of the anterolateral abdominal wall are the:
- Superior epigastric vessels and branches of the musculophrenic vessels, the terminal branches of the internal thoracic vessels.
- Inferior epigastric and deep circumflex iliac vessels from the external iliac vessels.
- Superficial circumflex iliac and superficial epigastric vessels from the femoral artery and great saphenous vein.
- Posterior intercostal vessels in the 11th intercostal space and anterior branches of subcostal vessels.

Incisional nerve injury. The inferior thoracic spinal nerves (T7–T12) and the iliohypogastric and ilioinguinal nerves (L1) approach the abdominal musculature separately to provide the multisegmental innervation of the abdominal muscles. Thus, they are distributed across the anterolateral abdominal wall, where they run oblique but mostly horizontal courses. They are susceptible to injury in surgical incisions or from trauma at any level of the abdominal wall. Injury to them may result in weakening of the muscles. In the inguinal region, such a weakness may predispose an individual to development of an inguinal hernia.

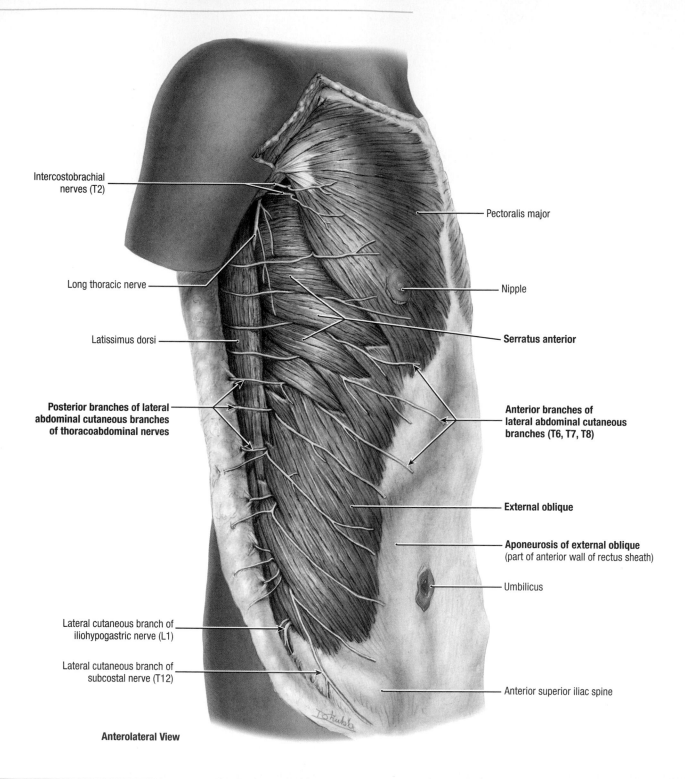

Intercostobrachial
nerves (T2)

Long thoracic nerve

Latissimus dorsi

**Posterior branches of lateral
abdominal cutaneous branches
of thoracoabdominal nerves**

Lateral cutaneous branch of
iliohypogastric nerve (L1)

Lateral cutaneous branch of
subcostal nerve (T12)

Pectoralis major

Nipple

Serratus anterior

**Anterior branches of
lateral abdominal cutaneous
branches (T6, T7, T8)**

External oblique

Aponeurosis of external oblique
(part of anterior wall of rectus sheath)

Umbilicus

Anterior superior iliac spine

Anterolateral View

| 4.6 | **Anterolateral Abdominal Wall, Superficial Dissection** |

The muscular portion of the external oblique muscle interdigitates with slips of the serratus anterior muscle, and the aponeurotic portion contributes to the anterior wall of the rectus sheath. The anterior and posterior branches of the lateral abdominal cutaneous branches of the thoracoabdominal nerves course superficially in the subcutaneous tissue.

- **Umbilical hernias** are usually small protrusions of extraperitoneal fat and/or peritoneum and omentum and sometimes bowel. They result from increased intraabdominal pressure in

the presence of weakness or incomplete closure of the anterior abdominal wall after ligation of the umbilical cord at birth, or may be acquired later, most commonly in women and obese people.

- The lines along which the fibers of the abdominal aponeurosis interlace (see Figs. 4.10A, D, & E) are also potential sites of herniation. These gaps may be congenital, the result of the stresses of obesity and aging, or the consequence of surgical or traumatic wounds.

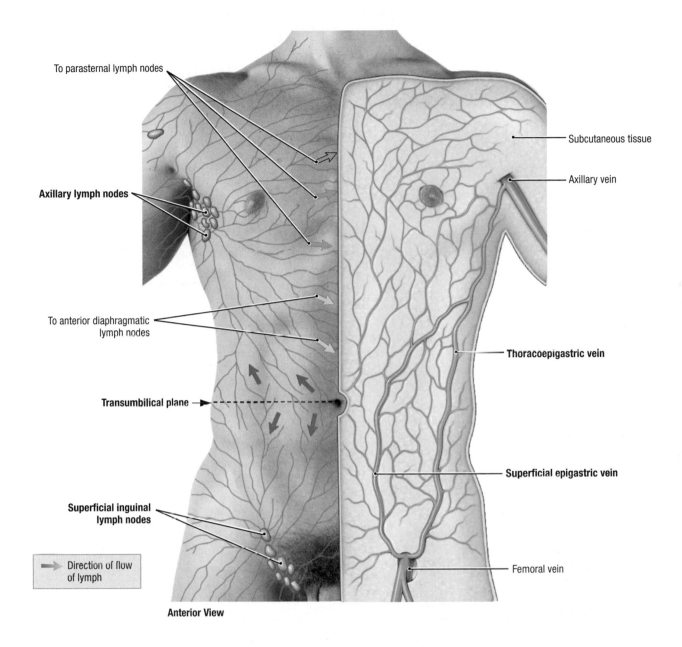

To parasternal lymph nodes

Axillary lymph nodes

To anterior diaphragmatic
lymph nodes

Transumbilical plane

**Superficial inguinal
lymph nodes**

Direction of flow
of lymph

Anterior View

Subcutaneous tissue

Axillary vein

Thoracoepigastric vein

Superficial epigastric vein

Femoral vein

Lymphatic Drainage and Subcutaneous (Superficial) Venous Drainage of Anterolateral Abdominal Wall   4.7

- The skin and subcutaneous tissue of the abdominal wall are served by an intricate subcutaneous venous plexus, draining superiorly to the internal thoracic vein medially and the lateral thoracic vein laterally, and inferiorly to the superficial and inferior epigastric veins, tributaries of the femoral and external iliac veins, respectively.
- Superficial lymphatic vessels accompany the subcutaneous veins; those superior to the transumbilical plane drain mainly to the axillary lymph nodes; however, a few drain to the parasternal lymph nodes. Superficial lymphatic vessels inferior to the transumbilical plane drain to the superficial inguinal lymph nodes.

- **Liposuction** is a surgical method for removing unwanted subcutaneous fat using a percutaneously placed suction tube and high vacuum pressure. The tubes are inserted subdermally through small skin incisions.
- When flow in the superior or inferior vena cava is obstructed, anastomoses between the tributaries of these systemic veins, such as the thoracoepigastric vein, may provide **collateral pathways** by which the obstruction may be bypassed, allowing blood to return to the heart. The veins become enlarged and tortuous.

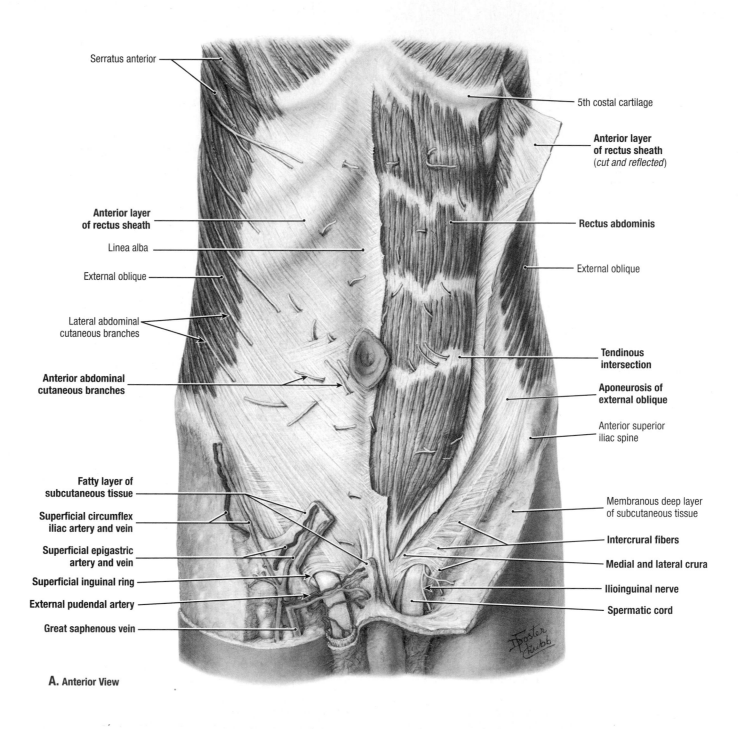

Serratus anterior

5th costal cartilage

Anterior layer of rectus sheath (*cut and reflected*)

Anterior layer of rectus sheath

Linea alba

Rectus abdominis

External oblique

External oblique

Lateral abdominal cutaneous branches

Tendinous intersection

Anterior abdominal cutaneous branches

Aponeurosis of external oblique

Anterior superior iliac spine

Fatty layer of subcutaneous tissue

Membranous deep layer of subcutaneous tissue

Superficial circumflex iliac artery and vein

Intercrural fibers

Superficial epigastric artery and vein

Medial and lateral crura

Superficial inguinal ring

Ilioinguinal nerve

External pudendal artery

Spermatic cord

Great saphenous vein

A. Anterior View

4.8   **Anterior Abdominal Wall**

A. Superficial dissection demonstrating relationship of cutaneous nerves and superficial vessels to musculoaponeurotic structures.
The anterior wall of the left rectus sheath is reflected, revealing the rectus abdominis muscle, segmented by tendinous intersections.

- After the T7–T12 spinal nerves supply the muscles, their anterior abdominal cutaneous branches emerge from the rectus abdominis muscle and pierce the anterior wall of its sheath.
- The three superficial inguinal branches of the femoral artery (superficial circumflex iliac artery, superficial epigastric artery,

and external pudendal artery) and the great saphenous vein lie in the fatty layer of subcutaneous tissue.
- The fibers of the inferior part of the external oblique aponeurosis separate into medial and lateral crura, which, with the intercrural fibers that unite them, form the superficial inguinal ring. The spermatic cord of the male (shown here), or round ligament of the female, exits the inguinal canal through the superficial inguinal ring along with the ilioinguinal nerve.

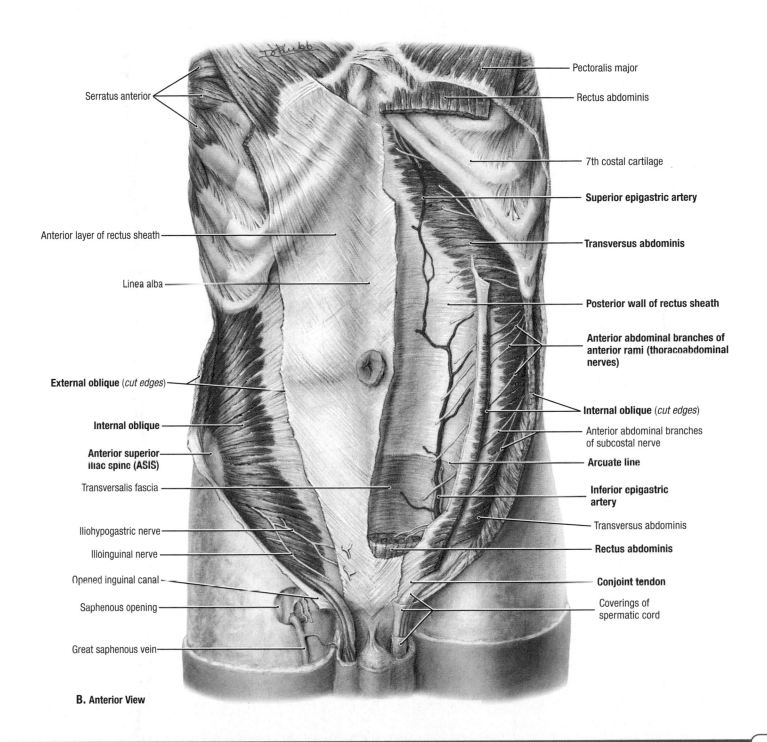

Serratus anterior

Anterior layer of rectus sheath

Linea alba

External oblique (*cut edges*)

Internal oblique

Anterior superior iliac spine (ASIS)

Transversalis fascia

Iliohypogastric nerve

Ilioinguinal nerve

Opened inguinal canal

Saphenous opening

Great saphenous vein

Pectoralis major

Rectus abdominis

7th costal cartilage

Superior epigastric artery

Transversus abdominis

Posterior wall of rectus sheath

Anterior abdominal branches of anterior rami (thoracoabdominal nerves)

Internal oblique (*cut edges*)

Anterior abdominal branches of subcostal nerve

Arcuate line

Inferior epigastric artery

Transversus abdominis

Rectus abdominis

Conjoint tendon

Coverings of spermatic cord

B. Anterior View

Anterior Abdominal Wall (*continued*)   **4.8**

B. Deep dissection. On the right side of the specimen, most of the external oblique muscle is excised. On the left, the internal oblique muscle is divided and the rectus abdominis muscle is excised, revealing the posterior wall of the rectus sheath.

- The fibers of the internal oblique muscle run horizontally at the level of the anterior superior iliac spine (ASIS), obliquely upward superior to the ASIS, and obliquely downward inferior to the ASIS.
- The arcuate line is at the level of the ASIS; inferior to the line, transversalis fascia lies immediately posterior to the rectus abdominis muscle.

- Initially, the anterior abdominal branches of the anterior rami course between the internal oblique and transversus abdominis muscles.
- The anastomosis between the superior and inferior epigastric arteries indirectly unites the subclavian artery of the upper limb to the external iliac arteries of the lower limb. The anastomosis can become functionally patent in response to slowly developing occlusion of the aorta.

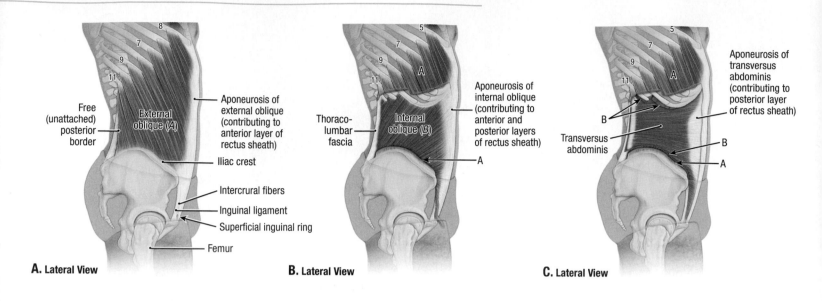

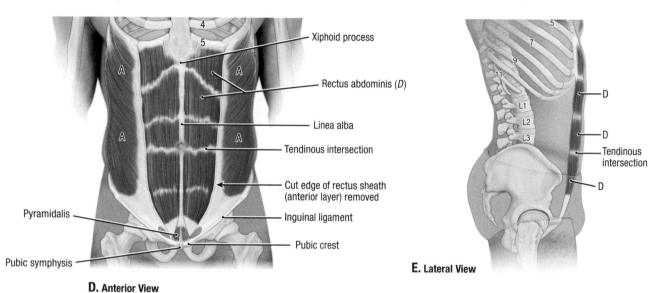

A. External oblique. B. Internal oblique. C. Transversus abdominis. D. and E. Rectus abdominis and pyramidalis.

4.9 Muscles of Anterolateral Abdominal Wall

A. External oblique. B. Internal oblique. C. Transversus abdominis. D. and E. Rectus abdominis and pyramidalis.

TABLE 4.1	Principal Muscles of Anterolateral Abdominal Wall			
Muscles[a]	Origin	Insertion	Innervation	Action(s)
External oblique (*Part A*)	External surfaces of 5th–12th ribs	Linea alba, pubic tubercle, and anterior half of iliac crest	Thoracoabdominal nerves (anterior rami of T7–T11) and subcostal nerve	Compresses and supports abdominal viscera; flexes and rotates trunk
Internal oblique (*Part B*)	Thoracolumbar fascia, anterior two thirds of iliac crest, and connective tissue deep to inguinal ligament	Inferior borders of 10th–12th ribs, linea alba, and pubis via conjoint tendon	Thoracoabdominal nerves (anterior rami of T7–T11), subcostal nerve, and first lumbar nerve	
Transversus abdominis (*Part C*)	Internal surfaces of 7th–12th costal cartilages, thoracolumbar fascia, iliac crest, and connective tissue deep to inguinal ligament (iliopsoas fascia)	Linea alba with aponeurosis of internal oblique, pubic crest, and pectin pubis via conjoint tendon		Compresses and supports abdominal viscera (with external oblique ipsilaterally, internal oblique contralaterally)
Rectus abdominis (*Part D*)	Pubic symphysis and pubic crest	Xiphoid process and 5th–7th costal cartilages	Thoracoabdominal nerves (T7–T11) and subcostal nerve	Flexes trunk and compresses abdominal viscera[b]; stabilizes and controls tilt of pelvis

[a]Approximately 80% of people have a *pyramidalis muscle*, which is located in the rectus sheath anterior to the most inferior part of the rectus abdominis. It extends from the pubic crest of the hip bone to the linea alba. This small muscle tenses the linea alba.
[b]In so doing, these muscles act as antagonists of the diaphragm to produce expiration.

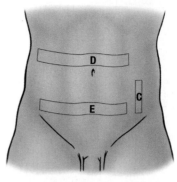

Anterior View Showing Location of Sections C–E

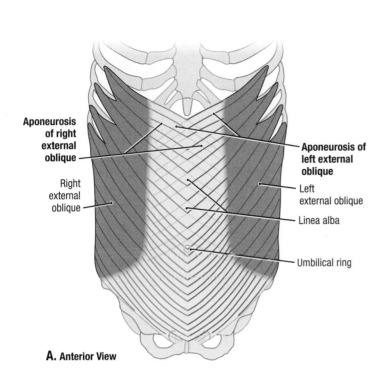

Aponeurosis of right external oblique

Aponeurosis of left external oblique

Right external oblique

Left external oblique

Linea alba

Umbilical ring

A. Anterior View

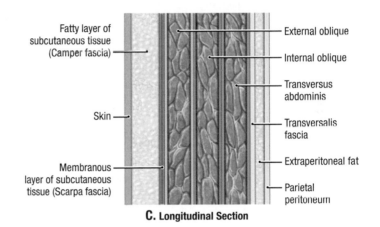

Fatty layer of subcutaneous tissue (Camper fascia)

External oblique

Internal oblique

Transversus abdominis

Skin

Transversalis fascia

Extraperitoneal fat

Membranous layer of subcutaneous tissue (Scarpa fascia)

Parietal peritoneum

C. Longitudinal Section

Aponeurosis of external oblique

Aponeurosis of internal oblique

External oblique

Linea alba

Internal oblique

B. Anterior View

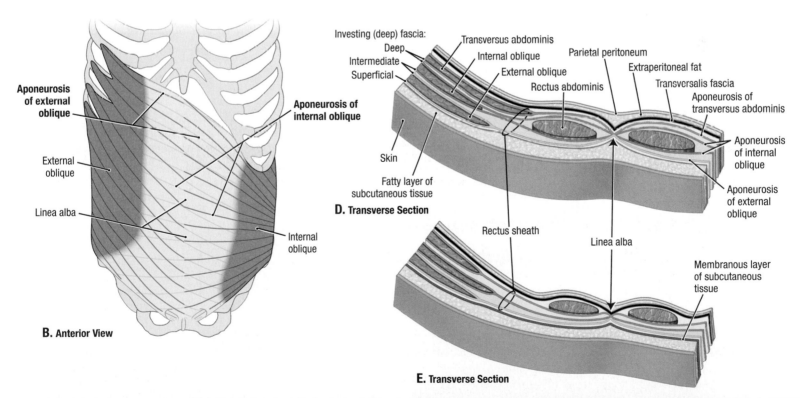

Investing (deep) fascia:
Deep
Intermediate
Superficial

Transversus abdominis

Internal oblique

Parietal peritoneum

External oblique

Extraperitoneal fat

Rectus abdominis

Transversalis fascia

Aponeurosis of transversus abdominis

Aponeurosis of internal oblique

Skin

Fatty layer of subcutaneous tissue

Aponeurosis of external oblique

D. Transverse Section

Rectus sheath

Linea alba

Membranous layer of subcutaneous tissue

E. Transverse Section

Structure of Anterolateral Abdominal Wall

4.10

A. Interdigitation of aponeuroses of right and left external oblique muscles. **B.** Interdigitation of aponeuroses of contralateral external and internal oblique muscles. **C–E.** Layers of abdominal wall and rectus sheath.

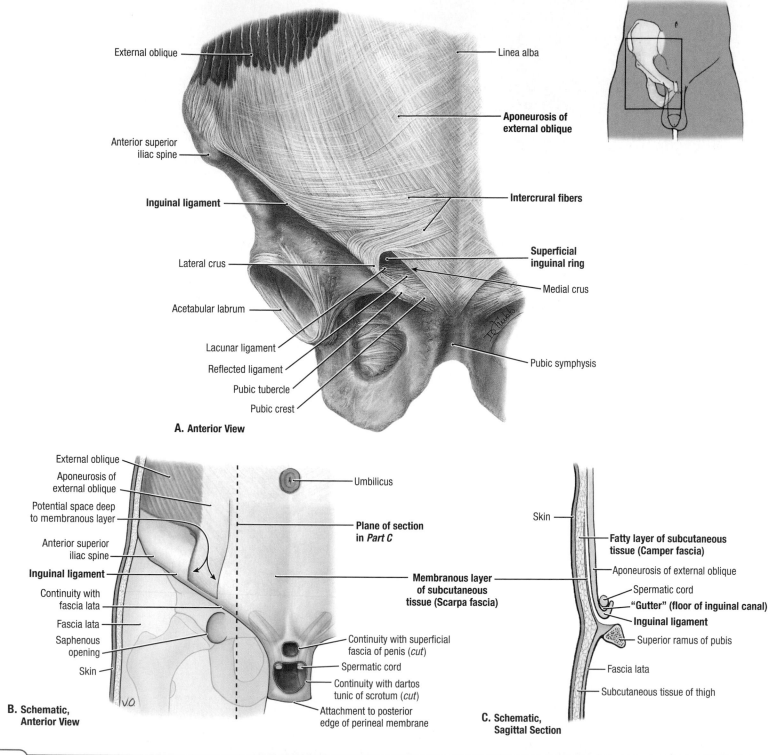

External oblique

Linea alba

Aponeurosis of external oblique

Anterior superior iliac spine

Inguinal ligament

Intercrural fibers

Lateral crus

Superficial inguinal ring

Medial crus

Acetabular labrum

Lacunar ligament

Reflected ligament

Pubic tubercle

Pubic crest

Pubic symphysis

A. Anterior View

External oblique

Aponeurosis of external oblique

Potential space deep to membranous layer

Anterior superior iliac spine

Inguinal ligament

Continuity with fascia lata

Fascia lata

Saphenous opening

Skin

Umbilicus

Plane of section in *Part C*

Membranous layer of subcutaneous tissue (Scarpa fascia)

Continuity with superficial fascia of penis (*cut*)

Spermatic cord

Continuity with dartos tunic of scrotum (*cut*)

Attachment to posterior edge of perineal membrane

B. Schematic, Anterior View

Skin

Fatty layer of subcutaneous tissue (Camper fascia)

Aponeurosis of external oblique

Spermatic cord

"Gutter" (floor of inguinal canal)

Inguinal ligament

Superior ramus of pubis

Fascia lata

Subcutaneous tissue of thigh

C. Schematic, Sagittal Section

| 4.11 | **Inguinal Region of Male (I)** |

A. Formations of aponeurosis of external oblique muscle. **B.** and **C.** Membranous (deep) layer of subcutaneous tissue. Inferior to the umbilicus, the subcutaneous tissue is composed of two layers: a superficial fatty layer and a deep membranous layer. Laterally, the membranous layer fuses with the fascia lata of the thigh about a finger's breadth inferior to the inguinal ligament. Medially, it fuses with the linea alba and pubic symphysis in the midline, and inferiorly, it continues as the membranous layer of the subcutaneous tissue of the perineum and penis and the dartos fascia of the scrotum. The inferior margin of the external oblique aponeurosis is thickened and turned internally forming the inguinal ligament. The superior surface of the in-turning inguinal ligament forms a shallow trough or "gutter" that is the floor of the inguinal canal.

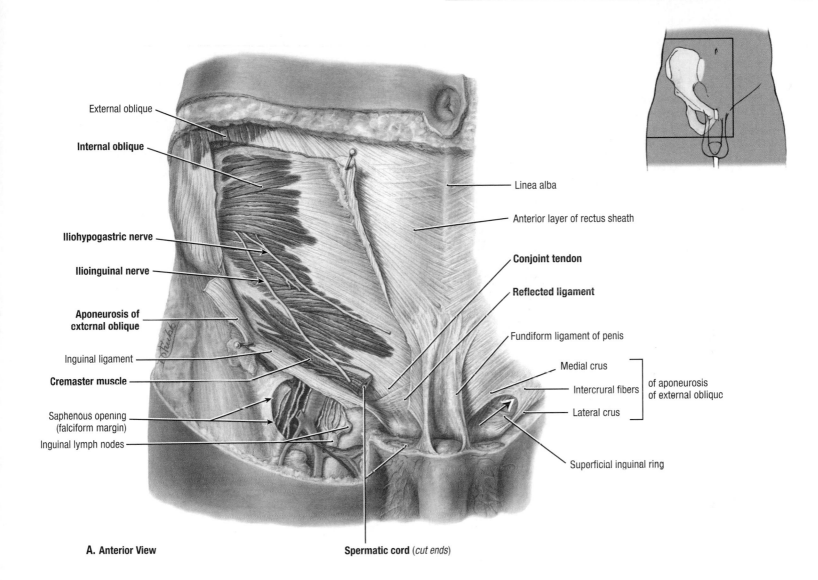

External oblique

Internal oblique

Iliohypogastric nerve

Ilioinguinal nerve

Aponeurosis of external oblique

Inguinal ligament

Cremaster muscle

Saphenous opening (falciform margin)

Inguinal lymph nodes

Linea alba

Anterior layer of rectus sheath

Conjoint tendon

Reflected ligament

Fundiform ligament of penis

Medial crus

Intercrural fibers — of aponeurosis of external oblique

Lateral crus

Superficial inguinal ring

Spermatic cord (*cut ends*)

A. Anterior View

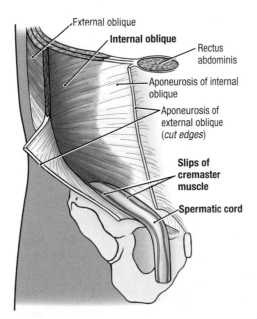

External oblique

Internal oblique

Rectus abdominis

Aponeurosis of internal oblique

Aponeurosis of external oblique (*cut edges*)

Slips of cremaster muscle

Spermatic cord

B. Anterior View

Inguinal Region of Male (II)

4.12

A. Internal oblique and cremaster muscle. Part of the aponeurosis of the external oblique muscle is cut away, and the spermatic cord is cut short. **B. Schematic.**

• The cremaster fascia covers the spermatic cord. Cremaster muscle is dispersed within the cremasteric fascia.

• The reflected ligament is formed by aponeurotic fibers of the external oblique muscle and lies anterior to the conjoint tendon. The conjoint tendon is formed by the fusion of the inferior most parts of the aponeurosis of the internal oblique and transversus abdominis muscles.

• The cutaneous branches of the iliohypogastric and ilioinguinal nerves (L1) course between the internal and external oblique muscles and must be avoided when an **appendectomy (gridiron) incision** is made in this region.

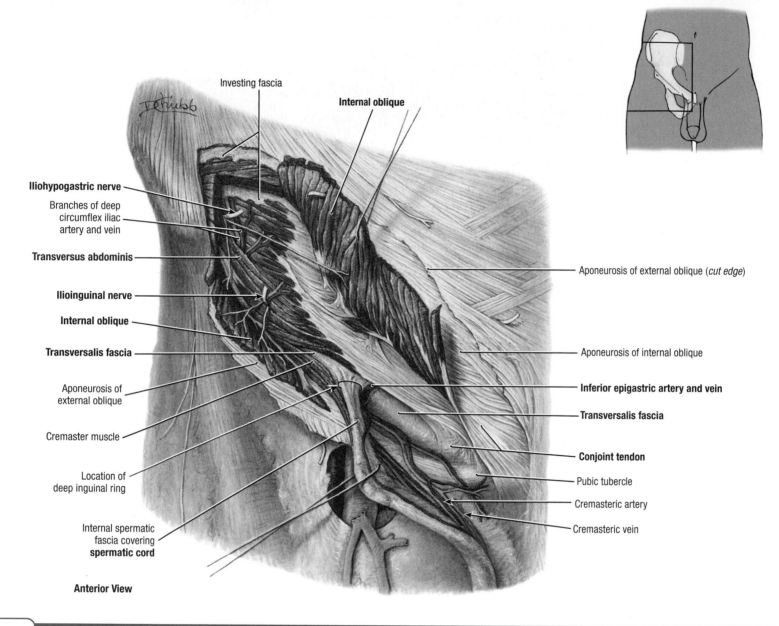

Investing fascia

Internal oblique

Iliohypogastric nerve

Branches of deep
circumflex iliac
artery and vein

Transversus abdominis

Ilioinguinal nerve

Internal oblique

Transversalis fascia

Aponeurosis of
external oblique

Cremaster muscle

Location of
deep inguinal ring

Internal spermatic
fascia covering
spermatic cord

Aponeurosis of external oblique (*cut edge*)

Aponeurosis of internal oblique

Inferior epigastric artery and vein

Transversalis fascia

Conjoint tendon

Pubic tubercle

Cremasteric artery

Cremasteric vein

Anterior View

4.13   Inguinal Region of Male (III)

The internal oblique muscle is reflected, and the spermatic cord is
retracted.

- The internal oblique muscle portion of the conjoint tendon is attached to the pubic crest, and the transversus abdominis portion
  to the pectineal line.

- The iliohypogastric and ilioinguinal nerves (L1) supply the internal oblique and transversus abdominis muscles.
- The transversalis fascia is evaginated to form the tubular internal
  spermatic fascia. The mouth of the tube, called the deep inguinal
  ring, is situated lateral to the inferior epigastric vessels.

TABLE 4.2	**Boundaries of Inguinal Canal**		
Boundary	**Deep Ring/Lateral Third**	**Middle Third**	**Lateral Third/Superficial Ring**
Posterior wall	Transversalis fascia	Transversalis fascia	Inguinal falx (conjoint tendon) plus reflected inguinal ligament
Anterior wall	Internal oblique plus lateral crus of aponeurosis of external oblique	Aponeurosis of external oblique (lateral crus and intercrural fibers)	Aponeurosis of external oblique (intercrural fibers), with fascia of external oblique continuing onto cord as external spermatic fascia
Roof	Transversalis fascia	Musculoaponeurotic arches of internal oblique and transversus abdominis	Medial crus of aponeurosis of external oblique
Floor	Iliopubic tract	Inguinal ligament	Lacunar ligament

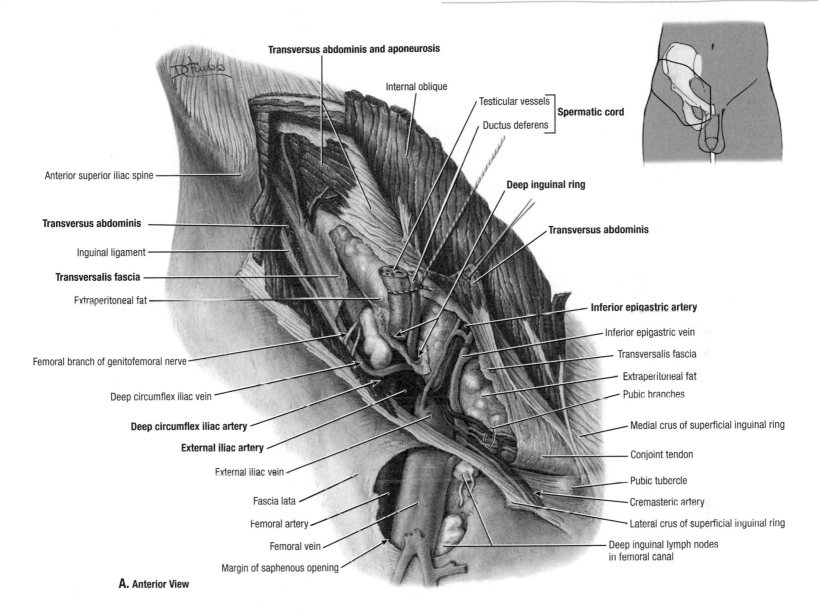

Transversus abdominis and aponeurosis

Internal oblique

Testicular vessels
Ductus deferens **Spermatic cord**

Anterior superior iliac spine

Deep inguinal ring

Transversus abdominis

Transversus abdominis

Inguinal ligament

Transversalis fascia

Extraperitoneal fat

Inferior epigastric artery

Inferior epigastric vein

Transversalis fascia

Femoral branch of genitofemoral nerve

Extraperitoneal fat

Deep circumflex iliac vein

Pubic branches

Deep circumflex iliac artery

Medial crus of superficial inguinal ring

External iliac artery

Conjoint tendon

External iliac vein

Pubic tubercle

Fascia lata

Cremasteric artery

Femoral artery

Lateral crus of superficial inguinal ring

Femoral vein

Deep inguinal lymph nodes
in femoral canal

Margin of saphenous opening

A. Anterior View

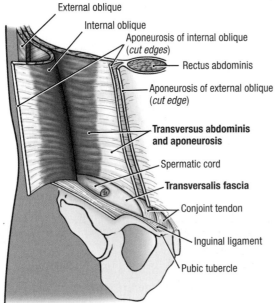

External oblique

Internal oblique

Aponeurosis of internal oblique
(*cut edges*)

Rectus abdominis

Aponeurosis of external oblique
(*cut edge*)

**Transversus abdominis
and aponeurosis**

Spermatic cord

Transversalis fascia

Conjoint tendon

Inguinal ligament

Pubic tubercle

B. Anterior View

Inguinal Region of Male (IV) | **4.14**

A. Deep inguinal ring. The inguinal part of the transversus abdominis muscle and transversalis fascia is partially cut away, the spermatic cord is excised, and the ductus deferens is retracted. **B. Schematic.**
• The deep inguinal ring is located superior to the inguinal ligament at the midpoint between the anterior superior iliac spine and pubic tubercle.
• The external iliac artery has two branches, the deep circumflex iliac and inferior epigastric arteries. Note also the cremasteric artery and pubic branch arising from the latter.

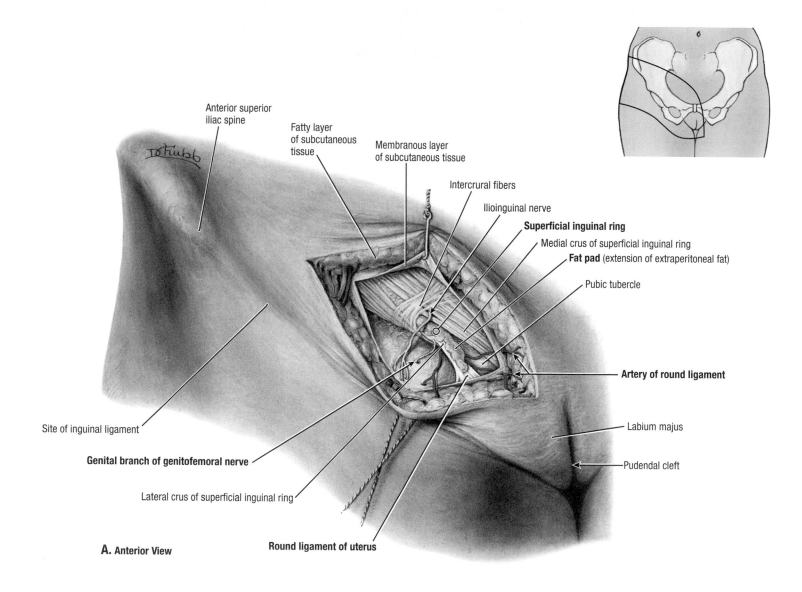

Anterior superior
iliac spine

Fatty layer
of subcutaneous
tissue

Membranous layer
of subcutaneous tissue

Intercrural fibers

Ilioinguinal nerve

Superficial inguinal ring

Medial crus of superficial inguinal ring

Fat pad (extension of extraperitoneal fat)

Pubic tubercle

Artery of round ligament

Labium majus

Pudendal cleft

Site of inguinal ligament

Genital branch of genitofemoral nerve

Lateral crus of superficial inguinal ring

Round ligament of uterus

A. Anterior View

4.15   **Inguinal Canal of Female**

A–D. Progressive dissections of female inguinal canal.
- The superficial inguinal ring is small (*Part A*). Passing through the superficial inguinal ring are the round ligament of the uterus, a closely applied fat pad, the genital branch of the genitofemoral nerve, and the artery of the round ligament of the uterus (*Part B*).
- The round ligament breaks up into strands as it leaves the inguinal canal and approaches the labium majus. The ilioinguinal nerve may also pass through the superficial inguinal ring (*Part C*).
- The external iliac artery and vein are exposed deep to the inguinal canal by excising the transversalis fascia (*Part D*).

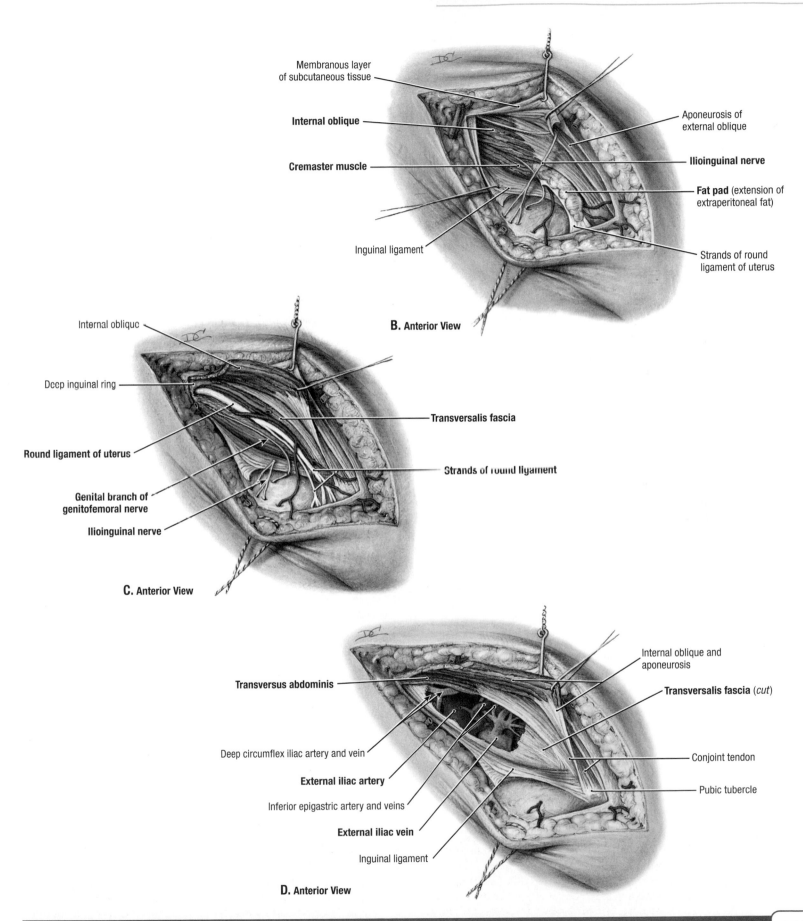

Membranous layer
of subcutaneous tissue

Internal oblique

Cremaster muscle

Inguinal ligament

Aponeurosis of
external oblique

Ilioinguinal nerve

Fat pad (extension of
extraperitoneal fat)

Strands of round
ligament of uterus

B. Anterior View

Internal oblique

Deep inguinal ring

Round ligament of uterus

**Genital branch of
genitofemoral nerve**

Ilioinguinal nerve

Transversalis fascia

Strands of round ligament

C. Anterior View

Transversus abdominis

Deep circumflex iliac artery and vein

External iliac artery

Inferior epigastric artery and veins

External iliac vein

Inguinal ligament

Internal oblique and
aponeurosis

Transversalis fascia (*cut*)

Conjoint tendon

Pubic tubercle

D. Anterior View

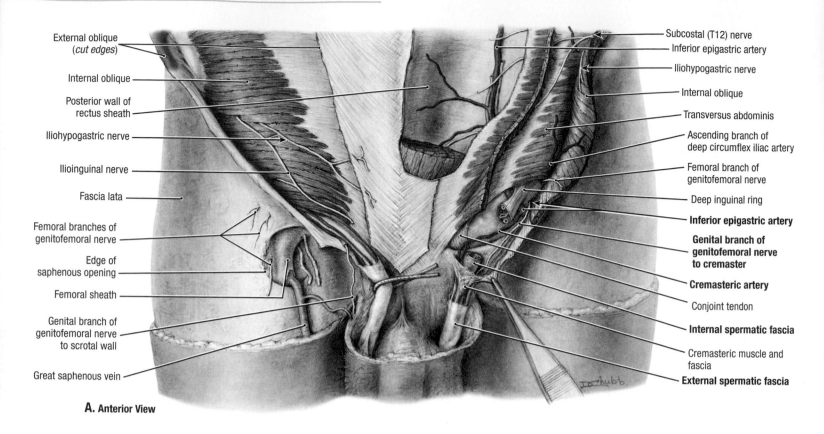

External oblique (*cut edges*)

Internal oblique

Posterior wall of rectus sheath

Iliohypogastric nerve

Ilioinguinal nerve

Fascia lata

Femoral branches of genitofemoral nerve

Edge of saphenous opening

Femoral sheath

Genital branch of genitofemoral nerve to scrotal wall

Great saphenous vein

Subcostal (T12) nerve

Inferior epigastric artery

Iliohypogastric nerve

Internal oblique

Transversus abdominis

Ascending branch of deep circumflex iliac artery

Femoral branch of genitofemoral nerve

Deep inguinal ring

Inferior epigastric artery

Genital branch of genitofemoral nerve to cremaster

Cremasteric artery

Conjoint tendon

Internal spermatic fascia

Cremasteric muscle and fascia

External spermatic fascia

A. Anterior View

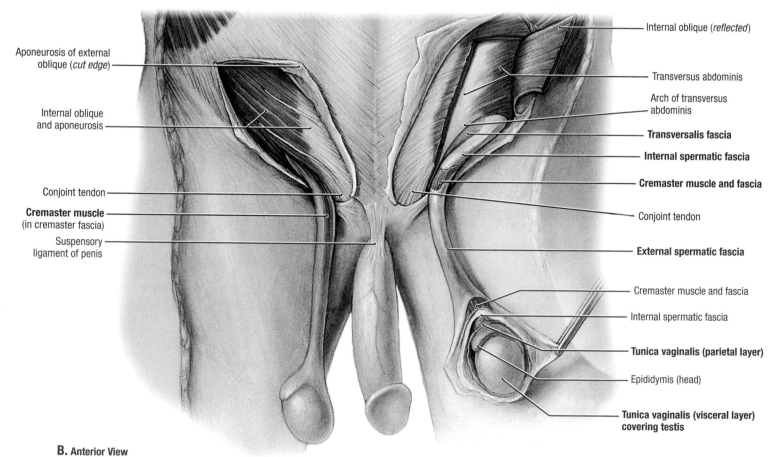

Aponeurosis of external oblique (*cut edge*)

Internal oblique and aponeurosis

Conjoint tendon

Cremaster muscle (in cremaster fascia)

Suspensory ligament of penis

Internal oblique (*reflected*)

Transversus abdominis

Arch of transversus abdominis

Transversalis fascia

Internal spermatic fascia

Cremaster muscle and fascia

Conjoint tendon

External spermatic fascia

Cremaster muscle and fascia

Internal spermatic fascia

Tunica vaginalis (parietal layer)

Epididymis (head)

Tunica vaginalis (visceral layer) covering testis

B. Anterior View

4.16 **Inguinal Canal, Spermatic Cord, and Testis**

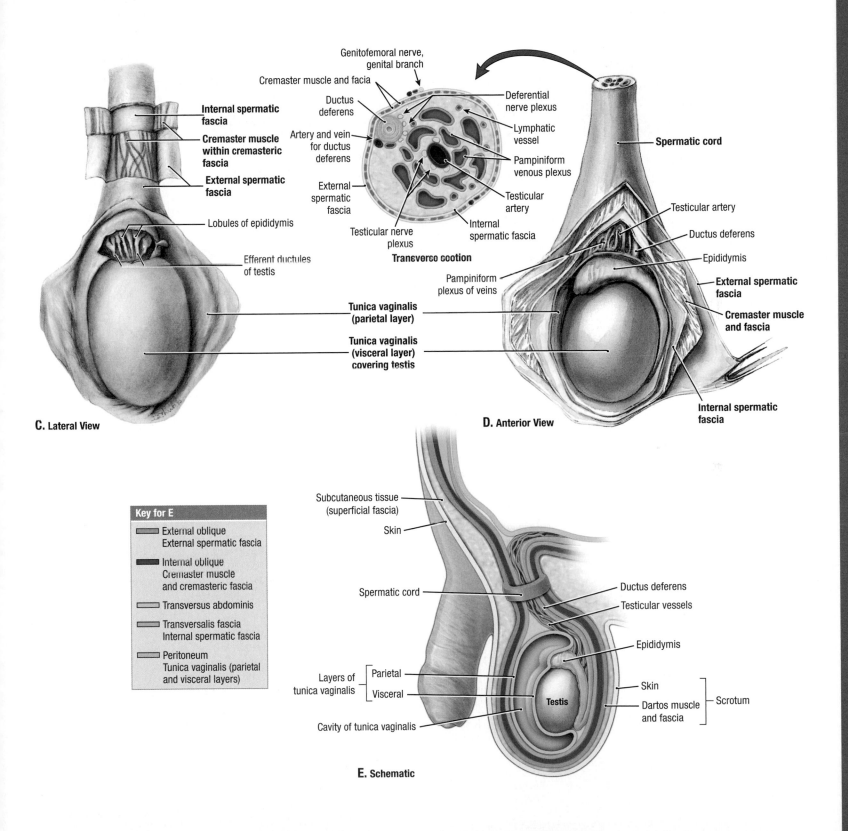

Genitofemoral nerve, genital branch

Cremaster muscle and facia

Ductus deferens

Artery and vein for ductus deferens

External spermatic fascia

Testicular nerve plexus

Transverse section

Deferential nerve plexus

Lymphatic vessel

Pampiniform venous plexus

Testicular artery

Internal spermatic fascia

Internal spermatic fascia

Cremaster muscle within cremasteric fascia

External spermatic fascia

Lobules of epididymis

Efferent ductules of testis

Pampiniform plexus of veins

Tunica vaginalis (parietal layer)

Tunica vaginalis (visceral layer) covering testis

C. Lateral View

Spermatic cord

Testicular artery

Ductus deferens

Epididymis

External spermatic fascia

Cremaster muscle and fascia

Internal spermatic fascia

D. Anterior View

Key for E

External oblique
External spermatic fascia

Internal oblique
Cremaster muscle
and cremasteric fascia

Transversus abdominis

Transversalis fascia
Internal spermatic fascia

Peritoneum
Tunica vaginalis (parietal
and visceral layers)

Subcutaneous tissue (superficial fascia)

Skin

Spermatic cord

Ductus deferens

Testicular vessels

Epididymis

Layers of tunica vaginalis — Parietal / Visceral

Cavity of tunica vaginalis

Testis

Skin

Dartos muscle and fascia

Scrotum

E. Schematic

A. Dissection of inguinal canal. **B.** Dissection of inguinal region and coverings of spermatic cord and testis. **C–E.** Coverings of spermatic cord and testis. The cavity of the tunica vaginalis is normally a potential space.

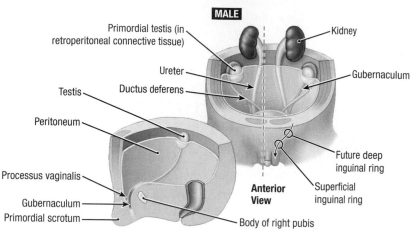

MALE

Primordial testis (in retroperitoneal connective tissue)

Kidney

Ureter

Gubernaculum

Ductus deferens

Testis

Peritoneum

Processus vaginalis

Gubernaculum

Primordial scrotum

Future deep inguinal ring

Anterior View

Superficial inguinal ring

Body of right pubis

Diagrammatic oblique sagittal section to right of midline (at *green dashed line*)

A. Seventh Week

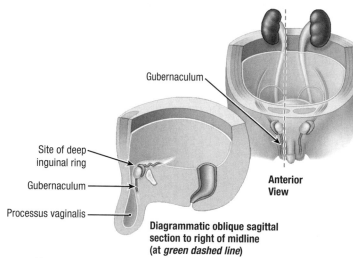

Gubernaculum

Site of deep inguinal ring

Gubernaculum

Processus vaginalis

Anterior View

Diagrammatic oblique sagittal section to right of midline (at *green dashed line*)

B. Seventh Month

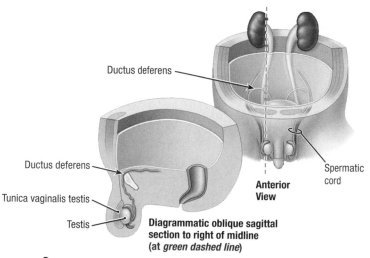

Ductus deferens

Ductus deferens

Tunica vaginalis testis

Testis

Spermatic cord

Anterior View

Diagrammatic oblique sagittal section to right of midline (at *green dashed line*)

C. Ninth Month

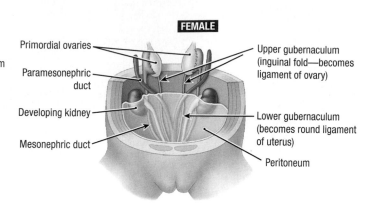

FEMALE

Primordial ovaries

Upper gubernaculum (inguinal fold—becomes ligament of ovary)

Paramesonephric duct

Developing kidney

Lower gubernaculum (becomes round ligament of uterus)

Mesonephric duct

Peritoneum

D. 2 Months

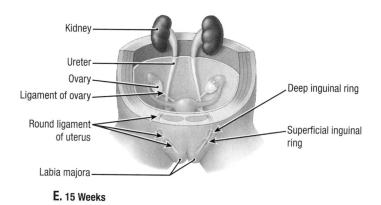

Kidney

Ureter

Ovary

Ligament of ovary

Deep inguinal ring

Round ligament of uterus

Superficial inguinal ring

Labia majora

E. 15 Weeks

4.17 Relocation of Gonads

The inguinal canals of females are narrower than those of males, and the canals in infants of both sexes are shorter and much less oblique than in adults.

The fetal testes relocate from the dorsal abdominal wall in the superior lumbar region to the deep inguinal rings during the 9th to 12th fetal weeks. This apparent migration probably results from the growth of the vertebral column and pelvis. The male gubernaculum, attached to the caudal pole of the testis and accompanied by an outpouching of peritoneum, the processus vaginalis, projects into the scrotum. The testis passes posterior to the processus vaginalis. The inferior remnant of the processus vaginalis forms the tunica vaginalis covering the testis. The ductus deferens, testicular vessels, nerves, and lymphatics accompany the testis. The descent of the testis into the scrotum usually occurs before or shortly after birth.

The fetal ovaries also relocate from the dorsal abdominal wall in the superior lumbar region during the 12th week but pass into the lesser pelvis. The female gubernaculum attaches to the caudal pole of the ovary and projects into the labia majora, attaching en route to the uterus; the part passing from the uterus to the ovary forms the ovarian ligament, and the remainder of it becomes the round ligament of the uterus. Because of the attachment of the ovarian ligaments to the uterus, the ovaries do not relocate to the inguinal region; however, the round ligament passes through the inguinal canal and attaches to the subcutaneous tissue of the labium majus.

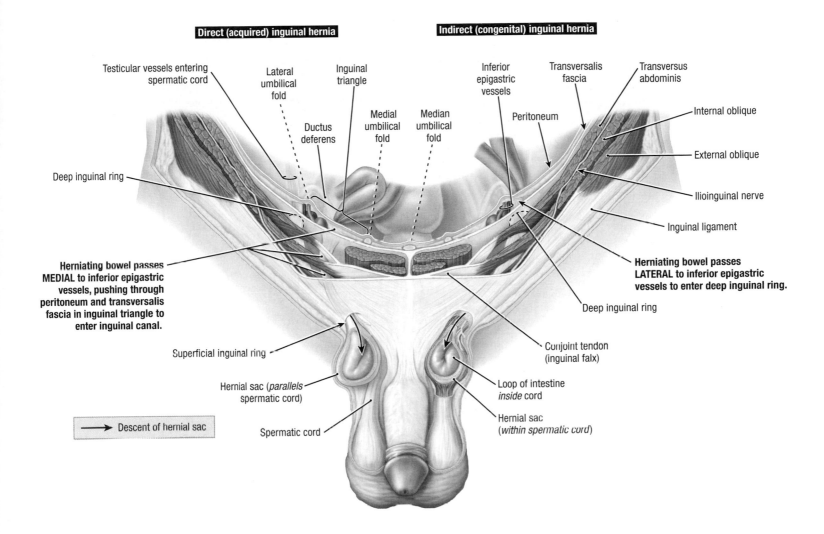

Direct (acquired) inguinal hernia — Indirect (congenital) inguinal hernia

Testicular vessels entering spermatic cord

Lateral umbilical fold

Inguinal triangle

Ductus deferens

Medial umbilical fold

Median umbilical fold

Inferior epigastric vessels

Peritoneum

Transversalis fascia

Transversus abdominis

Internal oblique

External oblique

Ilioinguinal nerve

Inguinal ligament

Deep inguinal ring

Herniating bowel passes MEDIAL to inferior epigastric vessels, pushing through peritoneum and transversalis fascia in inguinal triangle to enter inguinal canal.

Herniating bowel passes LATERAL to inferior epigastric vessels to enter deep inguinal ring.

Deep inguinal ring

Conjoint tendon (inguinal falx)

Superficial inguinal ring

Loop of intestine *inside* cord

Hernial sac (*parallels* spermatic cord)

Hernial sac (*within spermatic cord*)

→ Descent of hernial sac

Spermatic cord

Course of Direct and Indirect Inguinal Hernias

4.18

An **inguinal hernia** is a protrusion of parietal peritoneum and viscera, such as the small intestine, through the abdominal wall in the inguinal region. There are two major categories of inguinal hernia:

indirect and direct. More than two thirds are indirect hernias, most commonly occurring in males.

TABLE 4.3	**Characteristics of Inguinal Hernias**	
Characteristics	**Direct (Acquired)**	**Indirect (Congenital)**
Predisposing factors	Weakness of anterior abdominal wall in inguinal triangle (e.g., owing to distended superficial ring, narrow conjoint tendon, or attenuation of aponeurosis in males >40 years of age)	Patency of processus vaginalis (complete or at least of superior part) in younger persons, the great majority of whom are males
Frequency	Less common (one third to one fourth of inguinal hernias)	More common (two thirds to three fourths of inguinal hernias)
Coverings at exit from abdominal cavity	Peritoneum plus transversalis fascia (lies outside inner one or two fascial coverings, parallel to cord)	Peritoneum of persistent processus vaginalis plus all three fascial coverings of cord/round ligament
Course	Usually traverses only medial third of inguinal canal, external and parallel to vestige of processus vaginalis	Traverses inguinal canal (entire canal if it is sufficient size) within processus vaginalis
Exit from anterior abdominal wall	Via superficial ring, lateral to cord; rarely enters scrotum	Via superficial ring inside cord, commonly passing into scrotum/labium majus

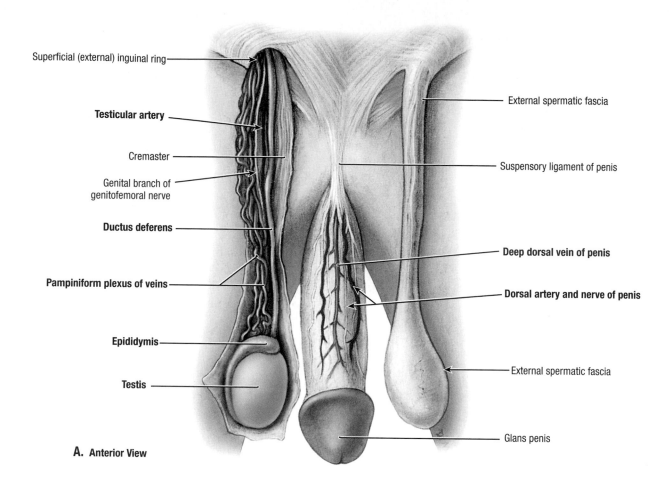

Superficial (external) inguinal ring

Testicular artery

Cremaster

Genital branch of genitofemoral nerve

Ductus deferens

Pampiniform plexus of veins

Epididymis

Testis

External spermatic fascia

Suspensory ligament of penis

Deep dorsal vein of penis

Dorsal artery and nerve of penis

External spermatic fascia

Glans penis

A. Anterior View

4.19 Spermatic Cord, Testis, and Epididymis

A. Dissection of spermatic cord. The subcutaneous tissue (dartos fascia) covering the penis has been removed and the deep fascia rendered transparent to demonstrate the median deep dorsal vein and the bilateral dorsal arteries and nerves of the penis. On the specimen's right, the coverings of the spermatic cord and testis are reflected, and the contents of the cord are separated. The testicular artery has been separated from the pampiniform plexus of veins that surrounds it as it courses parallel to the ductus deferens. Lymphatic vessels and autonomic nerve fibers (not shown) are also present. **B. Dissection of testis and epididymis.** The tunica vaginalis has been incised longitudinally to expose its cavity, surrounding the testis anteriorly and laterally, and extending between the testis and epididymis at the sinus of the epididymis. The epididymis is located posterolateral to the testis, that is, toward the right side of the right testis and the left side of the left testis. The appendices of the testis and epididymis may be observed in some specimens. These structures are small remnants of the embryonic genital (paramesonephric) duct.

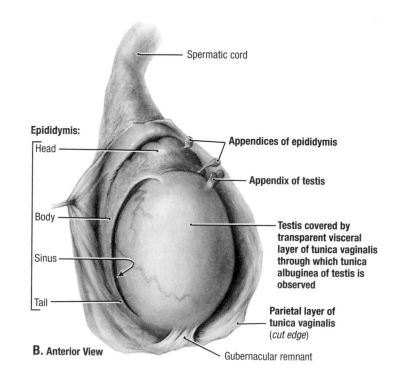

Spermatic cord

Epididymis:
Head

Body

Sinus

Tail

Appendices of epididymis

Appendix of testis

Testis covered by transparent visceral layer of tunica vaginalis through which tunica albuginea of testis is observed

Parietal layer of tunica vaginalis (*cut edge*)

Gubernacular remnant

B. Anterior View

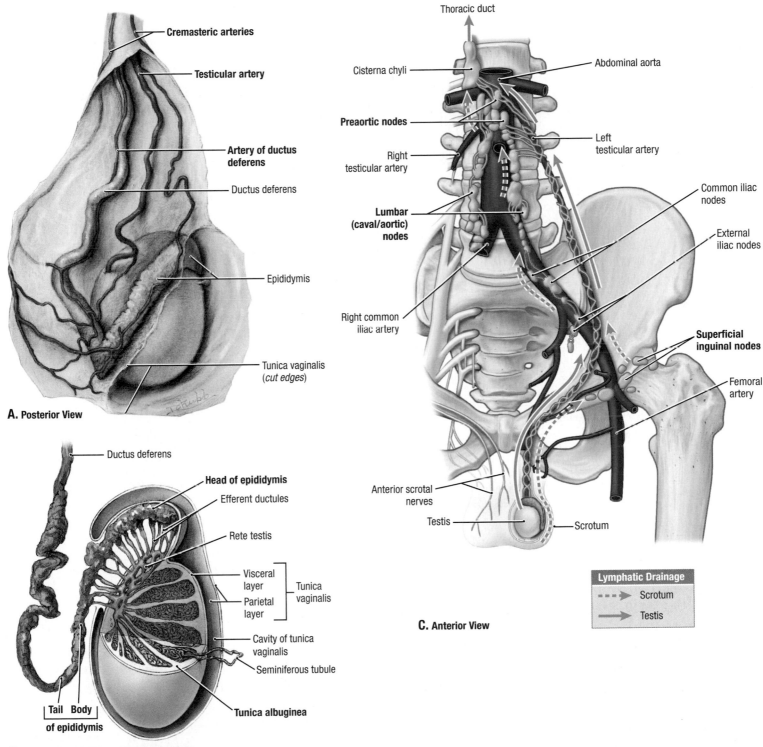

Cremasteric arteries

Testicular artery

Artery of ductus deferens

Ductus deferens

Epididymis

Tunica vaginalis (*cut edges*)

A. Posterior View

Thoracic duct

Cisterna chyli

Abdominal aorta

Preaortic nodes

Right testicular artery

Left testicular artery

Lumbar (caval/aortic) nodes

Common iliac nodes

External iliac nodes

Right common iliac artery

Superficial inguinal nodes

Femoral artery

Anterior scrotal nerves

Testis

Scrotum

Lymphatic Drainage	
⇢	Scrotum
→	Testis

C. Anterior View

Ductus deferens

Head of epididymis

Efferent ductules

Rete testis

Visceral layer — Tunica vaginalis

Parietal layer

Cavity of tunica vaginalis

Seminiferous tubule

Tail | Body of epididymis

Tunica albuginea

B. Longitudinal Section of Tunica Vaginalis; Testis Sectioned in Sagittal and Transverse Planes

Blood Supply and Lymphatic Drainage of Testis

4.20

A. Blood supply. **B.** Internal structure. **C.** Lymphatic drainage.

Because the testes relocate from the posterior abdominal wall into the scrotum during fetal development, their lymphatic drainage differs from that of the scrotum, which is an outpouching of the abdominal skin. Consequently, **cancer of the testis** metastasizes initially to the lumbar lymph nodes, and **cancer of the scrotum** metastasizes initially to the superficial inguinal lymph nodes.

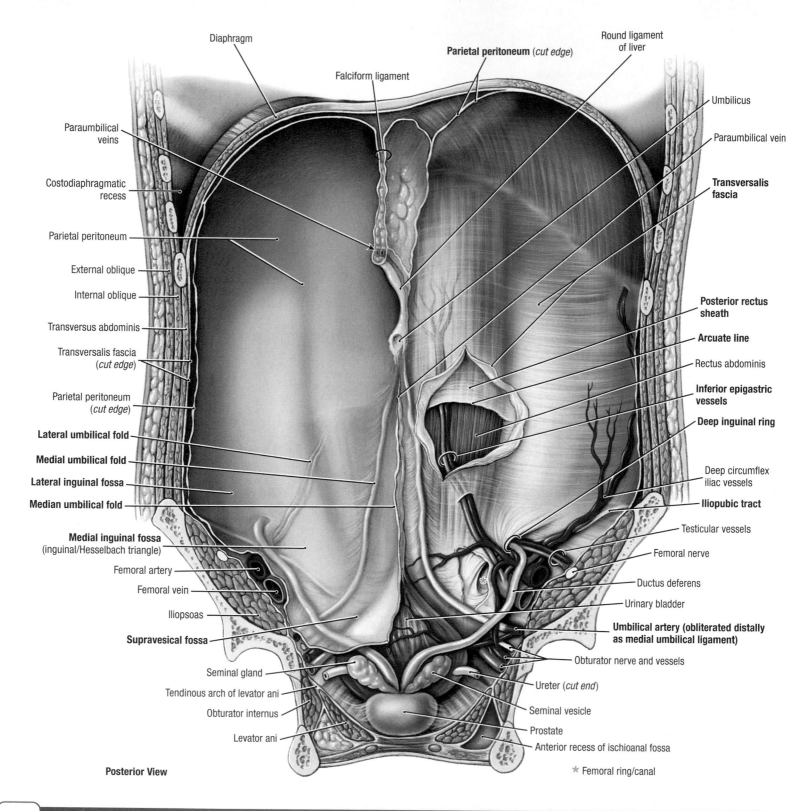

Diaphragm

Round ligament of liver

Parietal peritoneum (*cut edge*)

Falciform ligament

Paraumbilical veins

Costodiaphragmatic recess

Parietal peritoneum

External oblique

Internal oblique

Transversus abdominis

Transversalis fascia (*cut edge*)

Parietal peritoneum (*cut edge*)

Lateral umbilical fold

Medial umbilical fold

Lateral inguinal fossa

Median umbilical fold

Medial inguinal fossa (inguinal/Hesselbach triangle)

Femoral artery

Femoral vein

Iliopsoas

Supravesical fossa

Seminal gland

Tendinous arch of levator ani

Obturator internus

Levator ani

Umbilicus

Paraumbilical vein

Transversalis fascia

Posterior rectus sheath

Arcuate line

Rectus abdominis

Inferior epigastric vessels

Deep inguinal ring

Deep circumflex iliac vessels

Iliopubic tract

Testicular vessels

Femoral nerve

Ductus deferens

Urinary bladder

Umbilical artery (obliterated distally as medial umbilical ligament)

Obturator nerve and vessels

Ureter (*cut end*)

Seminal vesicle

Prostate

Anterior recess of ischioanal fossa

Posterior View

＊ Femoral ring/canal

| 4.21 | **Posterior Aspect of Anterolateral Abdominal Wall** |

Umbilical folds (median, medial, and lateral) are reflections of the parietal peritoneum that are raised from the body wall by underlying structures. The median umbilical fold extends from the urinary bladder to the umbilicus and covers the median umbilical ligament (the remnant of the urachus). The two medial umbilical folds cover the medial umbilical ligaments (occluded remnants of the fetal umbilical arteries). Two lateral umbilical folds cover the inferior epigastric vessels. The supravesical fossae are between the median and medial umbilical folds, the medial inguinal fossae (inguinal triangles) are between the medial and lateral umbilical folds, and the lateral inguinal fossae and deep inguinal rings are lateral to the lateral umbilical folds.

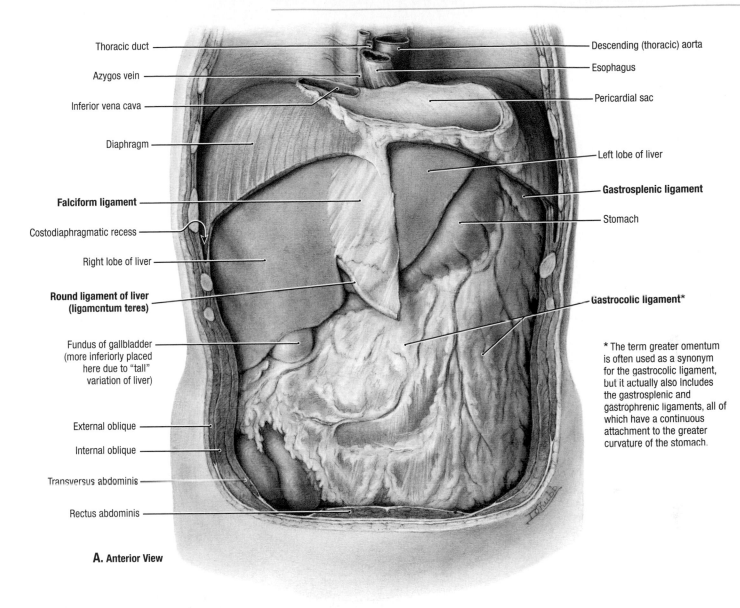

Thoracic duct

Azygos vein

Inferior vena cava

Diaphragm

Falciform ligament

Costodiaphragmatic recess

Right lobe of liver

**Round ligament of liver
(ligamentum teres)**

Fundus of gallbladder
(more inferiorly placed
here due to "tall"
variation of liver)

External oblique

Internal oblique

Transversus abdominis

Rectus abdominis

Descending (thoracic) aorta

Esophagus

Pericardial sac

Left lobe of liver

Gastrosplenic ligament

Stomach

Gastrocolic ligament*

* The term greater omentum
is often used as a synonym
for the gastrocolic ligament,
but it actually also includes
the gastrosplenic and
gastrophrenic ligaments, all of
which have a continuous
attachment to the greater
curvature of the stomach.

A. Anterior View

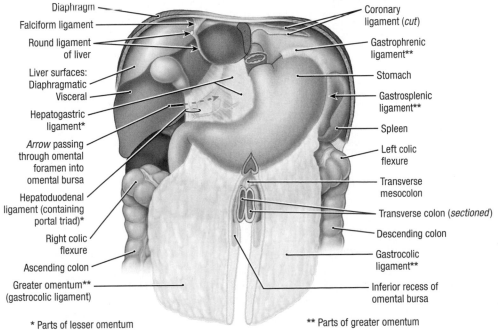

Diaphragm

Falciform ligament

Round ligament
of liver

Liver surfaces:
Diaphragmatic
Visceral

Hepatogastric
ligament*

Arrow passing
through omental
foramen into
omental bursa

Hepatoduodenal
ligament (containing
portal triad)*

Right colic
flexure

Ascending colon

Greater omentum**
(gastrocolic ligament)

Coronary
ligament (*cut*)

Gastrophrenic
ligament**

Stomach

Gastrosplenic
ligament**

Spleen

Left colic
flexure

Transverse
mesocolon

Transverse colon (*sectioned*)

Descending colon

Gastrocolic
ligament**

Inferior recess of
omental bursa

* Parts of lesser omentum

** Parts of greater omentum

B. Anterior View

**Abdominal Contents and
Peritoneum** **4.22**

A. Dissection. **B.** Components of
greater and lesser omentum.

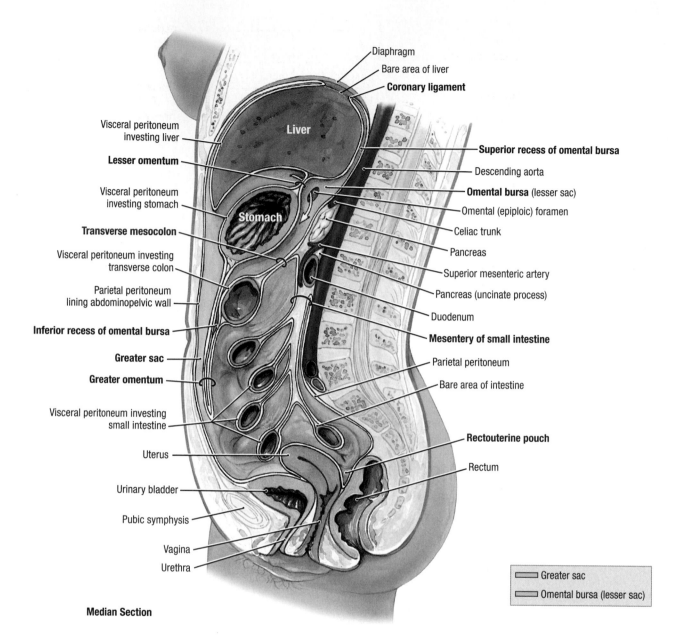

Diaphragm
Bare area of liver
Coronary ligament

Visceral peritoneum investing liver

Lesser omentum

Visceral peritoneum investing stomach

Transverse mesocolon

Visceral peritoneum investing transverse colon

Parietal peritoneum lining abdominopelvic wall

Inferior recess of omental bursa

Greater sac

Greater omentum

Visceral peritoneum investing small intestine

Uterus

Urinary bladder

Pubic symphysis

Vagina

Urethra

Liver

Stomach

Superior recess of omental bursa

Descending aorta

Omental bursa (lesser sac)

Omental (epiploic) foramen

Celiac trunk

Pancreas

Superior mesenteric artery

Pancreas (uncinate process)

Duodenum

Mesentery of small intestine

Parietal peritoneum

Bare area of intestine

Rectouterine pouch

Rectum

Greater sac

Omental bursa (lesser sac)

Median Section

4.23 Peritoneal Formations and Bare Areas

Various terms are used to describe the parts of the peritoneum that connect organs with other organs or to the abdominal wall and to describe the compartments and recesses that are formed as a consequence. The *arrow* passes through the omental (epiploic) foramen.

TABLE 4.4	Terms Used to Describe Parts of Peritoneum
Term	**Definition**
Peritoneal ligament	Double layer of peritoneum that connects an organ with another organ or to the abdominal wall.
Mesentery	Double layer of peritoneum that occurs as a result of the invagination of the peritoneum by one or more organs and constitutes a continuity of the visceral and parietal peritoneum.
Omentum	Double-layered extension of peritoneum passing from the proximal duodenum and/or stomach and to adjacent organs. The greater omentum extends from the greater curvature of the stomach and the proximal duodenum; the lesser omentum from the lesser curvature.
Bare area	Every organ must have an area, the bare area, that is not covered with visceral peritoneum, to allow the entrance and exit of neurovascular structures. Bare areas are formed in relation to the attachments of mesenteries, omenta, and ligaments. Named bare areas (e.g., bare area of liver) are especially extensive.

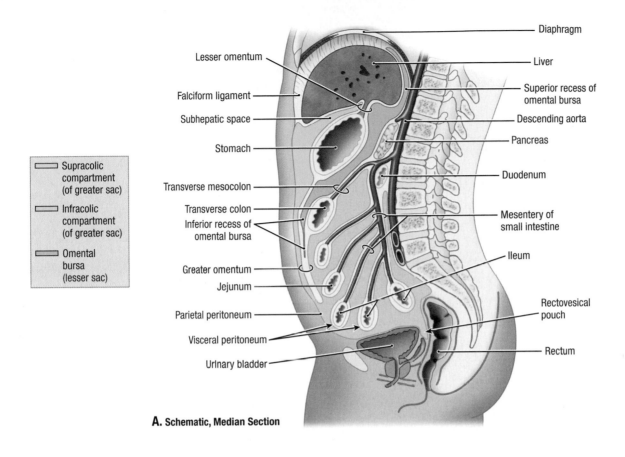

Diaphragm
Lesser omentum
Liver
Falciform ligament
Superior recess of omental bursa
Subhepatic space
Descending aorta
Stomach
Pancreas
Transverse mesocolon
Duodenum
Transverse colon
Inferior recess of omental bursa
Mesentery of small intestine
Greater omentum
Ileum
Jejunum
Parietal peritoneum
Rectovesical pouch
Visceral peritoneum
Rectum
Urlnary bladder

Supracolic compartment (of greater sac)
Infracolic compartment (of greater sac)
Omental bursa (lesser sac)

A. Schematic, Median Section

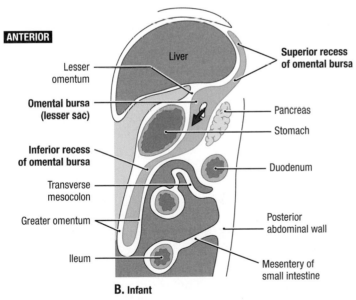

ANTERIOR
Liver
Lesser omentum
Superior recess of omental bursa
Omental bursa (lesser sac)
Pancreas
Stomach
Inferior recess of omental bursa
Duodenum
Transverse mesocolon
Greater omentum
Posterior abdominal wall
Ileum
Mesentery of small intestine

B. Infant

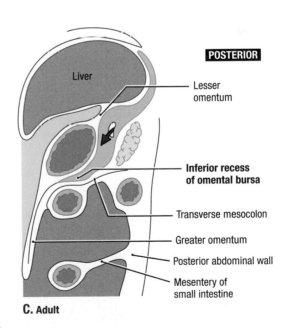

POSTERIOR
Liver
Lesser omentum
Inferior recess of omental bursa
Transverse mesocolon
Greater omentum
Posterior abdominal wall
Mesentery of small intestine

C. Adult

Schematic, Sagittal Sections

Subdivisions of Peritoneal Cavity

4.24

A. Schematic sagittal section. B. Omental bursa in infant. In an infant, the omental bursa (lesser sac) is an isolated part of the perito-neal cavity, lying posterior to the stomach and extending superiorly between the liver and diaphragm (superior recess of the omental bursa) and inferiorly between the layers of the greater omentum (inferior recess of the omental bursa). **C. Omental bursa in adult.** In an adult, after fusion of the layers of the greater omentum, the inferior recess of the omental bursa now extends inferiorly only as far as the transverse colon. The *red arrows* pass from the greater sac through the omental (epiploic) foramen into the omental bursa.

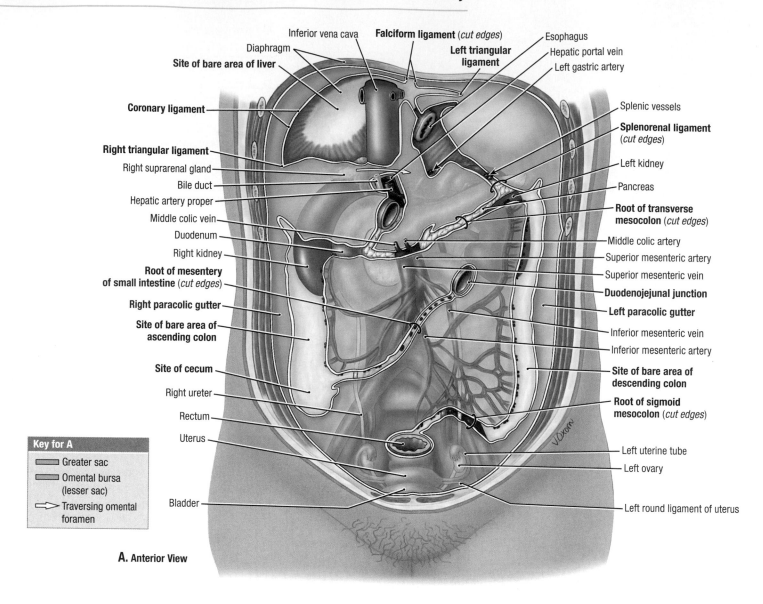

Inferior vena cava
Diaphragm
Site of bare area of liver
Coronary ligament
Right triangular ligament
Right suprarenal gland
Bile duct
Hepatic artery proper
Middle colic vein
Duodenum
Right kidney
Root of mesentery of small intestine (*cut edges*)
Right paracolic gutter
Site of bare area of ascending colon
Site of cecum
Right ureter
Rectum
Uterus
Bladder

Falciform ligament (*cut edges*)
Left triangular ligament
Esophagus
Hepatic portal vein
Left gastric artery
Splenic vessels
Splenorenal ligament (*cut edges*)
Left kidney
Pancreas
Root of transverse mesocolon (*cut edges*)
Middle colic artery
Superior mesenteric artery
Superior mesenteric vein
Duodenojejunal junction
Left paracolic gutter
Inferior mesenteric vein
Inferior mesenteric artery
Site of bare area of descending colon
Root of sigmoid mesocolon (*cut edges*)
Left uterine tube
Left ovary
Left round ligament of uterus

Key for A
	Greater sac
	Omental bursa (lesser sac)
⇨	Traversing omental foramen

A. Anterior View

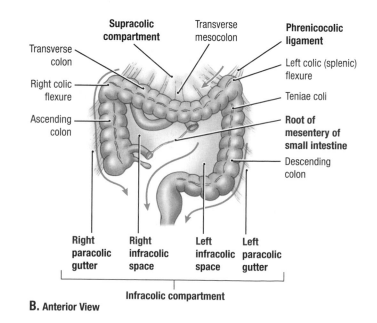

Supracolic compartment
Transverse mesocolon
Phrenicocolic ligament
Transverse colon
Left colic (splenic) flexure
Right colic flexure
Teniae coli
Ascending colon
Root of mesentery of small intestine
Descending colon

Right paracolic gutter
Right infracolic space
Left infracolic space
Left paracolic gutter

Infracolic compartment

B. Anterior View

4.25   **Posterior Wall of Peritoneal Cavity**

A. Roots of peritoneal reflections. The peritoneal reflections from the posterior abdominal wall (mesenteries and reflections surrounding bare areas of liver and secondarily retroperitoneal organs) have been cut at their roots, and the intraperitoneal and secondarily retroperitoneal viscera have been removed. The *white arrow* passes through the omental (epiploic) foramen. **B. Supracolic and infracolic compartments of greater sac.**

The infracolic spaces and paracolic gutters are of clinical importance because they determine the paths (*blue arrows*) for the **flow of ascitic fluid with changes in position,** and the spread of intraperitoneal infections.

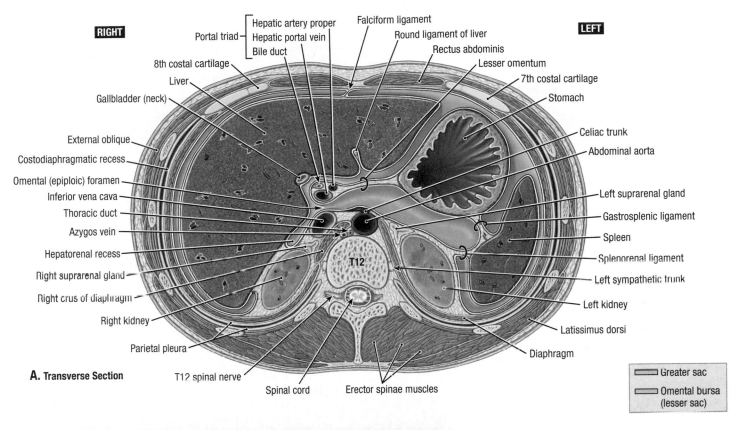

A. Transverse Section

RIGHT

Portal triad — Hepatic artery proper / Hepatic portal vein / Bile duct
Falciform ligament
Round ligament of liver
Rectus abdominis
8th costal cartilage
Lesser omentum
7th costal cartilage
Liver
Stomach
Gallbladder (neck)
Celiac trunk
External oblique
Abdominal aorta
Costodiaphragmatic recess
Omental (epiploic) foramen
Left suprarenal gland
Inferior vena cava
Gastrosplenic ligament
Thoracic duct
Spleen
Azygos vein
Splenorenal ligament
Hepatorenal recess
Left sympathetic trunk
Right suprarenal gland
Left kidney
Right crus of diaphragm
Right kidney
Latissimus dorsi
Parietal pleura
Diaphragm
T12 spinal nerve
Spinal cord
Erector spinae muscles

LEFT

T12

Greater sac
Omental bursa (lesser sac)

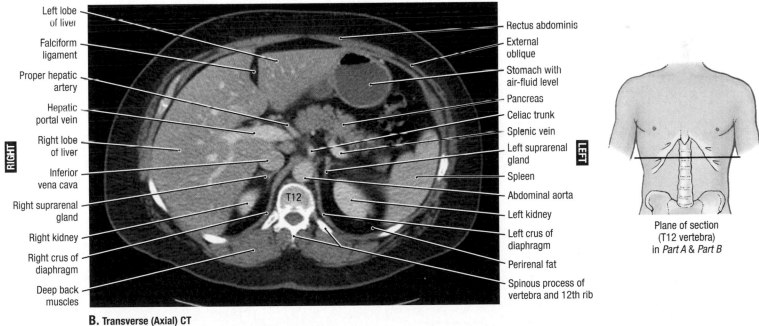

B. Transverse (Axial) CT

Left lobe of liver
Rectus abdominis
Falciform ligament
External oblique
Proper hepatic artery
Stomach with air-fluid level
Hepatic portal vein
Pancreas
Right lobe of liver
Celiac trunk
Splenic vein
Inferior vena cava
Left suprarenal gland
Right suprarenal gland
Spleen
Right kidney
Abdominal aorta
Right crus of diaphragm
Left kidney
Left crus of diaphragm
Deep back muscles
Perirenal fat
Spinous process of vertebra and 12th rib

RIGHT LEFT

T12

Plane of section (T12 vertebra) in *Part A* & *Part B*

Transverse Section and Axial CT Image through Greater Sac and Omental Bursa
4.26

- When bacterial contamination occurs or when the gut is traumatically penetrated or ruptured as the result of infection and inflammation, gas, fecal matter, and bacteria enter the peritoneal cavity. The result is infection and inflammation of the peritoneum, called **peritonitis**.
- Under certain pathological conditions such as peritonitis, the peritoneal cavity may be distended with abnormal fluid, **ascites**.

Widespread metastases (spread) of cancer cells to the abdominal viscera cause exudation (escape) of fluid that is often blood stained. Thus, the peritoneal cavity may be distended with several liters of abnormal fluid. Surgical puncture of the peritoneal cavity for the aspiration of drainage of fluid is called **paracentesis**.

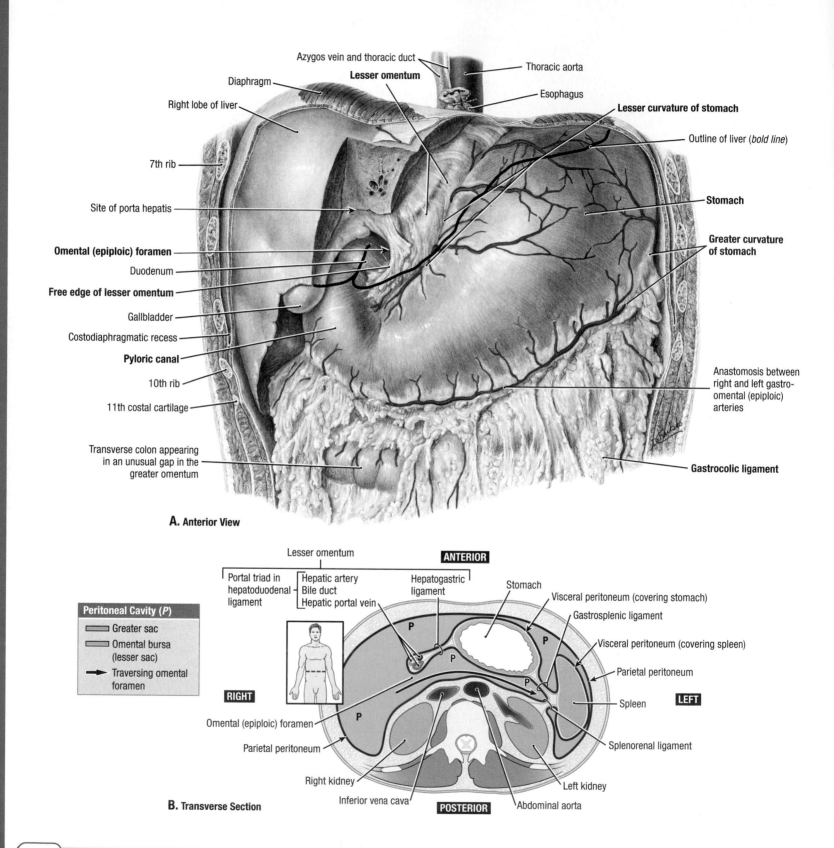

A. Anterior View

B. Transverse Section

4.27   Stomach and Omenta

A. Lesser and greater omenta. The stomach is inflated with air, and the left part of the liver is cut away. The gallbladder, followed superiorly, leads to the free margin of the lesser omentum and serves as a guide to the omental (epiploic) foramen, which lies posterior to that free margin. **B. Omental bursa (lesser sac), schematic transverse section.** *Arrow* is traversing omental foramen and bursa.

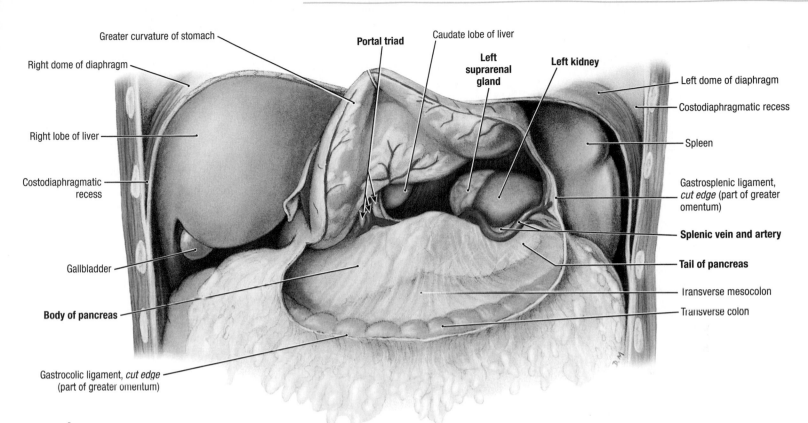

Greater curvature of stomach
Right dome of diaphragm
Right lobe of liver
Costodiaphragmatic recess
Gallbladder
Body of pancreas
Gastrocolic ligament, *cut edge* (part of greater omentum)
Portal triad
Caudate lobe of liver
Left suprarenal gland
Left kidney
Left dome of diaphragm
Costodiaphragmatic recess
Spleen
Gastrosplenic ligament, *cut edge* (part of greater omentum)
Splenic vein and artery
Tail of pancreas
Transverse mesocolon
Transverse colon

A. Anterior View

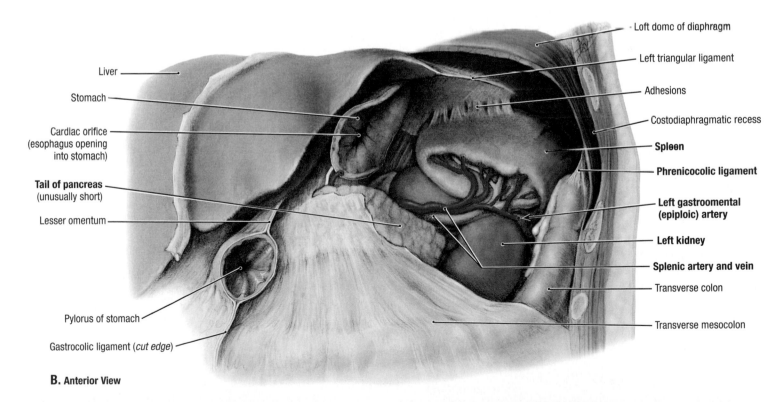

Liver
Stomach
Cardiac orifice (esophagus opening into stomach)
Tail of pancreas (unusually short)
Lesser omentum
Pylorus of stomach
Gastrocolic ligament (*cut edge*)
Left dome of diaphragm
Left triangular ligament
Adhesions
Costodiaphragmatic recess
Spleen
Phrenicocolic ligament
Left gastroomental (epiploic) artery
Left kidney
Splenic artery and vein
Transverse colon
Transverse mesocolon

B. Anterior View

Posterior Relationships of Omental Bursa (Lesser Sac)

4.28

A. Opened omental bursa. The greater omentum has been cut along the greater curvature of the stomach; the abdomen is reflected superiorly. Peritoneum of the posterior wall of the bursa is partially removed. **B. Stomach bed.** The stomach is excised.

Peritoneum covering the stomach bed and inferior part of the kidney and pancreas is largely removed. **Adhesions** binding intraperitoneal organs, such as the spleen to the diaphragm, are pathological but not unusual.

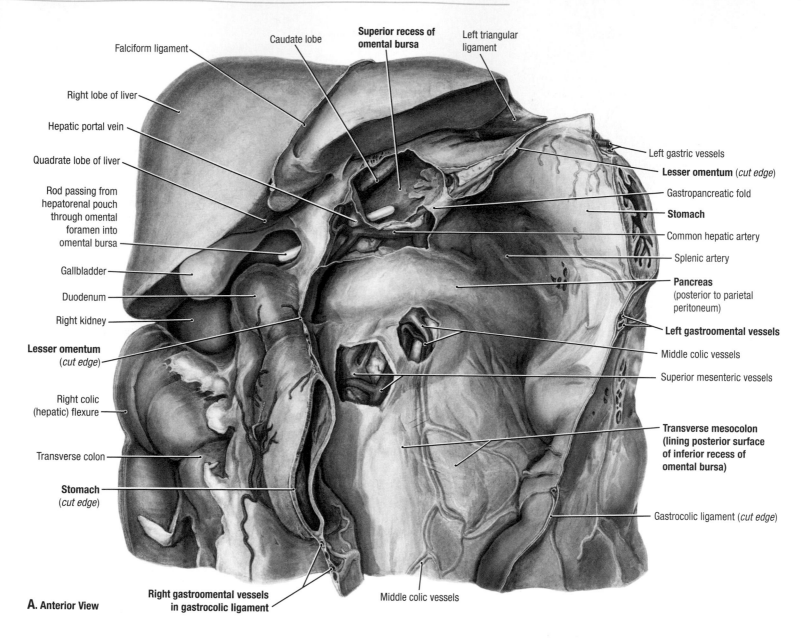

A. Anterior View

Falciform ligament

Caudate lobe

Superior recess of omental bursa

Left triangular ligament

Right lobe of liver

Hepatic portal vein

Quadrate lobe of liver

Rod passing from hepatorenal pouch through omental foramen into omental bursa

Gallbladder

Duodenum

Right kidney

Lesser omentum (*cut edge*)

Right colic (hepatic) flexure

Transverse colon

Stomach (*cut edge*)

Left gastric vessels

Lesser omentum (*cut edge*)

Gastropancreatic fold

Stomach

Common hepatic artery

Splenic artery

Pancreas (posterior to parietal peritoneum)

Left gastroomental vessels

Middle colic vessels

Superior mesenteric vessels

Transverse mesocolon (lining posterior surface of inferior recess of omental bursa)

Gastrocolic ligament (*cut edge*)

Right gastroomental vessels in gastrocolic ligament

Middle colic vessels

4.29 **Omental Bursa (Lesser Sac), Opened**

A. Dissection. B. Diagram indicating site of incision of stomach and greater omentum (*Part A*). The anterior wall of the omental bursa, consisting of the stomach, lesser omentum, anterior layer of the greater omentum, and vessels along the curvatures of the stomach, has been sectioned sagittally. The two halves have been retracted to the left and right: the body of the stomach on the left side and the pyloric part of the stomach and first part of the duodenum on the right. The right kidney forms the posterior wall of the hepatorenal pouch (part of greater sac), and the pancreas lies horizontally on the posterior wall of the main compartment of the omental bursa (lesser sac). The gastrocolic ligament forms the anterior wall and the lower part of the posterior wall of the inferior recess of the omental bursa. The transverse mesocolon forms the upper part of the posterior wall of the inferior recess of the omental bursa.

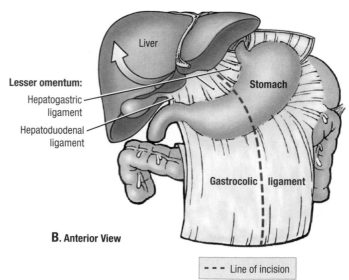

Liver

Lesser omentum:

Hepatogastric ligament

Hepatoduodenal ligament

Stomach

Gastrocolic ligament

B. Anterior View

- - - Line of incision

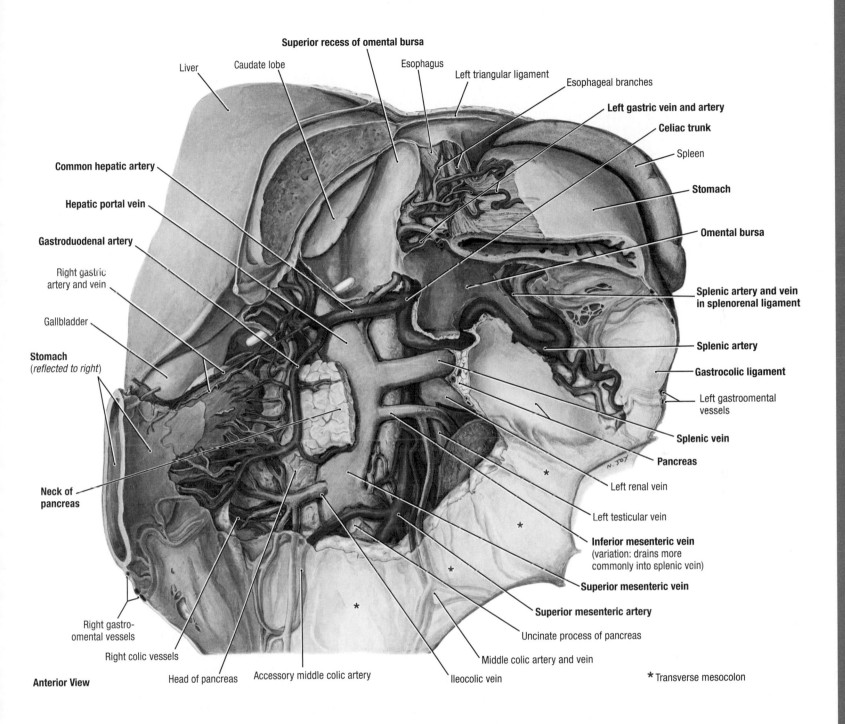

Superior recess of omental bursa

Liver   Caudate lobe   Esophagus

Left triangular ligament

Esophageal branches

Left gastric vein and artery

Celiac trunk

Spleen

Stomach

Common hepatic artery

Hepatic portal vein

Omental bursa

Gastroduodenal artery

Right gastric
artery and vein

**Splenic artery and vein
in splenorenal ligament**

Gallbladder

Splenic artery

Stomach
(reflected to right)

Gastrocolic ligament

Left gastroomental
vessels

Splenic vein

Pancreas

**Neck of
pancreas**

Left renal vein

Left testicular vein

Inferior mesenteric vein
(variation: drains more
commonly into splenic vein)

Superior mesenteric vein

Superior mesenteric artery

Right gastro-
omental vessels

Uncinate process of pancreas

Right colic vessels

Middle colic artery and vein

Head of pancreas   Accessory middle colic artery   Ileocolic vein

* Transverse mesocolon

Anterior View

Posterior Wall of Omental Bursa

4.30

The parietal peritoneum of the posterior wall of the omental bursa has been mostly removed, and a section of the pancreas has been excised. The rod passes through the omental foramen.

- The celiac trunk gives rise to the left gastric artery, the splenic artery that runs tortuously to the left, and the common hepatic artery that runs to the right, passing anterior to the hepatic portal vein.
- The hepatic portal vein is formed posterior to the neck of the pancreas by the union of the superior mesenteric and splenic

veins, with the inferior mesenteric vein joining at or near the angle of union.
- The left testicular vein usually drains into the left renal vein. Both are systemic veins.
- **Inflammation of the parietal peritoneum** can occur due to an enlarged organ or by the escape of fluid from an organ. The area becomes inflamed and causes pain over the affected region.
- **Rebound tenderness** is a pain that is elicited after pressure over the inflamed area is released.

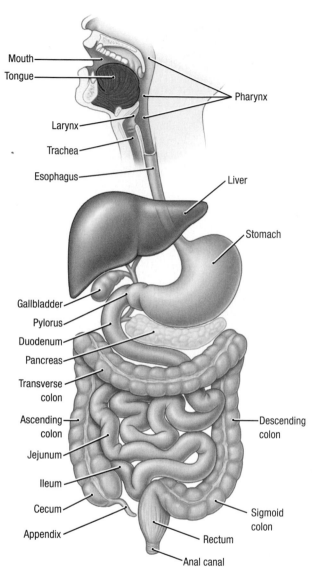

Mouth
Tongue
Pharynx
Larynx
Trachea
Esophagus
Liver
Stomach
Gallbladder
Pylorus
Duodenum
Pancreas
Transverse colon
Ascending colon
Descending colon
Jejunum
Ileum
Cecum
Sigmoid colon
Appendix
Rectum
Anal canal

A. Schematic, Anterior View; Medial View of Bisected Head

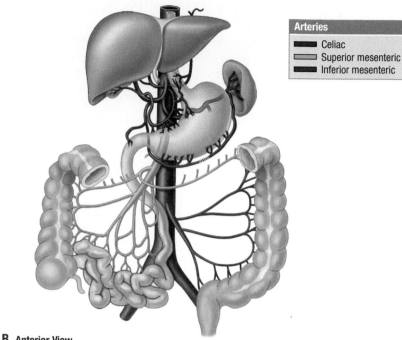

Arteries	
■	Celiac
□	Superior mesenteric
■	Inferior mesenteric

B. Anterior View

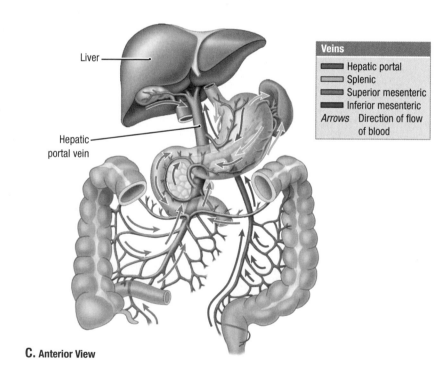

Liver
Hepatic portal vein

Veins	
■	Hepatic portal
□	Splenic
■	Superior mesenteric
■	Inferior mesenteric
Arrows	Direction of flow of blood

C. Anterior View

4.31 **Alimentary System**

A. Overview. The alimentary system extends from the lips to the anus. Associated organs include the liver, gallbladder, and pancreas.

B. Overview of arterial supply. C. Overview of portal venous drainage.

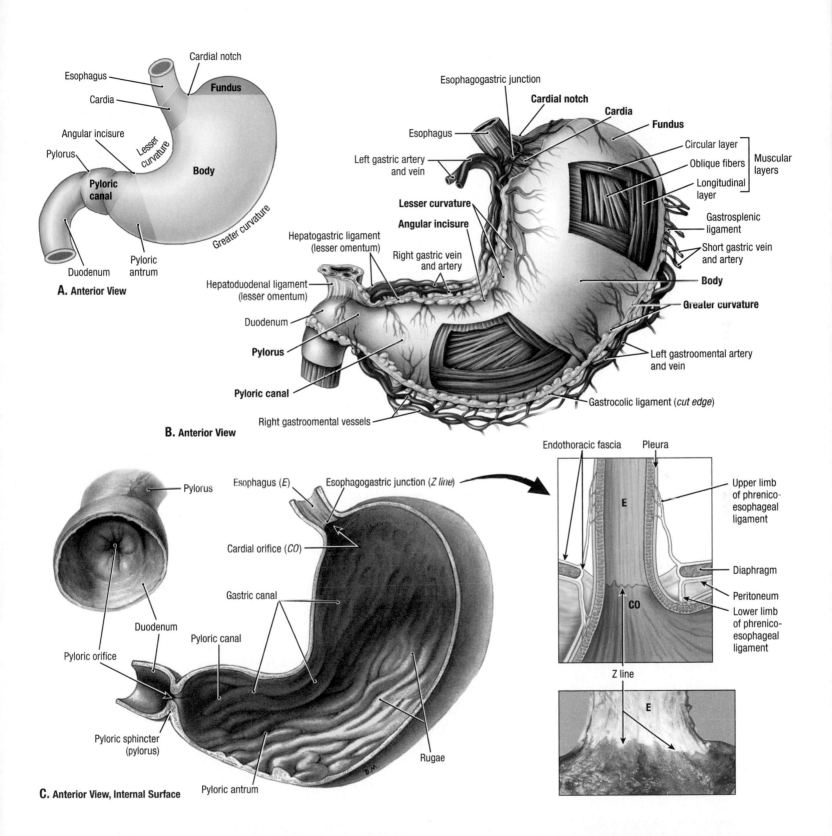

A. Anterior View

- Esophagus
- Cardial notch
- **Fundus**
- Cardia
- Angular incisure
- Pylorus
- Lesser curvature
- **Pyloric canal**
- **Body**
- Greater curvature
- Duodenum
- Pyloric antrum

B. Anterior View

- Esophagogastric junction
- **Cardial notch**
- **Cardia**
- Esophagus
- **Fundus**
- Left gastric artery and vein
- Circular layer
- Oblique fibers
- Longitudinal layer
- Muscular layers
- **Lesser curvature**
- **Angular incisure**
- Gastrosplenic ligament
- Short gastric vein and artery
- Hepatogastric ligament (lesser omentum)
- Right gastric vein and artery
- **Body**
- Hepatoduodenal ligament (lesser omentum)
- **Greater curvature**
- Duodenum
- **Pylorus**
- Left gastroomental artery and vein
- **Pyloric canal**
- Gastrocolic ligament (*cut edge*)
- Right gastroomental vessels

C. Anterior View, Internal Surface

- Pylorus
- Esophagus (*E*)
- Esophagogastric junction (*Z line*)
- Cardial orifice (*CO*)
- Duodenum
- Gastric canal
- Pyloric orifice
- Pyloric canal
- Pyloric sphincter (pylorus)
- Pyloric antrum
- Rugae

- Endothoracic fascia
- Pleura
- E
- Upper limb of phrenico-esophageal ligament
- Diaphragm
- CO
- Peritoneum
- Lower limb of phrenico-esophageal ligament
- Z line
- E

Stomach

A. Parts. B. External surface. C. Internal surface (mucous membrane), anterior wall removed. *Insets*: Left side of page—pylorus, viewed from the duodenum. Right side of page—details of the esophagogastric junction. The Z line is where the stratified squamous epithelium of the esophagus (*light portion in photograph*) changes to the simple columnar epithelium of the stomach (*dark portion*).

4.32

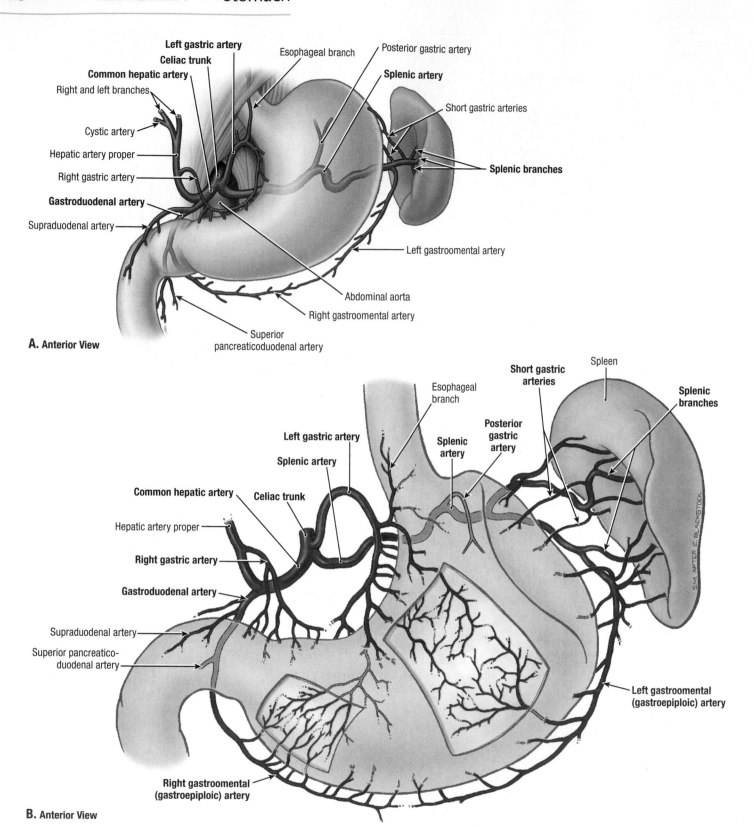

Left gastric artery
Celiac trunk
Common hepatic artery
Right and left branches
Cystic artery
Hepatic artery proper
Right gastric artery
Gastroduodenal artery
Supraduodenal artery
Esophageal branch
Posterior gastric artery
Splenic artery
Short gastric arteries
Splenic branches
Left gastroomental artery
Abdominal aorta
Right gastroomental artery
Superior pancreaticoduodenal artery

A. Anterior View

Esophageal branch
Short gastric arteries
Spleen
Splenic branches
Left gastric artery
Splenic artery
Splenic artery
Posterior gastric artery
Common hepatic artery
Celiac trunk
Hepatic artery proper
Right gastric artery
Gastroduodenal artery
Supraduodenal artery
Superior pancreatico-duodenal artery
Left gastroomental (gastroepiploic) artery
Right gastroomental (gastroepiploic) artery

B. Anterior View

4.33 Celiac Artery

A. Branches of celiac trunk. The celiac trunk is a branch of the abdominal aorta, arising immediately inferior to the aortic hiatus of the diaphragm (T12 vertebral level). The vessel is usually 1 to 2 cm long and divides into the left gastric, common hepatic, and splenic arteries. The celiac trunk supplies the liver, gallbladder, inferior esophagus, stomach, pancreas, spleen, and duodenum.

B. Arteries of stomach and spleen. The serous and muscular coats are removed from two areas of the stomach, revealing anastomotic networks in the submucous coat.

Five main sites where
esophagus is constricted:

1. Junction of pharynx
   and esophagus
   (in neck)

2. Aortic arch

3. Left main bronchus
   (at tracheal bifurcation)

4. Left atrium

5. Esophageal hiatus

POSTERIOR

ANTERIOR

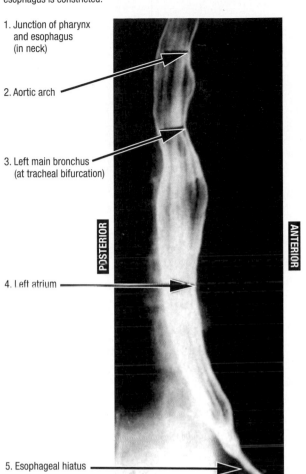

A. Lateral Barium Swallow Radiograph

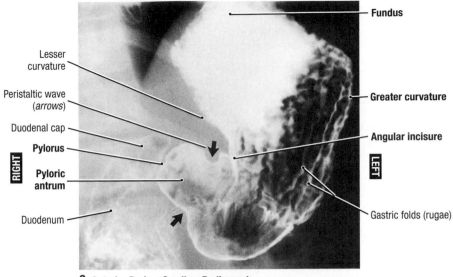

Lesser
curvature

Peristaltic wave
(*arrows*)

Duodenal cap

Pylorus

**Pyloric
antrum**

Duodenum

RIGHT

LEFT

Fundus

Greater curvature

Angular incisure

Gastric folds (rugae)

C. Anterior Barium Swallow Radiograph

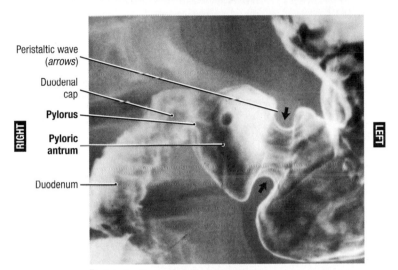

Peristaltic wave
(*arrows*)

Duodenal
cap

Pylorus

**Pyloric
antrum**

Duodenum

RIGHT

LEFT

D. Anterior Barium Swallow Radiograph

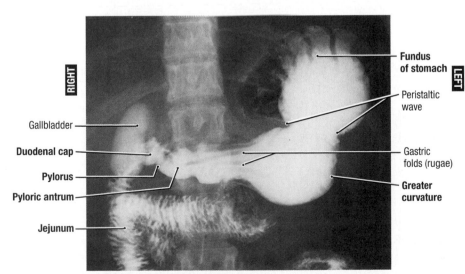

RIGHT

LEFT

Gallbladder

Duodenal cap

Pylorus

Pyloric antrum

Jejunum

**Fundus
of stomach**

Peristaltic
wave

Gastric
folds (rugae)

**Greater
curvature**

B. Anterior Barium Swallow Radiograph

Radiographs of Esophagus, Stomach, and Duodenum (Barium Swallow)

4.34

A. Five sites of normal esophageal constriction.
B. Stomach, small intestine, and gallbladder.
Note additional contrast medium in gallbladder.
C. Stomach and duodenum. **D.** Pyloric antrum
and duodenal cap.

Blockage of esophagus. The impressions
produced in the esophagus by adjacent structures are of clinical interest because of the slower
passage of substances at these sites. The impressions indicate where swallowed foreign objects
are most likely to lodge and where a stricture
may develop, for example, after the accidental
drinking of a caustic liquid, such as lye.

A hiatal (hiatus) hernia is a protrusion of a part
of the stomach into the mediastinum through the
esophageal hiatus of the diaphragm. The hernias
occur most often in people after middle age, possibly because of weakening of the muscular part of the
diaphragm and widening of the esophageal hiatus.

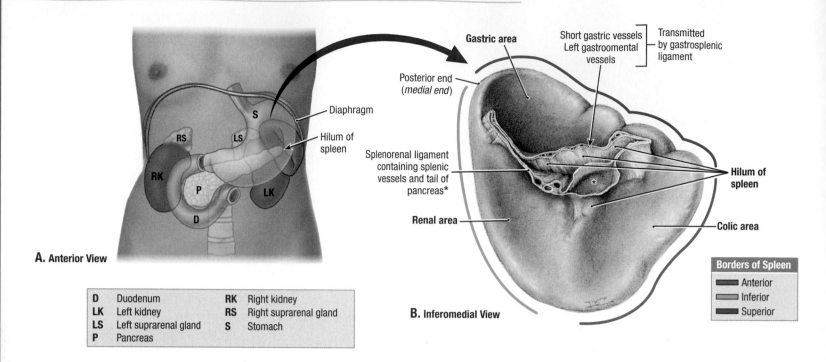

A. Anterior View

D	Duodenum	RK	Right kidney
LK	Left kidney	RS	Right suprarenal gland
LS	Left suprarenal gland	S	Stomach
P	Pancreas		

B. Inferomedial View

Borders of Spleen
- Anterior
- Inferior
- Superior

4.35   Spleen

A. Surface anatomy of spleen. The spleen lies superficially in the left upper abdominal quadrant between the 9th and 11th ribs.
B. Features of spleen. Note the impressions (colic, renal, and gastric areas) made by structures in contact with the spleen's visceral surface. Its superior border is notched.

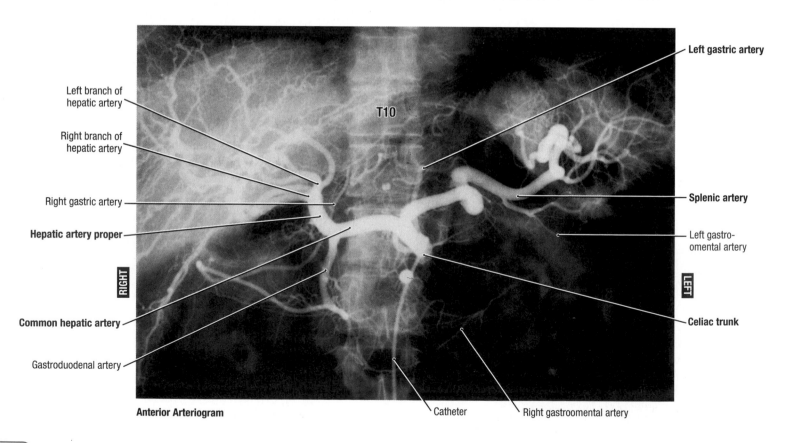

Anterior Arteriogram

4.36   Celiac Arteriogram

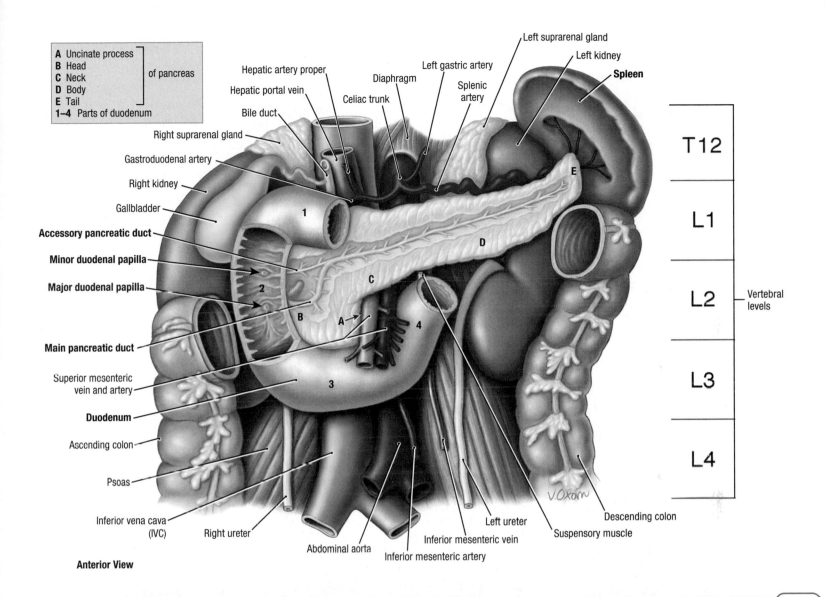

A Uncinate process
B Head
C Neck } of pancreas
D Body
E Tail
1–4 Parts of duodenum

Anterior View

Parts and Relationships of Pancreas and Duodenum **4.37**

Pancreas and duodenum *in situ.*

TABLE 4.5	**Parts and Relationships of Duodenum**					
Part of Duodenum	**Anterior**	**Posterior**	**Medial**	**Superior**	**Inferior**	**Vertebral Level**
Superior (1st) part	Peritoneum Gallbladder Quadrate lobe of liver	Bile duct Gastroduodenal artery Hepatic portal vein IVC		Neck of gallbladder	Neck of pancreas	Anterolateral to L1 vertebra
Descending (2nd) part	Transverse colon Transverse mesocolon Coils of small intestine	Hilum of right kidney Renal vessels Ureter Psoas major	Head of pancreas Pancreatic duct Bile duct			Right of L2–L3 vertebrae
Inferior (horizontal or 3rd) part	Superior mesenteric artery Superior mesenteric vein Coils of small intestine	Right psoas major IVC Aorta Right ureter		Head and uncinate process of pancreas Superior mesenteric artery and vein		Anterior to L3 vertebra
Ascending (4th) part	Beginning of root of mesentery Coils of jejunum	Left psoas major Left margin of aorta	Superior mesenteric artery and vein	Body of pancreas		Left of L3 vertebra

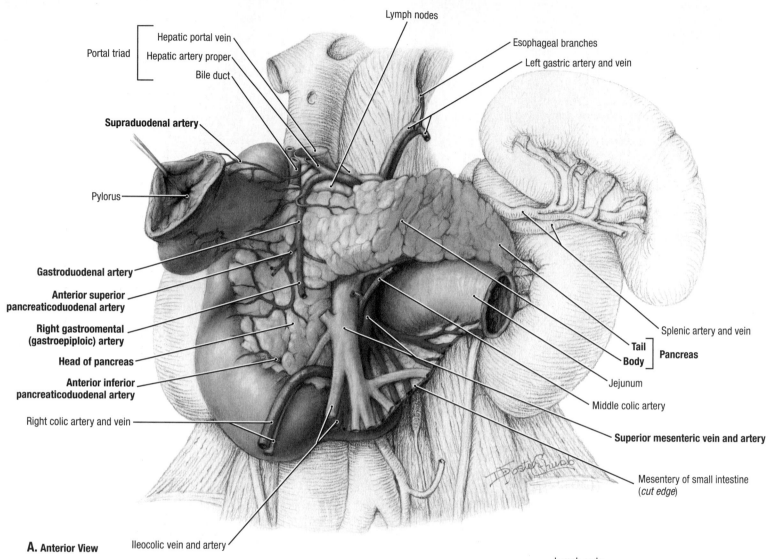

Lymph nodes

Portal triad
- Hepatic portal vein
- Hepatic artery proper
- Bile duct

Esophageal branches

Left gastric artery and vein

Supraduodenal artery

Pylorus

Gastroduodenal artery

Anterior superior pancreaticoduodenal artery

Right gastroomental (gastroepiploic) artery

Head of pancreas

Anterior inferior pancreaticoduodenal artery

Right colic artery and vein

Splenic artery and vein

Tail **Pancreas**
Body

Jejunum

Middle colic artery

Superior mesenteric vein and artery

Mesentery of small intestine (*cut edge*)

A. Anterior View

Ileocolic vein and artery

4.38 **Vascular Relationships of Pancreas and Duodenum**

A. Anterior relationships. The gastroduodenal artery descends anterior to the neck of the pancreas. **B. Posterior relationships.** The splenic artery and vein course on the posterior aspect of the pancreatic tail, which usually extends to the spleen. The pancreas "loops" around the right side of the superior mesenteric vessels so that its neck is anterior, its head is to the right, and its uncinate process is posterior to the vessels. The splenic and superior mesenteric veins unite posterior to the neck to form the hepatic portal vein. The bile duct descends in a fissure (opened up) in the posterior part of the head of the pancreas.

Most inflammatory erosions of the duodenal wall, **duodenal (peptic) ulcers,** are in the posterior wall of the superior (1st) part of the duodenum within 3 cm of the pylorus.

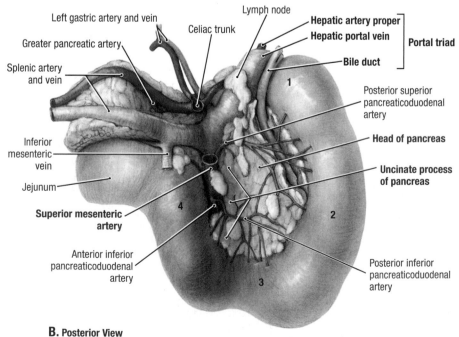

Left gastric artery and vein

Lymph node

Celiac trunk

Hepatic artery proper

Hepatic portal vein **Portal triad**

Bile duct

Greater pancreatic artery

Splenic artery and vein

Posterior superior pancreaticoduodenal artery

Head of pancreas

Uncinate process of pancreas

Inferior mesenteric vein

Jejunum

Superior mesenteric artery

Anterior inferior pancreaticoduodenal artery

Posterior inferior pancreaticoduodenal artery

B. Posterior View

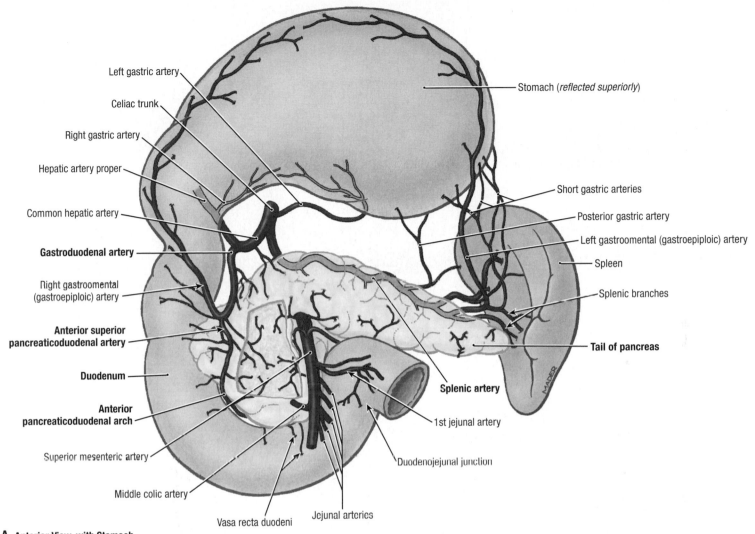

Left gastric artery

Celiac trunk

Right gastric artery

Hepatic artery proper

Common hepatic artery

Gastroduodenal artery

Right gastroomental (gastroepiploic) artery

Anterior superior pancreaticoduodenal artery

Duodenum

Anterior pancreaticoduodenal arch

Superior mesenteric artery

Middle colic artery

Vasa recta duodeni

Jejunal arteries

Stomach (*reflected superiorly*)

Short gastric arteries

Posterior gastric artery

Left gastroomental (gastroepiploic) artery

Spleen

Splenic branches

Tail of pancreas

Splenic artery

1st jejunal artery

Duodenojejunal junction

A. Anterior View, with Stomach Reflected Superiorly

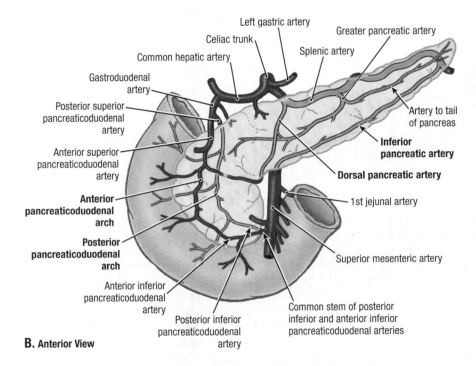

Left gastric artery

Celiac trunk

Common hepatic artery

Gastroduodenal artery

Posterior superior pancreaticoduodenal artery

Anterior superior pancreaticoduodenal artery

Anterior pancreaticoduodenal arch

Posterior pancreaticoduodenal arch

Anterior inferior pancreaticoduodenal artery

Posterior inferior pancreaticoduodenal artery

Greater pancreatic artery

Splenic artery

Artery to tail of pancreas

Inferior pancreatic artery

Dorsal pancreatic artery

1st jejunal artery

Superior mesenteric artery

Common stem of posterior inferior and anterior inferior pancreaticoduodenal arteries

B. Anterior View

Blood Supply to Pancreas, Duodenum, and Spleen

4.39

A. Celiac trunk and superior mesenteric artery.
B. Pancreatic and pancreaticoduodenal arteries.
- The anterior superior pancreaticoduodenal artery from the gastroduodenal artery and the anterior inferior pancreaticoduodenal artery of the superior mesenteric artery form the anterior pancreaticoduodenal arch anterior to the head of the pancreas. The posterior superior and posterior inferior branches of the same two arteries form the posterior pancreaticoduodenal arch posterior to the pancreas. The anterior and posterior inferior arteries often arise from a common stem.
- Arteries supplying the pancreas are derived from the common hepatic artery, gastroduodenal artery, pancreaticoduodenal arches, splenic artery, and superior mesenteric artery.

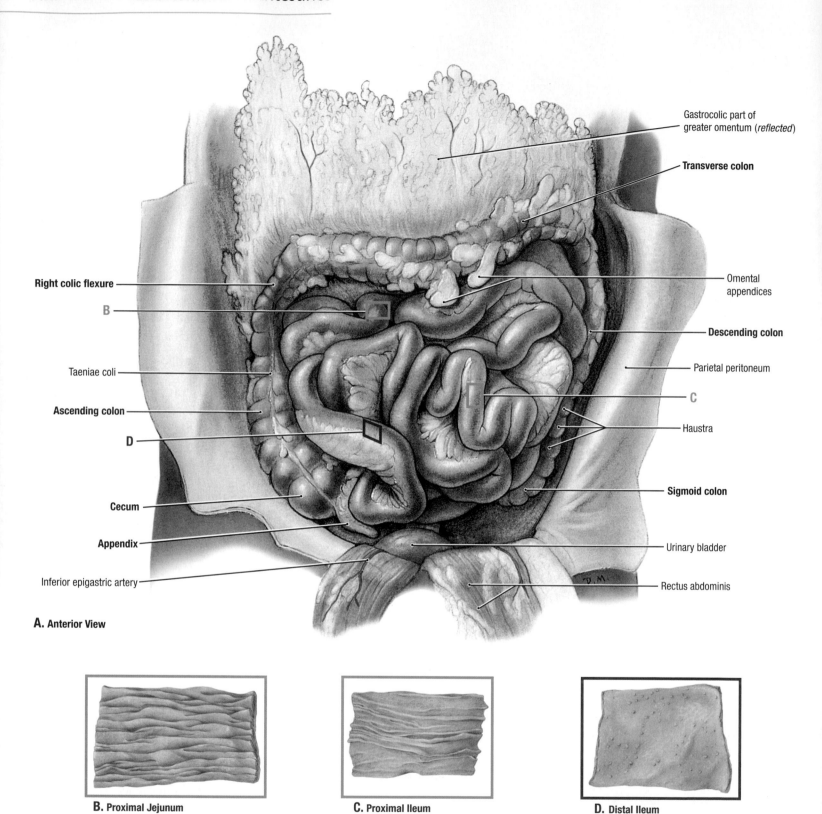

Gastrocolic part of
greater omentum (*reflected*)

Transverse colon

Right colic flexure

B

Omental
appendices

Descending colon

Taeniae coli

Parietal peritoneum

Ascending colon

C

D

Haustra

Cecum

Sigmoid colon

Appendix

Urinary bladder

Inferior epigastric artery

Rectus abdominis

A. Anterior View

B. Proximal Jejunum

C. Proximal Ileum

D. Distal Ileum

4.40   Intestines *In Situ*, Interior of Small Intestine

A. Intestines *in situ*, greater omentum reflected. The ileum
is reflected to expose the appendix. The appendix usually lies
posterior to the cecum (retrocecal) or, as in this case, projects over
the pelvic brim. The features of the large intestines are the taeniae
coli, haustra, and omental appendices. **B. Proximal jejunum.**

The circular folds are tall, closely packed, and commonly branched.
C. Proximal ileum. The circular folds are low and becoming sparse.
The caliber of the gut is reduced, and the wall is thinner. **D. Distal
ileum.** Circular folds are absent, and solitary lymph nodules stud
the wall.

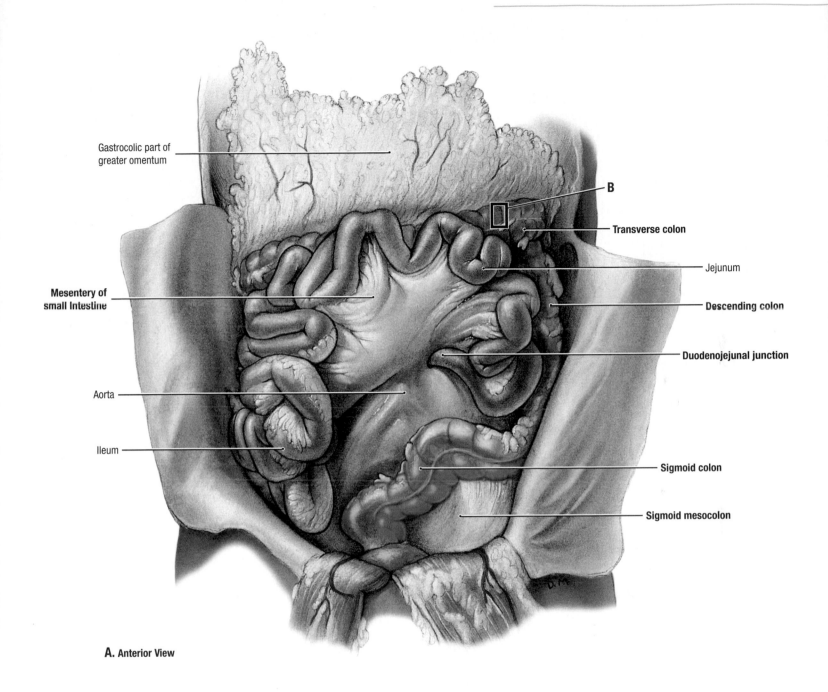

A. Anterior View

Gastrocolic part of greater omentum

Mesentery of small Intestine

Aorta

Ileum

B

Transverse colon

Jejunum

Descending colon

Duodenojejunal junction

Sigmoid colon

Sigmoid mesocolon

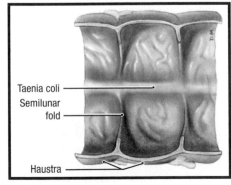

Taenia coli
Semilunar fold

Haustra

B. Transverse Colon

Sigmoid Mesocolon and Mesentery of Small Intestine, Interior of Transverse Colon

4.41

A. Sigmoid mesocolon and mesentery of small intestine.
- The duodenojejunal junction is situated to the left of the median plane.
- The mesentery of the small intestine fans out extensively from its short root to accommodate the length of jejunum and ileum (~6 m).
- The descending colon is the narrowest part of the large intestine and is retroperitoneal. The sigmoid colon has a mesentery, the sigmoid mesocolon; the sigmoid colon is continuous with the rectum at the point at which the sigmoid mesocolon ends.

B. Transverse colon. The semilunar folds and taeniae coli form prominent features on the smooth-surfaced internal wall.

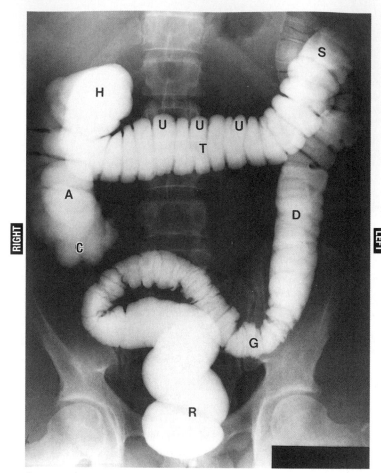

A. Posteroanterior Radiograph

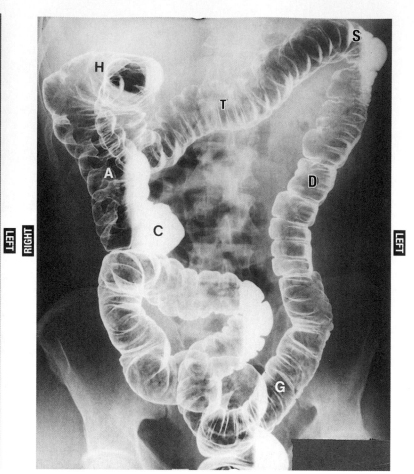

B. Posteroanterior Radiograph

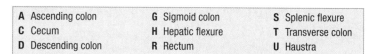

A	Ascending colon	**G**	Sigmoid colon	**S**	Splenic flexure
C	Cecum	**H**	Hepatic flexure	**T**	Transverse colon
D	Descending colon	**R**	Rectum	**U**	Haustra

4.42 Barium Enema and Colonoscopy of Colon

A. Single-contrast study. A barium enema has filled the colon.
B. Double-contrast study. Barium can be seen coating the walls
of the colon, which is distended with air, providing a vivid view
of the mucosal relief and haustra. **C. Endoscopy of colon.** The
interior of the colon can be observed with an elongated endoscope, usually a fiberoptic flexible colonoscope. The endoscope is a tube that inserts into the colon through the anus and
rectum. **D. Diverticulosis of colon.** Photograph taken through
a colonoscope. **E. Illustration of diverticula.** Diverticulosis is
a disorder in which multiple false diverticula (external evagina-
tions or outpocketings of the mucosa of the colon) develop
along the intestine. It primarily affects middle-aged and elderly
people. Diverticulosis is commonly (60%) found in the sigmoid
colon. Diverticula are subject to infection and rupture, leading
to **diverticulitis**, and they can distort and erode the nutrient
arteries, leading to hemorrhage.

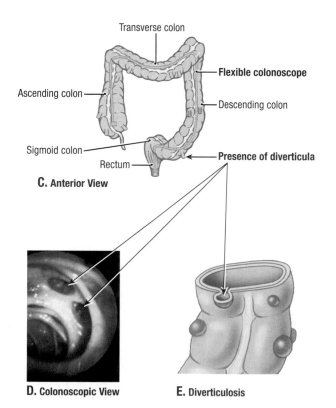

Transverse colon

Flexible colonoscope

Ascending colon

Descending colon

Sigmoid colon

Presence of diverticula

Rectum

C. Anterior View

D. Colonoscopic View

E. Diverticulosis

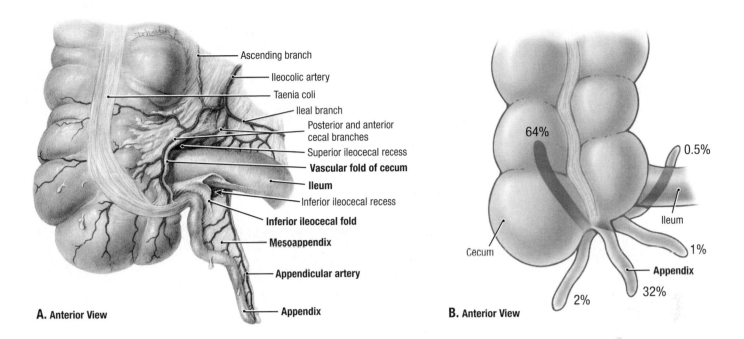

A. Anterior View

Ascending branch
Ileocolic artery
Taenia coli
Ileal branch
Posterior and anterior cecal branches
Superior ileocecal recess
Vascular fold of cecum
Ileum
Inferior ileocecal recess
Inferior ileocecal fold
Mesoappendix
Appendicular artery
Appendix

B. Anterior View

64%
0.5%
Ileum
1%
Appendix
32%
2%
Cecum

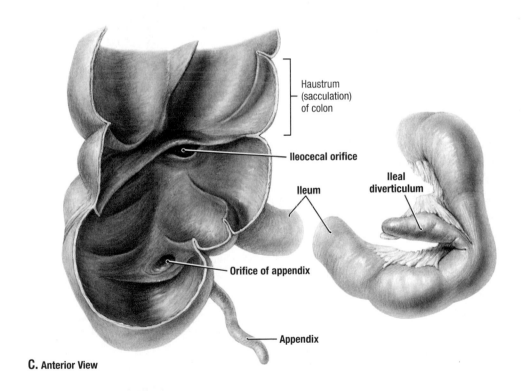

Haustrum (sacculation) of colon
Ileocecal orifice
Ileal diverticulum
Ileum
Orifice of appendix
Appendix

C. Anterior View

Ileocecal Region and Appendix

4.43

A. Blood supply. The appendicular artery is located in the free edge of the mesoappendix. The inferior ileocecal fold is bloodless, whereas the superior ileocecal fold is called the vascular fold of the cecum. **B. Approximate incidence of various positions of appendix. C. Interior of a dried cecum and ileal diverticulum** (of Meckel). This cecum was filled with air until dry, opened, and varnished. **Ileal diverticulum** is a congenital anomaly that occurs in 1% to 2% of persons. It is a pouchlike remnant (3 to 6 cm long) of the proximal part of the yolk stalk, typically within 50 cm of the ileocecal junction. It sometimes becomes inflamed and produces pain that may mimic that produced by appendicitis.

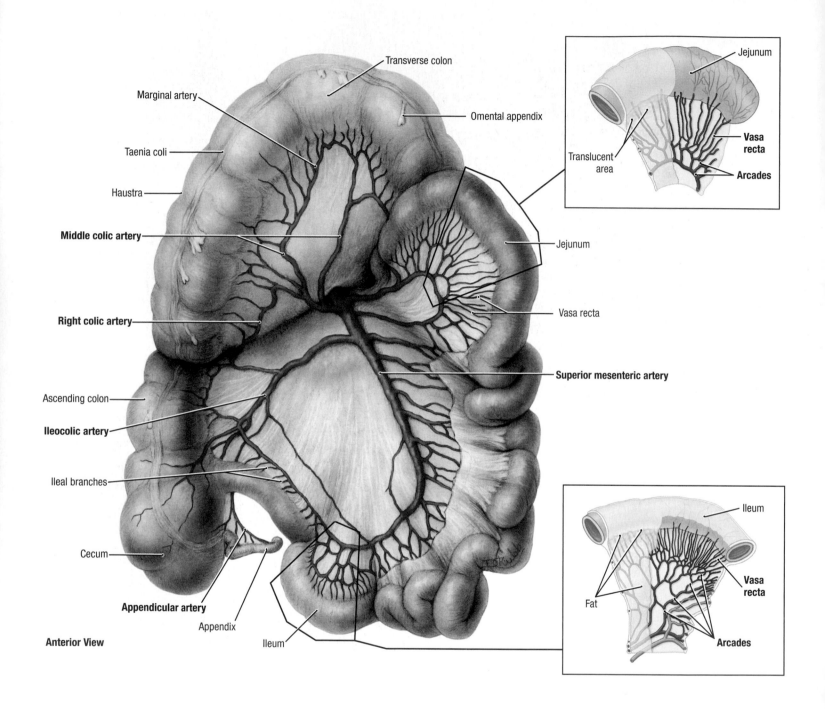

Transverse colon

Marginal artery

Omental appendix

Taenia coli

Haustra

Middle colic artery

Right colic artery

Ascending colon

Ileocolic artery

Ileal branches

Cecum

Appendicular artery

Appendix

Ileum

Anterior View

Jejunum

Translucent area

Vasa recta

Arcades

Jejunum

Vasa recta

Superior mesenteric artery

Ileum

Fat

Vasa recta

Arcades

4.44 Superior Mesenteric Artery and Arterial Arcades

The peritoneum is partially stripped off.
- The superior mesenteric artery ends by anastomosing with one of its own branches, the ileal branch of the ileocolic artery.
- On the *inset drawings* of jejunum and ileum, compare the diameter, thickness of wall, number of arterial arcades, long or short vasa recta, presence of translucent (fat-free) areas at the mesenteric border, and fat encroaching on the wall of the gut between the jejunum and ileum.

- **Acute inflammation of the appendix** is a common cause of an acute abdomen (severe abdominal pain arising suddenly). The pain of appendicitis usually commences as a vague pain in the periumbilical region because afferent pain fibers enter the spinal cord at the T10 level. Later, severe pain in the right lower quadrant results from irritation of the parietal peritoneum lining the posterior abdominal wall.

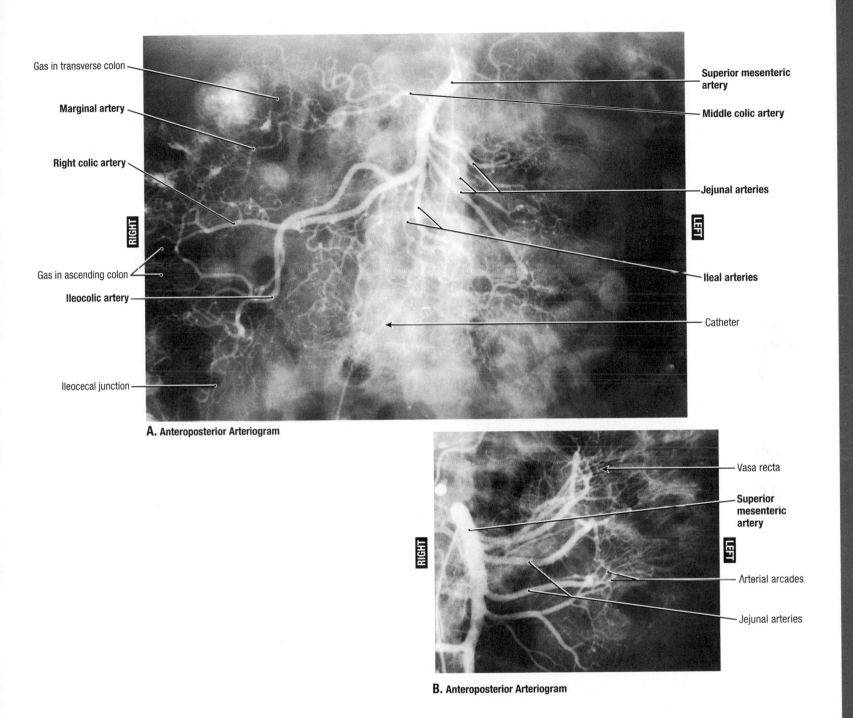

Gas in transverse colon

Marginal artery

Right colic artery

RIGHT

Gas in ascending colon

Ileocolic artery

Ileocecal junction

Superior mesenteric artery

Middle colic artery

Jejunal arteries

LEFT

Ileal arteries

Catheter

A. Anteroposterior Arteriogram

Vasa recta

Superior mesenteric artery

RIGHT

LEFT

Arterial arcades

Jejunal arteries

B. Anteroposterior Arteriogram

4.45

Superior Mesenteric Arteriograms

A. Branches of superior mesenteric artery. (Consult Fig. 4.44 to identify the branches.) **B. Enlargement to show jejunal arteries, arterial arcades, and vasa recta.**

- The branches of the superior mesenteric artery include, from its left side, 12 or more jejunal and ileal arteries that anastomose to form arcades from which vasa recta pass to the small intestine and, from its right side, the middle colic, ileocolic, and commonly (but not here) an independent right colic artery that anastomose to form a marginal artery that parallels the mesenteric border at the colon and from which vasa recta pass to the large intestine.

- **Occlusion of the vasa recta** by emboli results in ischemia of the part of the intestine concerned. If the ischemia is severe, necrosis of the involved segment results and ileus (obstruction of the intestine) of the paralytic type occurs. Ileus is accompanied by a severe colicky pain, along with abdominal distension, vomiting, and often fever and dehydration. If the condition is diagnosed early (e.g., using a superior mesenteric arteriogram), the obstructed part of the vessel may be cleared surgically.

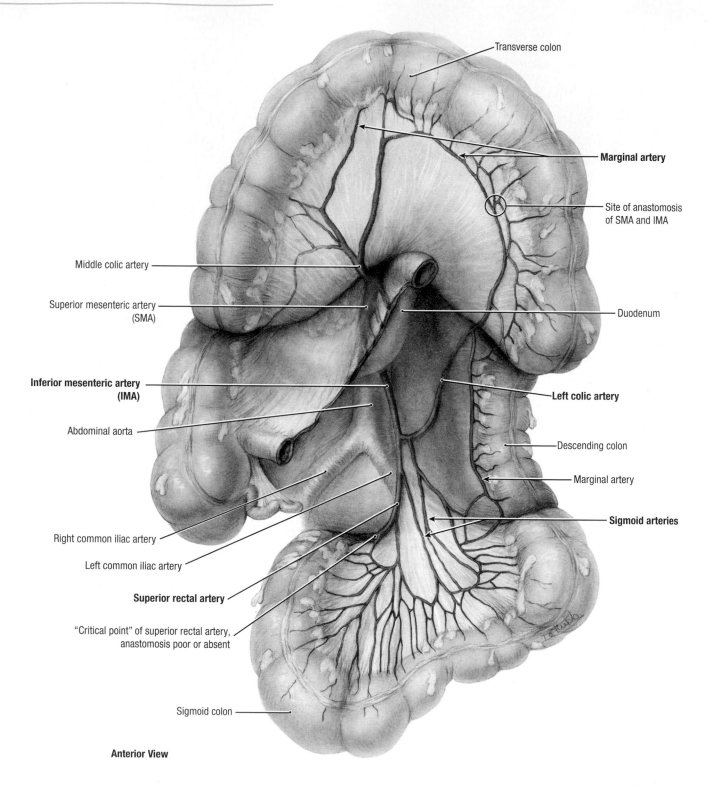

Transverse colon

Marginal artery

Site of anastomosis
of SMA and IMA

Middle colic artery

Superior mesenteric artery
(SMA)

Duodenum

**Inferior mesenteric artery
(IMA)**

Left colic artery

Abdominal aorta

Descending colon

Marginal artery

Right common iliac artery

Sigmoid arteries

Left common iliac artery

Superior rectal artery

"Critical point" of superior rectal artery,
anastomosis poor or absent

Sigmoid colon

Anterior View

4.46 **Inferior Mesenteric Artery**

The mesentery of the small intestine has been cut at its root.
- The inferior mesenteric artery arises posterior to the ascending part of the duodenum, about 4 cm superior to the bifurcation of the aorta; on crossing the left common iliac artery, it becomes the superior rectal artery.
- The branches of the inferior mesenteric artery include the left colic artery and several sigmoid arteries; the inferior two sigmoid arteries branch from the superior rectal artery.

- The point at which the last sigmoidal artery branches from the superior rectal artery is known as the "critical point" of the superior rectal artery; distal to this point, there are poor or no anastomotic connections between the superior rectal artery and the marginal artery.

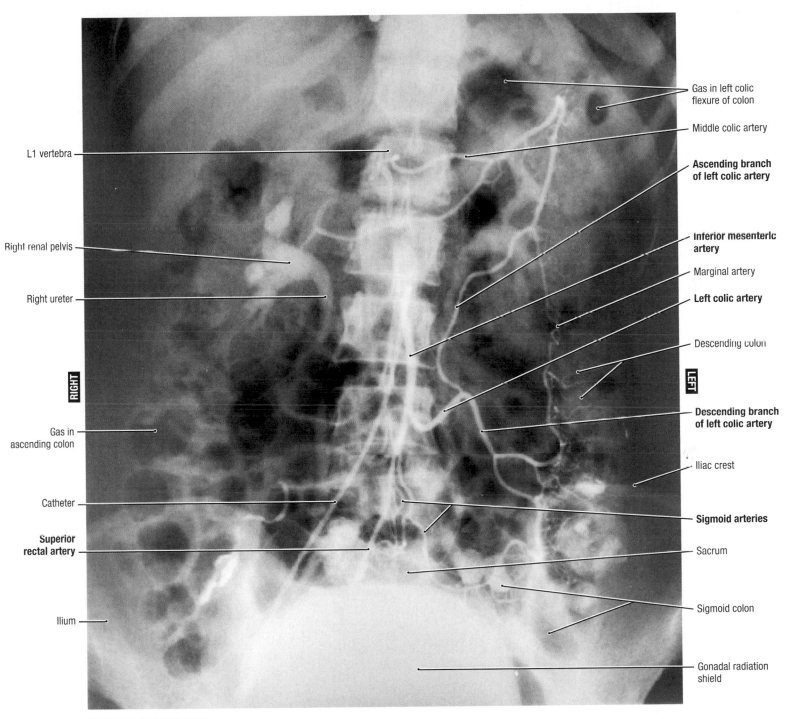

L1 vertebra

Right renal pelvis

Right ureter

RIGHT

Gas in ascending colon

Catheter

Superior rectal artery

Ilium

Gas in left colic flexure of colon

Middle colic artery

Ascending branch of left colic artery

Inferior mesenteric artery

Marginal artery

Left colic artery

Descending colon

LEFT

Descending branch of left colic artery

Iliac crest

Sigmoid arteries

Sacrum

Sigmoid colon

Gonadal radiation shield

Posteroanterior Arteriogram

Inferior Mesenteric Arteriogram

4.47

- The left colic artery courses to the left toward the descending colon and splits into ascending and descending branches.
- The sigmoid arteries, two to four in number, supply the sigmoid colon.
- The superior rectal artery, which is the continuation of the inferior mesenteric artery, supplies the rectum; the superior rectal anastomoses are formed by branches of the middle and inferior rectal arteries (from the internal iliac artery).

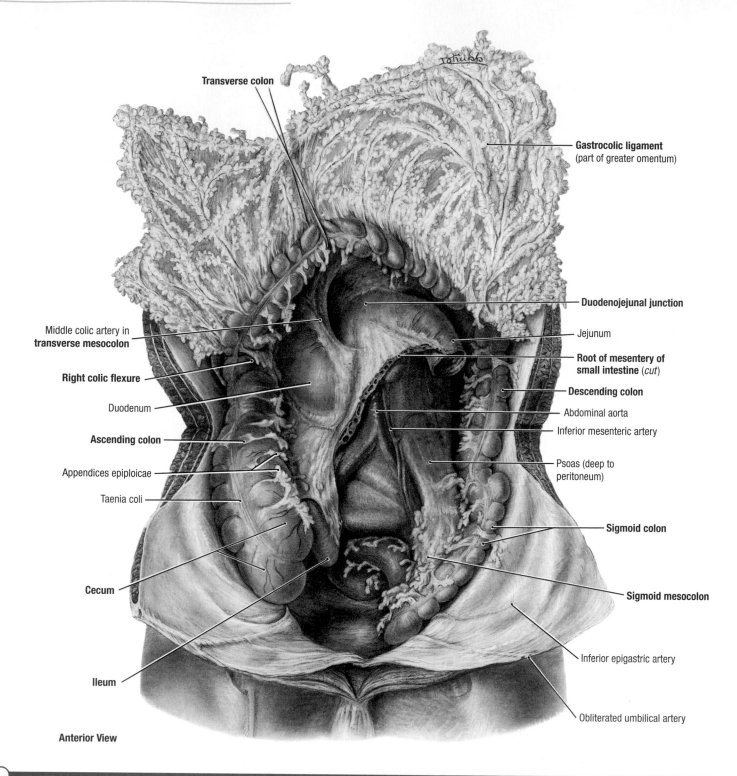

Transverse colon

Gastrocolic ligament
(part of greater omentum)

Middle colic artery in
transverse mesocolon

Duodenojejunal junction

Jejunum

Root of mesentery of
small intestine (*cut*)

Descending colon

Abdominal aorta

Inferior mesenteric artery

Right colic flexure

Duodenum

Ascending colon

Psoas (deep to
peritoneum)

Appendices epiploicae

Taenia coli

Sigmoid colon

Cecum

Sigmoid mesocolon

Inferior epigastric artery

Ileum

Obliterated umbilical artery

Anterior View

| **4.48** | **Peritoneum of Posterior Abdominal Cavity** |

The gastrocolic ligament is retracted superiorly, along with the transverse colon and transverse mesocolon. The appendix had been surgically removed. This dissection is continued in Figure 4.49.

- The root of the mesentery of the small intestine, approximately 15 to 20 cm in length, extends between the duodenojejunal junction and ileocecal junction.
- The large intestine forms 3½ sides of a square, "framing" the jejunum and ileum. On the right are the cecum and ascending colon,

superior is the transverse colon, on the left is the descending and sigmoid colon, and inferiorly is the sigmoid colon.

- **Chronic inflammation of the colon (ulcerative colitis, Crohn disease)** is characterized by severe inflammation and ulceration of the colon and rectum. In some patients, a colectomy is performed, during which the terminal ileum and colon as well as the rectum and anal canal are removed. An ileostomy is then constructed to establish an artificial cutaneous opening between the ileum and the skin of the anterolateral abdominal wall.

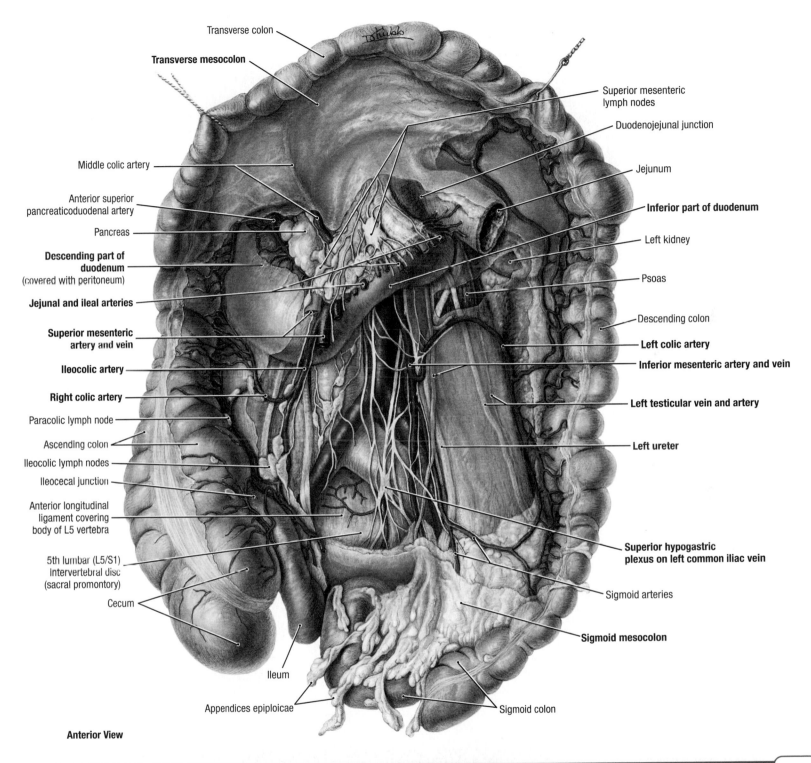

Transverse colon

Transverse mesocolon

Middle colic artery

Anterior superior
pancreaticoduodenal artery

Pancreas

**Descending part of
duodenum**
(covered with peritoneum)

Jejunal and ileal arteries

**Superior mesenteric
artery and vein**

Ileocolic artery

Right colic artery

Paracolic lymph node

Ascending colon

Ileocolic lymph nodes

Ileocecal junction

Anterior longitudinal
ligament covering
body of L5 vertebra

5th lumbar (L5/S1)
intervertebral disc
(sacral promontory)

Cecum

Ileum

Appendices epiploicae

Superior mesenteric
lymph nodes

Duodenojejunal junction

Jejunum

Inferior part of duodenum

Left kidney

Psoas

Descending colon

Left colic artery

Inferior mesenteric artery and vein

Left testicular vein and artery

Left ureter

**Superior hypogastric
plexus on left common iliac vein**

Sigmoid arteries

Sigmoid mesocolon

Sigmoid colon

Anterior View

Posterior Abdominal Cavity with Peritoneum Removed

4.49

The jejunal and ileal branches (cut) pass from the left side of the
superior mesenteric artery. The right colic artery here is a branch of
the ileocolic artery. This is the same specimen as in Figure 4.48.

- The duodenum is larger in diameter before crossing the superior
  mesenteric vessels and narrow afterward.
- On the right side, there are lymph nodes on the colon, paracolic
  nodes beside the colon, and nodes along the ileocolic artery, which
  drain into superior mesenteric nodes anterior to the pancreas.

- The intestines and intestinal vessels lie on a resectable plane
  (remnant of the embryological dorsal mesentery) anterior to that
  of the testicular vessels; these, in turn, lie anterior to the plane of
  the kidney, its vessels, and the ureter.
- The superior hypogastric plexus lies inferior to the bifurcation
  of the aorta and anterior to the left common iliac vein, the
  body of the L5–S1 lumbar vertebra, and the 5th intervertebral
  disc.

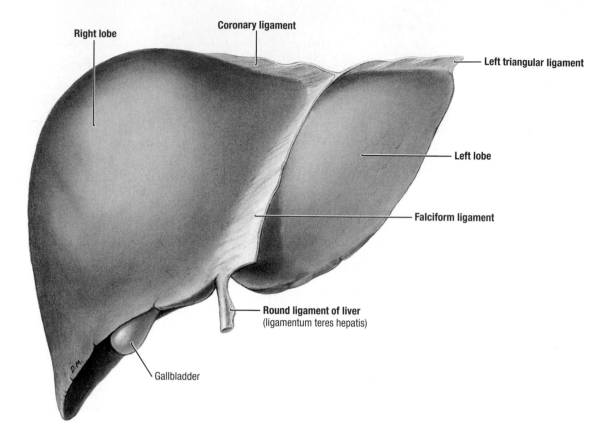

Right lobe

Coronary ligament

Left triangular ligament

Left lobe

Falciform ligament

Round ligament of liver
(ligamentum teres hepatis)

Gallbladder

A. Anterior View

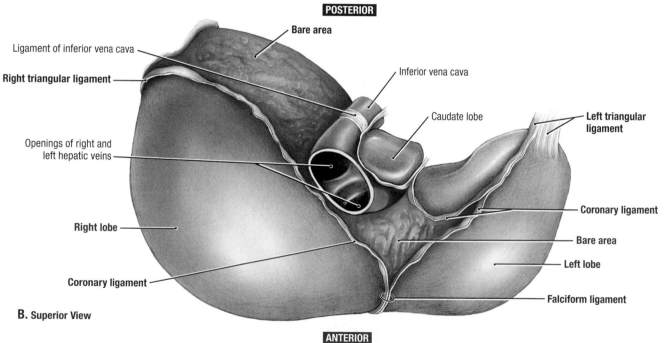

POSTERIOR

Bare area

Ligament of inferior vena cava

Right triangular ligament

Openings of right and
left hepatic veins

Inferior vena cava

Caudate lobe

**Left triangular
ligament**

Right lobe

Coronary ligament

Bare area

Left lobe

Coronary ligament

Falciform ligament

B. Superior View

ANTERIOR

4.50 **Diaphragmatic (Anterior and Superior) Surface of Liver**

A. Anterior surface of liver. The falciform ligament has been severed
close to its attachment to the diaphragm and anterior abdominal
wall. It demarcates the right and left lobes of the liver. The round ligament of the liver lies within the free edge of the falciform ligament.

B. Superior surface of liver. The two layers of peritoneum that form
the falciform ligament separate over the superior aspect (surrounding
the bare area) of the liver to form the superior layer of the coronary
ligament and the right and left triangular ligaments.

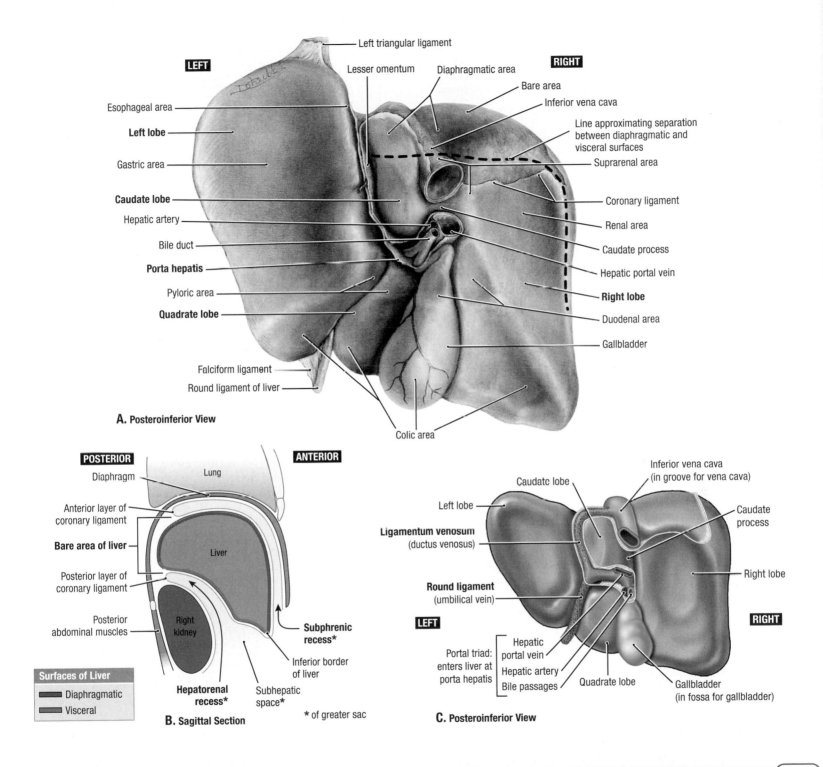

Left triangular ligament

LEFT

Esophageal area

Left lobe

Gastric area

Caudate lobe

Hepatic artery

Bile duct

Porta hepatis

Pyloric area

Quadrate lobe

Lesser omentum

Diaphragmatic area

RIGHT

Bare area

Inferior vena cava

Line approximating separation between diaphragmatic and visceral surfaces

Suprarenal area

Coronary ligament

Renal area

Caudate process

Hepatic portal vein

Right lobe

Duodenal area

Gallbladder

Falciform ligament

Round ligament of liver

A. Posteroinferior View

Colic area

POSTERIOR

Diaphragm

Lung

ANTERIOR

Anterior layer of coronary ligament

Bare area of liver

Posterior layer of coronary ligament

Liver

Posterior abdominal muscles

Right kidney

Subphrenic recess*

Inferior border of liver

Surfaces of Liver

■ Diaphragmatic
■ Visceral

Hepatorenal recess*

Subhepatic space***

* of greater sac

B. Sagittal Section

Caudate lobe

Left lobe

Ligamentum venosum
(ductus venosus)

Round ligament
(umbilical vein)

LEFT

Portal triad: enters liver at porta hepatis

Inferior vena cava (in groove for vena cava)

Caudate process

Right lobe

RIGHT

Hepatic portal vein

Hepatic artery

Bile passages

Quadrate lobe

Gallbladder (in fossa for gallbladder)

C. Posteroinferior View

4.51

Visceral (Posteroinferior) Surface of Liver

A. Isolated specimen demonstrating lobes and impressions of adjacent viscera. **B.** Hepatic surfaces and peritoneal recesses. **C.** Round ligament of liver and ligamentum venosum. The round ligament of liver includes the obliterated remains of the umbilical vein that carried well-oxygenated blood from the placenta to the fetus. The ligamentum venosum is the fibrous remnant of the fetal ductus venosus that shunted blood from the umbilical vein to the inferior vena cava by passing the liver. Hepatic tissue may be obtained for diagnostic purposes by **liver biopsy**. The needle puncture is commonly made through the right 10th intercostal space in the midaxillary line. Before the physician takes the biopsy, the person is asked to hold his or her breath in full expiration to minimize the costodiaphragmatic recess and to lessen the possibility of damaging the lung and contaminating the pleural cavity.

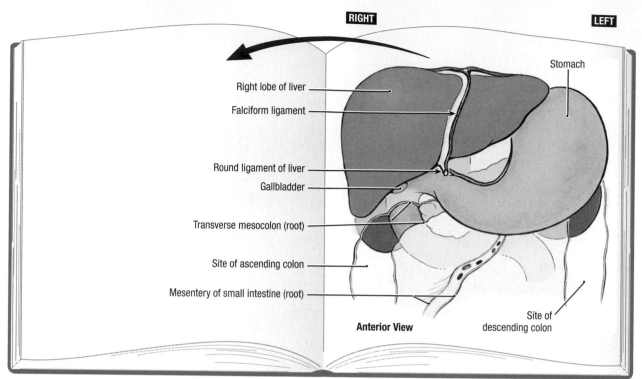

RIGHT LEFT

A. Open Book View

Stomach

Right lobe of liver

Falciform ligament

Round ligament of liver

Gallbladder

Transverse mesocolon (root)

Site of ascending colon

Mesentery of small intestine (root)

Site of descending colon

Anterior View

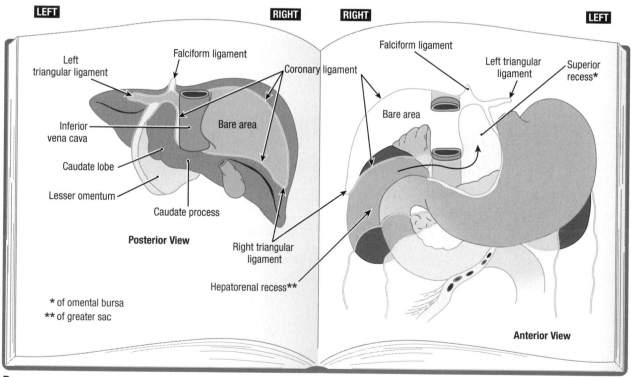

LEFT RIGHT RIGHT LEFT

Left triangular ligament

Falciform ligament

Coronary ligament

Falciform ligament

Left triangular ligament

Superior recess*

Bare area

Inferior vena cava

Bare area

Caudate lobe

Lesser omentum

Caudate process

Posterior View

Right triangular ligament

Hepatorenal recess**

* of omental bursa
** of greater sac

Anterior View

B. Open Book View

4.52 **Liver and Its Posterior Relations, Schematic**

A. Liver *in situ*. The jejunum, ileum, and the ascending, transverse, and descending colons have been removed. **B. Liver reflected showing its posterior relations.** The liver is drawn schematically on a page in a book, so that as the page is turned (*arrow* in *Part A*), the liver is reflected to the right to reveal its posterior surface, and on the facing page, the posterior relations that compose the bed of the liver are viewed. The *arrow* in *Part B* traverses the omental (epiploic) foramen to enter the omental bursa and its superior recess (*arrowhead*).

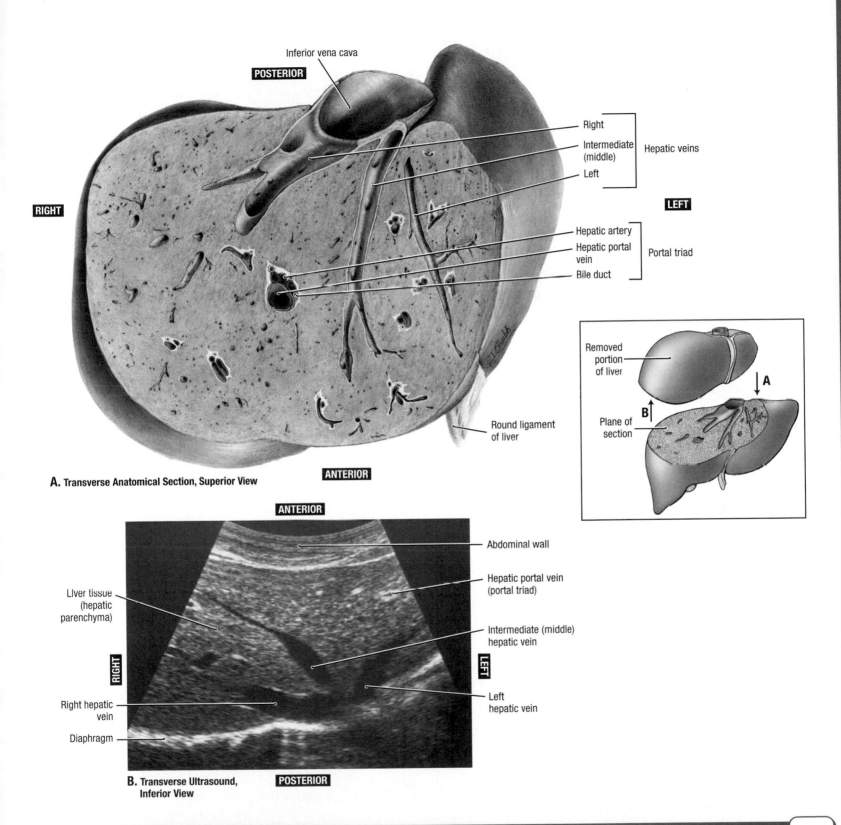

Inferior vena cava

POSTERIOR

Right
Intermediate (middle)
Left
} Hepatic veins

RIGHT

LEFT

Hepatic artery
Hepatic portal vein
Bile duct
} Portal triad

Round ligament of liver

A. Transverse Anatomical Section, Superior View

ANTERIOR

Removed portion of liver

Plane of section

A

B

ANTERIOR

Abdominal wall

Hepatic portal vein (portal triad)

Liver tissue (hepatic parenchyma)

Intermediate (middle) hepatic vein

RIGHT

LEFT

Right hepatic vein

Left hepatic vein

Diaphragm

B. Transverse Ultrasound, Inferior View

POSTERIOR

Hepatic Veins

4.53

A. Approximately horizontal section of liver with posterior aspect at top of page. Note the multiple perivascular fibrous capsules sectioned throughout the cut surface, each containing a portal triad (the hepatic portal vein, hepatic artery, bile ductules) plus lymph vessels. Interdigitating with these are branches of the three main hepatic veins (right, intermediate, and left), which, unaccompanied and lacking capsules, converge on the inferior vena cava. **B. Ultrasound scan.** The transducer was placed under the costal margin and directed posteriorly, producing an inverted image (*Part A*).

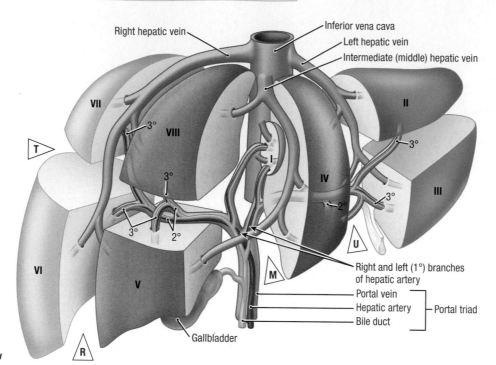

Right hepatic vein
Inferior vena cava
Left hepatic vein
Intermediate (middle) hepatic vein

VII
VIII
II
3°
3°
T
I
IV
III
3°
3°
3°
1° 2°
3°
2°
2°
U
VI
V
M
R

M Main portal fissure
R Right portal fissure
T Transverse hepatic plane
U Umbilical fissure
2° Secondary branches of portal triad structures
3° Tertiary branches of portal triad structures

Right and left (1°) branches of hepatic artery
Portal vein
Hepatic artery
Bile duct
Portal triad
Gallbladder

A. Anterior View

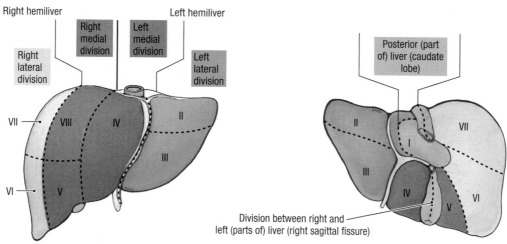

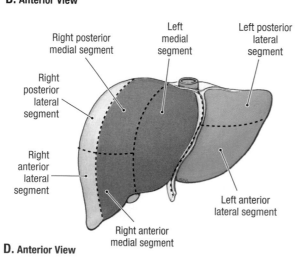

Right hemiliver   Left hemiliver

Right medial division   Left medial division

Right lateral division   Left lateral division

VII   VIII   IV   II

III

VI   V

B. Anterior View

Posterior (part of) liver (caudate lobe)

II   VII
I
III   VI
IV   V

Division between right and left (parts of) liver (right sagittal fissure)

C. Posteroinferior View

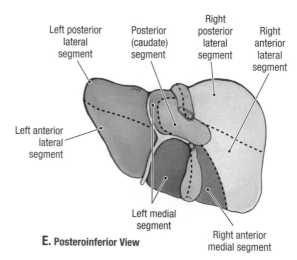

Right posterior medial segment   Left medial segment   Left posterior lateral segment

Right posterior lateral segment

Right anterior lateral segment

Right anterior medial segment

Left anterior lateral segment

D. Anterior View

Left posterior lateral segment   Posterior (caudate) segment   Right posterior lateral segment   Right anterior lateral segment

Left anterior lateral segment

Left medial segment

Right anterior medial segment

E. Posteroinferior View

4.54   **Hepatic Segmentation**

Hepatic Segmentation *(continued)* 4.54

Each segment is supplied by a secondary or tertiary branch of the hepatic artery, bile duct, and portal vein. The hepatic veins interdigitate between the portal triads and are intersegmental in that they drain adjacent segments. Since the right and left hepatic arteries and ducts and branches of the right and left portal veins do not communicate, it is possible to perform **hepatic lobectomies** (removal of the right or left part of the liver) and **segmentectomies**. Each segment can be identified numerically or by name (Table 4.6).

TABLE 4.6	Schema of Terminology for Subdivisions of Liver						
Anatomical Term	**Right Lobe**			**Left Lobe**		**Caudate Lobe**	
Functional/ surgical term[a]	Right (part of) liver [Right portal lobe[b]]			Left (part of) liver [Left portal lobe[c]]		Posterior (part of) liver	
	Right lateral division	Right medial division		Left medial division	Left lateral division	[Right caudate lobe[b]]	[Left caudate lobe[c]]
	Posterior lateral segment **Segment VII** [Posterior superior area]	Posterior medial segment **Segment VIII** [Anterior superior area]	[Medial superior area]		Lateral segment **Segment II** [Lateral superior area]	Posterior segment **Segment I**	
	Right anterior lateral segment **Segment VI** [Posterior inferior area]	Anterior medial segment **Segment V** [Anterior inferior area]	Left medial segment **Segment IV** [Medial inferior area = quadrate lobe]		Left anterior lateral segment **Segment III** [Lateral inferior area]		

[a]The labels in the table and figure above reflect the *Terminologia Anatomica: International Anatomical Terminology.* Previous terminology is in brackets.
[b,c]Under the schema of the previous terminology, the caudate lobe was divided into right and left halves, and [b]the right half of the caudate lobe was considered a subdivision of the right portal lobe; [c]the left half of the caudate lobe was considered a subdivision of the left portal lobe.

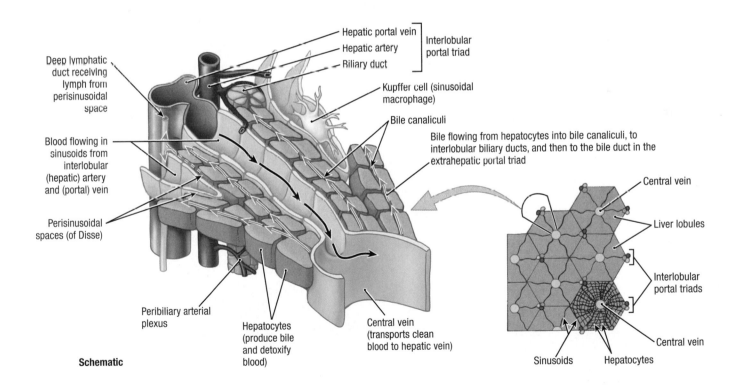

Deep lymphatic duct receiving lymph from perisinusoidal space

Blood flowing in sinusoids from interlobular (hepatic) artery and (portal) vein

Perisinusoidal spaces (of Disse)

Peribiliary arterial plexus

Hepatocytes (produce bile and detoxify blood)

Central vein (transports clean blood to hepatic vein)

Schematic

Hepatic portal vein
Hepatic artery
Biliary duct
} Interlobular portal triad

Kupffer cell (sinusoidal macrophage)

Bile canaliculi

Bile flowing from hepatocytes into bile canaliculi, to interlobular biliary ducts, and then to the bile duct in the extrahepatic portal triad

Central vein

Liver lobules

Interlobular portal triads

Central vein

Sinusoids   Hepatocytes

Flow of Blood and Bile in Liver 4.55

This small part of a liver lobule shows the components of the interlobular portal triad and the positioning of the sinusoids and bile canaliculi. The cut surface of the liver shows the hexagonal pattern of the lobules.

- With the exception of lipids, every substance absorbed by the alimentary tract is received first by the liver via the hepatic portal vein. In addition to its many metabolic activities, the liver stores glycogen and secretes bile.
- There is progressive destruction of hepatocytes in **cirrhosis of the liver** and replacement of them by fibrous tissue. This tissue surrounds the intrahepatic blood vessels and biliary ducts, making the liver firm and impeding circulation of blood through it.

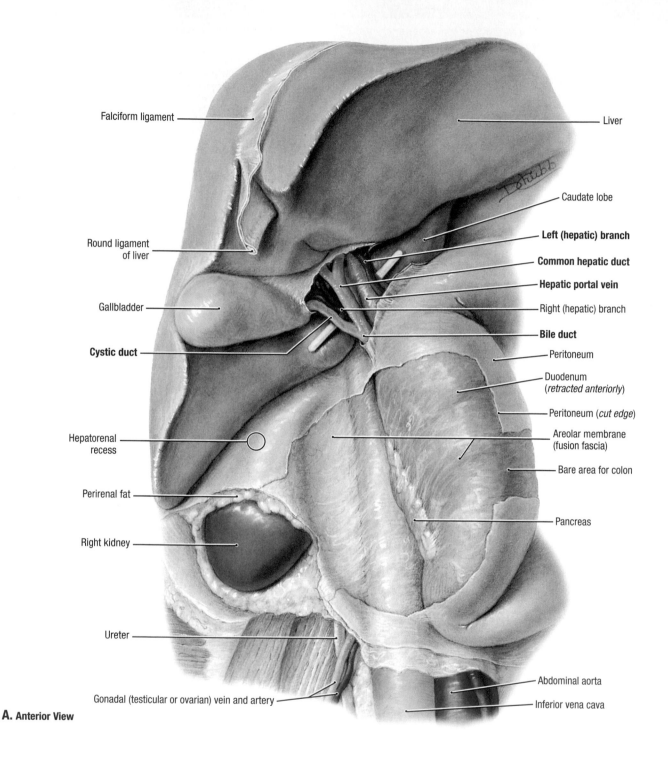

Falciform ligament

Liver

Caudate lobe

Left (hepatic) branch

Common hepatic duct

Round ligament
of liver

Hepatic portal vein

Right (hepatic) branch

Gallbladder

Bile duct

Cystic duct

Peritoneum

Duodenum
(*retracted anteriorly*)

Peritoneum (*cut edge*)

Hepatorenal
recess

Areolar membrane
(fusion fascia)

Bare area for colon

Perirenal fat

Pancreas

Right kidney

Ureter

Abdominal aorta

Gonadal (testicular or ovarian) vein and artery

Inferior vena cava

A. Anterior View

4.56   **Exposure of Portal Triad in Hepatoduodenal Ligament**

A. Anterior view of portal triad with duodenum retracted anteriorly. The hepatoduodenal ligament (hepatic pedicle) includes the portal triad consisting of the hepatic portal vein (posteriorly), the hepatic artery proper (ascending from the left), and the bile passages (descending to the right). Here, the hepatic artery proper is replaced by a left hepatic branch, arising directly from the common hepatic artery, and a right hepatic branch, arising from the superior mesenteric artery (a common variation). A rod traverses the omental (epiploic) foramen. The lesser omentum and transverse colon are removed, and the peritoneum is cut along the right border of the duodenum; this part of the duodenum is retracted anteriorly. The space opened up reveals two smooth areolar membranes (fusion fascia) normally applied to each other that are vestiges of the embryonic peritoneum originally covering these surfaces.

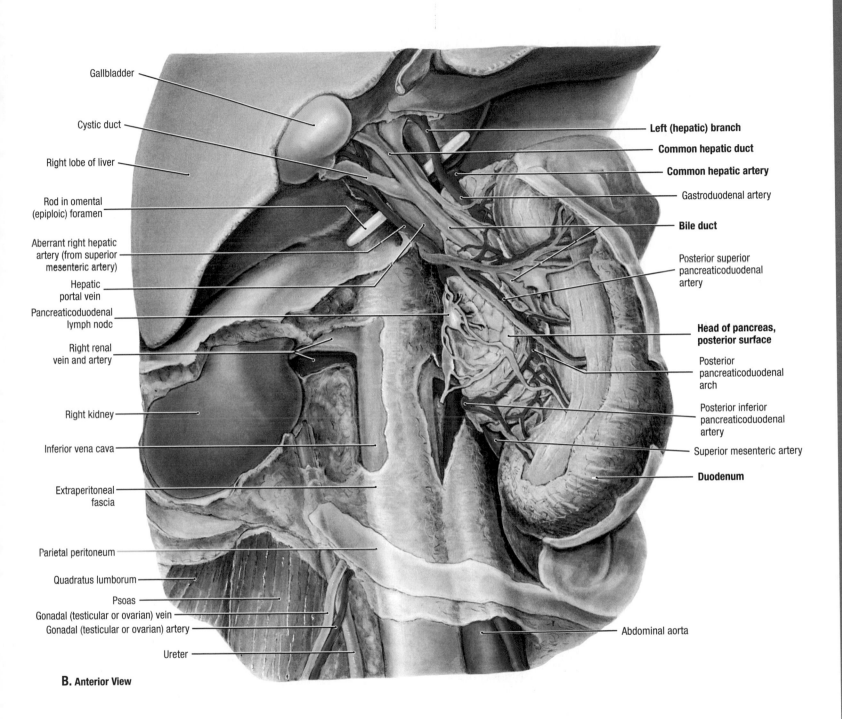

Gallbladder

Cystic duct

Right lobe of liver

Rod in omental
(epiploic) foramen

Aberrant right hepatic
artery (from superior
mesenteric artery)

Hepatic
portal vein

Pancreaticoduodenal
lymph node

Right renal
vein and artery

Right kidney

Inferior vena cava

Extraperitoneal
fascia

Parietal peritoneum

Quadratus lumborum

Psoas

Gonadal (testicular or ovarian) vein
Gonadal (testicular or ovarian) artery

Ureter

Left (hepatic) branch

Common hepatic duct

Common hepatic artery

Gastroduodenal artery

Bile duct

Posterior superior
pancreaticoduodenal
artery

**Head of pancreas,
posterior surface**

Posterior
pancreaticoduodenal
arch

Posterior inferior
pancreaticoduodenal
artery

Superior mesenteric artery

Duodenum

Abdominal aorta

B. Anterior View

Exposure of Portal Triad in Hepatoduodenal Ligament (continued)   4.56

B. Deep relationships of portal triad to surrounding viscera and vessels. Continuing the dissection, the secondarily retroperitoneal viscera (duodenum and head of the pancreas) are retracted anteriorly and to the left. The areolar membrane (fusion fascia) covering the posterior aspect of the pancreas and duodenum is largely removed, and that covering the anterior aspect of the great vessels is partly removed.

A common method for **reducing portal hypertension** is to divert blood from the portal venous system to the systemic venous system by creating a communication between the portal vein and the inferior vena cava (IVC). This **portacaval anastomosis** or **portosystemic shunt** may be created where these vessels lie close to each other posterior to the liver.

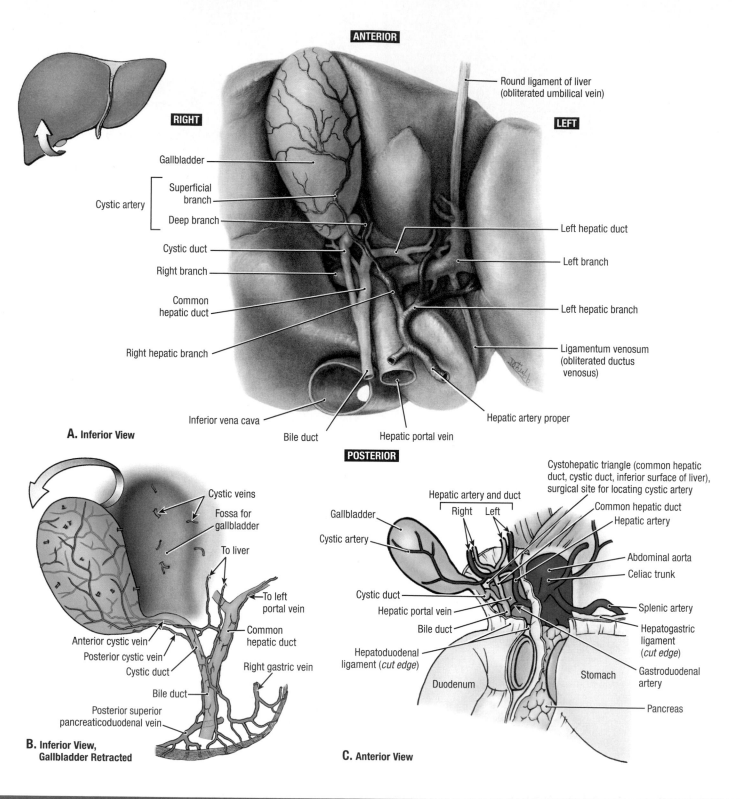

ANTERIOR

RIGHT

LEFT

Round ligament of liver
(obliterated umbilical vein)

Gallbladder

Cystic artery
  Superficial branch
  Deep branch

Cystic duct

Right branch

Common hepatic duct

Right hepatic branch

Left hepatic duct

Left branch

Left hepatic branch

Ligamentum venosum
(obliterated ductus venosus)

Inferior vena cava

Bile duct

Hepatic portal vein

Hepatic artery proper

A. Inferior View

POSTERIOR

Cystic veins

Fossa for gallbladder

To liver

To left portal vein

Common hepatic duct

Anterior cystic vein

Posterior cystic vein

Cystic duct

Bile duct

Right gastric vein

Posterior superior pancreaticoduodenal vein

B. Inferior View, Gallbladder Retracted

Cystohepatic triangle (common hepatic duct, cystic duct, inferior surface of liver), surgical site for locating cystic artery

Hepatic artery and duct
  Right   Left

Gallbladder

Cystic artery

Common hepatic duct

Hepatic artery

Abdominal aorta

Celiac trunk

Cystic duct

Hepatic portal vein

Bile duct

Hepatoduodenal ligament (*cut edge*)

Duodenum

Stomach

Splenic artery

Hepatogastric ligament (*cut edge*)

Gastroduodenal artery

Pancreas

C. Anterior View

4.57   **Gallbladder and Structures of Porta Hepatis**

A. Gallbladder, cystic artery, and extrahepatic bile ducts. The inferior border of the liver is elevated to demonstrate its visceral surface (as in orientation figure). **B. Venous drainage of gallbladder and extrahepatic ducts.** Most veins are tributaries of the hepatic portal vein, but some drain directly to the liver. **C. Portal triad within hepatoduodenal ligament** (free edge of lesser omentum).

Gallstones are concretions in the gallbladder or extrahepatic biliary ducts. The cystohepatic (hepatobiliary) triangle (Calot), between the common hepatic duct, cystic duct, and liver, is an important endoscopic landmark for locating the cystic artery during **cholecystectomy.**

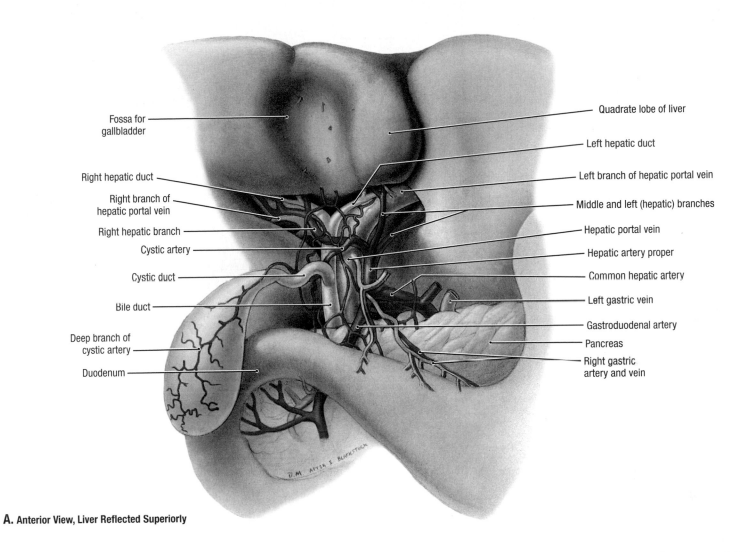

Fossa for gallbladder

Right hepatic duct

Right branch of hepatic portal vein

Right hepatic branch

Cystic artery

Cystic duct

Bile duct

Deep branch of cystic artery

Duodenum

Quadrate lobe of liver

Left hepatic duct

Left branch of hepatic portal vein

Middle and left (hepatic) branches

Hepatic portal vein

Hepatic artery proper

Common hepatic artery

Left gastric vein

Gastroduodenal artery

Pancreas

Right gastric artery and vein

A. Anterior View, Liver Reflected Superiorly

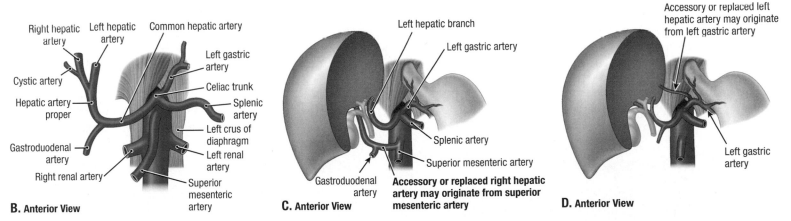

Right hepatic artery   Left hepatic artery   Common hepatic artery

Cystic artery

Hepatic artery proper

Gastroduodenal artery

Right renal artery

Left gastric artery

Celiac trunk

Splenic artery

Left crus of diaphragm

Left renal artery

Superior mesenteric artery

B. Anterior View

Left hepatic branch

Left gastric artery

Splenic artery

Superior mesenteric artery

Gastroduodenal artery

Accessory or replaced right hepatic artery may originate from superior mesenteric artery

C. Anterior View

Accessory or replaced left hepatic artery may originate from left gastric artery

Left gastric artery

D. Anterior View

Vessels in Porta Hepatis   **4.58**

A. Hepatic and cystic vessels. The liver is reflected superiorly. The gallbladder, freed from its bed or fossa, has remained nearly in its anatomical position, pulled slightly to the right. The deep branch of the cystic artery on the deep, or attached, surface of the gallbladder anastomoses with branches of the superficial branch of the cystic artery and sends twigs into the bed of the gallbladder. Veins (not all shown) accompany most arteries. **B. Typical pattern**

of branching of celiac trunk and hepatic arteries. **C. Aberrant (accessory or replaced) right hepatic artery. D. Aberrant left hepatic artery.**

Awareness of the variations in arteries and bile duct formation is important for surgeons when they ligate the cystic duct during **cholecystectomy** (removal of the gallbladder). (See Figs. 4.62, 4.63, and 4.64.)

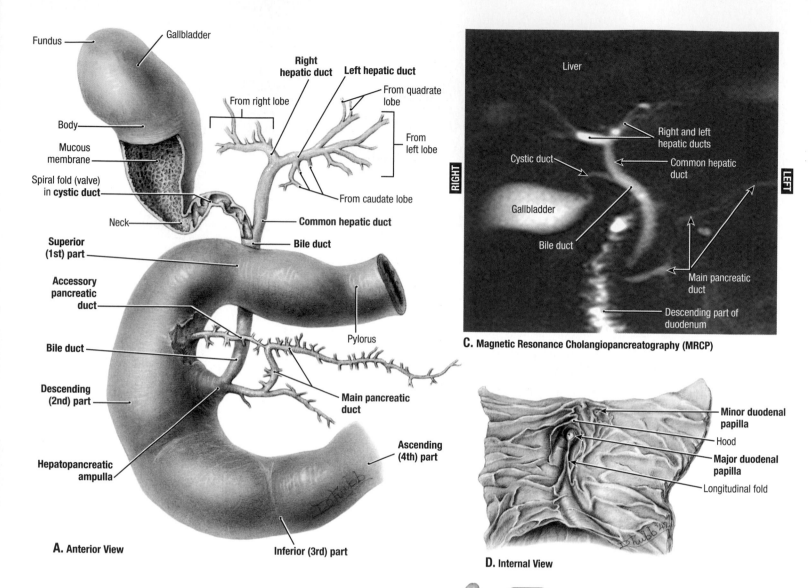

A. Anterior View

- Fundus
- Gallblader
- Body
- Mucous membrane
- Spiral fold (valve) in **cystic duct**
- Neck
- **Superior (1st) part**
- **Accessory pancreatic duct**
- **Bile duct**
- **Descending (2nd) part**
- **Hepatopancreatic ampulla**
- **Right hepatic duct**
- **Left hepatic duct**
- From right lobe
- From quadrate lobe
- From left lobe
- From caudate lobe
- **Common hepatic duct**
- **Bile duct**
- Pylorus
- **Main pancreatic duct**
- **Ascending (4th) part**
- **Inferior (3rd) part**

C. Magnetic Resonance Cholangiopancreatography (MRCP)

- Liver
- Right and left hepatic ducts
- Cystic duct
- Common hepatic duct
- Gallbladder
- Bile duct
- Main pancreatic duct
- Descending part of duodenum
- RIGHT
- LEFT

D. Internal View

- Minor duodenal papilla
- Hood
- Major duodenal papilla
- Longitudinal fold

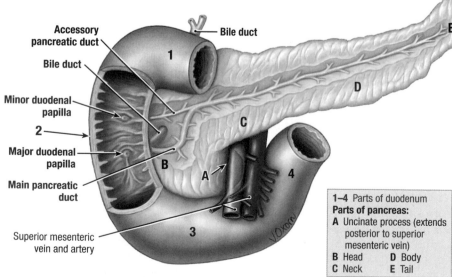

B. Anterior View, Wall Removed from 2nd Part of Duodenum

- Accessory pancreatic duct
- Bile duct
- Bile duct
- Minor duodenal papilla
- Major duodenal papilla
- Main pancreatic duct
- Superior mesenteric vein and artery

1–4 Parts of duodenum
Parts of pancreas:
A Uncinate process (extends posterior to superior mesenteric vein)
B Head
C Neck
D Body
E Tail

4.59 Bile and Pancreatic Ducts

A. and **B.** Extrahepatic bile passages and pancreatic ducts. **C.** Magnetic resonance cholangiopancreatography (MRCP) demonstrating bile and pancreatic ducts. The right and left hepatic ducts collect bile from the liver; the common hepatic duct unites with the cystic duct superior to the duodenum to form the bile duct, which descends posterior to the superior (1st) part of the duodenum. **D.** Interior of descending (2nd) part of duodenum. The bile duct joins the main pancreatic duct, forming the hepatopancreatic ampulla, which opens on the major duodenal papilla. This opening is the narrowest part of the biliary passages and is the common site for **impaction of a gallstone**. Gallstones may produce biliary colic (pain in the epigastric region). The accessory pancreatic duct opens on the minor duodenal papilla.

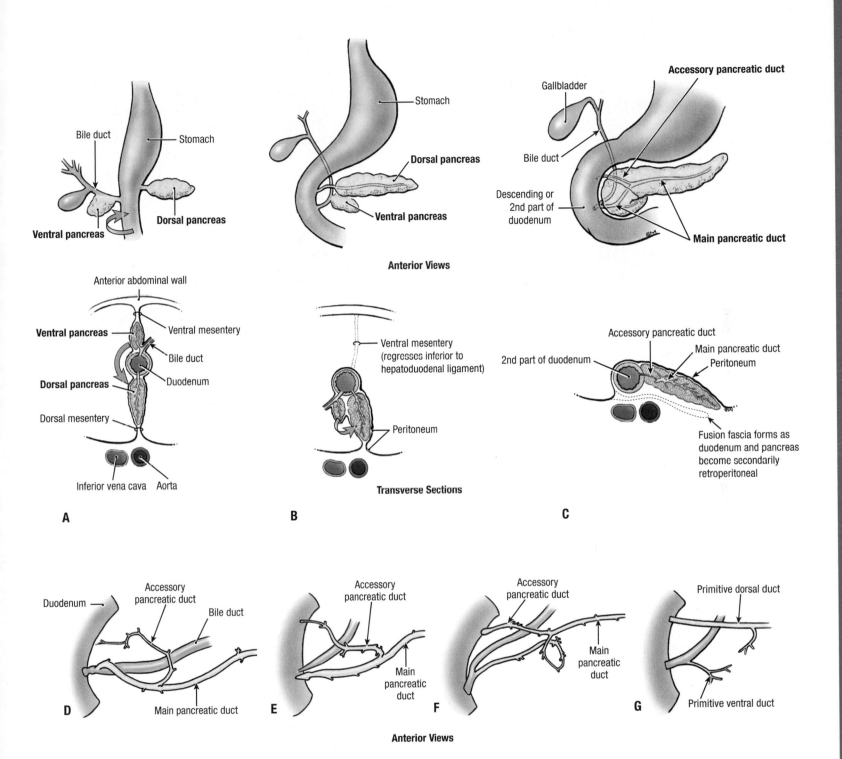

Stomach

Bile duct — Stomach

Dorsal pancreas

Ventral pancreas

Gallbladder

Accessory pancreatic duct

Bile duct

Dorsal pancreas

Ventral pancreas

Anterior Views

Descending or 2nd part of duodenum

Main pancreatic duct

Anterior abdominal wall

Ventral pancreas — Ventral mesentery

Bile duct

Dorsal pancreas — Duodenum

Dorsal mesentery

Inferior vena cava   Aorta

A

Ventral mesentery (regresses inferior to hepatoduodenal ligament)

Peritoneum

Transverse Sections

B

Accessory pancreatic duct

2nd part of duodenum

Main pancreatic duct

Peritoneum

Fusion fascia forms as duodenum and pancreas become secondarily retroperitoneal

C

Duodenum

Accessory pancreatic duct

Bile duct

Main pancreatic duct

D

Accessory pancreatic duct

Main pancreatic duct

E

Accessory pancreatic duct

Main pancreatic duct

F

Primitive dorsal duct

Primitive ventral duct

G

Anterior Views

Development and Variability of Pancreatic Ducts

4.60

A–C. Anterior views (*upper row*) and transverse sections (*middle row*) of stages in development of pancreas. **A.** Small, primitive ventral bud arises in common with bile duct, and a larger, primitive dorsal bud arises independently from duodenum. **B.** Second, or descending, part of duodenum rotates on its long axis, which brings ventral bud and bile duct posterior to dorsal bud. **C.** A connecting segment unites dorsal duct to ventral duct, whereupon duodenal end of dorsal duct atrophies, and direction of flow within it is reversed. **D–G. Common variations of pancreatic duct. D.** An accessory duct that has lost its connection with duodenum. **E.** An accessory duct that is large enough to relieve an obstructed main duct. **F.** An accessory duct that could probably substitute for main duct. **G.** A persisting primitive dorsal duct unconnected to primitive ventral duct.

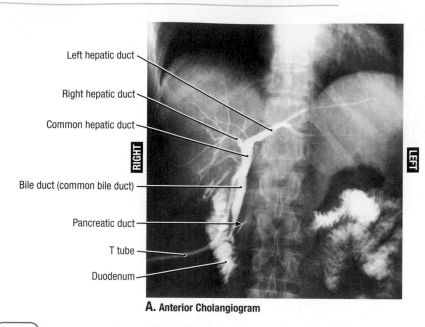

A. Anterior Cholangiogram

Left hepatic duct
Right hepatic duct
Common hepatic duct
RIGHT
LEFT
Bile duct (common bile duct)
Pancreatic duct
T tube
Duodenum

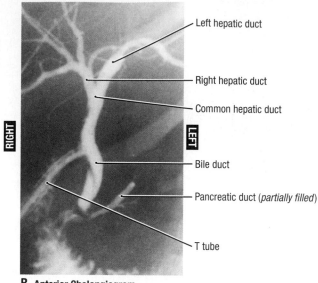

B. Anterior Cholangiogram

Left hepatic duct
Right hepatic duct
Common hepatic duct
RIGHT
LEFT
Bile duct
Pancreatic duct (*partially filled*)
T tube

4.61 **Radiographs of Biliary Passages**

After a cholecystectomy (removal of the gallbladder), contrast medium was injected with a T tube inserted into the bile passages. The biliary passages are visualized in the superior abdomen (*Part A*) and are more localized in *Part B*.

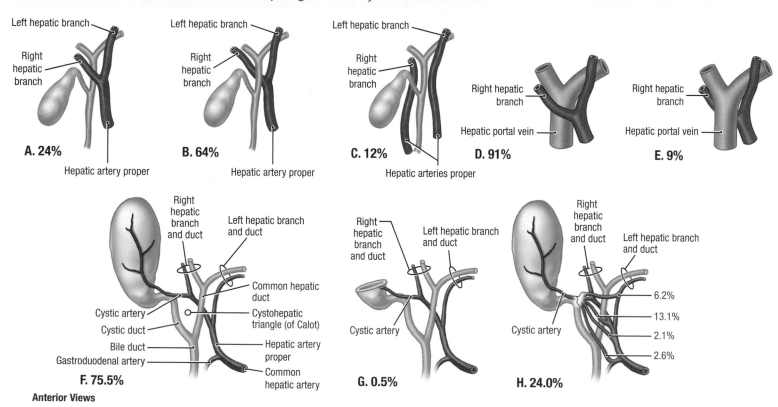

Left hepatic branch
Right hepatic branch
A. 24%
Hepatic artery proper

Left hepatic branch
Right hepatic branch
B. 64%
Hepatic artery proper

Left hepatic branch
Right hepatic branch
C. 12%
Hepatic arteries proper

Right hepatic branch
Hepatic portal vein
D. 91%

Right hepatic branch
Hepatic portal vein
E. 9%

Right hepatic branch and duct
Left hepatic branch and duct
Cystic artery
Cystic duct
Bile duct
Gastroduodenal artery
Common hepatic duct
Cystohepatic triangle (of Calot)
Hepatic artery proper
Common hepatic artery
F. 75.5%

Right hepatic branch and duct
Left hepatic branch and duct
Cystic artery
G. 0.5%

Right hepatic branch and duct
Left hepatic branch and duct
Cystic artery
6.2%
13.1%
2.1%
2.6%
H. 24.0%

Anterior Views

4.62 **Variations in Hepatic and Cystic Arteries**

A–H. Variations of hepatic and cystic arteries. In a study of 165 cadavers in Dr. Grant's laboratory, five patterns (*Parts A* to *E*) were observed. **A.** Right hepatic artery crossing anterior to bile passages, 24%. **B.** Right hepatic artery crossing posterior to bile passages, 64%. **C.** Aberrant artery arising from superior mesenteric artery, 12%. **D.** Cystic artery coursing anterior to portal vein. This occurred in 91% of specimens. **E.** Cystic artery coursing posterior to portal vein. This occurred in 9% of specimens. **F.** and **G.** Cystic artery arising from right hepatic artery. The cystic artery usually arises from the right hepatic artery in the angle between the common hepatic duct and cystic duct without crossing the common hepatic duct. **H.** Cystic artery arising on left side of biliary passages. The cystic artery almost always crosses anterior to the passages.

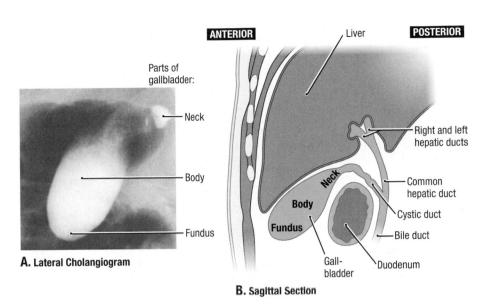

Parts of gallbladder:
— Neck
— Body
— Fundus

A. Lateral Cholangiogram

ANTERIOR   Liver   POSTERIOR

Neck

Body

Fundus

Gall-bladder

Right and left hepatic ducts

Common hepatic duct

Cystic duct

Bile duct

Duodenum

B. Sagittal Section

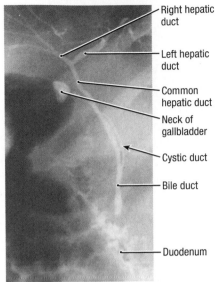

Right hepatic duct

Left hepatic duct

Common hepatic duct

Neck of gallbladder

Cystic duct

Bile duct

Duodenum

C. Lateral Cholangiogram

Gallbladder and Extrahepatic Biliary Ducts   4.63

A. Gallbladder demonstrated by endoscopic retrograde cholangiography (ERCP). **B.** Relationships to superior part of duodenum. **C.** ERCP of bile passages.

Endoscopic retrograde cholangiography (ERCP) is done by first passing a fiberoptic endoscope through the mouth, esophagus, and stomach. Then the duodenum is entered, and a cannula is inserted into the major duodenal papilla and advanced under fluoroscopic guidance into the duct of choice (bile duct or pancreatic duct) for injection of radiographic contrast medium.

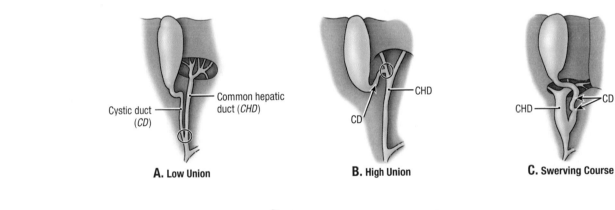

Cystic duct (CD)   Common hepatic duct (CHD)

A. Low Union

CHD   CD

B. High Union

CHD   CD

C. Swerving Course

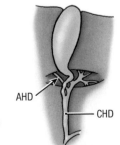

AHD   CHD

Inferior Views

D. Accessory Hepatic Duct (AHD)

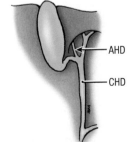

AHD   CHD

E. Accessory Hepatic Duct (AHD)

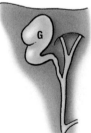

G

F. Folded Gallbladder (G)

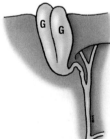

G   G

G. Double Gallbladder (G)

Variations of Cystic and Hepatic Ducts and Gallbladder   4.64

A–C. Common variations of cystic duct and common hepatic duct. The cystic duct usually lies on the right side of the common hepatic duct, joining it just above the superior (first) part of the duodenum, but this varies. **D.** and **E. Accessory biliary ducts.** Of 95 gallbladders and bile passages studied in Dr. Grant's laboratory, 7 had accessory ducts. **D.** Four of seven accessory ducts joined common hepatic duct near cystic duct. **E.** One of seven accessory ducts was an anastomosing duct connecting cystic with common hepatic duct. **F.** and **G. Gallbladder variations. F.** Folded gallbladder. **G.** Double gallbladder.

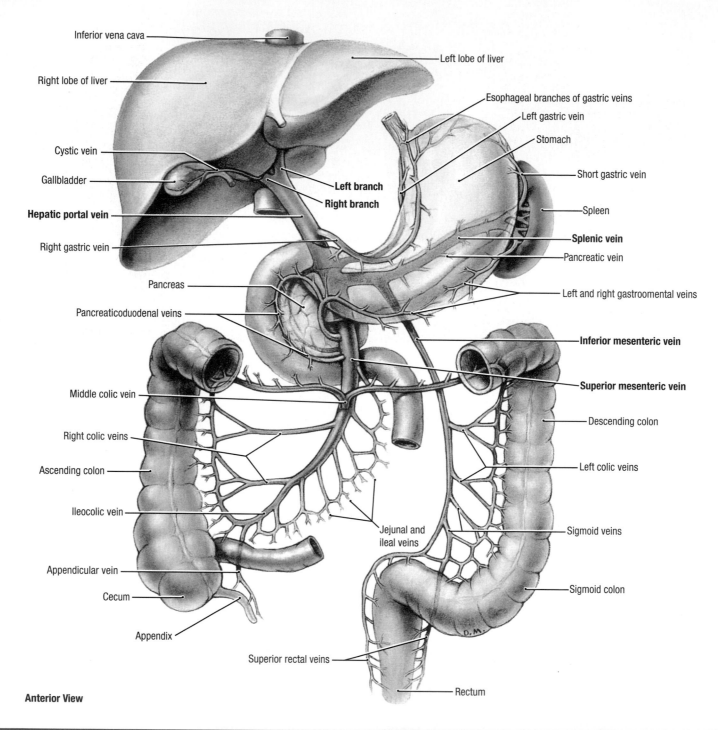

Inferior vena cava

Right lobe of liver

Cystic vein

Gallbladder

Hepatic portal vein

Right gastric vein

Pancreas

Pancreaticoduodenal veins

Middle colic vein

Right colic veins

Ascending colon

Ileocolic vein

Appendicular vein

Cecum

Appendix

Superior rectal veins

Left lobe of liver

Esophageal branches of gastric veins

Left gastric vein

Stomach

Short gastric vein

Left branch

Right branch

Spleen

Splenic vein

Pancreatic vein

Left and right gastroomental veins

Inferior mesenteric vein

Superior mesenteric vein

Descending colon

Left colic veins

Jejunal and ileal veins

Sigmoid veins

Sigmoid colon

Rectum

D.M.

Anterior View

4.65   Portal Venous System

- The hepatic portal vein drains venous blood from the gastrointestinal tract, spleen, pancreas, and gallbladder to the sinusoids of the liver; from here, the blood is conveyed to the systemic venous system by the hepatic veins that drain directly to the inferior vena cava.
- The hepatic portal vein forms posterior to the neck of the pancreas by the union of the superior mesenteric and splenic veins, with the inferior mesenteric vein joining at or near the angle of union.
- The splenic vein drains blood from the inferior mesenteric, left gastroomental (epiploic), short gastric, and pancreatic veins.

- The right gastroomental, pancreaticoduodenal, jejunal, ileal, right, and middle colic veins drain into the superior mesenteric vein.
- The inferior mesenteric vein commences in the rectal plexus as the superior rectal vein and, after crossing the common iliac vessels, becomes the inferior mesenteric vein; branches include the sigmoid and left colic veins.
- The hepatic portal vein divides into right and left branches at the porta hepatis. The left branch carries mainly, but not exclusively, blood from the inferior mesenteric, gastric, and splenic veins, and the right branch carries blood mainly from the superior mesenteric vein.

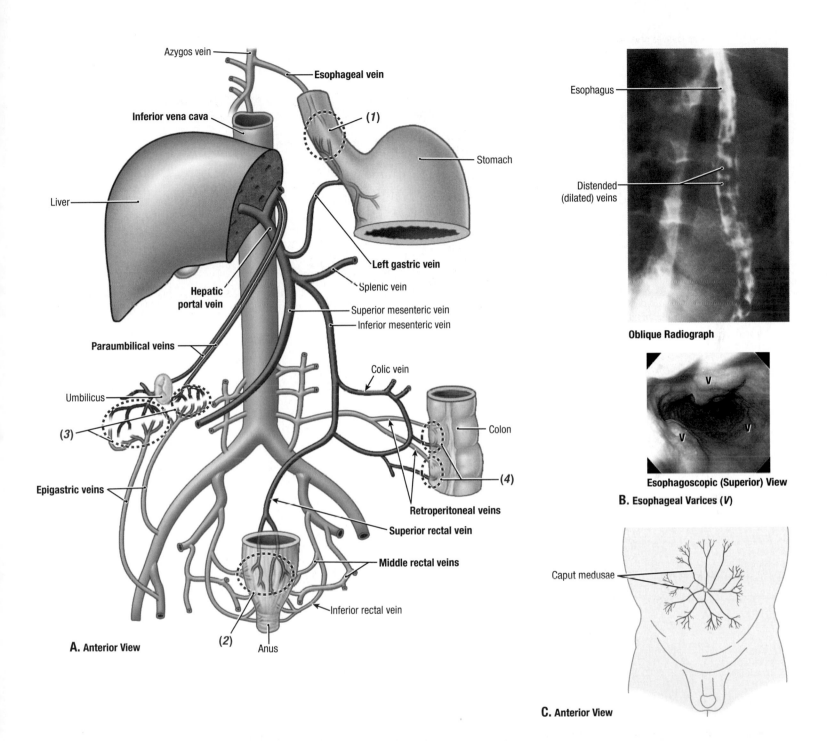

Azygos vein

Esophageal vein

Inferior vena cava

(1)

Stomach

Liver

Left gastric vein

Hepatic portal vein

Splenic vein

Superior mesenteric vein

Inferior mesenteric vein

Paraumbilical veins

Colic vein

Umbilicus

Colon

(3)

(4)

Epigastric veins

Retroperitoneal veins

Superior rectal vein

Middle rectal veins

Inferior rectal vein

A. Anterior View

(2) Anus

Esophagus

Distended (dilated) veins

Oblique Radiograph

V

V V

Esophagoscopic (Superior) View

B. Esophageal Varices (*V*)

Caput medusae

C. Anterior View

Portacaval System

4.66

A. Portacaval system. Portal tributaries (*dark blue*) and systemic tributaries (*light blue*) of portocaval anastomoses (*1–4*). In **portal hypertension** (as in hepatic cirrhosis), the portal blood cannot pass freely through the liver, and the portocaval anastomoses become engorged, dilated, or even varicose; as a consequence, these veins may rupture. The sites of the portocaval anastomosis shown are between (*1*) esophageal veins draining into the azygos vein (systemic) and left gastric vein (portal), which when dilated are esophageal varices; (*2*) the inferior and middle rectal veins, draining into the

inferior vena cava (systemic) and the superior rectal vein continuing as the inferior mesenteric vein (portal) (hemorrhoids result if the vessels are dilated); (*3*) paraumbilical veins (portal) and small epigastric veins of the anterior abdominal wall (systemic), which when varicose form "caput medusae" (so named because of the resemblance of the radiating veins to the serpents on the head of Medusa, a character in Greek mythology); and (*4*) twigs of colic veins (portal) anastomosing with systemic retroperitoneal veins.
B. Esophageal varices. C. Caput medusae.

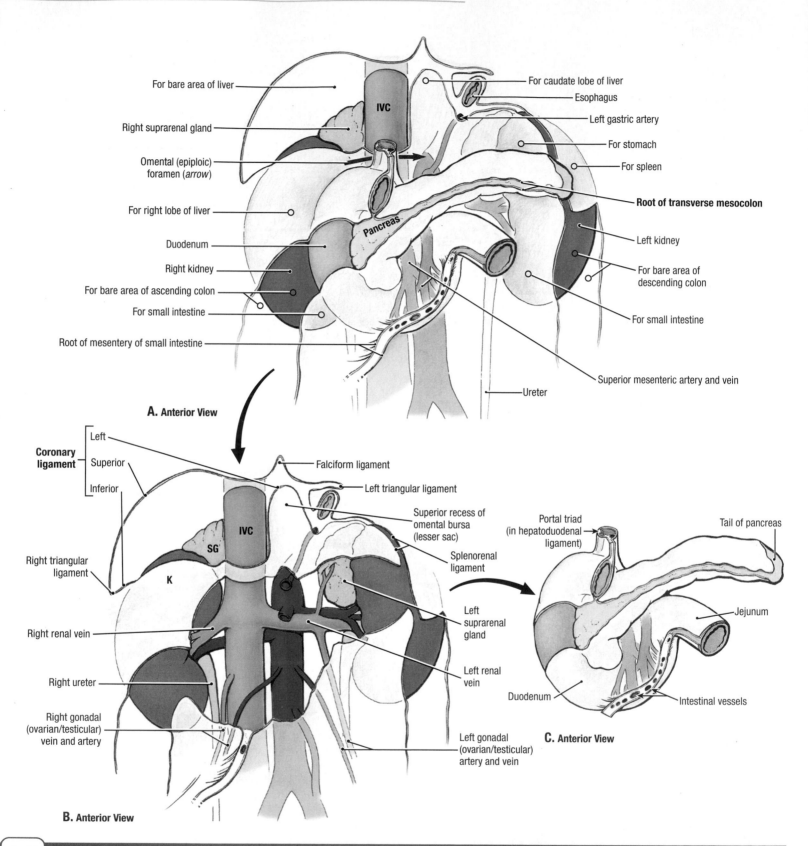

For bare area of liver

IVC

For caudate lobe of liver

Esophagus

Left gastric artery

Right suprarenal gland

For stomach

For spleen

Omental (epiploic)
foramen (*arrow*)

Root of transverse mesocolon

For right lobe of liver

Left kidney

Pancreas

Duodenum

Right kidney

For bare area of
descending colon

For bare area of ascending colon

For small intestine

For small intestine

Root of mesentery of small intestine

Superior mesenteric artery and vein

Ureter

A. Anterior View

Coronary
ligament
Left
Superior
Inferior

Falciform ligament

Left triangular ligament

Superior recess of
omental bursa
(lesser sac)

Portal triad
(in hepatoduodenal
ligament)

Tail of pancreas

IVC

SG

Splenorenal
ligament

Right triangular
ligament

K

Right renal vein

Left
suprarenal
gland

Jejunum

Right ureter

Left renal
vein

Duodenum

Intestinal vessels

Right gonadal
(ovarian/testicular)
vein and artery

C. Anterior View

Left gonadal
(ovarian/testicular)
artery and vein

B. Anterior View

4.67   Posterior Abdominal Viscera and Their Anterior Relations

A. Duodenum and pancreas *in situ*. Note the line of attachment of the root of the transverse mesocolon is to the body and tail of the pancreas. The viscera contacting specific regions are indicated by the term "for." The omental (epiploic) foramen is traversed by an *arrow*.

B. After removal of duodenum and pancreas. The three parts of the coronary ligament are attached to the diaphragm, except where the inferior vena cava (*IVC*), suprarenal gland (*SG*), and kidney (*K*) intervene. **C. Pancreas and duodenum removed from *Part A*.**

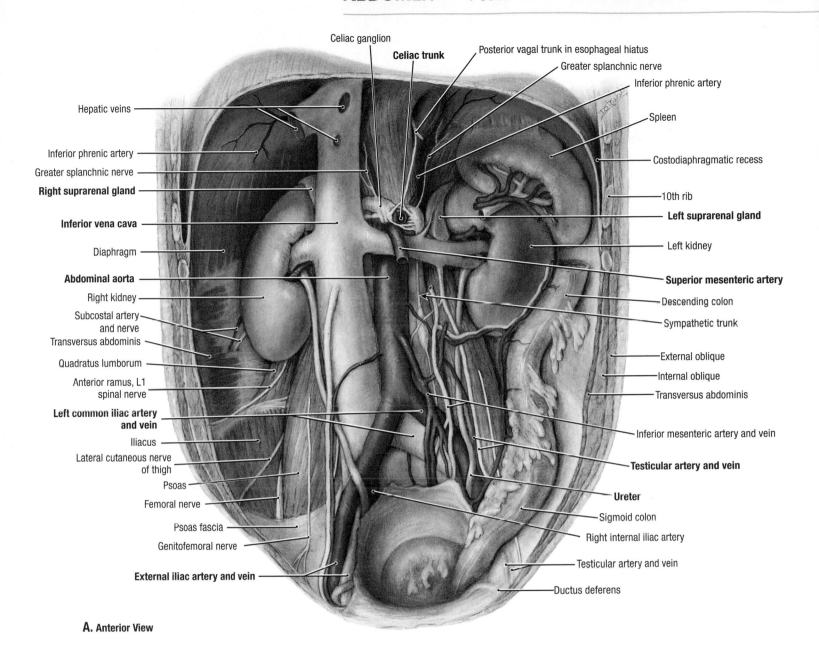

Celiac ganglion
Celiac trunk
Posterior vagal trunk in esophageal hiatus
Greater splanchnic nerve
Inferior phrenic artery
Hepatic veins
Spleen
Inferior phrenic artery
Greater splanchnic nerve
Costodiaphragmatic recess
Right suprarenal gland
10th rib
Left suprarenal gland
Inferior vena cava
Left kidney
Diaphragm
Abdominal aorta
Superior mesenteric artery
Right kidney
Descending colon
Subcostal artery and nerve
Sympathetic trunk
Transversus abdominis
Quadratus lumborum
External oblique
Anterior ramus, L1 spinal nerve
Internal oblique
Transversus abdominis
Left common iliac artery and vein
Inferior mesenteric artery and vein
Iliacus
Testicular artery and vein
Lateral cutaneous nerve of thigh
Psoas
Ureter
Femoral nerve
Sigmoid colon
Psoas fascia
Right internal iliac artery
Genitofemoral nerve
Testicular artery and vein
External iliac artery and vein
Ductus deferens

A. Anterior View

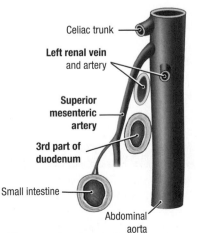

Celiac trunk
Left renal vein and artery
Superior mesenteric artery
3rd part of duodenum
Small intestine
Abdominal aorta

B. Lateral View (from Left)

Viscera and Vessels of Posterior Abdominal Wall `4.68`

A. Great vessels, kidneys, and suprarenal glands. **B.** Relationships of left renal vein and inferior (third) part of duodenum to aorta and superior mesenteric artery.

- The abdominal aorta is shorter and smaller in caliber than the inferior vena cava.
- The inferior mesenteric artery arises about 4 cm superior to the aortic bifurcation and crosses the left common iliac vessels to become the superior rectal artery.
- The left renal vein drains the left testis, left suprarenal gland, and left kidney; the renal arteries are posterior to the renal veins.
- The ureter crosses the external iliac artery just beyond the common iliac bifurcation.
- The testicular vessels cross anterior to the ureter and join the ductus deferens at the deep inguinal ring.
- The left renal vein and duodenum (and uncinate process of pancreas—not shown) pass between the aorta posteriorly and the superior mesenteric artery anteriorly; they may be compressed like nuts in a nutcracker (*Part B*).

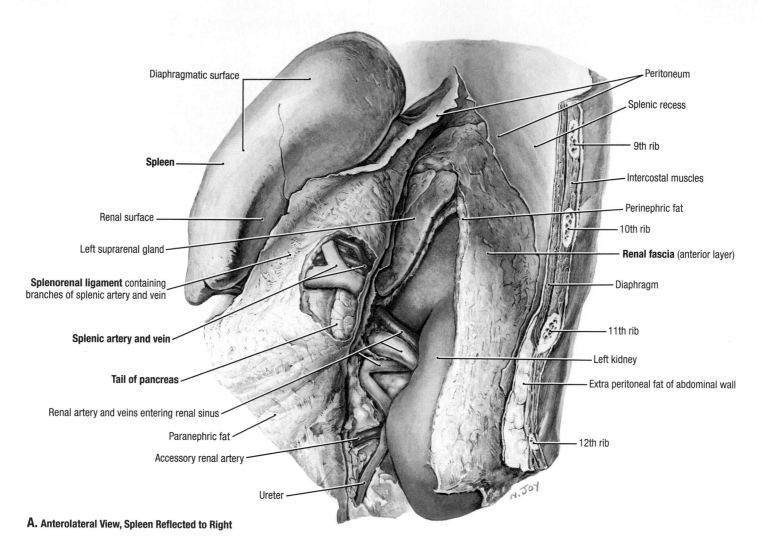

Diaphragmatic surface

Spleen

Renal surface

Left suprarenal gland

Splenorenal ligament containing
branches of splenic artery and vein

Splenic artery and vein

Tail of pancreas

Renal artery and veins entering renal sinus

Paranephric fat

Accessory renal artery

Ureter

Peritoneum

Splenic recess

9th rib

Intercostal muscles

Perinephric fat

10th rib

Renal fascia (anterior layer)

Diaphragm

11th rib

Left kidney

Extra peritoneal fat of abdominal wall

12th rib

A. Anterolateral View, Spleen Reflected to Right

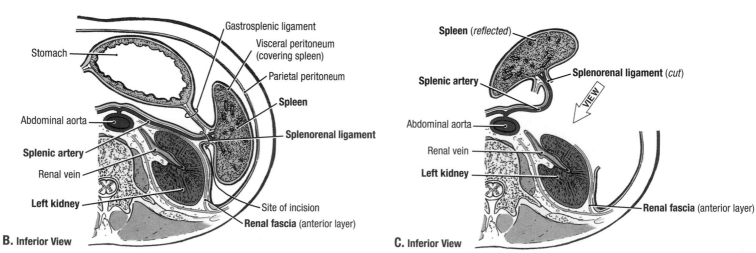

Gastrosplenic ligament

Visceral peritoneum
(covering spleen)

Parietal peritoneum

Stomach

Spleen

Splenorenal ligament

Abdominal aorta

Splenic artery

Renal vein

Left kidney

Site of incision

Renal fascia (anterior layer)

B. Inferior View

Spleen (reflected)

Splenic artery

Splenorenal ligament (cut)

VIEW

Abdominal aorta

Renal vein

Left kidney

Renal fascia (anterior layer)

C. Inferior View

4.69   **Exposure of Left Kidney and Suprarenal Gland**

**A. Dissection. B. Schematic section with spleen and splenorenal
ligament intact. C. Procedure used in *Part A* to expose kidney.**
The spleen and splenorenal ligament are reflected anteriorly, with
the splenic vessels and tail of the pancreas. Part of the renal fascia

of the kidney is removed. Note the proximity of the splenic vein
and left renal vein, enabling a **splenorenal shunt** to be established
surgically to relieve portal hypertension.

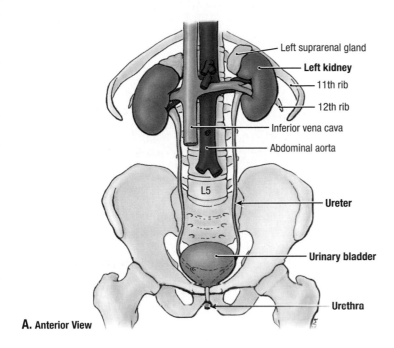

A. Anterior View

Left suprarenal gland
Left kidney
11th rib
12th rib
Inferior vena cava
Abdominal aorta
L5
Ureter
Urinary bladder
Urethra

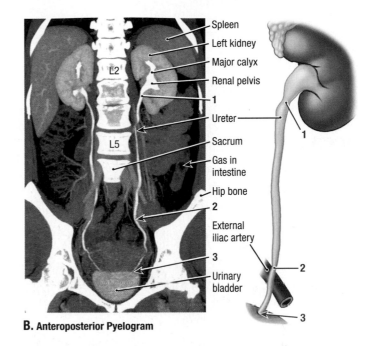

Spleen
Left kidney
Major calyx
Renal pelvis
1
Ureter
Sacrum
Gas in intestine
Hip bone
2
External iliac artery
3
Urinary bladder
L2
L5
1
2
3

B. Anteroposterior Pyelogram

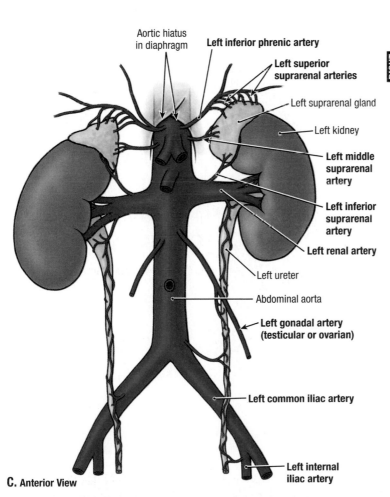

Aortic hiatus in diaphragm
Left inferior phrenic artery
Left superior suprarenal arteries
Left suprarenal gland
Left kidney
Left middle suprarenal artery
Left inferior suprarenal artery
Left renal artery
Left ureter
Abdominal aorta
Left gonadal artery (testicular or ovarian)
Left common iliac artery
Left internal iliac artery

C. Anterior View

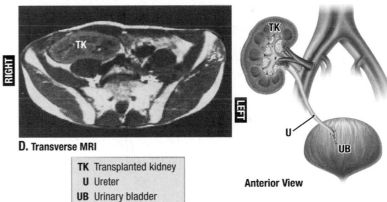

RIGHT
TK

LEFT
TK
U
UB

D. Transverse MRI

TK	Transplanted kidney
U	Ureter
UB	Urinary bladder

Anterior View

Kidneys and Suprarenal Glands 4.70

A. Overview of urinary system. B. Retrograde pyelogram.
Contrast medium was injected into the ureters from a flexible endoscope (urethroscope) in the bladder. Note the papillae bulging into the minor calices, which empty into a major calyx that opens, in turn, into the renal pelvis drained by the ureter. Sites at which relative constrictions in the ureters normally appear: (1) ureteropelvic junction, (2) crossing external iliac vessels or pelvic brim, and (3) as ureter traverses bladder wall. These constricted areas are potential sites of obstruction by ureteric (kidney) stones. **C. Arterial supply of suprarenal glands, kidneys, and ureters.**

 D. Renal transplantation. It is now an established operation for the treatment of selected cases of chronic renal failure. The kidney can be removed from the donor without damaging the suprarenal gland because of the weak septum of renal fascia that separates the kidney from this gland. The site for transplanting a kidney is in the iliac fossa of the greater pelvis. The renal artery and vein are joined to the external iliac artery and vein, respectively, and the ureter is sutured into the urinary bladder.

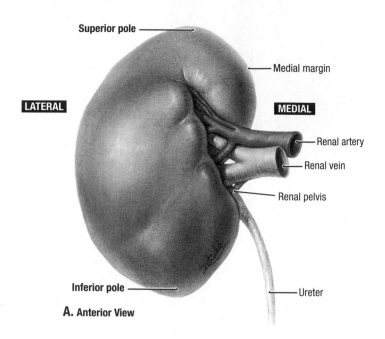

Superior pole

Medial margin

LATERAL

MEDIAL

Renal artery

Renal vein

Renal pelvis

Inferior pole

Ureter

A. Anterior View

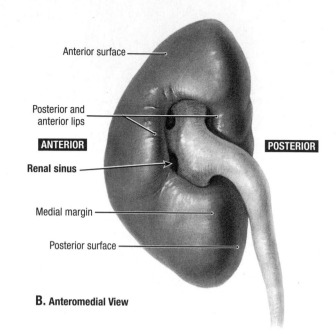

Anterior surface

Posterior and
anterior lips

ANTERIOR

POSTERIOR

Renal sinus

Medial margin

Posterior surface

B. Anteromedial View

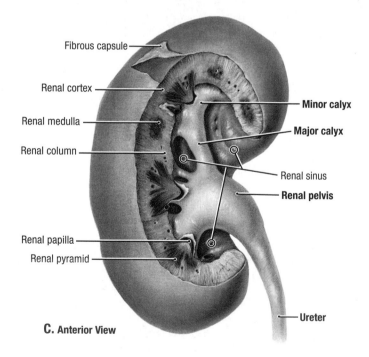

Fibrous capsule

Renal cortex

Renal medulla

Renal column

Renal papilla

Renal pyramid

Minor calyx

Major calyx

Renal sinus

Renal pelvis

Ureter

C. Anterior View

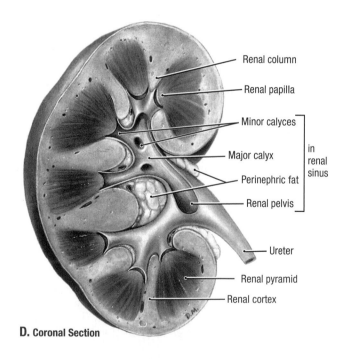

Renal column

Renal papilla

Minor calyces

Major calyx

Perinephric fat

Renal pelvis

in
renal
sinus

Ureter

Renal pyramid

Renal cortex

D. Coronal Section

4.71   **Structure of Kidney**

A. External features. The superior pole of the kidney is closer to the median plane than the inferior pole. Approximately 25% of kidneys may have a 2nd, 3rd, and even 4th accessory renal artery branching from the aorta. These multiple vessels enter through the renal sinus or at the superior or inferior pole (polar arteries). **B. Renal sinus.** The renal sinus is a vertical "pocket" opening on the medial side of the kidney. Tucked into the pocket are the renal pelvis and renal vessels in a matrix of perinephric fat. **C. Renal calices.** The anterior wall of the renal sinus has been cut away to expose the renal pelvis and the calices. **D. Internal features.** **Cysts in the kidney,** multiple or solitary, are common and usually benign findings during ultrasound examinations and dissection of cadavers. **Adult polycystic disease** of the kidneys, however, is an important cause of renal failure.

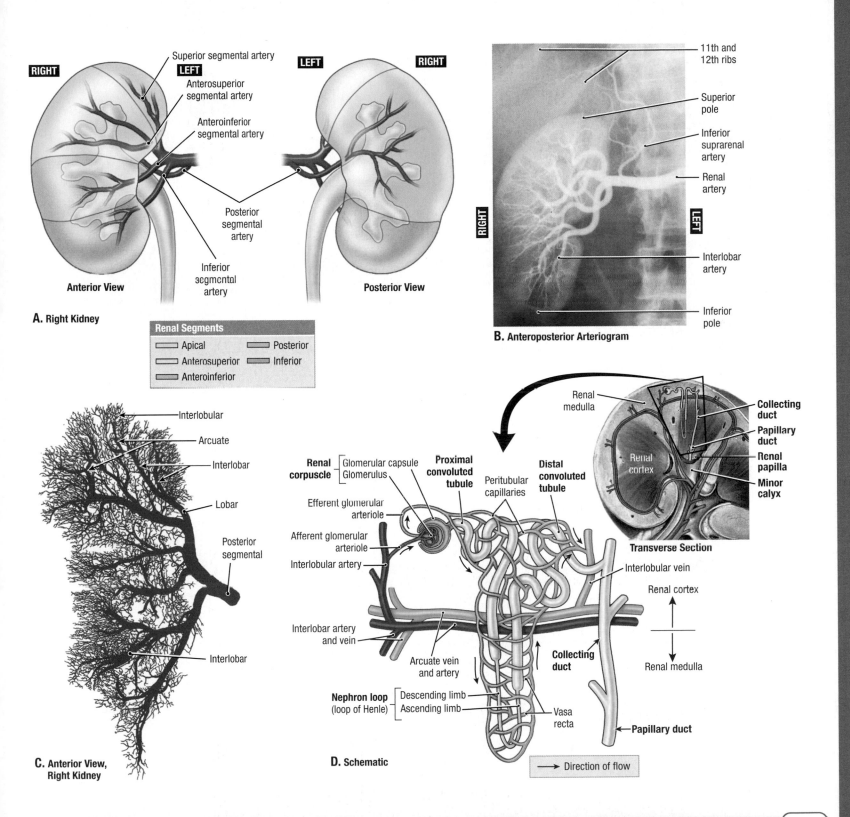

RIGHT   **LEFT**

Superior segmental artery

Anterosuperior segmental artery

Anteroinferior segmental artery

Posterior segmental artery

Inferior segmental artery

Anterior View

A. Right Kidney

LEFT   **RIGHT**

Posterior View

Renal Segments

Apical		Posterior	
Anterosuperior		Inferior	
Anteroinferior			

11th and 12th ribs

Superior pole

Inferior suprarenal artery

Renal artery

RIGHT   **LEFT**

Interlobar artery

Inferior pole

B. Anteroposterior Arteriogram

Interlobular

Arcuate

Interlobar

Lobar

Posterior segmental

Interlobar

C. Anterior View, Right Kidney

Renal medulla

Renal cortex

Transverse Section

Collecting duct

Papillary duct

Renal papilla

Minor calyx

Renal corpuscle [Glomerular capsule / Glomerulus]

Proximal convoluted tubule

Peritubular capillaries

Distal convoluted tubule

Efferent glomerular arteriole

Afferent glomerular arteriole

Interlobular artery

Interlobar artery and vein

Arcuate vein and artery

Nephron loop (loop of Henle) [Descending limb / Ascending limb]

Interlobular vein

Renal cortex

Renal medulla

Collecting duct

Vasa recta

Papillary duct

D. Schematic

→ Direction of flow

A. Segmental arteries. Segmental arteries do not anastomose significantly with other segmental arteries; they are end arteries. The area supplied by each segmented artery is an independent, surgically respectable unit or **renal segment**. **B.** Renal arteriogram. **C.** Corrosion cast of posterior segmental artery of kidney.

D. Structure of nephron. The nephron is the functional unit of the kidney consisting of a renal corpuscle, proximal tubule, nephron loop, and distal tubule. Papillary ducts open onto renal papillae, emptying into minor calices.

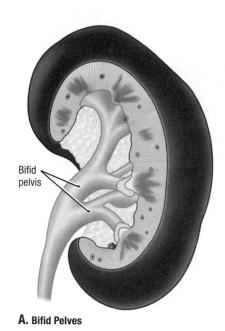

Bifid
pelvis

A. Bifid Pelves

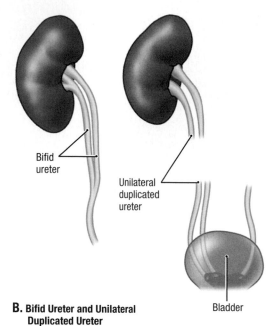

Bifid
ureter

Unilateral
duplicated
ureter

Bladder

B. Bifid Ureter and Unilateral
Duplicated Ureter

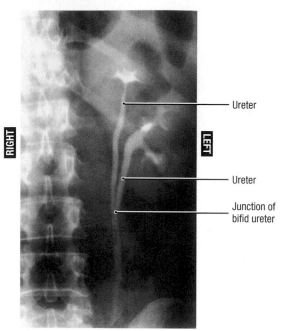

RIGHT

LEFT

Ureter

Ureter

Junction of
bifid ureter

C. Anteroposterior Pyelogram

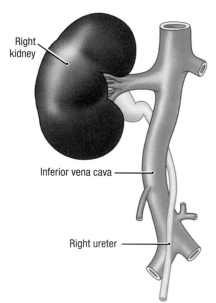

Right
kidney

Inferior vena cava

Right ureter

D. Retrocaval Ureter

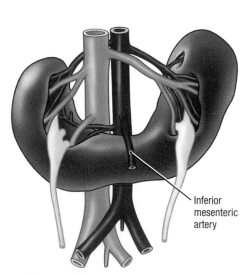

Inferior
mesenteric
artery

E. Horseshoe Kidney

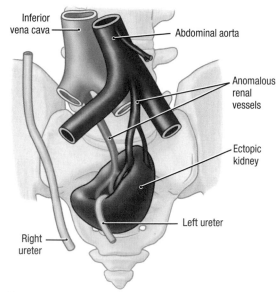

Inferior
vena cava

Abdominal aorta

Anomalous
renal
vessels

Ectopic
kidney

Right
ureter

Left ureter

F. Ectopic Pelvic Kidney

Anterior Views

| 4.73 | **Anomalies of Kidney and Ureter** |

A. Bifid pelves. The pelves are almost replaced by two long major calices, which extend outside the sinus. **B.** and **C. Duplicated, or bifid, ureters.** These can be unilateral or bilateral and complete or incomplete. **D. Retrocaval ureter.** The ureter courses posterior and then anterior to the inferior vena cava. **E. Horseshoe kidney.** The right and left kidneys are fused in the midline. **F. Ectopic pelvic kidney.** Pelvic kidneys have no fatty capsule and can be unilateral or bilateral. During childbirth, they may cause obstruction and suffer injury.

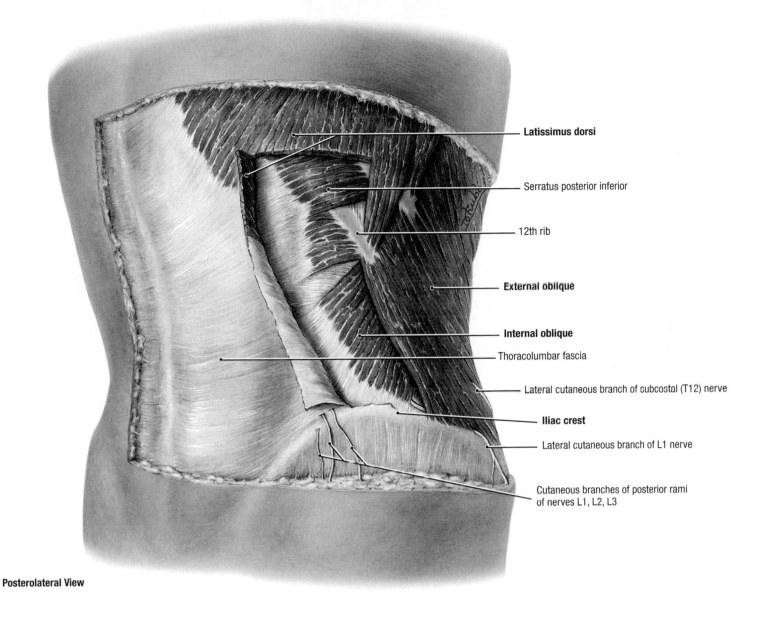

Latissimus dorsi

Serratus posterior inferior

12th rib

External oblique

Internal oblique

Thoracolumbar fascia

Lateral cutaneous branch of subcostal (T12) nerve

Iliac crest

Lateral cutaneous branch of L1 nerve

Cutaneous branches of posterior rami of nerves L1, L2, L3

Posterolateral View

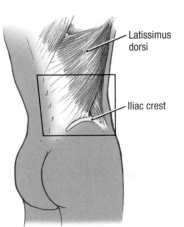

Latissimus dorsi

Iliac crest

Posterolateral Abdominal Wall: Exposure of Kidney (I)   4.74

The latissimus dorsi is partially reflected.
- The external oblique muscle has an oblique, free posterior border that extends from the tip of the 12th rib to the midpoint of the iliac crest.
- The internal oblique muscle extends posteriorly beyond the border of the external oblique muscle.

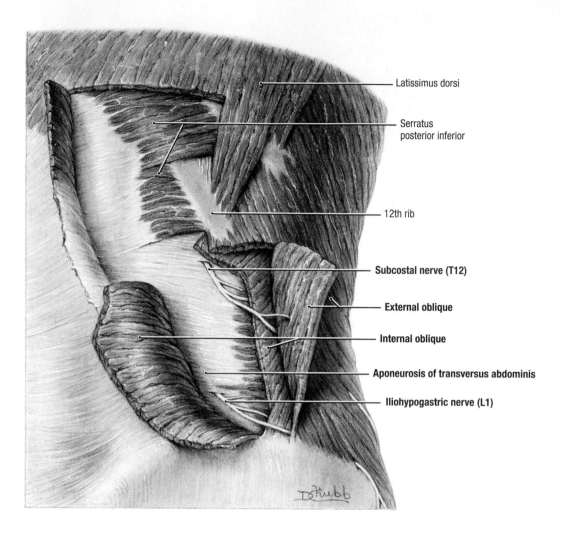

Latissimus dorsi

Serratus posterior inferior

12th rib

Subcostal nerve (T12)

External oblique

Internal oblique

Aponeurosis of transversus abdominis

Iliohypogastric nerve (L1)

Posterolateral View

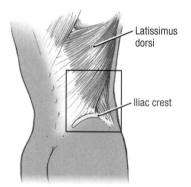

Latissimus dorsi

Iliac crest

4.75 Posterolateral Abdominal Wall: Exposure of Kidney (II)

The external oblique muscle is incised and reflected laterally, and the internal oblique muscle is incised and reflected medially; the transversus abdominis muscle and its posterior aponeurosis are exposed where pierced by the subcostal (T12) and iliohypogastric (L1) nerves. These nerves give off motor twigs and lateral cutaneous branches and continue anteriorly between the internal oblique and transversus abdominis muscles.

4.76 Posterolateral Abdominal Wall: Exposure of Kidney (III) and Renal Fascia (next page)

A. Dissection. The posterior aponeurosis of the transversus abdominis muscle is divided between the subcostal and iliohypogastric nerves and lateral to the oblique lateral border of the quadratus lumborum muscle; the retroperitoneal fat surrounding the kidney is exposed. **B. Renal fascia and retroperitoneal fat, schematic transverse section.** The renal fascia is within this fat; fat internal to the renal fascia is termed perinephric fat (perirenal fat capsule), and the fat immediately external is paranephric fat (pararenal fat body).

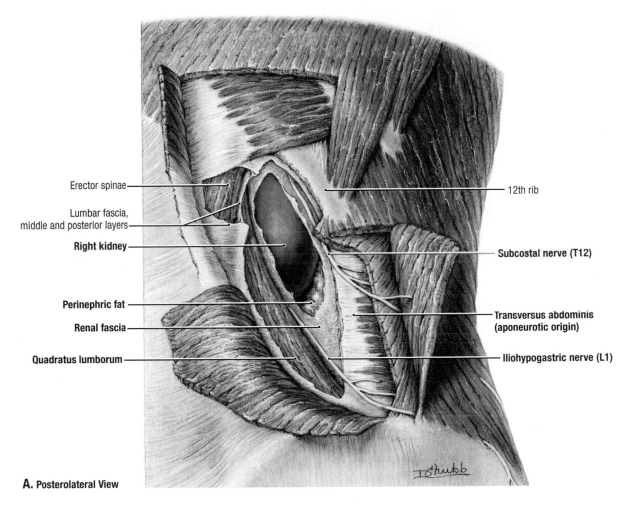

Erector spinae

Lumbar fascia,
middle and posterior layers

Right kidney

Perinephric fat

Renal fascia

Quadratus lumborum

12th rib

Subcostal nerve (T12)

**Transversus abdominis
(aponeurotic origin)**

Iliohypogastric nerve (L1)

A. Posterolateral View

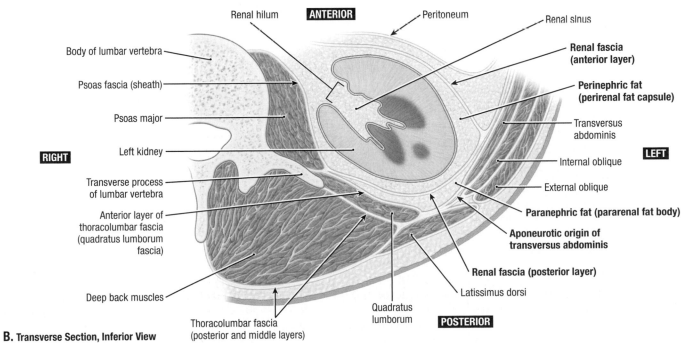

Renal hilum

ANTERIOR

Peritoneum

Renal sinus

Body of lumbar vertebra

**Renal fascia
(anterior layer)**

Psoas fascia (sheath)

**Perinephric fat
(perirenal fat capsule)**

Psoas major

Transversus
abdominis

RIGHT

Left kidney

LEFT

Internal oblique

Transverse process
of lumbar vertebra

External oblique

Anterior layer of
thoracolumbar fascia
(quadratus lumborum
fascia)

Paranephric fat (pararenal fat body)

**Aponeurotic origin of
transversus abdominis**

Renal fascia (posterior layer)

Deep back muscles

Latissimus dorsi

Quadratus
lumborum

POSTERIOR

Thoracolumbar fascia
(posterior and middle layers)

B. Transverse Section, Inferior View

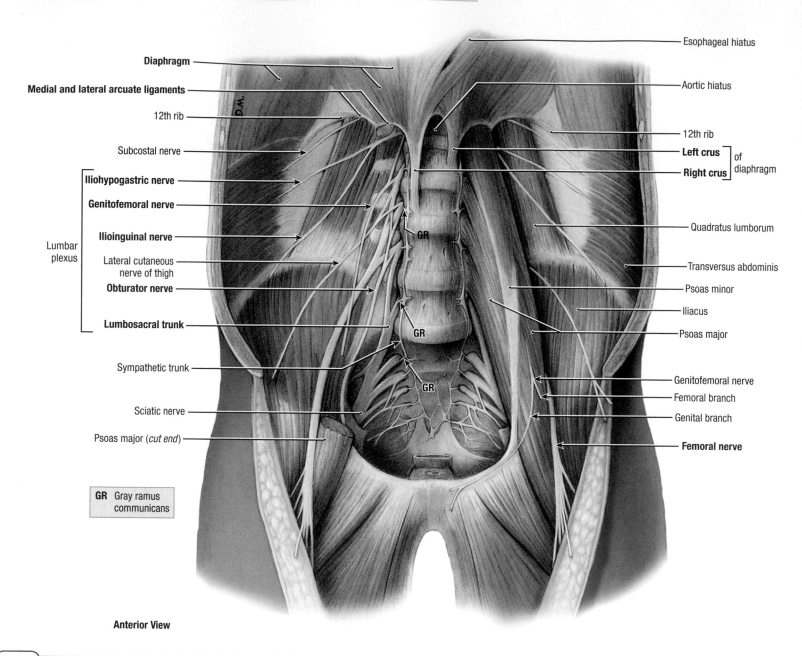

Esophageal hiatus

Diaphragm

Aortic hiatus

Medial and lateral arcuate ligaments

12th rib

12th rib

Subcostal nerve

Left crus } of diaphragm

Right crus

Iliohypogastric nerve

Genitofemoral nerve

Quadratus lumborum

Lumbar plexus

Ilioinguinal nerve

Lateral cutaneous nerve of thigh

Transversus abdominis

Obturator nerve

Psoas minor

Iliacus

Lumbosacral trunk

Psoas major

Sympathetic trunk

Genitofemoral nerve

Sciatic nerve

Femoral branch

Psoas major (*cut end*)

Genital branch

Femoral nerve

GR   Gray ramus communicans

Anterior View

4.77   **Lumbar Plexus and Vertebral Attachment of Diaphragm**

TABLE 4.7	Principal Muscles of Posterior Abdominal Wall			
Muscle	**Superior Attachments**	**Inferior Attachments**	**Innervation**	**Actions**
Psoas major*[a,b]*	Lateral aspects of T12–L5 vertebrae and intervening intervertebral discs; transverse processes of all lumbar vertebrae	By a strong tendon to lesser trochanter of femur	Anterior rami of lumbar nerves (**L1***[c]*, **L2***[c]*, L3)	Acting inferiorly with iliacus, it flexes hip joint; acting superiorly, it flexes vertebral column laterally; it is used to balance the trunk; during sitting, it acts inferiorly with iliacus to flex trunk
Iliacus*[a]*	Iliac crest, iliac fossa, ala of sacrum and anterior sacroiliac ligaments	Tendon of psoas major, lesser trochanter, and femur distal to it	Femoral nerve (**L2***[c]*, L3, L4)	
Quadratus lumborum	Medial half of inferior border of 12th rib and tips of lumbar transverse processes	Iliolumbar ligament and internal lip of iliac crest	Anterior rami of T12 and L1–L4 nerves	Extends and laterally flexes vertebral column; fixes 12th rib during inspiration

*[a]*Psoas major and iliacus muscles are often described together as the iliopsoas muscle when flexion of the hip joint is discussed.
*[b]*Psoas minor attaches proximally to the sides of bodies of T12–L1 vertebrae and intervertebral disc and distally to the pectineal line and iliopectineal eminence via the iliopectineal arch; it does not cross the hip joint. It is used to balance the trunk, in conjunction with psoas major. Innervation is from the anterior rami of lumbar nerves (L1, L2).
*[c]*Primary segment(s) of innervation are boldface type.

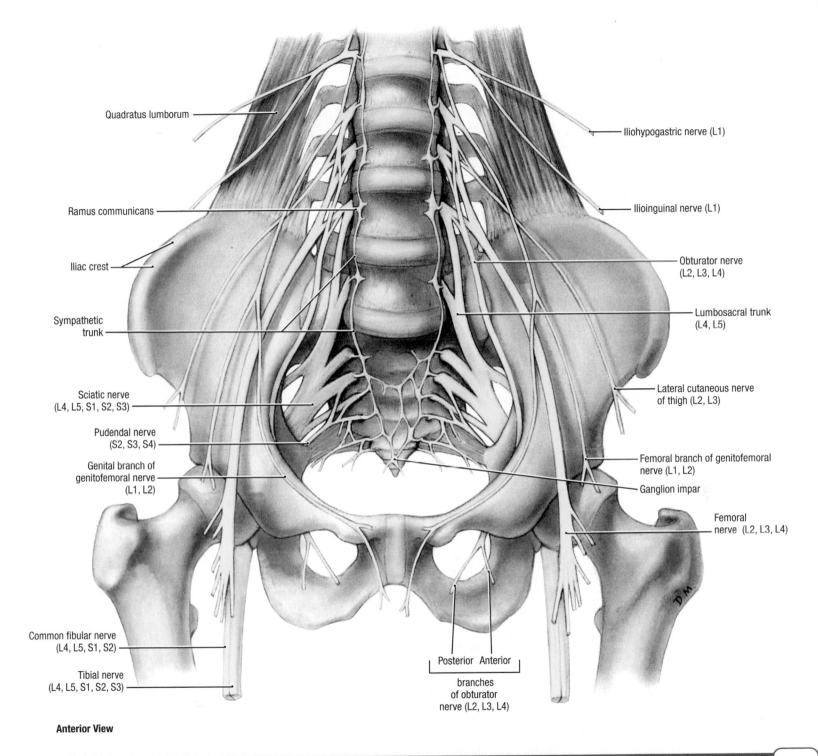

Quadratus lumborum

Ramus communicans

Iliac crest

Sympathetic trunk

Sciatic nerve (L4, L5, S1, S2, S3)

Pudendal nerve (S2, S3, S4)

Genital branch of genitofemoral nerve (L1, L2)

Common fibular nerve (L4, L5, S1, S2)

Tibial nerve (L4, L5, S1, S2, S3)

Iliohypogastric nerve (L1)

Ilioinguinal nerve (L1)

Obturator nerve (L2, L3, L4)

Lumbosacral trunk (L4, L5)

Lateral cutaneous nerve of thigh (L2, L3)

Femoral branch of genitofemoral nerve (L1, L2)

Ganglion impar

Femoral nerve (L2, L3, L4)

Posterior Anterior

branches of obturator nerve (L2, L3, L4)

Anterior View

Nerves of Lumbar Plexus

4.78

The lumbar plexus of nerves is composed of the anterior rami of L1–L4 nerves:

- Ilioinguinal and iliohypogastric nerves (L1) enter the abdomen posterior to the medial arcuate ligaments; they run between the transversus abdominis and internal oblique to supply the skin of the suprapubic and inguinal regions.
- Lateral cutaneous nerve of thigh (L2, L3) enters the thigh posterior to the inguinal ligament, just medial to the anterior superior iliac spine; it supplies the skin on the anterolateral surface of the thigh.

- Femoral nerve (L2–L4) emerges from the lateral border of the psoas; innervates the iliacus muscle and the extensor muscles of the knee.
- Genitofemoral nerve (L1, L2) pierces the anterior surface of the psoas major muscle; divides into femoral and genital branches.
- Obturator nerve (L2–L4) emerges from the medial border of the psoas to supply the adductor muscles of the thigh.
- Lumbosacral trunk (L4, L5) passes over the ala of the sacrum to join the sacral plexus.

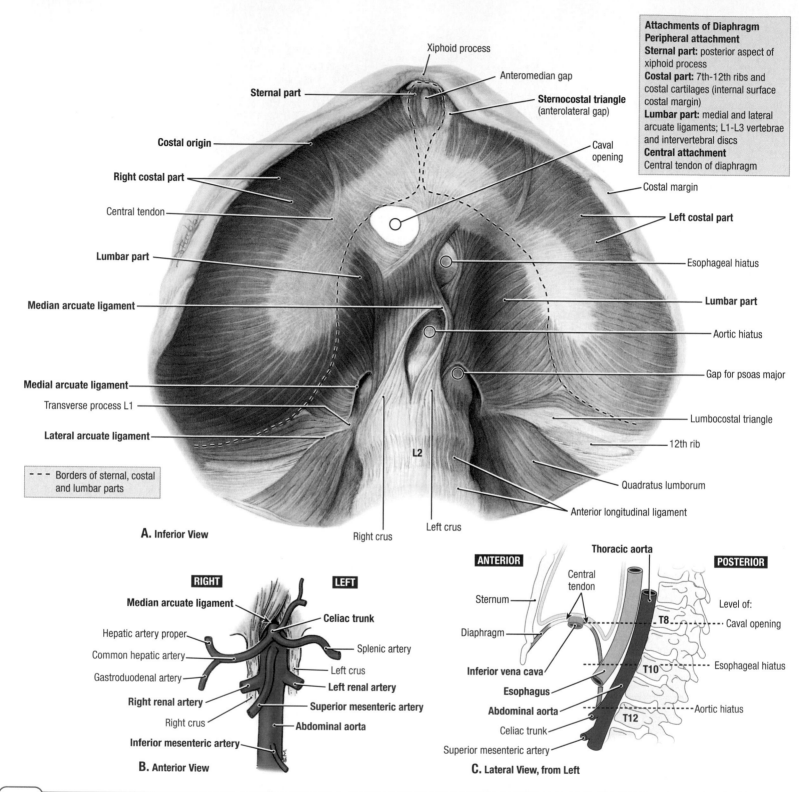

A. Inferior View

Attachments of Diaphragm
Peripheral attachment
Sternal part: posterior aspect of xiphoid process
Costal part: 7th-12th ribs and costal cartilages (internal surface costal margin)
Lumbar part: medial and lateral arcuate ligaments; L1-L3 vertebrae and intervertebral discs
Central attachment
Central tendon of diaphragm

- - - Borders of sternal, costal and lumbar parts

B. Anterior View

C. Lateral View, from Left

4.79   **Diaphragm**

A. Dissection. The clover-shaped central tendon is the aponeurotic insertion of the muscle. **Diaphragmatic hernia.** The diaphragm in this specimen fails to arise from the left lateral arcuate ligament, leaving a potential opening, the lumbocostal triangle, through which abdominal contents may be herniated into the thoracic cavity following a sudden increase in intrathoracic or intraabdominal pressure. A **hiatal hernia** is a protrusion of part of the stomach into the thorax through the esophageal hiatus. **B.** Median arcuate ligament and branches of aorta. **C. Openings of diaphragm.** There are three major openings: (1) the caval opening for the inferior vena cava, most anterior, at the T8 vertebral level to the right of the midline; (2) the esophageal hiatus, intermediate, at T10 level and to the left; and (3) the aortic hiatus, which allows the aorta to pass posterior to the vertebral attachment of the diaphragm in the midline at T12.

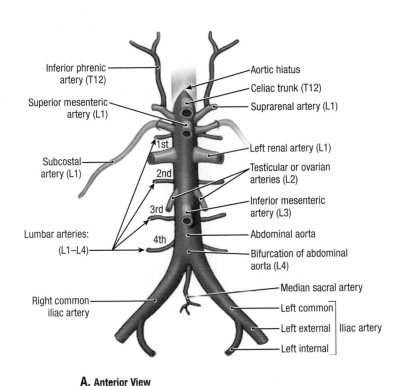

A. Anterior View

Inferior phrenic artery (T12)
Superior mesenteric artery (L1)
Subcostal artery (L1)
Lumbar arteries: (L1–L4)
1st
2nd
3rd
4th
Right common iliac artery

Aortic hiatus
Celiac trunk (T12)
Suprarenal artery (L1)
Left renal artery (L1)
Testicular or ovarian arteries (L2)
Inferior mesenteric artery (L3)
Abdominal aorta
Bifurcation of abdominal aorta (L4)
Median sacral artery
Left common
Left external } Iliac artery
Left internal

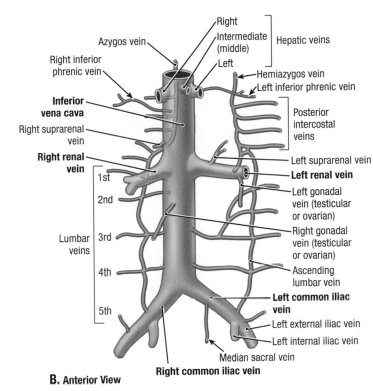

B. Anterior View

Azygos vein
Right inferior phrenic vein
Inferior vena cava
Right suprarenal vein
Right renal vein
Lumbar veins
1st
2nd
3rd
4th
5th
Right
Intermediate (middle) } Hepatic veins
Left
Hemiazygos vein
Left inferior phrenic vein
Posterior intercostal veins
Left suprarenal vein
Left renal vein
Left gonadal vein (testicular or ovarian)
Right gonadal vein (testicular or ovarian)
Ascending lumbar vein
Left common iliac vein
Left external iliac vein
Left internal iliac vein
Median sacral vein
Right common iliac vein

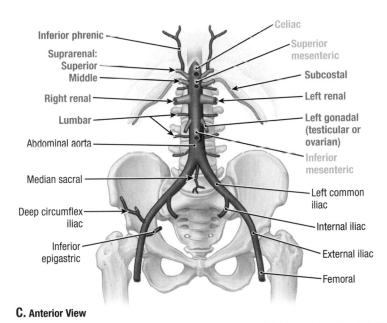

C. Anterior View

Inferior phrenic
Suprarenal:
Superior
Middle
Right renal
Lumbar
Abdominal aorta
Median sacral
Deep circumflex iliac
Inferior epigastric

Celiac
Superior mesenteric
Subcostal
Left renal
Left gonadal (testicular or ovarian)
Inferior mesenteric
Left common iliac
Internal iliac
External iliac
Femoral

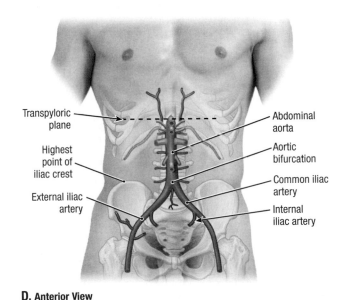

D. Anterior View

Transpyloric plane
Highest point of iliac crest
External iliac artery

Abdominal aorta
Aortic bifurcation
Common iliac artery
Internal iliac artery

Branches of Abdominal Aorta
Anterior midline   Lateral   Posterolateral

Abdominal Aorta and Inferior Vena Cava and Their Branches

4.80

A. Branches (and their vertebral levels) of abdominal aorta.
B. Tributaries of inferior vena cava (*IVC*). **C.** Arteries of posterior abdominal wall, branches of aorta. **D.** Surface anatomy.

Rupture of an aortic aneurysm (localized enlargement of the abdominal aorta) causes severe pain in the abdomen or back. If unrecognized, a ruptured aneurysm has a mortality of nearly 90% because of heavy blood loss. Surgeons can repair an aneurysm by opening it, inserting a prosthetic graft (such as one made of Dacron), and sewing the wall of the aneurysmal aorta over the graft to protect it. Aneurysms may also be treated by endovascular catheterization procedures.

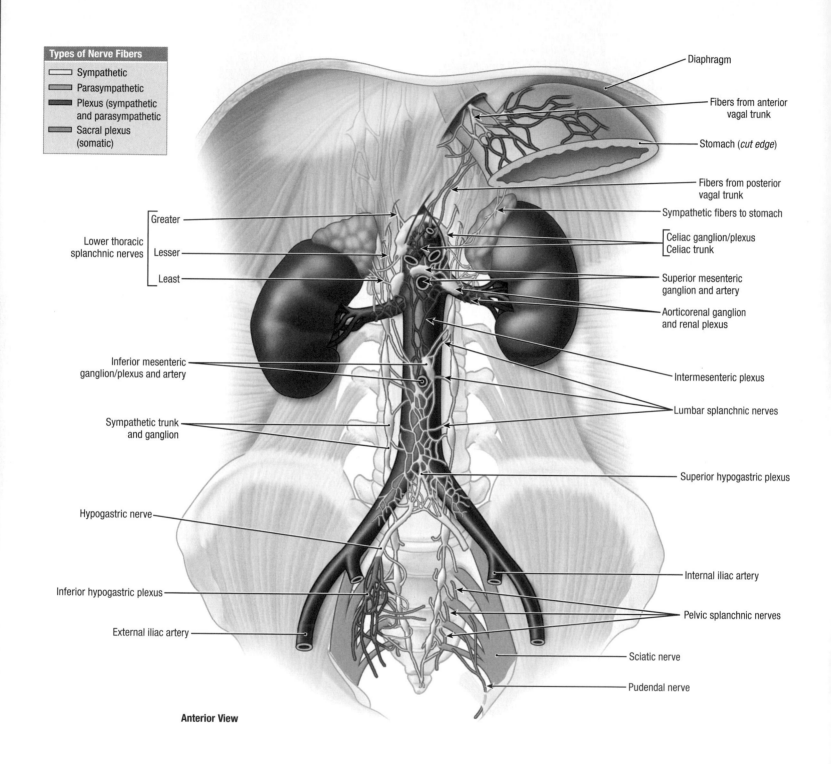

Types of Nerve Fibers
- ☐ Sympathetic
- ☐ Parasympathetic
- ☐ Plexus (sympathetic and parasympathetic
- ☐ Sacral plexus (somatic)

Diaphragm

Fibers from anterior vagal trunk

Stomach (*cut edge*)

Fibers from posterior vagal trunk

Sympathetic fibers to stomach

Celiac ganglion/plexus
Celiac trunk

Superior mesenteric ganglion and artery

Aorticorenal ganglion and renal plexus

Intermesenteric plexus

Lumbar splanchnic nerves

Superior hypogastric plexus

Internal iliac artery

Pelvic splanchnic nerves

Sciatic nerve

Pudendal nerve

Greater
Lesser
Least

Lower thoracic splanchnic nerves

Inferior mesenteric ganglion/plexus and artery

Sympathetic trunk and ganglion

Hypogastric nerve

Inferior hypogastric plexus

External iliac artery

Anterior View

4.81 Abdominopelvic Nerve Plexuses and Ganglia

The sympathetic part of the autonomic nervous system in the abdomen consists of:

- *Abdominopelvic splanchnic nerves* from the thoracic and abdominal sympathetic trunks.
- Prevertebral sympathetic ganglia.

- *Abdominal aortic plexus* and its extensions, the periarterial plexuses.

The plexuses are mixed, shared with the parasympathetic nervous system and visceral afferent fibers.

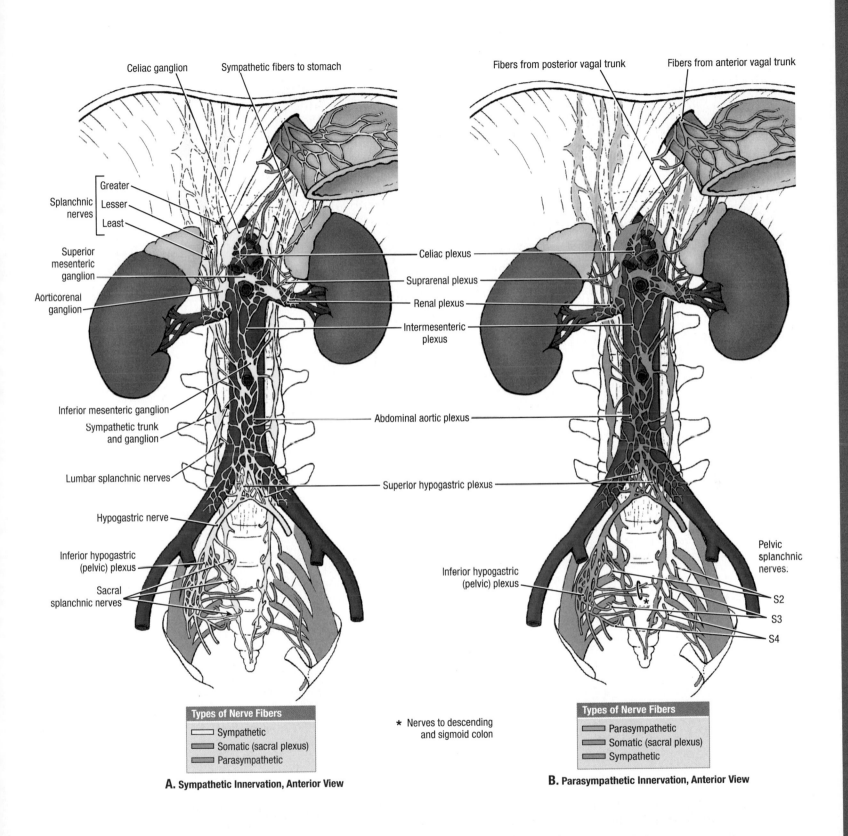

Celiac ganglion

Sympathetic fibers to stomach

Splanchnic nerves
- Greater
- Lesser
- Least

Superior mesenteric ganglion

Aorticorenal ganglion

Inferior mesenteric ganglion

Sympathetic trunk and ganglion

Lumbar splanchnic nerves

Hypogastric nerve

Inferior hypogastric (pelvic) plexus

Sacral splanchnic nerves

Fibers from posterior vagal trunk

Fibers from anterior vagal trunk

Celiac plexus

Suprarenal plexus

Renal plexus

Intermesenteric plexus

Abdominal aortic plexus

Superior hypogastric plexus

Inferior hypogastric (pelvic) plexus

Pelvic splanchnic nerves.

S2

S3

S4

* Nerves to descending and sigmoid colon

Types of Nerve Fibers
- ☐ Sympathetic
- ▨ Somatic (sacral plexus)
- ▨ Parasympathetic

A. Sympathetic Innervation, Anterior View

Types of Nerve Fibers
- ▨ Parasympathetic
- ▨ Somatic (sacral plexus)
- ▨ Sympathetic

B. Parasympathetic Innervation, Anterior View

A. Sympathetic. **B.** Parasympathetic.

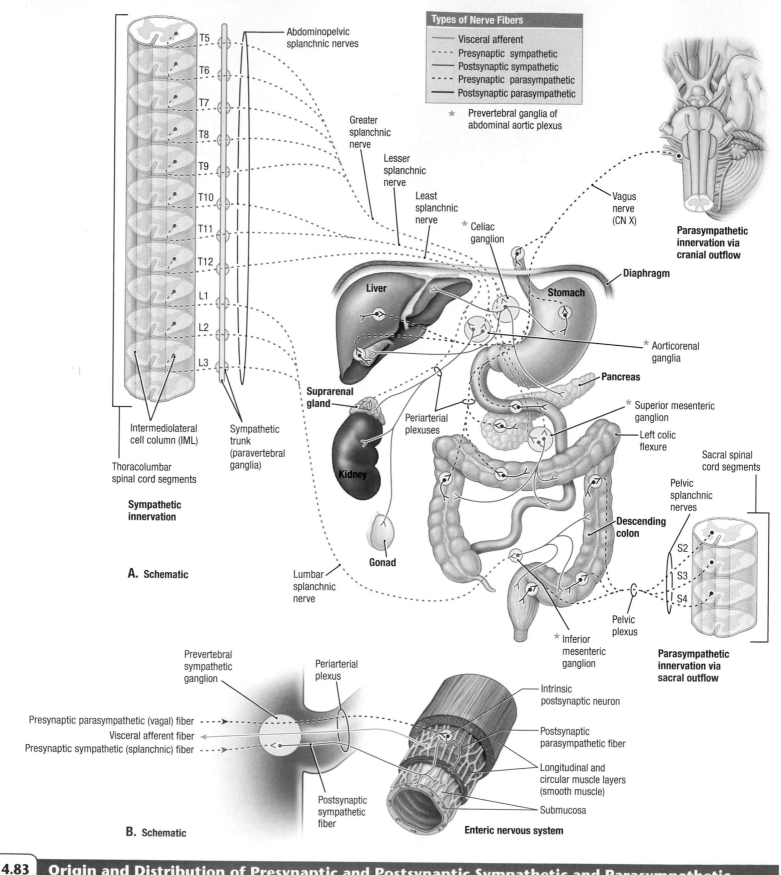

Types of Nerve Fibers

- —— Visceral afferent
- ----- Presynaptic sympathetic
- ----- Postsynaptic sympathetic
- ----- Presynaptic parasympathetic
- —— Postsynaptic parasympathetic

* Prevertebral ganglia of abdominal aortic plexus

T5
T6
T7
T8
T9
T10
T11
T12
L1
L2
L3

Abdominopelvic splanchnic nerves

Greater splanchnic nerve

Lesser splanchnic nerve

Least splanchnic nerve

Intermediolateral cell column (IML)

Sympathetic trunk (paravertebral ganglia)

Thoracolumbar spinal cord segments

Sympathetic innervation

A. Schematic

Lumbar splanchnic nerve

Vagus nerve (CN X)

Parasympathetic innervation via cranial outflow

* **Celiac ganglion**

Liver

Diaphragm

Stomach

* Aorticorenal ganglia

Pancreas

Suprarenal gland

Periarterial plexuses

* Superior mesenteric ganglion

Left colic flexure

Kidney

Descending colon

Sacral spinal cord segments

Pelvic splanchnic nerves

S2
S3
S4

Gonad

* Inferior mesenteric ganglion

Pelvic plexus

Parasympathetic innervation via sacral outflow

Prevertebral sympathetic ganglion

Periarterial plexus

Intrinsic postsynaptic neuron

Presynaptic parasympathetic (vagal) fiber

Visceral afferent fiber

Presynaptic sympathetic (splanchnic) fiber

Postsynaptic parasympathetic fiber

Longitudinal and circular muscle layers (smooth muscle)

Submucosa

Postsynaptic sympathetic fiber

Enteric nervous system

B. Schematic

4.83 **Origin and Distribution of Presynaptic and Postsynaptic Sympathetic and Parasympathetic Fibers, and Ganglia Involved in Supplying Abdominal Viscera**

A. Overview. **B.** Fibers supplying intrinsic plexuses of abdominal viscera.

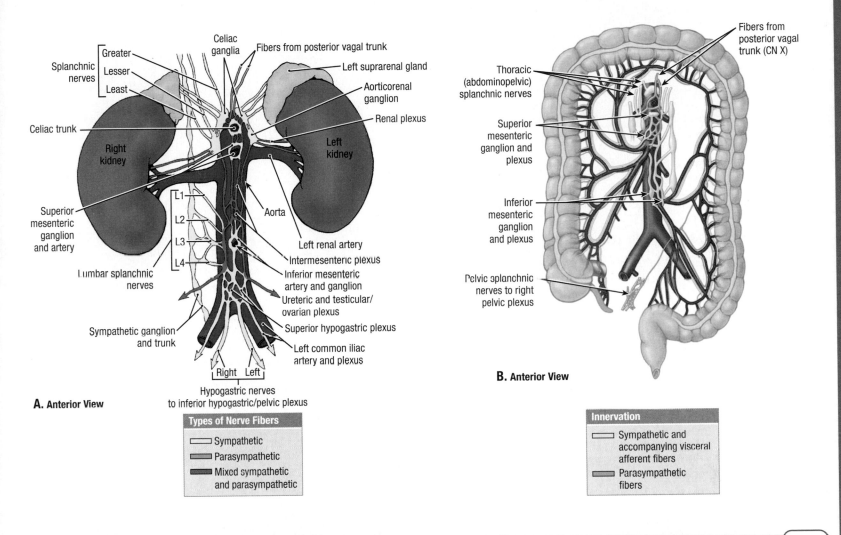

A. Anterior View

Splanchnic nerves — Greater, Lesser, Least

Celiac ganglia
Fibers from posterior vagal trunk
Left suprarenal gland
Aorticorenal ganglion
Renal plexus
Celiac trunk
Right kidney
Left kidney
Superior mesenteric ganglion and artery
L1, L2, L3, L4
Aorta
Left renal artery
Intermesenteric plexus
Inferior mesenteric artery and ganglion
Ureteric and testicular/ovarian plexus
Superior hypogastric plexus
Left common iliac artery and plexus
Lumbar splanchnic nerves
Sympathetic ganglion and trunk
Right   Left
Hypogastric nerves to inferior hypogastric/pelvic plexus

Types of Nerve Fibers
- ☐ Sympathetic
- ☐ Parasympathetic
- ☐ Mixed sympathetic and parasympathetic

B. Anterior View

Fibers from posterior vagal trunk (CN X)
Thoracic (abdominopelvic) splanchnic nerves
Superior mesenteric ganglion and plexus
Inferior mesenteric ganglion and plexus
Pelvic splanchnic nerves to right pelvic plexus

Innervation
- ☐ Sympathetic and accompanying visceral afferent fibers
- ☐ Parasympathetic fibers

Autonomic Nerve Supply to Abdomen and Pelvis   **4.84**

A. Abdominal nerve plexuses and ganglia. Sympathetic and parasympathetic nerves mingle in the tangle of nerve plexuses anterior to the aorta; both types of fibers reach their destinations by "piggybacking" on the branches of the abdominal aorta. This network of nerves is difficult to dissect.
B. Innervation of large intestine. Parasympathetic nerve fibers ascend from the inferior hypogastric plexuses to the colon distal to the left colic flexure.

TABLE 4.8   Splanchnic Nerve Innervation of Abdominal Viscera

Splanchnic Nerves	Autonomic Fiber Type[a]	System	Origin	Destination
A. Cardiopulmonary (cervical and upper thoracic)	Postsynaptic		Cervical and upper thoracic sympathetic trunk	Thoracic cavity (viscera superior to the level of diaphragm)

B. Abdominopelvic
  1. Lower thoracic
    a. Greater
    b. Lesser
    c. Least
  2. Lumbar
  3. Sacral
	Presynaptic	Sympathetic	Lower thoracic and abdominopelvic sympathetic trunk:
			1. Thoracic sympathetic trunk:
			  a. T5–T9 or T10 level
			  b. T10–T11 level
			  c. T12 level
			2. Abdominal sympathetic trunk
			3. Pelvic (sacral) sympathetic trunk
				Abdominopelvic cavity (prevertebral ganglia serving viscera and suprarenal glands inferior to the level of diaphragm)
				1. Abdominal prevertebral ganglia:
				  a. Celiac ganglia
				  b. Aorticorenal ganglia
				  c. and 2. Other abdominal prevertebral ganglia (superior and inferior mesenteric and of intermesenteric/hypogastric plexuses)
				3. Pelvic prevertebral ganglia

C. Pelvic	Presynaptic	Parasympathetic	Anterior rami of S2–S4 spinal nerves	Intrinsic ganglia of descending and sigmoid colon, rectum, and pelvic viscera

[a]Splanchnic and vagus nerves also convey visceral afferent fibers.

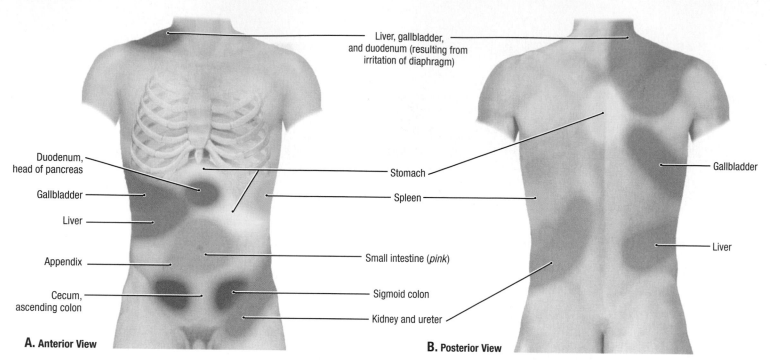

Liver, gallbladder, and duodenum (resulting from irritation of diaphragm)

Duodenum, head of pancreas

Gallbladder

Liver

Appendix

Cecum, ascending colon

Stomach

Spleen

Small intestine (*pink*)

Sigmoid colon

Kidney and ureter

Gallbladder

Liver

A. Anterior View

B. Posterior View

| 4.85 | **Surface Projections of Visceral Pain** |

A. and **B.** Sites of visceral referred pain. **C.** Approximate spinal cord segments and spinal sensory ganglia involved in sympathetic and visceral afferent (pain) innervation of abdominal viscera.

Pain is an unpleasant sensation associated with actual or potential tissue damage, mediated by specific nerve fibers to the brain, where its conscious appreciation may be modified. Organic pain arising from an organ such as the stomach varies from dull to severe; however, the pain is poorly localized. It radiates to the dermatome level served by the corresponding sensory ganglion, which receives the visceral afferent fibers from the organ concerned. **Visceral referred pain** from a gastric ulcer, for example, is referred to the epigastric region because the stomach is supplied by pain afferents that reach the T7 and T8 spinal (sensory) ganglia and spinal cord segments through the greater splanchnic nerve. The brain interprets the pain as though the irritation occurred in the skin of the epigastric region, which is also supplied by the same sensory ganglia and spinal cord segments.

Pain arising from the parietal peritoneum is of the somatic type and is usually severe. The site of its origin may be localized. The anatomical basis for this localization of pain is that the parietal peritoneum is supplied by somatic sensory fibers through thoracic nerves, whereas a viscus such as the appendix is supplied by visceral afferent fibers in the lesser splanchnic nerve. Inflamed parietal peritoneum is extremely sensitive to stretching. When digital pressure is applied to the anterolateral abdominal wall over the site of inflammation, the parietal peritoneum is stretched. When the fingers are suddenly removed, extreme localized pain is usually felt, known as **rebound tenderness**.

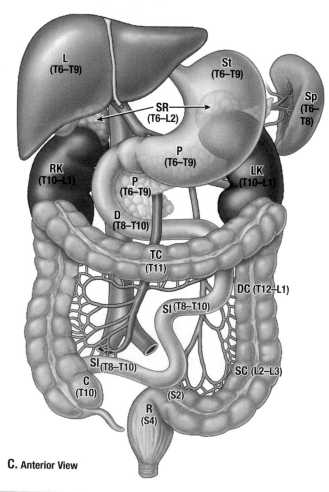

C. Anterior View

C	Cecum	**P**	Pancreas	**Sp**	Spleen
D	Duodenum	**R**	Rectum	**SR**	Suprarenal glands
DC	Descending colon	**RK**	Right kidney	**St**	Stomach
L	Liver	**SC**	Sigmoid colon	**TC**	Transverse colon
LK	Left kidney	**SI**	Small intestine		

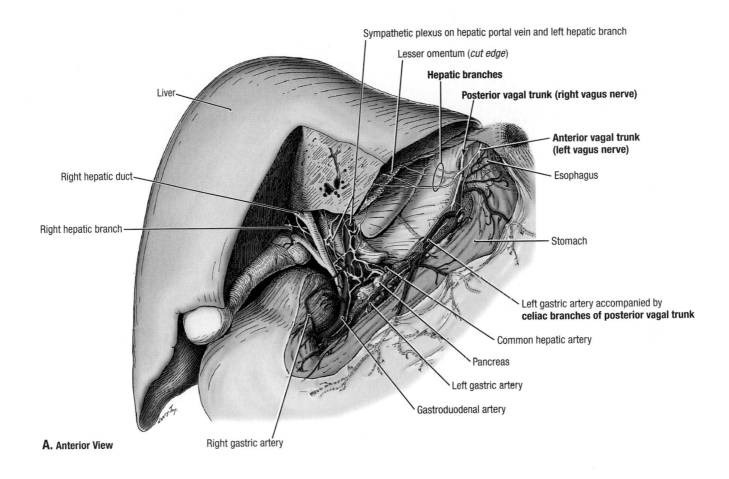

Sympathetic plexus on hepatic portal vein and left hepatic branch

Lesser omentum (*cut edge*)

Hepatic branches

Posterior vagal trunk (right vagus nerve)

Liver

**Anterior vagal trunk
(left vagus nerve)**

Esophagus

Right hepatic duct

Right hepatic branch

Stomach

Left gastric artery accompanied by
celiac branches of posterior vagal trunk

Common hepatic artery

Pancreas

Left gastric artery

Gastroduodenal artery

A. Anterior View

Right gastric artery

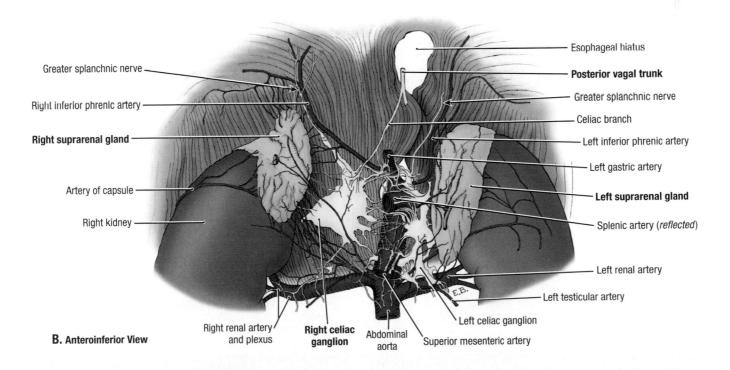

Esophageal hiatus

Greater splanchnic nerve

Posterior vagal trunk

Right inferior phrenic artery

Greater splanchnic nerve

Celiac branch

Right suprarenal gland

Left inferior phrenic artery

Left gastric artery

Artery of capsule

Left suprarenal gland

Right kidney

Splenic artery (*reflected*)

Left renal artery

Left testicular artery

Right renal artery
and plexus

**Right celiac
ganglion**

Abdominal
aorta

Superior mesenteric artery

Left celiac ganglion

B. Anteroinferior View

Vagus Nerves in Abdomen

4.86

A. Anterior and posterior vagal trunks. **B.** Celiac plexus and ganglia and suprarenal glands.

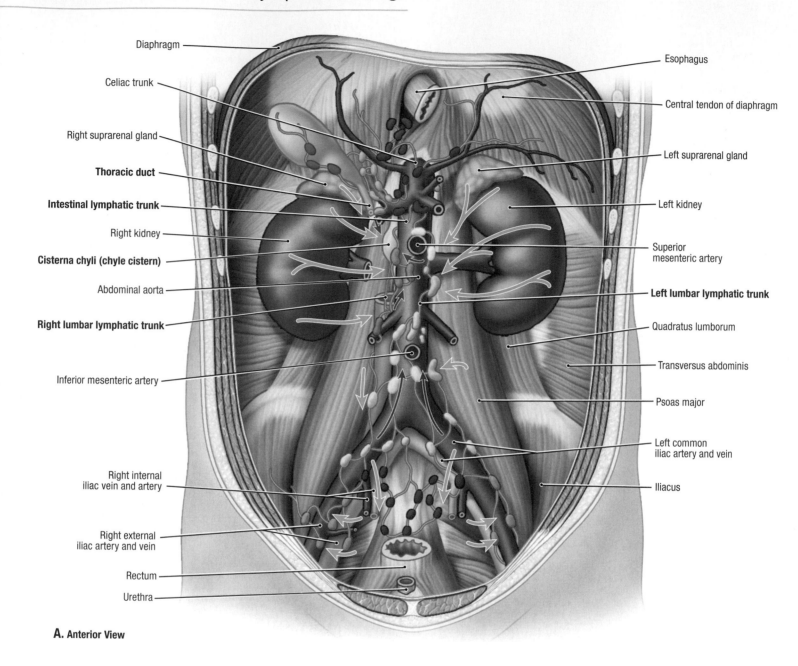

A. Anterior View

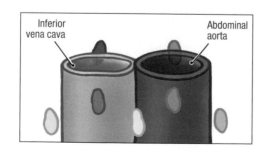

B. Anterior View

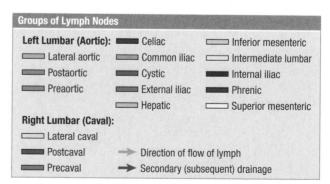

Groups of Lymph Nodes

Left Lumbar (Aortic):	Celiac	Inferior mesenteric
Lateral aortic	Common iliac	Intermediate lumbar
Postaortic	Cystic	Internal iliac
Preaortic	External iliac	Phrenic
	Hepatic	Superior mesenteric
Right Lumbar (Caval):		
Lateral caval		
Postcaval	⟶ Direction of flow of lymph	
Precaval	⟹ Secondary (subsequent) drainage	

4.87 ## Lymphatic Drainage of Suprarenal Glands, Kidneys, and Ureters

Lymphatic vessels from the suprarenal glands, kidneys, and upper ureters drain to the lumbar nodes. Lymphatic vessels from the middle part of the ureter usually drain into the **common iliac lymph nodes**, whereas vessels from its inferior part drain into the common, external, or internal **iliac lymph nodes**.

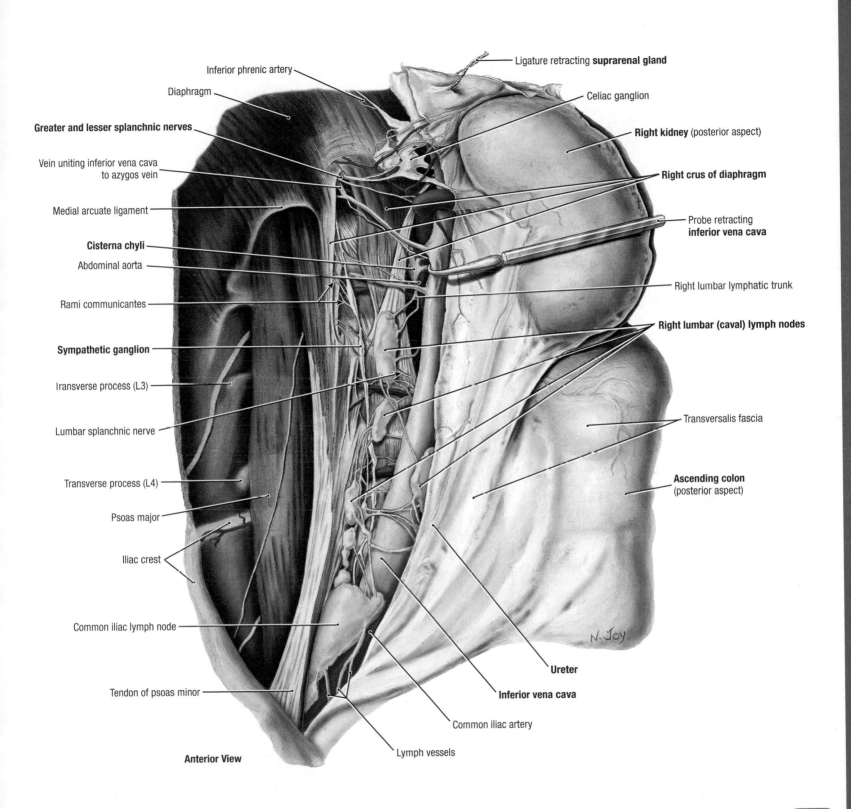

Inferior phrenic artery

Ligature retracting **suprarenal gland**

Diaphragm

Celiac ganglion

Greater and lesser splanchnic nerves

Right kidney (posterior aspect)

Vein uniting inferior vena cava to azygos vein

Right crus of diaphragm

Medial arcuate ligament

Probe retracting **inferior vena cava**

Cisterna chyli

Abdominal aorta

Right lumbar lymphatic trunk

Rami communicantes

Right lumbar (caval) lymph nodes

Sympathetic ganglion

Transverse process (L3)

Transversalis fascia

Lumbar splanchnic nerve

Transverse process (L4)

Ascending colon (posterior aspect)

Psoas major

Iliac crest

Common iliac lymph node

N. Joy

Tendon of psoas minor

Ureter

Inferior vena cava

Common iliac artery

Lymph vessels

Anterior View

Lumbar Lymph Nodes, Sympathetic Trunk, Nerves, and Ganglia

4.88

The right suprarenal gland, kidney, ureter, and colon are reflected to the left along with the transversalis fascia covering their posterior aspects. The inferior vena cava is pulled medially, and the third and fourth lumbar veins are removed. In this specimen, the greater and lesser splanchnic nerves, the sympathetic trunk, and a communicating vein pass through an unusually wide cleft in the right crus. The splanchnic nerves convey preganglionic fibers arising from the cell bodies in the (thoracolumbar) sympathetic trunk. The greater splanchnic nerve is from thoracic ganglia 5 to 9, and the lesser from thoracic ganglia 10 and 11.

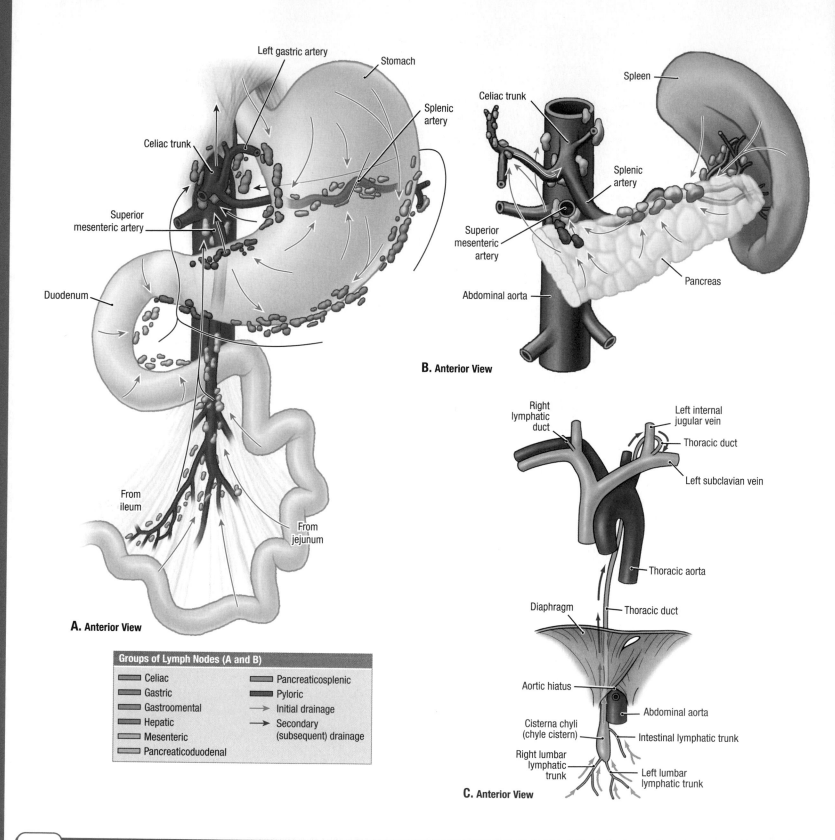

Left gastric artery

Stomach

Celiac trunk

Splenic artery

Superior mesenteric artery

Duodenum

From ileum

From jejunum

A. Anterior View

Celiac trunk

Spleen

Splenic artery

Superior mesenteric artery

Abdominal aorta

Pancreas

B. Anterior View

Right lymphatic duct

Left internal jugular vein

Thoracic duct

Left subclavian vein

Thoracic aorta

Diaphragm

Thoracic duct

Aortic hiatus

Abdominal aorta

Cisterna chyli (chyle cistern)

Intestinal lymphatic trunk

Right lumbar lymphatic trunk

Left lumbar lymphatic trunk

C. Anterior View

Groups of Lymph Nodes (A and B)

Celiac	Pancreaticosplenic
Gastric	Pyloric
Gastroomental	Initial drainage
Hepatic	Secondary
Mesenteric	(subsequent) drainage
Pancreaticoduodenal	

4.89 **Lymphatic Drainage**

**A. Stomach and small intestine. B. Spleen and pancreas.
C. Drainage from lumbar and intestinal lymphatic trunks.** The *arrows* indicate the direction of lymph flow; each group of lymph nodes is color-coded. Lymph from the abdominal nodes drains into the cisterna chyli, origin of the inferior end of the thoracic duct. The thoracic duct receives all lymph that forms inferior to the diaphragm and left upper quadrant (thorax and left upper limb) and empties into the junction of the left subclavian and left internal jugular veins.

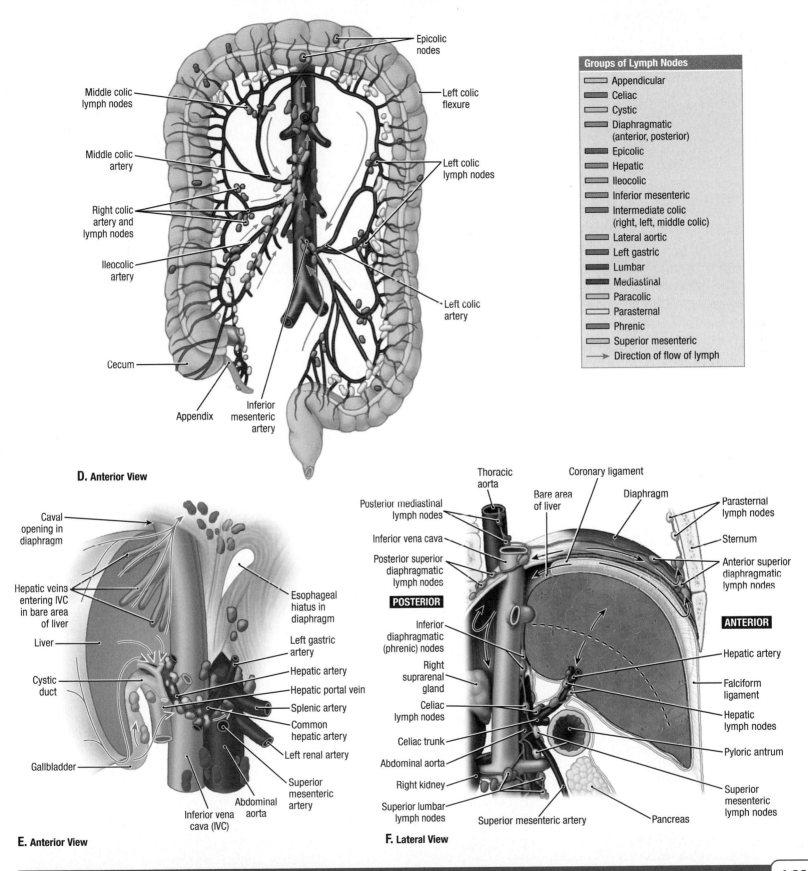

Epicolic nodes

Middle colic lymph nodes

Middle colic artery

Right colic artery and lymph nodes

Ileocolic artery

Cecum

Appendix

Inferior mesenteric artery

Left colic flexure

Left colic lymph nodes

Left colic artery

Groups of Lymph Nodes
- Appendicular
- Celiac
- Cystic
- Diaphragmatic (anterior, posterior)
- Epicolic
- Hepatic
- Ileocolic
- Inferior mesenteric
- Intermediate colic (right, left, middle colic)
- Lateral aortic
- Left gastric
- Lumbar
- Mediastinal
- Paracolic
- Parasternal
- Phrenic
- Superior mesenteric
→ Direction of flow of lymph

D. Anterior View

Caval opening in diaphragm

Hepatic veins entering IVC in bare area of liver

Liver

Cystic duct

Gallbladder

Inferior vena cava (IVC)

Abdominal aorta

Superior mesenteric artery

Left renal artery

Common hepatic artery

Splenic artery

Hepatic portal vein

Hepatic artery

Left gastric artery

Esophageal hiatus in diaphragm

E. Anterior View

Thoracic aorta

Coronary ligament

Bare area of liver

Diaphragm

Parasternal lymph nodes

Sternum

Anterior superior diaphragmatic lymph nodes

Posterior mediastinal lymph nodes

Inferior vena cava

Posterior superior diaphragmatic lymph nodes

POSTERIOR

Inferior diaphragmatic (phrenic) nodes

Right suprarenal gland

Celiac lymph nodes

Celiac trunk

Abdominal aorta

Right kidney

Superior lumbar lymph nodes

Superior mesenteric artery

Pancreas

ANTERIOR

Hepatic artery

Falciform ligament

Hepatic lymph nodes

Pyloric antrum

Superior mesenteric lymph nodes

F. Lateral View

D. Large intestine. E. Liver and gallbladder. F. Liver. Flow of lymph to diaphragmatic or visceral surfaces and to body wall indicated by *black arrows.*

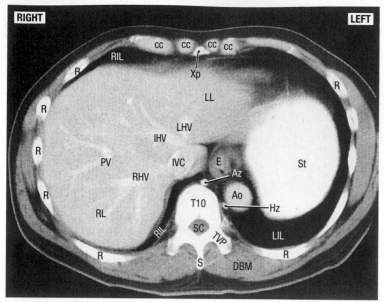

A. Transverse MRI

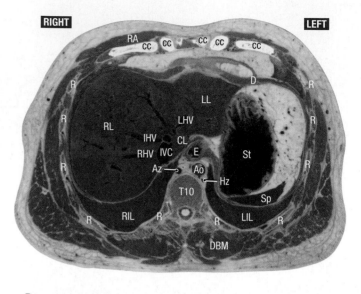

B. Transverse Section

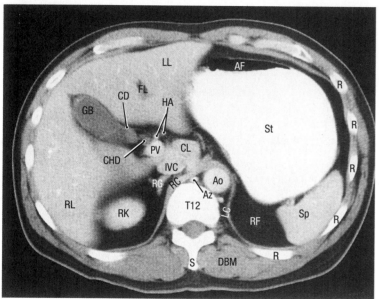

C. Transverse MRI

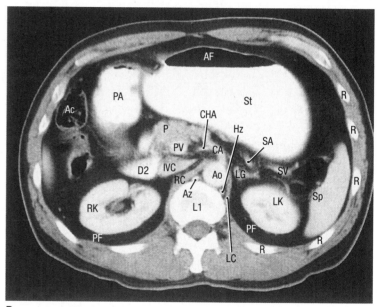

D. Transverse MRI

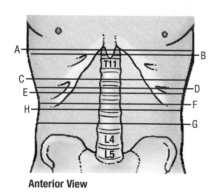

Anterior View

Key for A–H					
Ac	Ascending colon	**Dc**	Descending colon	**LG**	Left suprarenal gland
AF	Air-fluid level of stomach	**D2**	Descending part of duodenum	**LHV**	Left hepatic vein
Ao	Aorta	**D3**	Inferior part of duodenum	**LIL**	Left inferior lobe of lung
Az	Azygos vein	**E**	Esophagus	**LK**	Left kidney
CA	Celiac artery	**FL**	Falciform ligament	**LL**	Left lobe of liver
cc	Costal cartilage	**GB**	Gallbladder	**LRV**	Left renal vein
CD	Cystic duct	**HA**	Hepatic artery	**LU**	Left ureter
CHA	Common hepatic artery	**Hz**	Hemiazygos vein	**P**	Pancreas
CHD	Common hepatic duct	**IHV**	Intermediate hepatic vein	**PA**	Pyloric antrum of stomach
CL	Caudate lobe of liver	**IMV**	Inferior mesenteric vein	**PB**	Body of pancreas
D	Diaphragm	**IVC**	Inferior vena cava	**PC**	Portal confluence
DBM	Deep back muscles	**LC**	Left crus of diaphragm		

4.90 **Transverse (Axial) MRIs of Abdomen**

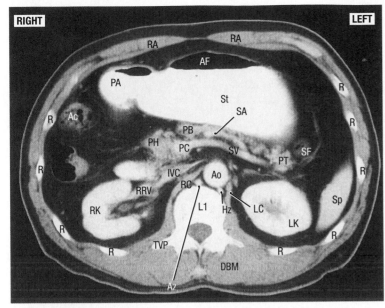

E. Transverse MRI

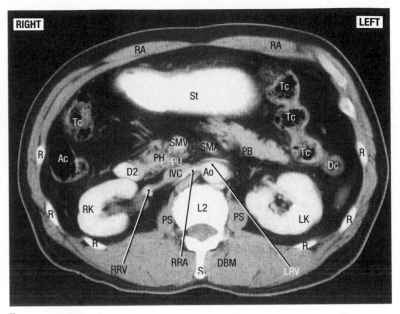

F. Transverse MRI

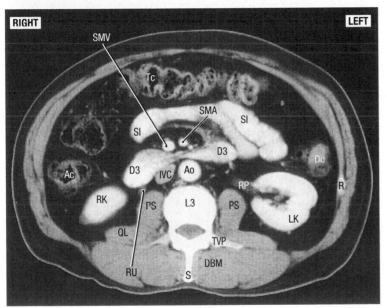

G. Transverse MRI

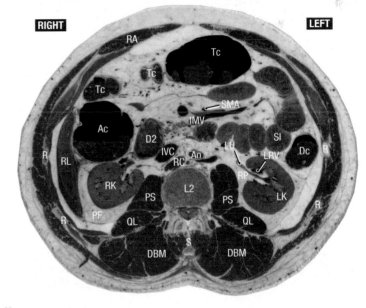

H. Transverse Section

Key for A–H (continued)					
PF	Perinephric fat	**RC**	Right crus of diaphragm	**RRV**	Right renal vein
PH	Head of pancreas	**RF**	Retroperitoneal fat	**RU**	Right ureter
PS	Psoas muscle	**RG**	Right suprarenal gland	**S**	Spinous process
PT	Tail of pancreas	**RHV**	Right hepatic vein	**SA**	Splenic artery
PU	Uncinate process of pancreas	**RIL**	Right inferior lobe of lung	**SC**	Spinal cord
PV	Hepatic portal vein	**RK**	Right kidney	**SF**	Splenic flexure
QL	Quadratus lumborum	**RL**	Right lobe of liver	**SI**	Small intestine
R	Rib	**RP**	Renal pelvis	**SMA**	Superior mesenteric artery
RA	Rectus abdominis	**RRA**	Right renal artery	**SMV**	Superior mesenteric vein

Sp	Spleen
St	Stomach
SV	Splenic vein
Tc	Transverse colon
TVP	Transverse process
Xp	Xiphoid process

Transverse (Axial) MRIs of Abdomen *(continued)*

4.90

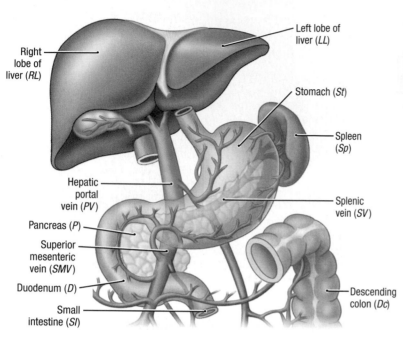

A. Anterior View (Formation of Portal Vein)

Right lobe of liver (*RL*)

Left lobe of liver (*LL*)

Stomach (*St*)

Spleen (*Sp*)

Hepatic portal vein (*PV*)

Splenic vein (*SV*)

Pancreas (*P*)

Superior mesenteric vein (*SMV*)

Duodenum (*D*)

Small intestine (*SI*)

Descending colon (*Dc*)

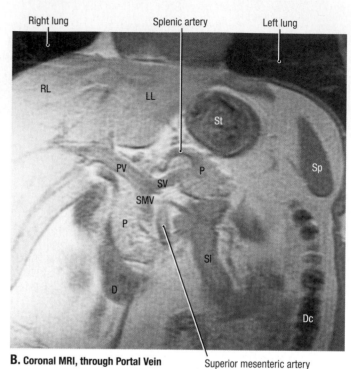

B. Coronal MRI, through Portal Vein

Right lung   Splenic artery   Left lung

Superior mesenteric artery

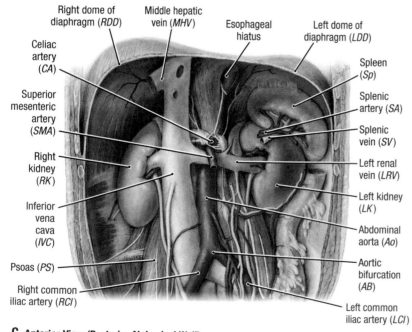

C. Anterior View (Posterior Abdominal Wall)

Right dome of diaphragm (*RDD*)

Middle hepatic vein (*MHV*)

Esophageal hiatus

Left dome of diaphragm (*LDD*)

Celiac artery (*CA*)

Spleen (*Sp*)

Superior mesenteric artery (*SMA*)

Splenic artery (*SA*)

Splenic vein (*SV*)

Right kidney (*RK*)

Left renal vein (*LRV*)

Left kidney (*LK*)

Inferior vena cava (*IVC*)

Abdominal aorta (*Ao*)

Psoas (*PS*)

Aortic bifurcation (*AB*)

Right common iliac artery (*RCI*)

Left common iliac artery (*LCI*)

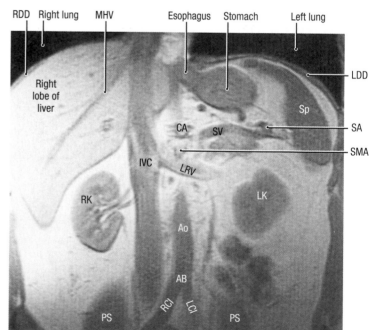

D. Coronal MRI, through Inferior Vena Cava

RDD   Right lung   MHV   Esophagus   Stomach   Left lung

Right lobe of liver   LDD

4.91 **Coronal MRIs of Abdomen**

A. Illustration of formation of hepatic portal vein. **B.** Coronal MRI through hepatic portal vein. **C.** Illustration of posterior abdominal wall. **D.** Coronal MRI through inferior vena cava and right and left kidneys.

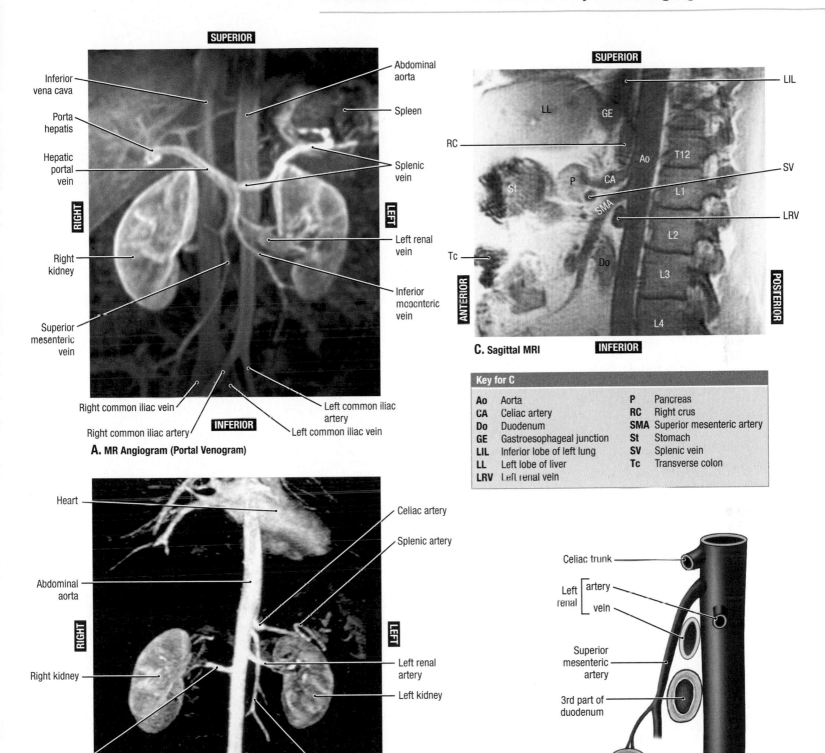

SUPERIOR

Inferior vena cava

Porta hepatis

Hepatic portal vein

RIGHT

Right kidney

Superior mesenteric vein

Abdominal aorta

Spleen

Splenic vein

LEFT

Left renal vein

Inferior mesenteric vein

Right common iliac vein

Right common iliac artery

INFERIOR

Left common iliac artery

Left common iliac vein

A. MR Angiogram (Portal Venogram)

SUPERIOR

LIL

LL   GE

RC

Ao   T12

SV

P   CA

St   L1

SMA   LRV

ANTERIOR

Tc   Do   L2

L3

POSTERIOR

L4

INFERIOR

C. Sagittal MRI

Key for C

Ao	Aorta	**P**	Pancreas
CA	Celiac artery	**RC**	Right crus
Do	Duodenum	**SMA**	Superior mesenteric artery
GE	Gastroesophageal junction	**St**	Stomach
LIL	Inferior lobe of left lung	**SV**	Splenic vein
LL	Left lobe of liver	**Tc**	Transverse colon
LRV	Left renal vein		

Heart

Abdominal aorta

RIGHT

Right kidney

Right renal artery

Celiac artery

Splenic artery

LEFT

Left renal artery

Left kidney

Right common iliac artery

Left common iliac vein

Superior mesenteric artery

B. MR Angiogram of Aorta and Its Branches

Celiac trunk

Left renal   artery   vein

Superior mesenteric artery

3rd part of duodenum

Small intestine

Aorta

D. Lateral View (from Left)

MR Angiograms and Sagittal MRI of Abdomen

A. Magnetic resonance (MR) angiogram (portal venogram) demonstrating tributaries and formation of hepatic portal vein. **B.** MR angiogram of aorta and branches. **C.** Sagittal MRI (magnetic resonance imaging) through aorta showing relationships of celiac and superior mesenteric arteries to surrounding structures. **D.** Schematic of relationships of superior mesenteric artery.

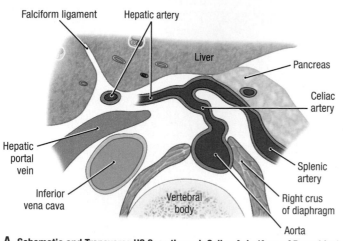

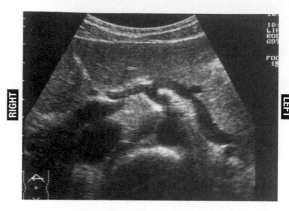

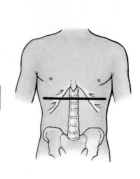

A. Schematic and Transverse US Scan through Celiac Axis (Area of Branching)

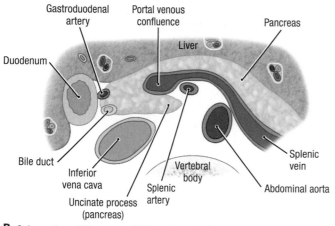

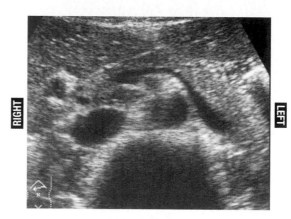

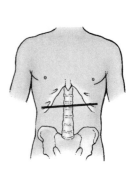

B. Schematic and Transverse US Scan through Splenic View

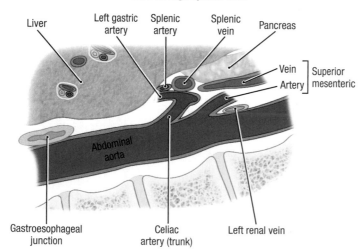

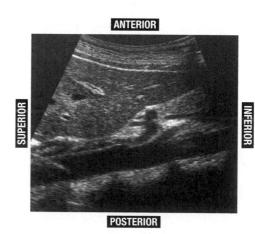

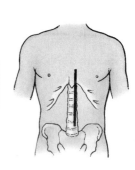

C. Schematic and Midsagittal US Scan through Abdominal Aorta

4.93 **Ultrasound (US) Scans of Abdomen**

A. Transverse ultrasound scan through celiac artery (axis). **B.** Transverse ultrasound scan through pancreas. **C.** and **D.** Sagittal ultrasound scans through aorta, celiac trunk, and superior mesenteric artery (*Part D* with Doppler). **E.** Transverse ultrasound scan at hilum of left kidney with left renal artery and vein (with Doppler). **F.** Sagittal ultrasound scan of right kidney.

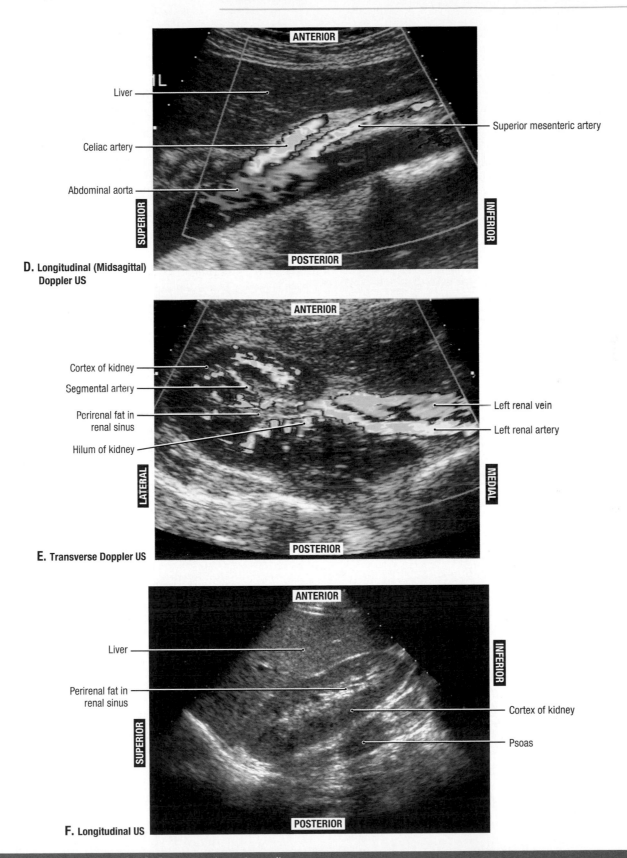

D. Longitudinal (Midsagittal) Doppler US

Labels: Liver, Celiac artery, Abdominal aorta, Superior mesenteric artery. Orientation: ANTERIOR, SUPERIOR, INFERIOR, POSTERIOR

E. Transverse Doppler US

Labels: Cortex of kidney, Segmental artery, Perirenal fat in renal sinus, Hilum of kidney, Left renal vein, Left renal artery. Orientation: ANTERIOR, LATERAL, MEDIAL, POSTERIOR

F. Longitudinal US

Labels: Liver, Perirenal fat in renal sinus, Cortex of kidney, Psoas. Orientation: ANTERIOR, SUPERIOR, INFERIOR, POSTERIOR

Ultrasound (US) Scans of Abdomen *(continued)*

4.93

A major advantage of ultrasonography is its ability to produce real-time images, demonstrating motion of structures and flow within blood vessels. In Doppler ultrasonography (*Part D* and *Part E*), the shifts in frequency between emitted ultrasonic waves and their echoes are used to measure the velocities of moving objects. This technique is based on the principle of the Doppler effect. Blood flow through vessels is displayed in color, superimposed on the two-dimensional cross-sectional image (slow flow: *blue*, fast flow: *orange*).

CHAPTER 5

PELVIS AND PERINEUM

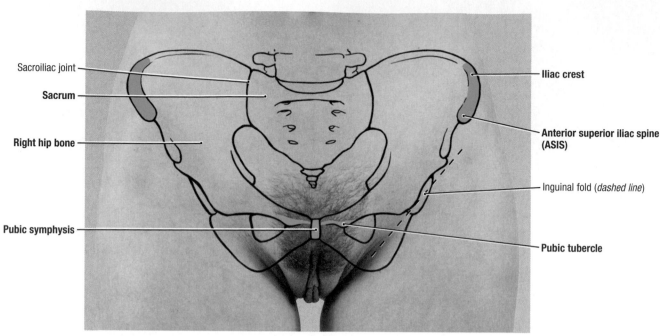

Sacroiliac joint

Sacrum

Right hip bone

Pubic symphysis

Iliac crest

Anterior superior iliac spine (ASIS)

Inguinal fold (*dashed line*)

Pubic tubercle

A. Anterior View

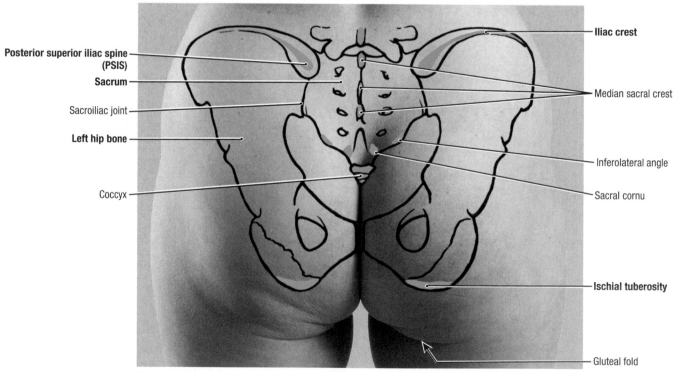

Posterior superior iliac spine (PSIS)

Sacrum

Sacroiliac joint

Left hip bone

Coccyx

Iliac crest

Median sacral crest

Inferolateral angle

Sacral cornu

Ischial tuberosity

Gluteal fold

B. **Posterior View**

5.1 | Surface Anatomy of Female Pelvic Girdle

The pelvic girdle (bony pelvis) is a basin-shaped ring of three bones (right and left hip bones and sacrum) that connects the vertebral column to the femora. Palpable features (*green*) should be symmetrical across the midline. The female pelvic girdle is relatively wider and shallower than that of the male, related to its additional roles of bearing the weight of the gravid uterus in late **pregnancy** and allowing passage of the fetus through the pelvic outlet during childbirth (parturition). **A. Palpable features (*green*) of anterior aspect of pelvic girdle.** The hip bones are joined anteriorly at the pubic symphysis. The presence of a thick overlying pubic fat pad forming the mons pubis may interfere with palpation of the pubic tubercles and symphysis. **B. Palpable features (*green*) of posterior aspect of pelvic girdle.** Posteriorly, the hip bones articulate with the sacrum at the sacroiliac joints.

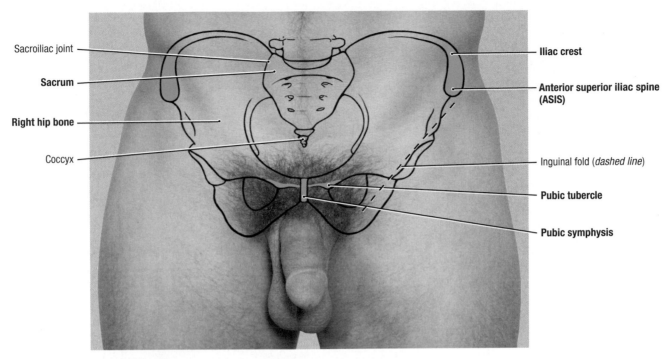

Sacroiliac joint

Sacrum

Right hip bone

Coccyx

Iliac crest

Anterior superior iliac spine (ASIS)

Inguinal fold (*dashed line*)

Pubic tubercle

Pubic symphysis

A. Anterior View

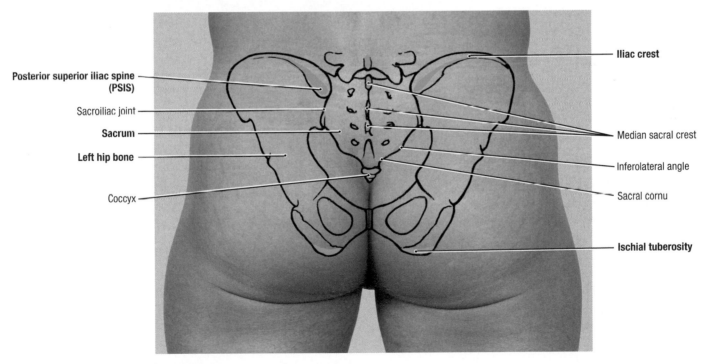

Posterior superior iliac spine (PSIS)

Sacroiliac joint

Sacrum

Left hip bone

Coccyx

Iliac crest

Median sacral crest

Inferolateral angle

Sacral cornu

Ischial tuberosity

B. Posterior View

Surface Anatomy of Male Pelvic Girdle
5.2

A. Palpable features of anterior aspect of pelvic girdle. The anterior third of the iliac crests are subcutaneous and usually easily palpable. The remainder of the crests may also be palpable, depending on the thickness of the overlying subcutaneous tissue (fat). The inguinal ligament spans between the palpable anterior superior iliac spine (ASIS) and pubic tubercle, located superior to the lateral and medial ends of the inguinal fold. **B. Palpable features of posterior aspect of pelvic girdle.** The posterior superior iliac spine (PSIS) is usually palpable and often lies deep to a visible dimple, indicating the S2 vertebral level. The ischial tuberosities may be palpated when the hip joint is flexed.

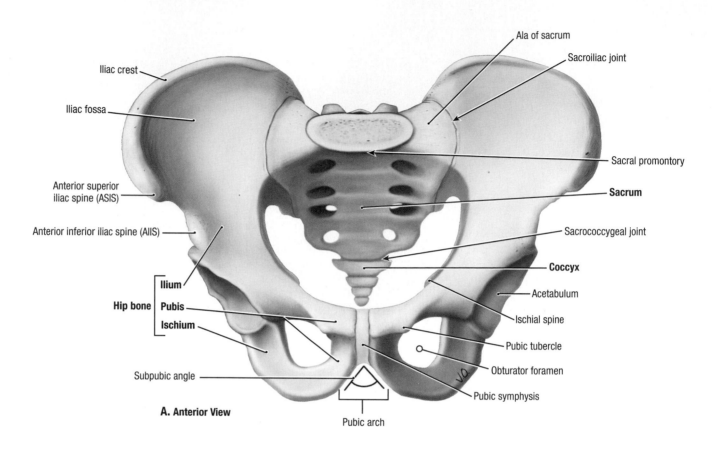

A. Anterior View

- Iliac crest
- Iliac fossa
- Anterior superior iliac spine (ASIS)
- Anterior inferior iliac spine (AIIS)

Hip bone
- **Ilium**
- **Pubis**
- **Ischium**

- Subpubic angle
- Pubic arch

- Ala of sacrum
- Sacroiliac joint
- Sacral promontory
- **Sacrum**
- Sacrococcygeal joint
- **Coccyx**
- Acetabulum
- Ischial spine
- Pubic tubercle
- Obturator foramen
- Pubic symphysis

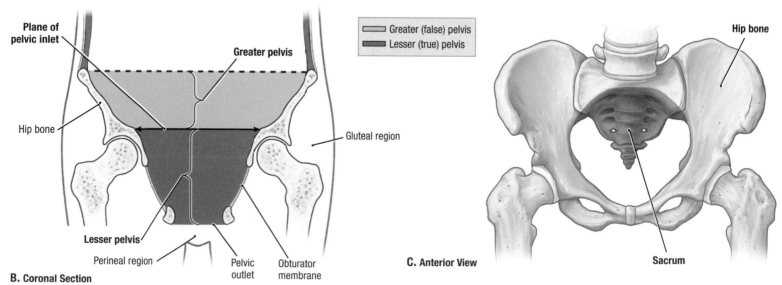

B. Coronal Section

- **Plane of pelvic inlet**
- **Greater pelvis**
- Hip bone
- **Lesser pelvis**
- Perineal region
- Pelvic outlet
- Obturator membrane

- Greater (false) pelvis
- Lesser (true) pelvis

- Gluteal region

C. Anterior View

- Hip bone
- **Sacrum**

5.3 | Bones and Divisions of Pelvis

A. Bones of pelvis. The three bones composing the pelvis are the pubis, ischium, and ilium. **B.** and **C. Lesser and greater pelvis, schematics.** The plane of the pelvic inlet (*double-headed arrow* in

Part B) separates the greater pelvis (part of the abdominal cavity) from the lesser pelvis (pelvic cavity). *Dashed line*, superior extent of greater pelvis.

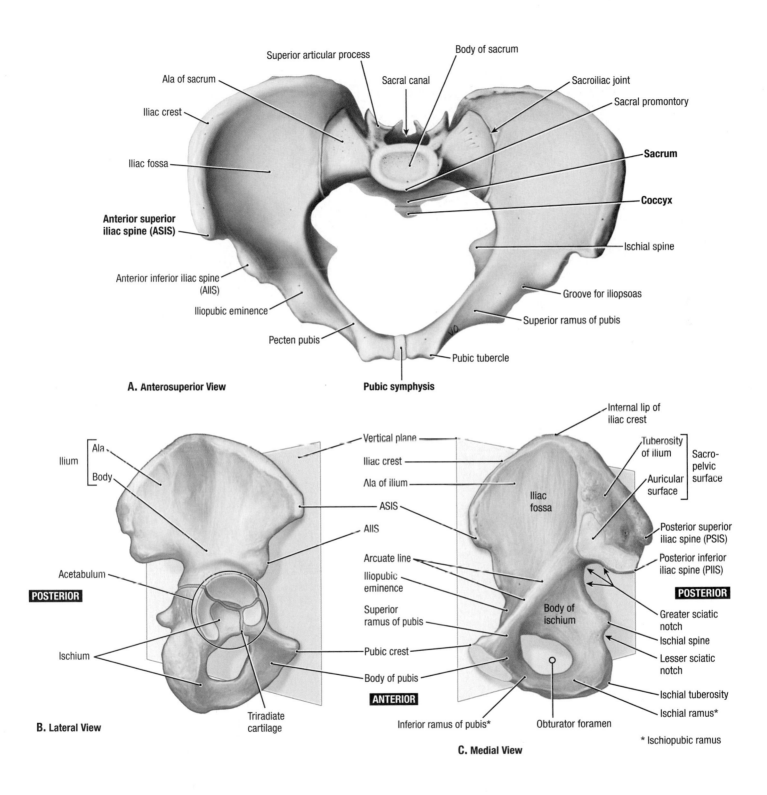

Superior articular process

Body of sacrum

Ala of sacrum

Sacral canal

Sacroiliac joint

Iliac crest

Sacral promontory

Iliac fossa

Sacrum

Coccyx

**Anterior superior
iliac spine (ASIS)**

Ischial spine

Anterior inferior iliac spine
(AIIS)

Groove for iliopsoas

Iliopubic eminence

Superior ramus of pubis

Pecten pubis

Pubic tubercle

Pubic symphysis

A. Anterosuperior View

Ilium { Ala / Body }

Internal lip of
iliac crest

Vertical plane

Tuberosity
of ilium

Sacro-
pelvic
surface

Iliac crest

Ala of ilium

Iliac
fossa

Auricular
surface

ASIS

AIIS

Posterior superior
iliac spine (PSIS)

Acetabulum

Arcuate line

Posterior inferior
iliac spine (PIIS)

Iliopubic
eminence

POSTERIOR

POSTERIOR

Superior
ramus of pubis

Body of
ischium

Greater sciatic
notch

Ischium

Pubic crest

Ischial spine

Body of pubis

Lesser sciatic
notch

ANTERIOR

Ischial tuberosity

Triradiate
cartilage

Inferior ramus of pubis*

Obturator foramen

Ischial ramus*

B. Lateral View

* Ischiopubic ramus

C. Medial View

Pelvis, Anatomical Position

5.4

A. Pelvic girdle. B. Placement of hip bone in anatomical position. In the anatomical position, (1) the anterior superior iliac spine (*ASIS*) and the anterior aspect of the pubis lie in the same vertical plane and (2) the sacrum is located superiorly, the coccyx posteriorly, and the pubic symphysis anteroinferiorly. **C. Features of hip bone.**

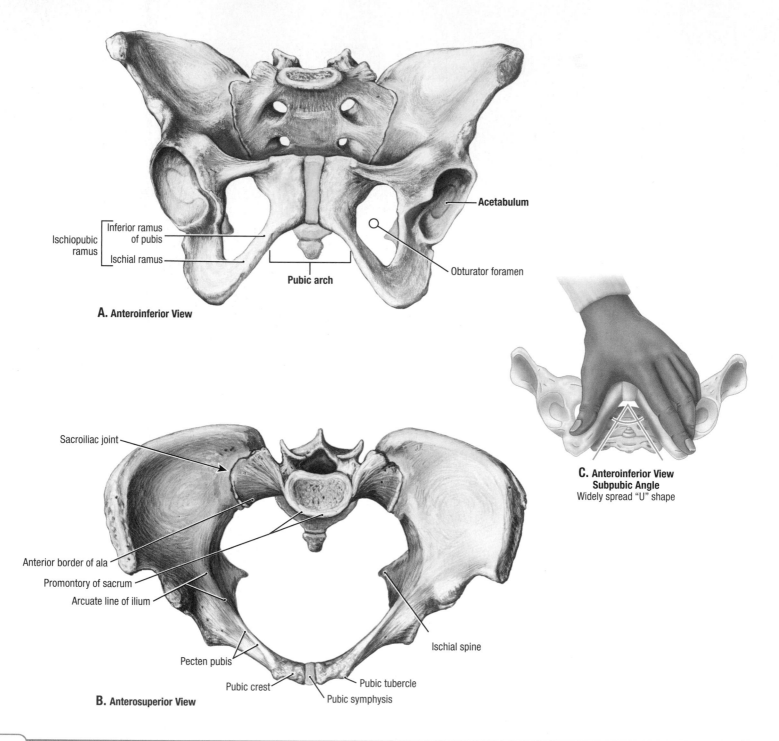

A. Anteroinferior View

Ischiopubic ramus
Inferior ramus of pubis
Ischial ramus
Pubic arch
Acetabulum
Obturator foramen

Sacroiliac joint
Anterior border of ala
Promontory of sacrum
Arcuate line of ilium
Pecten pubis
Pubic crest
Pubic symphysis
Pubic tubercle
Ischial spine

B. Anterosuperior View

C. Anteroinferior View
Subpubic Angle
Widely spread "U" shape

5.5   **Female Pelvic Girdle**

TABLE 5.1	Differences between Female and Male Pelves	
Bony Pelvis	**Female**	**Male**
General structure	Thinner and lighter	Thicker and heavier
Greater pelvis (pelvis major)	Shallower	Deeper
Lesser pelvis (pelvis minor)	Wider and shallower, cylindrical	Narrower and deeper, tapering
Pelvic inlet (superior pelvic aperture)	More oval or rounded, wider	Heart shaped, narrower
Sacrum/coccyx	Less curved	More curved

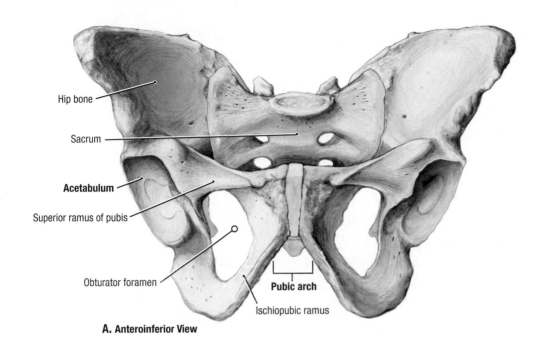

Hip bone

Sacrum

Acetabulum

Superior ramus of pubis

Obturator foramen

Pubic arch

Ischiopubic ramus

A. Anteroinferior View

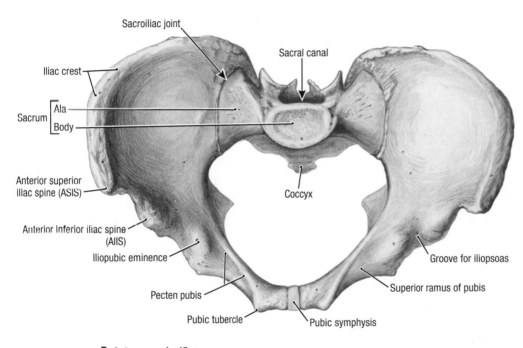

Sacroiliac joint

Sacral canal

Iliac crest

Sacrum
- Ala
- Body

Anterior superior
iliac spine (ASIS)

Anterior Inferior iliac spine
(AIIS)

Iliopubic eminence

Pecten pubis

Pubic tubercle

Coccyx

Groove for iliopsoas

Superior ramus of pubis

Pubic symphysis

B. Anterosuperior View

C. Anteroinferior View
Subpubic Angle
Narrow "V" shape

Male Pelvic Girdle   **5.6**

TABLE 5.1	Differences between Female and Male Pelves *(continued)*	
Bony Pelvis	**Female**	**Male**
Pelvic outlet (inferior pelvic aperture)	Comparatively large	Comparatively small
Pubic arch and subpubic angle	Wider	Narrower
Obturator foramen	Oval	Round
Acetabulum	Small	Large

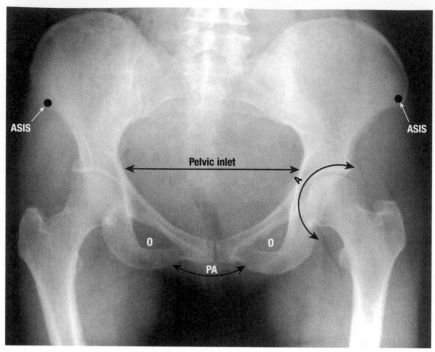

A. Anteroposterior Radiograph, Female Pelvis

A	Acetabulum	O	Obturator foramen
ASIS	Anterior superior iliac spine	**PA**	Pubic arch

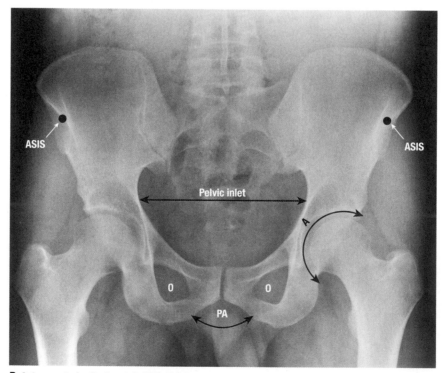

B. Anteroposterior Radiograph, Male Pelvis

5.7   **Radiographs of Pelvis**

A. Female. B. Male. Some of the main differences of female and male pelves are listed in Table 5.1. The radiographs highlight some of these differences.

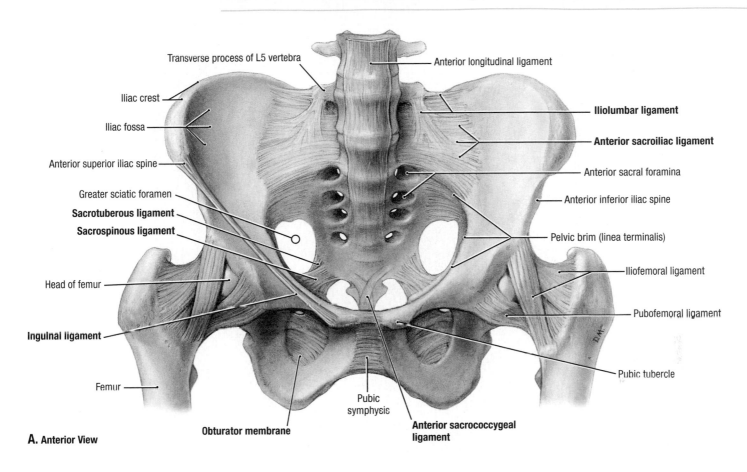

Transverse process of L5 vertebra

Iliac crest

Iliac fossa

Anterior superior iliac spine

Greater sciatic foramen

Sacrotuberous ligament

Sacrospinous ligament

Head of femur

Inguinal ligament

Femur

Anterior longitudinal ligament

Iliolumbar ligament

Anterior sacroiliac ligament

Anterior sacral foramina

Anterior inferior iliac spine

Pelvic brim (linea terminalis)

Iliofemoral ligament

Pubofemoral ligament

Pubic tubercle

Pubic symphysis

Obturator membrane

Anterior sacrococcygeal ligament

A. Anterior View

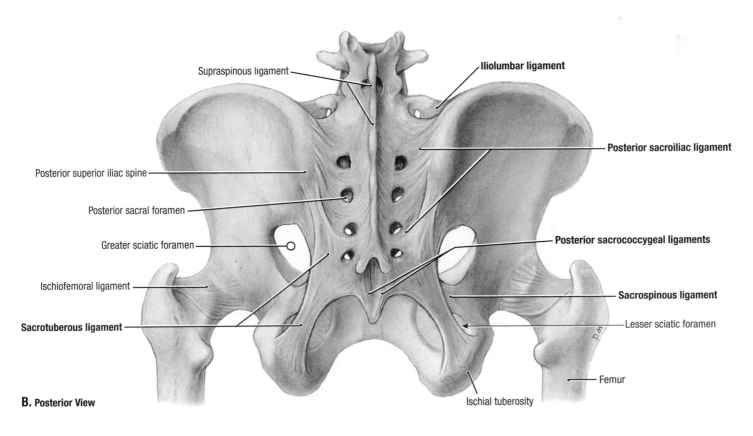

Supraspinous ligament

Iliolumbar ligament

Posterior superior iliac spine

Posterior sacral foramen

Greater sciatic foramen

Ischiofemoral ligament

Sacrotuberous ligament

Posterior sacroiliac ligament

Posterior sacrococcygeal ligaments

Sacrospinous ligament

Lesser sciatic foramen

Femur

Ischial tuberosity

B. Posterior View

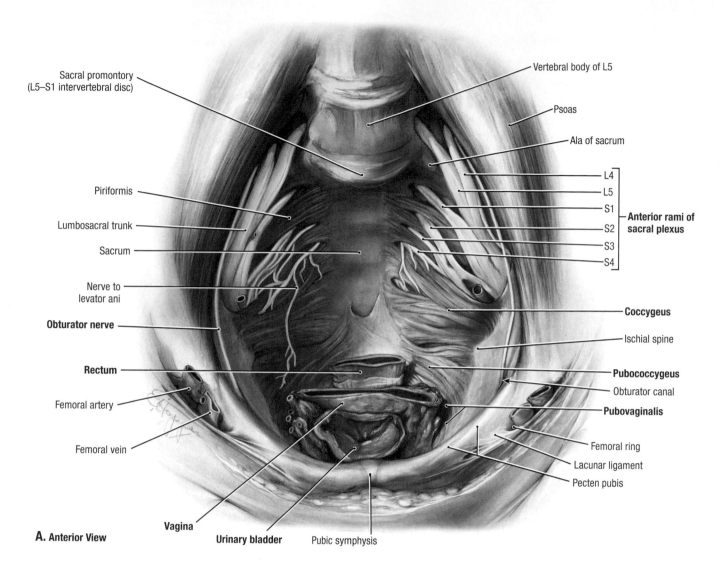

Sacral promontory
(L5–S1 intervertebral disc)

Piriformis

Lumbosacral trunk

Sacrum

Nerve to
levator ani

Obturator nerve

Rectum

Femoral artery

Femoral vein

Vagina

A. Anterior View

Urinary bladder   Pubic symphysis

Vertebral body of L5

Psoas

Ala of sacrum

L4
L5
S1   **Anterior rami of
S2   sacral plexus**
S3
S4

Coccygeus

Ischial spine

Pubococcygeus

Obturator canal

Pubovaginalis

Femoral ring

Lacunar ligament

Pecten pubis

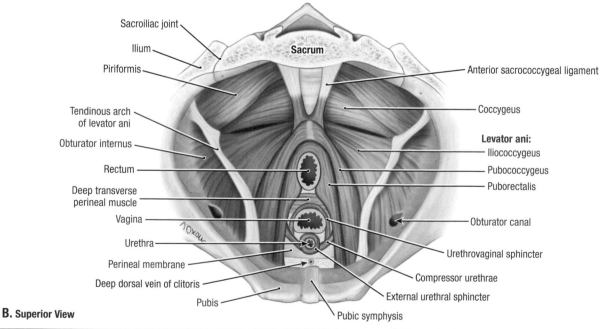

Sacroiliac joint

Ilium

Piriformis

Tendinous arch
of levator ani

Obturator internus

Rectum

Deep transverse
perineal muscle

Vagina

Urethra

Perineal membrane

Deep dorsal vein of clitoris

Pubis

B. Superior View

Sacrum

Anterior sacrococcygeal ligament

Coccygeus

Levator ani:
Iliococcygeus

Pubococcygeus

Puborectalis

Obturator canal

Urethrovaginal sphincter

Compressor urethrae

External urethral sphincter

Pubic symphysis

5.9   **Floor and Walls of Female Pelvis**

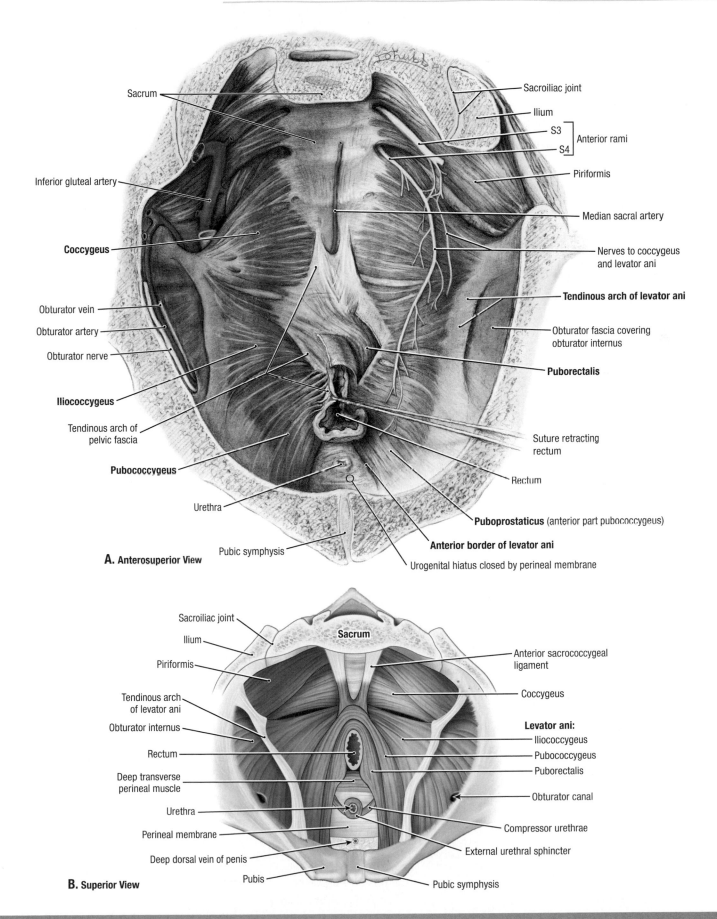

Sacrum

Inferior gluteal artery

Coccygeus

Obturator vein

Obturator artery

Obturator nerve

Iliococcygeus

Tendinous arch of pelvic fascia

Pubococcygeus

Urethra

Pubic symphysis

A. Anterosuperior View

Sacroiliac joint

Ilium

S3
S4 } Anterior rami

Piriformis

Median sacral artery

Nerves to coccygeus and levator ani

Tendinous arch of levator ani

Obturator fascia covering obturator internus

Puborectalis

Suture retracting rectum

Rectum

Puboprostaticus (anterior part pubococcygeus)

Anterior border of levator ani

Urogenital hiatus closed by perineal membrane

Sacroiliac joint

Ilium

Piriformis

Tendinous arch of levator ani

Obturator internus

Rectum

Deep transverse perineal muscle

Urethra

Perineal membrane

Deep dorsal vein of penis

B. Superior View

Pubis

Sacrum

Anterior sacrococcygeal ligament

Coccygeus

Levator ani:
Iliococcygeus
Pubococcygeus
Puborectalis

Obturator canal

Compressor urethrae

External urethral sphincter

Pubic symphysis

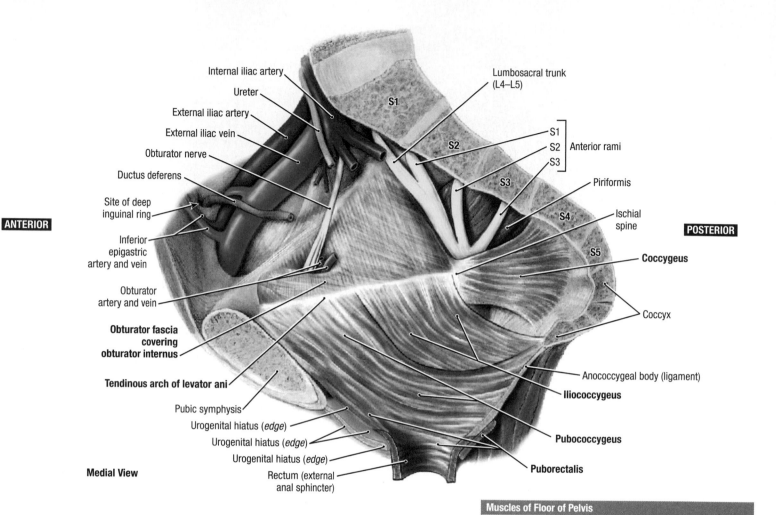

Medial View

Internal iliac artery
Ureter
External iliac artery
External iliac vein
Obturator nerve
Ductus deferens
Site of deep inguinal ring
ANTERIOR
Inferior epigastric artery and vein
Obturator artery and vein
Obturator fascia covering obturator internus
Tendinous arch of levator ani
Pubic symphysis
Urogenital hiatus (*edge*)
Urogenital hiatus (*edge*)
Urogenital hiatus (*edge*)
Rectum (external anal sphincter)

Lumbosacral trunk (L4–L5)
S1
S2
S1
S2
S3
Anterior rami
S3
Piriformis
Ischial spine
POSTERIOR
S4
S5
Coccygeus
Coccyx
Anococcygeal body (ligament)
Iliococcygeus
Pubococcygeus
Puborectalis

Muscles of Floor of Pelvis

Pelvic diaphragm (PD) = Levator ani (LA) + Coccygeus (C)
(PD = LA + C)

Levator ani (LA) = Pubococcygeus (PC) + Iliococcygeus (IC)
(LA = PC + IC)

Pubococcygeus (PC ♀) = Puborectalis (PR) + Pubovaginalis (PV)
(PC = PR + PV ♀)

Pubococcygeus (PC ♂) = Puborectalis (PR) + Puboprostaticus (PP)
(PC = PR + PP ♂)   (Levator prostatae)

5.11 Muscles of Pelvic Diaphragm

The pelvis has been bisected in the median plane. The pelvic floor is formed by the funnel- or bowl-shaped pelvic diaphragm. The funnel shape can be seen in a medial view.

TABLE 5.2 Muscles of Pelvic Walls and Floor

Boundary	Muscle	Proximal Attachment	Distal Attachment	Innervation	Main Action
Lateral wall	Obturator internus	Pelvic surfaces of ilium and ischium, obturator membrane	Greater trochanter of femur	Nerve to obturator internus (L5, S1, S2)	Rotates hip joint laterally; assists in holding head of femur in acetabulum
Posterolateral wall	Piriformis	Pelvic surface of S2–S4 segments, superior margin of greater sciatic notch, sacrotuberous ligament		Anterior rami of S1 and S2	Rotates hip joint laterally; abducts hip joint; assists in holding head of femur in acetabulum
Floor	Levator ani (pubococcygeus, puborectalis, and iliococcygeus)	Body of pubis, tendinous arch of obturator fascia, ischial spine	Perineal body, coccyx, anococcygeal ligament, walls of prostate or vagina, rectum, and anal canal	Nerve to levator ani (branches of S4), inferior anal (rectal) nerve, and coccygeal plexus	Forms most of pelvic diaphragm that helps support pelvic viscera and resists increases in intraabdominal pressure
	Coccygeus (ischiococcygeus)	Ischial spine	Inferior end of sacrum and coccyx	Branches of S4 and S5 spinal nerves	Forms small part of pelvic diaphragm that supports pelvic viscera; flexes sacrococcygeal joints

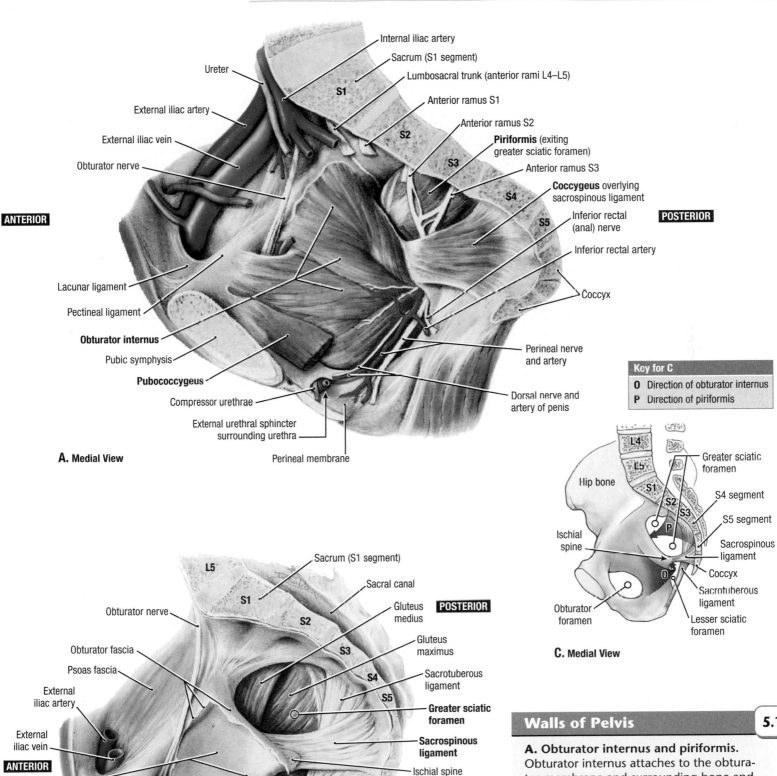

A. Medial View

Internal iliac artery
Sacrum (S1 segment)
Lumbosacral trunk (anterior rami L4–L5)
Anterior ramus S1
Anterior ramus S2
Piriformis (exiting greater sciatic foramen)
Anterior ramus S3
Coccygeus overlying sacrospinous ligament
Inferior rectal (anal) nerve
Inferior rectal artery
Coccyx
Perineal nerve and artery
Dorsal nerve and artery of penis

Ureter
External iliac artery
External iliac vein
Obturator nerve
ANTERIOR
Lacunar ligament
Pectineal ligament
Obturator internus
Pubic symphysis
Pubococcygeus
Compressor urethrae
External urethral sphincter surrounding urethra
Perineal membrane

POSTERIOR

Key for C
O   Direction of obturator internus
P   Direction of piriformis

C. Medial View

L4
L5
S1
S2
S3
Hip bone
Ischial spine
Obturator foramen
Greater sciatic foramen
S4 segment
S5 segment
Sacrospinous ligament
Coccyx
Sacrotuberous ligament
Lesser sciatic foramen

B. Medial View

Obturator nerve
Obturator fascia
Psoas fascia
External iliac artery
External iliac vein
ANTERIOR
Ischium
Obturator canal
Pubis
Pubic symphysis
Obturator membrane
Inferior pubic ligament
Lesser sciatic notch

Sacrum (S1 segment)
Sacral canal
Gluteus medius
POSTERIOR
Gluteus maximus
Sacrotuberous ligament
Greater sciatic foramen
Sacrospinous ligament
Ischial spine
Tip of coccyx
Sacrotuberous ligament
Lesser sciatic foramen
Gluteus maximus
Ischial tuberosity
L5
S1
S2
S3
S4
S5

Walls of Pelvis   5.12

A. Obturator internus and piriformis. Obturator internus attaches to the obturator membrane and surrounding bone and exits the lesser pelvis through the lesser sciatic foramen. Piriformis lies on the posterolateral pelvic wall and leaves the lesser pelvis through the greater sciatic foramen. **B. Obturator membrane, obturator internus removed.** On the lateral pelvic wall, the obturator foramen is closed by the obturator membrane except for the obturator canal. **C. Course of obturator internus and piriformis.**

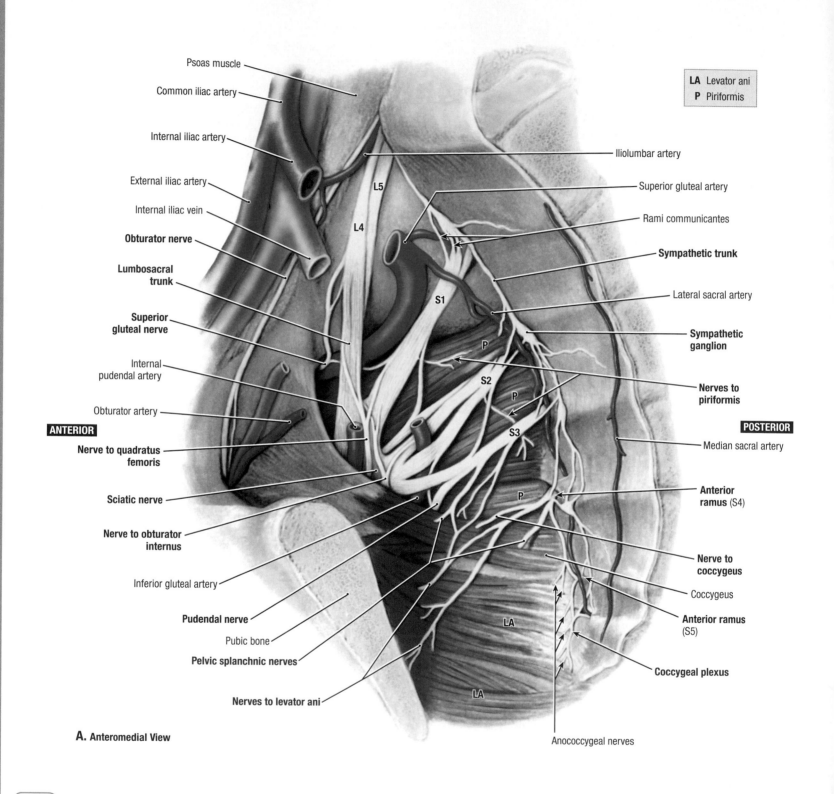

| LA | Levator ani |
| P | Piriformis |

Psoas muscle

Common iliac artery

Internal iliac artery

External iliac artery

Internal iliac vein

Obturator nerve

Lumbosacral trunk

Superior gluteal nerve

Internal pudendal artery

Obturator artery

ANTERIOR

Nerve to quadratus femoris

Sciatic nerve

Nerve to obturator internus

Inferior gluteal artery

Pudendal nerve

Pubic bone

Pelvic splanchnic nerves

Nerves to levator ani

L5

L4

S1

P

S2

P

S3

P

LA

LA

Iliolumbar artery

Superior gluteal artery

Rami communicantes

Sympathetic trunk

Lateral sacral artery

Sympathetic ganglion

Nerves to piriformis

POSTERIOR

Median sacral artery

Anterior ramus (S4)

Nerve to coccygeus

Coccygeus

Anterior ramus (S5)

Coccygeal plexus

Anococcygeal nerves

A. Anteromedial View

5.13   **Sacral and Coccygeal Nerve Plexuses**

A. Dissection.
- The sympathetic trunk or its ganglia send rami communicantes to each sacral and coccygeal nerve.
- The anterior ramus from L4 joins that of L5 to form the lumbosacral trunk.

- The sciatic nerve arises from anterior rami of L4, L5, S1, S2, and S3; the pudendal nerve from S2, S3, and S4; and the coccygeal plexus from S4, S5, and coccygeal segments.

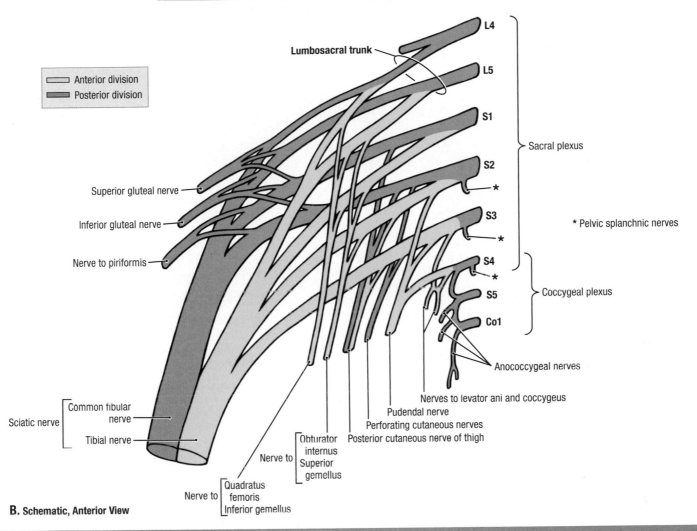

Anterior division
Posterior division

L4
L5
Lumbosacral trunk
S1
S2
*
S3
*
S4
*
S5
Co1

Sacral plexus

* Pelvic splanchnic nerves

Coccygeal plexus

Superior gluteal nerve
Inferior gluteal nerve
Nerve to piriformis

Anococcygeal nerves
Nerves to levator ani and coccygeus
Pudendal nerve
Perforating cutaneous nerves
Posterior cutaneous nerve of thigh

Sciatic nerve
Common fibular nerve
Tibial nerve

Obturator internus
Superior gemellus
Nerve to

Nerve to
Quadratus femoris
Inferior gemellus

B. Schematic, Anterior View

Sacral and Coccygeal Nerve Plexuses (continued)

5.13

B. Branches of anterior and posterior divisions of sacral and coccygeal plexuses.

TABLE 5.3   Nerves of Sacral and Coccygeal Plexuses

Nerve	Origin	Distribution
Sciatic: 1. Common fibular	L4, L5, S1, S2	Articular branches to hip joint and muscular branches to flexors of knee joint in thigh and all muscles in leg and foot
2. Tibial	L4, L5, S1, S2, S3	
3. Superior gluteal	L4, L5, S1	Gluteus medius and gluteus minimus muscles
4. Nerve to quadratus femoris and inferior gemellus	L4, L5, S1	Quadratus femoris and inferior gemellus muscles
5. Inferior gluteal	L5, S1, S2	Gluteus maximus muscle
6. Nerve to obturator internus and superior gemellus	L5, S1, S2	Obturator internus and superior gemellus muscles
7. Nerve to piriformis	S1, S2	Piriformis muscle
8. Posterior cutaneous nerve of thigh	S1, S2, S3	Cutaneous branches to buttock and uppermost medial and posterior surfaces of thigh
9. Perforating cutaneous	S2, S3	Cutaneous branches to medial part of buttock
10. Pudendal	S2, S3, S4	Structures in perineum; sensory to genitalia; muscular branches to perineal muscles, external urethral sphincter, and external anal sphincter
11. Pelvic splanchnic	S2, S3, S4	Pelvic viscera via inferior hypogastric and pelvic plexuses
12. Nerves to levator ani and coccygeus	S3, S4	Levator ani and coccygeus muscles
13. Anococcygeal nerve	S4, S5, Co1	Penetrate coccygeal attachments of sacrospinous/sacrotuberous ligaments to supply overlying skin

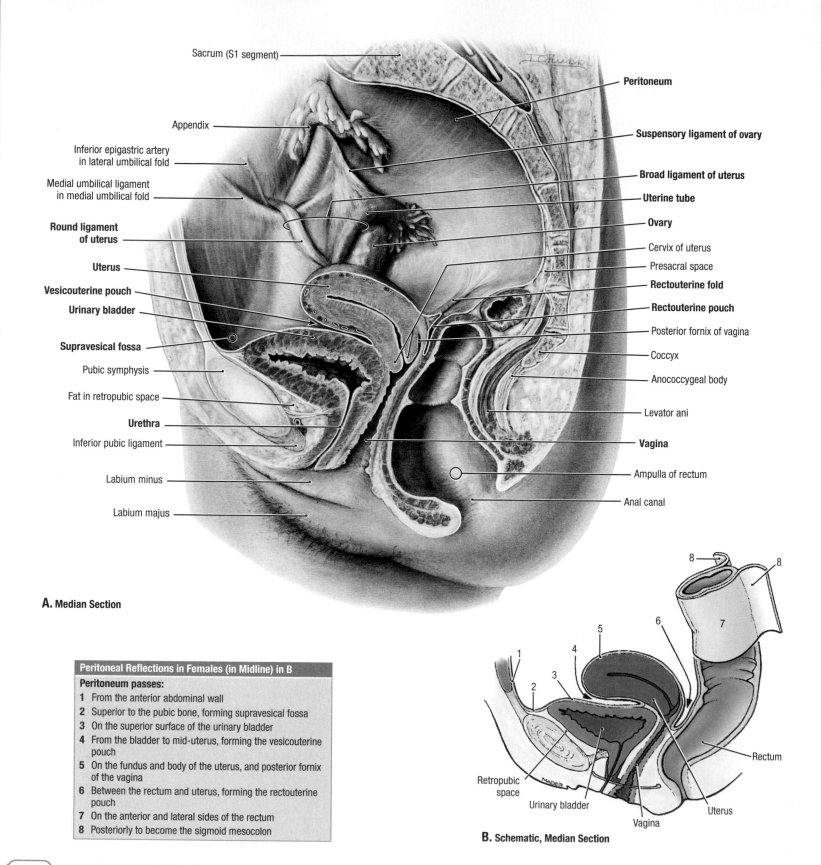

A. Median Section

Peritoneal Reflections in Females (in Midline) in B
Peritoneum passes:
1 From the anterior abdominal wall
2 Superior to the pubic bone, forming supravesical fossa
3 On the superior surface of the urinary bladder
4 From the bladder to mid-uterus, forming the vesicouterine pouch
5 On the fundus and body of the uterus, and posterior fornix of the vagina
6 Between the rectum and uterus, forming the rectouterine pouch
7 On the anterior and lateral sides of the rectum
8 Posteriorly to become the sigmoid mesocolon

B. Schematic, Median Section

5.14 **Peritoneum Covering Female Pelvic Organs**

A. Organs *in situ* **with peritoneal reflections. B. Schematic of peritoneal reflections.** The level of the supravesical fossa changes with filling and emptying of bladder.

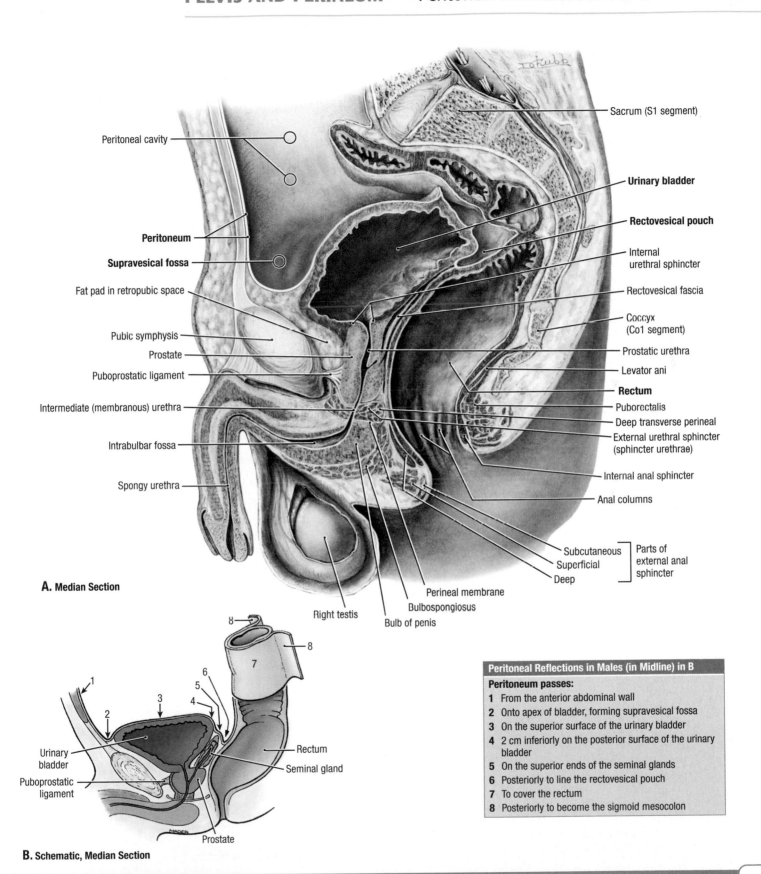

Peritoneal cavity

Peritoneum

Supravesical fossa

Fat pad in retropubic space

Pubic symphysis

Prostate

Puboprostatic ligament

Intermediate (membranous) urethra

Intrabulbar fossa

Spongy urethra

Sacrum (S1 segment)

Urinary bladder

Rectovesical pouch

Internal urethral sphincter

Rectovesical fascia

Coccyx (Co1 segment)

Prostatic urethra

Levator ani

Rectum

Puborectalis

Deep transverse perineal

External urethral sphincter (sphincter urethrae)

Internal anal sphincter

Anal columns

Subcutaneous
Superficial
Deep

Parts of external anal sphincter

Perineal membrane

Bulbospongiosus

Right testis

Bulb of penis

A. Median Section

8

8

7

6

5

4

3

2

1

Urinary bladder

Puboprostatic ligament

Prostate

Rectum

Seminal gland

B. Schematic, Median Section

Peritoneal Reflections in Males (in Midline) in B
Peritoneum passes:
1 From the anterior abdominal wall
2 Onto apex of bladder, forming supravesical fossa
3 On the superior surface of the urinary bladder
4 2 cm inferiorly on the posterior surface of the urinary bladder
5 On the superior ends of the seminal glands
6 Posteriorly to line the rectovesical pouch
7 To cover the rectum
8 Posteriorly to become the sigmoid mesocolon

Peritoneum Covering Male Pelvic Organs   **5.15**

A. Organs *in situ*. The urinary bladder is distended and displaced posteriorly in this specimen, not anteriorly as is usual, forming a broad and deep supravesical fossa even when the bladder is full.

B. Peritoneum covering male pelvic organs. Typically, the location of supravesical fossa changes with filling and emptying of bladder.

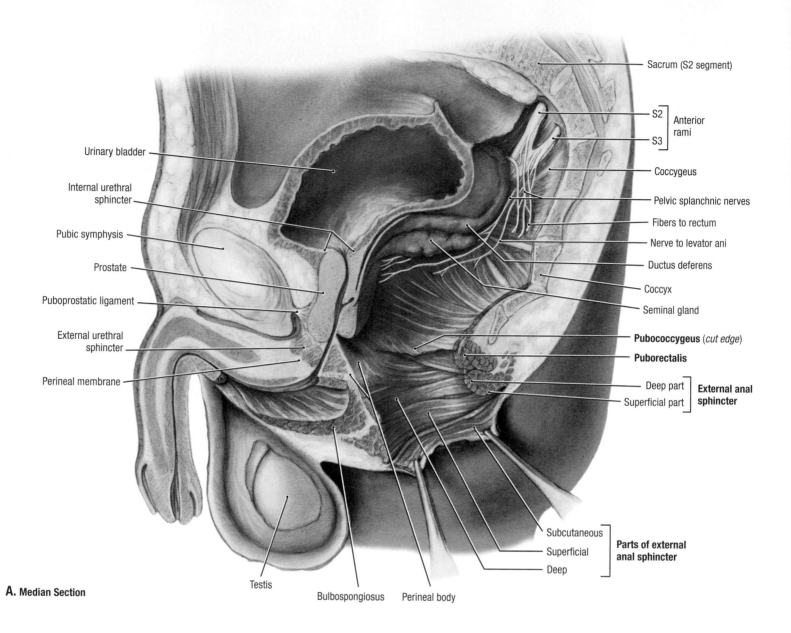

Urinary bladder

Internal urethral
sphincter

Pubic symphysis

Prostate

Puboprostatic ligament

External urethral
sphincter

Perineal membrane

Sacrum (S2 segment)

S2 ⎤
     ⎬ Anterior
S3 ⎦   rami

Coccygeus

Pelvic splanchnic nerves

Fibers to rectum

Nerve to levator ani

Ductus deferens

Coccyx

Seminal gland

Pubococcygeus (*cut edge*)

Puborectalis

Deep part ⎤ **External anal**
Superficial part ⎦ **sphincter**

Subcutaneous ⎤ **Parts of external**
Superficial ⎬ **anal sphincter**
Deep ⎦

Testis

Bulbospongiosus   Perineal body

A. Median Section

5.16   Anal Sphincters and Anal Canal

A. Levator ani, in right half of hemisected pelvis.
- The subcutaneous fibers of the external anal sphincter and overlying skin are reflected with forceps. The pubococcygeus muscle is cut to reveal the anal canal, to which it is, in part, attached.
- The **external anal sphincter** is a large voluntary sphincter that forms a broad band on each side of the inferior two thirds of the anal canal. This sphincter blends superiorly with the puborectalis muscle and has subcutaneous, superficial, and deep parts.

B. Puborectalis.
- The most medial part of the levator ani/pubococcygeus muscle, the puborectalis, forms a U-shaped muscular "sling" around the anorectal junction, which maintains the anorectal (perineal) flexure.

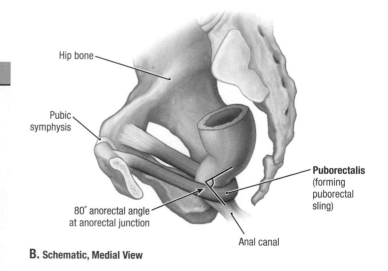

Hip bone

Pubic
symphysis

80° anorectal angle
at anorectal junction

Puborectalis
(forming
puborectal
sling)

Anal canal

B. Schematic, Medial View

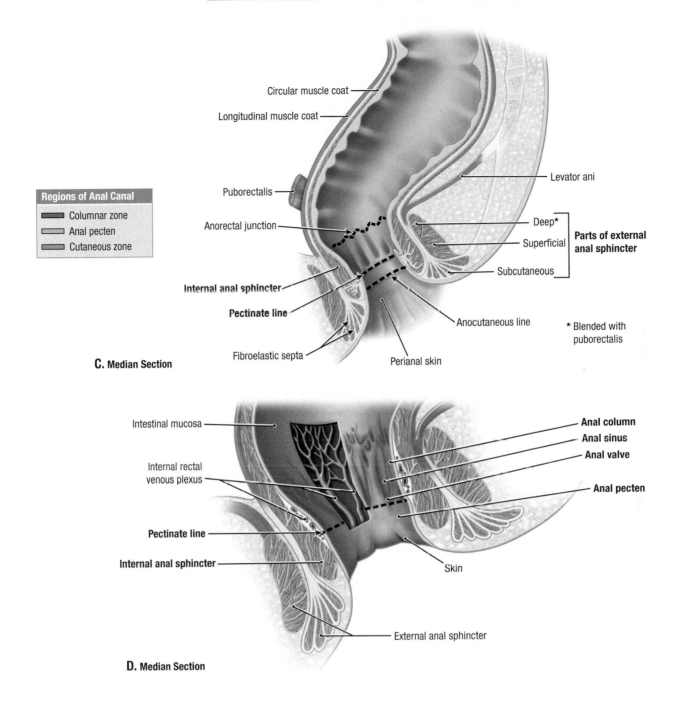

Regions of Anal Canal
- ▬ Columnar zone
- ▭ Anal pecten
- ▬ Cutaneous zone

Circular muscle coat

Longitudinal muscle coat

Puborectalis

Anorectal junction

Internal anal sphincter

Pectinate line

Fibroelastic septa

C. Median Section

Levator ani

Deep*

Superficial

Parts of external anal sphincter

Subcutaneous

Anocutaneous line

Perianal skin

* Blended with puborectalis

Intestinal mucosa

Internal rectal venous plexus

Pectinate line

Internal anal sphincter

External anal sphincter

Anal column

Anal sinus

Anal valve

Anal pecten

Skin

D. Median Section

Anal Sphincters and Anal Canal (continued)   5.16

C. External and internal anal sphincters.
- The internal anal sphincter is a thickening of the inner, circular muscular coat of the anal canal.
- The external anal sphincter has three often indistinct continuous zones: deep, superficial, and subcutaneous; the deep part intermingles with the puborectalis muscle posteriorly.
- The longitudinal muscle layer of the rectum separates the internal and external anal sphincters and terminates in the subcutaneous tissue and skin around the anus.

D. Features of anal canal.
- The anal columns are 5 to 10 vertical folds of mucosa separated by anal sinuses and valves; they contain portions of the rectal venous plexus.

- The pecten is a smooth area of hairless stratified epithelium that lies between the anal valves superiorly and the inferior border of the internal anal sphincter inferiorly.
- The pectinate line is an irregular line at the base of the anal valves where the intestinal mucosa is continuous with the pecten; this indicates the junction of the superior part of the anal canal (derived from embryonic hindgut) and the inferior part of the anal canal (derived from the anal pit [proctodeum]). Innervation is visceral proximal to the line and somatic distally; lymphatic drainage is to the pararectal nodes proximally and to the superficial inguinal nodes distally.

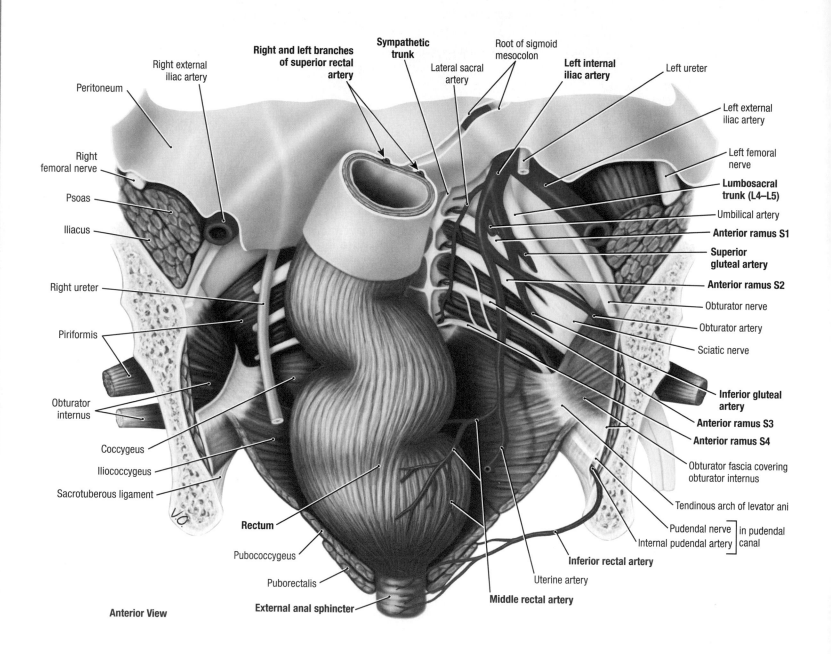

Right external
iliac artery

Peritoneum

Right
femoral nerve

Psoas

Iliacus

Right ureter

Piriformis

Obturator
internus

Coccygeus

Iliococcygeus

Sacrotuberous ligament

Rectum

Pubococcygeus

Puborectalis

External anal sphincter

**Right and left branches
of superior rectal
artery**

**Sympathetic
trunk**

Lateral sacral
artery

Root of sigmoid
mesocolon

**Left internal
iliac artery**

Left ureter

Left external
iliac artery

Left femoral
nerve

**Lumbosacral
trunk (L4–L5)**

Umbilical artery

Anterior ramus S1

**Superior
gluteal artery**

Anterior ramus S2

Obturator nerve

Obturator artery

Sciatic nerve

**Inferior gluteal
artery**

Anterior ramus S3

Anterior ramus S4

Obturator fascia covering
obturator internus

Tendinous arch of levator ani

Pudendal nerve ⎤ in pudendal
Internal pudendal artery ⎦ canal

Inferior rectal artery

Uterine artery

Middle rectal artery

Anterior View

5.17 | **Rectum, Anal Canal, and Neurovascular Structures of Posterior Pelvis**

The pelvis is coronally bisected anterior to the rectum and anal
canal. The superior gluteal artery often passes posteriorly between
the anterior rami of L5 and S1, and the inferior gluteal artery
between S2 and S3.

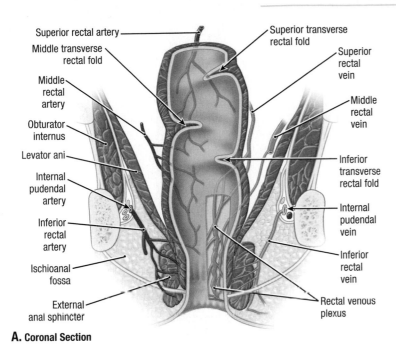

Superior rectal artery
Middle transverse rectal fold
Middle rectal artery
Obturator internus
Levator ani
Internal pudendal artery
Inferior rectal artery
Ischioanal fossa
External anal sphincter

Superior transverse rectal fold
Superior rectal vein
Middle rectal vein
Inferior transverse rectal fold
Internal pudendal vein
Inferior rectal vein
Rectal venous plexus

A. Coronal Section

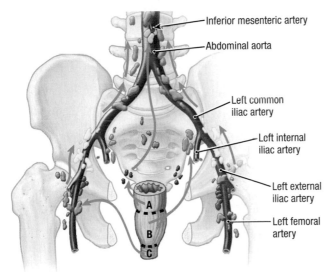

Inferior mesenteric artery
Abdominal aorta
Left common iliac artery
Left internal iliac artery
Left external iliac artery
Left femoral artery

A
B
C

B. Anterior View

Key for B

A Superior half of rectum
B Inferior half of rectum
C Anal canal

☐ Lumbar
☐ Inferior mesenteric
☐ Common iliac
☐ Internal iliac
☐ External iliac
☐ Superficial inguinal
☐ Deep inguinal
☐ Sacral
→ Direction of flow of lymph

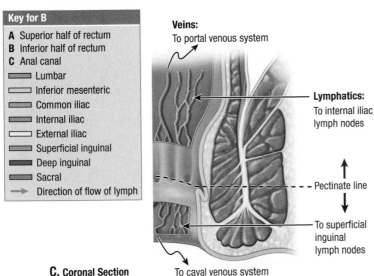

Veins:
To portal venous system

Lymphatics:
To internal iliac lymph nodes

- - Pectinate line

To superficial inguinal lymph nodes

To caval venous system

C. Coronal Section

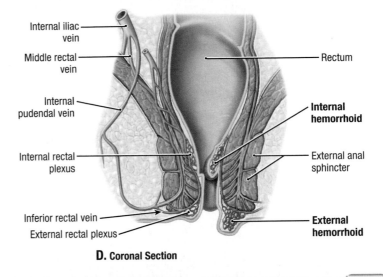

Internal iliac vein
Middle rectal vein
Internal pudendal vein
Internal rectal plexus
Inferior rectal vein
External rectal plexus

Rectum
Internal hemorrhoid
External anal sphincter
External hemorrhoid

D. Coronal Section

Drainage of Rectum Vasculature and Lymphatic   5.18

A. Arterial and venous drainage. **B.** Lymphatic drainage. **C.** Venous and lymphatic drainage superior and inferior to pectinate line. **D.** Hemorrhoids. **Internal hemorrhoids** (piles) are prolapses of rectal mucosa containing the normally dilated veins of the internal rectal venous plexus. Internal hemorrhoids are thought to result from a breakdown of the muscularis mucosae, a smooth muscle layer deep to the mucosa. Internal hemorrhoids that prolapse through the anal canal are often compressed by the contracted sphincters, impeding blood flow. As a result, they tend to strangulate and ulcerate. Because of the presence of abundant arteriovenous anastomoses, bleeding from internal hemorrhoids is characteristically bright red. The current practice is to treat only prolapsed, ulcerated internal hemorrhoids.

External hemorrhoids are thromboses (blood clots) in the veins of the external rectal venous plexus and are covered by skin. Predisposing factors for hemorrhoids include pregnancy, chronic constipation, and any disorder that impedes venous return including increased intraabdominal pressure. The superior rectal vein drains into the inferior mesenteric vein, whereas the middle and inferior rectal veins drain through the systemic system into the inferior vena cava. Any abnormal increase in pressure in the valveless portal system or veins of the trunk may cause enlargement of the superior rectal veins, resulting in an increase in blood flow or stasis in the internal rectal venous plexus. In **portal hypertension** that occurs in relation to **hepatic cirrhosis**, the portacaval anastomosis (e.g., esophageal) may become varicose and rupture. Note that the veins of the rectal plexuses normally appear varicose (dilated and tortuous), even in newborns, and that internal hemorrhoids occur most commonly in the absence of portal hypertension.

Regarding pain from and the treatment of hemorrhoids, note that the anal canal superior to the pectinate line is visceral; thus, it is innervated by visceral afferent pain fibers, so that an incision or needle insertion into this region is painless. Internal hemorrhoids are not painful and can be treated without anesthesia. Inferior to the pectinate line, the anal canal is somatic, supplied by the inferior anal (rectal) nerves containing somatic sensory fibers. Therefore, it is sensitive to painful stimuli (e.g., to the prick of a hypodermic needle). External hemorrhoids can be painful but often resolve in a few days.

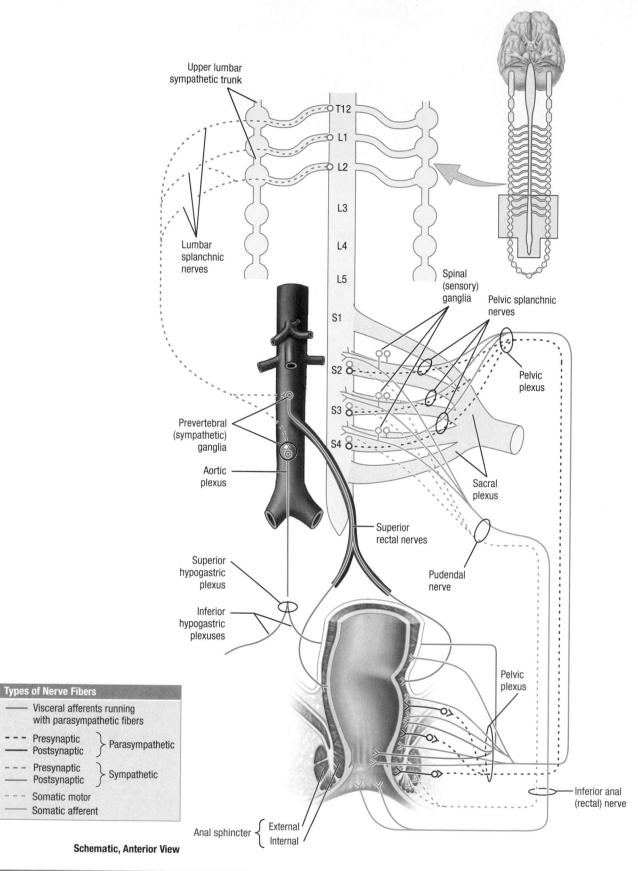

Upper lumbar
sympathetic trunk

Lumbar
splanchnic
nerves

T12
L1
L2
L3
L4
L5
S1
S2
S3
S4

Spinal
(sensory)
ganglia

Pelvic splanchnic
nerves

Pelvic
plexus

Prevertebral
(sympathetic)
ganglia

Aortic
plexus

Sacral
plexus

Superior
rectal nerves

Superior
hypogastric
plexus

Inferior
hypogastric
plexuses

Pudendal
nerve

Pelvic
plexus

Inferior anal
(rectal) nerve

Types of Nerve Fibers

——— Visceral afferents running
      with parasympathetic fibers

- - - Presynaptic   ⎫
——— Postsynaptic   ⎬ Parasympathetic

- - - Presynaptic   ⎫
——— Postsynaptic   ⎬ Sympathetic

- - - Somatic motor
——— Somatic afferent

Anal sphincter ⎰ External
               ⎱ Internal

Schematic, Anterior View

5.19   **Innervation of Rectum and Anal Canal**

The lumbar and pelvic spinal nerves and hypogastric plexuses have been retracted laterally for clarity.

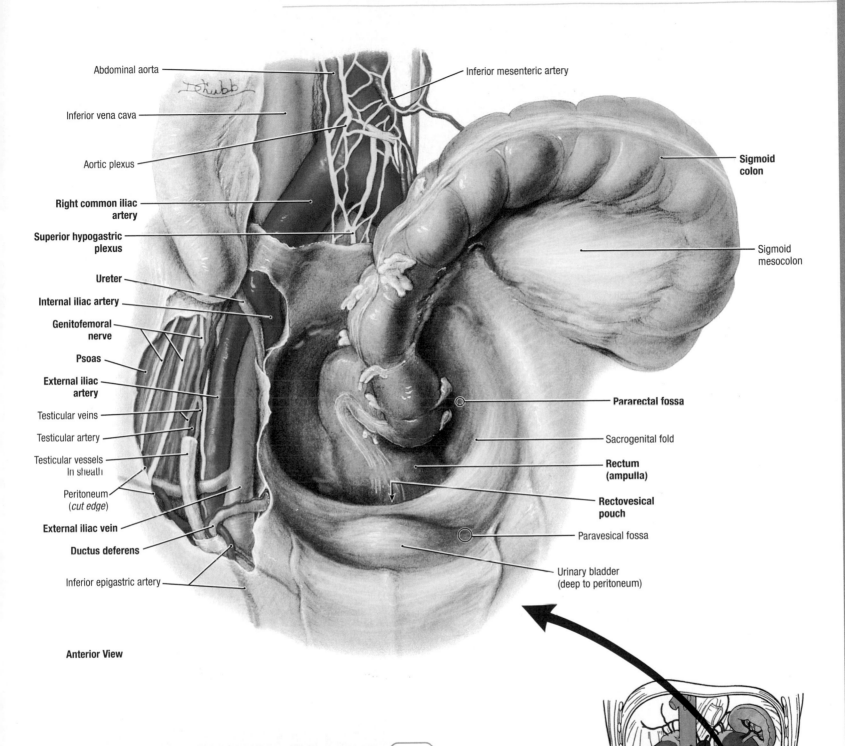

Abdominal aorta

Inferior mesenteric artery

Inferior vena cava

Aortic plexus

Sigmoid colon

Right common iliac artery

Superior hypogastric plexus

Sigmoid mesocolon

Ureter

Internal iliac artery

Genitofemoral nerve

Psoas

External iliac artery

Pararectal fossa

Sacrogenital fold

Testicular veins

Testicular artery

Rectum (ampulla)

Testicular vessels in sheath

Peritoneum (*cut edge*)

Rectovesical pouch

External iliac vein

Paravesical fossa

Ductus deferens

Urinary bladder (deep to peritoneum)

Inferior epigastric artery

Anterior View

Rectum *In Situ*   5.20

- The sigmoid colon begins at the left pelvic brim and becomes the rectum anterior to the third sacral segment in the midline.
- The superior hypogastric plexus lies inferior to the bifurcation of the aorta and anterior to the left common iliac vein.
- The ureter adheres to the external aspect of the peritoneum, crosses the external iliac vessels, and descends anterior to the internal iliac artery. The ductus deferens and its artery also adhere to the peritoneum, cross the external iliac vessels, and then hook around the inferior epigastric artery to join the other components of the spermatic cord.
- The genitofemoral nerve lies on the psoas.

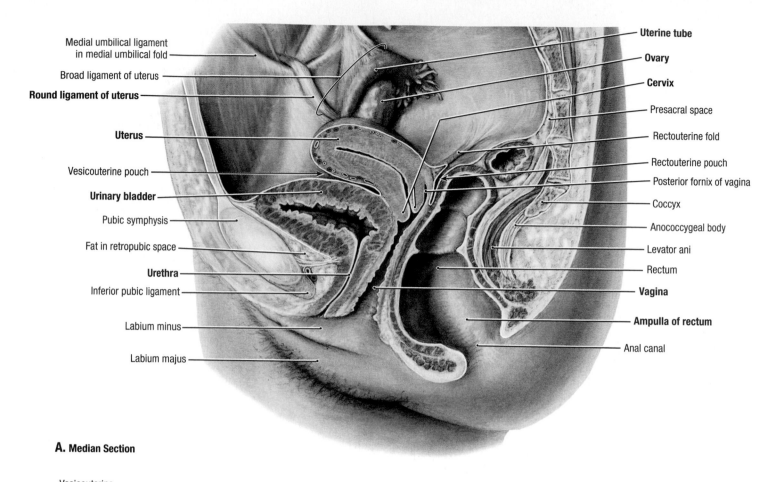

A. Median Section

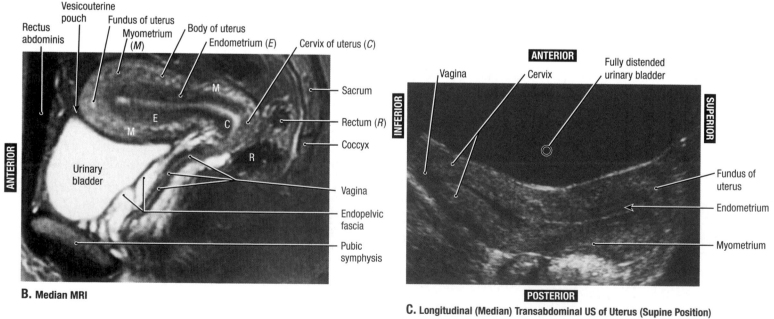

B. Median MRI

C. Longitudinal (Median) Transabdominal US of Uterus (Supine Position)

5.21   Female Pelvic Organs *In Situ*

A. Median section. The adult uterus is typically *anteverted* (tipped anterosuperiorly relative to the axis of the vagina) and *anteflexed* (flexed or bent anteriorly relative to the cervix, creating the *angle of flexion*) so that its mass lies over the bladder. The cervix, opening on the anterior wall of the vagina, has a short, round, anterior lip and a long, thin, posterior lip. **B. Midsagittal MRI of uterus. C. Median (transabdominal) ultrasound image.** The urinary bladder is distended to displace the loops of bowel from the pelvis.

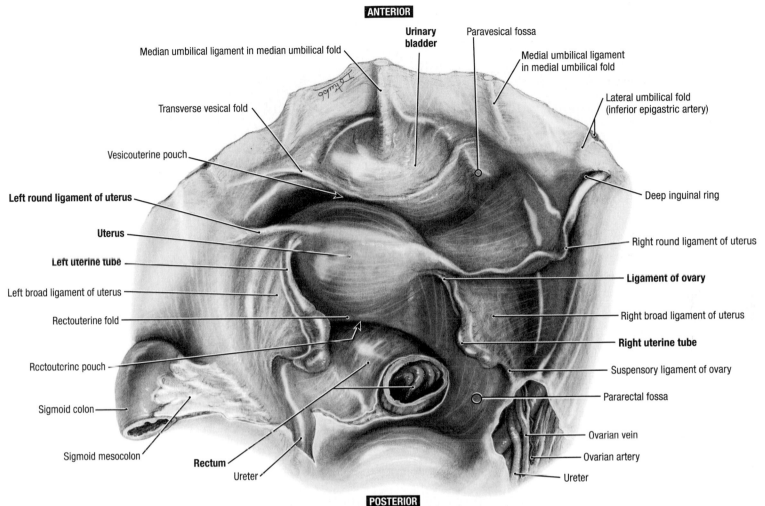

ANTERIOR

Median umbilical ligament in median umbilical fold

Urinary bladder

Paravesical fossa

Medial umbilical ligament in medial umbilical fold

Transverse vesical fold

Lateral umbilical fold (inferior epigastric artery)

Vesicouterine pouch

Deep inguinal ring

Left round ligament of uterus

Right round ligament of uterus

Uterus

Ligament of ovary

Left uterine tube

Left broad ligament of uterus

Right broad ligament of uterus

Rectouterine fold

Right uterine tube

Rectouterine pouch

Suspensory ligament of ovary

Pararectal fossa

Sigmoid colon

Ovarian vein

Ovarian artery

Sigmoid mesocolon

Ureter

Rectum

Ureter

POSTERIOR

D. Superior View

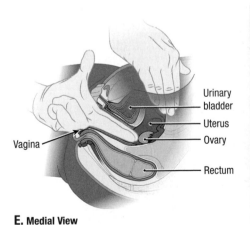

E. Medial View

Urinary bladder

Uterus

Ovary

Rectum

Vagina

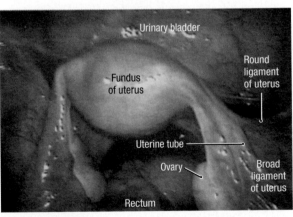

F. Laparoscopic View

Urinary bladder

Fundus of uterus

Round ligament of uterus

Uterine tube

Broad ligament of uterus

Ovary

Rectum

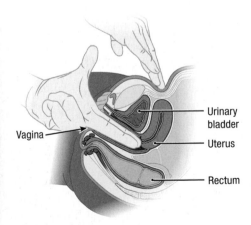

G. Medial View

Urinary bladder

Uterus

Rectum

Vagina

5.21

Female Pelvic Organs *In Situ* (continued)

D. True pelvis with peritoneum intact, viewed from above. The uterus is usually asymmetrically placed. The round ligament of the female takes the same subperitoneal course as the ductus deferens of the male. **E. Bimanual palpation of uterine adnexa** (accessory structures, e.g., ovaries). **F. Laparoscopy.** This procedure involves inserting a laparoscope into the peritoneal cavity through a small incision below the umbilicus. Insufflation of inert gas creates a pneumoperitoneum to provide space to visualize the pelvic organs. Additional openings (ports) can be made to introduce other instruments for manipulation or to enable therapeutic procedures (e.g., ligation of the uterine tubes). **G. Bimanual palpation of uterus.**

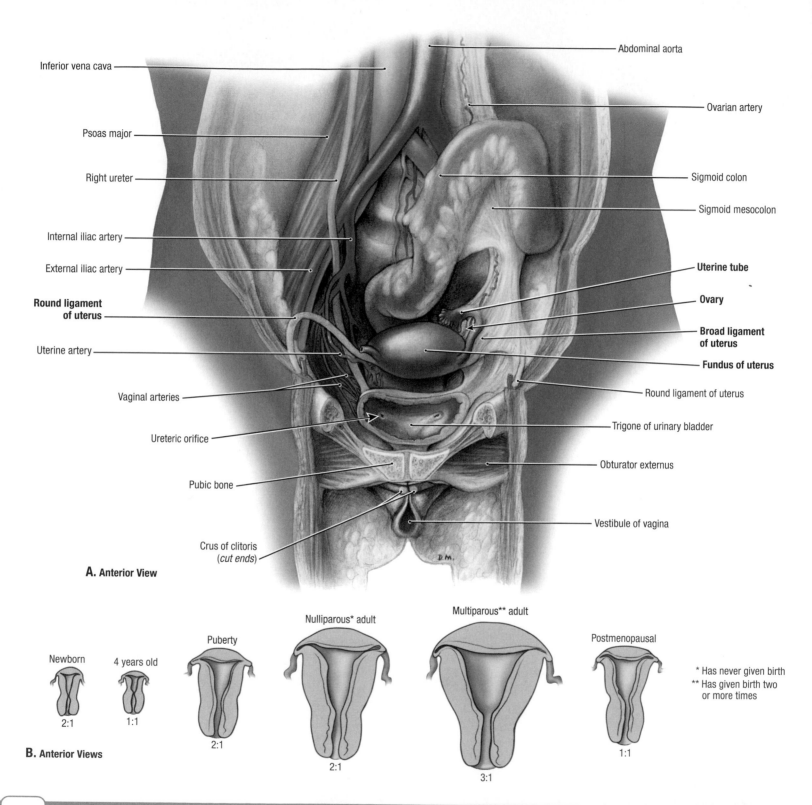

Inferior vena cava

Psoas major

Right ureter

Internal iliac artery

External iliac artery

Round ligament of uterus

Uterine artery

Vaginal arteries

Ureteric orifice

Pubic bone

Crus of clitoris (*cut ends*)

Abdominal aorta

Ovarian artery

Sigmoid colon

Sigmoid mesocolon

Uterine tube

Ovary

Broad ligament of uterus

Fundus of uterus

Round ligament of uterus

Trigone of urinary bladder

Obturator externus

Vestibule of vagina

A. Anterior View

Newborn

4 years old

Puberty

Nulliparous* adult

Multiparous** adult

Postmenopausal

* Has never given birth
** Has given birth two or more times

2:1

1:1

2:1

2:1

3:1

1:1

B. Anterior Views

5.22 Female Genital Organs

A. Dissection. Part of the pubic bones, the anterior aspect of the bladder, and—on the specimen's right side—the uterine tube, ovary, broad ligament, and peritoneum covering the lateral wall of the pelvis have been removed. **B. Lifetime changes in uterine size**

and proportion (body to cervical ratio, e.g., 2:1). All these stages represent normal anatomy for the particular age and reproductive status of the woman.

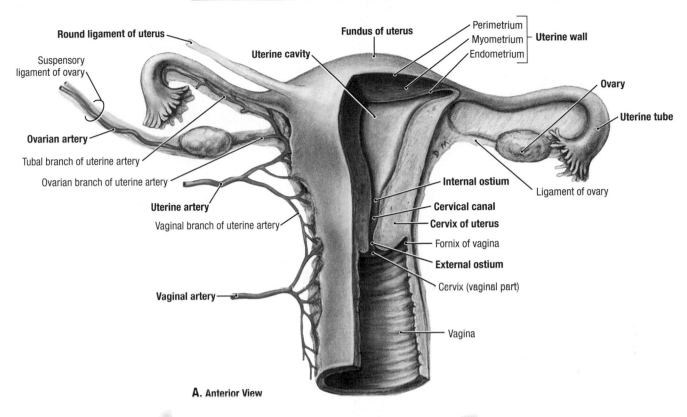

Round ligament of uterus

Suspensory
ligament of ovary

Ovarian artery

Tubal branch of uterine artery

Ovarian branch of uterine artery

Uterine artery

Vaginal branch of uterine artery

Vaginal artery

Fundus of uterus

Uterine cavity

Perimetrium
Myometrium
Endometrium
Uterine wall

Ovary

Uterine tube

Internal ostium

Ligament of ovary

Cervical canal

Cervix of uterus

Fornix of vagina

External ostium

Cervix (vaginal part)

Vagina

A. Anterior View

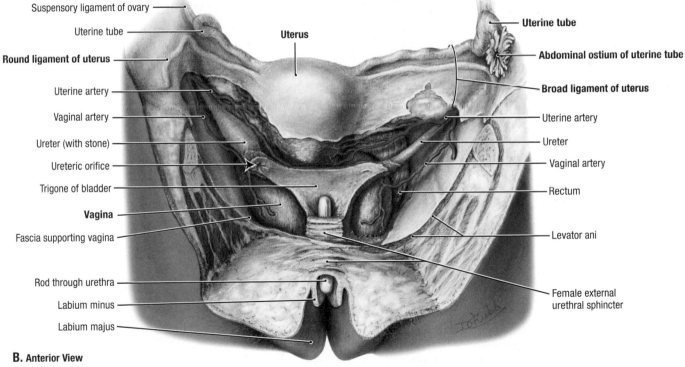

Suspensory ligament of ovary

Uterine tube

Round ligament of uterus

Uterine artery

Vaginal artery

Ureter (with stone)

Ureteric orifice

Trigone of bladder

Vagina

Fascia supporting vagina

Rod through urethra

Labium minus

Labium majus

Uterus

Uterine tube

Abdominal ostium of uterine tube

Broad ligament of uterus

Uterine artery

Ureter

Vaginal artery

Rectum

Levator ani

Female external
urethral sphincter

B. Anterior View

Uterus and Its Adnexa

5.23

A. Blood supply. On the specimen's left side, part of the uterine wall with the round ligament and the vaginal wall have been cut away to expose the cervix, uterine cavity, and thick muscular wall of the uterus, the myometrium. On the specimen's right side, the ovarian artery (from the aorta) and uterine artery (from the internal iliac) supply the ovary, uterine tube, and uterus and anastomose in the broad ligament along the lateral aspect of the uterus. The uterine artery sends a uterine branch to supply the uterine body and fundus and a vaginal branch to supply the cervix and vagina.

B. Uterus and broad ligament. The pubic bones and bladder, trigone excepted, are removed, as a continued dissection from Figure 5.22A.

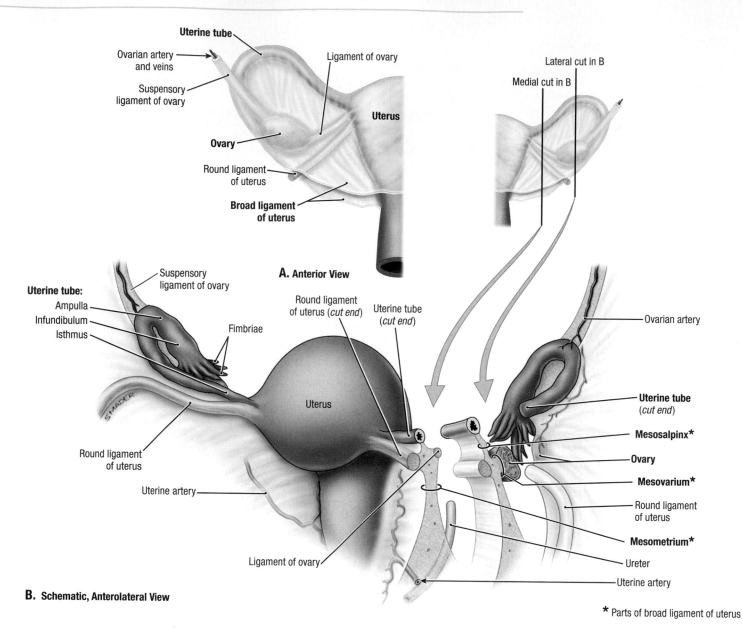

A. Anterior View

B. Schematic, Anterolateral View

* Parts of broad ligament of uterus

5.24 Uterus and Broad Ligament

A. Uterus, ovary, and broad ligament. B. Parts of broad ligament. Two paramedian sections ("cuts") in *Part B* show "mesenteries" with the prefix meso-. "Salpinx" is the Greek word for trumpet or tube, and "metro" for uterus. The mesentery of the uterus and uterine tube is called the broad ligament. The major part of the broad ligament, the *mesometrium*, is attached to the uterus. A smaller part of the broad ligament, the mesovarium, runs posteriorly to attach to each ovary. The ovary is also attached to the uterus by the ligament of the ovary and near the pelvic brim by the suspensory ligament of the ovary containing the ovarian vessels and nerves. The part of the broad ligament superior to the level of the mesovarium is called the *mesosalpinx*.
C. Hysterectomy (excision of the uterus). This procedure is performed through the lower anterior abdominal wall or through the vagina. Because the uterine artery crosses superior to the ureter near the lateral fornix of the vagina, the ureter is in danger of being inadvertently clamped or severed when the uterine artery is tied off during a hysterectomy.

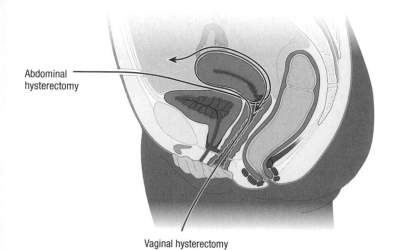

C. Schematic, Median Section

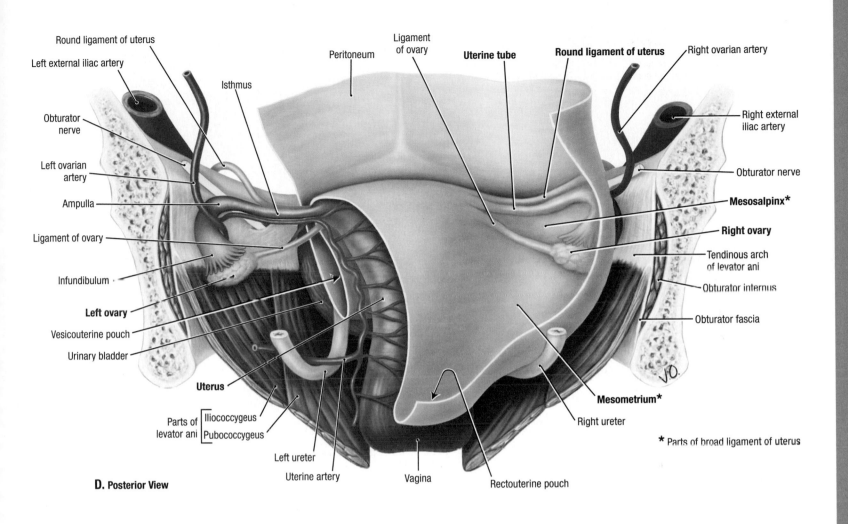

Round ligament of uterus

Left external iliac artery

Isthmus

Obturator nerve

Left ovarian artery

Ampulla

Ligament of ovary

Infundibulum

Left ovary

Vesicouterine pouch

Urinary bladder

Uterus

Parts of levator ani { Iliococcygeus | Pubococcygeus }

Left ureter

Uterine artery

D. Posterior View

Peritoneum

Ligament of ovary

Uterine tube

Round ligament of uterus

Right ovarian artery

Right external iliac artery

Obturator nerve

Mesosalpinx*

Right ovary

Tendinous arch of levator ani

Obturator internus

Obturator fascia

Mesometrium*

Right ureter

Vagina

Rectouterine pouch

* Parts of broad ligament of uterus

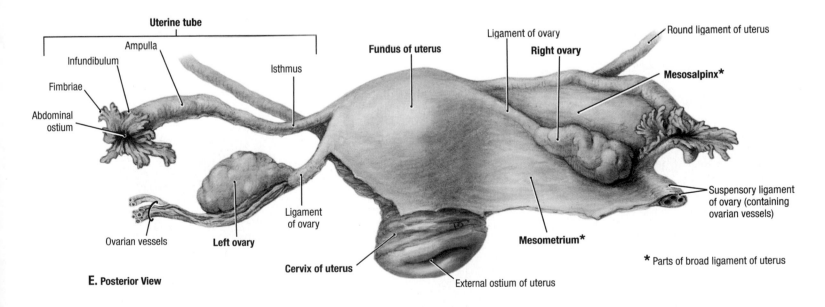

Uterine tube

Ampulla

Infundibulum

Isthmus

Fimbriae

Fundus of uterus

Ligament of ovary

Right ovary

Round ligament of uterus

Mesosalpinx*

Abdominal ostium

Suspensory ligament of ovary (containing ovarian vessels)

Ovarian vessels

Left ovary

Ligament of ovary

Mesometrium*

Cervix of uterus

External ostium of uterus

* Parts of broad ligament of uterus

E. Posterior View

D. Uterus *in situ*. E. Uterus and adnexa, removed from cadaver.

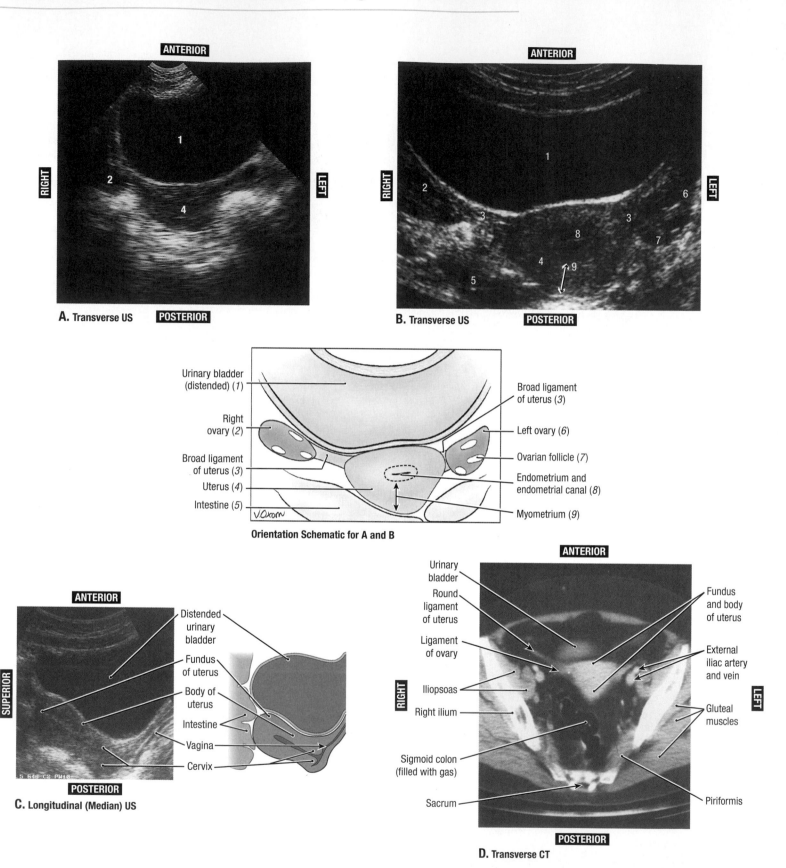

A. Transverse US

B. Transverse US

Orientation Schematic for A and B

Urinary bladder (distended) (1)
Right ovary (2)
Broad ligament of uterus (3)
Uterus (4)
Intestine (5)
Broad ligament of uterus (3)
Left ovary (6)
Ovarian follicle (7)
Endometrium and endometrial canal (8)
Myometrium (9)

C. Longitudinal (Median) US

Distended urinary bladder
Fundus of uterus
Body of uterus
Intestine
Vagina
Cervix

D. Transverse CT

Urinary bladder
Round ligament of uterus
Ligament of ovary
Iliopsoas
Right ilium
Sigmoid colon (filled with gas)
Sacrum
Fundus and body of uterus
External iliac artery and vein
Gluteal muscles
Piriformis

5.25 **Imaging of Uterus and Uterine Adnexa**

A. and **B. Transverse (axial) ultrasound images. C. Longitudinal ultrasound image.** Temporary retroversion and retroflexion result when a fully distended urinary bladder temporarily retroverts the uterus and decreases the angle of flexion. **D. Transverse (axial) CT.**

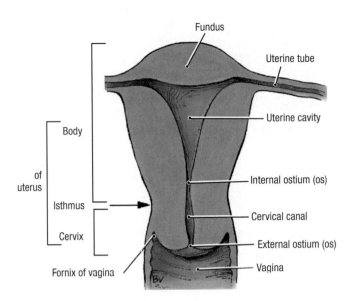

A. Coronal Section, Normal Uterus

Fundus
Uterine tube
Uterine cavity
Body
of uterus
Internal ostium (os)
Isthmus
Cervical canal
Cervix
External ostium (os)
Fornix of vagina
Vagina

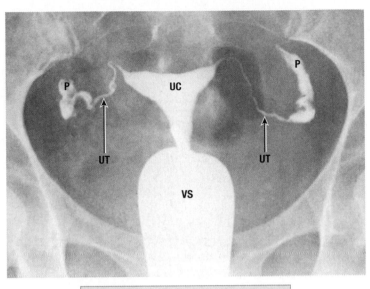

| P | Peritoneal cavity | UT | Uterine tube |
| UC | Uterine cavity | VS | Vaginal speculum |

B. Anteroposterior Hysterosalpingogram, Normal Uterus

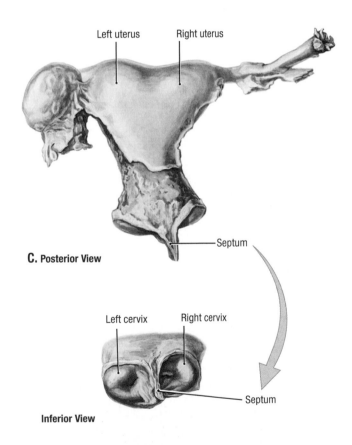

Left uterus   Right uterus

Septum

C. Posterior View

Left cervix   Right cervix

Septum

Inferior View

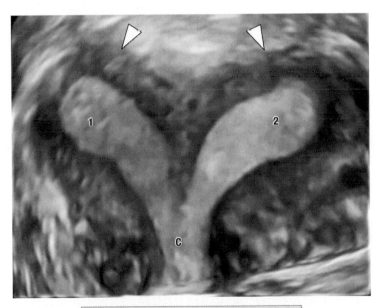

| 1 and 2 | Uterine cavities | C | Cervical canal |
| ▷ | Two horns of uterus | | |

D. Coronal MRI Reconstructed Image

Radiograph of Uterus and Uterine Tubes (Hysterosalpingogram)

5.26

A. Parts of uterus and superior vagina. B. Hysterosalpingography. During this procedure, radiopaque material is injected into the uterus through external os of the uterus. If normal, contrast medium travels through the triangular uterine cavity and uterine tubes and passes into the pararectal fossae of the peritoneal cavity.

The female genital tract is in direct communication with the peritoneal cavity and is, therefore, a potential pathway for the spread of an infection from the vagina and uterus. **C. Illustration of duplicated uterus. D. Bicornuate ("two-horned") uterus, 3D reconstruction.**

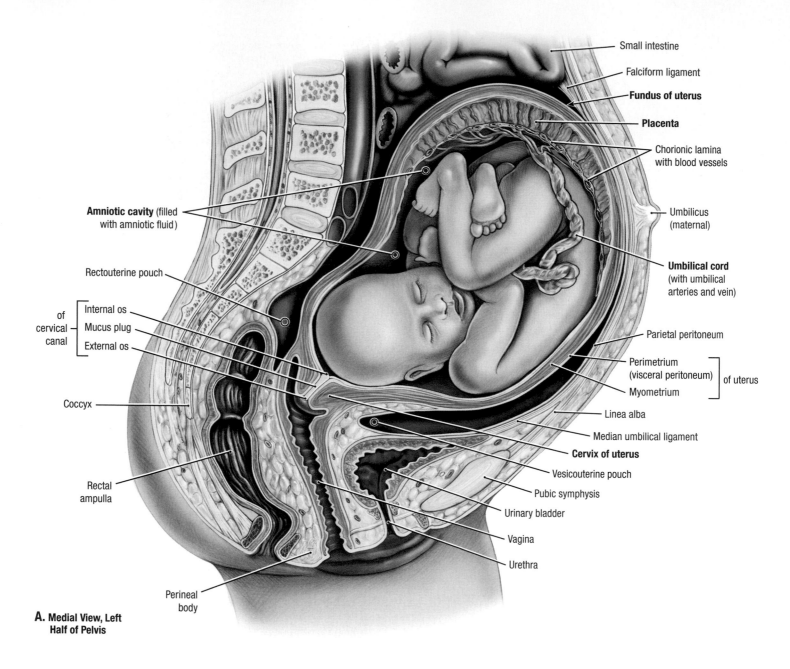

Small intestine

Falciform ligament

Fundus of uterus

Placenta

Chorionic lamina
with blood vessels

Umbilicus
(maternal)

Umbilical cord
(with umbilical
arteries and vein)

Parietal peritoneum

Perimetrium
(visceral peritoneum)   of uterus

Myometrium

Linea alba

Median umbilical ligament

Cervix of uterus

Vesicouterine pouch

Pubic symphysis

Urinary bladder

Vagina

Urethra

Amniotic cavity (filled
with amniotic fluid)

Rectouterine pouch

of   Internal os
cervical   Mucus plug
canal   External os

Coccyx

Rectal
ampulla

Perineal
body

**A. Medial View, Left
Half of Pelvis**

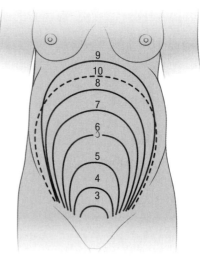

B. Anterior View

| 5.27 | **Pregnant Uterus** |

**A. Median section; fetus is intact. B. Monthly changes in size of
uterus during pregnancy.** Over the 9 months of pregnancy, the
gravid uterus expands greatly to accommodate the fetus, becoming larger and increasingly thin walled. At the end of pregnancy, the
fetus "drops," as the head becomes engaged in the lesser pelvis.
The uterus becomes nearly membranous, with the fundus dropping
below its highest level (achieved in the ninth month), at which time
it extends superiorly to the costal margin, occupying most of the
abdominopelvic cavity.

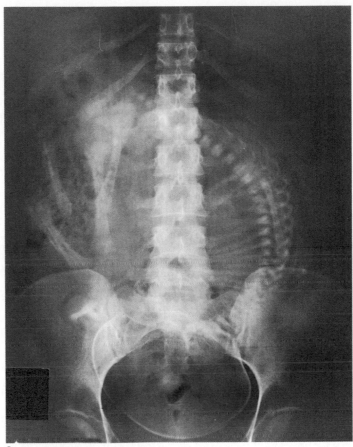

C. Anteroposterior Radiograph

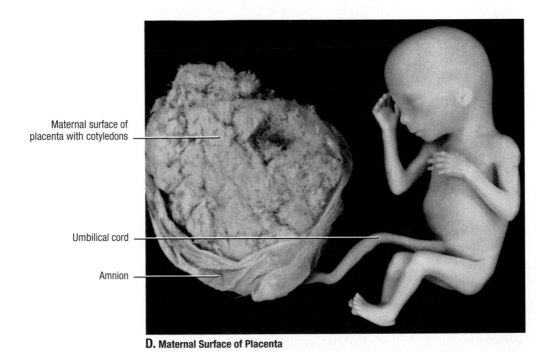

Maternal surface of
placenta with cotyledons

Umbilical cord

Amnion

D. Maternal Surface of Placenta

C. Radiograph of fetus. **D.** Photograph of an 18-week-old fetus connected to placenta by umbilical cord.

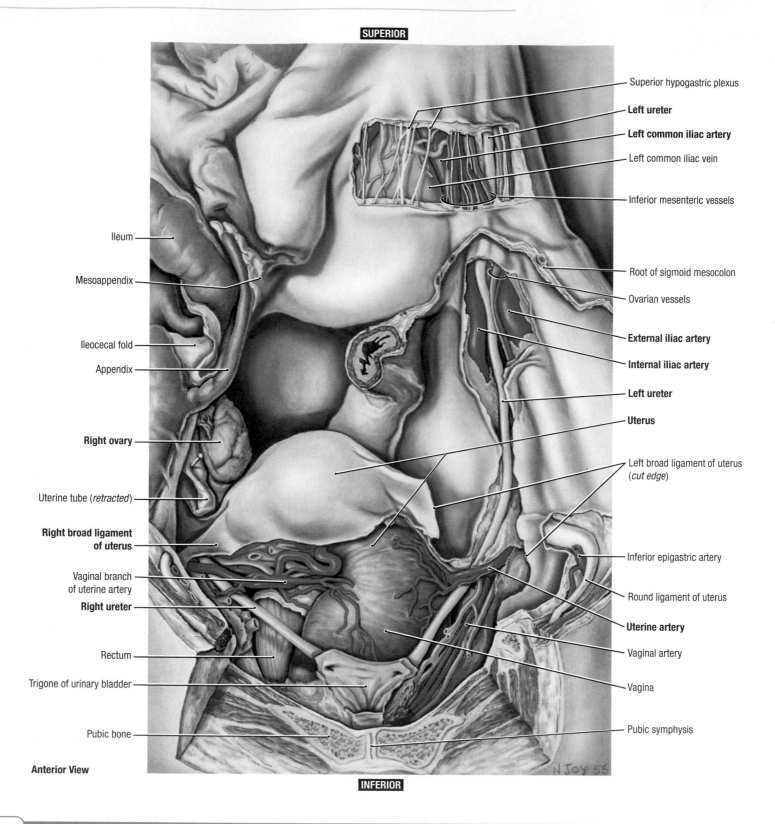

SUPERIOR

Superior hypogastric plexus

Left ureter

Left common iliac artery

Left common iliac vein

Inferior mesenteric vessels

Ileum

Mesoappendix

Root of sigmoid mesocolon

Ovarian vessels

Ileocecal fold

External iliac artery

Appendix

Internal iliac artery

Left ureter

Uterus

Right ovary

Left broad ligament of uterus (*cut edge*)

Uterine tube (*retracted*)

Right broad ligament of uterus

Inferior epigastric artery

Vaginal branch of uterine artery

Round ligament of uterus

Right ureter

Uterine artery

Rectum

Vaginal artery

Trigone of urinary bladder

Vagina

Pubic bone

Pubic symphysis

Anterior View

N.JOY 55

INFERIOR

5.28 Ureter and Relationship to Uterine Artery

- Most of the pubic symphysis and most of the bladder (except the trigone) have been removed.
- The left ureter is crossed by the ovarian vessels and nerves; the apex of the inverted V-shaped root of the sigmoid mesocolon is situated anterior to the left ureter.

- The left ureter crosses the external iliac artery at the bifurcation of the common iliac artery and then descends anterior to the internal iliac artery; its course is subperitoneal from where it enters the pelvis to where it passes deep to the broad ligament and is crossed by the uterine artery. **Injury of the ureter** may occur in this region when the uterine artery is ligated and cut during hysterectomy.

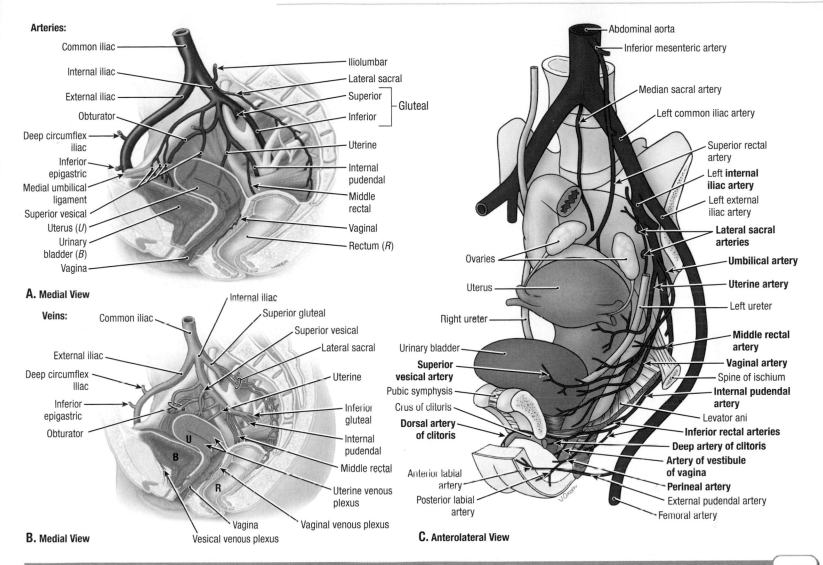

Arteries:

Common iliac — Internal iliac — External iliac — Obturator — Deep circumflex iliac — Inferior epigastric — Medial umbilical ligament — Superior vesical — Uterus (U) — Urinary bladder (B) — Vagina

Iliolumbar — Lateral sacral — Superior — Inferior] Gluteal — Uterine — Internal pudendal — Middle rectal — Vaginal — Rectum (R)

A. Medial View

Veins:

Common iliac — External iliac — Deep circumflex Iliac — Inferior epigastric — Obturator

Internal iliac — Superior gluteal — Superior vesical — Lateral sacral — Uterine — Inferior gluteal — Internal pudendal — Middle rectal — Uterine venous plexus — Vaginal venous plexus — Vagina — Vesical venous plexus

U — B — R

B. Medial View

Abdominal aorta — Inferior mesenteric artery — Median sacral artery — Left common iliac artery — Superior rectal artery — **Left internal iliac artery** — Left external iliac artery — **Lateral sacral arteries** — **Umbilical artery** — **Uterine artery** — Left ureter — **Middle rectal artery** — **Vaginal artery** — Spine of ischium — **Internal pudendal artery** — Levator ani — **Inferior rectal arteries** — **Deep artery of clitoris** — **Artery of vestibule of vagina** — **Perineal artery** — External pudendal artery — Femoral artery

Ovaries — Uterus — Right ureter — Urinary bladder — **Superior vesical artery** — Pubic symphysis — Crus of clitoris — **Dorsal artery of clitoris** — Anterior labial artery — Posterior labial artery

C. Anterolateral View

Arteries and Veins of Female Pelvis

5.29

TABLE 5.4 Arteries of Female Pelvis (Derivatives of Internal Iliac Artery [IIA], Branching Pattern Highly Variable)

Artery	Origin	Course	Distribution
Anterior division of IIA	IIA	Passes anteriorly along lateral wall of pelvis, dividing into visceral and obturator arteries	Pelvic viscera and muscles of superior medial thigh and perineum
Patent umbilical	Anterior div. IIA	Short pelvic course, gives off multiple superior vesical arteries	Superior aspect of urinary bladder
Obturator		Runs anteroinferiorly on lateral pelvic wall	Pelvic muscles, ilium, femoral head, medial thigh
Uterine		Runs anteromedially between broad and cardinal ligaments; crosses ureter superiorly to lateral aspect of uterine cervix	Uterus, ligaments of uterus, medial parts of uterine tube and ovary, and superior vagina
Vaginal	Anterior division IIA	Divides into vaginal and inferior vesical branches	Vaginal branch: lower vagina, vestibular bulb, and adjacent rectum; inferior vesical branch: fundus of urinary bladder
Middle rectal		Descends in pelvis to inferior part of rectum	Inferior part of rectum
Internal pudendal		Exits pelvis via greater sciatic foramen and enters perineum (ischioanal fossa) via lesser sciatic foramen	Main artery to perineum including muscles of anal canal and perineum, skin and urogenital triangle and erectile bodies
Posterior division of IIA	IIA	Passes posteriorly and gives rise to parietal branches	Pelvic wall and gluteal region
Iliolumbar	Posterior division IIA	Ascends anterior to sacroiliac joint and posterior to common iliac vessels and psoas major muscle	Iliacus, psoas major, quadratus lumborum muscles, and cauda equina in vertebral canal
Lateral sacral		Runs on anteromedial aspect of piriformis muscle	Piriformis and erector spinae muscles, structures in sacral canal
Ovarian	Abdominal aorta	Crosses pelvic brim and descends in suspensory ligament to ovary	Abdominal and/or pelvic ureter, ovary, and ampullary end of uterine tube

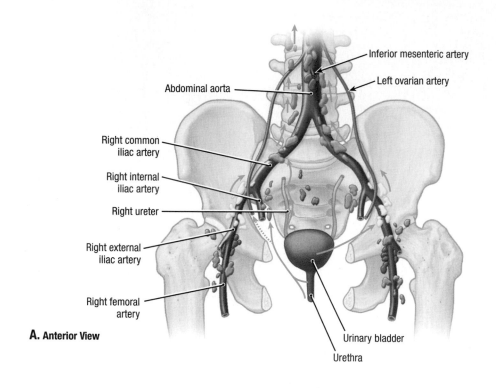

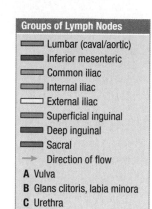

Inferior mesenteric artery

Abdominal aorta

Left ovarian artery

Right common iliac artery

Right internal iliac artery

Right ureter

Right external iliac artery

Right femoral artery

A. Anterior View

Urinary bladder

Urethra

Groups of Lymph Nodes

Lumbar (caval/aortic)
Inferior mesenteric
Common iliac
Internal iliac
External iliac
Superficial inguinal
Deep inguinal
Sacral
→ Direction of flow
A Vulva
B Glans clitoris, labia minora
C Urethra

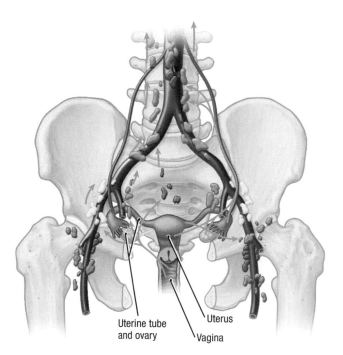

Uterine tube and ovary

Uterus

Vagina

B. Anterior View

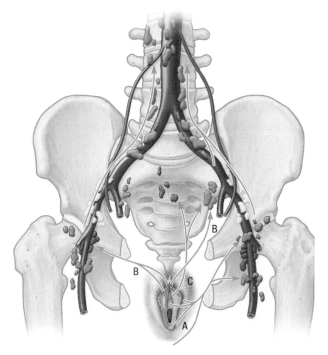

B

B

C

A

C. Anterior View

5.30 **Lymphatic Drainage of Female Pelvis and Perineum**

A. Pelvic urinary system. **B.** Internal genital organs. **C.** Vulva.

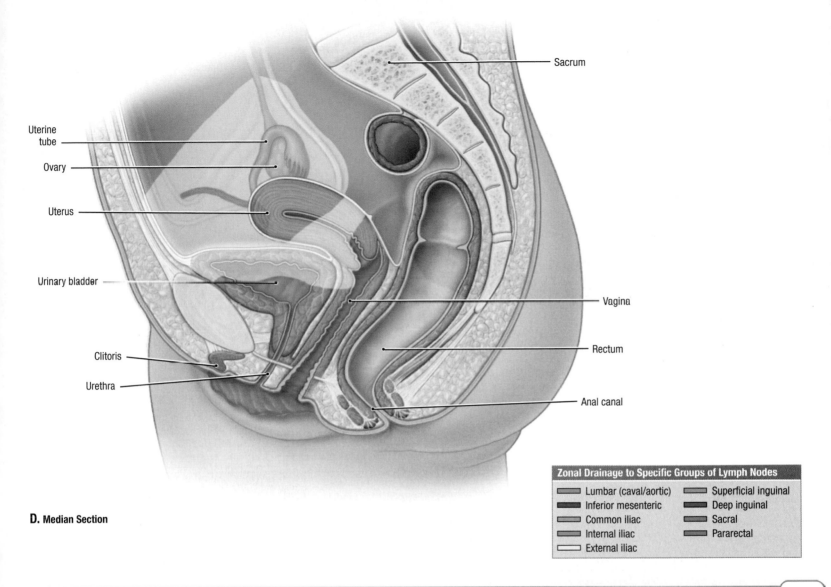

Sacrum

Uterine tube

Ovary

Uterus

Urinary bladder

Clitoris

Urethra

Vagina

Rectum

Anal canal

D. Median Section

Zonal Drainage to Specific Groups of Lymph Nodes	
Lumbar (caval/aortic)	Superficial inguinal
Inferior mesenteric	Deep inguinal
Common iliac	Sacral
Internal iliac	Pararectal
External iliac	

Lymphatic Drainage of Female Pelvis and Perineum (continued)   **5.30**

D. Zones of lymphatic drainage of pelvis and perineum initially draining to specific groups of regional nodes.

TABLE 5.5   Lymphatic Drainage of Structures of Female Pelvis and Perineum

Lymph Node Group	Structures Typically Draining to Lymph Node Group
Lumbar	Gonads and associated structures (along ovarian vessels), ovary, uterine tube (except isthmus and intra-uterine parts), fundus of uterus, common iliac nodes
Inferior mesenteric	Superiormost rectum, sigmoid colon, descending colon, pararectal nodes
Common iliac	External and internal iliac lymph nodes
Internal iliac	Inferior pelvic structures, deep perineal structures, sacral nodes, base of bladder, inferior pelvic ureter, anal canal (above pectinate line), inferior rectum, middle and upper vagina, cervix, body of uterus, sacral nodes
External iliac	Anterosuperior pelvic structures, deep inguinal nodes, superior bladder, superior pelvic ureter, upper vagina, cervix, lower body of uterus
Superficial inguinal	Lower limb, superficial drainage of inferolateral quadrant of trunk, including anterior abdominal wall inferior to umbilicus, gluteal region, superolateral uterus (near attachment of round ligament), skin of perineum including vulva, ostium of vagina (inferior to hymen), prepuce of clitoris, perianal skin, anal canal inferior to pectinate line
Deep inguinal	Glans of clitoris, superficial inguinal nodes
Sacral	Posteroinferior pelvic structures, inferior rectum, inferior vagina
Pararectal	Superior rectum

Types of Nerve Fibers

——	Visceral afferents running with parasympathetic fibers
– – – Presynaptic	} Parasympathetic
—— Postsynaptic	
——	Visceral afferents running with sympathetic fibers
– – – Presynaptic	} Sympathetic
—— Postsynaptic	
– – –	Somatic motor
——	Somatic afferent

5.31 **Innervation of Female Pelvic Viscera**

- Pelvic splanchnic nerves (S2–S4) supply parasympathetic motor fibers to the uterus and vagina (and vasodilator fibers to the erectile tissue of the clitoris and bulb of the vestibule; not shown).
- Presynaptic sympathetic fibers pass through the lumbar splanchnic nerves to synapse in prevertebral ganglia; the postsynaptic fibers travel through the superior and inferior hypogastric plexuses to reach the pelvic viscera.
- Visceral afferent fibers conducting pain from intraperitoneal viscera travel with the sympathetic fibers to the T12–L2 spinal ganglia. Visceral afferent fibers conducting pain from subperitoneal viscera travel with parasympathetic fibers to the S2–S4 spinal ganglia.
- Somatic sensation from the opening of the vagina also passes to the S2–S4 spinal ganglia via the pudendal nerve.
- Muscular contractions of the uterus are hormonally induced.

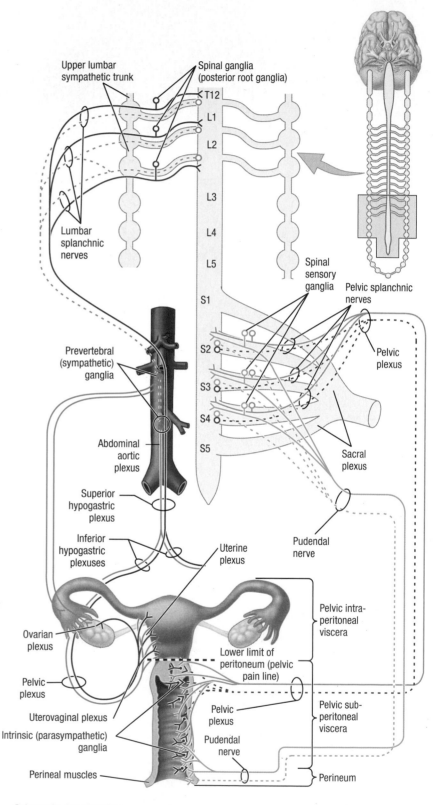

Schematic, Anterior View

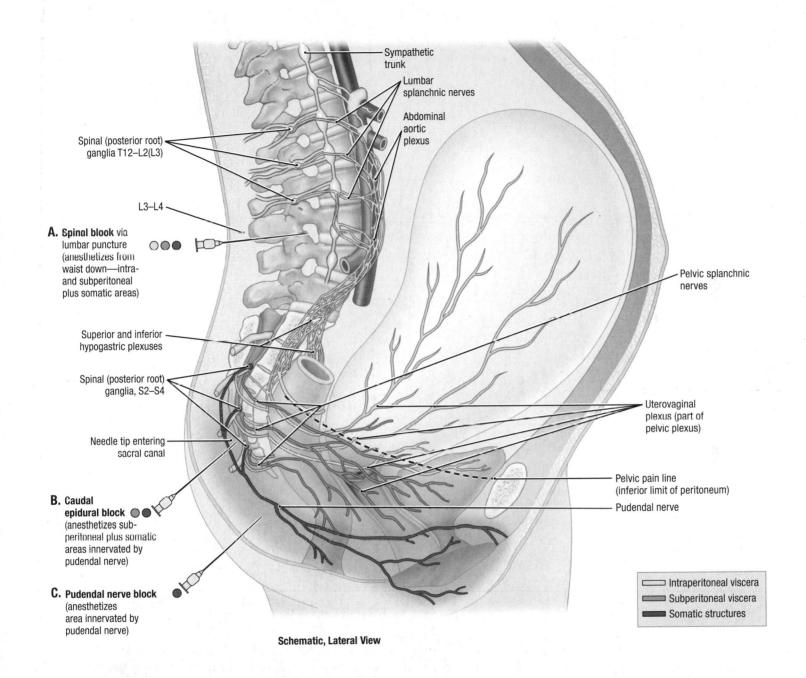

Sympathetic trunk

Lumbar splanchnic nerves

Abdominal aortic plexus

Spinal (posterior root) ganglia T12–L2(L3)

L3–L4

A. Spinal block via lumbar puncture (anesthetizes from waist down—intra- and subperitoneal plus somatic areas)

Superior and inferior hypogastric plexuses

Spinal (posterior root) ganglia, S2–S4

Needle tip entering sacral canal

B. Caudal epidural block (anesthetizes sub- peritoneal plus somatic areas innervated by pudendal nerve)

C. Pudendal nerve block (anesthetizes area innervated by pudendal nerve)

Pelvic splanchnic nerves

Uterovaginal plexus (part of pelvic plexus)

Pelvic pain line (inferior limit of peritoneum)

Pudendal nerve

Intraperitoneal viscera
Subperitoneal viscera
Somatic structures

Schematic, Lateral View

Innervation of Pelvic Viscera, Obstetrical Nerve Blocks   5.32

- A **spinal block** (*Part A*), in which the anesthetic agent is intro- duced with a needle into the spinal subarachnoid space at the L3–L4 vertebral level, produces complete anesthesia inferior to approximately the waist level. The perineum, pelvic floor, and birth canal are anesthetized, and motor and sensory functions of the entire lower limbs, as well as sensation of uterine contrac- tions, are temporarily eliminated.
- With the **caudal epidural block** (*Part B*), the anesthetic agent is administered using an indwelling catheter in the sacral canal.

The entire birth canal, pelvic floor, and most of the perineum are anesthetized, but the lower limbs are not usually affected. The mother is aware of her uterine contractions.
- A **pudendal nerve block** (*Part C*) is a peripheral nerve block that provides local anesthesia over the S2–S4 dermatomes (most of the perineum) and the inferior quarter of the vagina. It does not block pain from the superior birth canal (uterine cervix and superior vagina), so the mother is able to feel uterine contractions.

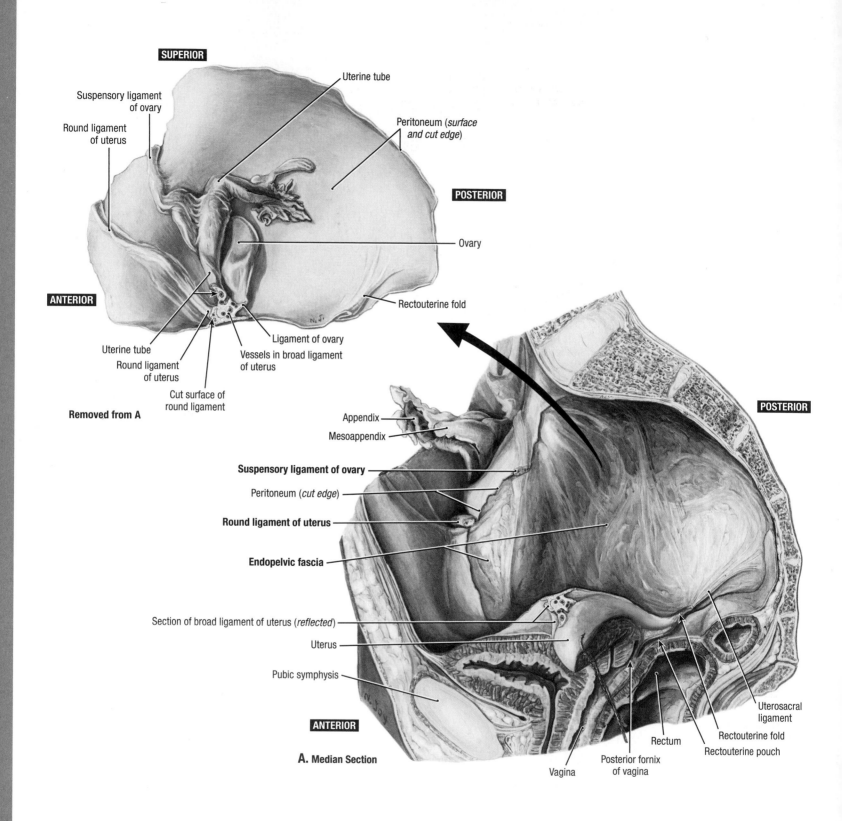

SUPERIOR

Suspensory ligament of ovary

Round ligament of uterus

Uterine tube

Peritoneum (*surface and cut edge*)

POSTERIOR

Ovary

ANTERIOR

Rectouterine fold

Uterine tube

Round ligament of uterus

Cut surface of round ligament

Ligament of ovary

Vessels in broad ligament of uterus

Removed from A

Appendix

Mesoappendix

Suspensory ligament of ovary

Peritoneum (*cut edge*)

Round ligament of uterus

Endopelvic fascia

Section of broad ligament of uterus (*reflected*)

Uterus

Pubic symphysis

ANTERIOR

A. Median Section

Vagina

Posterior fornix of vagina

Rectum

POSTERIOR

Uterosacral ligament

Rectouterine fold

Rectouterine pouch

5.33 **Serial Dissection of Autonomic Nerves of Female Pelvis**

A. Broad ligament and peritoneum of lateral wall pelvic cavity have been removed to expose endopelvic fascia.

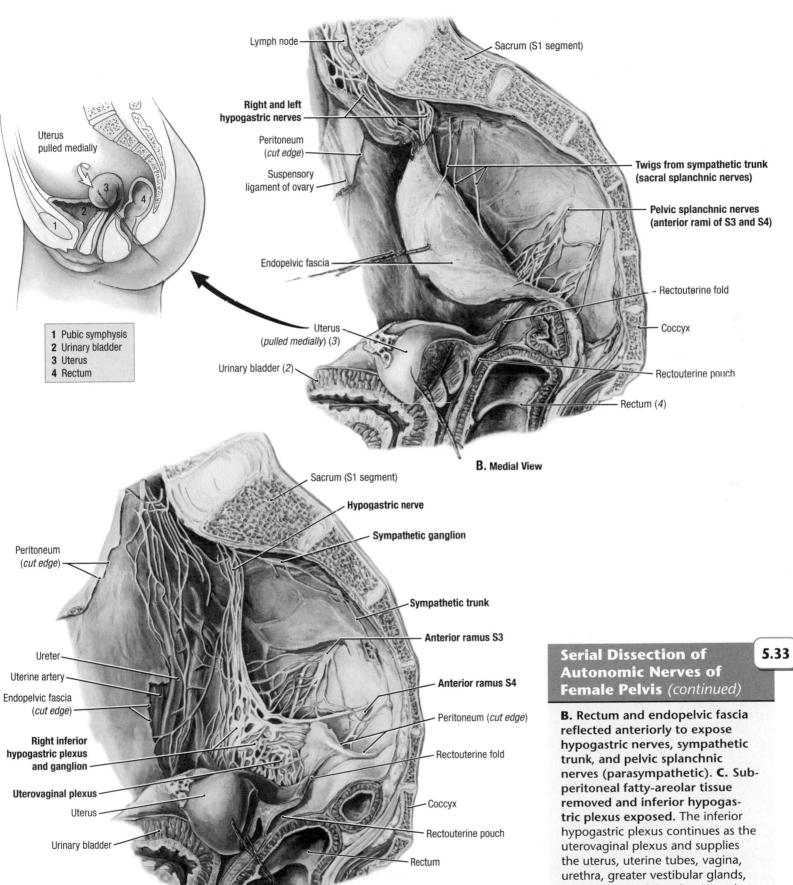

Uterus pulled medially

1 Pubic symphysis
2 Urinary bladder
3 Uterus
4 Rectum

Lymph node

Right and left hypogastric nerves

Peritoneum (*cut edge*)

Suspensory ligament of ovary

Endopelvic fascia

Uterus (*pulled medially*) (*3*)

Urinary bladder (*2*)

Sacrum (S1 segment)

Twigs from sympathetic trunk (sacral splanchnic nerves)

Pelvic splanchnic nerves (anterior rami of S3 and S4)

Rectouterine fold

Coccyx

Rectouterine pouch

Rectum (*4*)

B. Medial View

Peritoneum (*cut edge*)

Ureter

Uterine artery

Endopelvic fascia (*cut edge*)

Right inferior hypogastric plexus and ganglion

Uterovaginal plexus

Uterus

Urinary bladder

Sacrum (S1 segment)

Hypogastric nerve

Sympathetic ganglion

Sympathetic trunk

Anterior ramus S3

Anterior ramus S4

Peritoneum (*cut edge*)

Rectouterine fold

Coccyx

Rectouterine pouch

Rectum

C. Medial View

5.33

Serial Dissection of Autonomic Nerves of Female Pelvis (*continued*)

B. Rectum and endopelvic fascia reflected anteriorly to expose hypogastric nerves, sympathetic trunk, and pelvic splanchnic nerves (parasympathetic). **C.** Subperitoneal fatty-areolar tissue removed and inferior hypogastric plexus exposed. The inferior hypogastric plexus continues as the uterovaginal plexus and supplies the uterus, uterine tubes, vagina, urethra, greater vestibular glands, erectile tissue of the clitoris, and bulb of the vestibule.

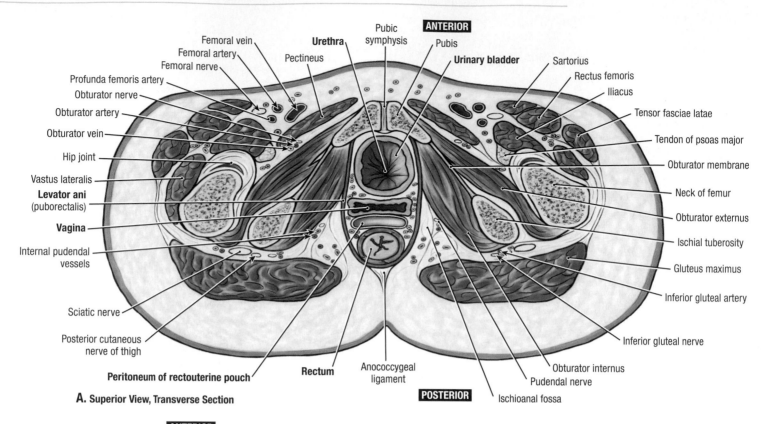

A. Superior View, Transverse Section

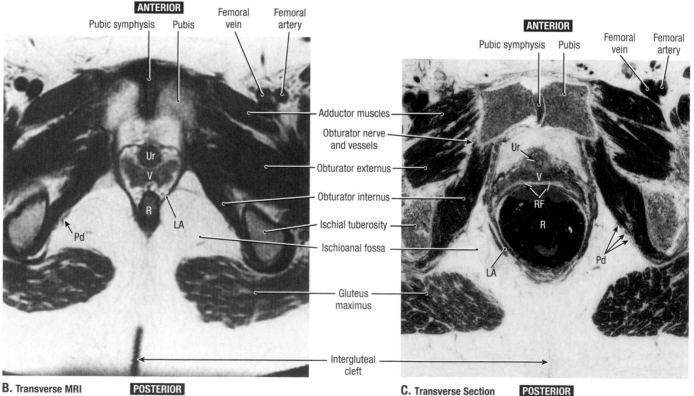

B. Transverse MRI

C. Transverse Section

Key for B and C

LA	Levator ani
Pd	Pudendal nerve and vessels
R	Rectum
RF	Rectouterine fold
Ur	Urethra
V	Vagina

5.34   **Transverse Sections and MRIs through Female Pelvis**

A. Transverse section through ischial tuberosities, bladder, vagina, rectum, and rectouterine pouch.
B. Transverse (axial) MRI. **C.** Sectioned specimen.

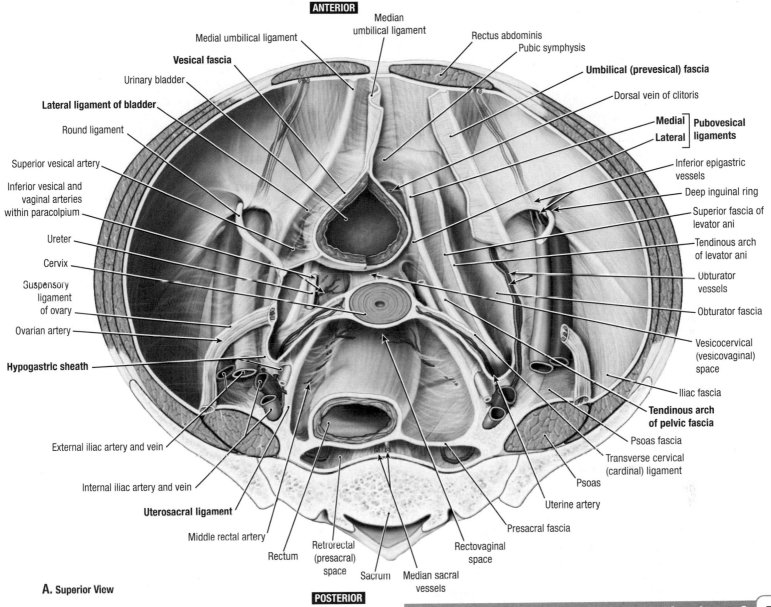

ANTERIOR

Median umbilical ligament

Medial umbilical ligament

Rectus abdominis

Pubic symphysis

Vesical fascia

Urinary bladder

Umbilical (prevesical) fascia

Dorsal vein of clitoris

Lateral ligament of bladder

Medial } **Pubovesical**
Lateral } **ligaments**

Round ligament

Inferior epigastric vessels

Superior vesical artery

Deep inguinal ring

Inferior vesical and vaginal arteries within paracolpium

Superior fascia of levator ani

Ureter

Tendinous arch of levator ani

Cervix

Obturator vessels

Suspensory ligament of ovary

Obturator fascia

Ovarian artery

Vesicocervical (vesicovaginal) space

Hypogastric sheath

Iliac fascia

Tendinous arch of pelvic fascia

External iliac artery and vein

Psoas fascia

Transverse cervical (cardinal) ligament

Internal iliac artery and vein

Psoas

Uterosacral ligament

Uterine artery

Middle rectal artery

Presacral fascia

Rectum

Rectovaginal space

Retrorectal (presacral) space

Sacrum

Median sacral vessels

A. Superior View

POSTERIOR

Tendinous arch of pelvic fascia

ANTERIOR

Pubic symphysis

Retropubic space (opened)

Pubovesical ligament

Urinary bladder

Vesical fascia

Tendinous arch of levator ani

Cervix

Transverse cervical ligament

Rectouterine pouch

Uterosacral (rectouterine ligament)

Rectum

Rectal fascia

Sacrum

Presacral space (opened)

B. Superior View

Pelvic Fascia and Supporting Mechanism of Cervix and Upper Vagina **5.35**

A. Greater and lesser pelvis demonstrating pelvic viscera and endopelvic fascia. **B.** Schematic of fascial ligaments and areolar spaces at level of tendinous arch of pelvic fascia.

- Note the parietal pelvic fascia covering the obturator internus and levator ani muscles and the visceral pelvic fasciae are continuous where the organs penetrate the pelvic floor, forming a tendinous arch of pelvic fascia bilaterally.
- The endopelvic fascia lies between, and is continuous with, both visceral and parietal layers of pelvic fascia. The loose, areolar portions of the endopelvic fascia have been removed; the fibrous, condensed portions remain. Note the condensation of this fascia into the hypogastric sheath, containing the vessels to the pelvic viscera, the ureters, and (in the male) the ductus deferens.
- Observe the ligamentous extensions of the hypogastric sheath: the lateral ligament of the urinary bladder, the transverse cervical ligament at the base of the broad ligament, and a less prominent lamina posteriorly containing the middle rectal vessels.

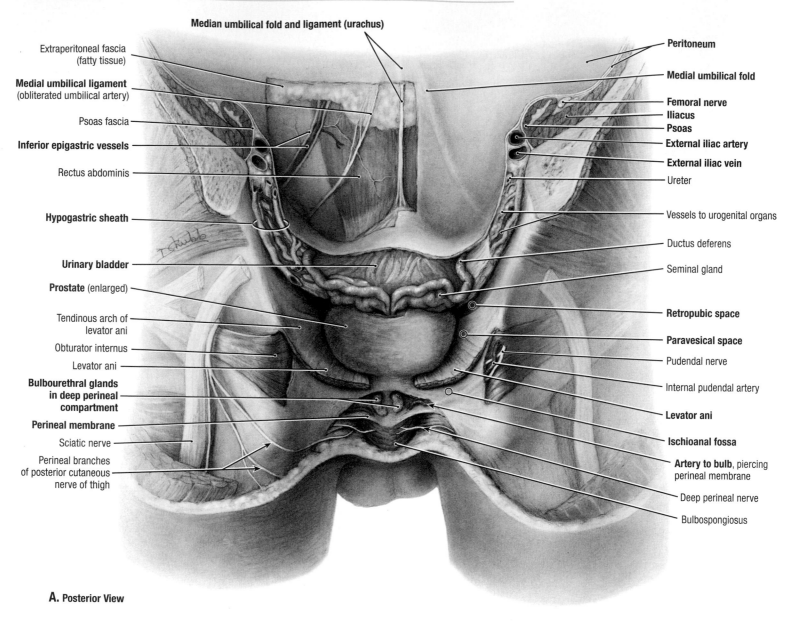

Median umbilical fold and ligament (urachus)

Extraperitoneal fascia (fatty tissue)

Medial umbilical ligament (obliterated umbilical artery)

Psoas fascia

Inferior epigastric vessels

Rectus abdominis

Hypogastric sheath

Urinary bladder

Prostate (enlarged)

Tendinous arch of levator ani

Obturator internus

Levator ani

Bulbourethral glands in deep perineal compartment

Perineal membrane

Sciatic nerve

Perineal branches of posterior cutaneous nerve of thigh

Peritoneum

Medial umbilical fold

Femoral nerve
Iliacus
Psoas
External iliac artery
External iliac vein
Ureter

Vessels to urogenital organs

Ductus deferens

Seminal gland

Retropubic space

Paravesical space

Pudendal nerve

Internal pudendal artery

Levator ani

Ischioanal fossa

Artery to bulb, piercing perineal membrane

Deep perineal nerve

Bulbospongiosus

A. Posterior View

5.36 Posterior Approach to Anterior Pelvic and Perineal Structures and Spaces

A. Dissection. The rectovesical septum and all pelvic and perineal structures posterior to it have been removed. **B. Schematic coronal section through anterior pelvis demonstrating pelvic fascia.**

- The inferior epigastric artery and accompanying veins enter the rectus sheath, covered posteriorly with peritoneum to form the lateral umbilical fold.
- The medial umbilical fold is formed by peritoneum overlying the medial umbilical ligament (obliterated umbilical artery).
- The median umbilical fold is formed by the median umbilical ligament (urachus).
- Near the bladder, the ureter accompanies a "leash" of internal iliac vessels and derivatives within the hypogastric sheath, a fibro-areolar structure.

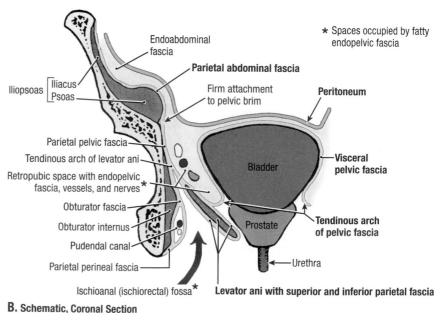

Endoabdominal fascia

Iliopsoas [Iliacus / Psoas]

Parietal abdominal fascia

Firm attachment to pelvic brim

Parietal pelvic fascia

Tendinous arch of levator ani

Retropubic space with endopelvic fascia, vessels, and nerves *

Obturator fascia

Obturator internus

Pudendal canal

Parietal perineal fascia

Ischioanal (ischiorectal) fossa *

* Spaces occupied by fatty endopelvic fascia

Peritoneum

Bladder

Visceral pelvic fascia

Prostate

Tendinous arch of pelvic fascia

Urethra

Levator ani with superior and inferior parietal fascia

B. Schematic, Coronal Section

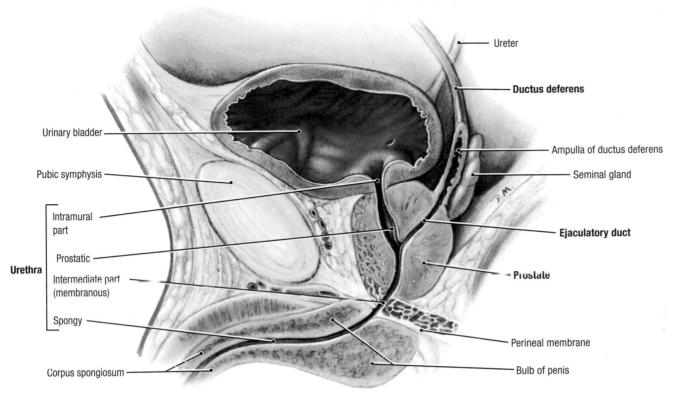

A. Median Section

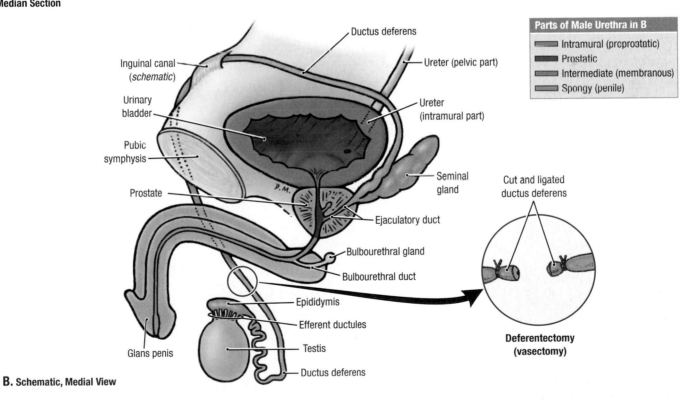

B. Schematic, Medial View

Parts of Male Urethra in B	
	Intramural (preprostatic)
	Prostatic
	Intermediate (membranous)
	Spongy (penile)

Deferentectomy (vasectomy)

Urinary Bladder, Prostate, Seminal Glands, and Ductus Deferens   5.37

A. Dissection. The ejaculatory duct (~2 cm in length) is formed by the union of the ductus deferens and duct of the seminal gland; it passes anteriorly and inferiorly through the substance of the prostate to enter the prostatic urethra. **B. Overview of urogenital system, schematic.** The common method of sterilizing males is a **deferentectomy**, popularly called vasectomy. During this procedure, part of the ductus deferens is ligated and/or excised through an incision in the superior part of the scrotum. Hence, the subsequent ejaculated fluid contains no sperms.

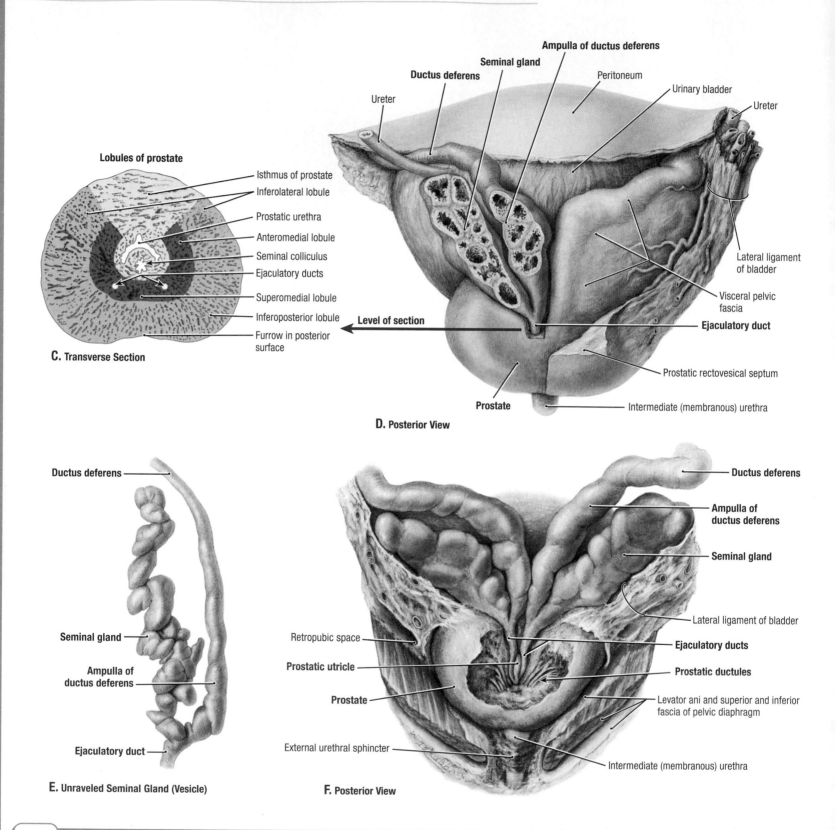

Lobules of prostate

Isthmus of prostate
Inferolateral lobule
Prostatic urethra
Anteromedial lobule
Seminal colliculus
Ejaculatory ducts
Superomedial lobule
Inferoposterior lobule
Furrow in posterior surface

C. Transverse Section

Ureter
Ductus deferens
Seminal gland
Ampulla of ductus deferens
Peritoneum
Urinary bladder
Ureter

Lateral ligament of bladder

Visceral pelvic fascia

Level of section

Ejaculatory duct

Prostate

Prostatic rectovesical septum

Intermediate (membranous) urethra

D. Posterior View

Ductus deferens

Seminal gland

Ampulla of ductus deferens

Ejaculatory duct

E. Unraveled Seminal Gland (Vesicle)

Ductus deferens

Ampulla of ductus deferens

Seminal gland

Lateral ligament of bladder

Ejaculatory ducts

Prostatic ductules

Levator ani and superior and inferior fascia of pelvic diaphragm

Intermediate (membranous) urethra

Retropubic space
Prostatic utricle
Prostate
External urethral sphincter

F. Posterior View

5.37   **Urinary Bladder, Prostate, Seminal Glands, and Ductus Deferens** *(continued)*

C. and **D.** **Bladder, ductus deferens, seminal glands (vesicles), and lobules of prostate.** The left seminal gland and ampulla of the ductus deferens are dissected and opened; part of the prostate is cut away to expose the ejaculatory duct. **E. Seminal gland unraveled.** The gland is a tortuous tube with numerous dilatations. The

ampulla of the ductus deferens has similar dilatations. **F. Prostate, dissected posteriorly.** The ejaculatory duct enters the prostatic urethra on the seminal colliculus. The prostatic utricle lies between the ends of the two ejaculatory ducts. The prostatic ductules mostly open onto the prostatic sinus.

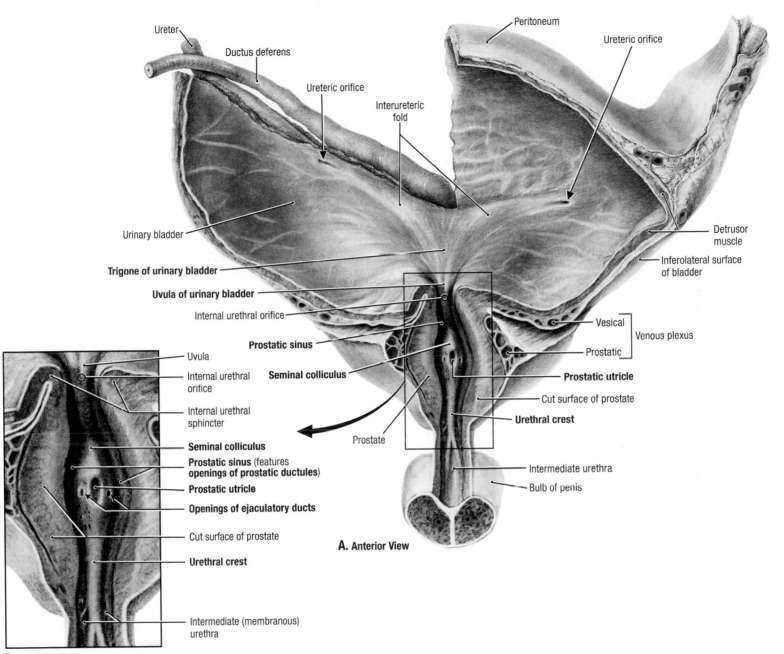

Ureter

Ductus deferens

Ureteric orifice

Interureteric fold

Peritoneum

Ureteric orifice

Urinary bladder

Trigone of urinary bladder

Uvula of urinary bladder

Internal urethral orifice

Prostatic sinus

Seminal colliculus

Detrusor muscle

Inferolateral surface of bladder

Vesical

Prostatic

Venous plexus

Prostatic utricle

Cut surface of prostate

Urethral crest

Prostate

Intermediate urethra

Bulb of penis

A. Anterior View

Uvula

Internal urethral orifice

Internal urethral sphincter

Seminal colliculus

Prostatic sinus (features openings of prostatic ductules)

Prostatic utricle

Openings of ejaculatory ducts

Cut surface of prostate

Urethral crest

Intermediate (membranous) urethra

B. Anterior View

Interior of Male Urinary Bladder and Prostatic Urethra

A. Dissection. The anterior walls of the bladder, prostate, and urethra were cut away. **B. Features of prostatic urethra.**

- The mucous membrane is smooth over the trigone of the urinary bladder (triangular region demarcated by ureteric and internal urethral orifices) but folded elsewhere, especially when the bladder is empty.
- The opening of the vestigial prostatic utricle is in the seminal colliculus on the urethral crest; there is an orifice of an ejaculatory duct on each side of the prostatic utricle. The prostatic fascia encloses the prostatic venous plexus.

The prostate is of considerable medical interest because enlargement or **benign hyperplasia of the prostate (BHP)** is common

after middle age, affecting virtually every male who lives long enough. An enlarged prostate projects into the urinary bladder and impedes urination by distorting the prostatic urethra. The middle lobule usually enlarges the most and obstructs the internal urethral orifice. The more the person strains, the more the valve-like prostatic mass occludes the urethra.

BHP is a common cause of urethral obstruction, leading to **nocturia** (needing to void during the night), **dysuria** (difficulty and/or pain during urination), and **urgency** (sudden desire to void). BHP also increases the risk of bladder infections (**cystitis**) as well as kidney damage.

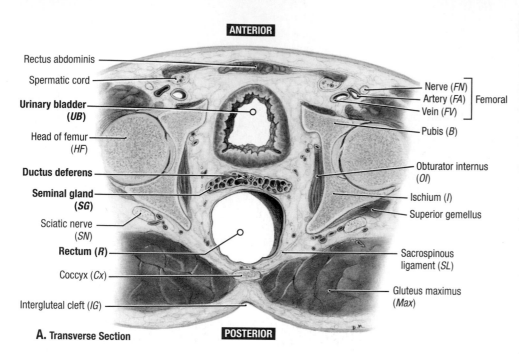

ANTERIOR

Rectus abdominis

Spermatic cord

Urinary bladder (UB)

Head of femur (HF)

Ductus deferens

Seminal gland (SG)

Sciatic nerve (SN)

Rectum (R)

Coccyx (Cx)

Intergluteal cleft (IG)

Nerve (FN)
Artery (FA) } Femoral
Vein (FV)

Pubis (B)

Obturator internus (OI)

Ischium (I)

Superior gemellus

Sacrospinous ligament (SL)

Gluteus maximus (Max)

A. Transverse Section

POSTERIOR

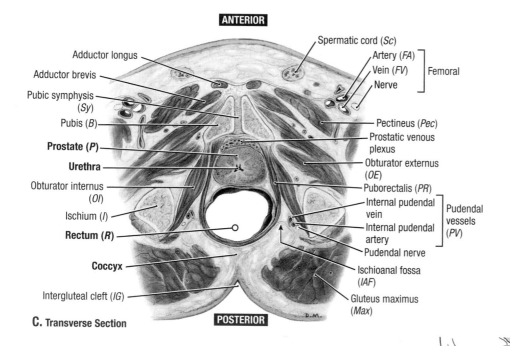

ANTERIOR

Adductor longus

Adductor brevis

Pubic symphysis (Sy)

Pubis (B)

Prostate (P)

Urethra

Obturator internus (OI)

Ischium (I)

Rectum (R)

Coccyx

Intergluteal cleft (IG)

Spermatic cord (Sc)

Artery (FA)
Vein (FV) } Femoral
Nerve

Pectineus (Pec)

Prostatic venous plexus

Obturator externus (OE)

Puborectalis (PR)

Internal pudendal vein
Internal pudendal artery } Pudendal vessels (PV)

Pudendal nerve

Ischioanal fossa (IAF)

Gluteus maximus (Max)

C. Transverse Section

POSTERIOR

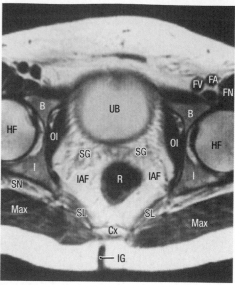

B. Transverse MRI

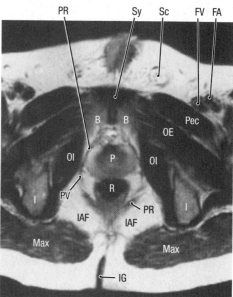

D. Transverse MRI

5.39 Male Pelvis, Transverse Sections and MRI

A. and **B.** Transverse section and MRI through urinary bladder, seminal gland, and rectum. **C.** and **D.** Transverse section and MRI through prostate and rectum. **E.** Digital rectal examination.

The prostate is examined for enlargement and tumors (focal masses or asymmetry) by **digital rectal examination**. A full bladder offers resistance, holding the gland in place and making it more readily palpable. The malignant prostate feels hard and often irregular.

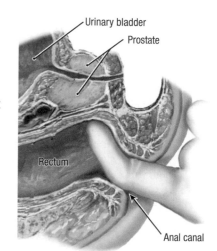

Urinary bladder

Prostate

Rectum

Anal canal

E. Median Section

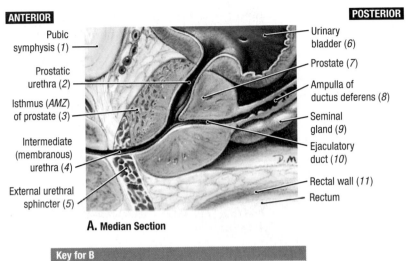

ANTERIOR   **POSTERIOR**

Pubic symphysis (1)

Prostatic urethra (2)

Isthmus (AMZ) of prostate (3)

Intermediate (membranous) urethra (4)

External urethral sphincter (5)

Urinary bladder (6)

Prostate (7)

Ampulla of ductus deferens (8)

Seminal gland (9)

Ejaculatory duct (10)

Rectal wall (11)

Rectum

A. Median Section

Key for B	
12	Site of transducer in rectum
13	Concretions surrounding distended and collapsed urethra
14	Calcification in seminal colliculus

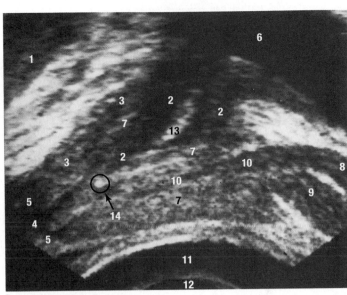

B. **Longitudinal (Median) US**

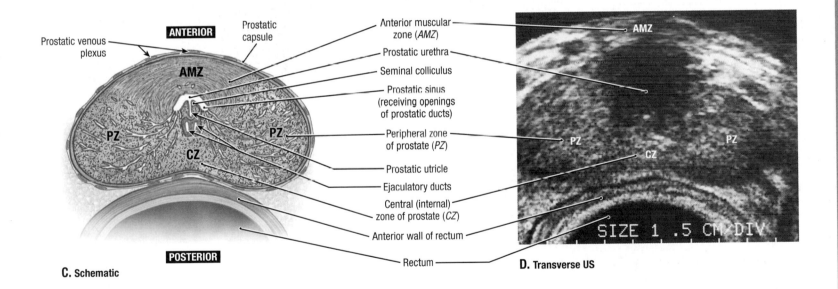

Prostatic venous plexus

ANTERIOR   Prostatic capsule

Prostatic capsule

AMZ

PZ   PZ

CZ

POSTERIOR

C. Schematic

Anterior muscular zone (AMZ)

Prostatic urethra

Seminal colliculus

Prostatic sinus (receiving openings of prostatic ducts)

Peripheral zone of prostate (PZ)

Prostatic utricle

Ejaculatory ducts

Central (internal) zone of prostate (CZ)

Anterior wall of rectum

Rectum

D. Transverse US

AMZ

PZ   PZ

CZ

SIZE 1 .5 CM/DIV

Transrectal Ultrasound (US) Scans of Male Pelvis

5.40

A. and **B. Longitudinal (median) scan. C.** and **D. Transverse scan.** The probe was inserted into the rectum to scan the anteriorly located prostate. The ducts of the glands in the peripheral zone open into the prostatic sinuses, whereas the ducts of the glands in the central (internal) zone open into the prostatic sinuses and onto the seminal colliculus.

Because of the close relationship of the prostate to the prostatic urethra, obstructions of the urethra may be relieved endoscopically. The instrument is inserted transurethrally through the external urethral orifice and spongy urethra into the prostatic urethra. All or part of the

prostate, or just the hypertrophied part, is removed by **transurethral resection of the prostate (TURP)**. In more serious cases, the entire prostate is removed along with the seminal glands, ejaculatory ducts, and terminal parts of the deferent ducts (**radical prostatectomy**).

TURP and improved operative techniques (laparoscopic or robotic surgery) attempt to preserve the nerves and blood vessels associated with the capsule of the prostate and adjacent to the seminal vesicles as they pass to and from the penis, increasing the possibility for patients to retain sexual function after surgery as well as restoring normal urinary control.

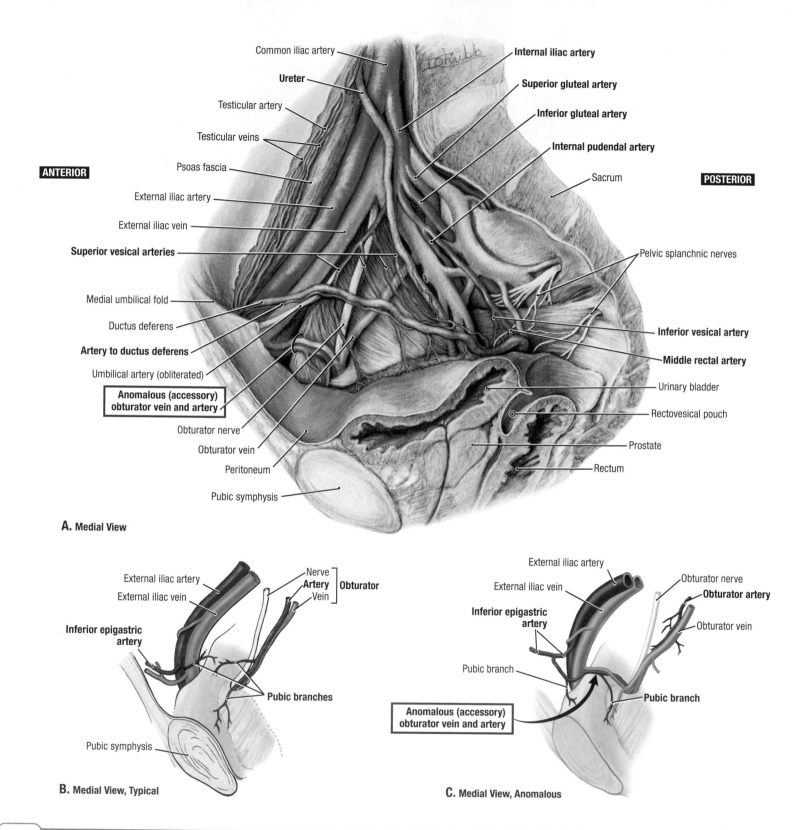

A. Medial View

Common iliac artery

Ureter

Testicular artery

Testicular veins

Psoas fascia

ANTERIOR

External iliac artery

External iliac vein

Superior vesical arteries

Medial umbilical fold

Ductus deferens

Artery to ductus deferens

Umbilical artery (obliterated)

Anomalous (accessory) obturator vein and artery

Obturator nerve

Obturator vein

Peritoneum

Pubic symphysis

Internal iliac artery

Superior gluteal artery

Inferior gluteal artery

Internal pudendal artery

Sacrum

POSTERIOR

Pelvic splanchnic nerves

Inferior vesical artery

Middle rectal artery

Urinary bladder

Rectovesical pouch

Prostate

Rectum

B. Medial View, Typical

External iliac artery

External iliac vein

Inferior epigastric artery

Nerve

Artery   **Obturator**

Vein

Pubic branches

Pubic symphysis

C. Medial View, Anomalous

External iliac artery

External iliac vein

Inferior epigastric artery

Pubic branch

Anomalous (accessory) obturator vein and artery

Obturator nerve

Obturator artery

Obturator vein

Pubic branch

5.41   **Pelvic Vessels *In Situ*, Lateral Pelvic Wall**

A. Dissection of lateral pelvic wall. The ureter crosses the external iliac artery at its origin (common iliac bifurcation), and the ductus deferens crosses the external iliac artery at its termination (deep inguinal ring). In this specimen, an anomalous (accessory) obturator artery branches from the inferior epigastric artery. **B. Typical obturator artery. C. Anomalous obturator artery.** Surgeons performing hernia repairs must keep this common variation (also shown in *Part A*) in mind.

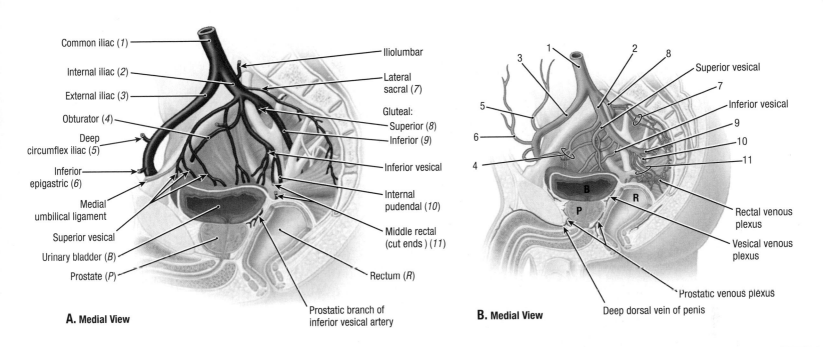

A. Medial View

B. Medial View

Arteries and Veins of Male Pelvis

5.42

A. Arteries. **B.** Veins.

The neurovascular structures of the pelvis lie extraperitoneally. When dissecting from the pelvic cavity toward the pelvic walls,

the pelvic arteries are encountered first, followed by the associated pelvic veins, and then the somatic nerves of the pelvis.

TABLE 5.6	Arteries of Male Pelvis[a]		
Artery	**Origin**	**Course**	**Distribution**
Internal iliac	Common iliac artery	Passes medially over pelvic brim and descends into pelvic cavity; often forms anterior and posterior divisions	Main blood supply to pelvic organs, gluteal muscles, and perineum
Anterior division of internal iliac artery	Internal iliac artery	Passes laterally along lateral wall of pelvis, dividing into visceral, obturator, and internal pudendal arteries	Pelvic viscera, perineum, and muscles of superior medial thigh
Umbilical	Anterior division of internal iliac artery	Short pelvic course; gives off superior vesical arteries and then obliterates, becoming medial umbilical ligament	Urinary bladder and, in some males, ductus deferens
Superior vesical	Patent part of umbilical artery	Usually multiple; pass to superior aspect of urinary bladder	Superior aspect of urinary bladder and distal ureter
Artery to ductus deferens	Superior or inferior vesical artery	Runs subperitoneally to ductus deferens	Ductus deferens
Obturator	Anterior division of internal iliac artery	Runs anteroinferiorly on lateral pelvic wall	Pelvic muscles, nutrient artery to head of femur and medial compartment of thigh
Inferior vesical		Passes subperitoneally giving rise to prostatic artery and occasionally the artery to the ductus deferens	Inferior aspect of urinary bladder, pelvic ureter, seminal glands, and prostate
Middle rectal		Descends in pelvis to rectum	Seminal glands, prostate, and inferior part of rectum
Internal pudendal		Exits pelvis through greater sciatic foramen and enters perineum via lesser sciatic foramen	Main artery to perineum, including muscles and skin of anal and urogenital triangles; erectile bodies
Posterior division of internal iliac artery	Internal iliac artery	Passes posteriorly and gives rise to parietal branches	Pelvic wall and gluteal region
Iliolumbar	Posterior division of internal iliac artery	Ascends anterior to sacroiliac joint and posterior to common iliac vessels and psoas major	Iliacus, psoas major, quadratus lumborum muscles, and cauda equina in vertebral canal
Lateral sacral (superior and inferior)		Run on anteromedial aspect of piriformis to send branches into pelvic sacral foramina	Piriformis muscle, structures in sacral canal and erector spinae muscles
Testicular (gonadal)	Abdominal aorta	Descends retroperitoneally; traverses inguinal canal and enters scrotum	Abdominal ureter, testis, and epididymis

[a]Branching of internal iliac artery is highly variable.

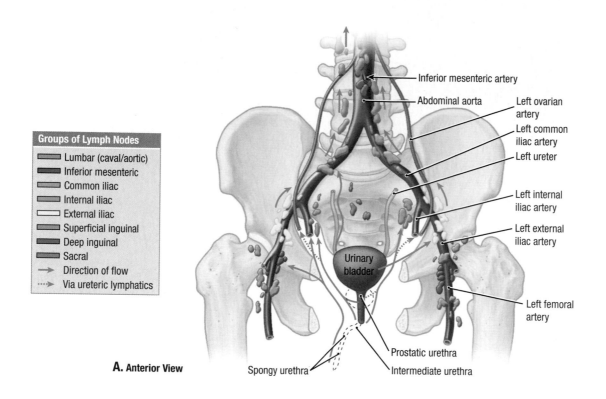

Groups of Lymph Nodes

- Lumbar (caval/aortic)
- Inferior mesenteric
- Common iliac
- Internal iliac
- External iliac
- Superficial inguinal
- Deep inguinal
- Sacral
- → Direction of flow
- ⤍ Via ureteric lymphatics

Inferior mesenteric artery
Abdominal aorta
Left ovarian artery
Left common iliac artery
Left ureter
Left internal iliac artery
Left external iliac artery
Urinary bladder
Left femoral artery
Prostatic urethra
Intermediate urethra
Spongy urethra

A. Anterior View

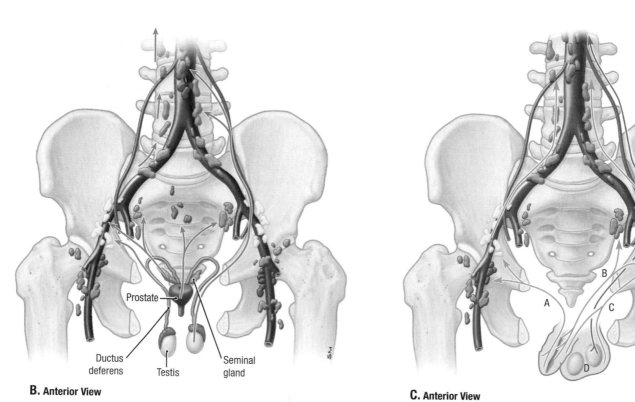

Prostate
Ductus deferens
Testis
Seminal gland

B. Anterior View

Key for C: Path for Lymph Flow from

- **A** Glans penis
- **B** Spongy urethra
- **C** Skin of body of penis/scrotum
- **D** Testis

C. Anterior View

A. Pelvic urinary system. **B.** Internal genital organs. **C.** Penis, spongy urethra, scrotum, and testis.

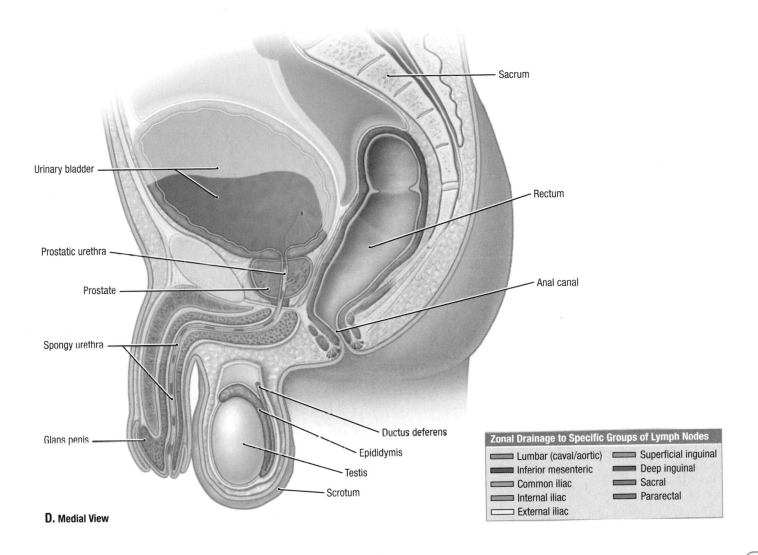

Urinary bladder

Prostatic urethra

Prostate

Spongy urethra

Glans penis

Sacrum

Rectum

Anal canal

Ductus deferens

Epididymis

Testis

Scrotum

D. Medial View

Zonal Drainage to Specific Groups of Lymph Nodes

- Lumbar (caval/aortic)
- Inferior mesenteric
- Common iliac
- Internal iliac
- External iliac
- Superficial inguinal
- Deep inguinal
- Sacral
- Pararectal

Lymphatic Drainage of Male Pelvis and Perineum (continued)   **5.43**

D. Zones of lymphatic drainage of pelvis and perineum.

TABLE 5.7	Lymphatic Drainage of Male Pelvis and Perineum
Lymph Node Group	**Structures Typically Draining to Lymph Node Group**
Lumbar	Gonads and associated structures (including testicular vessels), urethra, testis, epididymis, common iliac nodes
Inferior mesenteric nodes	Superiormost rectum, sigmoid colon, descending colon, pararectal nodes
Common iliac nodes	External and internal iliac lymph nodes
Internal iliac nodes	Inferior pelvic structures, deep perineal structures, sacral nodes, prostatic urethra, prostate, base of bladder, inferior part of pelvic ureter, inferior part of seminal glands, cavernous bodies, anal canal (above pectinate line), inferior rectum
External iliac nodes	Anterosuperior pelvic structures, deep inguinal nodes, superior aspect of bladder, superior part of pelvic ureter, upper part of seminal gland, pelvic part of ductus deferens, intermediate and spongy urethra
Superficial inguinal nodes	Lower limb, superficial drainage of inferolateral quadrant of trunk, including anterior abdominal wall inferior to umbilicus, gluteal region, superficial perineal structures, skin of perineum including skin and prepuce of penis, scrotum, perianal skin, anal canal inferior to pectinate line
Deep inguinal nodes	Glans of penis, distal spongy urethra, superficial inguinal nodes
Sacral nodes	Posteroinferior pelvic structures, inferior rectum
Pararectal nodes	Superior rectum

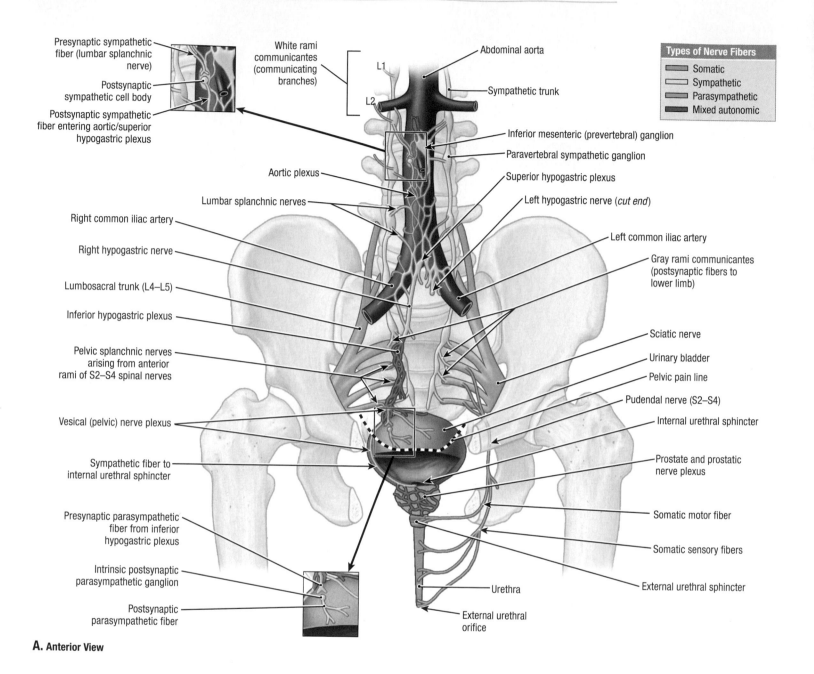

Types of Nerve Fibers

- Somatic
- Sympathetic
- Parasympathetic
- Mixed autonomic

Presynaptic sympathetic fiber (lumbar splanchnic nerve)

Postsynaptic sympathetic cell body

Postsynaptic sympathetic fiber entering aortic/superior hypogastric plexus

White rami communicantes (communicating branches)

Abdominal aorta

Sympathetic trunk

Inferior mesenteric (prevertebral) ganglion

Paravertebral sympathetic ganglion

Aortic plexus

Superior hypogastric plexus

Lumbar splanchnic nerves

Left hypogastric nerve (*cut end*)

Right common iliac artery

Left common iliac artery

Right hypogastric nerve

Gray rami communicantes (postsynaptic fibers to lower limb)

Lumbosacral trunk (L4–L5)

Inferior hypogastric plexus

Sciatic nerve

Pelvic splanchnic nerves arising from anterior rami of S2–S4 spinal nerves

Urinary bladder

Pelvic pain line

Pudendal nerve (S2–S4)

Vesical (pelvic) nerve plexus

Internal urethral sphincter

Sympathetic fiber to internal urethral sphincter

Prostate and prostatic nerve plexus

Presynaptic parasympathetic fiber from inferior hypogastric plexus

Somatic motor fiber

Intrinsic postsynaptic parasympathetic ganglion

Somatic sensory fibers

Postsynaptic parasympathetic fiber

External urethral sphincter

Urethra

External urethral orifice

L1

L2

A. Anterior View

5.44 **Innervation of Male Pelvis and Perineum**

A. Overview.

TABLE 5.8	Effect of Sympathetic and Parasympathetic Stimulation on Urinary Tract, Genital System, and Rectum	
Organ, Tract, or System	**Effect of Sympathetic Stimulation**	**Effect of Parasympathetic Stimulation**
Urinary tract	Vasoconstriction of renal vessels slows urine formation; internal sphincter of male bladder contracted to prevent retrograde ejaculation and maintain urinary continence	Inhibits contraction of internal sphincter of bladder in males; contracts detrusor muscle of the bladder wall causing urination
Genital system	Causes ejaculation and vasoconstriction resulting in remission of erection	Produces engorgement (erection) of erectile tissues of the external genitals
Rectum	Maintains tonus of internal anal sphincter; inhibits peristalsis of rectum	Rectal contraction (peristalsis) for defecation; inhibition of contraction of internal anal sphincter

The parasympathetic system is restricted in its distribution to the head, neck, and body cavities (except for erectile tissues of genitalia); otherwise, parasympathetic fibers are never found in the body wall and limbs. Sympathetic fibers, by comparison, are distributed to all vascularized portions of the body.

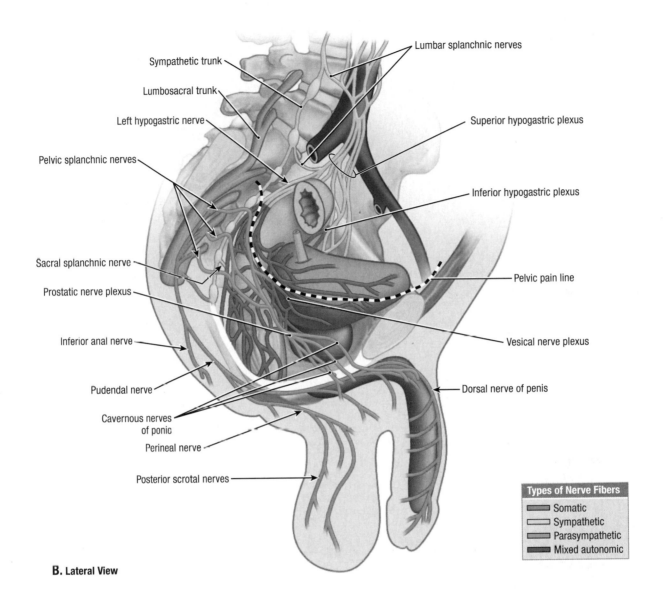

Lumbar splanchnic nerves

Sympathetic trunk

Lumbosacral trunk

Left hypogastric nerve

Superior hypogastric plexus

Pelvic splanchnic nerves

Inferior hypogastric plexus

Sacral splanchnic nerve

Pelvic pain line

Prostatic nerve plexus

Inferior anal nerve

Vesical nerve plexus

Pudendal nerve

Dorsal nerve of penis

Cavernous nerves
of ponic

Perineal nerve

Posterior scrotal nerves

Types of Nerve Fibers	
	Somatic
	Sympathetic
	Parasympathetic
	Mixed autonomic

B. Lateral View

Innervation of Male Pelvis and Perineum (*continued*)   **5.44**

B. Innervation of prostate and external genitalia.

- The primary function of the sacral sympathetic trunks is to provide postsynaptic fibers to the sacral plexus for sympathetic innervation of the lower limb.
- The periarterial plexuses of the ovarian, superior rectal, and internal iliac arteries are minor routes by which sympathetic fibers enter the pelvis. Their primary function is vasomotion of the arteries they accompany.
- The hypogastric plexuses (superior and inferior) are networks of sympathetic and visceral afferent nerve fibers.
- The superior hypogastric plexus carries fibers conveyed to and from the aortic (intermesenteric) plexus by the L3 and L4 splanchnic nerves. The superior hypogastric plexus divides into right and left hypogastric nerves that merge with the parasympathetic pelvic splanchnic nerves to form the inferior hypogastric plexuses.

- The fibers of the inferior hypogastric plexuses continue to the pelvic viscera on which they form pelvic plexuses (e.g., prostatic nerve plexus).
- The pelvic splanchnic nerves convey presynaptic parasympathetic fibers from the S2–S4 spinal cord segments, which make up the sacral outflow of the parasympathetic system.
- Visceral afferents conveying unconscious reflex sensation follow the course of the parasympathetic fibers retrogradely to the spinal sensory ganglia of S2–S4, as do those transmitting pain sensations from the viscera inferior to the pelvic pain line (structures that do not contact the peritoneum plus the distal sigmoid colon and rectum). Visceral afferent fibers conducting pain from structures superior to the pelvic pain line (structures in contact with the peritoneum, except for the distal sigmoid colon and rectum) follow the sympathetic fibers retrogradely to inferior thoracic and superior lumbar spinal ganglia.

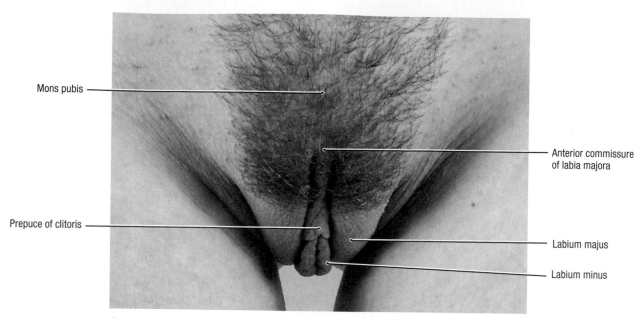

Mons pubis

Anterior commissure
of labia majora

Prepuce of clitoris

Labium majus

Labium minus

A. Anterior View

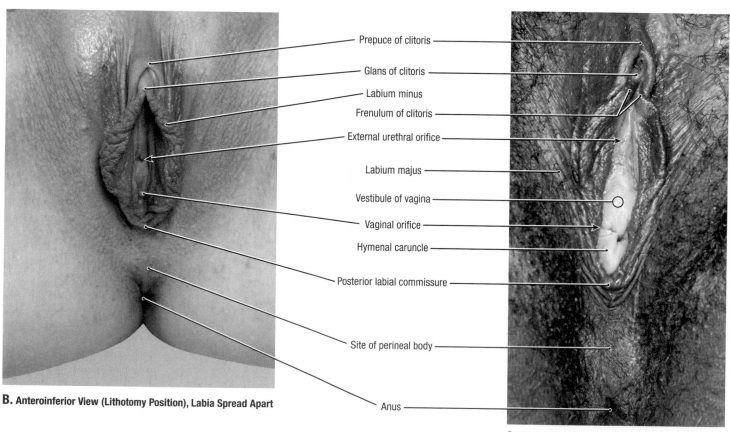

Prepuce of clitoris

Glans of clitoris

Labium minus

Frenulum of clitoris

External urethral orifice

Labium majus

Vestibule of vagina

Vaginal orifice

Hymenal caruncle

Posterior labial commissure

Site of perineal body

Anus

B. Anteroinferior View (Lithotomy Position), Labia Spread Apart

C. Inferior View, Labia Spread Apart

5.45 **Surface Anatomy of Female Perineum**

A. External genitalia (pudendum; vulva), standing position. **B.** and **C.** Vestibule of vagina and external urethral and vaginal orifices opening into it (recumbent position).

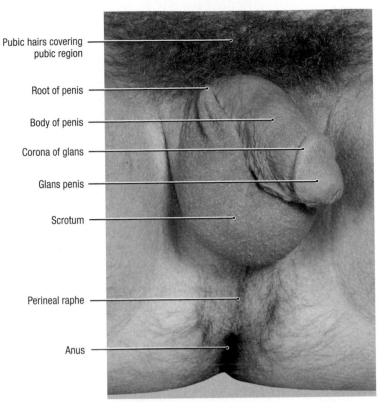

Pubic hairs covering pubic region

Root of penis

Body of penis

Corona of glans

Glans penis

Scrotum

Perineal raphe

Anus

B. Inferior View

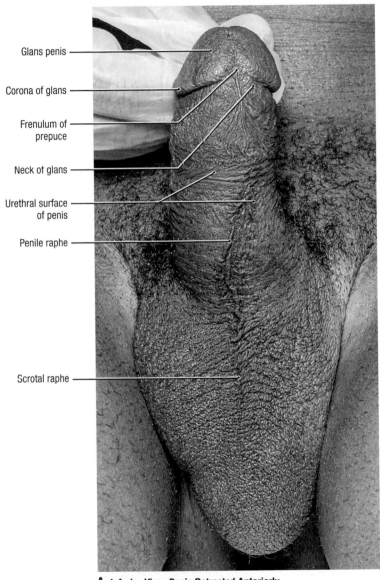

Glans penis

Corona of glans

Frenulum of prepuce

Neck of glans

Urethral surface of penis

Penile raphe

Scrotal raphe

A. Inferior View, Penis Retracted Anteriorly

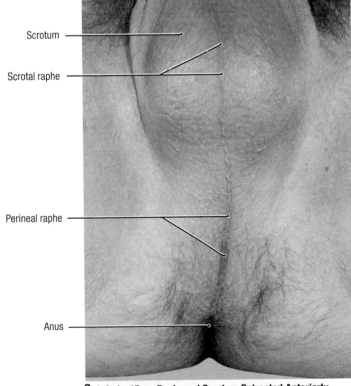

Scrotum

Scrotal raphe

Perineal raphe

Anus

C. Inferior View, Penis and Scrotum Retracted Anteriorly

Surface Anatomy of Male Perineum   **5.46**

A. Surface anatomy of circumcised penis. **B.** Penis and scrotum. **C.** Center of male perineal region.

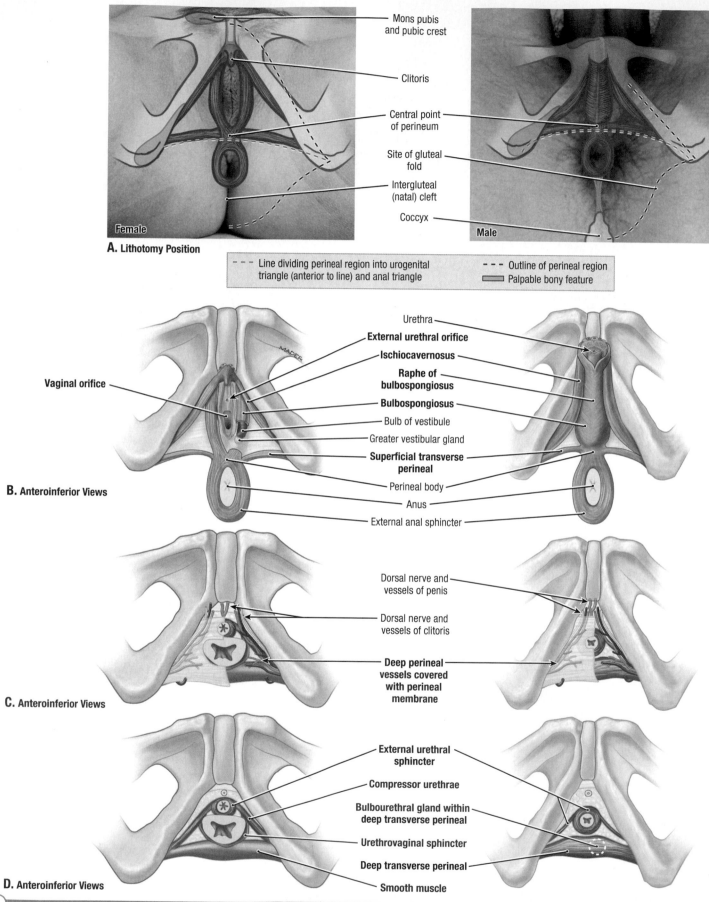

Mons pubis
and pubic crest

Clitoris

Central point
of perineum

Site of gluteal
fold

Intergluteal
(natal) cleft

Coccyx

Female

Male

A. Lithotomy Position

- - - Line dividing perineal region into urogenital
triangle (anterior to line) and anal triangle

- - - Outline of perineal region

Palpable bony feature

Urethra

External urethral orifice

Ischiocavernosus

**Raphe of
bulbospongiosus**

Vaginal orifice

Bulbospongiosus

Bulb of vestibule

Greater vestibular gland

**Superficial transverse
perineal**

Perineal body

B. Anteroinferior Views

Anus

External anal sphincter

Dorsal nerve and
vessels of penis

Dorsal nerve and
vessels of clitoris

**Deep perineal
vessels covered
with perineal
membrane**

C. Anteroinferior Views

External urethral
sphincter

Compressor urethrae

Bulbourethral gland within
deep transverse perineal

Urethrovaginal sphincter

Deep transverse perineal

D. Anteroinferior Views

Smooth muscle

5.47 **Layers of Perineum**

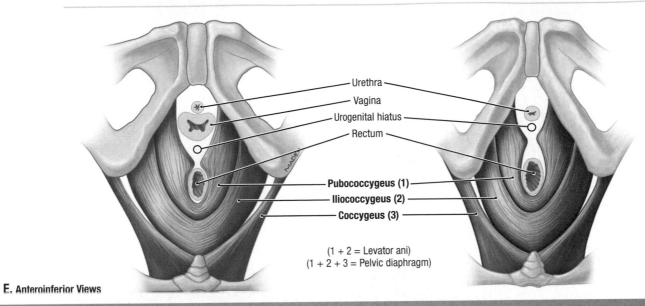

Urethra
Vagina
Urogenital hiatus
Rectum

Pubococcygeus (1)
Iliococcygeus (2)
Coccygeus (3)

(1 + 2 = Levator ani)
(1 + 2 + 3 = Pelvic diaphragm)

E. Anteroinferior Views

Layers of Perineum *(continued)*   5.47

A–E. Layers are shown from superficial to deep.

TABLE 5.9   Muscles of Perineum

Muscle	Origin	Course and Insertion	Innervation	Main Action
External anal sphincter	Skin and fascia surrounding anus; coccyx via anococcygeal ligament	Passes around lateral aspects of anal canal; insertion into perineal body	Inferior anal (rectal) nerve, a branch of pudendal nerve (S2–S4)	Constricts anal canal during peristalsis, resisting defecation; supports and fixes perineal body and pelvic floor
Bulbosponglosus	*Male:* median raphe on ventral surface of bulb of penis; perineal body	*Male:* surrounds lateral aspects of bulb of penis and most proximal part of body of penis, inserting into perineal membrane, dorsal aspect of corpora spongiosum and cavernosa, and fascia of bulb of penis	Muscular (deep) branch of perineal nerve, a branch of the pudendal nerve (S2–S4)	*Male:* supports and fixes perineal body/pelvic floor; compresses bulb of penis to expel last drops of urine/semen; assists erection by compressing outflow via deep perineal vein and by pushing blood from bulb into body of penis
	Female: perineal body	*Female:* passes on each side of lower vagina, enclosing bulb and greater vestibular gland; inserts onto pubic arch and fascia of corpora cavernosa of clitoris		*Female:* supports and fixes perineal body/pelvic floor; "sphincter" of vagina; assists in erection of clitoris (and perhaps bulb of vestibule); compresses greater vestibular gland
Ischiocavernosus	Internal surface of ischiopubic ramus and ischial tuberosity	Embraces crus of penis or clitoris, inserting onto the inferior and medial aspects of the crus and to the perineal membrane medial to the crus		Maintains erection of penis or clitoris by compressing outflow veins and pushing blood from the root of penis or clitoris into the body of penis or clitoris
Superficial transverse perineal	Internal surface of ischiopubic ramus and ischial tuberosity	Passes along inferior aspect of posterior border of perineal membrane to perineal body		Supports and fixes perineal body (pelvic floor) to support abdominopelvic viscera and resist increased intraabdominal pressure
Deep transverse perineal (male only)		Passes along superior aspect of posterior border of perineal membrane to perineal body, and external anal sphincter	Muscular (deep) branch of perineal nerve	
Smooth muscle (female only)	Ischiopubic rami	Passes to lateral wall of urethra and vagina	Autonomic nerves	Quantity of smooth muscle increases with age; function uncertain
External urethral sphincter		Surrounds urethra superior to perineal membrane; in males, also ascends anterior aspect of prostate	Dorsal nerve of penis or clitoris, terminal branch of pudendal nerve (S2–S4)	Compresses urethra to maintain urinary continence
Compressor urethrae (females only)	Internal surface of ischiopubic ramus	Continuous with external urethral sphincter		Compresses urethra; with pelvic diaphragm assists in elongation of urethra
Urethrovaginal sphincter (females only)	Anterior side of urethra	Continuous with compressor urethrae; extends posteriorly on lateral wall of urethra and vagina to interdigitate with fibers from opposite side of perineal body	Dorsal nerve of clitoris, terminal branch of pudendal nerve (S2–S4)	Compresses urethra and vagina

Oelrich TM. The urethral sphincter muscle in the male. *Am J Anat* 1980;158:229–246.
Oelrich TM. The striated urogenital sphincter muscle in the female. *Anat Rec* 1983;205:223–232.
Mirilas P, Skandalakis JE. Urogenital diaphragm: an erroneous concept casting its shadow over the sphincter urethrae and deep perineal space. *J Am Coll Surg* 2004;198:279–290.
DeLancey JO. Correlative study of paraurethral anatomy. *Obstet Gynecol* 1986;68:91–97.

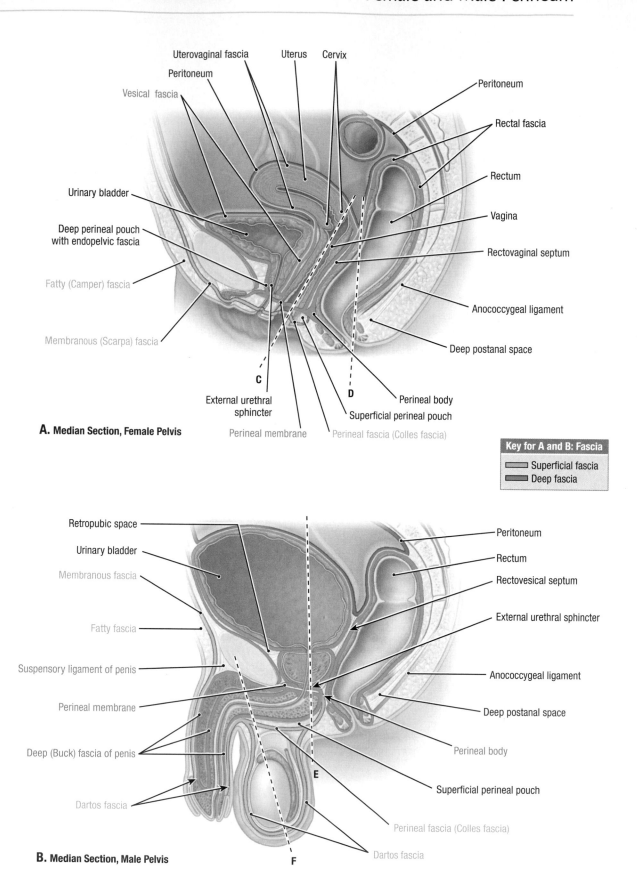

Uterovaginal fascia
Uterus
Cervix
Peritoneum
Vesical fascia
Peritoneum
Rectal fascia
Rectum
Urinary bladder
Vagina
Deep perineal pouch with endopelvic fascia
Rectovaginal septum
Fatty (Camper) fascia
Anococcygeal ligament
Membranous (Scarpa) fascia
Deep postanal space
C
D
Perineal body
External urethral sphincter
Superficial perineal pouch
Perineal membrane
Perineal fascia (Colles fascia)

A. Median Section, Female Pelvis

Key for A and B: Fascia
Superficial fascia
Deep fascia

Retropubic space
Peritoneum
Urinary bladder
Rectum
Membranous fascia
Rectovesical septum
Fatty fascia
External urethral sphincter
Suspensory ligament of penis
Anococcygeal ligament
Perineal membrane
Deep postanal space
Deep (Buck) fascia of penis
Perineal body
E
Superficial perineal pouch
Dartos fascia
Perineal fascia (Colles fascia)
F
Dartos fascia

B. Median Section, Male Pelvis

5.48 **Fasciae of Female and Male Perineum**

A. Fasciae of female perineum. **B.** Fasciae of male perineum.

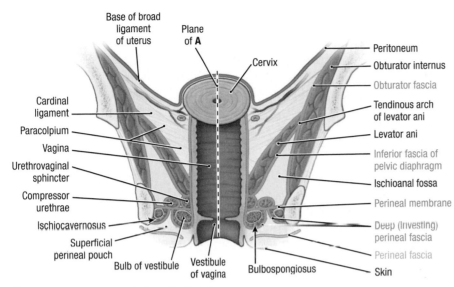

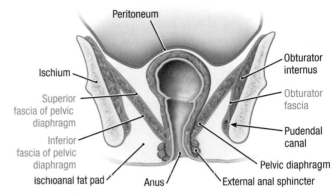

C. Coronal Section in Plane Indicated in *Part A*

D. Coronal Section in Plane Indicated in *Part A*

Fascia

| ▭ Superficial fascia | ▬ Deep fascia |

Key for F

CP	Corpora cavernosa penis
DV	Deep dorsal vein
PB	Pubic bones
PS	Pubic symphysis
SU	Spongy urethra

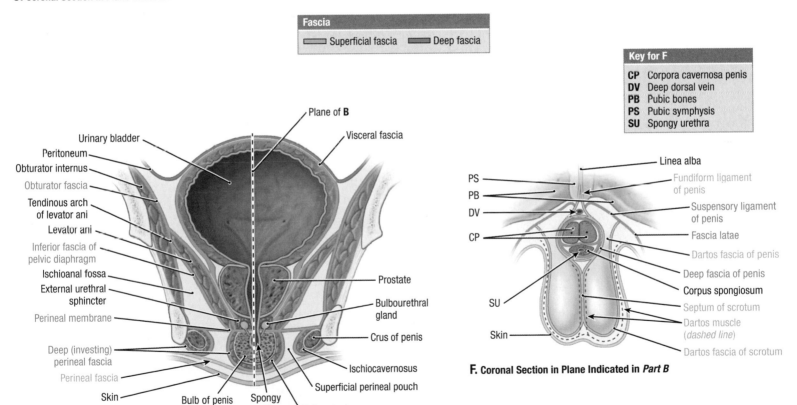

E. Coronal Section in Plane Indicated in *Part B*

F. Coronal Section in Plane Indicated in *Part B*

C. and D. Fasciae as seen on coronal sections of female pelvis. E. and F. Fasciae as seen on coronal sections of male pelvis.

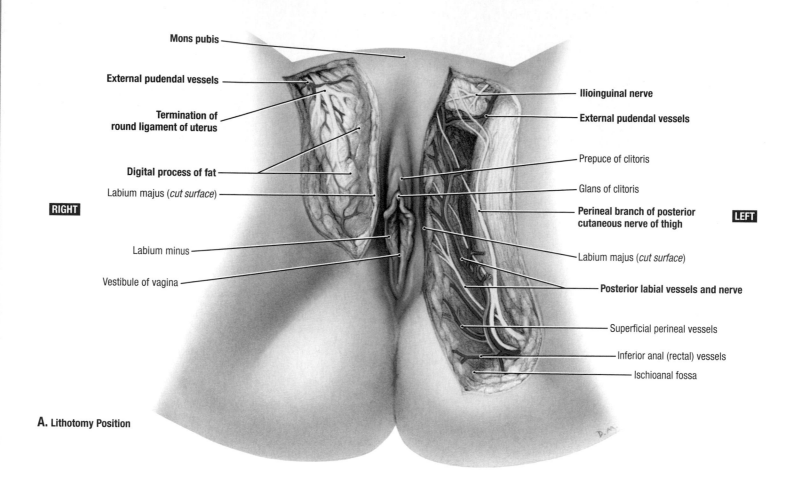

Mons pubis

External pudendal vessels

Termination of
round ligament of uterus

Digital process of fat

Labium majus (*cut surface*)

RIGHT

Labium minus

Vestibule of vagina

Ilioinguinal nerve

External pudendal vessels

Prepuce of clitoris

Glans of clitoris

**Perineal branch of posterior
cutaneous nerve of thigh**

LEFT

Labium majus (*cut surface*)

Posterior labial vessels and nerve

Superficial perineal vessels

Inferior anal (rectal) vessels

Ischioanal fossa

A. Lithotomy Position

5.49 **Female Perineum (I)**

A. Superficial dissection.
On the right side of the specimen:
- A long digital process of fat lies deep to the fatty subcutaneous tissue and descends into the labium majus.
- The round ligament of the uterus ends as a branching band of fascia that spreads out superficial to the fatty digital process.

On the left side of the specimen:
- Most of the fatty digital process is removed.
- The mons pubis is the rounded fatty prominence anterior to the pubic symphysis and bodies of the pubic bones.
- The posterior labial vessels and nerves (S2, S3) are joined by the perineal branch of the posterior cutaneous nerve of thigh (S1, S2, S3) and run anterior to the mons pubis. At the mons pubis, the vessels anastomose with the external pudendal vessels, and the nerves overlap in supply with the ilioinguinal nerve (L1).

B. Cutaneous zones of innervation.

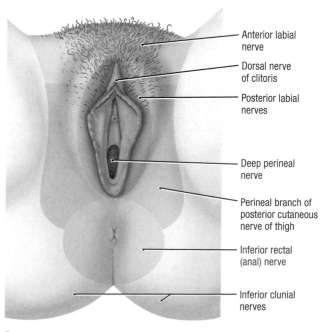

Anterior labial
nerve

Dorsal nerve
of clitoris

Posterior labial
nerves

Deep perineal
nerve

Perineal branch of
posterior cutaneous
nerve of thigh

Inferior rectal
(anal) nerve

Inferior clunial
nerves

B. Lithotomy Position

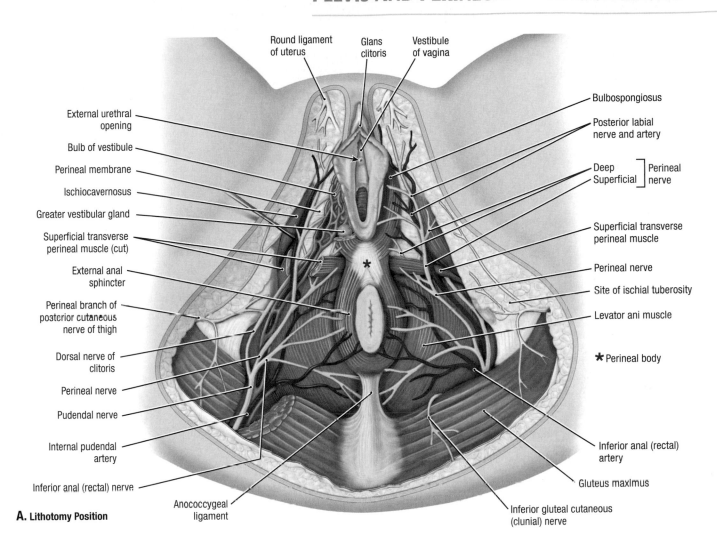

Round ligament of uterus

Glans clitoris

Vestibule of vagina

External urethral opening

Bulb of vestibule

Perineal membrane

Ischiocavernosus

Greater vestibular gland

Superficial transverse perineal muscle (cut)

External anal sphincter

Perineal branch of posterior cutaneous nerve of thigh

Dorsal nerve of clitoris

Perineal nerve

Pudendal nerve

Internal pudendal artery

Inferior anal (rectal) nerve

Bulbospongiosus

Posterior labial nerve and artery

Deep / Superficial } Perineal nerve

Superficial transverse perineal muscle

Perineal nerve

Site of ischial tuberosity

Levator ani muscle

★ Perineal body

Inferior anal (rectal) artery

Gluteus maximus

Anococcygeal ligament

Inferior gluteal cutaneous (clunial) nerve

A. Lithotomy Position

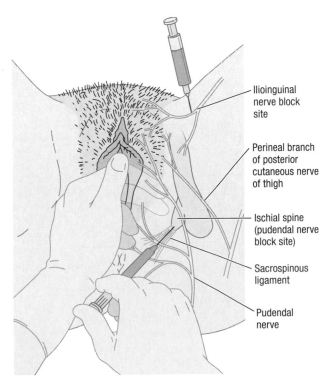

Ilioinguinal nerve block site

Perineal branch of posterior cutaneous nerve of thigh

Ischial spine (pudendal nerve block site)

Sacrospinous ligament

Pudendal nerve

B. Inferior View (Lithotomy Position)

Female Perineum (II)   5.50

A. Dissection of perineal nerves. The anterior aspect of the perineum is supplied by anterior labial nerves, derived from the ilioinguinal nerve and genital branch of the genitofemoral nerve. The pudendal nerve is the main nerve of the perineum. Posterior labial nerves, derived from the superficial perineal nerve, supply most of the vulva. The deep perineal nerve supplies the orifice of the vagina and superficial perineal muscles, and the dorsal nerve of the clitoris supplies deep perineal muscles and sensations to the clitoris. The inferior anal (rectal) nerve, also from the pudendal nerve, innervates the external anal sphincter and the perianal skin. The lateral perineum is supplied by the perineal branch of the posterior cutaneous nerve of the thigh. **B. Pudendal nerve block anesthesia.** To relieve the pain experienced during childbirth, **pudendal nerve block anesthesia** may be performed by injecting a local anesthetic agent into the tissue surrounding the pudendal nerve, near the ischial spine. A pudendal nerve block does not abolish sensations from the anterior and lateral parts of the perineum. Therefore, **an anesthetic block of the ilioinguinal and/or perineal branch of the posterior cutaneous nerve of the thigh** may also need to be performed.

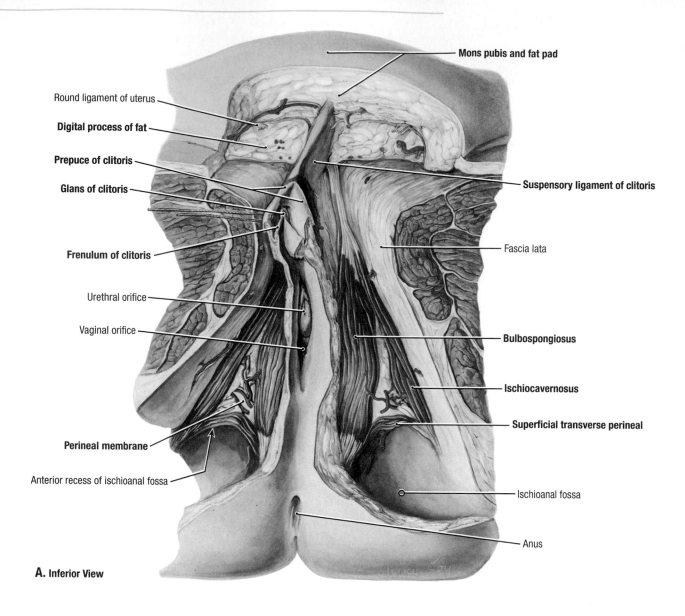

Round ligament of uterus

Digital process of fat

Prepuce of clitoris

Glans of clitoris

Frenulum of clitoris

Urethral orifice

Vaginal orifice

Perineal membrane

Anterior recess of ischioanal fossa

Mons pubis and fat pad

Suspensory ligament of clitoris

Fascia lata

Bulbospongiosus

Ischiocavernosus

Superficial transverse perineal

Ischioanal fossa

Anus

A. Inferior View

| **5.51** | **Female Perineum (III)** |

A. Dissection. **B.** Clitoris in context of vulva.

- Note the thickness of the subcutaneous fatty tissue of the mons pubis and the encapsulated digital process of fat deep to this. The suspensory ligament of the clitoris descends from the linea alba.
- Anteriorly, each labium minus forms two laminae or folds: The lateral laminae of the labia pass on each side of the glans clitoris and unite, forming a hood that partially or completely covers the glans, the prepuce (foreskin) of the clitoris. The medial laminae of the labia merge posterior to the glans, forming the frenulum of the clitoris.
- The bulbospongiosus muscle overlies the bulb of the vestibule and the great vestibular gland. In the male, the muscles of the two sides are united by a median raphe; in the female, the orifice of the vagina separates the right from the left.

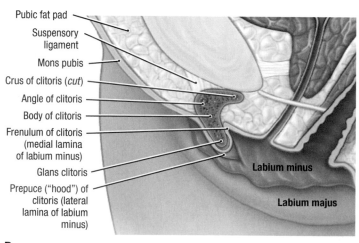

Pubic fat pad

Suspensory ligament

Mons pubis

Crus of clitoris (*cut*)

Angle of clitoris

Body of clitoris

Frenulum of clitoris (medial lamina of labium minus)

Glans clitoris

Prepuce ("hood") of clitoris (lateral lamina of labium minus)

Labium minus

Labium majus

B. Median Section

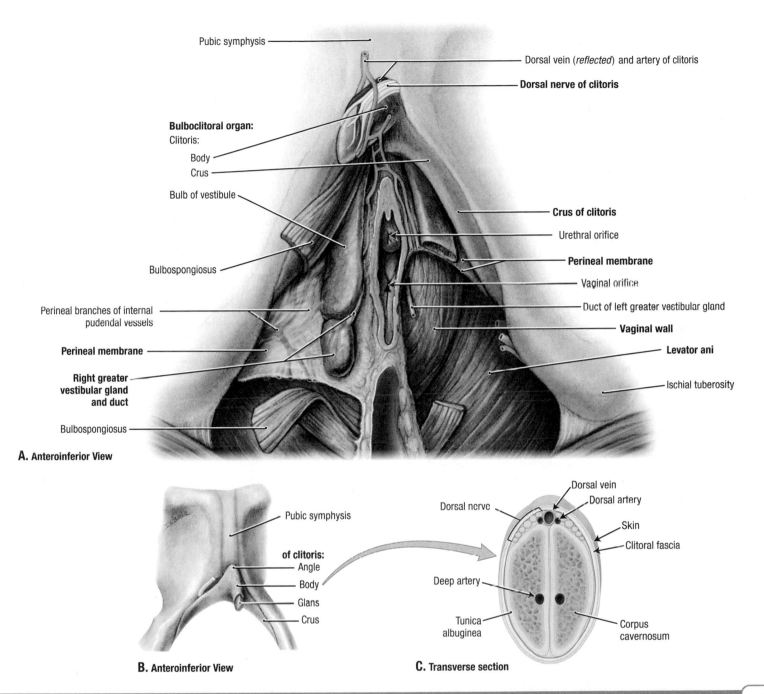

Pubic symphysis

Dorsal vein (*reflected*) and artery of clitoris

Dorsal nerve of clitoris

Bulboclitoral organ:
Clitoris:

Body

Crus

Bulb of vestibule

Crus of clitoris

Urethral orifice

Perineal membrane

Vaginal orifice

Bulbospongiosus

Perineal branches of internal
pudendal vessels

Duct of left greater vestibular gland

Vaginal wall

Perineal membrane

Levator ani

**Right greater
vestibular gland
and duct**

Ischial tuberosity

Bulbospongiosus

A. Anteroinferior View

Pubic symphysis

of clitoris:
Angle
Body
Glans
Crus

Dorsal vein
Dorsal artery
Dorsal nerve

Skin
Clitoral fascia

Deep artery

Tunica
albuginea

Corpus
cavernosum

B. Anteroinferior View

C. Transverse section

Female Perineum (IV)

5.52

A. Deeper dissection demonstrating bulboclitoral organ. **B.** Clitoris.
C. Transverse section of body of clitoris.
In *Part A*:
- The bulbospongiosus muscle is reflected on the right side and removed on the left side; the posterior portion of the bulb of the vestibule and the greater vestibular gland have been removed on the left side.
- The glans and body of the clitoris is displaced to the right so that the distribution of the dorsal vessels and nerve of the clitoris can be seen.
- Homologues of the bulb of the penis, the bulbs of the vestibule exist as two masses of elongated erectile tissue that lie along the sides of the vaginal orifice; veins connect the bulbs of the vestibule to the glans of the clitoris.

- On the specimen's right side, the greater vestibular gland is situated at the posterior end of the bulb; both structures are covered by bulbospongiosus muscle.
- On the specimen's left side, the bulb, gland, and perineal membrane are cut away, thereby revealing the external aspect of the vaginal wall.
In *Part B*:
- The body of the clitoris, composed of two crura (corpora cavernosa), is capped by the glans.
In *Part C*:
- Note the ovoid shape of the corpora cavernosa and the large fasciculated dorsal nerve of the clitoris.

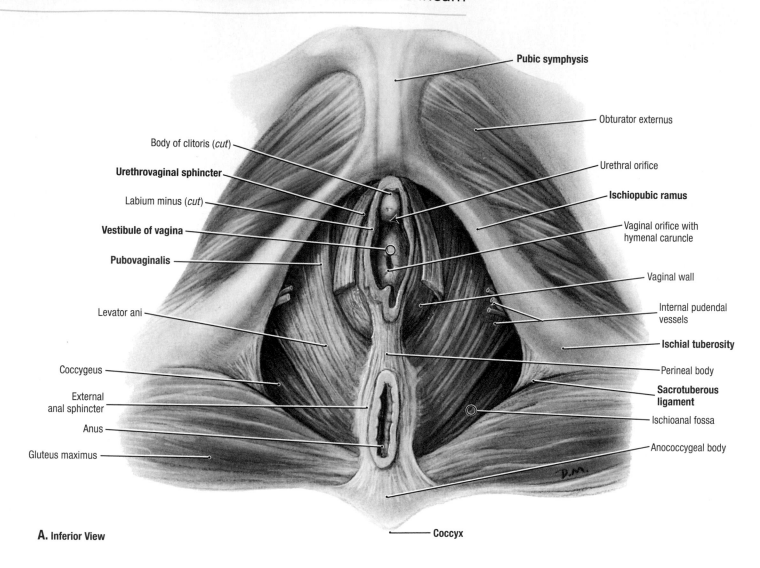

Pubic symphysis

Obturator externus

Body of clitoris (*cut*)

Urethral orifice

Urethrovaginal sphincter

Ischiopubic ramus

Labium minus (*cut*)

Vaginal orifice with hymenal caruncle

Vestibule of vagina

Pubovaginalis

Vaginal wall

Levator ani

Internal pudendal vessels

Ischial tuberosity

Coccygeus

Perineal body

External anal sphincter

Sacrotuberous ligament

Anus

Ischioanal fossa

Gluteus maximus

Anococcygeal body

A. Inferior View

Coccyx

5.53 Female Perineum (V)

A. Deep perineal compartment. The perineal membrane and smooth muscle corresponding in position to the deep transverse perineal muscle in the male have been removed.

- The most anterior and medial part of the levator ani muscle, the pubovaginalis, passes posterior to the vaginal orifice.
- The urethrovaginal sphincter, part of the external urethral sphincter of the female, rests on the urethra and straddles the vagina.
- The labia minora (cut short here) bound the vestibule of the vagina.

B. Urogenital and anal triangles. The osseoligamentous boundaries of the diamond-shaped perineum are the pubic symphysis, ischiopubic rami, ischial tuberosities, sacrotuberous ligaments, and coccyx. For descriptive purposes, a transverse line connecting the ischial tuberosities subdivides the diamond into urogenital and anal triangles.

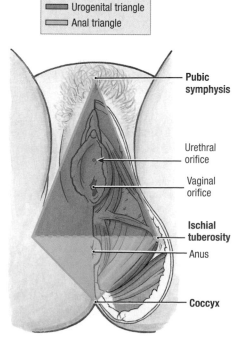

Urogenital triangle
Anal triangle

Pubic symphysis

Urethral orifice

Vaginal orifice

Ischial tuberosity

Anus

Coccyx

B. Lithotomy Position

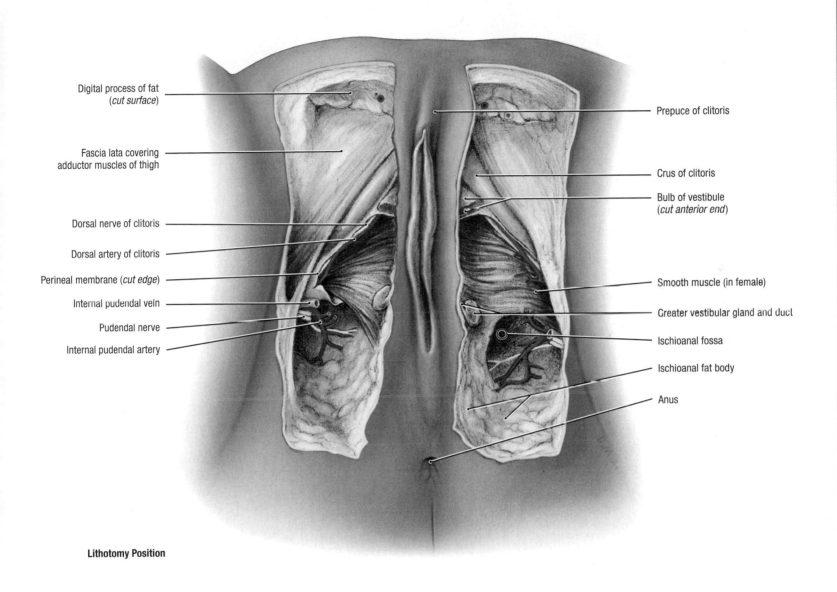

Digital process of fat
(*cut surface*)

Fascia lata covering
adductor muscles of thigh

Dorsal nerve of clitoris

Dorsal artery of clitoris

Perineal membrane (*cut edge*)

Internal pudendal vein

Pudendal nerve

Internal pudendal artery

Prepuce of clitoris

Crus of clitoris

Bulb of vestibule
(*cut anterior end*)

Smooth muscle (in female)

Greater vestibular gland and duct

Ischioanal fossa

Ischioanal fat body

Anus

Lithotomy Position

Female Perineum (VI)

5.54

This is a different dissection than the previous series, with the vulva undissected centrally but the perineum dissected deeply on each side. Although most of the perineal membrane and bulbs of the vestibule have been removed, the greater vestibular glands (structures of the superficial perineal compartment) have been left in place. The development and extent of the smooth muscle layer corresponding in position to the voluntary deep transverse perineal muscles of the male are highly variable, being relatively extensive in this case, blending centrally with voluntary fibers of the external urethral sphincter and the perineal body.

The greater vestibular glands are usually not palpable but are so when infected. Occlusion of the vestibular gland duct can predispose the individual to **infection of the vestibular gland**. The gland is the site or origin of most **vulvar adenocarcinomas** (cancers). **Bartholinitis**, inflammation of the greater vestibular (Bartholin) glands, may result from a number of pathogenic organisms. Infected glands may enlarge to a diameter of 4 to 5 cm and impinge on the wall of the rectum. Occlusion of the vestibular gland duct without infection can result in the accumulation of mucin (**Bartholin cyst**).

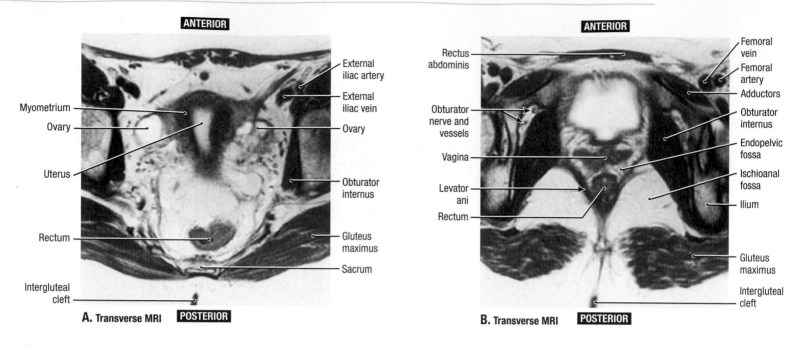

ANTERIOR

Myometrium

Ovary

Uterus

Rectum

Intergluteal cleft

External iliac artery

External iliac vein

Ovary

Obturator internus

Gluteus maximus

Sacrum

A. Transverse MRI **POSTERIOR**

ANTERIOR

Rectus abdominis

Obturator nerve and vessels

Vagina

Levator ani

Rectum

Femoral vein

Femoral artery

Adductors

Obturator internus

Endopelvic fossa

Ischioanal fossa

Ilium

Gluteus maximus

Intergluteal cleft

B. Transverse MRI **POSTERIOR**

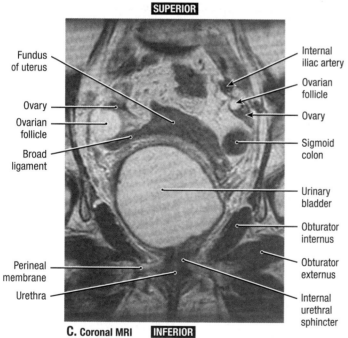

SUPERIOR

Fundus of uterus

Ovary

Ovarian follicle

Broad ligament

Perineal membrane

Urethra

Internal iliac artery

Ovarian follicle

Ovary

Sigmoid colon

Urinary bladder

Obturator internus

Obturator externus

Internal urethral sphincter

C. Coronal MRI **INFERIOR**

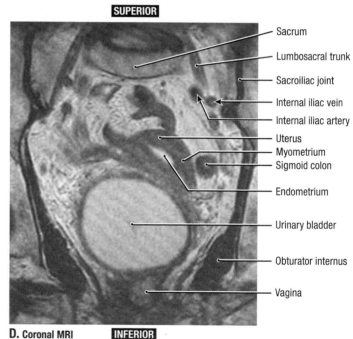

SUPERIOR

Sacrum

Lumbosacral trunk

Sacroiliac joint

Internal iliac vein

Internal iliac artery

Uterus

Myometrium

Sigmoid colon

Endometrium

Urinary bladder

Obturator internus

Vagina

D. Coronal MRI **INFERIOR**

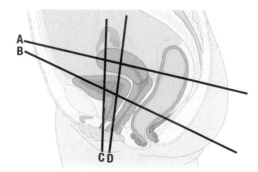

A

B

C D

5.55 **Imaging of Female Pelvis and Perineum**

A. and **B.** Transverse (axial) MRIs of female pelvis. **C.** and **D.** Coronal MRIs. **E–H.** Transverse anatomical sections and corresponding MRIs of female perineum.

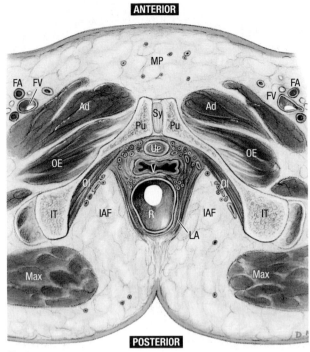

E. Transverse Section

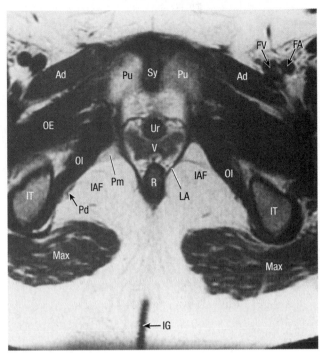

F. Transverse MRI

AC	Anal canal	**LA**	Levator ani	**PR**	Puborectalis
Ad	Adductor muscles	**LM**	Labium majus	**Pu**	Pubic bone
CC	Crus of clitoris	**Max**	Gluteus maximus	**QF**	Quadratus femoris
FA	Femoral artery	**MP**	Mons pubis	**R**	Rectum
FV	Femoral vein	**OE**	Obturator externus	**Sy**	Pubic symphysis
IAF	Ischioanal fossa	**OI**	Obturator internus	**Ur**	Urethra
IG	Intergluteal cleft	**Pd**	Pudendal canal	**V**	Vagina
IPR	Ischiopubic ramus	**Pec**	Pectineus	**Ve**	Vestibule of the vagina
IT	Ischial tuberosity	**Pm**	Perineal membrane		

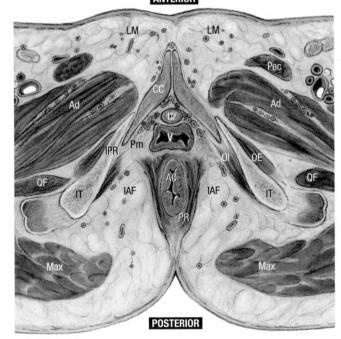

G. Transverse Section

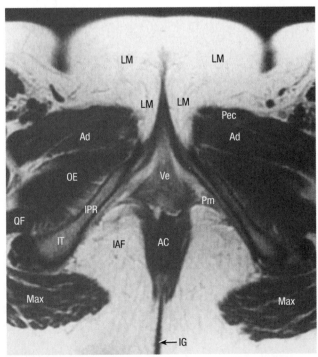

H. Transverse MRI

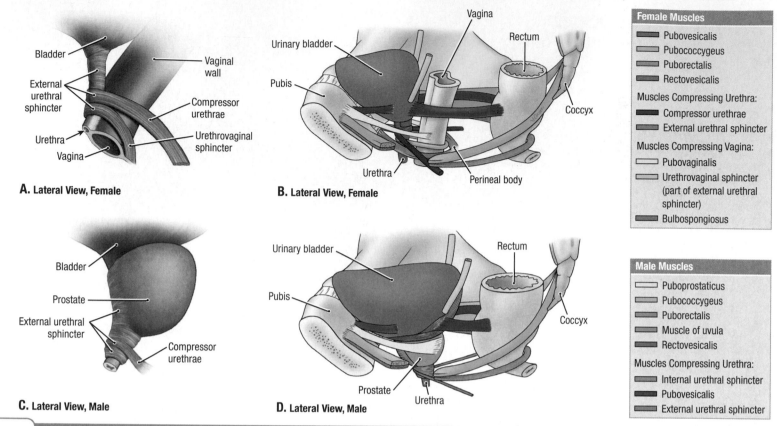

A. Lateral View, Female

Bladder
External urethral sphincter
Urethra
Vagina
Vaginal wall
Compressor urethrae
Urethrovaginal sphincter

B. Lateral View, Female

Urinary bladder
Pubis
Vagina
Rectum
Coccyx
Urethra
Perineal body

C. Lateral View, Male

Bladder
Prostate
External urethral sphincter
Compressor urethrae

D. Lateral View, Male

Urinary bladder
Pubis
Rectum
Coccyx
Prostate
Urethra

Female Muscles
- Pubovesicalis
- Pubococcygeus
- Puborectalis
- Rectovesicalis

Muscles Compressing Urethra:
- Compressor urethrae
- External urethral sphincter

Muscles Compressing Vagina:
- Pubovaginalis
- Urethrovaginal sphincter (part of external urethral sphincter)
- Bulbospongiosus

Male Muscles
- Puboprostaticus
- Pubococcygeus
- Puborectalis
- Muscle of uvula
- Rectovesicalis

Muscles Compressing Urethra:
- Internal urethral sphincter
- Pubovesicalis
- External urethral sphincter

5.56 **Supporting and Compressor/Sphincteric Muscles of Pelvis**

A. Female. **B.** Female urethral sphincters. **C.** Male. **D.** Male urethral sphincters.

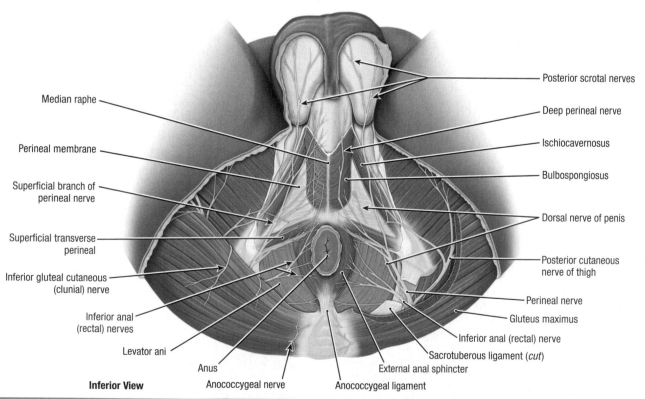

Median raphe
Perineal membrane
Superficial branch of perineal nerve
Superficial transverse perineal
Inferior gluteal cutaneous (clunial) nerve
Inferior anal (rectal) nerves
Levator ani
Anus
Anococcygeal nerve

Posterior scrotal nerves
Deep perineal nerve
Ischiocavernosus
Bulbospongiosus
Dorsal nerve of penis
Posterior cutaneous nerve of thigh
Perineal nerve
Gluteus maximus
Inferior anal (rectal) nerve
Sacrotuberous ligament (*cut*)
External anal sphincter
Anococcygeal ligament

Inferior View

5.57 **Dissection of Male Perineum (I)**

A. Superficial dissection.

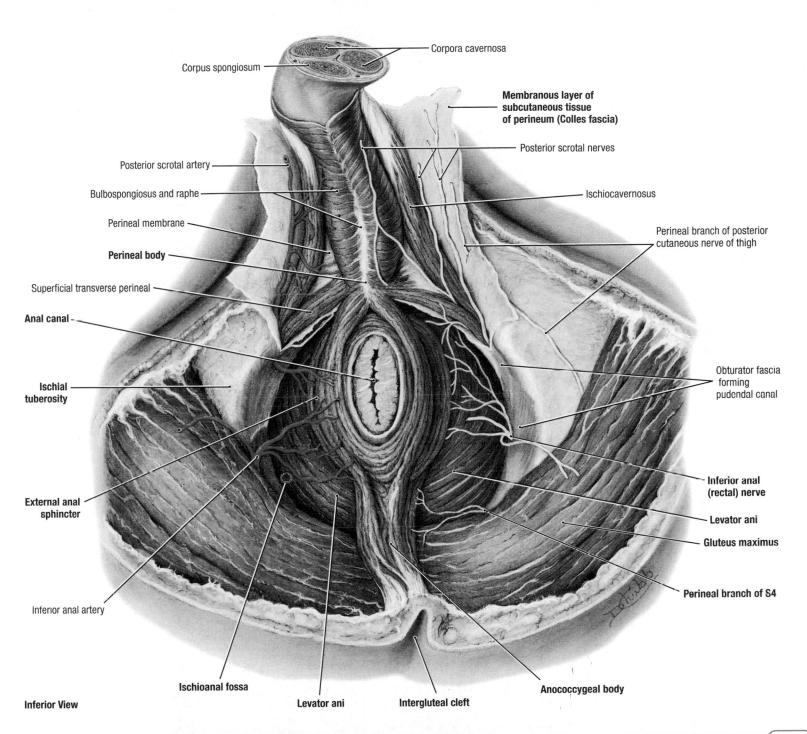

Corpora cavernosa

Corpus spongiosum

Membranous layer of subcutaneous tissue of perineum (Colles fascia)

Posterior scrotal nerves

Posterior scrotal artery

Bulbospongiosus and raphe

Ischiocavernosus

Perineal membrane

Perineal body

Perineal branch of posterior cutaneous nerve of thigh

Superficial transverse perineal

Anal canal

Ischial tuberosity

Obturator fascia forming pudendal canal

External anal sphincter

Inferior anal (rectal) nerve

Levator ani

Gluteus maximus

Inferior anal artery

Perineal branch of S4

Ischioanal fossa

Levator ani

Intergluteal cleft

Anococcygeal body

Inferior View

Dissection of Male Perineum (II)

5.58

B. Deeper dissection.
- The membranous layer of subcutaneous tissue of the perineum was incised and reflected, opening the subcutaneous perineal compartment (pouch) in which the cutaneous nerves course.
- The perineal membrane is exposed between the three paired muscles of the superficial compartment; although not evident here, the muscles are individually ensheathed with investing fascia.
- The anal canal is surrounded by the external anal sphincter. The superficial fibers of the sphincter anchor the anal canal anteriorly to the perineal body and posteriorly, via the anococcygeal body (ligament), to the coccyx and skin of the intergluteal cleft.

- Ischioanal (ischiorectal) fossae, from which fat bodies have been removed, lie on each side of the external anal sphincter. The fossae are also bound medially and superiorly by the levator ani, laterally by the ischial tuberosities and obturator internus fascia, and posteriorly by the gluteus maximus overlying the sacrotuberous ligaments. An anterior recess of each ischioanal fossa extends superior to the perineal membrane.
- In the lateral wall of the fossa, the inferior anal (rectal) nerve emerges from the pudendal canal and, with the perineal branch of S4, supplies the voluntary external anal sphincter and perianal skin; most cutaneous twigs have been removed.

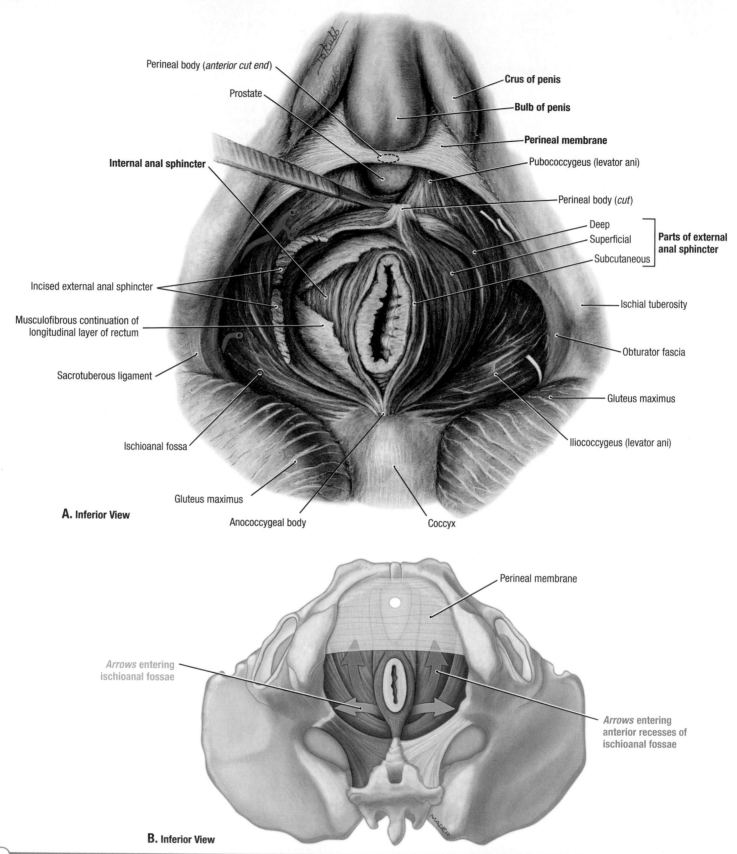

Perineal body (*anterior cut end*)

Prostate

Crus of penis

Bulb of penis

Perineal membrane

Internal anal sphincter

Pubococcygeus (levator ani)

Perineal body (*cut*)

Deep
Superficial   **Parts of external anal sphincter**
Subcutaneous

Incised external anal sphincter

Ischial tuberosity

Musculofibrous continuation of longitudinal layer of rectum

Obturator fascia

Sacrotuberous ligament

Gluteus maximus

Ischioanal fossa

Iliococcygeus (levator ani)

Gluteus maximus

Anococcygeal body

Coccyx

A. Inferior View

Perineal membrane

Arrows entering ischioanal fossae

Arrows entering anterior recesses of ischioanal fossae

B. Inferior View

5.59   Dissection of Male Perineum (III)

A. Parts of external anal sphincter. On the left side, the superficial and deep parts of the external anal sphincter were incised and reflected; the underlying musculofibrous continuation of the outer longitudinal layer of the muscular layer of the rectum is cut to reveal thickening of the inner circular layer that comprises the internal anal sphincter. **B. Relationships of ischioanal fossae.**

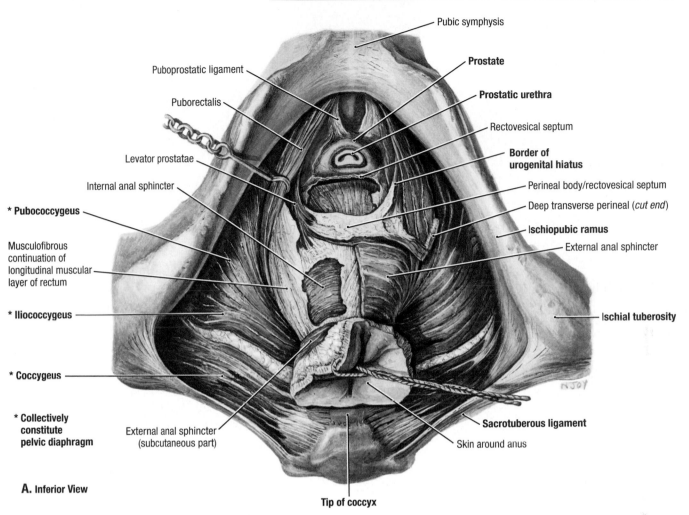

Pubic symphysis

Puboprostatic ligament

Puborectalis

Levator prostatae

Internal anal sphincter

* **Pubococcygeus**

Musculofibrous
continuation of
longitudinal muscular
layer of rectum

* **Iliococcygeus**

* **Coccygeus**

* **Collectively
constitute
pelvic diaphragm**

External anal sphincter
(subcutaneous part)

Prostate

Prostatic urethra

Rectovesical septum

**Border of
urogenital hiatus**

Perineal body/rectovesical septum

Deep transverse perineal (*cut end*)

Ischiopubic ramus

External anal sphincter

Ischial tuberosity

Sacrotuberous ligament

Skin around anus

Tip of coccyx

A. Inferior View

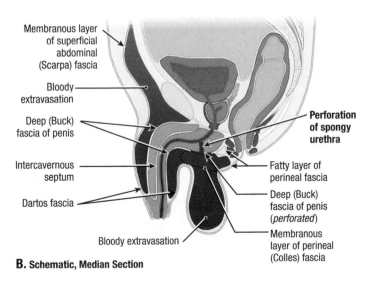

Membranous layer
of superficial
abdominal
(Scarpa) fascia

Bloody
extravasation

Deep (Buck)
fascia of penis

Intercavernous
septum

Dartos fascia

Bloody extravasation

**Perforation
of spongy
urethra**

Fatty layer of
perineal fascia

Deep (Buck)
fascia of penis
(*perforated*)

Membranous
layer of perineal
(Colles) fascia

B. Schematic, Median Section

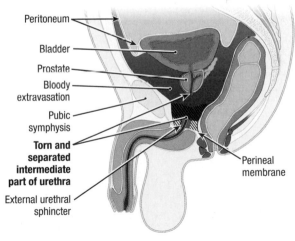

Peritoneum

Bladder

Prostate

Bloody
extravasation

Pubic
symphysis

**Torn and
separated
intermediate
part of urethra**

External urethral
sphincter

Perineal
membrane

C. Schematic, Median Section

Dissection of Male Perineum (IV)

5.60

**A. Parts of levator ani. B. Rupture of spongy urethra in bulb
of penis.** This results in extravasation (abnormal passage) of urine
into the subcutaneous perineal compartment. Attachments of the
membranous layer of subcutaneous tissue determine the direction
and restrictions of flow of the extravasated urine. Urine and blood
may pass deep to the continuations of the membranous layer in
the scrotum, penis, and inferior abdominal wall. Urine cannot pass
laterally and inferiorly into the thighs because the membranous
layer fuses with the fascia lata or posteriorly into the anal triangle
due to continuity with the perineal membrane and perineal body.
C. Rupture of intermediate part of urethra. This results in
extravasation of urine and blood into the deep perineal compartment. The fluid may pass superiorly through the urogenital hiatus
and distribute extraperitoneally around the prostate and bladder.

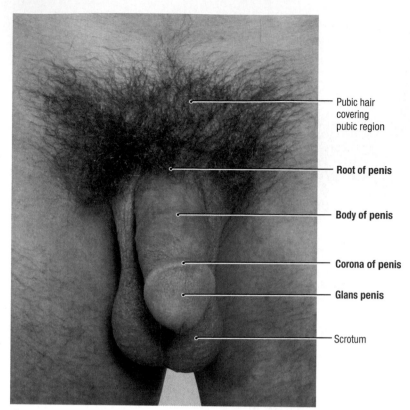

Pubic hair
covering
pubic region

Root of penis

Body of penis

Corona of penis

Glans penis

Scrotum

A. Anterior View

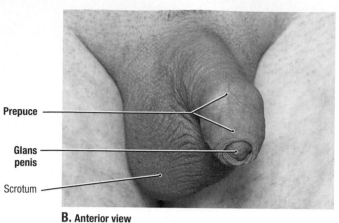

Prepuce

Glans penis

Scrotum

B. Anterior view

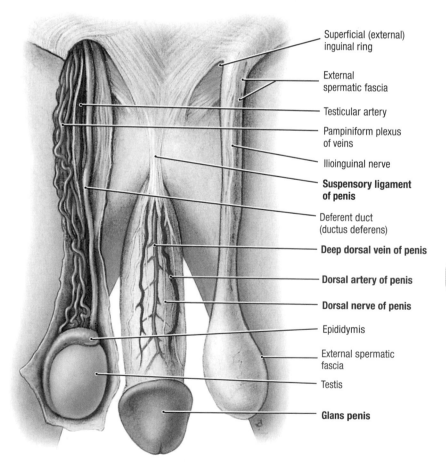

Superficial (external)
inguinal ring

External
spermatic fascia

Testicular artery

Pampiniform plexus
of veins

Ilioinguinal nerve

**Suspensory ligament
of penis**

Deferent duct
(ductus deferens)

Deep dorsal vein of penis

Dorsal artery of penis

Dorsal nerve of penis

Epididymis

External spermatic
fascia

Testis

Glans penis

C. Anterior View

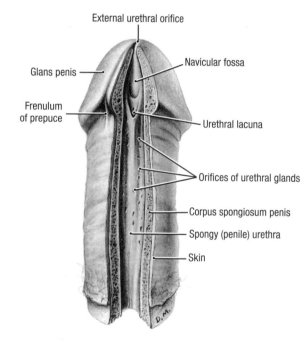

External urethral orifice

Navicular fossa

Glans penis

Frenulum
of prepuce

Urethral lacuna

Orifices of urethral glands

Corpus spongiosum penis

Spongy (penile) urethra

Skin

D. Urethral Aspect of Distal Penis

5.61   **Glans, Prepuce, and
Neurovascular Bundle of Penis**

**A. Surface anatomy, penis circumcised.
B. Uncircumcised penis. C. Vessels and
nerves of penis and contents of spermatic
cord.** The superficial and deep fasciae covering
the penis are removed to expose the midline
deep dorsal vein and the bilateral dorsal arteries
and nerves of the penis. **D. Spongy urethra,
interior.** A longitudinal incision was made on
the urethral surface of the penis and carried
through the floor of the urethra, allowing a
view of the dorsal surface of the interior of the
urethra.

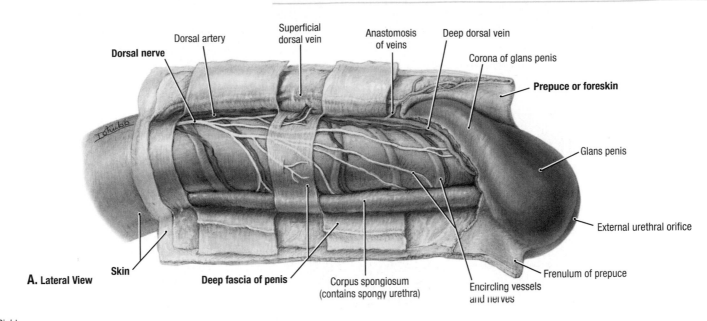

Dorsal artery
Superficial dorsal vein
Anastomosis of veins
Deep dorsal vein
Corona of glans penis
Dorsal nerve
Prepuce or foreskin
Glans penis
External urethral orifice
Frenulum of prepuce
Encircling vessels and nerves
Corpus spongiosum (contains spongy urethra)
Deep fascia of penis
Skin
A. Lateral View

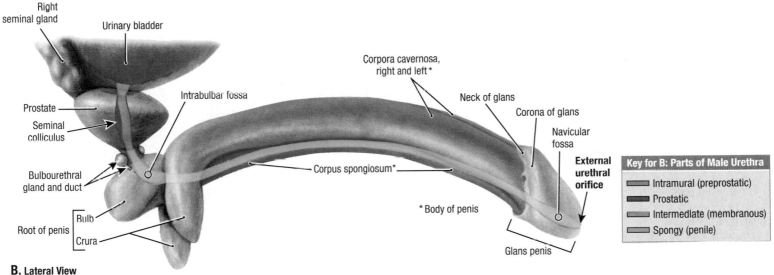

Right seminal gland
Urinary bladder
Corpora cavernosa, right and left *
Neck of glans
Corona of glans
Navicular fossa
Prostate
Intrabulbar fossa
Seminal colliculus
External urethral orifice
Bulbourethral gland and duct
Corpus spongiosum*
Bulb
Crura
Root of penis
* Body of penis
Glans penis

Key for B: Parts of Male Urethra	
	Intramural (preprostatic)
	Prostatic
	Intermediate (membranous)
	Spongy (penile)

B. Lateral View

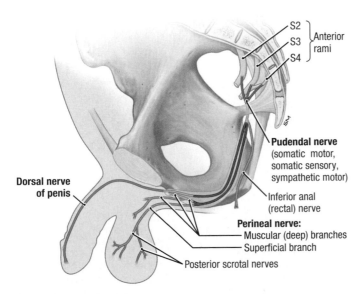

S2
S3
S4
Anterior rami

Dorsal nerve of penis

Pudendal nerve (somatic motor, somatic sensory, sympathetic motor)

Inferior anal (rectal) nerve

Perineal nerve:
Muscular (deep) branches
Superficial branch

Posterior scrotal nerves

C. Schematic, Medial View

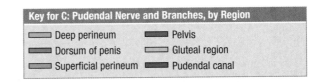

Key for C: Pudendal Nerve and Branches, by Region	
Deep perineum	Pelvis
Dorsum of penis	Gluteal region
Superficial perineum	Pudendal canal

Urethra, Layers, and Nerves of Penis 5.62

A. Dissection. The skin, subcutaneous tissue, and deep fascia of the penis and prepuce are reflected separately. **B. Parts of male urethra. C. Distribution of pudendal nerve, right hemipelvis.** Five regions transversed by the nerve are demonstrated.

An uncircumcised prepuce covers all or most of the glans penis. The prepuce is usually sufficiently elastic to allow retraction over the glans. In some males, it is tight and cannot be retracted easily (phimosis), if at all. Secretions (smegma) may accumulate in the preputial sac, located between the glans penis and prepuce, causing irritation. **Circumcision** exposes most, or all, of the glans.

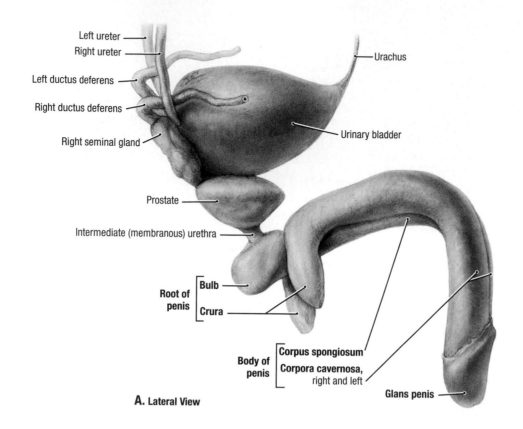

Left ureter
Right ureter
Left ductus deferens
Right ductus deferens
Right seminal gland
Prostate
Intermediate (membranous) urethra
Root of penis { **Bulb** / **Crura**
Body of penis { **Corpus spongiosum** / **Corpora cavernosa, right and left**

Urachus
Urinary bladder
Glans penis

A. Lateral View

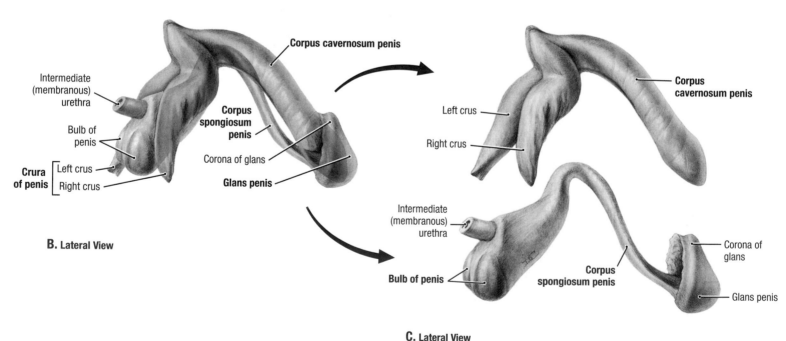

Corpus cavernosum penis

Intermediate (membranous) urethra
Bulb of penis
Crura of penis { **Left crus** / **Right crus**
Corpus spongiosum penis
Corona of glans
Glans penis

Corpus cavernosum penis
Left crus
Right crus

Intermediate (membranous) urethra
Bulb of penis
Corpus spongiosum penis
Corona of glans
Glans penis

B. Lateral View

C. Lateral View

5.63   Male Urogenital System, Erectile Bodies

A. Pelvic components of genital and urinary tracts and erectile bodies of perineum. **B.** Dissection of male erectile bodies (corpora cavernosa and corpus spongiosum). **C.** Corpus spongiosum and corpora cavernosa, separated. The erectile bodies are flexed where the penis is suspended by the suspensory ligament of the penis from the pubic symphysis. The corpus spongiosum extends posteriorly as the bulb of the penis and terminates anteriorly as the glans.

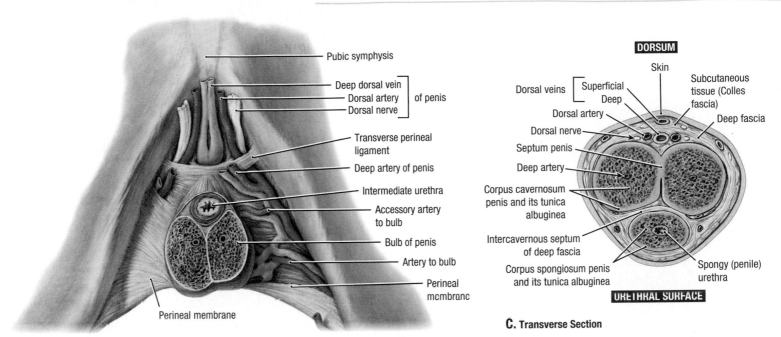

Pubic symphysis
Deep dorsal vein
Dorsal artery } of penis
Dorsal nerve
Transverse perineal ligament
Deep artery of penis
Intermediate urethra
Accessory artery to bulb
Bulb of penis
Artery to bulb
Perineal membrane
Perineal membrane

A. Anteroinferior View

DORSUM
Skin
Dorsal veins { Superficial / Deep
Subcutaneous tissue (Colles fascia)
Dorsal artery
Deep fascia
Dorsal nerve
Septum penis
Deep artery
Corpus cavernosum penis and its tunica albuginea
Intercavernous septum of deep fascia
Corpus spongiosum penis and its tunica albuginea
Spongy (penile) urethra
URETHRAL SURFACE

C. Transverse Section

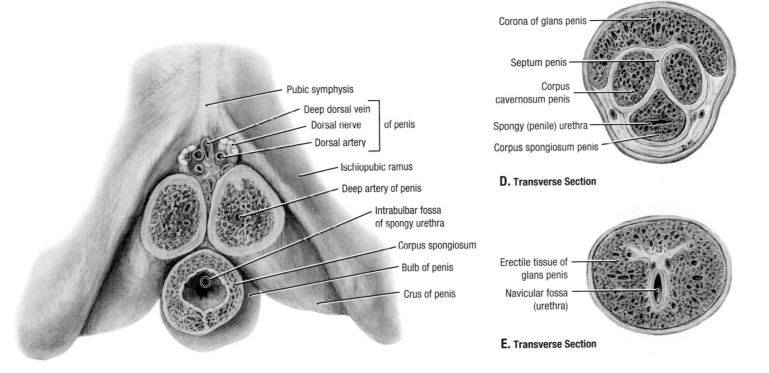

Pubic symphysis
Deep dorsal vein
Dorsal nerve } of penis
Dorsal artery
Ischiopubic ramus
Deep artery of penis
Intrabulbar fossa of spongy urethra
Corpus spongiosum
Bulb of penis
Crus of penis

B. Anteroinferior View

Corona of glans penis
Septum penis
Corpus cavernosum penis
Spongy (penile) urethra
Corpus spongiosum penis

D. Transverse Section

Erectile tissue of glans penis
Navicular fossa (urethra)

E. Transverse Section

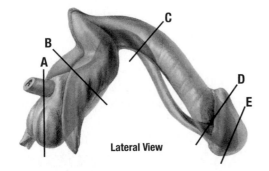

Lateral View

Cross Sections of Penis **5.64**

A. Transverse section through bulb of penis with crura removed. The bulb is cut posterior to the entry of the intermediate urethra. On the left side, the perineal membrane is partially removed, opening the deep perineal compartment. **B.** Crura and bulb of penis sectioned obliquely. The spongy urethra is dilated within the bulb of the penis. **C.** Transverse section through body of penis. **D.** Transverse section through proximal part of glans penis. **E.** Transverse section through distal part of glans penis.

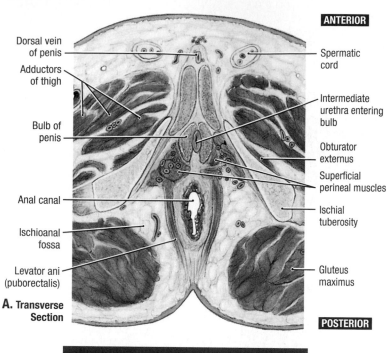

ANTERIOR

Dorsal vein of penis

Adductors of thigh

Bulb of penis

Anal canal

Ischioanal fossa

Levator ani (puborectalis)

Spermatic cord

Intermediate urethra entering bulb

Obturator externus

Superficial perineal muscles

Ischial tuberosity

Gluteus maximus

POSTERIOR

A. Transverse Section

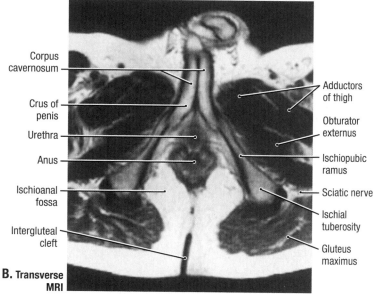

Corpus cavernosum

Crus of penis

Urethra

Anus

Ischioanal fossa

Intergluteal cleft

Adductors of thigh

Obturator externus

Ischiopubic ramus

Sciatic nerve

Ischial tuberosity

Gluteus maximus

B. Transverse MRI

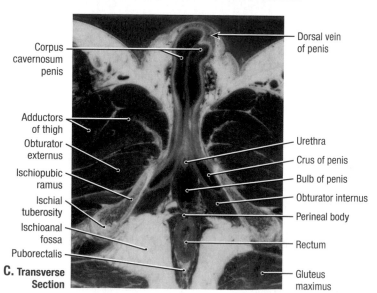

Corpus cavernosum penis

Adductors of thigh

Obturator externus

Ischiopubic ramus

Ischial tuberosity

Ischioanal fossa

Puborectalis

Dorsal vein of penis

Urethra

Crus of penis

Bulb of penis

Obturator internus

Perineal body

Rectum

Gluteus maximus

C. Transverse Section

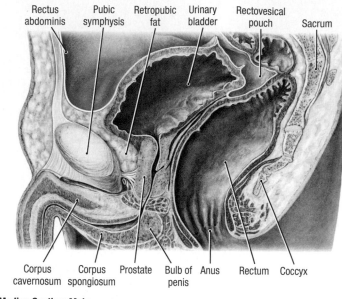

Rectus abdominis

Pubic symphysis

Retropubic fat

Urinary bladder

Rectovesical pouch

Sacrum

Corpus cavernosum

Corpus spongiosum

Prostate

Bulb of penis

Anus

Rectum

Coccyx

D. Median Section, Male

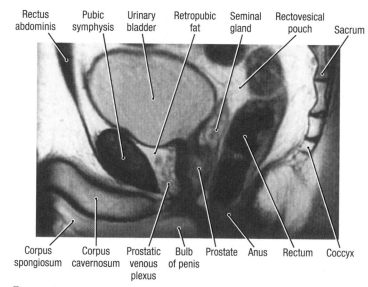

Rectus abdominis

Pubic symphysis

Urinary bladder

Retropubic fat

Seminal gland

Rectovesical pouch

Sacrum

Corpus spongiosum

Corpus cavernosum

Prostatic venous plexus

Bulb of penis

Prostate

Anus

Rectum

Coccyx

E. Median MRI, Prostate

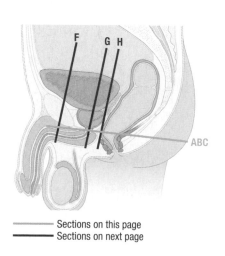

F   G   H

ABC

Sections on this page
Sections on next page

5.65   Imaging of Male Pelvis and Perineum

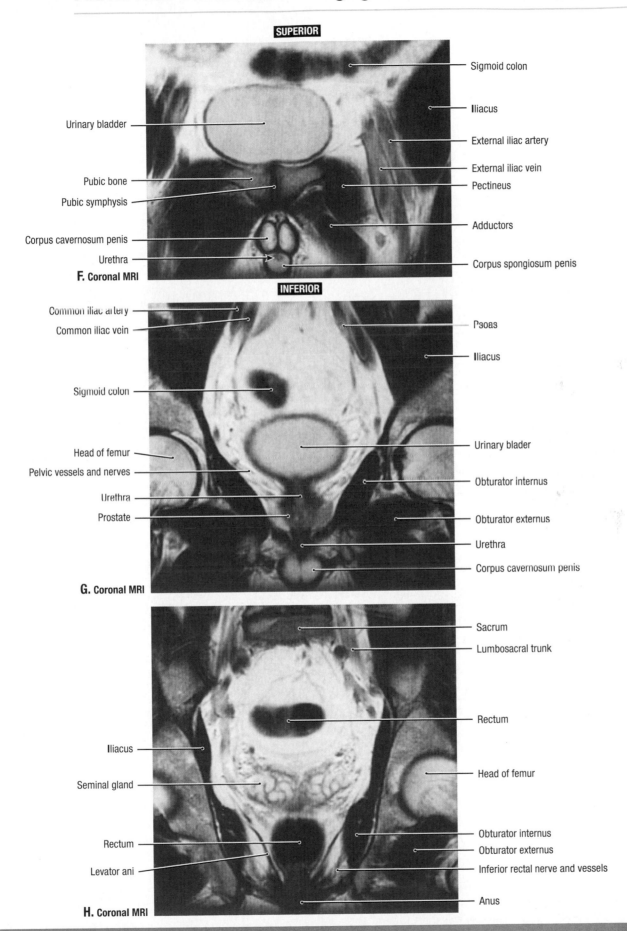

SUPERIOR

Urinary bladder

Pubic bone
Pubic symphysis

Corpus cavernosum penis
Urethra

F. Coronal MRI

Sigmoid colon

Iliacus

External iliac artery

External iliac vein
Pectineus

Adductors

Corpus spongiosum penis

INFERIOR

Common iliac artery
Common iliac vein

Sigmoid colon

Head of femur
Pelvic vessels and nerves

Urethra
Prostate

G. Coronal MRI

Psoas

Iliacus

Urinary blader

Obturator internus

Obturator externus

Urethra

Corpus cavernosum penis

Iliacus

Seminal gland

Rectum
Levator ani

H. Coronal MRI

Sacrum
Lumbosacral trunk

Rectum

Head of femur

Obturator internus
Obturator externus
Inferior rectal nerve and vessels

Anus

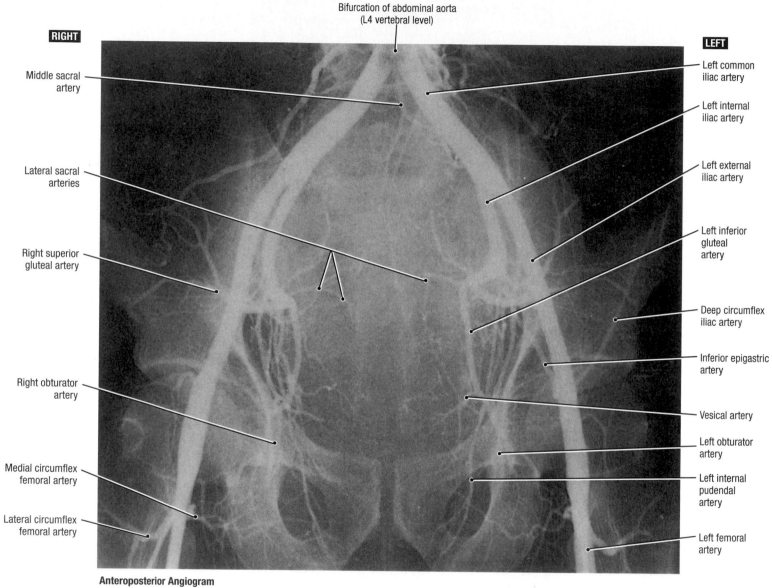

Bifurcation of abdominal aorta
(L4 vertebral level)

RIGHT

LEFT

Middle sacral
artery

Lateral sacral
arteries

Right superior
gluteal artery

Right obturator
artery

Medial circumflex
femoral artery

Lateral circumflex
femoral artery

Left common
iliac artery

Left internal
iliac artery

Left external
iliac artery

Left inferior
gluteal
artery

Deep circumflex
iliac artery

Inferior epigastric
artery

Vesical artery

Left obturator
artery

Left internal
pudendal
artery

Left femoral
artery

Anteroposterior Angiogram

5.66   Pelvic Angiography

Radiopaque dye released into the aorta of this male patient entered the branches of the external and internal iliac arteries at the time this radiograph was produced.

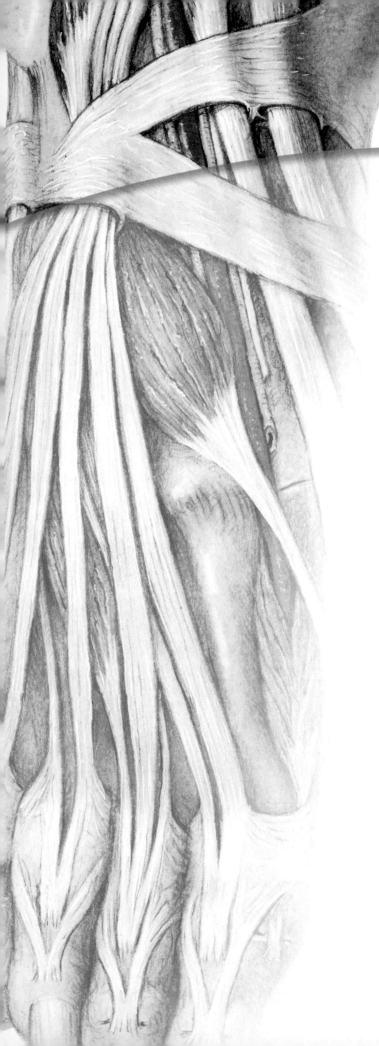

CHAPTER 6

LOWER LIMB

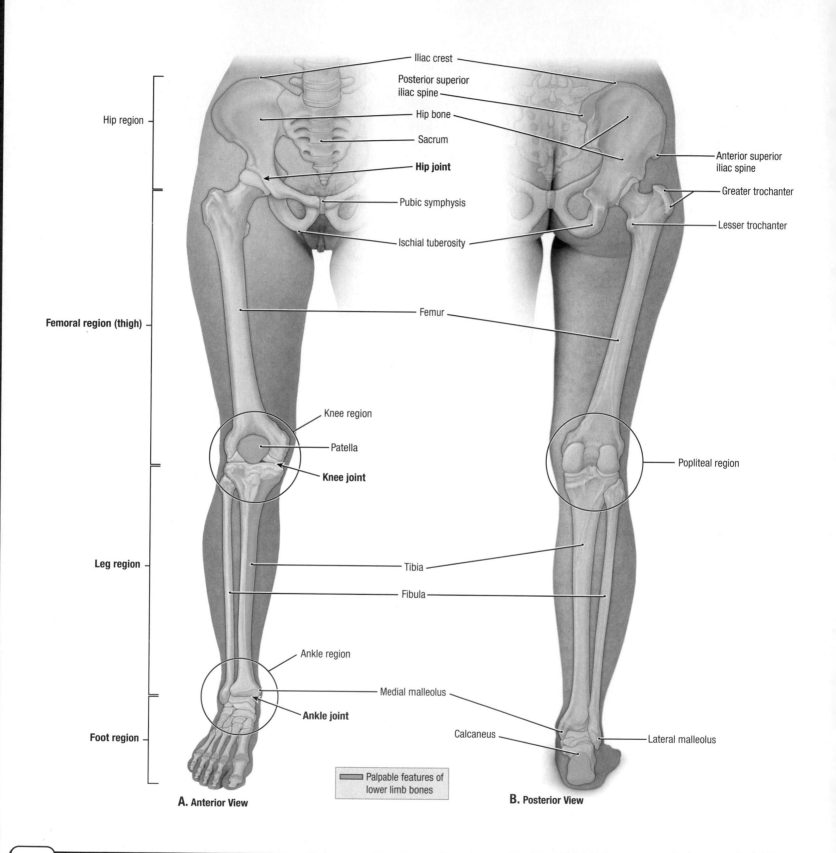

Iliac crest

Posterior superior iliac spine

Hip bone

Sacrum

Hip joint

Pubic symphysis

Ischial tuberosity

Anterior superior iliac spine

Greater trochanter

Lesser trochanter

Hip region

Femoral region (thigh)

Femur

Knee region

Patella

Knee joint

Popliteal region

Leg region

Tibia

Fibula

Ankle region

Medial malleolus

Ankle joint

Calcaneus

Lateral malleolus

Foot region

Palpable features of lower limb bones

A. Anterior View

B. Posterior View

6.1   **Regions, Bones, and Major Joints of Lower Limb**

The hip bones meet anteriorly at the pubic symphysis and articulate with the sacrum posteriorly. The femur articulates with the hip bone proximally and the tibia distally. The tibia and fibula are the bones of the leg that join the foot at the ankle.

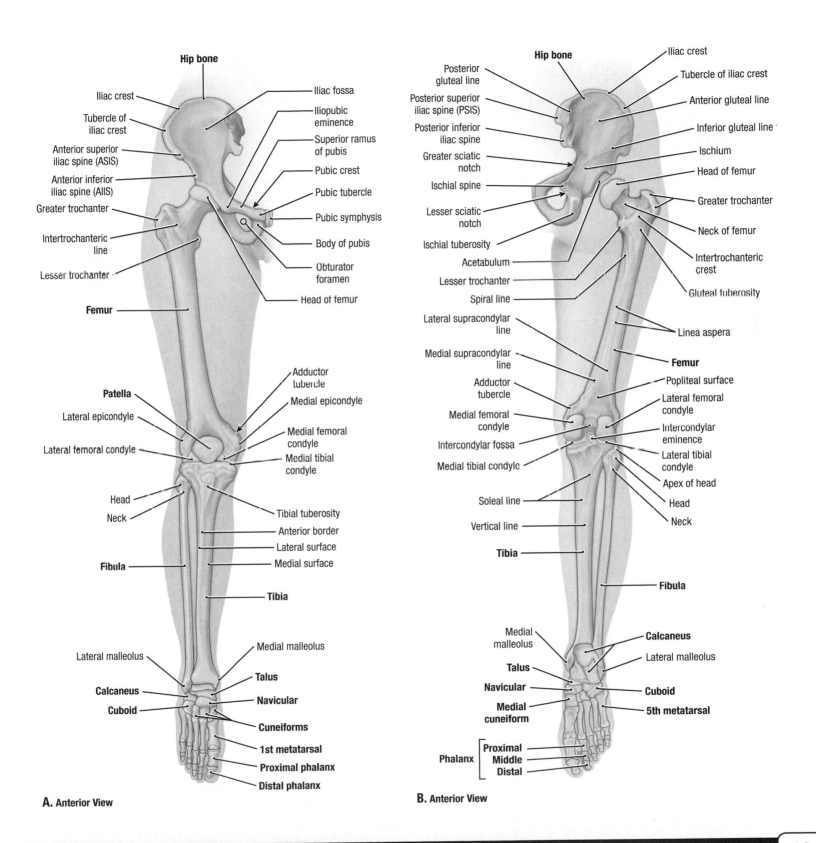

A. Anterior View

Hip bone
Iliac crest
Tubercle of iliac crest
Anterior superior iliac spine (ASIS)
Anterior inferior iliac spine (AIIS)
Greater trochanter
Intertrochanteric line
Lesser trochanter
Femur
Iliac fossa
Iliopubic eminence
Superior ramus of pubis
Pubic crest
Pubic tubercle
Pubic symphysis
Body of pubis
Obturator foramen
Head of femur
Patella
Lateral epicondyle
Lateral femoral condyle
Head
Neck
Fibula
Tibia
Adductor tubercle
Medial epicondyle
Medial femoral condyle
Medial tibial condyle
Tibial tuberosity
Anterior border
Lateral surface
Medial surface
Lateral malleolus
Calcaneus
Cuboid
Medial malleolus
Talus
Navicular
Cuneiforms
1st metatarsal
Proximal phalanx
Distal phalanx

B. Anterior View

Hip bone
Posterior gluteal line
Posterior superior iliac spine (PSIS)
Posterior inferior iliac spine
Greater sciatic notch
Ischial spine
Lesser sciatic notch
Ischial tuberosity
Acetabulum
Lesser trochanter
Spiral line
Lateral supracondylar line
Medial supracondylar line
Adductor tubercle
Medial femoral condyle
Intercondylar fossa
Medial tibial condyle
Soleal line
Vertical line
Tibia
Iliac crest
Tubercle of iliac crest
Anterior gluteal line
Inferior gluteal line
Ischium
Head of femur
Greater trochanter
Neck of femur
Intertrochanteric crest
Gluteal tuberosity
Linea aspera
Femur
Popliteal surface
Lateral femoral condyle
Intercondylar eminence
Lateral tibial condyle
Apex of head
Head
Neck
Fibula
Medial malleolus
Talus
Navicular
Medial cuneiform
Phalanx — Proximal, Middle, Distal
Calcaneus
Lateral malleolus
Cuboid
5th metatarsal

Features of Bones of Lower Limb

6.2

The foot is in full plantar flexion. The hip joint is disarticulated in *Part B* to demonstrate the acetabulum of the hip bone and the entire head of the femur. (See also regional treatments of bones and joints of thigh, leg, and foot in this chapter, and for hip bone, see Pelvic Girdle in Chapter 5.)

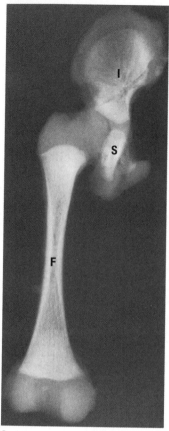

A. Anteroposterior Radiograph

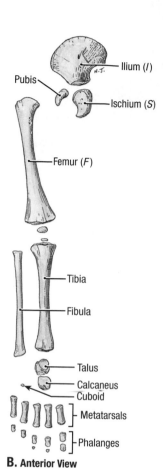

Ilium (*I*)
Pubis
Ischium (*S*)
Femur (*F*)
Tibia
Fibula
Talus
Calcaneus
Cuboid
Metatarsals
Phalanges

B. Anterior View

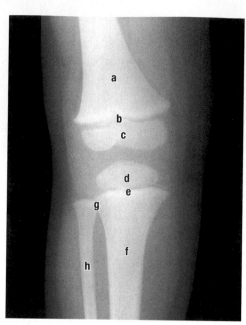

C. Anteroposterior Radiograph

Key for C		
Femur:	**Tibia:**	**Fibula:**
a Diaphysis	d Epiphysis	h Shaft
b Epiphyseal plate	e Epiphyseal plate	
c Epiphysis	f Shaft	
	g Proximal tibiofibular joint	

6.3   Postnatal Lower Limb Development

A. and **C. Normal postmortem specimens of newborns.** Bony (*white*) and cartilaginous (*gray*) components. **B. Ossified portions of bones of lower limb at birth.** The hip bone can be divided into three primary parts: ilium, ischium, and pubis. The diaphyses (bodies) of the long bones are well ossified. Some epiphyses (growth plates) and tarsal bones have begun to ossify. **D. Foot of child age 4.**

Dislocated epiphysis of femoral head. In older children and adolescents (10 to 17 years of age), the epiphysis of the femoral head may slip away from the femoral neck because of weakness of the epiphyseal plate. This injury may be caused by acute trauma or repetitive microtraumas that place increased shearing stress on the epiphysis, especially with abduction and lateral rotation.

Fractures involving epiphyseal plates. The primary ossification center for the superior end of the tibia appears shortly after birth and joins the shaft of the tibia during adolescence (usually 16 to 18 years of age). Tibial fractures in children are more serious if they involve the epiphyseal plates because continued normal growth of bone may be jeopardized. Disruption of the epiphyseal plate at the tibial tuberosity may cause inflammation of the tuberosity and chronic recurring pain during adolescence (Osgood-Schlatter disease), especially in young athletes.

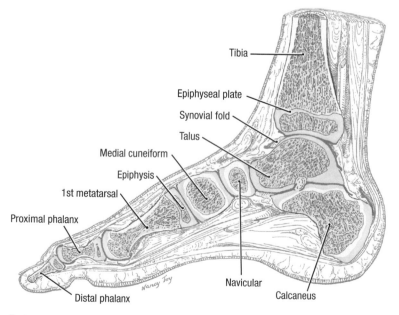

Tibia
Epiphyseal plate
Synovial fold
Talus
Medial cuneiform
Epiphysis
1st metatarsal
Proximal phalanx
Distal phalanx
Navicular
Calcaneus

D. Sagittal Section

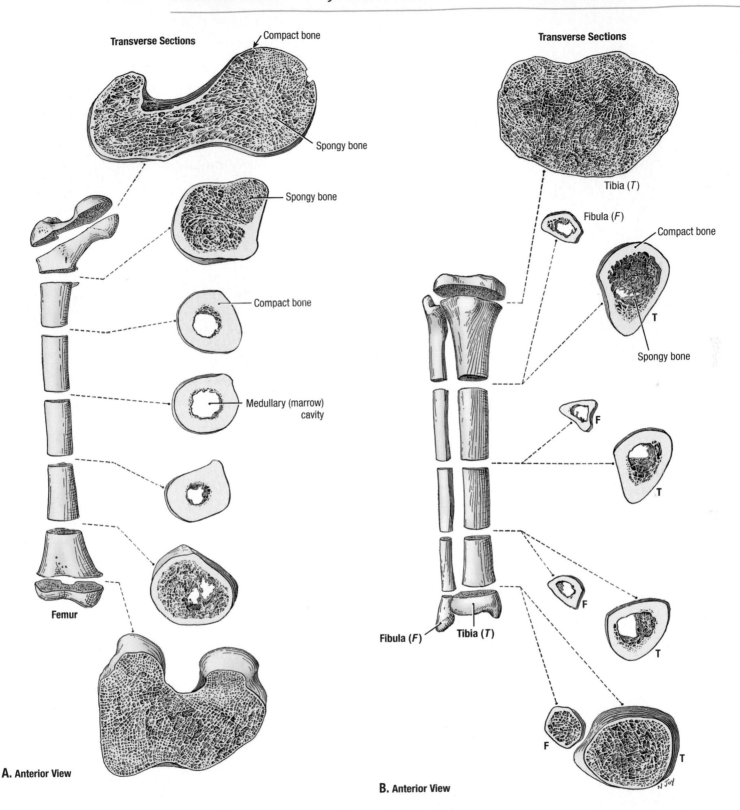

Transverse Sections

Compact bone

Spongy bone

Spongy bone

Compact bone

Medullary (marrow) cavity

Femur

A. Anterior View

Transverse Sections

Tibia (*T*)

Fibula (*F*)

Compact bone

Spongy bone

T

F

T

F

T

Fibula (*F*)   Tibia (*T*)

F   *T*

B. Anterior View

Transverse Sections through Femur, Tibia, and Fibula

6.4

A. Femur. B. Tibia and fibula. Note the differences in thickness of the compact and spongy bone and in the width of the medullary (marrow) cavity. Compact and spongy bones are distinguished by the relative amount of solid matter and by the number and size of the spaces they contain. All bones have a superficial thin layer of compact bone around a central mass of spongy bone, except where the latter is replaced by the medullary (marrow) cavity. Within the medullary cavity of adult bones and between the spicules (trabeculae) of spongy bone, yellow (fatty) or red (blood cell and platelet-forming) bone marrow or both are found. This is significant for MRIs where the compact bone is seen as a thin black line surrounding the whiter spongy bone with its abundant fatty marrow.

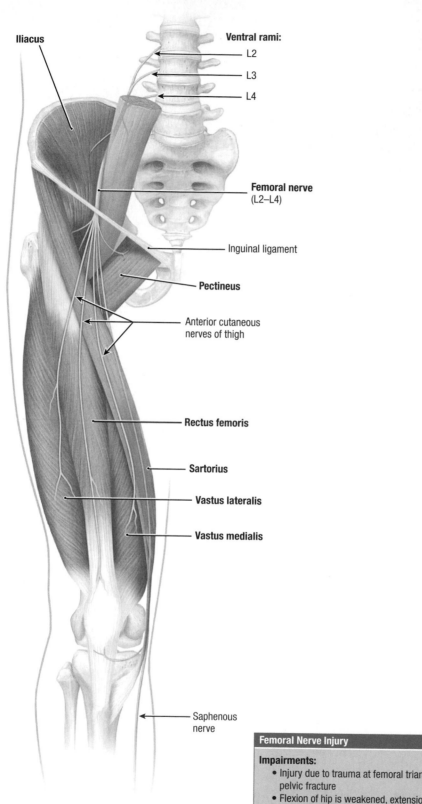

Iliacus

Ventral rami:
- L2
- L3
- L4

Femoral nerve
(L2–L4)

Inguinal ligament

Pectineus

Anterior cutaneous
nerves of thigh

Rectus femoris

Sartorius

Vastus lateralis

Vastus medialis

Saphenous
nerve

A. Anterior View

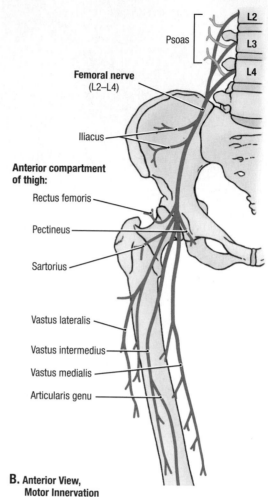

Psoas

Femoral nerve
(L2–L4)

L2
L3
L4

Iliacus

**Anterior compartment
of thigh:**

Rectus femoris

Pectineus

Sartorius

Vastus lateralis

Vastus intermedius

Vastus medialis

Articularis genu

B. Anterior View,
Motor Innervation

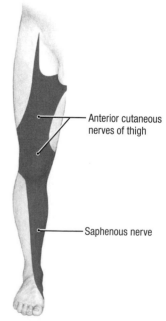

Anterior cutaneous
nerves of thigh

Saphenous nerve

C. Anterior View,
Cutaneous Innervation

Femoral Nerve Injury

Impairments:
- Injury due to trauma at femoral triangle; pelvic fracture
- Flexion of hip is weakened, extension of knee is lost, sensory loss on anterior thigh and medial leg, loss of knee joint reflex

6.5   **Overview of Innervation of Lower Limb: Femoral Nerve**

A. Overview. **B.** Motor innervation. **C.** Cutaneous innervation.

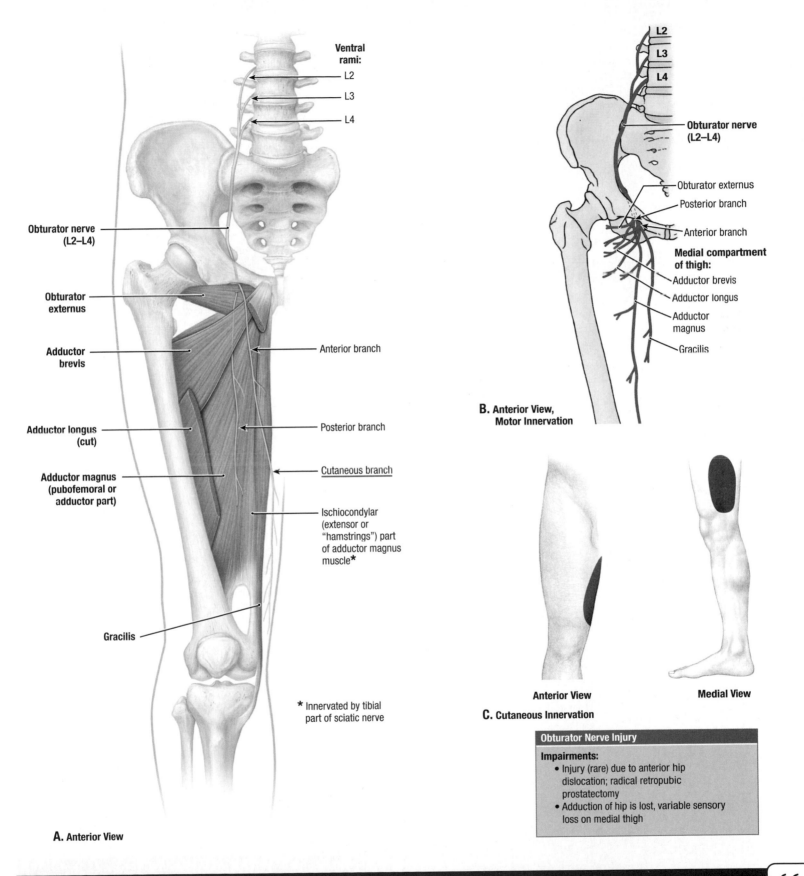

Ventral rami:
- L2
- L3
- L4

Obturator nerve (L2–L4)

Obturator externus

Adductor brevis

Adductor longus (cut)

Adductor magnus (pubofemoral or adductor part)

Anterior branch

Posterior branch

Cutaneous branch

Ischiocondylar (extensor or "hamstrings") part of adductor magnus muscle*

Gracilis

* Innervated by tibial part of sciatic nerve

A. Anterior View

L2
L3
L4

Obturator nerve (L2–L4)

Obturator externus
Posterior branch
Anterior branch

Medial compartment of thigh:
Adductor brevis
Adductor longus
Adductor magnus
Gracilis

B. Anterior View, Motor Innervation

Anterior View   Medial View

C. Cutaneous Innervation

Obturator Nerve Injury

Impairments:
- Injury (rare) due to anterior hip dislocation; radical retropubic prostatectomy
- Adduction of hip is lost, variable sensory loss on medial thigh

Overview of Innervation of Lower Limb: Obturator Nerve

6.6

A. Overview. **B.** Motor innervation. **C.** Cutaneous innervation.

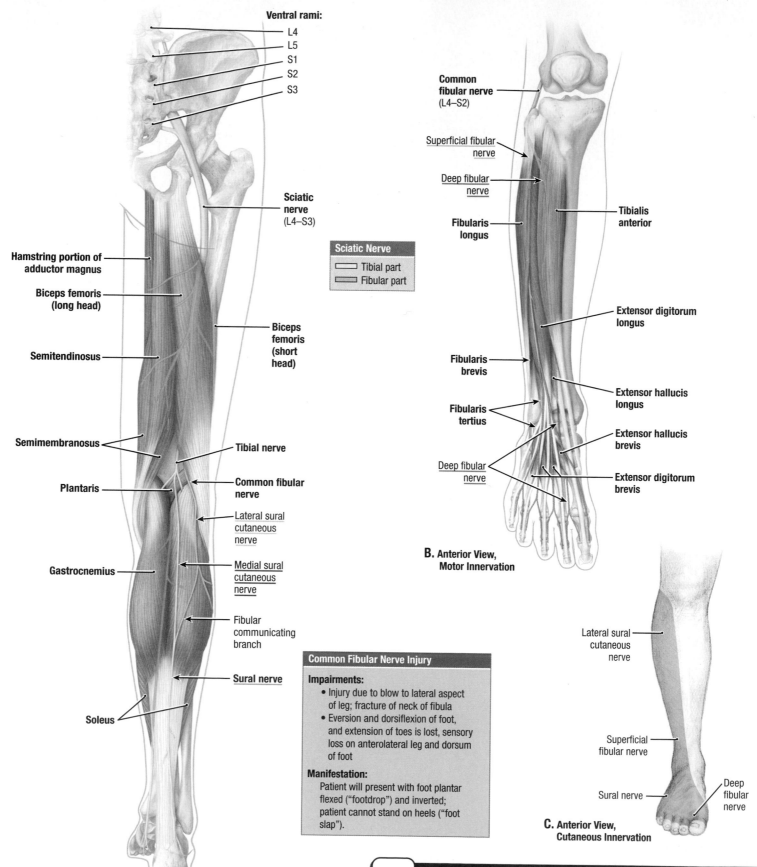

Ventral rami:
L4
L5
S1
S2
S3

Common fibular nerve (L4–S2)

Superficial fibular nerve

Deep fibular nerve

Sciatic nerve (L4–S3)

Tibialis anterior

Fibularis longus

Sciatic Nerve

| | Tibial part |
| | Fibular part |

Hamstring portion of adductor magnus

Biceps femoris (long head)

Semitendinosus

Biceps femoris (short head)

Extensor digitorum longus

Fibularis brevis

Extensor hallucis longus

Fibularis tertius

Extensor hallucis brevis

Semimembranosus

Tibial nerve

Plantaris

Common fibular nerve

Deep fibular nerve

Extensor digitorum brevis

Lateral sural cutaneous nerve

B. Anterior View, Motor Innervation

Gastrocnemius

Medial sural cutaneous nerve

Fibular communicating branch

Lateral sural cutaneous nerve

Sural nerve

Common Fibular Nerve Injury

Impairments:
- Injury due to blow to lateral aspect of leg; fracture of neck of fibula
- Eversion and dorsiflexion of foot, and extension of toes is lost, sensory loss on anterolateral leg and dorsum of foot

Manifestation:
Patient will present with foot plantar flexed ("footdrop") and inverted; patient cannot stand on heels ("foot slap").

Superficial fibular nerve

Soleus

Sural nerve

Deep fibular nerve

C. Anterior View, Cutaneous Innervation

A. Posterior View

6.7   **Overview of Innervation of Lower Limb: Sciatic and Common Fibular Nerves**

A. and **B.** Overview. **C.** Cutaneous innervation.

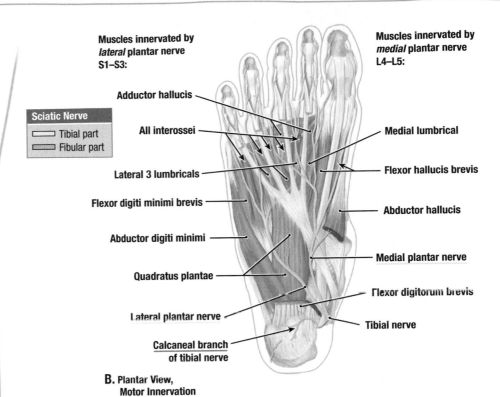

Muscles innervated by *lateral* plantar nerve S1–S3:

Muscles innervated by *medial* plantar nerve L4–L5:

Adductor hallucis

Sciatic Nerve
☐	Tibial part
☐	Fibular part

All interossei

Medial lumbrical

Lateral 3 lumbricals

Flexor hallucis brevis

Flexor digiti minimi brevis

Abductor hallucis

Abductor digiti minimi

Medial plantar nerve

Quadratus plantae

Flexor digitorum brevis

Lateral plantar nerve

Tibial nerve

Calcaneal branch of tibial nerve

B. Plantar View, Motor Innervation

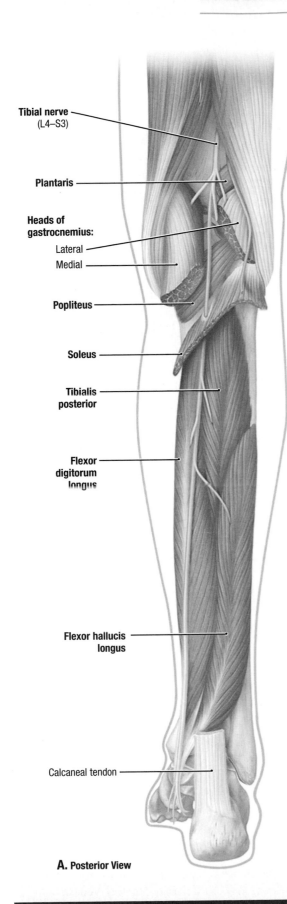

Tibial nerve (L4–S3)

Plantaris

Heads of gastrocnemius:
Lateral
Medial

Popliteus

Soleus

Tibialis posterior

Flexor digitorum longus

Flexor hallucis longus

Calcaneal tendon

A. Posterior View

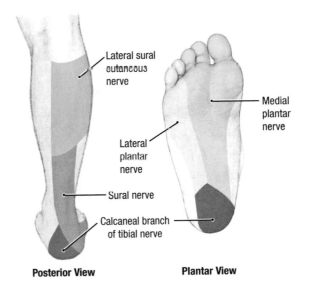

Lateral sural cutaneous nerve

Medial plantar nerve

Lateral plantar nerve

Sural nerve

Calcaneal branch of tibial nerve

Posterior View

Plantar View

C. Cutaneous Innervation

Tibial Nerve Injury in Popliteal Fossa

Impairments:
- Trauma at popliteal fossa
- Inversion of foot is weakened, plantarflexion of foot is lost, sensory loss on sole of foot

Manifestation:
Patient will present with foot dorsiflexed and everted; patient cannot stand on toes.

Overview of Innervation of Lower Limb: Sciatic and Tibial Nerves   **6.8**

A. and **B.** Overview of motor innervation. **C.** Cutaneous innervation.

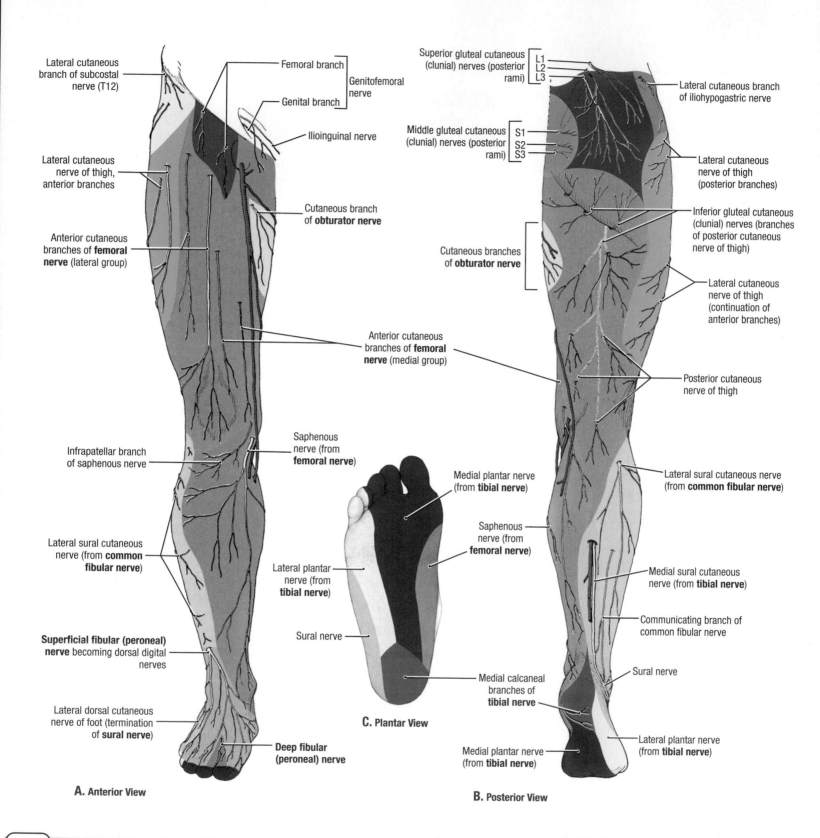

Lateral cutaneous branch of subcostal nerve (T12)

Femoral branch

Genitofemoral nerve

Genital branch

Ilioinguinal nerve

Lateral cutaneous nerve of thigh, anterior branches

Cutaneous branch of **obturator nerve**

Anterior cutaneous branches of **femoral nerve** (lateral group)

Anterior cutaneous branches of **femoral nerve** (medial group)

Infrapatellar branch of saphenous nerve

Saphenous nerve (from **femoral nerve**)

Lateral sural cutaneous nerve (from **common fibular nerve**)

Superficial fibular (peroneal) nerve becoming dorsal digital nerves

Lateral dorsal cutaneous nerve of foot (termination of **sural nerve**)

Deep fibular (peroneal) nerve

A. Anterior View

Superior gluteal cutaneous (clunial) nerves (posterior rami)   L1 L2 L3

Lateral cutaneous branch of iliohypogastric nerve

Middle gluteal cutaneous (clunial) nerves (posterior rami)   S1 S2 S3

Lateral cutaneous nerve of thigh (posterior branches)

Inferior gluteal cutaneous (clunial) nerves (branches of posterior cutaneous nerve of thigh)

Cutaneous branches of **obturator nerve**

Lateral cutaneous nerve of thigh (continuation of anterior branches)

Posterior cutaneous nerve of thigh

Lateral sural cutaneous nerve (from **common fibular nerve**)

Medial sural cutaneous nerve (from **tibial nerve**)

Communicating branch of common fibular nerve

Sural nerve

Lateral plantar nerve (from **tibial nerve**)

Medial plantar nerve (from **tibial nerve**)

Medial calcaneal branches of **tibial nerve**

B. Posterior View

Medial plantar nerve (from **tibial nerve**)

Lateral plantar nerve (from tibial nerve)

Sural nerve

Medial calcaneal branches of **tibial nerve**

C. Plantar View

6.9   **Cutaneous Nerves of Lower Limb**

Cutaneous nerves in the subcutaneous tissue supply the skin of the lower limb. In the posterior view, the medial sural cutaneous nerve (*sural* is Latin for calf) is joined between the popliteal fossa and posterior aspect of the ankle by a communicating branch of the lateral sural cutaneous nerve to form the sural nerve. The level of the junction is variable and is low in this specimen.

TABLE 6.1	**Cutaneous Nerves of Lower Limb**		
Nerve	**Origin (Contributing Spinal Nerves)**	**Course**	**Distribution to Skin of Lower Limb**
Subcostal (lateral cutaneous branch)	T12 anterior ramus	Descends over iliac crest	Hip region inferior to anterior part of iliac crest and anterior to greater trochanter
Iliohypogastric	Lumbar plexus (L1; occasionally T12)	Parallels iliac crest	Lateral cutaneous branch supplies superolateral quadrant of buttock
Ilioinguinal	Lumbar plexus (L1; occasionally T12)	Passes through inguinal canal	Inguinal fold; femoral branch supplies skin over medial femoral triangle
Genitofemoral	Lumbar plexus (L1–L2)	Descends anterior surface of psoas major	Femoral branch supplies skin over lateral part of femoral triangle; genital branch supplies anterior scrotum or labia majora
Lateral cutaneous nerve of thigh	Lumbar plexus (L2–L3)	Passes deep to inguinal ligament, ~1 cm medial to anterior superior iliac spine	Skin on anterior and lateral aspects of thigh
Anterior cutaneous branches	Lumbar plexus via femoral nerve (L2–L4)	Arise in femoral triangle; pierce fascia lata along the path of sartorius muscle	Skin of anterior and medial aspects of thigh
Cutaneous branch of obturator nerve	Lumbar plexus via obturator nerve (L2–L4)	Following its descent between adductors longus and brevis, obturator nerve pierces fascia lata to reach the skin of thigh	Variable area of skin of middle part of medial thigh
Posterior cutaneous nerve of thigh	Sacral plexus (S1–S3)	Enters gluteal region via greater sciatic foramen deep to gluteus maximus; then descends deep to fascia lata; terminal branches pierce fascia lata	Skin of posterior thigh and popliteal fossa
Saphenous nerve	Lumbar plexus via femoral nerve (L3–L4)	Traverses adductor canal but does not pass through adductor hiatus	Skin on medial side of leg and foot
Superficial fibular nerve	Common fibular nerve (L4–S1)	After supplying fibular muscles, perforates deep fascia of leg	Skin of anterolateral leg and dorsum of foot
Deep fibular nerve	Common fibular nerve (L5)	After supplying muscles on dorsum of foot, pierces deep fascia superior to heads of 1st and 2nd metatarsals	Skin of web between great and 2nd toes
Sural nerve	Tibial and common fibular nerves (S1–S2)	Medial sural cutaneous branch of tibial nerve and lateral sural cutaneous branch of common fibular nerve merge at varying levels on posterior leg	Skin of posterolateral leg and lateral margin of foot
Medial plantar nerve	Tibial nerve (L4–L5)	Passes between first and second layers of plantar muscles	Skin of medial side of sole, and plantar aspect, sides, and nail beds of medial 3½ toes
Lateral plantar nerve	Tibial nerve (S1–S2)	Passes between first and second layers of plantar muscles	Skin of lateral sole, and plantar aspect, sides, and nail beds of lateral 1½ toes
Calcaneal nerves	Tibial and sural nerves (S1–S2)	Branch over calcaneal tuberosity	Skin of heel
Superior gluteal cutaneous (clunial) nerves	L1–L3 posterior rami	Course laterally/inferiorly in subcutaneous tissue	Skin overlying superior and central parts of buttock
Middle gluteal cutaneous (clunial) nerves	S1–S3 posterior rami	From dorsal sacral foramina; enter overlying subcutaneous tissue	Skin of medial buttock and intergluteal cleft
Inferior gluteal cutaneous (clunial) nerves	Posterior cutaneous nerve of thigh (S2–S3)	Arise deep to gluteus maximus; emerge from beneath inferior border of muscle	Skin of inferior buttock (overlying gluteal fold)

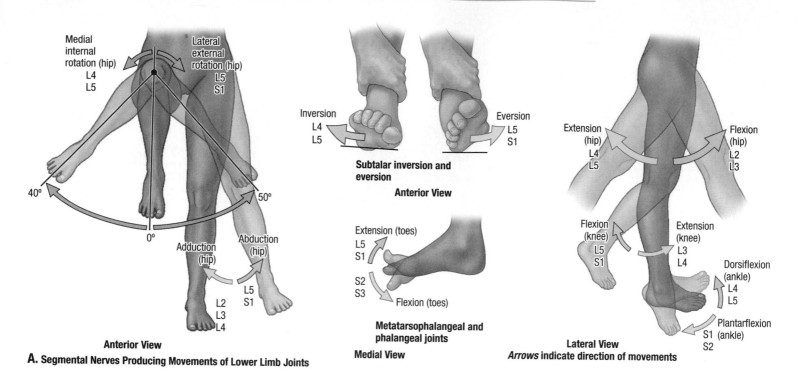

A. Segmental Nerves Producing Movements of Lower Limb Joints

Subtalar inversion and eversion
Anterior View

Metatarsophalangeal and phalangeal joints
Medial View

Lateral View
Arrows indicate direction of movements

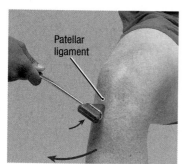

B. Quadriceps Reflex

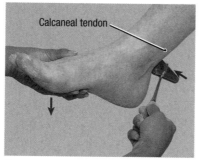

C. Calcaneal Tendon Reflex

Myotatic (Deep Tendon) Reflex	Spinal Cord Segments Tested
Quadriceps (knee jerk)	L3–L4
Calcaneal (Achilles; ankle jerk)	S1–S2

⟶ Direction of movement

6.10 Myotomes and Deep Tendon Reflexes

A. Myotomes. Somatic motor (general somatic efferent) fibers transmit impulses to skeletal (voluntary) muscles. The unilateral muscle mass receiving innervation from the somatic motor fibers conveyed by a single spinal nerve is a myotome. Each skeletal muscle is usually innervated by the somatic motor fibers of several spinal nerves; therefore, the muscle myotome will consist of several segments. The muscle myotomes have been grouped by joint movement to facilitate clinical testing. **B. Myotatic (deep tendon) reflexes.** A myotatic (stretch) reflex is an involuntary contraction of a muscle in response to being stretched. Deep tendon reflexes (e.g., "knee jerk") are monosynaptic stretch reflexes that are elicited by briskly tapping the tendon with a reflex hammer. Each tendon reflex is mediated by specific spinal nerves. Stretch reflexes control muscle tone (e.g., in antigravity, muscles that keep the body upright against gravity).

TABLE 6.2 Nerve Root (Anterior Ramus) Lesions

Compressed Nerve Root	Dermatome Affected	Muscles Affected	Weakened Movement/Deficit	Nerve and Reflex Involved
L4	L4: medial surface of leg; big toe	Quadriceps	Extension of knee	Femoral nerve Weak (decreased) knee jerk
L5	L5: lateral surface of leg; dorsum of foot	Tibialis anterior Extensor hallucis longus Extensor digitorum longus	Dorsiflexion of ankle (patient cannot stand on heels) Extension of toes	Common fibular nerve No reflex loss
S1	S1: posterior surface of lower limb; little toe	Gastrocnemius Soleus	Plantar flexion of ankle (patient cannot stand on toes) Flexion of toes	Tibial nerve Weak (decreased) ankle jerk

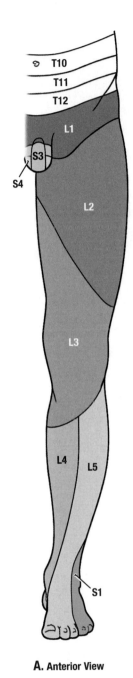

A. Anterior View

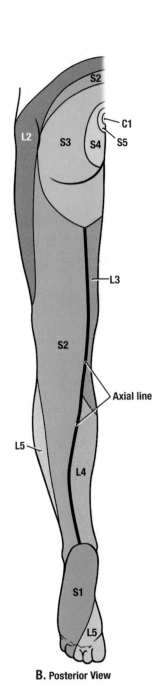

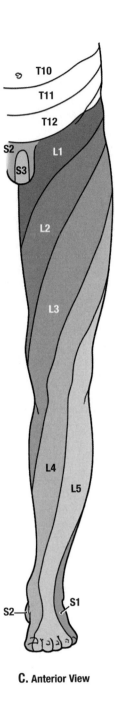

B. Posterior View

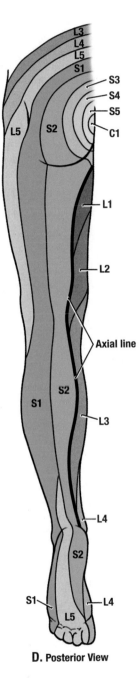

C. Anterior View

D. Posterior View

Dermatomes of Lower Limb

6.11

The dermatomal, or segmental, pattern of distribution of sensory nerve fibers persists despite the merging of spinal nerves in plexus formation during development. Two different dermatome maps are commonly used. **A.** and **B. Dermatome pattern of lower limb according to Foerster** (1933). The Foerster schema is preferred by many because of its correlation with clinical findings.

C. and **D. Dermatome pattern of lower limb according to Keegan and Garrett** (1948). This map is preferred by others for its aesthetic uniformity and obvious correlation with development. Although depicted as distinct zones, adjacent dermatomes overlap considerably, except along the axial line.

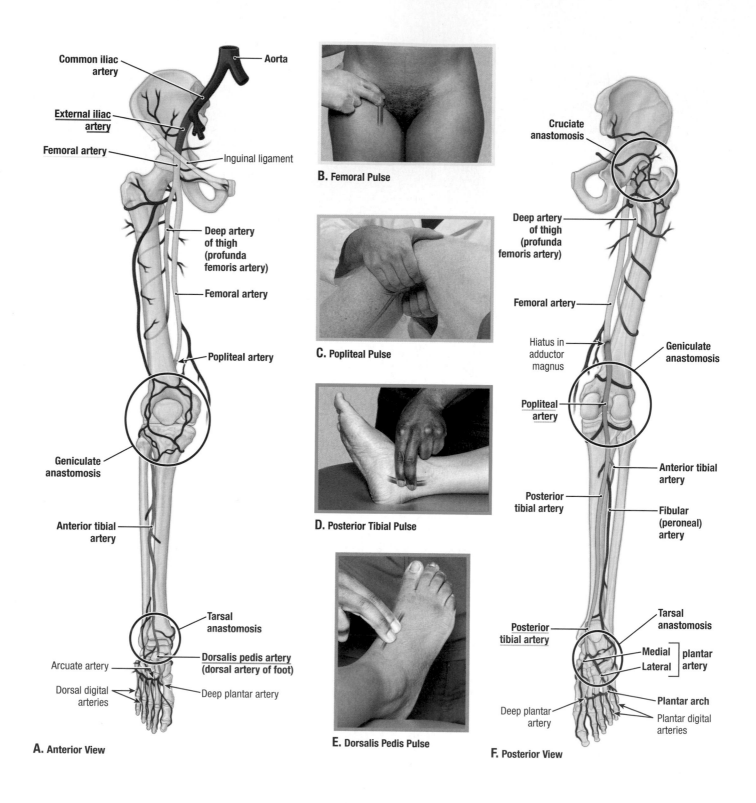

A. Anterior View

B. Femoral Pulse

C. Popliteal Pulse

D. Posterior Tibial Pulse

E. Dorsalis Pedis Pulse

F. Posterior View

6.12 **Arteries, Arterial Anastomoses, and Palpation Sites of Pulses of Lower Limb**

A. and **F.** Overview. **B–E.** Sites of palpation of pulses of upper limb. The arteries often anastomose or communicate to form networks to ensure blood supply distal to the joint throughout the range of movement (cruciate, geniculate, and tarsal anastomoses). If a main channel is slowly occluded, the smaller alternate channels can usually increase in size, providing a **collateral circulation** that ensures the blood supply to structures distal to the blockage.

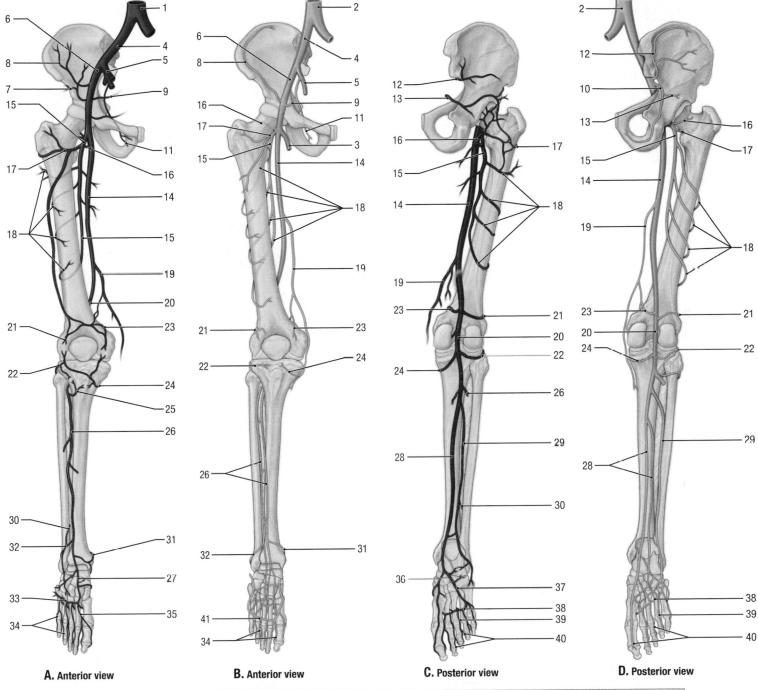

A. Anterior view   **B.** Anterior view   **C.** Posterior view   **D.** Posterior view

1	Aorta	**11**	Obturator	**21**	Superior lateral genicular	**31**	Medial malleolar
2	Inferior vena cava	**12**	Superior gluteal	**22**	Inferior lateral genicular	**32**	Lateral malleolar
3	Great saphenous vein	**13**	Inferior gluteal	**23**	Superior medial genicular	**33**	Arcuate artery
4	Common iliac	**14**	Femoral	**24**	Inferior medial genicular	**34**	Dorsal digital
5	Internal iliac	**15**	Deep artery/vein of thigh	**25**	Anterior tibial recurrent artery	**35**	1st dorsal metatarsal artery
6	External iliac	**16**	Medial circumflex femoral	**26**	Anterior tibial	**36**	Medial plantar artery
7	Superficial circumflex iliac	**17**	Lateral circumflex femoral	**27**	Dorsalis pedis artery	**37**	Lateral plantar artery
8	Deep circumflex iliac	**18**	Perforating	**28**	Posterior tibial	**38**	Plantar arch
9	Inferior epigastric	**19**	Descending genicular	**29**	Fibular	**39**	Plantar metatarsal
10	Internal pudendal vein	**20**	Popliteal	**30**	Perforating branch, fibular artery	**40**	Plantar digital
						41	Dorsal venous arch

Overview of Arterial Supply and Deep Venous Drainage of Lower Limb   **6.13**

A. and **C.** Arteries. **B.** and **D.** Deep veins.

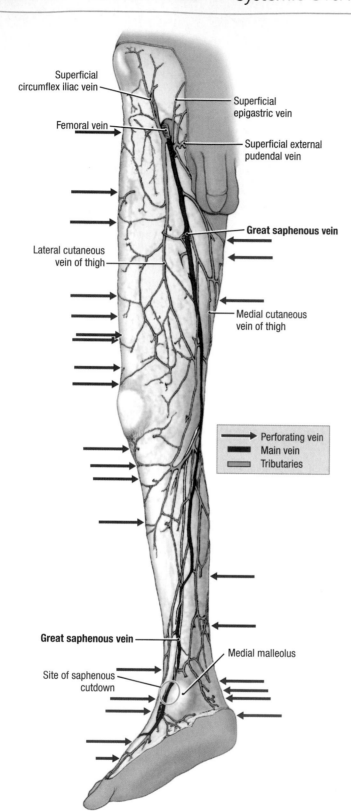

Superficial
circumflex iliac vein

Superficial
epigastric vein

Femoral vein

Superficial external
pudendal vein

Great saphenous vein

Lateral cutaneous
vein of thigh

Medial cutaneous
vein of thigh

→ Perforating vein
▬ Main vein
▭ Tributaries

Great saphenous vein

Medial malleolus

Site of saphenous
cutdown

A. Anteromedial View

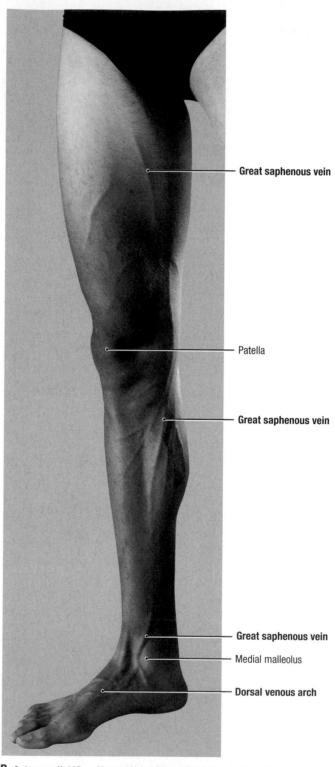

Great saphenous vein

Patella

Great saphenous vein

Great saphenous vein

Medial malleolus

Dorsal venous arch

B. Anteromedial View, Normal Veins Distended Following Exercise

6.14   Superficial Veins of Lower Limb: Great Saphenous Vein

A. Dissection. **B.** Surface anatomy.

Highly anastomotic veins, largely unaccompanied by arteries, are abundant in the subcutaneous tissue, draining deeply via multiple perforating veins.

Saphenous cut down. The great saphenous vein can be located by making a skin incision anterior to the medial malleolus. This procedure is used to insert a cannula for prolonged administration of blood, electrolytes, drugs, etc.

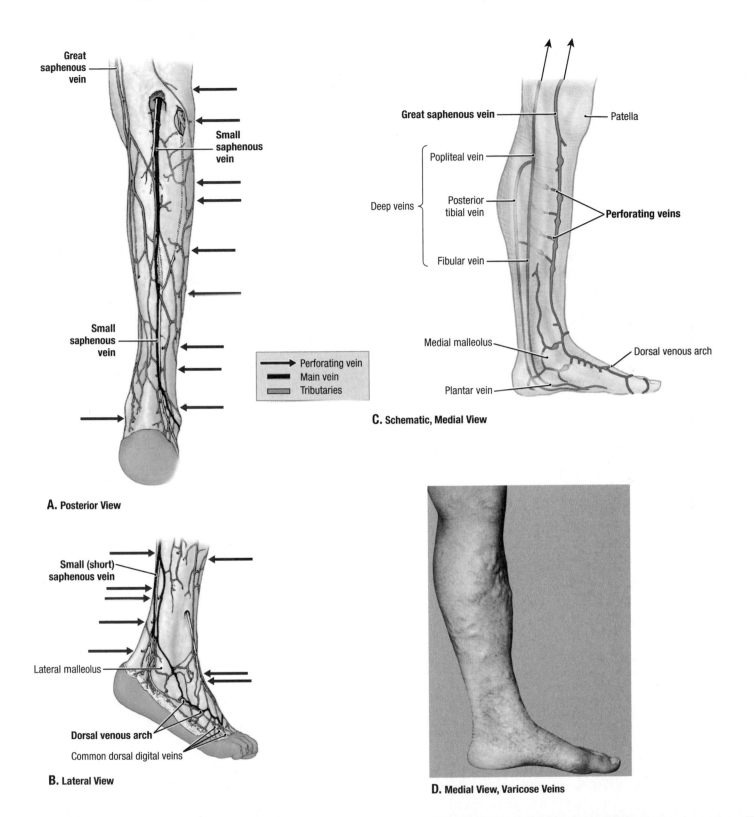

Great saphenous vein

Small saphenous vein

Small saphenous vein

Perforating vein
Main vein
Tributaries

A. Posterior View

Small (short) saphenous vein

Lateral malleolus

Dorsal venous arch

Common dorsal digital veins

B. Lateral View

Great saphenous vein — Patella

Popliteal vein

Deep veins { Posterior tibial vein

Perforating veins

Fibular vein

Medial malleolus — Dorsal venous arch

Plantar vein

C. Schematic, Medial View

D. Medial View, Varicose Veins

Superficial Veins of Lower Limb: Small Saphenous Vein

6.15

A. and **B. Dissections. C. Schematic of drainage of superficial veins.** Blood is shunted from the superficial veins (e.g., great saphenous vein) to the deep veins (e.g., fibular and posterior tibial veins) via perforating veins that penetrate the deep fascia. Muscular compression of deep veins assists return of blood to the heart against gravity. **D.** Varicose veins. Varicose veins form when either the deep fascia or the valves of the perforating veins are incompetent. This allows the muscular compression that normally propels blood toward the heart to push blood from the deep to the superficial veins. Consequently, superficial veins become enlarged and tortuous.

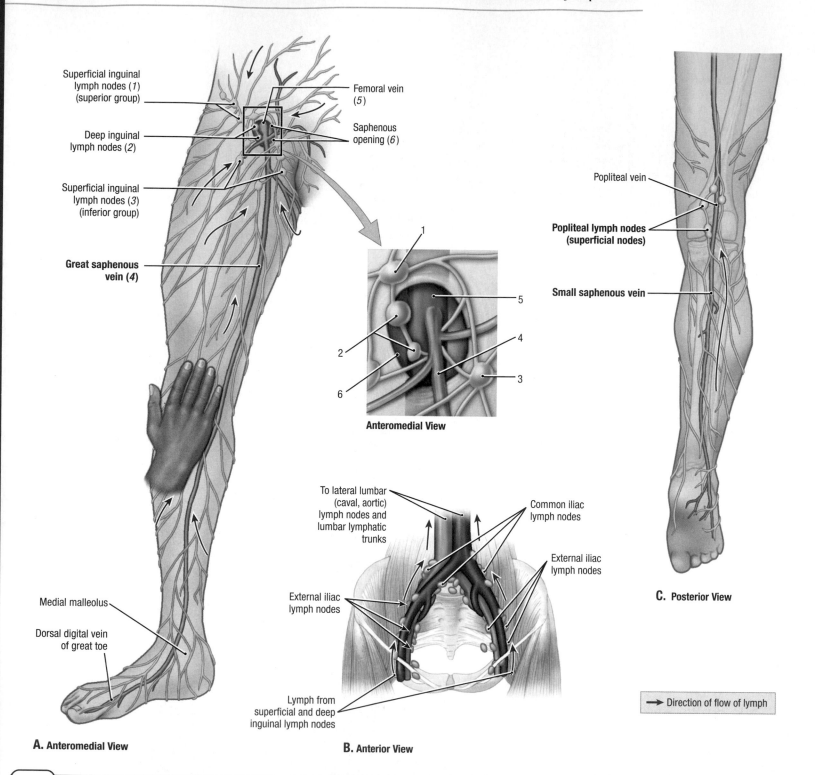

Superficial inguinal
lymph nodes (1)
(superior group)

Deep inguinal
lymph nodes (2)

Superficial inguinal
lymph nodes (3)
(inferior group)

**Great saphenous
vein (4)**

Medial malleolus

Dorsal digital vein
of great toe

A. Anteromedial View

Femoral vein
(5)

Saphenous
opening (6)

Anteromedial View

To lateral lumbar
(caval, aortic)
lymph nodes and
lumbar lymphatic
trunks

External iliac
lymph nodes

Lymph from
superficial and deep
inguinal lymph nodes

B. Anterior View

Common iliac
lymph nodes

External iliac
lymph nodes

Popliteal vein

**Popliteal lymph nodes
(superficial nodes)**

Small saphenous vein

C. Posterior View

→ Direction of flow of lymph

6.16 **Superficial Lymphatic Drainage of Lower Limb**

A. Anterior and medial aspects. **B.** Drainage of inguinal lymph nodes. **C.** Posterior aspect.

The superficial lymphatic vessels accompany the saphenous veins and their tributaries in the superficial fascia. The lymphatic vessels along the great saphenous vein drain into the superficial inguinal lymph nodes; those along the small saphenous vein drain into the popliteal lymph nodes. Lymph from the superficial inguinal nodes drains to the deep inguinal and external iliac nodes. Lymph from the popliteal nodes ascends through deep lymphatic vessels accompanying the deep blood vessels to the deep inguinal nodes. Note that the great saphenous vein lies anterior to the medial malleolus and a hand's breadth posterior to the medial border of the patella. **Lymph nodes enlarge** when diseased. Abrasions and minor sepsis, caused by pathogenic micro-organisms or their toxins, may produce slight enlargement of the superficial inguinal nodes (lymphadenopathy) in otherwise healthy people. Malignancies (e.g., of the external genitalia and uterus) and perineal abscesses also result in enlargement of these nodes.

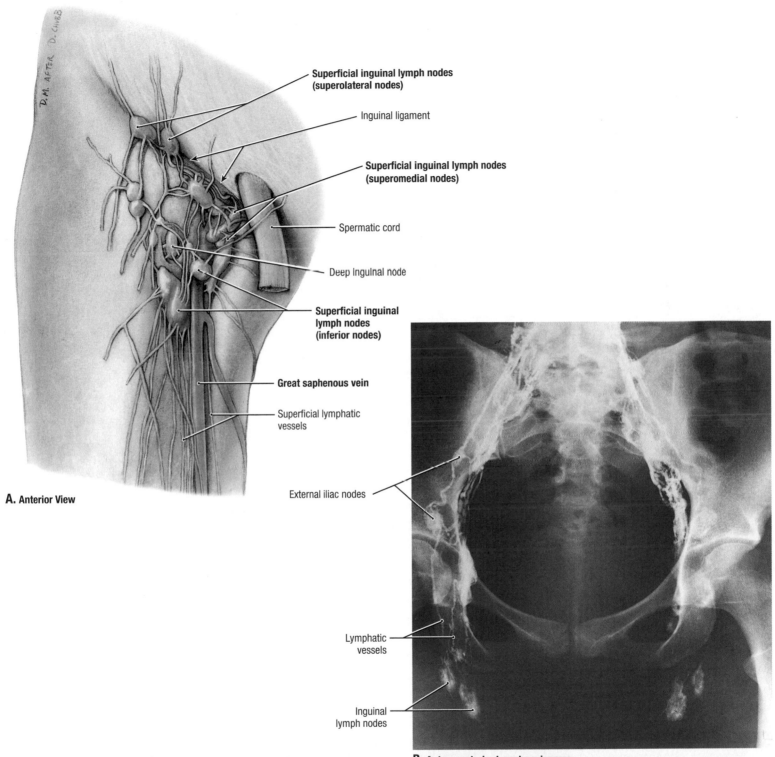

Superficial inguinal lymph nodes
(superolateral nodes)

Inguinal ligament

Superficial inguinal lymph nodes
(superomedial nodes)

Spermatic cord

Deep inguinal node

Superficial inguinal
lymph nodes
(inferior nodes)

Great saphenous vein

Superficial lymphatic
vessels

A. Anterior View

External iliac nodes

Lymphatic
vessels

Inguinal
lymph nodes

B. Anteroposterior Lymphangiogram

Inguinal Lymph Nodes   6.17

A. Dissection. **B.** Lymphangiogram.
- Observe the arrangement of the nodes: a proximal chain parallel to the inguinal ligament (superolateral and superomedial superficial inguinal lymph nodes) and a distal chain on the sides of the

great saphenous vein (inferior superficial inguinal lymph nodes). Efferent vessels leave these nodes and pass deep to the inguinal ligament to enter the deep inguinal and external iliac nodes.
- Note the anastomosis between the lymph vessels.

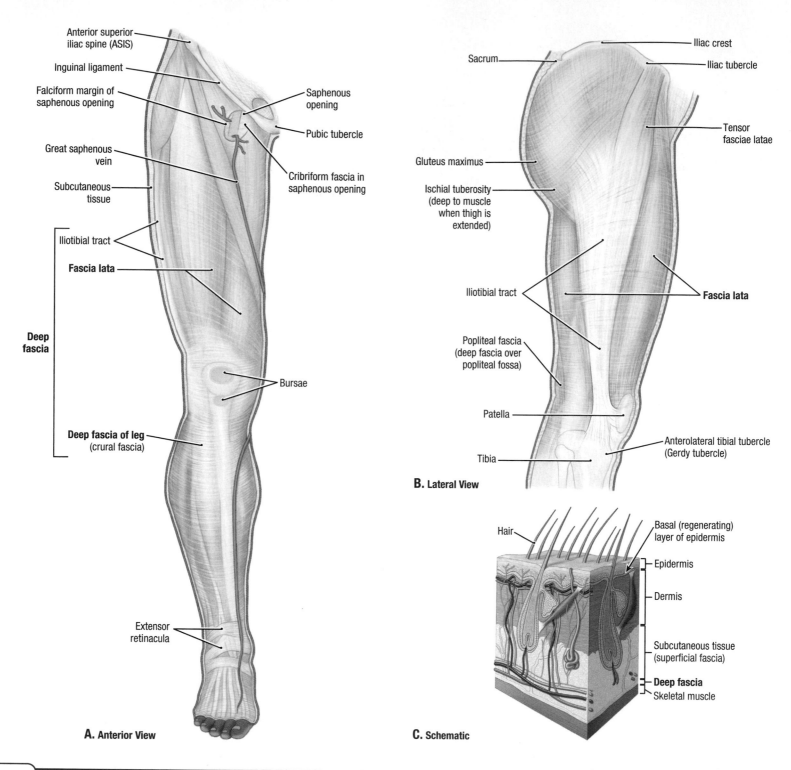

A. Anterior View

- Anterior superior iliac spine (ASIS)
- Inguinal ligament
- Falciform margin of saphenous opening
- Great saphenous vein
- Subcutaneous tissue
- Iliotibial tract
- **Fascia lata**
- **Deep fascia**
- **Deep fascia of leg** (crural fascia)
- Extensor retinacula
- Saphenous opening
- Pubic tubercle
- Cribriform fascia in saphenous opening
- Bursae

B. Lateral View

- Sacrum
- Gluteus maximus
- Ischial tuberosity (deep to muscle when thigh is extended)
- Iliotibial tract
- Popliteal fascia (deep fascia over popliteal fossa)
- Patella
- Tibia
- Iliac crest
- Iliac tubercle
- Tensor fasciae latae
- **Fascia lata**
- Anterolateral tibial tubercle (Gerdy tubercle)

C. Schematic

- Hair
- Basal (regenerating) layer of epidermis
- Epidermis
- Dermis
- Subcutaneous tissue (superficial fascia)
- **Deep fascia**
- Skeletal muscle

6.18 **Fascia and Musculofascial Compartments of Lower Limb**

A. Deep fascia of lower limb. Anterior skin and subcutaneous tissue have been removed to reveal the deep fascia of the thigh (fascia lata) and leg (crural fascia). **B. Iliotibial (IT) tract.** Lateral skin and subcutaneous tissue have been removed to reveal the fascia lata. The fascia lata is thick laterally and forms the IT tract. The iliotibial tract serves as a common aponeurosis for the gluteus maximus and tensor fasciae latae muscles. One of the most common causes of lateral knee pain in endurance athletes (e.g., runners, cyclers, hikers) is **iliotibial tract (band) syndrome (ITBS)**. Friction of the IT tract against the lateral epicondyle of the femur with flexion and extension of the knee (e.g., during running) may result in the inflammation of the IT tract over the lateral aspect of the knee or its attachment to the dorsolateral tubercle (Gerdy tubercle). ITBS may also occur in the hip region, especially in older individuals. **C. Relationship of deep fascia to skin and subcutaneous tissue.**

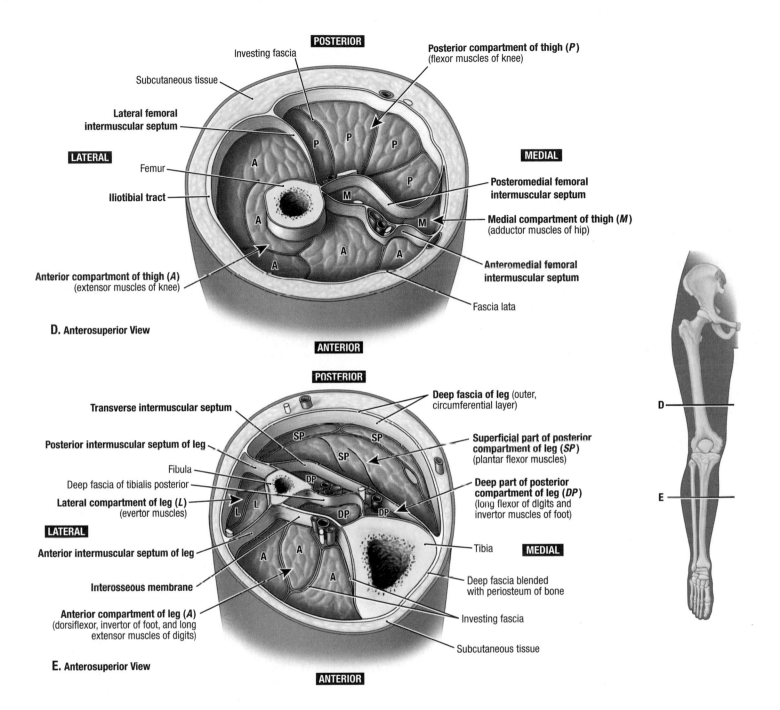

POSTERIOR

Investing fascia

Subcutaneous tissue

Lateral femoral
intermuscular septum

LATERAL

Femur

Iliotibial tract

Anterior compartment of thigh (*A*)
(extensor muscles of knee)

Posterior compartment of thigh (*P*)
(flexor muscles of knee)

MEDIAL

**Posteromedial femoral
intermuscular septum**

Medial compartment of thigh (*M*)
(adductor muscles of hip)

**Anteromedial femoral
intermuscular septum**

Fascia lata

D. Anterosuperior View

ANTERIOR

POSTERIOR

Transverse intermuscular septum

Posterior intermuscular septum of leg

Fibula

Deep fascia of tibialis posterior

Lateral compartment of leg (*L*)
(evertor muscles)

LATERAL

Anterior intermuscular septum of leg

Interosseous membrane

Anterior compartment of leg (*A*)
(dorsiflexor, invertor of foot, and long
extensor muscles of digits)

Deep fascia of leg (outer,
circumferential layer)

**Superficial part of posterior
compartment of leg (*SP*)**
(plantar flexor muscles)

**Deep part of posterior
compartment of leg (*DP*)**
(long flexor of digits and
invertor muscles of foot)

Tibia

MEDIAL

Deep fascia blended
with periosteum of bone

Investing fascia

Subcutaneous tissue

E. Anterosuperior View

ANTERIOR

Fascia and Musculofascial Compartments of Lower Limb (*continued*)   **6.18**

D. Transverse section of fascial compartments of thigh.
E. Transverse section of fascial compartments of leg. The
fascial compartments contain muscles that generally perform
common functions and share common innervation and contain the spread of infection. Although both thigh and leg have
anterior and posterior compartments, the thigh also includes a
medial compartment, and the leg, a lateral compartment. Trauma
to muscles and/or vessels in the compartments may produce
hemorrhage, edema, and inflammation of the muscles. Because

the septa, deep fascia, and bony attachments firmly bound the
compartments, increased volume resulting from these processes
raises intracompartmental pressure. In **compartment syndromes**,
structures within or distal to the compressed area become ischemic and may become permanently injured (e.g., compression of
capillary beds results in denervation and consequent paralysis of
muscles). A **fasciotomy** (incision of bounding fascia or septum)
may be performed to relieve the pressure in the compartment
and restore circulation.

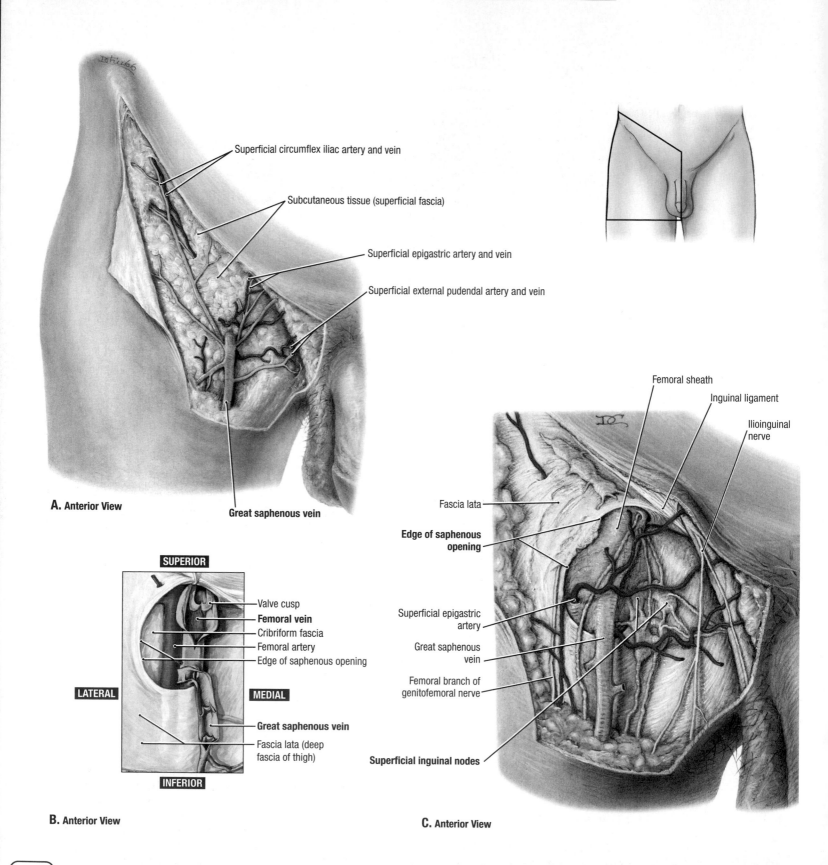

Superficial circumflex iliac artery and vein

Subcutaneous tissue (superficial fascia)

Superficial epigastric artery and vein

Superficial external pudendal artery and vein

Femoral sheath

Inguinal ligament

Ilioinguinal nerve

Fascia lata

Edge of saphenous opening

Superficial epigastric artery

Great saphenous vein

Femoral branch of genitofemoral nerve

Superficial inguinal nodes

A. Anterior View

Great saphenous vein

SUPERIOR

Valve cusp
Femoral vein
Cribriform fascia
Femoral artery
Edge of saphenous opening

LATERAL   MEDIAL

Great saphenous vein

Fascia lata (deep fascia of thigh)

INFERIOR

B. Anterior View

C. Anterior View

6.19   Superficial Inguinal Vessels and Saphenous Opening

A. Superficial inguinal vessels. The arteries are branches of the femoral artery, and the veins are tributaries of the great saphenous vein.

B. Valves of proximal part of femoral and great saphenous veins.
C. Saphenous opening.

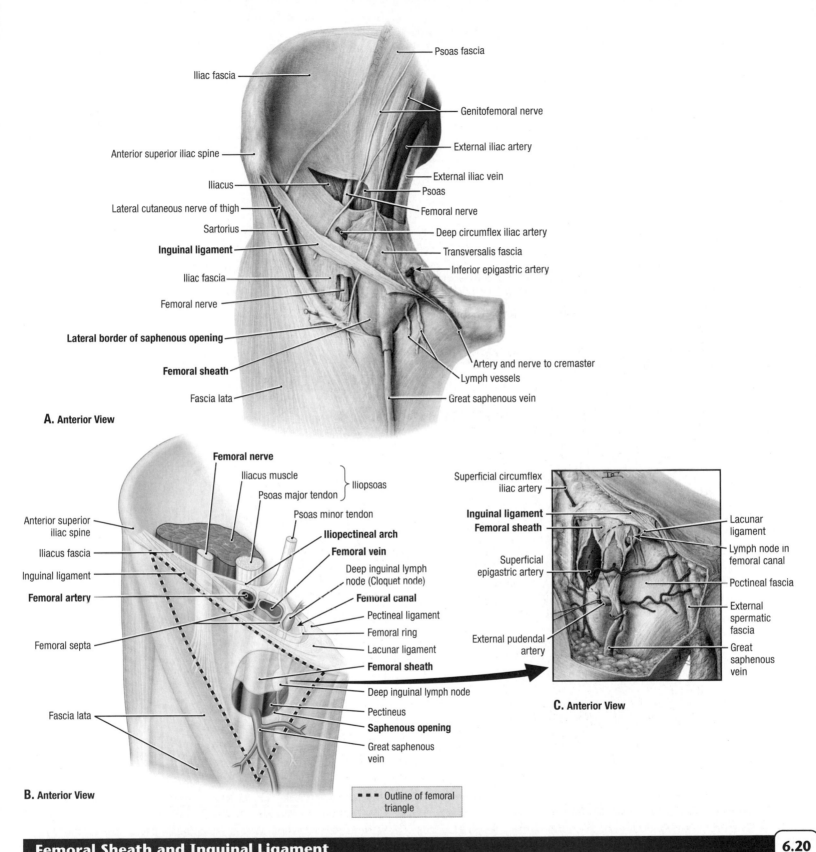

A. Anterior View

Psoas fascia

Iliac fascia

Genitofemoral nerve

Anterior superior iliac spine

External iliac artery

Iliacus

External iliac vein

Lateral cutaneous nerve of thigh

Psoas

Sartorius

Femoral nerve

Inguinal ligament

Deep circumflex iliac artery

Iliac fascia

Transversalis fascia

Femoral nerve

Inferior epigastric artery

Lateral border of saphenous opening

Femoral sheath

Artery and nerve to cremaster

Lymph vessels

Fascia lata

Great saphenous vein

B. Anterior View

Femoral nerve

Iliacus muscle

Psoas major tendon

Iliopsoas

Psoas minor tendon

Anterior superior iliac spine

Iliopectineal arch

Iliacus fascia

Femoral vein

Inguinal ligament

Deep inguinal lymph node (Cloquet node)

Femoral artery

Femoral canal

Pectineal ligament

Femoral ring

Femoral septa

Lacunar ligament

Femoral sheath

Deep inguinal lymph node

Fascia lata

Pectineus

Saphenous opening

Great saphenous vein

- - - Outline of femoral triangle

C. Anterior View

Superficial circumflex iliac artery

Inguinal ligament

Femoral sheath

Lacunar ligament

Lymph node in femoral canal

Superficial epigastric artery

Pectineal fascia

External spermatic fascia

External pudendal artery

Great saphenous vein

Femoral Sheath and Inguinal Ligament

6.20

A. Dissection. B. Schematic. The femoral sheath contains the femoral artery, vein, and lymph vessels, but the femoral nerve, lying posterior to the iliacus fascia, is outside the femoral sheath. **C. Femoral sheath and femoral ring.** The three compartments of the femoral sheath are for the femoral artery, vein, and femoral canal. The femoral canal has a small proximal opening at its abdominal end, the femoral ring, closed by extraperitoneal fatty tissue.

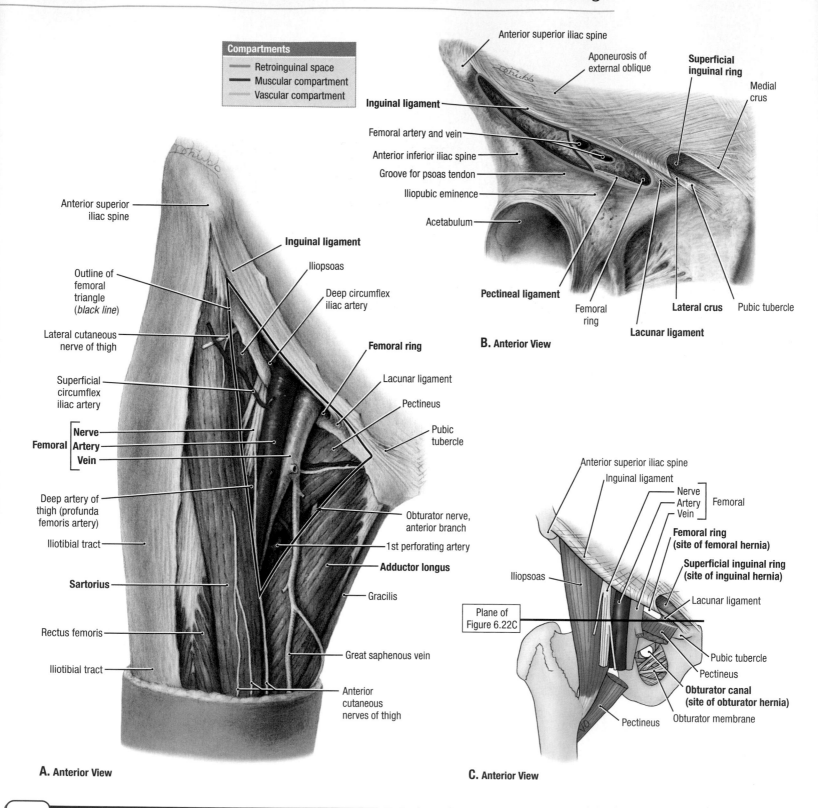

Compartments
— Retroinguinal space
— Muscular compartment
— Vascular compartment

Anterior superior iliac spine

Outline of femoral triangle (*black line*)

Lateral cutaneous nerve of thigh

Superficial circumflex iliac artery

Femoral — **Nerve** — **Artery** — **Vein**

Deep artery of thigh (profunda femoris artery)

Iliotibial tract

Sartorius

Rectus femoris

Iliotibial tract

Inguinal ligament
Iliopsoas
Deep circumflex iliac artery
Femoral ring
Lacunar ligament
Pectineus
Pubic tubercle
Obturator nerve, anterior branch
1st perforating artery
Adductor longus
Gracilis
Great saphenous vein
Anterior cutaneous nerves of thigh

A. Anterior View

Anterior superior iliac spine
Aponeurosis of external oblique
Superficial inguinal ring
Medial crus
Inguinal ligament
Femoral artery and vein
Anterior inferior iliac spine
Groove for psoas tendon
Iliopubic eminence
Acetabulum
Pectineal ligament
Femoral ring
Lacunar ligament
Lateral crus
Pubic tubercle

B. Anterior View

Anterior superior iliac spine
Inguinal ligament
Nerve
Artery — Femoral
Vein
Femoral ring (site of femoral hernia)
Superficial inguinal ring (site of inguinal hernia)
Iliopsoas
Lacunar ligament
Plane of Figure 6.22C
Pubic tubercle
Pectineus
Obturator canal (site of obturator hernia)
Pectineus
Obturator membrane

C. Anterior View

6.21 **Structures Passing to/from Femoral Triangle via Retroinguinal Passage**

A. Dissection. The boundaries of the femoral triangle are the inguinal ligament superiorly (base of triangle), the medial border of the sartorius (lateral side), and the lateral border of the adductor longus (medial side). The point at which the lateral and medial sides converge inferiorly forms the apex. The femoral triangle is bisected by the femoral vessels. **B. Retroinguinal space and muscular and vascular compartments deep to inguinal ligament. C. Structures** passing deep to inguinal ligament. The iliopsoas muscle; the femoral nerve, artery, and vein; and the lymphatic vessels draining the inguinal nodes pass deep to the inguinal ligament to enter the anterior thigh or return to the trunk. Three potential sites for **hernia formation** are indicated. **Pulsations of the femoral artery** can be felt distal to the inguinal ligament, midway between the anterior superior iliac spine and the pubic symphysis (the midinguinal point).

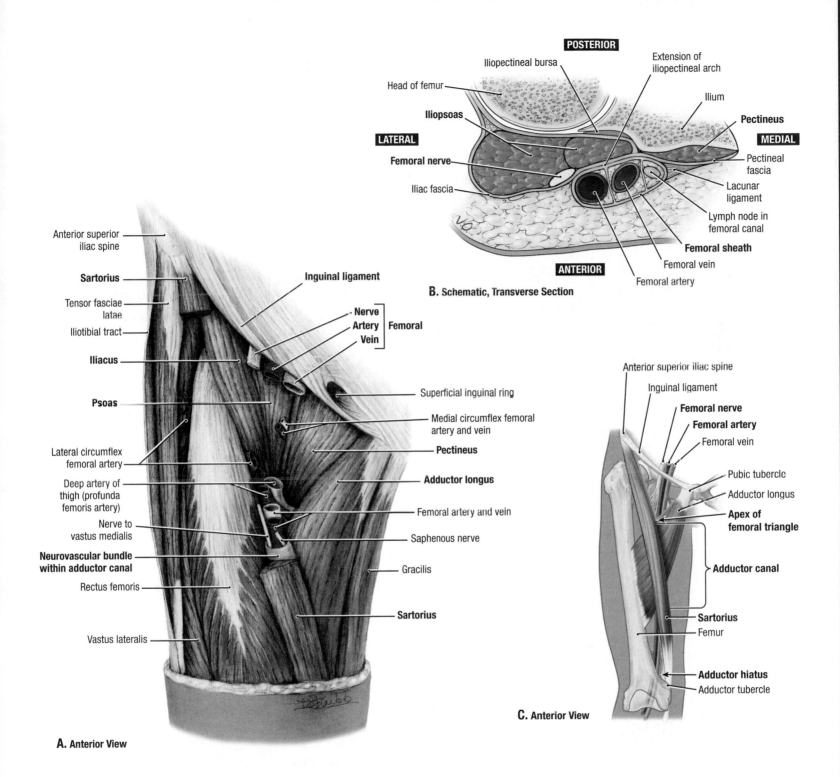

POSTERIOR

Iliopectineal bursa

Extension of iliopectineal arch

Head of femur

Ilium

Iliopsoas

Pectineus

LATERAL

MEDIAL

Femoral nerve

Pectineal fascia

Iliac fascia

Lacunar ligament

Lymph node in femoral canal

Femoral sheath

Femoral vein

ANTERIOR

Femoral artery

B. Schematic, Transverse Section

Anterior superior iliac spine

Sartorius

Inguinal ligament

Tensor fasciae latae

Nerve
Artery **Femoral**
Vein

Iliotibial tract

Iliacus

Superficial inguinal ring

Psoas

Medial circumflex femoral artery and vein

Lateral circumflex femoral artery

Pectineus

Deep artery of thigh (profunda femoris artery)

Adductor longus

Nerve to vastus medialis

Femoral artery and vein

Neurovascular bundle within adductor canal

Saphenous nerve

Rectus femoris

Gracilis

Vastus lateralis

Sartorius

A. Anterior View

Anterior superior iliac spine

Inguinal ligament

Femoral nerve

Femoral artery

Femoral vein

Pubic tubercle

Adductor longus

Apex of femoral triangle

Adductor canal

Sartorius

Femur

Adductor hiatus

Adductor tubercle

C. Anterior View

Boundaries and Floor of Femoral Canal and Retroinguinal Passage

6.22

A. Dissection. Portions of the sartorius muscle, femoral vessels, and femoral nerve have been removed revealing the floor of the femoral triangle, formed by the iliopsoas laterally and the pectineus medially. At the apex of the triangle, the femoral vessels, saphenous nerve, and the nerve to the vastus medialis pass deep to the sartorius into the adductor (subsartorial) canal. **B. Transverse section of femoral triangle at level of head of femur.** The iliopsoas and femoral nerve traverse the retroinguinal passage and femoral triangle in a fascial sheath separate from the femoral vessels, which are contained within the femoral sheath (see Fig. 6.21C for level of section). **C. Schematic of course of femoral vessels.** The adductor canal extends from the apex of the femoral triangle to the adductor hiatus by which the vessels enter and leave the popliteal fossa.

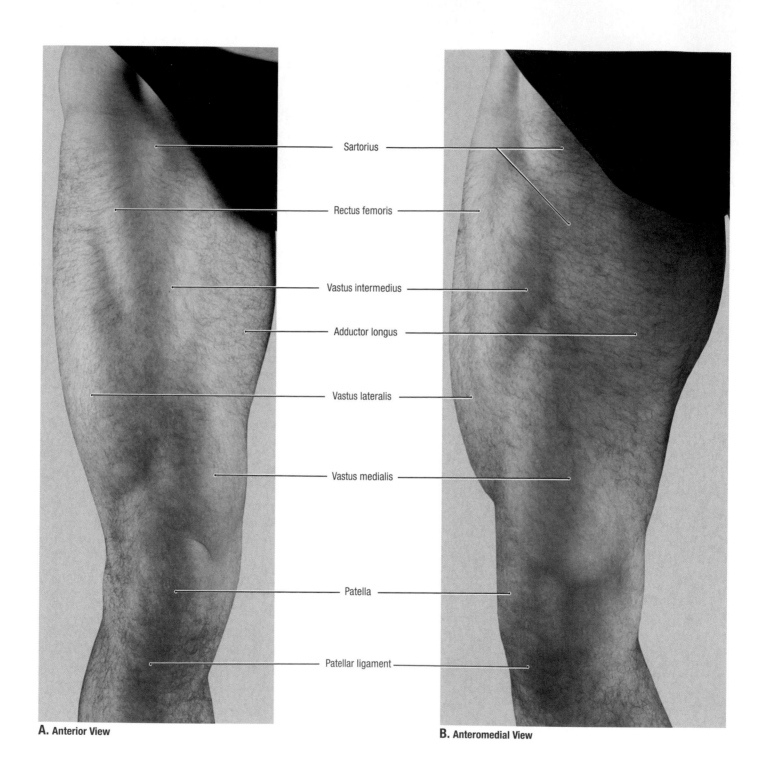

Sartorius

Rectus femoris

Vastus intermedius

Adductor longus

Vastus lateralis

Vastus medialis

Patella

Patellar ligament

A. Anterior View

B. Anteromedial View

6.23   **Surface Anatomy of Anterior and Medial Aspects of Thigh**

Patellar tendinitis (jumper's knee) is caused by continuous over-loading of the knee extensor mechanism, resulting in microtears of the tendon. The most vulnerable site is where the patellar ligament (tendon) attaches to the patella. This overuse injury can result in degeneration and tearing of the tendon.

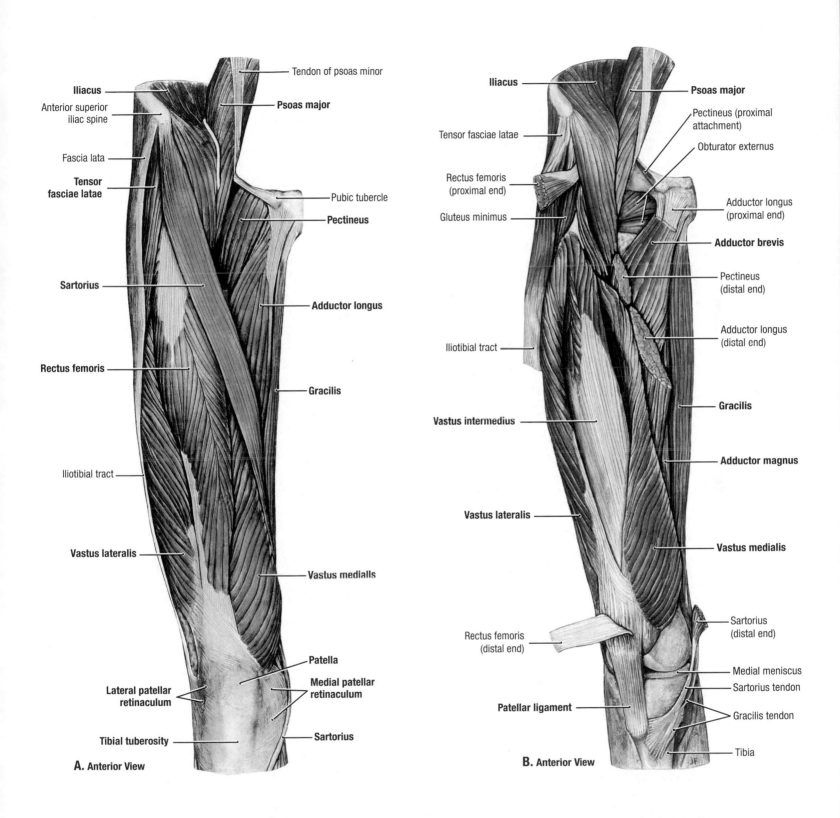

A. Anterior View

Tendon of psoas minor
Iliacus
Anterior superior iliac spine
Psoas major
Fascia lata
Tensor fasciae latae
Pubic tubercle
Pectineus
Sartorius
Adductor longus
Rectus femoris
Gracilis
Iliotibial tract
Vastus lateralis
Vastus medialis
Lateral patellar retinaculum
Patella
Medial patellar retinaculum
Tibial tuberosity
Sartorius

B. Anterior View

Iliacus
Psoas major
Tensor fasciae latae
Pectineus (proximal attachment)
Obturator externus
Rectus femoris (proximal end)
Gluteus minimus
Adductor longus (proximal end)
Adductor brevis
Pectineus (distal end)
Adductor longus (distal end)
Iliotibial tract
Gracilis
Vastus intermedius
Adductor magnus
Vastus lateralis
Vastus medialis
Sartorius (distal end)
Rectus femoris (distal end)
Medial meniscus
Sartorius tendon
Patellar ligament
Gracilis tendon
Tibia

Anterior and Medial Thigh Muscles, Superficial and Deep Dissections

6.24

A. Superficial dissection. B. Deep dissection. The central portions of the muscle bellies of the sartorius, rectus femoris, pectineus, and adductor longus muscles have been removed. **Weakness of** **the vastus medialis or vastus lateralis,** resulting from arthritis or trauma to the knee joint, for example, can result in abnormal patellar movement and loss of joint stability.

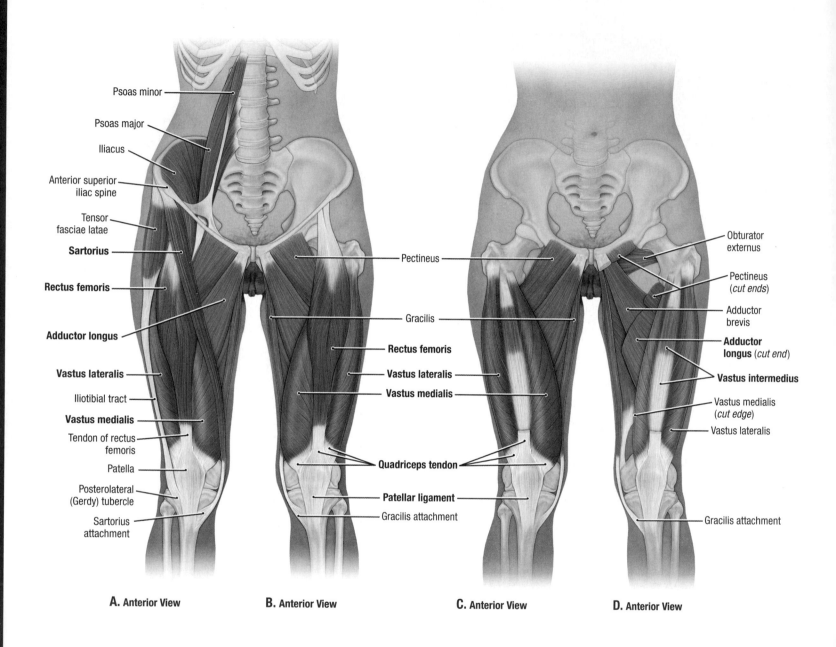

Psoas minor

Psoas major

Iliacus

Anterior superior
iliac spine

Tensor
fasciae latae

Sartorius

Rectus femoris

Adductor longus

Vastus lateralis

Iliotibial tract

Vastus medialis

Tendon of rectus
femoris

Patella

Posterolateral
(Gerdy) tubercle

Sartorius
attachment

Pectineus

Gracilis

Rectus femoris

Vastus lateralis

Vastus medialis

Quadriceps tendon

Patellar ligament

Gracilis attachment

Obturator
externus

Pectineus
(*cut ends*)

Adductor
brevis

**Adductor
longus** (*cut end*)

Vastus intermedius

Vastus medialis
(*cut edge*)

Vastus lateralis

Gracilis attachment

A. Anterior View   **B. Anterior View**   **C. Anterior View**   **D. Anterior View**

6.25   Anterior and Medial Thigh Muscles, Schematics

A–D. Sequential views from superficial to deep.

A "hip pointer," which is a **contusion of the iliac crest**, usually occurs at its anterior part (e.g., where the sartorius attaches to the anterior superior iliac spine). This is one of the most common injuries to the hip region, usually occurring in association with collision sports. Contusions cause bleeding from ruptured capillaries and infiltration of blood into the muscles, tendons, and other soft tissues. The term *hip pointer* may also refer to avulsion of bony muscle attachments, for example, of the sartorius or rectus femoris from the anterior superior or inferior iliac spines or of the iliopsoas from the lesser trochanter of the femur. However, these injuries should be called **avulsion fractures**.

A person with a **paralyzed quadriceps** cannot extend the leg against resistance and usually presses on the distal end of the thigh during walking to prevent inadvertent flexion of the knee joint.

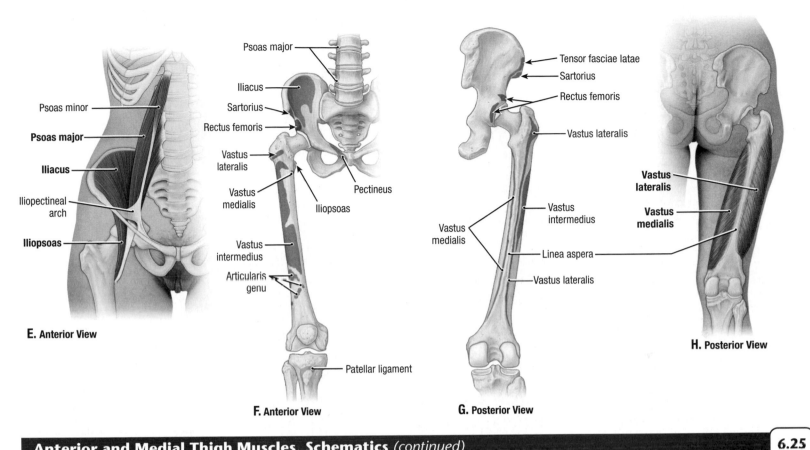

E. **Anterior View**

F. **Anterior View**

G. **Posterior View**

H. **Posterior View**

Anterior and Medial Thigh Muscles, Schematics (*continued*)   **6.25**

E. Iliopsoas. F. and G. Attachments of anterior muscles of thigh. H. Posterior attachment of vastus medialis and lateralis.

TABLE 6.3	Muscles of Anterior Thigh			
Muscle	**Proximal Attachment**[a]	**Distal Attachment**[a]	**Innervation**[b]	**Main Actions**
Iliopsoas Psoas major	Lateral aspects of T12–L5 vertebrae and intervening intervertebral discs; transverse processes of all çlumbar vertebrae	By a strong tendon to lesser trochanter of femur	Anterior rami of lumbar nerves (**L1**, **L2**, L3)	Acting inferiorly with iliacus, it flexes hip joint; acting superiorly, it flexes vertebral column laterally; it is used to balance the trunk; during sitting, it acts inferiorly with iliacus to flex the trunk
Iliacus	Iliac crest, iliac fossa, ala of sacrum and anterior sacroiliac ligaments	Tendon of psoas major, lesser trochanter, and femur distal to it	Femoral nerve (L2, L3, **L4**)	
Tensor fasciae latae	Anterior superior iliac spine and anterior part of iliac crest	Iliotibial tract that attaches to lateral condyle of tibia	Superior gluteal (L4, L5)	Abducts and medially rotates hip joint; helps to keep knee extended; stabilizes trunk on thigh
Sartorius	Anterior superior iliac spine and superior part of notch inferior to it	Superior part of medial surface of tibia (as part of pes anserinus)	Femoral nerve (L2, L3)	Flexes, abducts, and laterally rotates hip joint; flexes knee joint[c]
Quadriceps femoris Rectus femoris	Anterior inferior iliac spine and ilium superior to acetabulum	Base of patella and by patellar ligament to tibial tuberosity; medial and lateral vasti also attach to tibia and patella via aponeuroses (medial and lateral patellar retinacula)	Femoral nerve (L2, **L3**, **L4**)	Extends knee joint; rectus femoris also steadies hip joint and helps iliopsoas to flex hip joint
Vastus lateralis	Greater trochanter and lateral lip of linea aspera of femur			
Vastus medialis	Intertrochanteric line and medial lip of linea aspera of femur			
Vastus intermedius	Anterior and lateral surfaces of body of femur			

[a]See also Figure 6.25 for muscle attachments.
[b]Numbers indicate spinal cord segmental innervation of nerves (e.g., L1, L2, and L3 indicate that nerves supplying psoas major are derived from first three lumbar segments of the spinal cord; boldface type [e.g., **L1**, **L2**] indicates main segmental innervation). Damage to one or more of these spinal cord segments or to motor nerve roots arising from these segments results in paralysis of the muscles concerned.
[c]Four actions of sartorius (L. *sartor*, tailor) produce the once-common cross-legged sitting position used by tailors—hence the name.

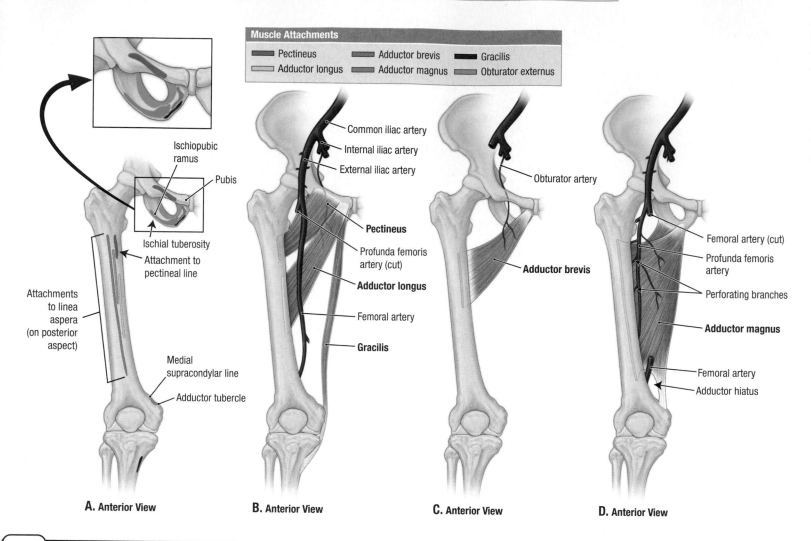

Muscle Attachments

- Pectineus
- Adductor longus
- Adductor brevis
- Adductor magnus
- Gracilis
- Obturator externus

Common iliac artery
Internal iliac artery
External iliac artery
Obturator artery

Ischiopubic ramus
Pubis
Ischial tuberosity
Attachment to pectineal line
Attachments to linea aspera (on posterior aspect)
Medial supracondylar line
Adductor tubercle

Pectineus
Profunda femoris artery (cut)
Adductor longus
Femoral artery
Gracilis

Adductor brevis

Femoral artery (cut)
Profunda femoris artery
Perforating branches
Adductor magnus
Femoral artery
Adductor hiatus

A. Anterior View   **B. Anterior View**   **C. Anterior View**   **D. Anterior View**

6.26 Attachments of Muscles of Medial Aspect of Thigh

A. Overview of attachments. **B.** Pectineus, adductor longus, and gracilis. **C.** Adductor brevis. **D.** Adductor magnus.

TABLE 6.4   Muscles of Medial Thigh

Muscle	Proximal Attachment	Distal Attachment[a]	Innervation[b]	Main Actions
Pectineus	Superior pubic ramus	Pectineal line of femur, just inferior to lesser trochanter	Femoral nerve (L2 and L3) may receive a branch from obturator nerve	Adducts and flexes hip joint; assists with medial rotation of hip joint
Adductor longus	Body of pubis inferior to pubic crest	Middle third of linea aspera of femur	Obturator nerve (L2, **L3**, and L4)	Adducts hip joint
Adductor brevis	Body of pubis and inferior pubic ramus	Pectineal line and proximal part of linea aspera of femur	Obturator nerve (L2, **L3**, and L4)	Adducts hip joint and, to some extent, flexes it
Adductor magnus	Inferior pubic ramus, ramus of ischium (adductor part), and ischial tuberosity	Gluteal tuberosity, linea aspera, medial supracondylar line (adductor part), and adductor tubercle of femur (hamstring part)	*Adductor part:* obturator nerve (L2, **L3**, and **L4**) *Hamstring part:* tibial part of sciatic nerve (**L4**)	Adducts hip joint; its adductor part also flexes hip joint, and its hamstring part extends it
Gracilis	Body of pubis and inferior pubic ramus	Superior part of medial surface of tibia	Obturator nerve (**L2** and L3)	Adducts hip joint, flexes knee joint, and helps rotate it medially
Obturator externus	Margins of obturator foramen and obturator membrane	Trochanteric fossa of femur	Obturator nerve (L3 and **L4**)	Laterally rotates hip joint; steadies head of femur in acetabulum

Collectively, the first five muscles listed are the adductors of the thigh, but their actions are more complex (e.g., they act as flexors of the hip joint during flexion of the knee joint and are active during walking).
[a]See Figure 6.25 for muscle attachments.
[b]See Table 6.2 for explanation of segmental innervation. Numbers indicate spinal cord segmental innervation of nerves (e.g., L2, L3, and L4 indicate that the obturator nerve supplying adductor longus is derived from lumbar segments of the spinal cord; boldface type [**L3**] indicates main segmental innervation). Damage to one or more of these spinal cord segments or to motor nerve roots arising from these segments results in paralysis of the muscles concerned.

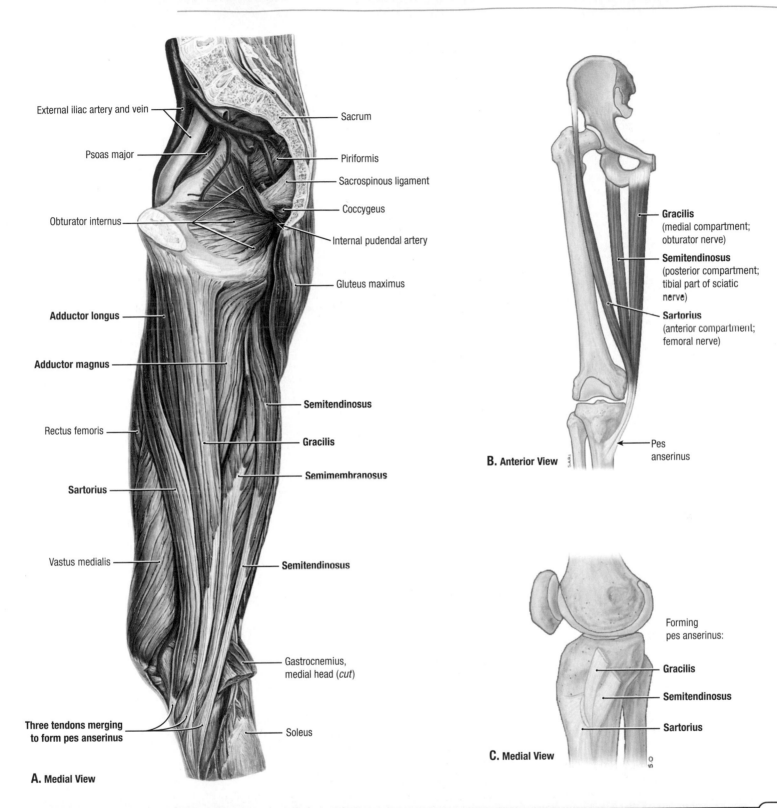

External iliac artery and vein

Psoas major

Obturator internus

Adductor longus

Adductor magnus

Rectus femoris

Sartorius

Vastus medialis

Three tendons merging to form pes anserinus

A. Medial View

Sacrum

Piriformis

Sacrospinous ligament

Coccygeus

Internal pudendal artery

Gluteus maximus

Semitendinosus

Gracilis

Semimembranosus

Semitendinosus

Gastrocnemius, medial head (*cut*)

Soleus

Gracilis
(medial compartment; obturator nerve)

Semitendinosus
(posterior compartment; tibial part of sciatic nerve)

Sartorius
(anterior compartment; femoral nerve)

Pes anserinus

B. Anterior View

Forming pes anserinus:

Gracilis

Semitendinosus

Sartorius

C. Medial View

Muscles of Medial Aspect of Thigh

6.27

A. Dissection. B. Muscular tripod. The sartorius, gracilis, and semitendinosus muscles form an inverted tripod arising from three different components of the hip bone. These muscles course within three different compartments, perform three different functions, and are innervated by three different nerves yet share a common distal attachment. **C. Distal attachment of sartorius, gracilis, and semitendinosus muscles.** All three tendons become thin and aponeurotic and are collectively referred to as the pes anserinus.

The gracilis is a relatively weak member of the adductor group and hence can be removed without noticeable loss of its actions on the leg. Surgeons often **transplant the gracilis,** or part of it, with its nerve and blood vessels to replace a damaged muscle, in the hand, for example.

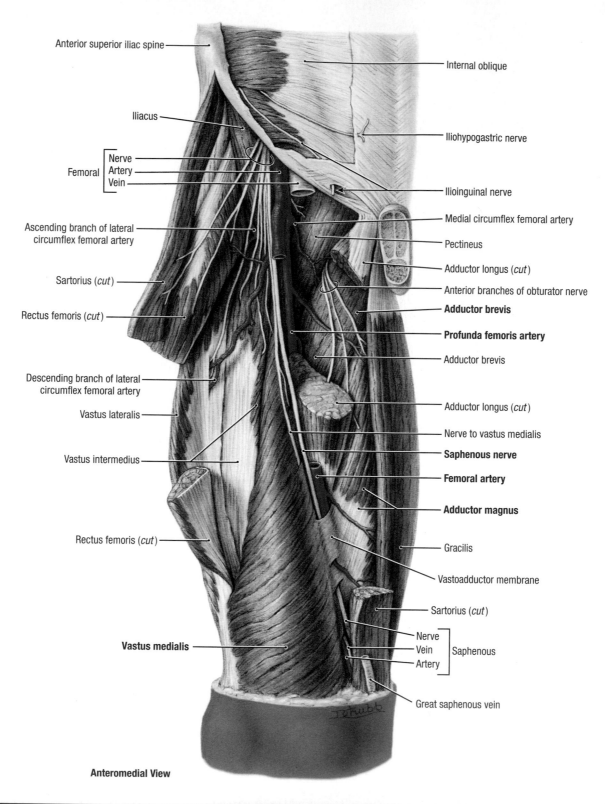

Anterior superior iliac spine

Internal oblique

Iliacus

Iliohypogastric nerve

Femoral {
Nerve
Artery
Vein
}

Ilioinguinal nerve

Ascending branch of lateral circumflex femoral artery

Medial circumflex femoral artery

Pectineus

Sartorius (*cut*)

Adductor longus (*cut*)

Anterior branches of obturator nerve

Rectus femoris (*cut*)

Adductor brevis

Profunda femoris artery

Adductor brevis

Descending branch of lateral circumflex femoral artery

Adductor longus (*cut*)

Vastus lateralis

Nerve to vastus medialis

Saphenous nerve

Vastus intermedius

Femoral artery

Adductor magnus

Rectus femoris (*cut*)

Gracilis

Vastoadductor membrane

Sartorius (*cut*)

Vastus medialis

Nerve
Vein
Artery
} Saphenous

Great saphenous vein

Anteromedial View

6.28   Anteromedial Aspect of Thigh

- The limb is rotated laterally.
- The femoral nerve breaks up into multiple nerves on entering the thigh.
- The femoral artery lies between two motor territories: that of the obturator nerve, which is medial, and that of the femoral nerve, which is lateral.

- The nerve to the vastus medialis muscle and the saphenous nerve accompany the femoral artery into the adductor canal.
- The deep artery of thigh (profunda femoris artery) is the largest branch of the femoral artery and the chief artery to the thigh.

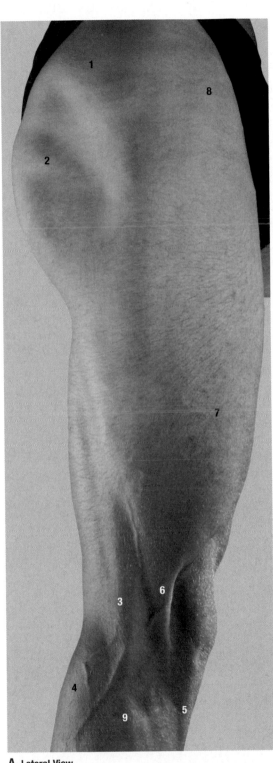

A. Lateral View

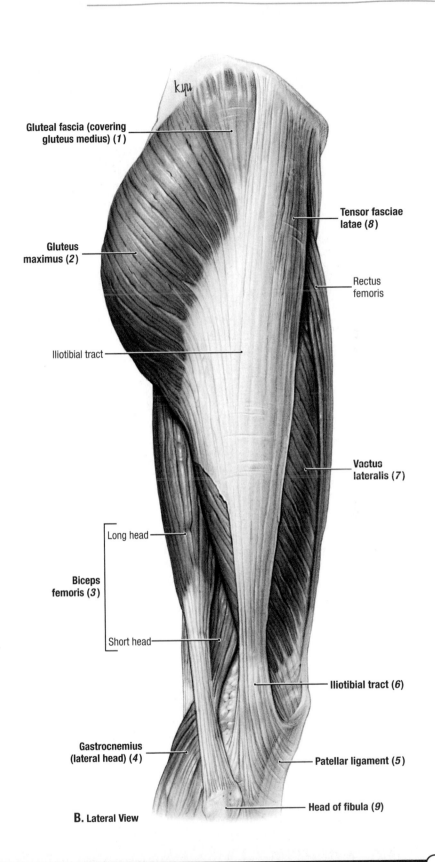

Gluteal fascia (covering gluteus medius) (*1*)

Gluteus maximus (*2*)

Iliotibial tract

Biceps femoris (*3*)
- Long head
- Short head

Gastrocnemius (lateral head) (*4*)

Tensor fasciae latae (*8*)

Rectus femoris

Vastus lateralis (*7*)

Iliotibial tract (*6*)

Patellar ligament (*5*)

Head of fibula (*9*)

B. Lateral View

Lateral Aspect of Thigh

6.29

A. Surface anatomy. Numbers refer to structures labeled in *Part B*.
B. Dissection. The iliotibial tract, a thickening of the fascia lata, serves as a tendon of attachment for the gluteus maximus and tensor fasciae latae. It attaches distally to the anterolateral (Gerdy) tubercle of the lateral condyle of the tibia.

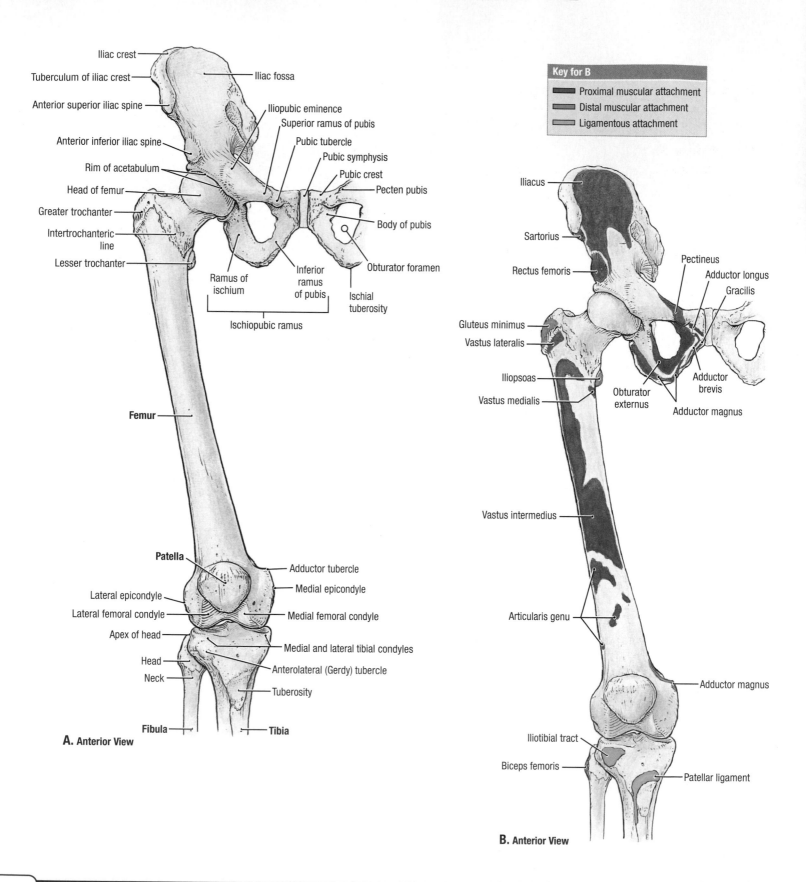

Key for B

- ▬ Proximal muscular attachment
- ▬ Distal muscular attachment
- ▬ Ligamentous attachment

A. Anterior View

Iliac crest
Tuberculum of iliac crest
Anterior superior iliac spine
Anterior inferior iliac spine
Rim of acetabulum
Head of femur
Greater trochanter
Intertrochanteric line
Lesser trochanter
Femur
Iliac fossa
Iliopubic eminence
Superior ramus of pubis
Pubic tubercle
Pubic symphysis
Pubic crest
Pecten pubis
Body of pubis
Obturator foramen
Ramus of ischium
Inferior ramus of pubis
Ischial tuberosity
Ischiopubic ramus

Patella
Lateral epicondyle
Lateral femoral condyle
Apex of head
Head
Neck
Fibula
Adductor tubercle
Medial epicondyle
Medial femoral condyle
Medial and lateral tibial condyles
Anterolateral (Gerdy) tubercle
Tuberosity
Tibia

B. Anterior View

Iliacus
Sartorius
Rectus femoris
Gluteus minimus
Vastus lateralis
Iliopsoas
Vastus medialis
Pectineus
Adductor longus
Gracilis
Obturator externus
Adductor brevis
Adductor magnus
Vastus intermedius
Articularis genu
Adductor magnus
Iliotibial tract
Biceps femoris
Patellar ligament

6.30   **Bones of Thigh and Proximal Leg**

A. Bony features. **B.** Muscle attachment sites.

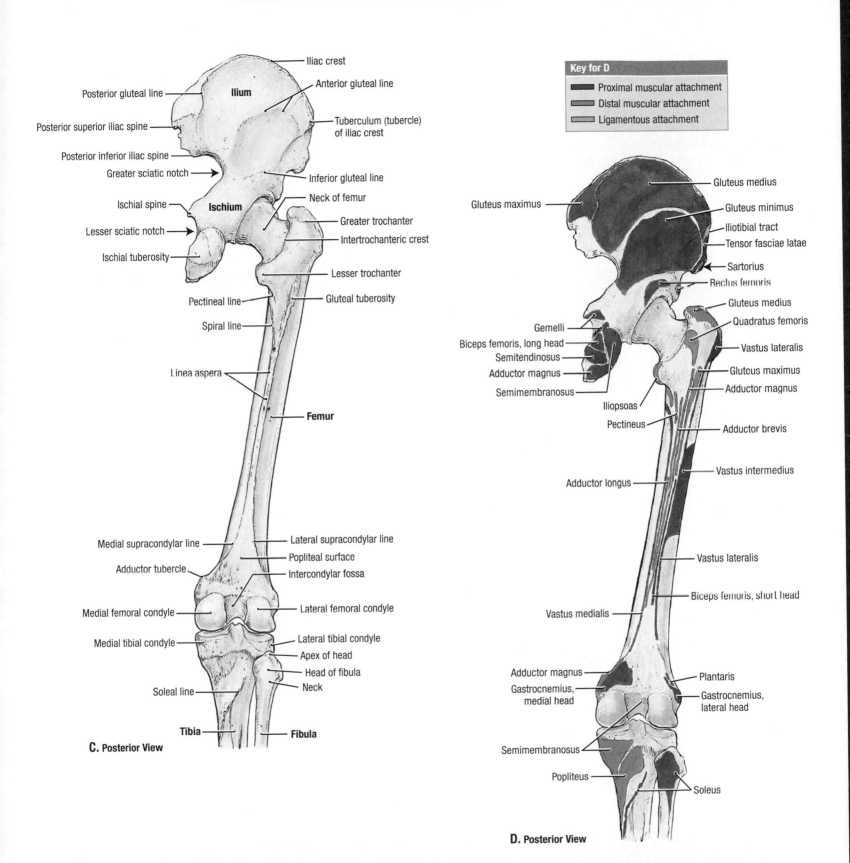

Key for D

■ Proximal muscular attachment
■ Distal muscular attachment
□ Ligamentous attachment

Iliac crest

Anterior gluteal line

Posterior gluteal line

Ilium

Posterior superior iliac spine

Tuberculum (tubercle) of iliac crest

Posterior inferior iliac spine

Greater sciatic notch

Inferior gluteal line

Ischial spine

Ischium

Neck of femur

Lesser sciatic notch

Greater trochanter

Intertrochanteric crest

Ischial tuberosity

Lesser trochanter

Pectineal line

Gluteal tuberosity

Spiral line

Linea aspera

Femur

Medial supracondylar line

Lateral supracondylar line

Adductor tubercle

Popliteal surface

Intercondylar fossa

Medial femoral condyle

Lateral femoral condyle

Medial tibial condyle

Lateral tibial condyle

Apex of head

Head of fibula

Soleal line

Neck

Tibia

Fibula

C. Posterior View

Gluteus maximus

Gluteus medius

Gluteus minimus

Iliotibial tract

Tensor fasciae latae

Sartorius

Rectus femoris

Gemelli

Gluteus medius

Biceps femoris, long head

Quadratus femoris

Semitendinosus

Vastus lateralis

Adductor magnus

Gluteus maximus

Semimembranosus

Adductor magnus

Iliopsoas

Pectineus

Adductor brevis

Vastus intermedius

Adductor longus

Vastus lateralis

Biceps femoris, short head

Vastus medialis

Adductor magnus

Plantaris

Gastrocnemius, medial head

Gastrocnemius, lateral head

Semimembranosus

Popliteus

Soleus

D. Posterior View

Bones of Thigh and Proximal Leg *(continued)*

6.30

C. Bony features. **D.** Muscle attachment sites.

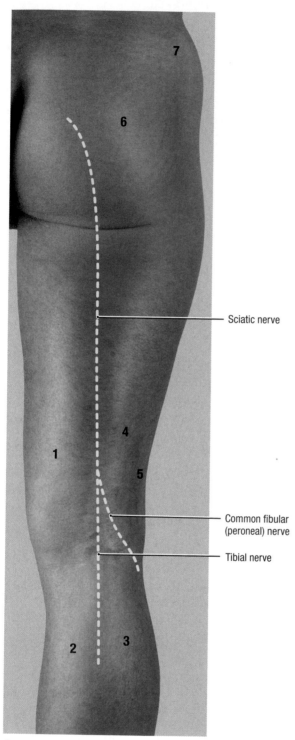

A. Posterior View

Sciatic nerve

Common fibular
(peroneal) nerve

Tibial nerve

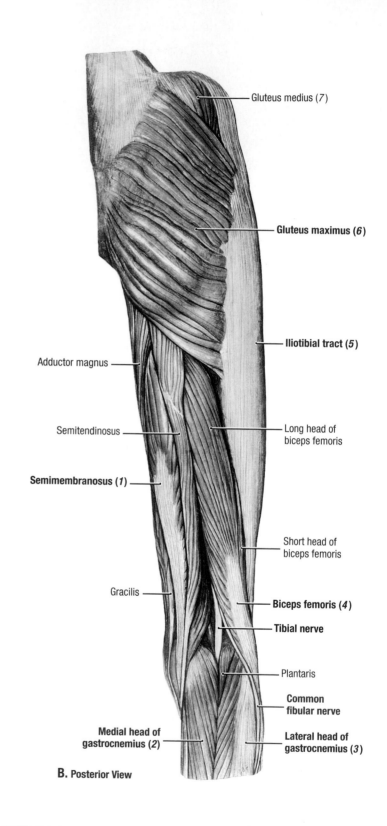

Gluteus medius (*7*)

Gluteus maximus (*6*)

Iliotibial tract (*5*)

Adductor magnus

Semitendinosus

Long head of
biceps femoris

Semimembranosus (*1*)

Short head of
biceps femoris

Gracilis

Biceps femoris (*4*)

Tibial nerve

Plantaris

**Common
fibular nerve**

Medial head of
gastrocnemius (*2*)

**Lateral head of
gastrocnemius (*3*)**

B. Posterior View

| 6.31 | **Muscles of Gluteal Region and Posterior Thigh** |

A. Surface anatomy. Numbers refer to structures labeled in *Part B.*
B. Superficial dissection. Muscles of gluteal region and posterior thigh (hamstring muscles consist of semimembranosus, semitendinosus, and biceps femoris).

Hamstring strains (pulled and/or torn hamstrings) are common in running, jumping, and quick-start sports. The muscular exertion required to excel in these sports may tear part of the proximal attachments of the hamstrings from the ischial tuberosity.

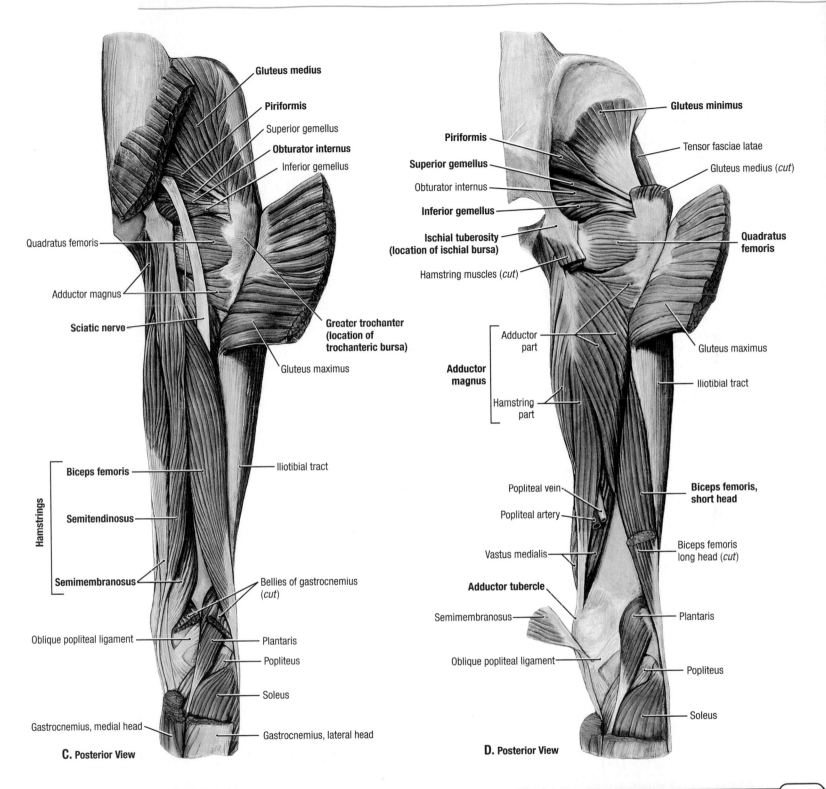

Gluteus medius

Piriformis

Superior gemellus

Obturator internus

Inferior gemellus

Quadratus femoris

Adductor magnus

Sciatic nerve

Greater trochanter
(location of
trochanteric bursa)

Gluteus maximus

Iliotibial tract

Biceps femoris

Hamstrings

Semitendinosus

Semimembranosus

Oblique popliteal ligament

Plantaris

Popliteus

Soleus

Gastrocnemius, medial head

Bellies of gastrocnemius
(cut)

Gastrocnemius, lateral head

C. Posterior View

Gluteus minimus

Tensor fasciae latae

Gluteus medius (cut)

Piriformis

Superior gemellus

Obturator internus

Inferior gemellus

Ischial tuberosity
(location of ischial bursa)

Hamstring muscles (cut)

**Quadratus
femoris**

Adductor
part

**Adductor
magnus**

Hamstring
part

Gluteus maximus

Iliotibial tract

Popliteal vein

Popliteal artery

Vastus medialis

Adductor tubercle

Semimembranosus

Oblique popliteal ligament

**Biceps femoris,
short head**

Biceps femoris
long head (cut)

Plantaris

Popliteus

Soleus

D. Posterior View

Muscles of Gluteal Region and Posterior Thigh (continued)   **6.31**

C. Muscles of gluteal region and posterior thigh with gluteus maximus reflected. D. Adductor magnus muscle. The adductor magnus has two parts: one belongs to the adductor group, innervated by the obturator nerve, and the other to the hamstring group, innervated by the tibial portion of the sciatic nerve. The trochanteric bursa separates the superior fibers of the gluteus maximus from the greater trochanter of the femur, and the ischial bursa separates the inferior part of the gluteus maximus from the ischial tuberosity.

Diffuse deep pain in the lateral thigh region (e.g., during stair climbing) may be caused by **trochanteric bursitis**. It is characterized by point tenderness over the greater trochanter, with pain radiating along the iliotibial tract. **Ischial bursitis** results from excessive friction between the ischial bursae and ischial tuberosities (e.g., as from cycling).

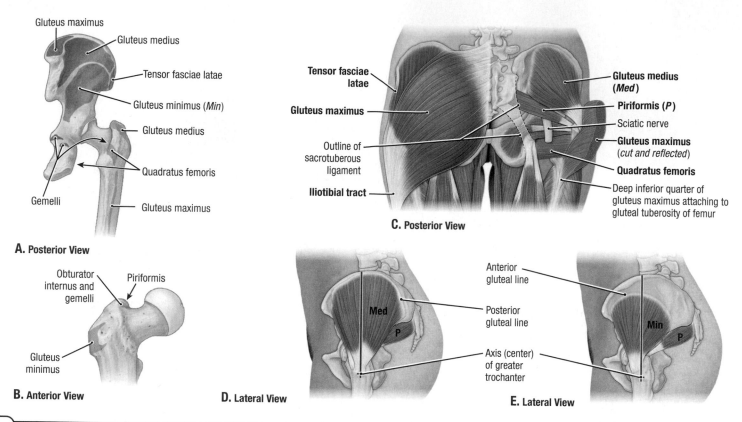

A. Posterior View

B. Anterior View

D. Lateral View

C. Posterior View

E. Lateral View

6.32   **Muscles of Gluteal Region**

A. and **B.** Attachments. **C.** Gluteus maximus and tensor fasciae latae. **D.** Gluteus medius. **E.** Gluteus minimus.

TABLE 6.5	Muscles of Gluteal Region			
Muscle	**Proximal Attachment[a] (Red)**	**Distal Attachment[a] (Blue)**	**Innervation[b]**	**Main Actions**
Gluteus maximus	Ilium posterior to posterior gluteal line, dorsal surface of sacrum and coccyx, sacrotuberous ligament	Iliotibial tract that inserts into lateral condyle of tibia; lower, deep fibers to gluteal tuberosity	Inferior gluteal nerve (L5, **S1, S2**)	Extends hip joint and assists in lateral rotation; steadies thigh and assists in raising trunk from flexed position
Gluteus medius	External surface of ilium between anterior and posterior gluteal lines; gluteal fascia	Lateral surface of greater trochanter of femur	Superior gluteal nerve (**L5**, S1)	Abducts and medially rotates hip joint[c]; keeps pelvis level when opposite leg is off ground and advances pelvis during swing phase of gait
Gluteus minimus	External surface of ilium between anterior and inferior gluteal lines	Anterior surface of greater trochanter of femur		
Tensor fasciae latae (TFL)	Anterior superior iliac spine and iliac crest	Iliotibial tract that attaches to lateral condyle (Gerdy tubercle) of tibia	Superiopr gluteal nerve (L4, L5)	Abducts and medially rotates hip joint; helps to keep knee extended; stabilizes trunk on thigh
Piriformis	Anterior surface of sacrum and sacrotuberous ligament	Superior border of greater trochanter of femur	Anterior rami of S1 and S2	Laterally rotate extended hip joint and abduct flexed hip joint; steady femoral head in acetabulum
Obturator internus	Pelvic surface of obturator membrane and surrounding bones	Medial surface (trochanteric fossa) of greater trochanter of femur by common tendons	Nerve to obturator internus (L5, S1)	
Superior gemellus	Ischial spine			
Inferior gemellus	Ischial tuberosity			
Quadratus femoris	Lateral border of ischial tuberosity	Quadrate tubercle on intertrochanteric crest of femur	Nerve to quadratus femoris (L5, S1)	Laterally rotates hip joint,[d] steadies femoral head in acetabulum

[a]See Figure 6.25 for muscle attachments.
[b]Numbers indicate spinal cord segmental innervation of nerves (e.g., L5, S1, and S2 indicate that the inferior gluteal nerve supplying gluteus maximus is derived from three segments of the spinal cord; boldface type [S1, S2] indicates main segmental innervation). Damage to one or more of these spinal cord segments or to motor nerve roots arising from these segments results in paralysis of the muscles concerned.
[c]Gluteus medius and minimus: Anterior fibers medially rotate hip joint and posterior fibers laterally rotate hip joint.
[d]There are six lateral rotators of the hip joint: piriformis, obturator internus, gemelli (superior and inferior), quadratus femoris, and obturator externus. These muscles also stabilize the hip joint.

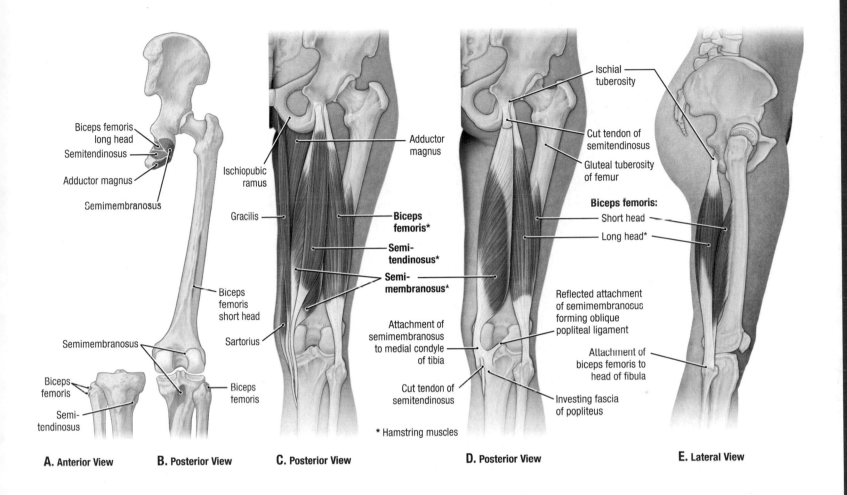

Biceps femoris
long head

Semitendinosus

Adductor magnus

Semimembranosus

Biceps
femoris
short head

Semimembranosus

Biceps
femoris

Semi-
tendinosus

A. Anterior View

Ischiopubic
ramus

Gracilis

Biceps
femoris
short head

Sartorius

Biceps
femoris

B. Posterior View

Adductor
magnus

**Biceps
femoris***

**Semi-
tendinosus***

**Semi-
membranosus***

Attachment of
semimembranosus
to medial condyle
of tibia

Cut tendon of
semitendinosus

* Hamstring muscles

C. Posterior View

Ischial
tuberosity

Cut tendon of
semitendinosus

Gluteal tuberosity
of femur

Biceps femoris:

Short head

Long head*

Reflected attachment
of semimembranosus
forming oblique
popliteal ligament

Attachment of
biceps femoris to
head of fibula

Investing fascia
of popliteus

D. Posterior View

Biceps femoris:
Short head
Long head*

Attachment of
biceps femoris to
head of fibula

E. Lateral View

Muscles of Posterior Thigh (I–III)   6.33

A. Attachments. **B.** Superficial layer. **C.** Intermediate layer. **D.** Deep layer.

TABLE 6.6	Muscles of Posterior Thigh (Hamstring)			
Muscle[a]	**Proximal Attachment[a] (Red)**	**Distal Attachment[a] (Blue)**	**Innervation[b]**	**Main Actions**
Semitendinosus	Ischial tuberosity	Medial surface of superior part of tibia	Tibial division of sciatic nerve (L5, S1, and S2)	Extend hip joint; flex knee joint and rotate it medially; when hip and knee joints are flexed, can extend trunk
Semimembranosus		Posterior part of medial condyle of tibia; reflected attachment forms oblique popliteal ligament to lateral femoral condyle		
Biceps femoris	*Long head:* ischial tuberosity *Short head:* linea aspera and lateral supracondylar line of femur	Lateral side of head of fibula; tendon is split at this site by fibular collateral ligament of knee	*Long head:* tibial division of sciatic nerve (L5, S1, and S2) *Short head:* common fibular (peroneal) division of sciatic nerve (L5, S1, and S2)	Flexes knee joint and rotates it laterally; extends hip joint (e.g., when initiating a walking gait)

[a]See Figure 6.25 for muscle attachments.
[b]See Table 6.2 for explanation of segmental innervation.

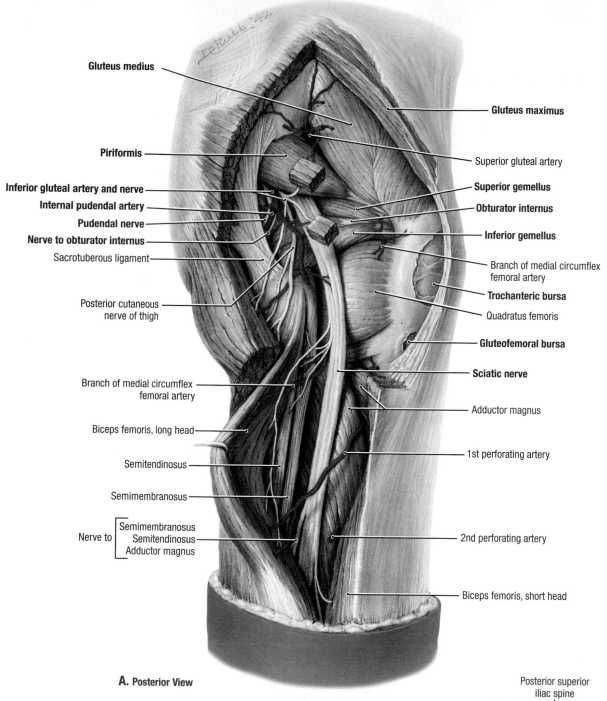

Gluteus medius

Gluteus maximus

Piriformis

Superior gluteal artery

Inferior gluteal artery and nerve

Superior gemellus

Internal pudendal artery

Obturator internus

Pudendal nerve

Inferior gemellus

Nerve to obturator internus

Sacrotuberous ligament

Branch of medial circumflex femoral artery

Trochanteric bursa

Posterior cutaneous nerve of thigh

Quadratus femoris

Gluteofemoral bursa

Branch of medial circumflex femoral artery

Sciatic nerve

Adductor magnus

Biceps femoris, long head

1st perforating artery

Semitendinosus

Semimembranosus

Nerve to [Semimembranosus / Semitendinosus / Adductor magnus]

2nd perforating artery

Biceps femoris, short head

A. Posterior View

6.34 Muscles of Gluteal Region and Posterior Thigh (IV)

A. Dissection. The gluteus maximus muscle is split superiorly and inferiorly, and the middle part is excised; two cubes remain to identify its nerve. The gluteus maximus is the only muscle to cover the greater trochanter; it is aponeurotic and has underlying bursae where it glides on the trochanter (trochanteric bursa) and the aponeurosis of the vastus lateralis muscle (gluteofemoral bursa). **B. Intragluteal injection.** Injections can be made safely only into the superolateral part of the buttock to avoid injury to the sciatic and gluteal nerves. This site has a rich vascular network from the superior gluteal vessels that lie between the gluteus medius and minimus muscles.

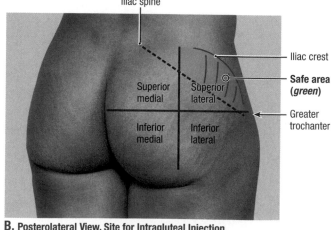

Posterior superior iliac spine

Iliac crest

Safe area (*green*)

Superior medial

Superior lateral

Greater trochanter

Inferior medial

Inferior lateral

B. Posterolateral View, Site for Intragluteal Injection

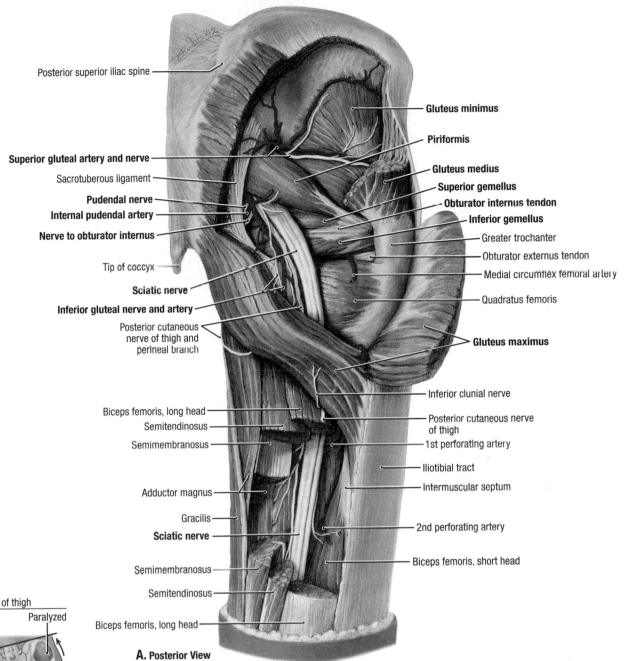

Posterior superior iliac spine

Gluteus minimus

Piriformis

Superior gluteal artery and nerve

Gluteus medius

Sacrotuberous ligament

Superior gemellus

Obturator internus tendon

Pudendal nerve

Inferior gemellus

Internal pudendal artery

Greater trochanter

Nerve to obturator internus

Obturator externus tendon

Tip of coccyx

Medial circumflex femoral artery

Sciatic nerve

Quadratus femoris

Inferior gluteal nerve and artery

Posterior cutaneous
nerve of thigh and
perineal branch

Gluteus maximus

Inferior clunial nerve

Biceps femoris, long head

Posterior cutaneous nerve
of thigh

Semitendinosus

1st perforating artery

Semimembranosus

Iliotibial tract

Intermuscular septum

Adductor magnus

Gracilis

Sciatic nerve

2nd perforating artery

Semimembranosus

Biceps femoris, short head

Semitendinosus

Biceps femoris, long head

A. Posterior View

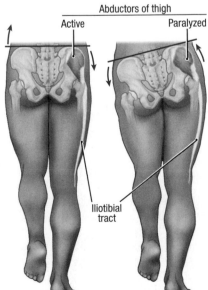

Abductors of thigh

Active

Paralyzed

Iliotibial
tract

B. Posterior View   **C. Posterior View**

Muscles of Gluteal Region and Posterior Thigh (V)

6.35

A. Dissection. The proximal three quarters of the gluteus maximus muscle are reflected, and parts of the gluteus medius and the three hamstring muscles are excised. The superior gluteal vessels and nerves emerge superior to the piriformis muscle; all other vessels and nerves emerge inferior to it. **B. Role of hip abductors in stabilizing pelvis.** When the weight is borne by one limb, the muscles on the supported side fix the pelvis so that it does not sag to the unsupported side, keeping the pelvis level. **C. Pelvic tilt due to paralysis of hip abductors.** When the right **abductors are paralyzed**, owing to a lesion of the right superior gluteal nerve, fixation by these muscles is lost and the pelvis tilts to the unsupported left side (positive Trendelenburg sign).

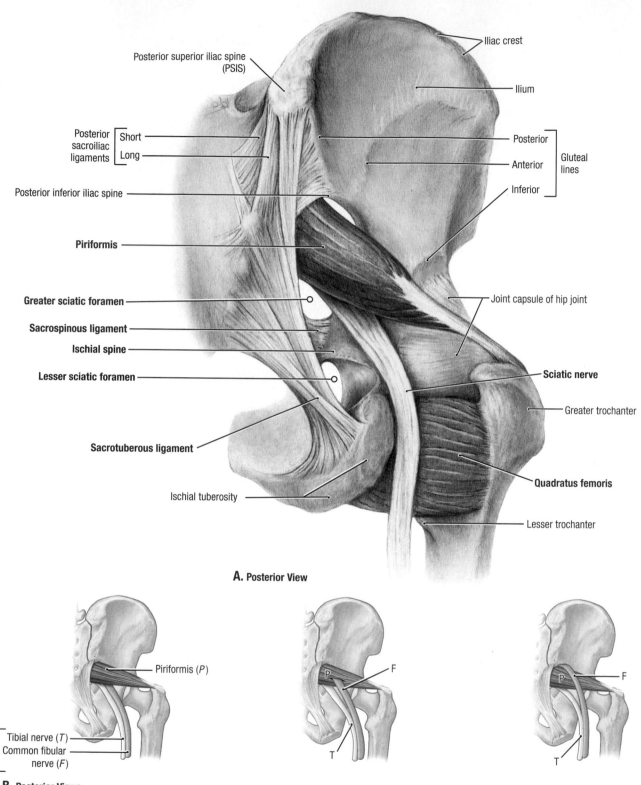

Posterior superior iliac spine (PSIS)

Iliac crest

Ilium

Posterior sacroiliac ligaments
Short
Long

Posterior inferior iliac spine

Piriformis

Greater sciatic foramen

Sacrospinous ligament

Ischial spine

Lesser sciatic foramen

Sacrotuberous ligament

Ischial tuberosity

Posterior
Anterior
Inferior
Gluteal lines

Joint capsule of hip joint

Sciatic nerve

Greater trochanter

Quadratus femoris

Lesser trochanter

A. Posterior View

Piriformis (*P*)

Sciatic nerve
Tibial nerve (*T*)
Common fibular nerve (*F*)

P
F

T

P
F

T

B. Posterior Views

6.36   **Lateral Rotators of Hip, Sciatic Nerve, and Ligaments of Gluteal Region**

A. **Piriformis and quadratus femoris. B.** **Relationship of sciatic nerve to piriformis muscle.** Of 640 limbs studied in Dr. Grant's laboratory, in 87%, the tibial and fibular (peroneal) divisions passed inferior to the piriformis (*left*); in 12.2%, the fibular (peroneal) division passed through the piriformis (*center*); and in 0.5%, the fibular (peroneal) division passed superior to the piriformis (*right*).

Sciatic nerve block. Sensation conveyed by the sciatic nerve can be blocked by injecting an anesthetic agent a few centimeters inferior to the midpoint of the line joining the *PSIS* and the superior border of the greater trochanter. Paresthesia radiates to the foot because of anesthesia of the plantar nerves, which are terminal branches of the tibial nerve derived from the sciatic nerve.

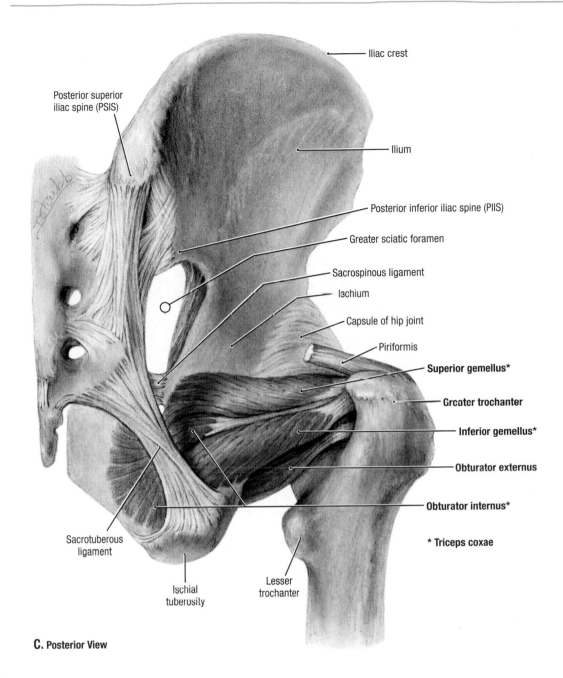

Iliac crest

Posterior superior iliac spine (PSIS)

Ilium

Posterior inferior iliac spine (PIIS)

Greater sciatic foramen

Sacrospinous ligament

Ischium

Capsule of hip joint

Piriformis

Superior gemellus*

Greater trochanter

Inferior gemellus*

Obturator externus

Obturator internus*

* Triceps coxae

Sacrotuberous ligament

Ischial tuberosity

Lesser trochanter

C. Posterior View

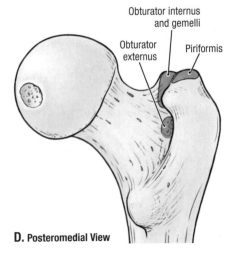

Obturator internus and gemelli

Obturator externus

Piriformis

D. Posteromedial View

Lateral Rotators of Hip, Sciatic Nerve, and Ligaments of Gluteal Region *(continued)* | 6.36

C. Obturator internus, obturator externus, and superior and inferior gemelli. **D.** Muscle attachments of posterior aspect of proximal femur.

- The obturator internus is located partly in the pelvis, where it covers most of the lateral wall of the lesser pelvis. It leaves the pelvis through the lesser sciatic foramen, makes a right-angle turn, becomes tendinous, and receives the distal attachments of the gemelli before attaching to the medial surface of the greater trochanter (trochanteric fossa).
- The obturator externus extends from the external surface of the obturator membrane and surrounding bone of the pelvis to the trochanteric fossa, passing directly under the acetabulum and neck of the femur.
- **Common fibular nerve compression at piriformis.** In the approximately 12% of people in whom the common fibular division of the sciatic nerve passes through the piriformis, this muscle may compress the nerve.

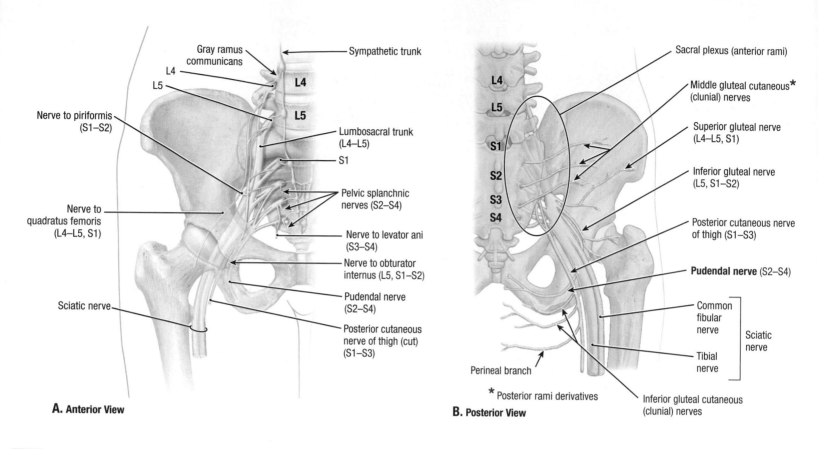

A. Anterior View

B. Posterior View

* Posterior rami derivatives

6.37   Nerves of Gluteal Region

The muscles of the gluteal region are innervated by the sacral plexus.

TABLE 6.7	Nerves of Gluteal Region		
Nerve	**Origin**	**Course**	**Distribution in Gluteal Region**
Gluteal cutaneous (clunial) nerves (superior, middle, and inferior)	*Superior:* posterior rami of L1–L3 nerves *Middle:* posterior rami of S1–S3 nerves *Inferior:* posterior cutaneous nerve of thigh	*Superior nerves* cross iliac crest; *middle nerves* exit through posterior sacral foramina and enter gluteal region; *inferior nerves* curve around inferior border of gluteus maximus	Gluteal region as far laterally as greater trochanter
Sciatic	Sacral plexus (L4–S3)	Exits pelvis via greater sciatic foramen inferior to piriformis to enter gluteal region	No muscles in gluteal region
Posterior cutaneous nerve of thigh	Sacral plexus (S1–S3)	Exits pelvis via greater sciatic foramen inferior to piriformis, emerges from inferior border of gluteus maximus coursing deep to fascia lata	Skin of buttock via inferior cluneal branches, skin over posterior thigh and popliteal fossa; skin of lateral perineum and upper medial thigh via perineal branch
Superior gluteal	Anterior rami of L4–S1 nerves	Exits pelvis via greater sciatic foramen superior to piriformis; courses between gluteus medius and minimus	Gluteus medius, gluteus minimus, and tensor fasciae latae
Inferior gluteal	Anterior rami of L5–S2 nerves	Exits pelvis via greater sciatic foramen inferior to piriformis, dividing into multiple branches	Gluteus maximus
Nerve to quadratus femoris	Anterior rami of L4–S1 nerves	Exits pelvis via greater sciatic foramen deep to sciatic nerve	Posterior hip joint, inferior gemellus, and quadratus femoris
Pudendal	Anterior rami of S2–S4 nerves	Exits pelvis via greater sciatic foramen inferior to piriformis; descends posterior to sacrospinous ligament; enters perineum (pudendal canal) through lesser sciatic foramen	No structures in gluteal region (supplies most of perineum)
Nerve to obturator internus	Anterior rami of L5–S2 nerves	Exits pelvis via greater sciatic foramen inferior to piriformis; descends posterior to ischial spine; enters lesser sciatic foramen and passes to obturator internus	Superior gemellus and obturator internus

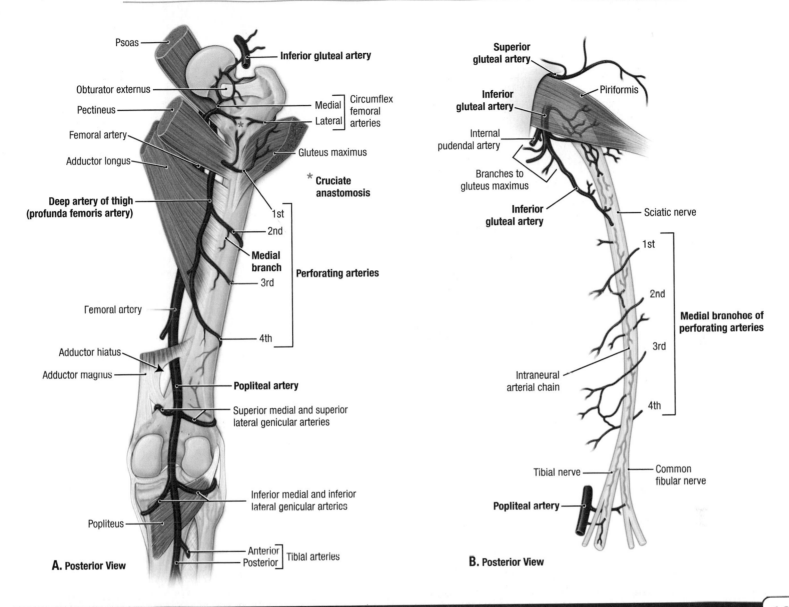

A. Posterior View

- Psoas
- **Inferior gluteal artery**
- Obturator externus
- Pectineus
- Medial ⎱ Circumflex
- Lateral ⎰ femoral arteries
- Femoral artery
- Adductor longus
- Gluteus maximus
- **Deep artery of thigh (profunda femoris artery)**
- * **Cruciate anastomosis**
- 1st
- 2nd
- **Medial branch**
- **Perforating arteries**
- 3rd
- Femoral artery
- 4th
- Adductor hiatus
- Adductor magnus
- **Popliteal artery**
- Superior medial and superior lateral genicular arteries
- Inferior medial and inferior lateral genicular arteries
- Popliteus
- Anterior ⎱ Tibial arteries
- Posterior ⎰

B. Posterior View

- **Superior gluteal artery**
- Piriformis
- **Inferior gluteal artery**
- Internal pudendal artery
- Branches to gluteus maximus
- **Inferior gluteal artery**
- Sciatic nerve
- 1st
- 2nd
- **Medial branches of perforating arteries**
- 3rd
- Intraneural arterial chain
- 4th
- Tibial nerve
- Common fibular nerve
- **Popliteal artery**

Arteries of Gluteal Region and Posterior Thigh   6.38

TABLE 6.8	Arteries of Gluteal Region and Posterior Thigh		
Artery	**Origin**	**Course**	**Distribution**
Superior gluteal	Internal iliac	Enters gluteal region through greater sciatic foramen superior to piriformis; divides into superficial and deep branches; anastomoses with inferior gluteal and medial circumflex femoral arteries	*Superficial branch:* superior gluteus maximus *Deep branch:* runs between gluteus medius and minimus, supplying both and tensor fasciae latae
Inferior gluteal		Enters gluteal region through greater sciatic foramen inferior to piriformis; descends on medial side of sciatic nerve; anastomoses with superior gluteal artery and participates in cruciate anastomosis of thigh	Inferior gluteus maximus, obturator internus, quadratus femoris, and superior parts of hamstring muscles
Internal pudendal		Enters gluteal region through greater sciatic foramen; descends posterior to ischial spine; exits gluteal region via lesser sciatic foramen to perineum	No structures in gluteal region (supplies external genitalia and muscles in perineal region)
Perforating arteries	Deep artery of thigh (profunda femoris artery) (may arise from femoral)	Perforate aponeurotic portion of adductor magnus attachment and medial intermuscular septum to enter and supply muscular branches to posterior compartment; then pierce lateral intermuscular septum to enter posterolateral aspect of anterior compartment	Hamstring muscles in posterior compartment; posterior portion of vastus lateralis in anterior compartment; femur (via femoral nutrient arteries); reinforce arterial supply of sciatic nerve
Lateral circumflex femoral		Passes laterally deep to sartorius and rectus femoris; enters gluteal region	Anterior part of gluteal region
Medial circumflex femoral		Passes medially and posteriorly between pectineus and iliopsoas; enters gluteal region	Supplies most blood to head and neck of femur; hip region

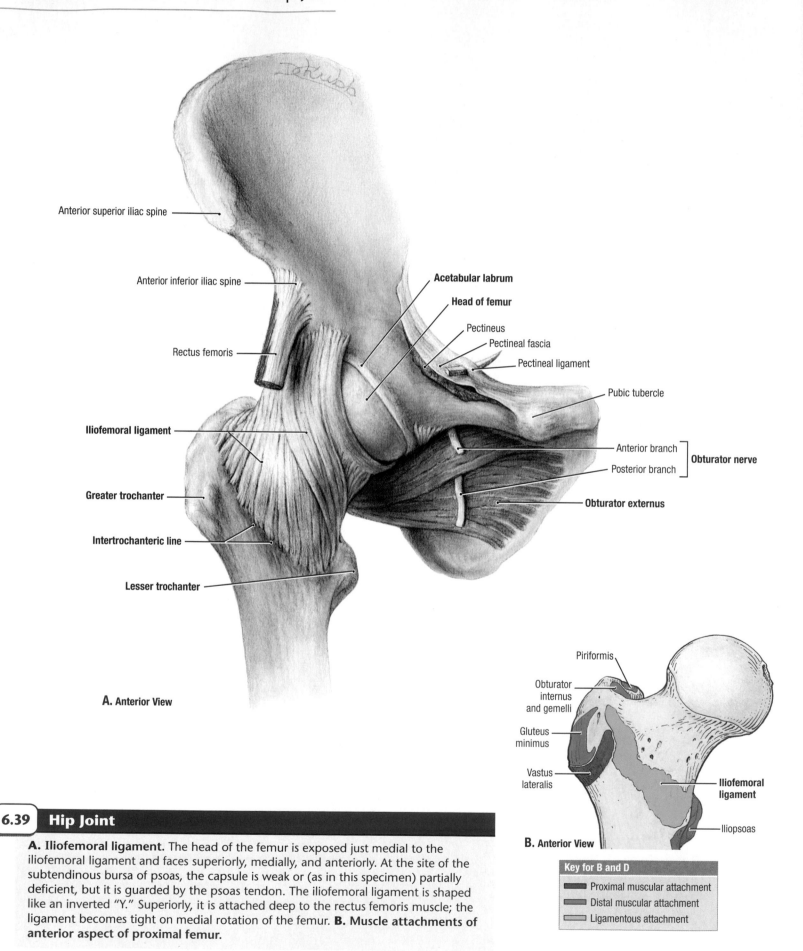

Anterior superior iliac spine

Anterior inferior iliac spine

Rectus femoris

Iliofemoral ligament

Greater trochanter

Intertrochanteric line

Lesser trochanter

Acetabular labrum

Head of femur

Pectineus

Pectineal fascia

Pectineal ligament

Pubic tubercle

Anterior branch

Posterior branch

Obturator nerve

Obturator externus

A. Anterior View

Piriformis

Obturator internus and gemelli

Gluteus minimus

Vastus lateralis

Iliofemoral ligament

Iliopsoas

B. Anterior View

| 6.39 | **Hip Joint** |

A. Iliofemoral ligament. The head of the femur is exposed just medial to the iliofemoral ligament and faces superiorly, medially, and anteriorly. At the site of the subtendinous bursa of psoas, the capsule is weak or (as in this specimen) partially deficient, but it is guarded by the psoas tendon. The iliofemoral ligament is shaped like an inverted "Y." Superiorly, it is attached deep to the rectus femoris muscle; the ligament becomes tight on medial rotation of the femur. **B.** Muscle attachments of anterior aspect of proximal femur.

Key for B and D

- ▬ Proximal muscular attachment
- ▬ Distal muscular attachment
- ▬ Ligamentous attachment

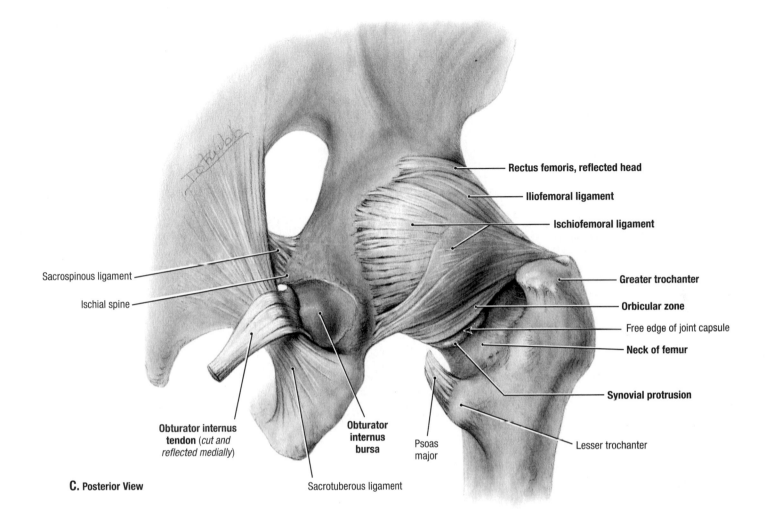

Rectus femoris, reflected head

Iliofemoral ligament

Ischiofemoral ligament

Sacrospinous ligament

Ischial spine

Greater trochanter

Orbicular zone

Free edge of joint capsule

Neck of femur

Synovial protrusion

Obturator internus tendon (*cut and reflected medially*)

Obturator internus bursa

Psoas major

Lesser trochanter

Sacrotuberous ligament

C. Posterior View

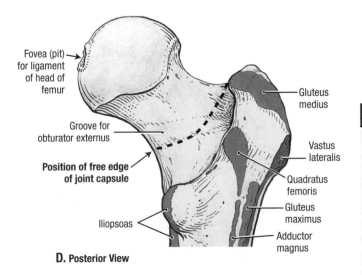

Fovea (pit) for ligament of head of femur

Groove for obturator externus

Position of free edge of joint capsule

Iliopsoas

Gluteus medius

Vastus lateralis

Quadratus femoris

Gluteus maximus

Adductor magnus

D. Posterior View

Hip Joint (*continued*) 6.39

C. Ischiofemoral ligament. The fibers of the capsule spiral to become taut during extension and medial rotation of the femur. The synovial membrane protrudes inferior to the fibrous capsule and forms a bursa for the tendon of the obturator externus muscle. Note the large subtendinous bursa of the obturator internus at the lesser sciatic notch, where the tendon turns 90 degrees to attach to the greater trochanter. **D. Muscle attachments onto posterior aspect of proximal femur.**

Osteoarthritis of the hip joint, characterized by pain, edema, limitation of motion, and erosion of articular cartilage, is a common cause of disability. During **hip replacement**, a metal prosthesis anchored to the person's femur by bone cement replaces the femoral head and neck. A plastic socket cemented to the hip bone replaces the acetabulum.

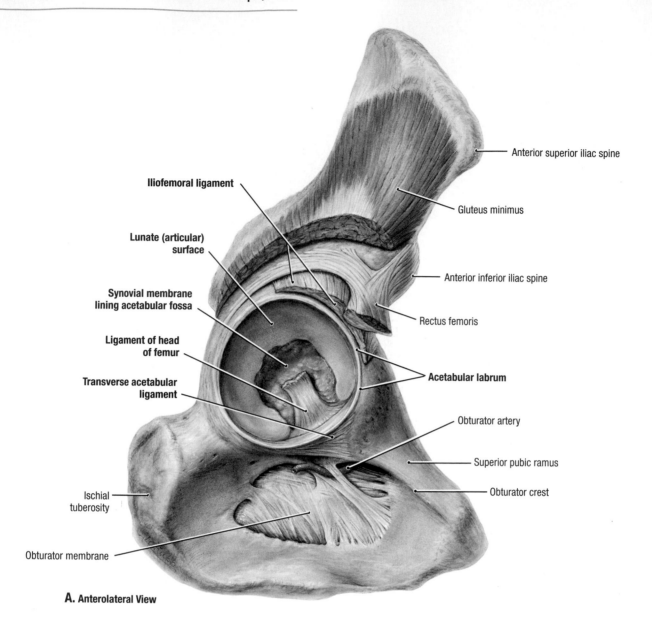

Iliofemoral ligament

Lunate (articular) surface

Synovial membrane lining acetabular fossa

Ligament of head of femur

Transverse acetabular ligament

Ischial tuberosity

Obturator membrane

Anterior superior iliac spine

Gluteus minimus

Anterior inferior iliac spine

Rectus femoris

Acetabular labrum

Obturator artery

Superior pubic ramus

Obturator crest

A. Anterolateral View

6.40 Acetabular Region

A. Dissection of acetabulum. **B.** Muscle attachments of acetabular region.

In *Part A*:
- The transverse acetabular ligament bridges the acetabular notch.
- The acetabular labrum is attached to the acetabular rim and transverse acetabular ligament and forms a complete ring around the head of the femur.
- The ligament of the head of the femur lies between the head of the femur and the acetabulum. These fibers are attached superiorly to the pit (fovea) on the head of the femur and inferiorly to the transverse acetabular ligament and the margins of the acetabular notch. The artery of the ligament of the head of the femur passes through the acetabular notch and into the ligament of the head of the femur.

In *Part B*:
- The adductor muscles of the thigh attach proximally to the pubic bone, ischiopubic ramus, and ischial tuberosity.
- The hamstring muscles have proximal attachment to the ischial tuberosity deep to the gluteus maximus.

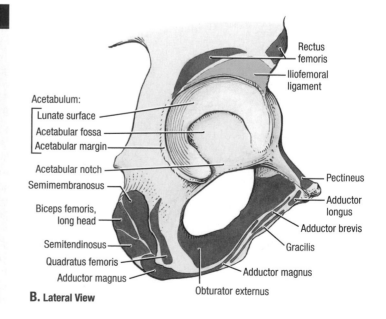

Rectus femoris

Iliofemoral ligament

Acetabulum:
Lunate surface
Acetabular fossa
Acetabular margin

Acetabular notch

Semimembranosus

Biceps femoris, long head

Semitendinosus

Quadratus femoris

Adductor magnus

Pectineus

Adductor longus

Adductor brevis

Gracilis

Adductor magnus

Obturator externus

B. Lateral View

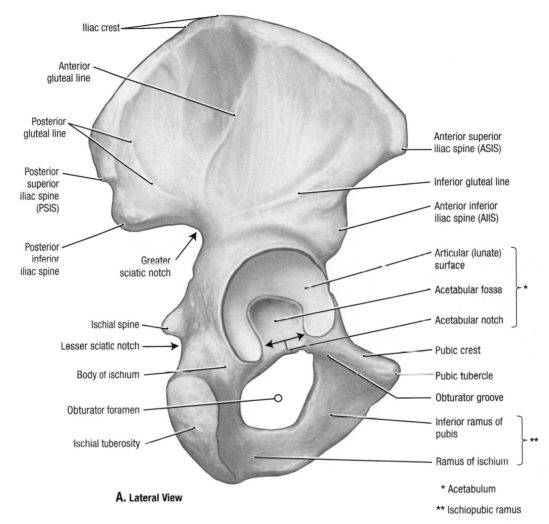

Iliac crest

Anterior
gluteal line

Posterior
gluteal line

Posterior
superior
iliac spine
(PSIS)

Posterior
inferior
iliac spine

Greater
sciatic notch

Ischial spine

Lesser sciatic notch

Body of ischium

Obturator foramen

Ischial tuberosity

Anterior superior
iliac spine (ASIS)

Inferior gluteal line

Anterior inferior
iliac spine (AIIS)

Articular (lunate)
surface

Acetabular fossa

Acetabular notch

Pubic crest

Pubic tubercle

Obturator groove

Inferior ramus of
pubis

Ramus of ischium

* Acetabulum

** Ischiopubic ramus

A. Lateral View

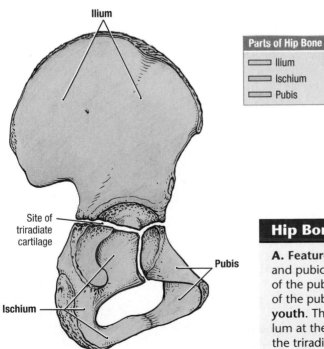

Ilium

Site of
triradiate
cartilage

Pubis

Ischium

B. Lateral View

Parts of Hip Bone

- Ilium
- Ischium
- Pubis

Hip Bone

6.41

A. Features of lateral aspect. In the anatomical position, the anterior superior iliac spine and pubic tubercle are in the same coronal plane, and the ischial spine and superior end of the pubic symphysis are in the same horizontal plane; the internal aspect of the body of the pubis faces superiorly, and the acetabulum faces inferolaterally. **B. Hip bone in youth.** The three parts of the hip bone (ilium, ischium, and pubis) meet in the acetabulum at the triradiate synchondrosis. One or more primary centers of ossification appear in the triradiate cartilage at approximately the 12th year. Secondary centers of ossification appear along the length of the iliac crest, at the anterior inferior iliac spine, the ischial tuberosity, and the pubic symphysis at about puberty; fusion is usually complete by age 23.

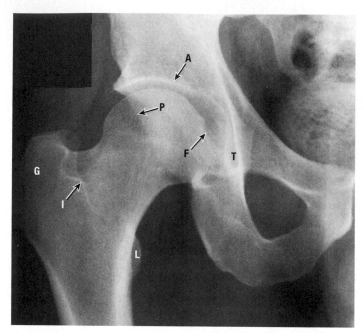

A. Anteroposterior Radiograph

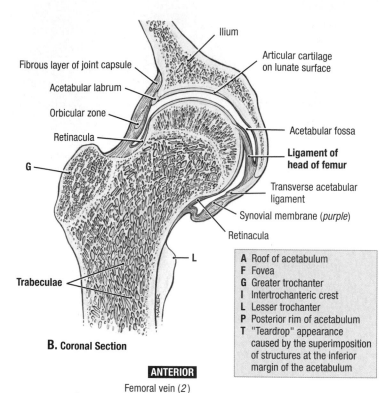

B. Coronal Section

A	Roof of acetabulum
F	Fovea
G	Greater trochanter
I	Intertrochanteric crest
L	Lesser trochanter
P	Posterior rim of acetabulum
T	"Teardrop" appearance caused by the superimposition of structures at the inferior margin of the acetabulum

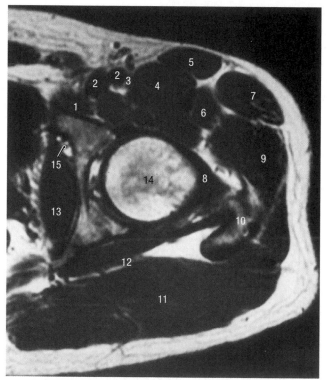

C. Transverse MRI

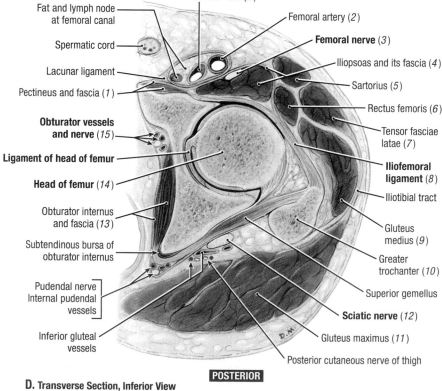

D. Transverse Section, Inferior View

6.42   **Radiograph and Transverse MRI of Hip Joint**

A. Radiograph. The "teardrop" appearance is caused by the super-imposition of structures at the inferior margin of the acetabulum.

B. Coronal section. C. MRI. Numbers refer to structures labeled in *Part D*. **D. Transverse section.**

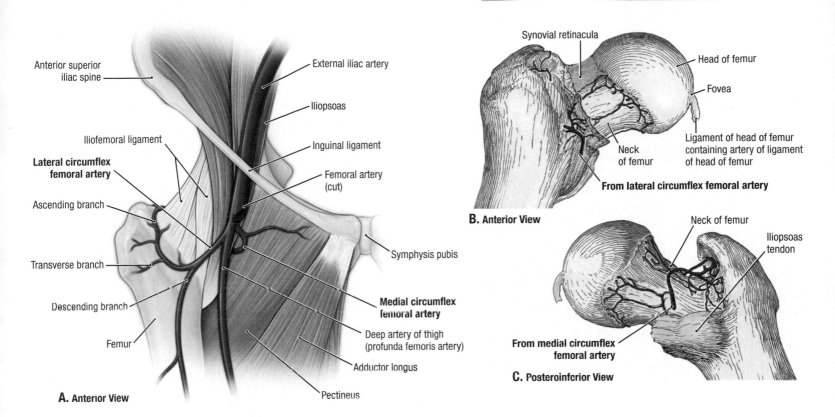

Anterior superior
iliac spine

External iliac artery

Iliopsoas

Iliofemoral ligament

Inguinal ligament

**Lateral circumflex
femoral artery**

Femoral artery
(cut)

Ascending branch

Symphysis pubis

Transverse branch

**Medial circumflex
femoral artery**

Descending branch

Deep artery of thigh
(profunda femoris artery)

Femur

Adductor longus

Pectineus

A. Anterior View

Synovial retinacula

Head of femur

Fovea

Neck
of femur

Ligament of head of femur
containing artery of ligament
of head of femur

From lateral circumflex femoral artery

B. Anterior View

Neck of femur

Iliopsoas
tendon

**From medial circumflex
femoral artery**

C. Posteroinferior View

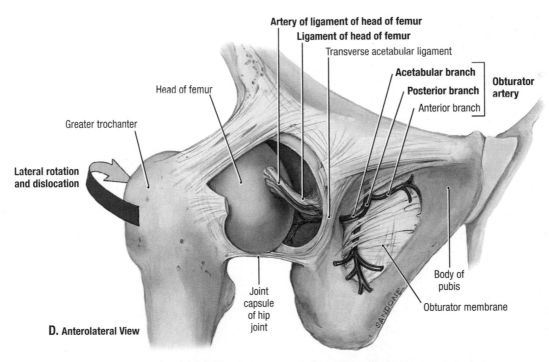

Artery of ligament of head of femur
Ligament of head of femur
Transverse acetabular ligament

Acetabular branch

**Obturator
artery**

Posterior branch

Anterior branch

Head of femur

Greater trochanter

**Lateral rotation
and dislocation**

Body of
pubis

Joint
capsule
of hip
joint

Obturator membrane

D. Anterolateral View

Blood Supply to Head of Femur

6.43

A. Medial and lateral circumflex femoral arteries in femoral triangle. **B.** Branches of lateral circumflex femoral artery. **C.** Branches of medial circumflex femoral artery. **D.** Obturator artery. The artery of the ligament of the head of the femur is a branch of the acetabular artery and can be seen traveling in the ligament to the head of the femur.

Fractures of the femoral neck often disrupt the blood supply to the head of the femur. The medial circumflex femoral artery supplies most of the blood to the head and neck of the femur and is often torn when the femoral neck is fractured. In some cases, the blood supplied by the artery of the ligament of the head may be the only blood received by the proximal fragment of the femoral head, which may be inadequate. If the blood vessels are ruptured, the fragment of bone may receive no blood and undergo aseptic avascular necrosis.

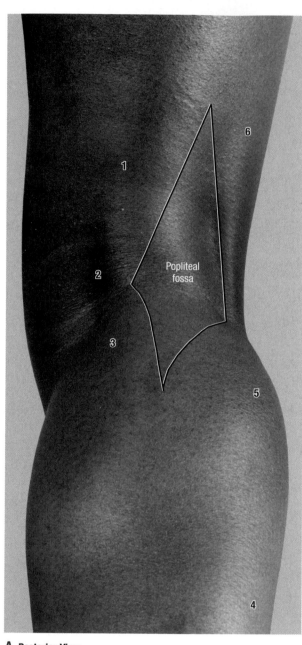

A. Posterior View

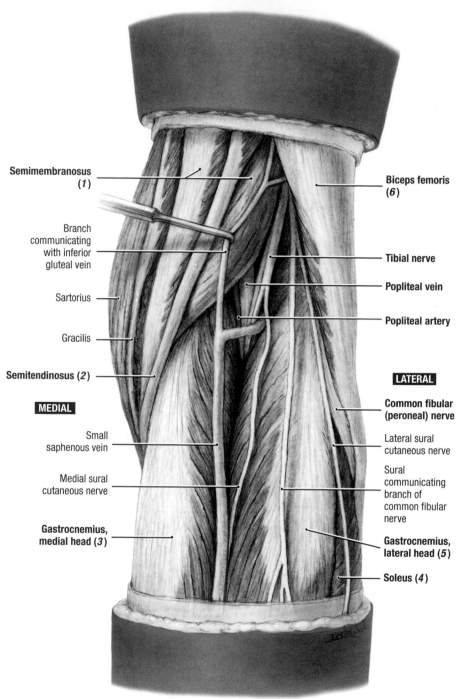

Semimembranosus (**1**)

Branch communicating with inferior gluteal vein

Sartorius

Gracilis

Semitendinosus (2)

MEDIAL

Small saphenous vein

Medial sural cutaneous nerve

Gastrocnemius, medial head (3)

Biceps femoris (6)

Tibial nerve

Popliteal vein

Popliteal artery

LATERAL

Common fibular (peroneal) nerve

Lateral sural cutaneous nerve

Sural communicating branch of common fibular nerve

Gastrocnemius, lateral head (5)

Soleus (4)

B. Posterior View

6.44   **Popliteal Fossa**

A. Surface anatomy. Numbers refer to structures labeled in *Part B*.
B. Superficial dissection.
    Because the popliteal artery is deep in the popliteal fossa, it may be difficult to feel the **popliteal pulse**. Palpation of this pulse is

commonly performed by placing the person in the prone position with the knee flexed to relax the popliteal fascia and hamstrings. The pulsations are best felt in the inferior part of the fossa. Weakening or loss of the popliteal pulse is a sign of femoral artery obstruction.

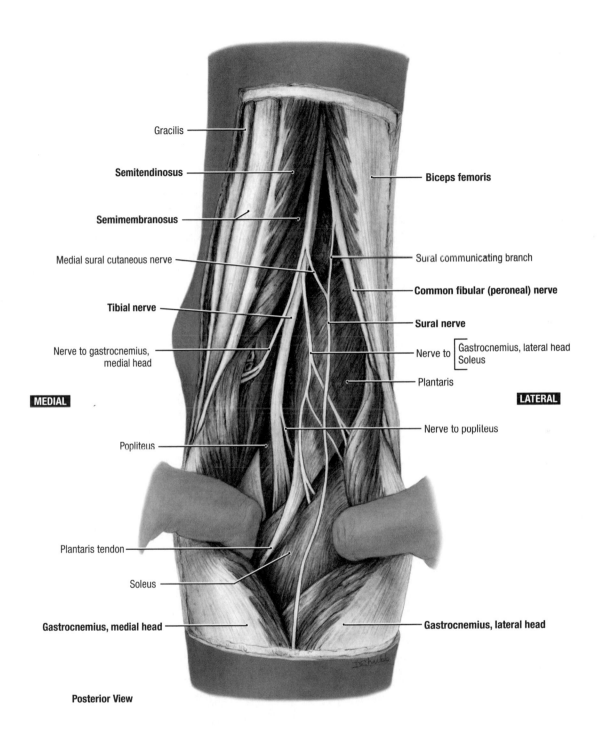

Gracilis

Semitendinosus

Semimembranosus

Medial sural cutaneous nerve

Tibial nerve

Nerve to gastrocnemius, medial head

MEDIAL

Popliteus

Plantaris tendon

Soleus

Gastrocnemius, medial head

Biceps femoris

Sural communicating branch

Common fibular (peroneal) nerve

Sural nerve

Nerve to [Gastrocnemius, lateral head / Soleus]

Plantaris

LATERAL

Nerve to popliteus

Gastrocnemius, lateral head

Posterior View

Nerves of Popliteal Fossa

6.45

The two heads of the gastrocnemius muscle are separated. A cutaneous branch of the tibial nerve joins a communicating branch of the common fibular (peroneal) nerve to form the sural nerve. In this specimen, the junction is high; usually it is 5 to 8 cm proximal to the ankle.

All motor branches in this region emerge from the tibial nerve, one branch from its medial side and the others from its lateral side; hence, it is safer to dissect on the medial side.

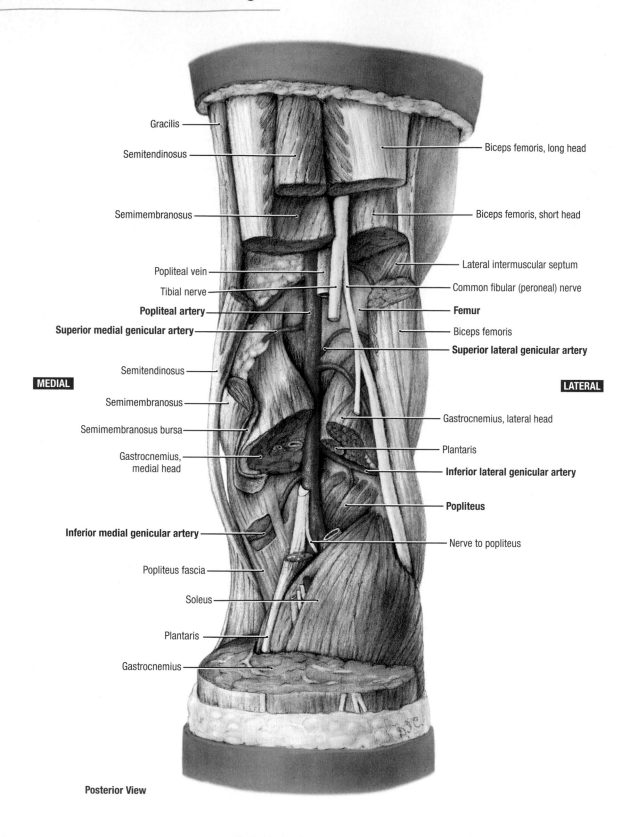

Gracilis

Semitendinosus

Semimembranosus

Popliteal vein

Tibial nerve

Popliteal artery

Superior medial genicular artery

Semitendinosus

MEDIAL

Semimembranosus

Semimembranosus bursa

Gastrocnemius, medial head

Inferior medial genicular artery

Popliteus fascia

Soleus

Plantaris

Gastrocnemius

Biceps femoris, long head

Biceps femoris, short head

Lateral intermuscular septum

Common fibular (peroneal) nerve

Femur

Biceps femoris

Superior lateral genicular artery

LATERAL

Gastrocnemius, lateral head

Plantaris

Inferior lateral genicular artery

Popliteus

Nerve to popliteus

Posterior View

6.46 Deep Dissection of Popliteal Fossa

The common fibular (peroneal) nerve follows the posterior border of the biceps femoris muscle, formed centrally by the fibrous capsule of the knee joint. The popliteal artery lies on the floor of the popliteal fossa. The floor is formed by the femur, capsule of the knee joint, and popliteus muscle and fascia. The popliteal artery gives off genicular branches that also lie on the floor of the fossa. A **popliteal aneurysm** (abnormal dilation of all or part of the popliteal artery) usually causes edema (swelling) and pain in the popliteal fossa. If the femoral artery has to be ligated, blood can bypass the occlusion through the genicular anastomosis and reach the popliteal artery distal to the ligation.

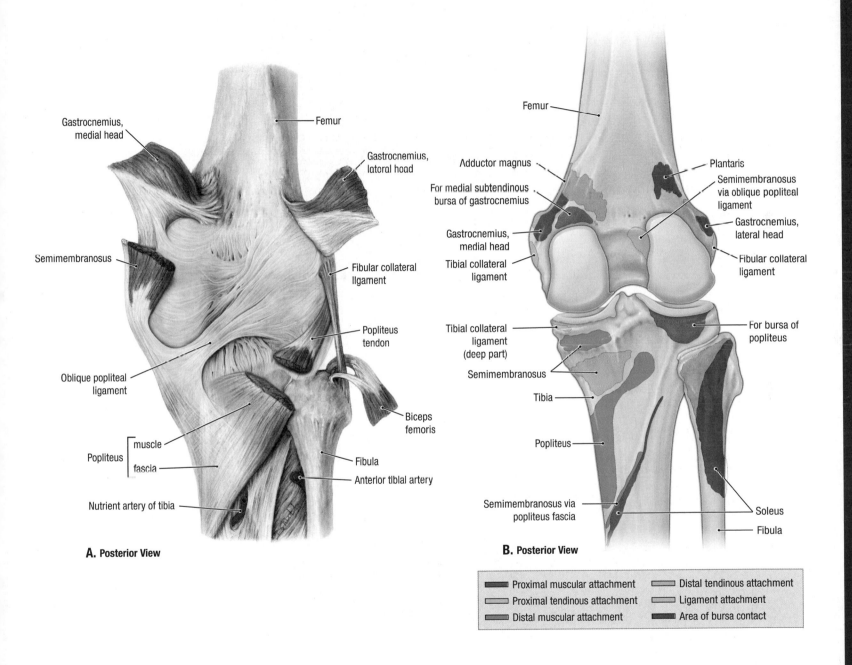

Gastrocnemius, medial head
Femur
Gastrocnemius, lateral head
Semimembranosus
Fibular collateral ligament
Popliteus tendon
Oblique popliteal ligament
Biceps femoris
Popliteus [muscle
fascia]
Fibula
Anterior tibial artery
Nutrient artery of tibia

A. Posterior View

Femur
Adductor magnus
Plantaris
For medial subtendinous bursa of gastrocnemius
Semimembranosus via oblique popliteal ligament
Gastrocnemius, medial head
Gastrocnemius, lateral head
Tibial collateral ligament
Fibular collateral ligament
Tibial collateral ligament (deep part)
For bursa of popliteus
Semimembranosus
Tibia
Popliteus
Semimembranosus via popliteus fascia
Soleus
Fibula

B. Posterior View

▬ Proximal muscular attachment	▭ Distal tendinous attachment
▭ Proximal tendinous attachment	▭ Ligament attachment
▬ Distal muscular attachment	▬ Area of bursa contact

Floor of Popliteal Fossa

6.47

A. Knee joint capsule and related structures. **B.** Attachment of muscles of popliteal region. Lighter tones are secondary attachments.

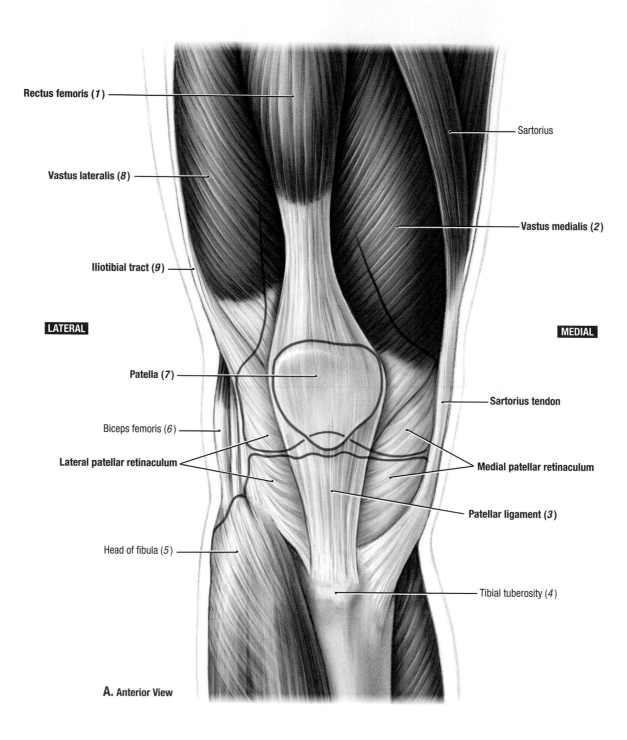

Rectus femoris (*1*)

Vastus lateralis (*8*)

Iliotibial tract (*9*)

LATERAL

Patella (*7*)

Biceps femoris (*6*)

Lateral patellar retinaculum

Head of fibula (*5*)

Sartorius

Vastus medialis (*2*)

MEDIAL

Sartorius tendon

Medial patellar retinaculum

Patellar ligament (*3*)

Tibial tuberosity (*4*)

A. Anterior View

6.48 **Anterior Aspect of Knee**

A. Distal thigh and knee regions. Note that the tendons of the four parts of the quadriceps unite to form the quadriceps tendon, a broad band that attaches to the patella. The patellar ligament, a continuation of the quadriceps tendon, attaches the patella to the tibial tuberosity. The lateral and medial patellar retinacula, formed largely by continuation of the iliotibial tract and investing fascia of the vasti muscles, maintains alignment of the patella and patellar ligament. The retinacula also form the anterolateral and anteromedial portions of the fibrous layer of the joint capsule of the knee.

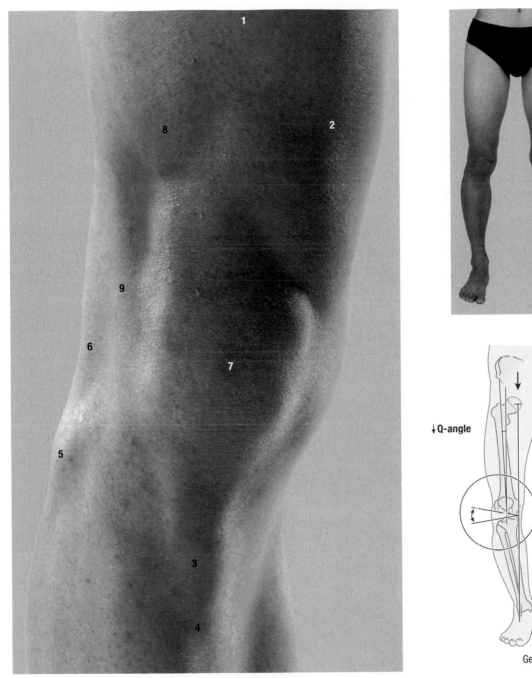

B. Anterior View

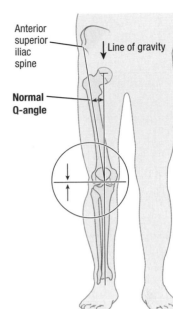

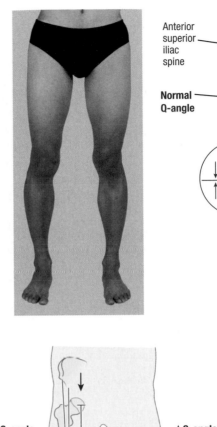

Anterior
superior
iliac
spine

↓ Line of gravity

**Normal
Q-angle**

Normal alignment

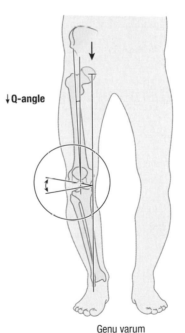

↓ Q-angle

↑ Q-angle

Genu varum

Genu valgum

C. Anterior Views

Anterior Aspect of Knee (continued)

6.48

B. Surface anatomy. Numbers refer to structures labeled in *Part A.* The femur is placed diagonally within the thigh, whereas the tibia is almost vertical within the leg, creating an angle at the knee between the long axes of the bones. The angle between the two bones, referred to clinically as the **Q-angle**, is assessed by drawing a line from the anterior superior iliac spine to the middle of the patella and extrapolating a second (vertical) line passing through the middle of the patella and tibial tuberosity. The Q-angle is typically greater in adult females, owing to their wider pelves.

C. Genu valgum and genu varum. A medial angulation of the leg in relation to the thigh, in which the femur is abnormally vertical and the Q-angle is small, is a deformity called **genu varum** (bowleg) that causes unequal weight bearing resulting in arthrosis (destruction of knee cartilages) and an overstressed fibular collateral ligament. A lateral angulation of the leg (large Q-angle, >17 degrees) in relation to the thigh is called **genu valgum** (knock-knee). This results in excess stress and degeneration of the lateral structures of the knee joint.

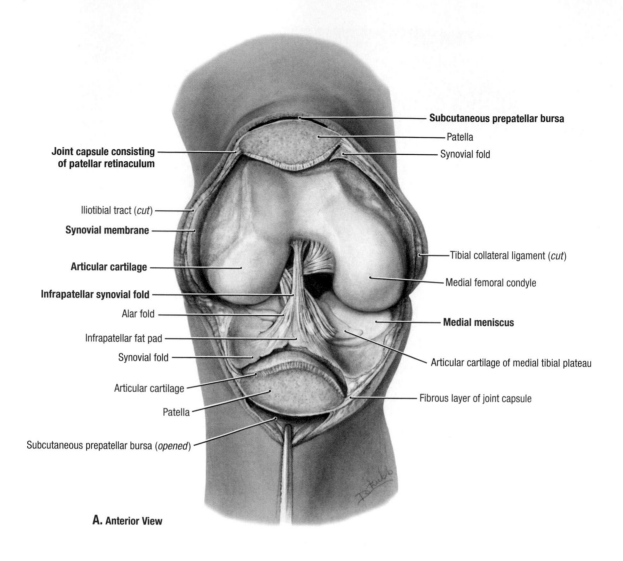

Subcutaneous prepatellar bursa

Patella

Synovial fold

Joint capsule consisting of patellar retinaculum

Iliotibial tract (*cut*)

Synovial membrane

Articular cartilage

Infrapatellar synovial fold

Alar fold

Infrapatellar fat pad

Synovial fold

Articular cartilage

Patella

Subcutaneous prepatellar bursa (*opened*)

Tibial collateral ligament (*cut*)

Medial femoral condyle

Medial meniscus

Articular cartilage of medial tibial plateau

Fibrous layer of joint capsule

A. Anterior View

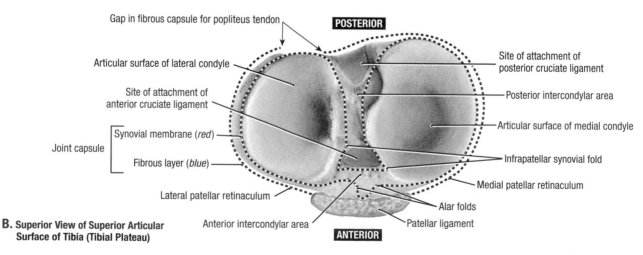

Gap in fibrous capsule for popliteus tendon

POSTERIOR

Articular surface of lateral condyle

Site of attachment of anterior cruciate ligament

Joint capsule

Synovial membrane (*red*)

Fibrous layer (*blue*)

Lateral patellar retinaculum

Anterior intercondylar area

Site of attachment of posterior cruciate ligament

Posterior intercondylar area

Articular surface of medial condyle

Infrapatellar synovial fold

Medial patellar retinaculum

Alar folds

Patellar ligament

ANTERIOR

B. Superior View of Superior Articular Surface of Tibia (Tibial Plateau)

6.49 Fibrous Layer and Synovial Membrane of Joint Capsule

A. Dissection. B. Attachment of layers of joint capsule to tibia.
The fibrous layer (*blue dotted line*) and synovial membrane (*red dotted line*) are adjacent on each side, but they part company centrally to accommodate intercondylar and infrapatellar structures that are intracapsular (inside the fibrous layer) but extra-articular (excluded from the articular cavity by synovial membrane).

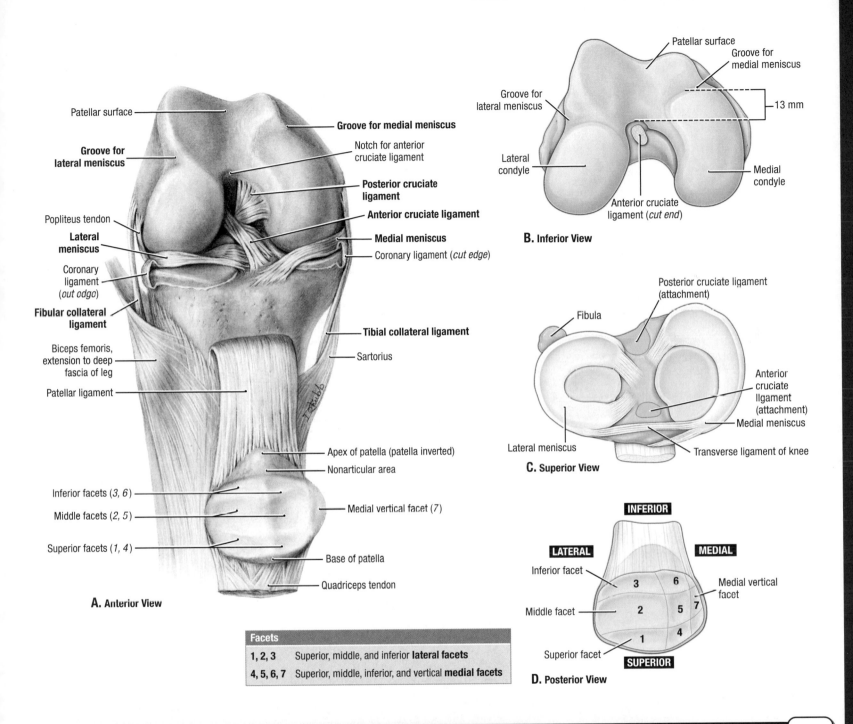

A. Anterior View

Patellar surface
Groove for lateral meniscus
Popliteus tendon
Lateral meniscus
Coronary ligament (*out odgo*)
Fibular collateral ligament
Biceps femoris, extension to deep fascia of leg
Patellar ligament
Inferior facets (*3, 6*)
Middle facets (*2, 5*)
Superior facets (*1, 4*)

Groove for medial meniscus
Notch for anterior cruciate ligament
Posterior cruciate ligament
Anterior cruciate ligament
Medial meniscus
Coronary ligament (*cut edge*)
Tibial collateral ligament
Sartorius
Apex of patella (patella inverted)
Nonarticular area
Medial vertical facet (*7*)
Base of patella
Quadriceps tendon

B. Inferior View

Patellar surface
Groove for medial meniscus
Groove for lateral meniscus
13 mm
Lateral condyle
Medial condyle
Anterior cruciate ligament (*cut end*)

C. Superior View

Posterior cruciate ligament (attachment)
Fibula
Anterior cruciate ligament (attachment)
Medial meniscus
Lateral meniscus
Transverse ligament of knee

D. Posterior View

INFERIOR
LATERAL
MEDIAL
Inferior facet
Medial vertical facet
Middle facet
Superior facet
SUPERIOR

Facets	
1, 2, 3	Superior, middle, and inferior **lateral facets**
4, 5, 6, 7	Superior, middle, inferior, and vertical **medial facets**

Articular Surfaces and Ligaments of Knee Joint

6.50

A. Flexed knee joint with patella reflected. There are indentations on the sides of the femoral condyles at the junction of the patellar and tibial articular areas. The lateral tibial articular area is shorter than the medial one. The notch at the anterolateral part of the intercondylar notch is for the anterior cruciate ligament on full extension. **B. Distal femur. C. Tibial plateaus. D. Articular surfaces of patella.** The three paired facets (superior, middle, and inferior) on the posterior surface of the patella articulate with the patellar surface of the femur successively during (1) extension, (2) slight flexion, (3) flexion, and the most medial vertical facet on the patella (4) articulates during full flexion with the crescentic facet on the medial margin of the

intercondylar notch of the femur. Note that the patella has been reflected inferiorly in *Part A* and removed and inverted in *Part D* to show the posterior surface.

When **patellar dislocation** occurs, it nearly always dislocates laterally. The tendency toward lateral dislocation is normally counterbalanced by the medial, more horizontal pull of the powerful vastus medialis. In addition, the more anterior projection of the lateral femoral condyle and deeper slope for the large lateral patellar facet provide a mechanical deterrent to lateral dislocation. An imbalance of the lateral pull and the mechanisms resisting it result in abnormal tracking of the patella within the patellar groove and chronic patellar pain, even if actual dislocation does not occur.

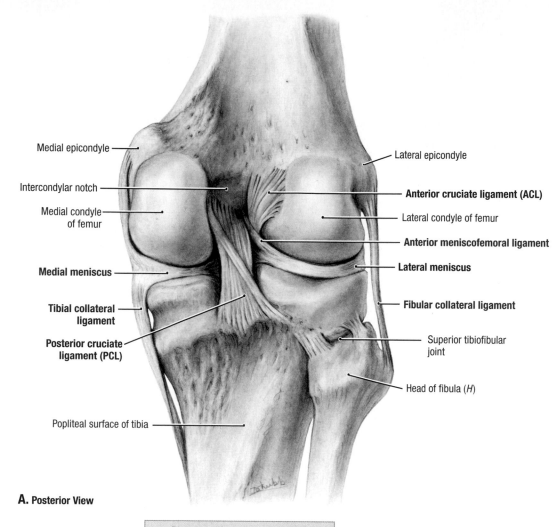

Medial epicondyle

Intercondylar notch

Medial condyle of femur

Medial meniscus

Tibial collateral ligament

Posterior cruciate ligament (PCL)

Popliteal surface of tibia

Lateral epicondyle

Anterior cruciate ligament (ACL)

Lateral condyle of femur

Anterior meniscofemoral ligament

Lateral meniscus

Fibular collateral ligament

Superior tibiofibular joint

Head of fibula (H)

A. Posterior View

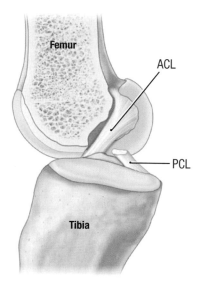

Femur

PCL

H

Tibia

ACL

B. Lateral View

Posterior Cruciate Ligament (PCL)

Prevents the femur from sliding anteriorly on the tibia, particularly when the knee is flexed

Femur

ACL

PCL

Tibia

C. Medial View

Anterior Cruciate Ligament (ACL)

Prevents the femur from sliding posteriorly on the tibia, preventing hyperextension of the knee, and limits medial rotation of the femur when the foot is planted (leg is fixed)

→ Direction of force applied by examiner

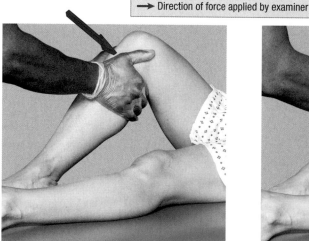

D. Posterior Drawer Sign (PCL)

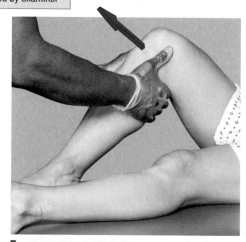

E. Anterior Drawer Sign (ACL)

6.51 **Ligaments of Knee Joint**

A. Posterior aspect of joint. **B.** Posterior cruciate ligament (PCL). **C.** Anterior cruciate ligament (ACL). In each illustration, half the femur is sagittally sectioned and removed with the proximal part of the corresponding cruciate ligament. **D.** Posterior cruciate ligament testing. **E.** Anterior cruciate ligament testing. Injury to the knee joint is frequently caused by a blow to the lateral side of the extended knee or excessive lateral twisting of the flexed knee, which disrupts the tibial collateral ligament and concomitantly tears and/or detaches the medial meniscus from the joint capsule. The ACL, which serves as a pivot for rotary movements of the knee, is taut during flexion and may also tear subsequent to the rupture of the tibial collateral ligament.

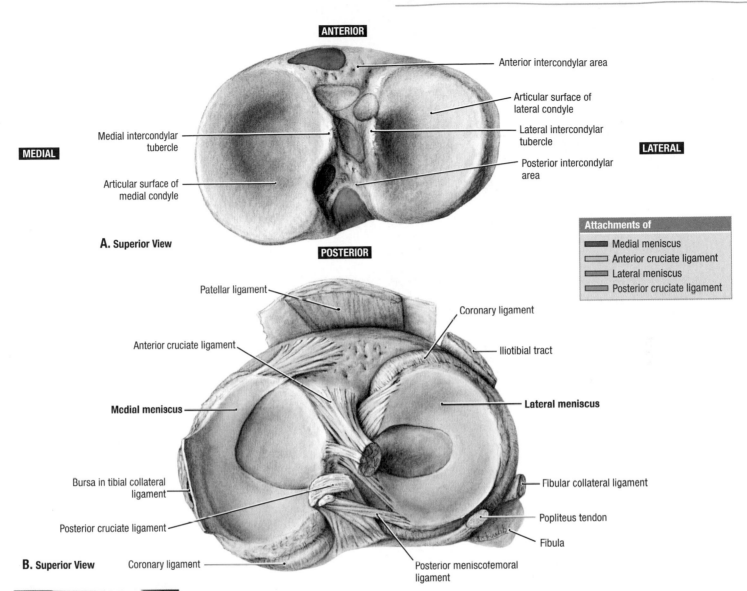

ANTERIOR

Anterior intercondylar area

Articular surface of lateral condyle

MEDIAL

Medial intercondylar tubercle

Lateral intercondylar tubercle

LATERAL

Posterior intercondylar area

Articular surface of medial condyle

A. Superior View

POSTERIOR

Attachments of	
	Medial meniscus
	Anterior cruciate ligament
	Lateral meniscus
	Posterior cruciate ligament

Patellar ligament

Coronary ligament

Anterior cruciate ligament

Iliotibial tract

Medial meniscus

Lateral meniscus

Bursa in tibial collateral ligament

Fibular collateral ligament

Posterior cruciate ligament

Popliteus tendon

Fibula

B. Superior View

Coronary ligament

Posterior meniscofemoral ligament

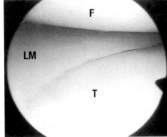

F

LM

T

Normal lateral meniscus

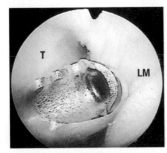

T

LM

Trimming torn lateral meniscus

C. Femoral Condyle (F), Tibial Plateau (T), Lateral Meniscus (LM)

Cruciate Ligaments and Menisci

6.52

A. Attachments sites on tibia. **B.** Menisci *in situ*.

- The lateral tibial condyle is flatter, shorter from anterior to posterior, and more circular. The medial condyle is concave, longer from anterior to posterior, and more oval.
- The menisci conform to the shapes of the surfaces on which they rest. Because the horns of the lateral meniscus are attached close together and its coronary ligament is slack, this meniscus can slide anteriorly and posteriorly on the (flat) condyle; because the horns of the medial meniscus are attached further apart, its movements on the (concave) condyle are restricted.

C. Arthroscopy of knee joint.

Arthroscopy is an endoscopic examination that allows visualization of the interior of the knee joint cavity with minimal disruption of tissue. The arthroscope and one (or more) additional cannula(e) are inserted through tiny incisions, known as portals. The second cannula is for passage of specialized tools. This technique allows removal of torn menisci, loose bodies in the joint such as bone chips, and debridement (the excision of devitalized articular cartilaginous material). Ligament repair or replacement may also be performed using an arthroscope.

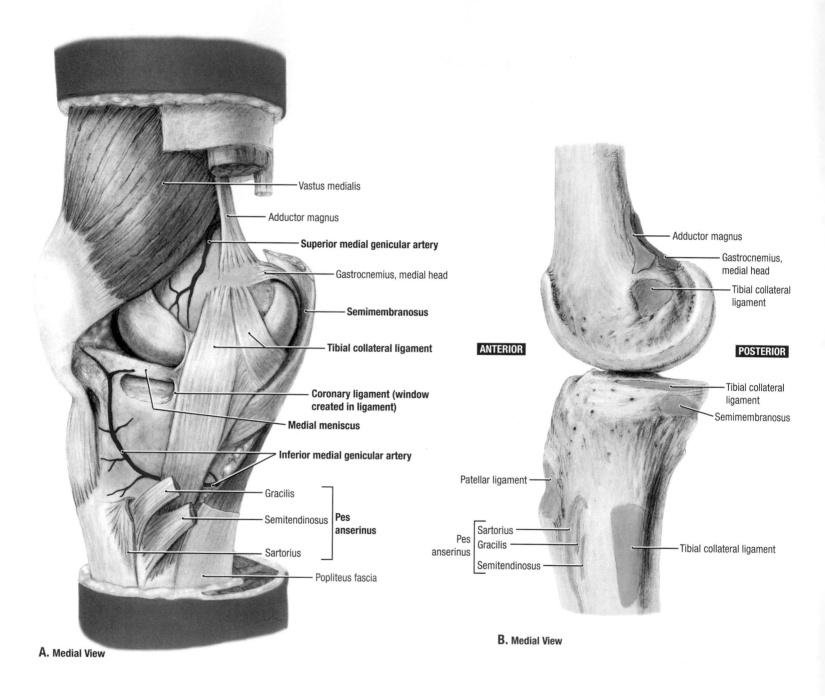

Vastus medialis

Adductor magnus

Superior medial genicular artery

Gastrocnemius, medial head

Semimembranosus

Tibial collateral ligament

Coronary ligament (window created in ligament)

Medial meniscus

Inferior medial genicular artery

Gracilis

Semitendinosus — **Pes anserinus**

Sartorius

Popliteus fascia

A. Medial View

Adductor magnus

Gastrocnemius, medial head

Tibial collateral ligament

ANTERIOR   POSTERIOR

Tibial collateral ligament

Semimembranosus

Patellar ligament

Pes anserinus
Sartorius
Gracilis
Semitendinosus

Tibial collateral ligament

B. Medial View

6.53   **Medial Aspect of Knee**

A. Dissection. The band-like part of the tibial collateral ligament attaches to the medial epicondyle of the femur, bridges superficial to the insertion of the semimembranosus muscle, and crosses the medial inferior genicular artery. Distally, the ligament is crossed by the three tendons forming the pes anserinus (sartorius, gracilis, and semitendinosus). **B. Muscle and ligament attachment sites.**

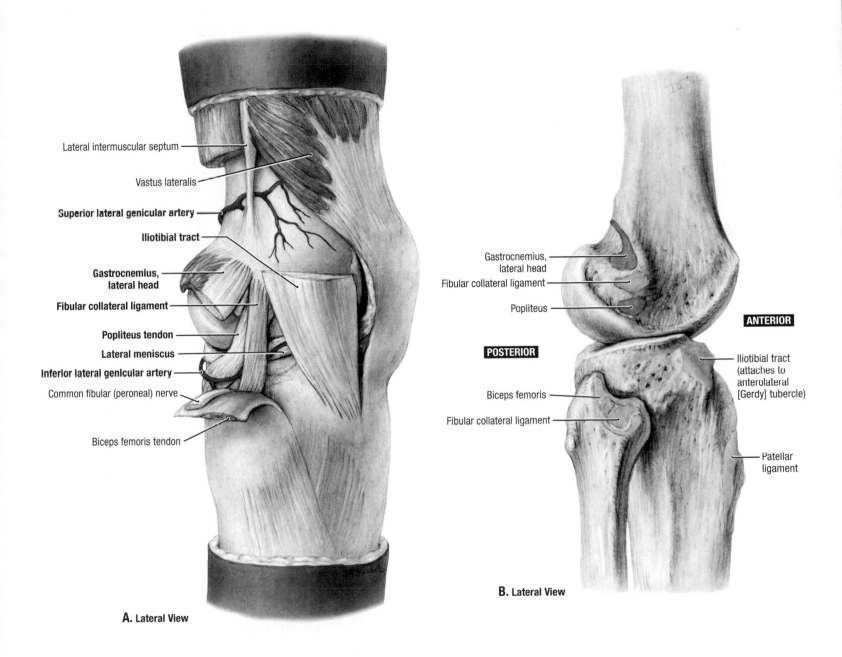

Lateral intermuscular septum

Vastus lateralis

Superior lateral genicular artery

Iliotibial tract

Gastrocnemius, lateral head

Fibular collateral ligament

Popliteus tendon

Lateral meniscus

Inferior lateral genicular artery

Common fibular (peroneal) nerve

Biceps femoris tendon

A. Lateral View

Gastrocnemius, lateral head

Fibular collateral ligament

Popliteus

POSTERIOR

ANTERIOR

Biceps femoris

Fibular collateral ligament

Iliotibial tract (attaches to anterolateral [Gerdy] tubercle)

Patellar ligament

B. Lateral View

Lateral Aspect of Knee

6.54

A. Dissection. Three structures arise from the lateral epicondyle and are uncovered by reflecting the biceps femoris tendon: The gastrocnemius muscle is posterosuperior; the popliteus muscle is anteroinferior; and the fibular collateral ligament is in between, crossing superficial to the popliteus muscle. The lateral inferior genicular artery courses along the lateral meniscus. **B. Muscle and ligament attachments.**

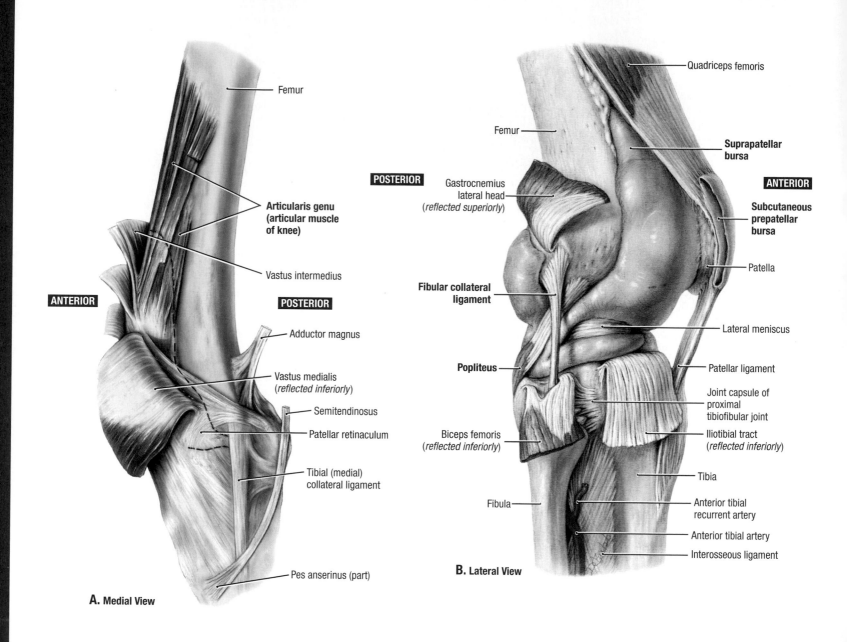

Femur

Articularis genu (articular muscle of knee)

Vastus intermedius

ANTERIOR

POSTERIOR

Adductor magnus

Vastus medialis (*reflected inferiorly*)

Semitendinosus

Patellar retinaculum

Tibial (medial) collateral ligament

Pes anserinus (part)

A. Medial View

POSTERIOR

Gastrocnemius lateral head (*reflected superiorly*)

Fibular collateral ligament

Popliteus

Biceps femoris (*reflected inferiorly*)

Fibula

Quadriceps femoris

Femur

Suprapatellar bursa

ANTERIOR

Subcutaneous prepatellar bursa

Patella

Lateral meniscus

Patellar ligament

Joint capsule of proximal tibiofibular joint

Iliotibial tract (*reflected inferiorly*)

Tibia

Anterior tibial recurrent artery

Anterior tibial artery

Interosseous ligament

B. Lateral View

6.55 | **Articularis Genu and Bursae of Knee Region**

A. Articularis genu (articular muscle of knee). This muscle lies deep to vastus intermedius muscle and consists of fibers arising from the anterior surface of the femur proximally and attaching into the synovial membrane distally. The articularis genu pulls the synovial membrane of the suprapatellar bursa (*dashed line*) superiorly during extension of the knee so that it will not be caught between the patella and femur within the knee joint. **B. Lateral aspect of knee.** Latex was injected into the articular cavity and fixed with acetic acid. The distended synovial membrane was exposed and cleaned. The gastrocnemius muscle was reflected proximally, and the biceps femoris muscle and the iliotibial tract were reflected distally. The extent of the synovial capsule: superiorly, it rises superior to the pa-tella, where it rests on a layer of fat that allows it to glide freely with

movements of the joint—this superior part is called the suprapatel-lar bursa; posteriorly, it rises as high as the origin of the gastroc-nemius muscle; laterally, it curves inferior to the lateral femoral epicondyle, where the popliteus tendon and fibular collateral ligament are attached; and inferiorly, it bulges inferior to the lateral meniscus, overlapping the tibia (the coronary ligament is removed to show this). **Prepatellar bursitis** (housemaid's knee) is usually a friction bursitis caused by friction between the skin and the patella. The suprapatellar bursa communicates with the articular cavity of the knee joint; consequently, abrasions or penetrating wounds su-perior to the patella may result in **suprapatellar bursitis** caused by bacteria entering the bursa from the torn skin. The infection may spread to the knee joint. **C. Posterior aspect of knee.**

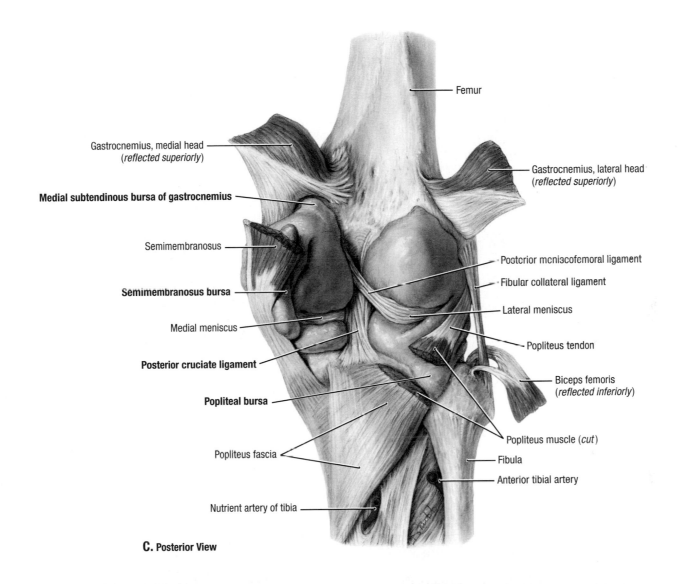

Femur

Gastrocnemius, medial head
(*reflected superiorly*)

Gastrocnemius, lateral head
(*reflected superiorly*)

Medial subtendinous bursa of gastrocnemius

Semimembranosus

Posterior meniscofemoral ligament

Fibular collateral ligament

Semimembranosus bursa

Lateral meniscus

Medial meniscus

Popliteus tendon

Posterior cruciate ligament

Biceps femoris
(*reflected inferiorly*)

Popliteal bursa

Popliteus muscle (*cut*)

Popliteus fascia

Fibula

Anterior tibial artery

Nutrient artery of tibia

C. Posterior View

Articularis Genu and Bursae of Knee Region (*continued*)   **6.55**

TABLE 6.9	Bursae around Knee	
Bursa	**Location**	**Structural Features or Functions**
Suprapatellar	Located between femur and tendon of quadriceps femoris	Held in position by articular muscle of knee; superior extension of synovial cavity of knee joint
Popliteus	Located between tendon of popliteus and lateral condyle of tibia	Opens into synovial cavity of knee joint, inferior to lateral meniscus
Anserine	Separates tendons of sartorius, gracilis, and semitendinosus from tibia and tibial collateral ligament	Area where tendons of these muscles attach to tibia (pes anserinus) resembles the foot of a goose (L. *pes*, foot; L. *anser*, goose)
Medial subtendinous bursa of gastrocnemius	Lies deep to proximal attachment of tendon of medial head of gastrocnemius	Extension of synovial cavity of knee joint
Semimembranosus	Located between medial head of gastrocnemius and semimembranosus tendon	Related to the distal attachment of semimembranosus
Subcutaneous prepatellar	Lies between skin and anterior surface of patella	Allows free movement of skin over patella during movements of leg
Subcutaneous infrapatellar	Located between skin and tibial tuberosity	Helps knee to withstand pressure when kneeling[a]
Deep infrapatellar	Lies between patellar ligament and anterior surface of tibia	Separated from knee joint by infrapatellar fat pad[a]

[a]See Figure 6.59.

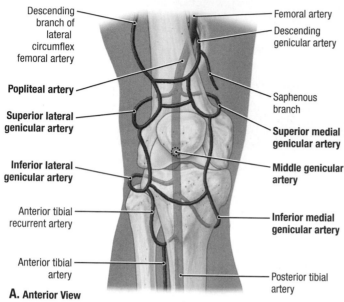

A. Anterior View

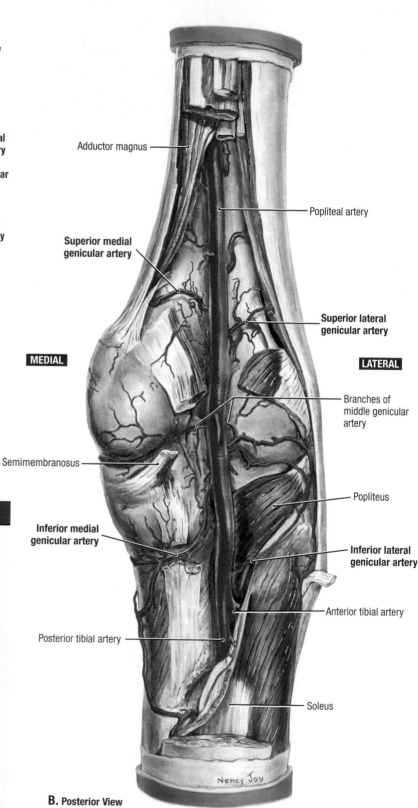

B. Posterior View

6.56　Anastomoses around Knee

A. Genicular anastomosis on anterior aspect of knee. **B.** Popliteal artery in popliteal fossa.

- The popliteal artery runs from the adductor hiatus (in the adductor magnus muscle) proximally to the inferior border of the popliteus muscle distally, where it bifurcates into the anterior and posterior tibial arteries.
- The three anterior relations of the popliteal artery include the femur, joint capsule of the knee, and the popliteus muscle.
- The genicular arteries participate in the formation of the periarticular genicular anastomosis, a network of vessels surrounding the knee that provides collateral circulation capable of maintaining blood supply to the leg during full knee flexion, which may kink the popliteal artery.
- Five genicular branches of the popliteal artery supply the capsule and ligaments of the knee joint. The genicular arteries are the superior lateral, superior medial, middle, inferior lateral, and inferior medial genicular arteries.
- Other contributors are the descending genicular artery, a branch of the femoral artery, superomedially; descending branch of the lateral circumflex femoral artery, superolaterally; and anterior tibial recurrent artery, a branch of the anterior tibial artery, inferolaterally.

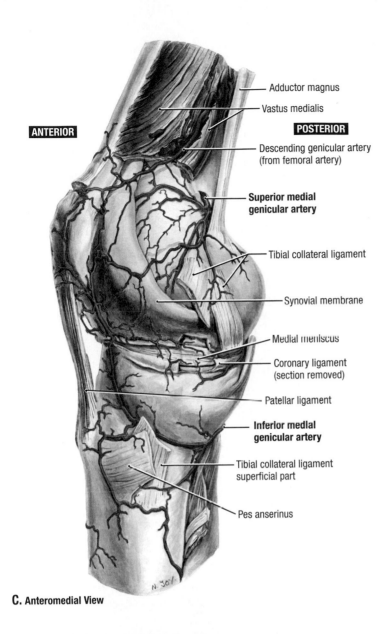

C. Anteromedial View

- Adductor magnus
- Vastus medialis

ANTERIOR

POSTERIOR

- Descending genicular artery (from femoral artery)
- **Superior medial genicular artery**
- Tibial collateral ligament
- Synovial membrane
- Medial meniscus
- Coronary ligament (section removed)
- Patellar ligament
- **Inferior medial genicular artery**
- Tibial collateral ligament superficial part
- Pes anserinus

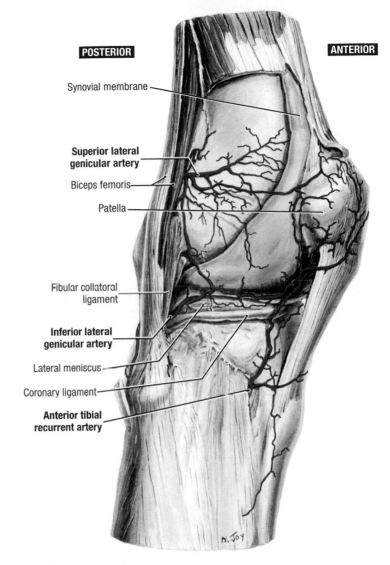

E. Anterolateral View

POSTERIOR

ANTERIOR

- Synovial membrane
- **Superior lateral genicular artery**
- Biceps femoris
- Patella
- Fibular collateral ligament
- **Inferior lateral genicular artery**
- Lateral meniscus
- Coronary ligament
- **Anterior tibial recurrent artery**

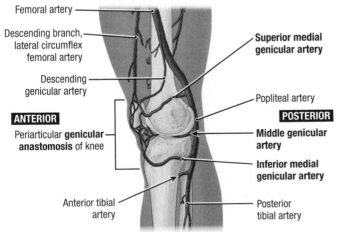

D. Medial View

- Femoral artery
- Descending branch, lateral circumflex femoral artery
- Descending genicular artery

ANTERIOR

- Periarticular **genicular anastomosis** of knee
- Anterior tibial artery
- **Superior medial genicular artery**
- Popliteal artery

POSTERIOR

- **Middle genicular artery**
- **Inferior medial genicular artery**
- Posterior tibial artery

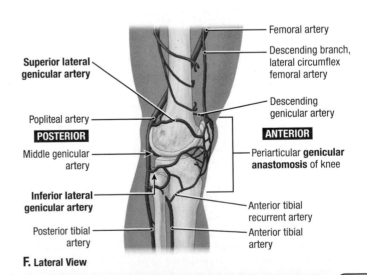

F. Lateral View

- Femoral artery
- Descending branch, lateral circumflex femoral artery
- Descending genicular artery
- **Superior lateral genicular artery**
- Popliteal artery

POSTERIOR

ANTERIOR

- Middle genicular artery
- **Inferior lateral genicular artery**
- Posterior tibial artery
- Periarticular **genicular anastomosis** of knee
- Anterior tibial recurrent artery
- Anterior tibial artery

Anastomoses around Knee (continued)

6.56

C. and **D.** Medial aspect of knee showing superior and inferior medial genicular arteries. **E.** and **F.** Lateral aspect of knee showing superior and inferior lateral genicular arteries.

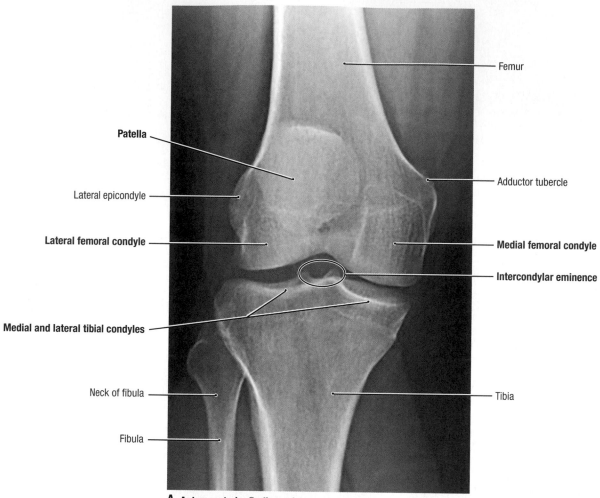

A. Anteroposterior Radiograph

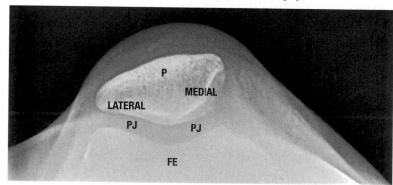

B. Skyline (Merchant) Radiograph (Knee in Flexion)

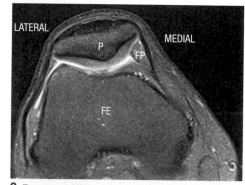

C. Transverse MRI

6.57   Imaging of Knee and Patellofemoral Articulation

A. Anteroposterior radiograph of knee. **B.** Radiograph of patella (knee joint flexed). **C.** Transverse MRI showing patellofemoral joint. *FE,* femur; *FP,* fat pad; *P,* patella; *PJ,* patellofemoral joint.

Pain deep to the patella often results from excessive running; hence, this type of pain is often called "runner's knee." The pain results from repetitive microtrauma caused by abnormal tracking of the patella relative to the patellar surface of the femur, a condition known as the **patellofemoral syndrome**. This syndrome may also result from a direct blow to the patella and from osteoarthritis of the patellofemoral compartment (degenerative wear and tear of articular cartilages). In some cases, strengthening of the vastus medialis corrects patellofemoral dysfunction. This muscle tends to prevent lateral dislocation of the patella resulting from the Q-angle because the vastus medialis attaches to and pulls on the medial border of the patella. Hence, weakness of the vastus medialis predisposes the individual to patellofemoral dysfunction and patellar dislocation.

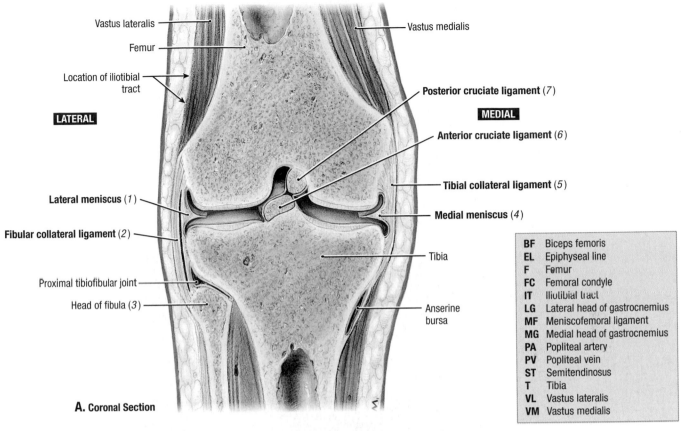

Vastus lateralis
Femur
Location of iliotibial tract

LATERAL

Lateral meniscus (*1*)
Fibular collateral ligament (*2*)
Proximal tibiofibular joint
Head of fibula (*3*)

Vastus medialis

Posterior cruciate ligament (*7*)

MEDIAL

Anterior cruciate ligament (*6*)
Tibial collateral ligament (*5*)
Medial meniscus (*4*)
Tibia
Anserine bursa

A. Coronal Section

BF	Biceps femoris
EL	Epiphyseal line
F	Femur
FC	Femoral condyle
IT	Iliotibial tract
LG	Lateral head of gastrocnemius
MF	Meniscofemoral ligament
MG	Medial head of gastrocnemius
PA	Popliteal artery
PV	Popliteal vein
ST	Semitendinosus
T	Tibia
VL	Vastus lateralis
VM	Vastus medialis

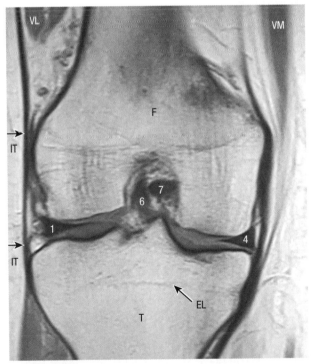

B. Coronal MRI

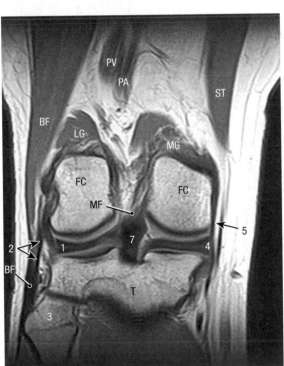

C. Coronal MRI

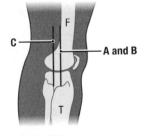

Lateral View

Coronal Section and MRI of Knee

A. Section through intercondylar notch of femur, tibia, and fibula. **B.** MRI through intercondylar notch of femur and tibia.

C. MRI through femoral condyles, tibia, and fibula. Numbers in MRIs refer to structures in *Part A.*

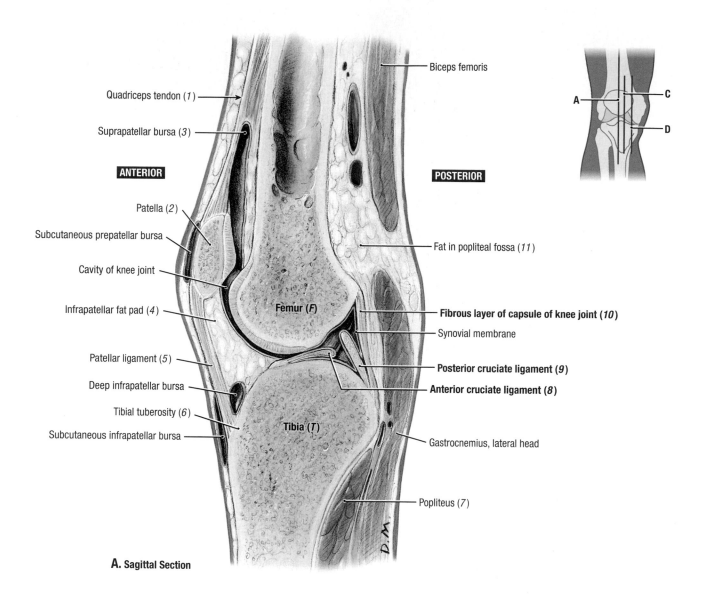

Quadriceps tendon (*1*)

Suprapatellar bursa (*3*)

ANTERIOR

Patella (*2*)

Subcutaneous prepatellar bursa

Cavity of knee joint

Infrapatellar fat pad (*4*)

Patellar ligament (*5*)

Deep infrapatellar bursa

Tibial tuberosity (*6*)

Subcutaneous infrapatellar bursa

Biceps femoris

POSTERIOR

Fat in popliteal fossa (*11*)

Femur (F)

Fibrous layer of capsule of knee joint (*10*)

Synovial membrane

Posterior cruciate ligament (*9*)

Anterior cruciate ligament (*8*)

Tibia (T)

Gastrocnemius, lateral head

Popliteus (*7*)

A. Sagittal Section

6.59   Sagittal Section and Imaging of Knee

A. Illustration of section through lateral aspect of intercondylar notch of femur.

Fractures of the distal end of the femur, or lacerations of the anterior thigh, may involve the suprapatellar bursa and result in infection of the knee joint. When the knee joint is infected and inflamed, the amount of synovial fluid may increase. **Joint effusions**, the escape of fluid from blood or lymphatic vessels, result in increased amounts of fluid in the joint cavity. Because the suprapatellar bursa is a superior continuation of the synovial cavity of the knee

joint, fullness of the thigh in the region of the bursa may indicate increased synovial fluid. This bursa can be aspirated to remove the fluid for examination. Direct **aspiration of the knee joint** is usually performed with the patient sitting on a table with the knee flexed. The joint is approached laterally, using three bony points as landmarks for needle insertion: the anterolateral tibial (Gerdy) tubercle, the lateral epicondyle of the femur, and the apex of the patella. In addition, this triangular area also is used for drug injection for treating pathology of the knee joint.

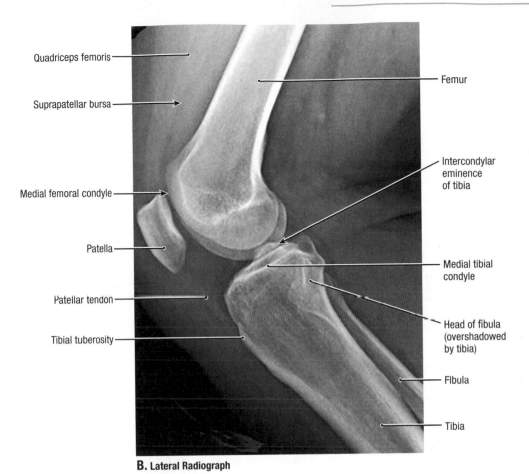

Quadriceps femoris

Suprapatellar bursa

Medial femoral condyle

Patella

Patellar tendon

Tibial tuberosity

Femur

Intercondylar eminence of tibia

Medial tibial condyle

Head of fibula (overshadowed by tibia)

Fibula

Tibia

AM	Anterior horn of medial meniscus
F	Femur
MG	Medial head of gastrocnemius
PF	Prefemoral fat
PM	Posterior horn of medial meniscus
PV	Popliteal vessels
SF	Suprapatellar fat
SM	Semimembranosus
ST	Semitendinosus
T	Tibia
VM	Vastus medialis

B. Lateral Radiograph

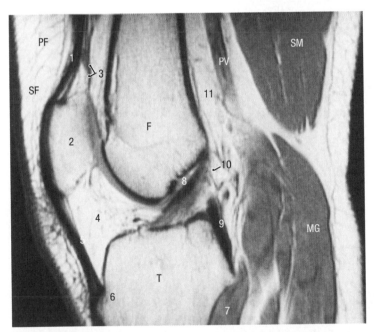

C. Sagittal MRI

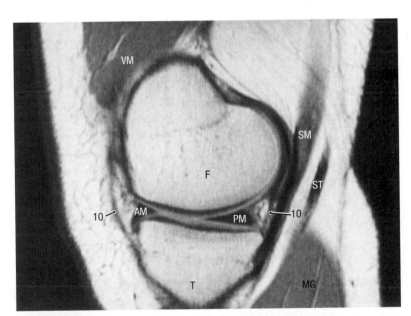

D. Sagittal MRI

Sagittal Section and Imaging of Knee *(continued)*

6.59

B. Lateral radiograph of flexed knee. The fabella is an inconsistent sesamoid bone in the lateral head of gastrocnemius muscle. **C.** MRI through medial aspect of intercondylar notch of femur showing cruciate ligaments. **D.** MRI through medial femoral and tibial condyles. Numbers in MRIs refer to structures labeled in *Part A.*

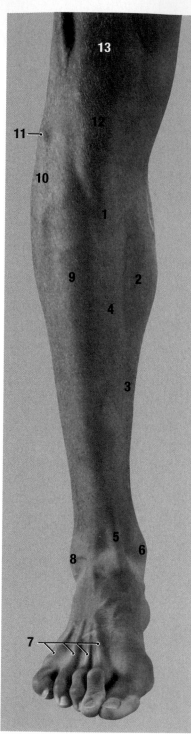

A. Anterior View

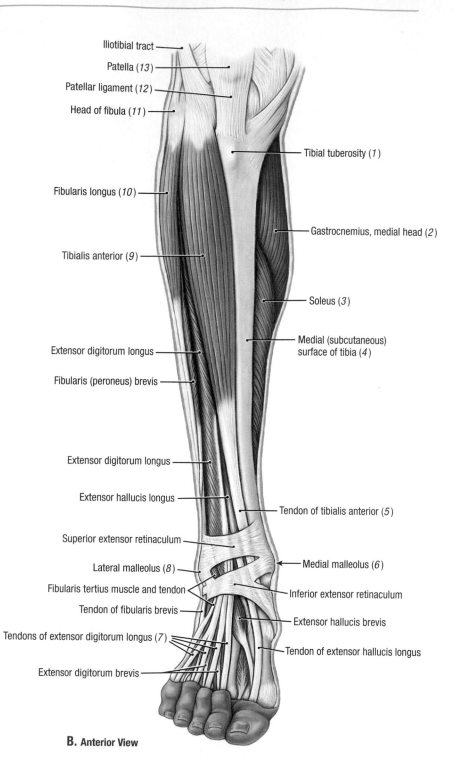

Iliotibial tract
Patella (*13*)
Patellar ligament (*12*)
Head of fibula (*11*)
Tibial tuberosity (*1*)
Fibularis longus (*10*)
Gastrocnemius, medial head (*2*)
Tibialis anterior (*9*)
Soleus (*3*)
Extensor digitorum longus
Medial (subcutaneous) surface of tibia (*4*)
Fibularis (peroneus) brevis
Extensor digitorum longus
Extensor hallucis longus
Tendon of tibialis anterior (*5*)
Superior extensor retinaculum
Lateral malleolus (*8*)
Medial malleolus (*6*)
Fibularis tertius muscle and tendon
Inferior extensor retinaculum
Tendon of fibularis brevis
Extensor hallucis brevis
Tendons of extensor digitorum longus (*7*)
Extensor digitorum brevis
Tendon of extensor hallucis longus

B. Anterior View

6.60 Anterior Leg: Superficial Muscles

A. Surface anatomy. Numbers refer to structures labeled in *Part B*.
B. Dissection. The muscles of the anterior compartment are ankle dorsiflexors/toe extensors. They are active in walking as they concentrically contract to raise the forefoot to clear the ground during the swing phase of the gait cycle and eccentrically contract to lower the forefoot to the ground after the heel strike of the stance phase.

Shin splints, edema, and pain in the area of the distal third of the tibia result from repetitive microtrauma of the anterior compartment muscles, especially the tibialis anterior. This produces a mild form of **anterior compartment syndrome**. The pain commonly occurs during traumatic injury or athletic overexertion of the muscles. Edema and muscle-tendon inflammation causes swelling that reduces blood flow to the muscles. Swollen ischemic muscles are painful and tender to pressure.

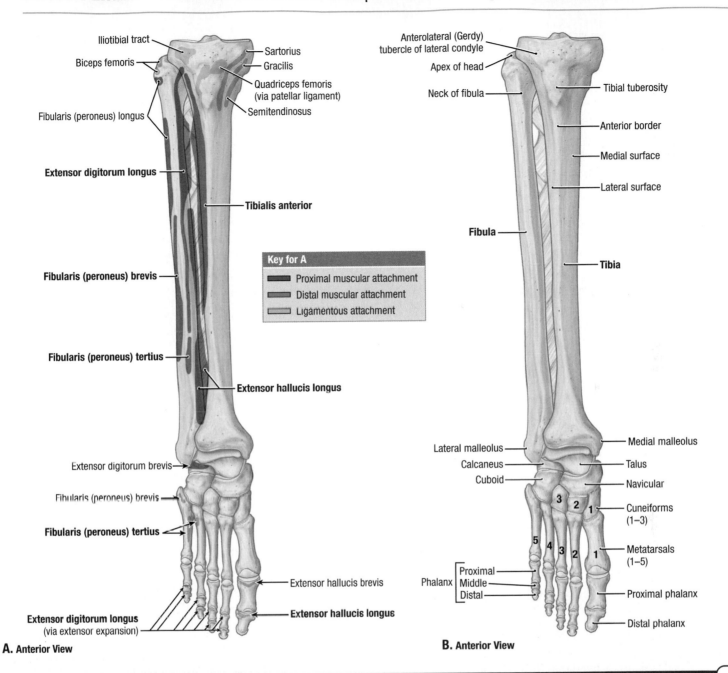

A. Anterior View

B. Anterior View

Anterior Leg and Dorsum of Foot: Features of Bones and Muscle Attachments   **6.61**

A. Attachments. **B.** Features of bones.

TABLE 6.10	Muscles of Anterior Compartment of Leg			
Muscle	**Proximal Attachment**	**Distal Attachment**	**Innervation**[a]	**Main Actions**
Tibialis anterior	Lateral condyle and superior half of lateral surface of tibia	Medial and inferior surfaces of medial cuneiform and base of 1st metatarsal	Deep fibular (peroneal) nerve (L4–L5)	Dorsiflexes ankle joint and inverts foot
Extensor hallucis longus	Middle part of anterior surface of fibula and interosseous membrane	Dorsal aspect of base of distal phalanx of great toe (hallux)		Extends great toe and dorsiflexes ankle joint
Extensor digitorum longus	Lateral condyle of tibia and superior three fourths of anterior surface of interosseous membrane	Middle and distal phalanges of lateral four digits	Deep fibular (peroneal) nerve (L5–S1)	Extends lateral four digits and dorsiflexes ankle joint
Fibularis (peroneus) tertius	Inferior third of anterior surface of fibula and interosseous membrane	Dorsum of base of 5th metatarsal		Dorsiflexes ankle joint and aids in eversion of foot

[a]See Table 6.3 for explanation of segmental innervation.

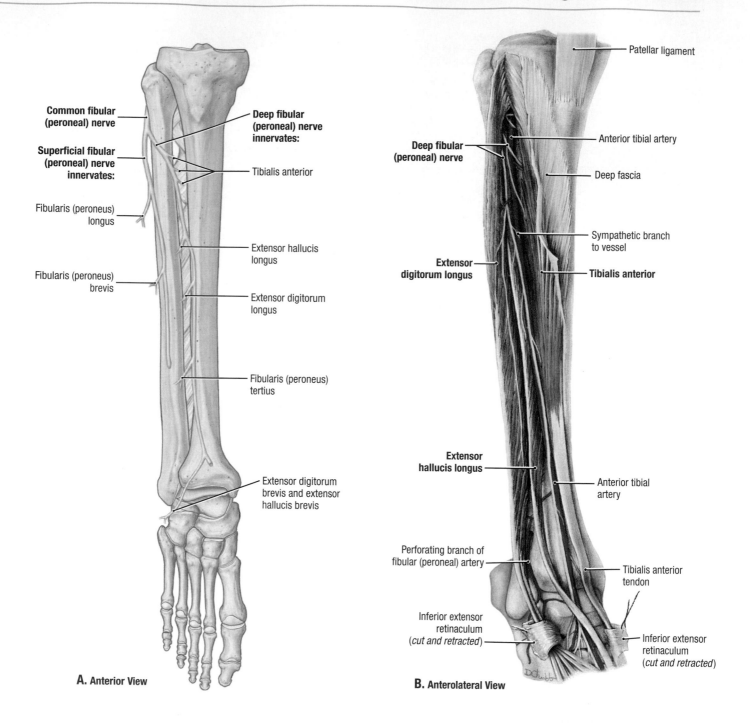

Common fibular (peroneal) nerve

Superficial fibular (peroneal) nerve innervates:

Deep fibular (peroneal) nerve innervates:

Tibialis anterior

Fibularis (peroneus) longus

Fibularis (peroneus) brevis

Extensor hallucis longus

Extensor digitorum longus

Fibularis (peroneus) tertius

Extensor digitorum brevis and extensor hallucis brevis

A. Anterior View

Patellar ligament

Deep fibular (peroneal) nerve

Anterior tibial artery

Deep fascia

Sympathetic branch to vessel

Extensor digitorum longus

Tibialis anterior

Extensor hallucis longus

Anterior tibial artery

Perforating branch of fibular (peroneal) artery

Tibialis anterior tendon

Inferior extensor retinaculum (*cut and retracted*)

Inferior extensor retinaculum (*cut and retracted*)

B. Anterolateral View

6.62 **Anterior Leg: Muscles, Nerves, and Vessels**

TABLE 6.11	Common, Superficial, and Deep Fibular (Peroneal) Nerves		
Nerve	**Origin**	**Course**	**Distribution/Structure(s) Supplied**
Common fibular	Sciatic nerve	Forms as sciatic nerve bifurcates at the apex of popliteal fossa and follows medial border of biceps femoris; winds around neck of fibula, dividing into superficial and deep fibular nerves	Skin on lateral part of posterior aspect of leg via the lateral sural cutaneous nerve; lateral aspect of knee joint via its articular branch
Superficial fibular	Common fibular nerve	Arises deep to fibularis longus and descends in lateral compartment of leg; pierces crural fascia at distal third of leg to become cutaneous	Fibularis longus and brevis and skin on distal third of anterolateral surface of leg and dorsum of foot
Deep fibular	Common fibular nerve	Arises deep to fibularis longus; passes through extensor digitorum longus, descends on interosseous membrane, and continues on dorsum of foot	Anterior muscles of leg, dorsum of foot, and skin of first interdigital cleft; dorsal aspect of joints crossed via articular branches

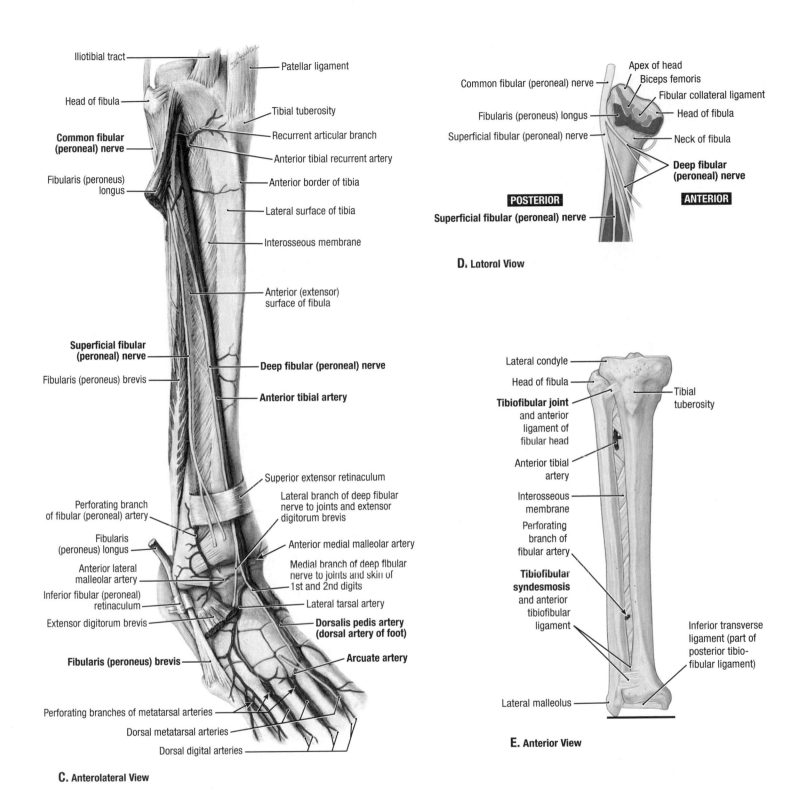

Iliotibial tract

Head of fibula

Common fibular (peroneal) nerve

Fibularis (peroneus) longus

Superficial fibular (peroneal) nerve

Fibularis (peroneus) brevis

Perforating branch of fibular (peroneal) artery

Fibularis (peroneus) longus

Anterior lateral malleolar artery

Inferior fibular (peroneal) retinaculum

Extensor digitorum brevis

Fibularis (peroneus) brevis

Perforating branches of metatarsal arteries

Dorsal metatarsal arteries

Dorsal digital arteries

Patellar ligament

Tibial tuberosity

Recurrent articular branch

Anterior tibial recurrent artery

Anterior border of tibia

Lateral surface of tibia

Interosseous membrane

Anterior (extensor) surface of fibula

Deep fibular (peroneal) nerve

Anterior tibial artery

Superior extensor retinaculum

Lateral branch of deep fibular nerve to joints and extensor digitorum brevis

Anterior medial malleolar artery

Medial branch of deep fibular nerve to joints and skin of 1st and 2nd digits

Lateral tarsal artery

Dorsalis pedis artery (dorsal artery of foot)

Arcuate artery

C. Anterolateral View

Common fibular (peroneal) nerve

Fibularis (peroneus) longus

Superficial fibular (peroneal) nerve

POSTERIOR

Superficial fibular (peroneal) nerve

Apex of head

Biceps femoris

Fibular collateral ligament

Head of fibula

Neck of fibula

Deep fibular (peroneal) nerve

ANTERIOR

D. Lateral View

Lateral condyle

Head of fibula

Tibiofibular joint and anterior ligament of fibular head

Anterior tibial artery

Interosseous membrane

Perforating branch of fibular artery

Tibiofibular syndesmosis and anterior tibiofibular ligament

Lateral malleolus

Tibial tuberosity

Inferior transverse ligament (part of posterior tibio-fibular ligament)

E. Anterior View

A. Overview of motor innervation. B. Deep dissection of anterior compartment of leg. The muscles are separated to display anterior tibial artery and deep fibular nerve. **C. Neurovascular** structures of lateral compartment and dorsum of foot. **D. Relations of common fibular nerve and branches to proximal fibula. E. Interosseous membrane.**

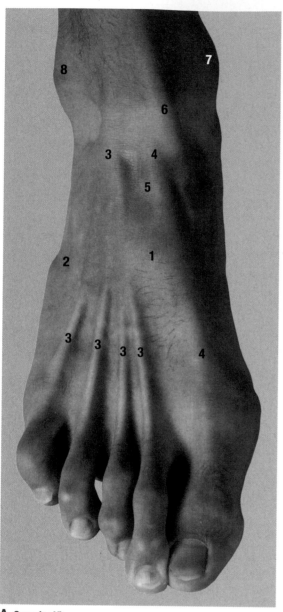

A. Superior View

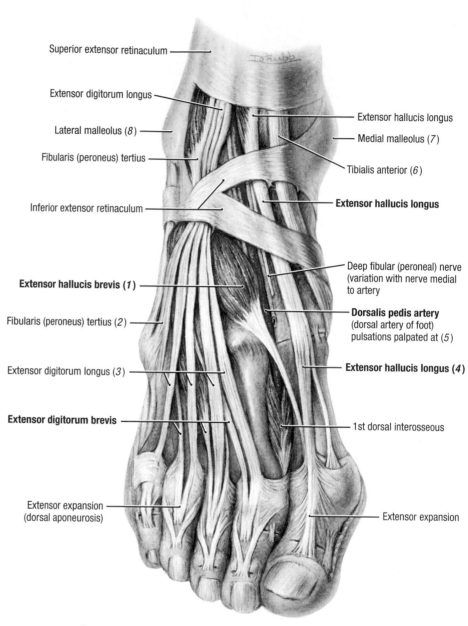

Superior extensor retinaculum

Extensor digitorum longus

Lateral malleolus (8)

Fibularis (peroneus) tertius

Inferior extensor retinaculum

Extensor hallucis brevis (1)

Fibularis (peroneus) tertius (2)

Extensor digitorum longus (3)

Extensor digitorum brevis

Extensor expansion
(dorsal aponeurosis)

Extensor hallucis longus

Medial malleolus (7)

Tibialis anterior (6)

Extensor hallucis longus

Deep fibular (peroneal) nerve
(variation with nerve medial
to artery

Dorsalis pedis artery
(dorsal artery of foot)
pulsations palpated at (5)

Extensor hallucis longus (4)

1st dorsal interosseous

Extensor expansion

B. Superior View

6.63 **Dorsum of Foot**

A. Surface anatomy. Numbers refer to structures labeled in *Part B*.
B. Dissection. The dorsal vein of foot and deep fibular nerve are cut.

At the ankle, the dorsalis pedis artery (dorsal artery of foot) and deep fibular nerve lie midway between the malleoli. On the dorsum of the foot, the dorsal artery of foot is crossed by the extensor hallucis brevis muscle and disappears between the two heads of the first dorsal interosseous muscle.

Clinically, knowing the location of the belly of the extensor digitorum brevis is important for distinguishing this muscle from abnormal edema. Contusion and tearing of the muscle fibers and

associated blood vessels result in a **hematoma in extensor digitorum brevis**, producing edema anteromedial to the lateral malleolus. Most people who have not seen this inflamed muscle assume they have a severely sprained ankle.

The **dorsalis pedis pulse** may be palpated with the feet slightly dorsiflexed. The pulse is usually easy to palpate because the dorsal arteries of the foot are subcutaneous and pass along a line from the extensor retinaculum to a point just lateral to the extensor hallucis longus tendon. A diminished or absent dorsalis pedis pulse usually suggests vascular insufficiency resulting from arterial disease.

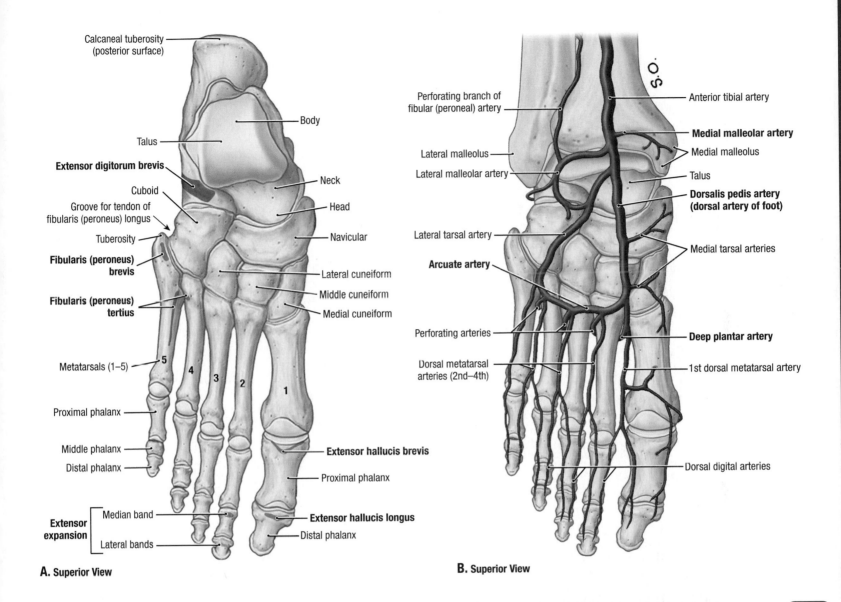

A. Superior View

B. Superior View

Muscle Attachments and Arteries of Dorsum of Foot

6.64

A. Attachments. **B.** Arterial supply.

TABLE 6.12	Arterial Supply to Dorsum of Foot		
Artery	**Origin**	**Course**	**Distribution**
Dorsalis pedis (dorsal artery of foot)	Continuation of anterior tibial artery distal to talocrural joint	Descends anteromedially to 1st interosseous space and divides into deep plantar and arcuate arteries	
Lateral tarsal artery		Runs an arched course laterally beneath extensor digitorum brevis to anastomose with branches of arcuate artery	Dorsal surface of hind foot
Arcuate artery	From dorsalis pedis artery (dorsal artery of foot)	Runs laterally from 1st interosseous space across bases of lateral four metatarsals, deep to extensor tendons	
Deep plantar artery		Passes to sole of foot and joins plantar arch	Sole of foot
Metatarsal arteries: 1st	From deep plantar artery	Run between metatarsals to clefts of toes where each vessel divides into two dorsal digital arteries	Dorsal surface of forefoot
2nd to 4th	From arcuate artery	Perforating arteries connect to plantar arch and plantar metatarsal arteries.	
Dorsal digital arteries	From metatarsal arteries	Pass to sides of adjoining digits	Proximal dorsal digits

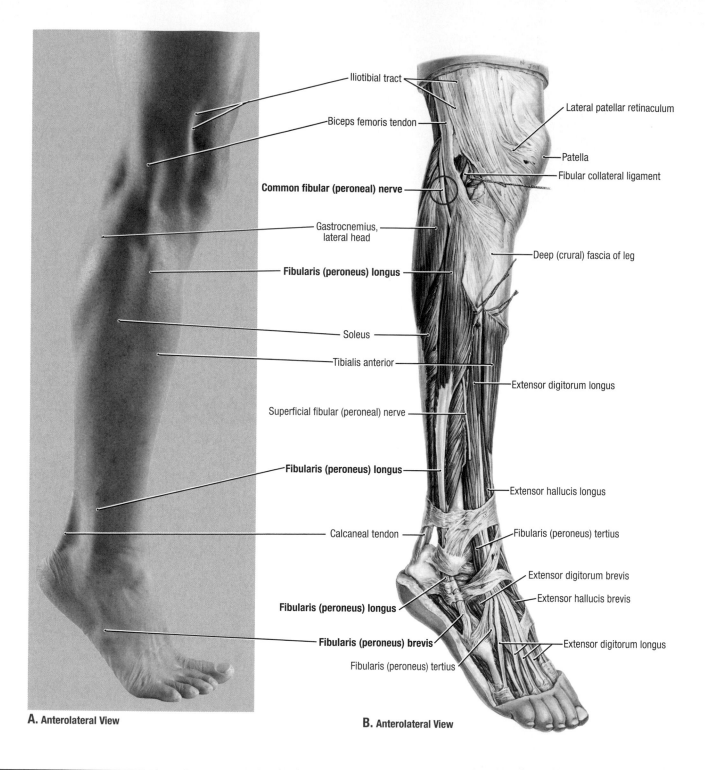

Iliotibial tract

Biceps femoris tendon

Common fibular (peroneal) nerve

Gastrocnemius, lateral head

Fibularis (peroneus) longus

Soleus

Tibialis anterior

Superficial fibular (peroneal) nerve

Fibularis (peroneus) longus

Calcaneal tendon

Fibularis (peroneus) longus

Fibularis (peroneus) brevis

Fibularis (peroneus) tertius

Lateral patellar retinaculum

Patella

Fibular collateral ligament

Deep (crural) fascia of leg

Extensor digitorum longus

Extensor hallucis longus

Fibularis (peroneus) tertius

Extensor digitorum brevis

Extensor hallucis brevis

Extensor digitorum longus

A. Anterolateral View

B. Anterolateral View

6.65 Lateral Leg and Foot: Muscles

A. Surface anatomy. **B.** Dissection.
- The two fibular (peroneal) muscles both attach to two thirds of the fibula, the fibularis (peroneus) longus muscle to the proximal two thirds, and the fibularis (peroneus) brevis muscle to the distal two thirds. Where they overlap, the fibularis brevis muscle lies anteriorly.
- The fibularis (peroneus) longus muscle enters the foot by hooking around the cuboid and traveling medially to the base of the 1st metatarsal and medial cuneiform.

- **Common fibular (peroneal) nerve lesion.** The nerve lies in contact with the neck of the fibula deep to the fibularis longus muscle, where it is vulnerable to injury (*red circle*). This injury may have serious implications because the nerve supplies the extensor and everter muscle groups, with loss of function resulting in **footdrop** (inability to dorsiflex the ankle) and difficulty in everting the foot.

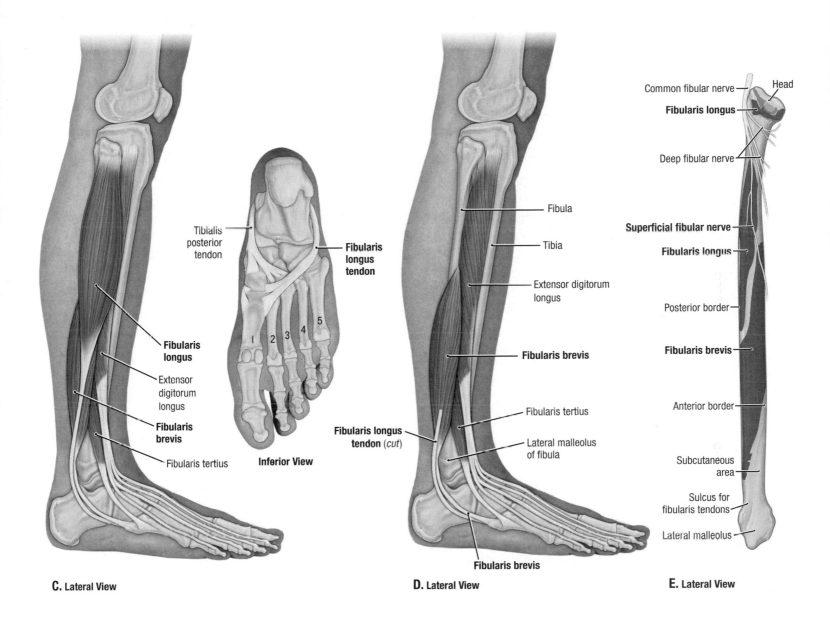

C. Lateral View

Inferior View

D. Lateral View

E. Lateral View

Lateral Leg and Foot: Muscles *(continued)* **6.65**

C. Fibularis (peroneus) longus. **D.** Fibularis (peroneus) brevis. **E.** Attachments sites on fibula.

TABLE 6.13	Muscles of Lateral Compartment of Leg			
Muscle	**Proximal Attachment**	**Distal Attachment**	**Innervation**[a]	**Main Actions**
Fibularis (peroneus) longus	Head and superior two thirds of lateral surface of fibula	Base of 1st metatarsal and medial cuneiform	Superficial fibular (peroneal) nerve (L5, S1, and S2)	Evert foot and weakly plantar flex ankle joint reflexively resist inadvertent inversion of foot
Fibularis (peroneus) brevis	Inferior two thirds of lateral surface of fibula	Dorsal surface of tuberosity on lateral side of base of 5th metatarsal		

[a]See Table 6.2 for explanation of segmental innervation.

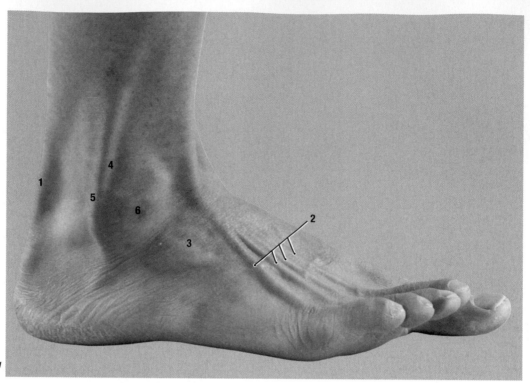

A. Lateral View

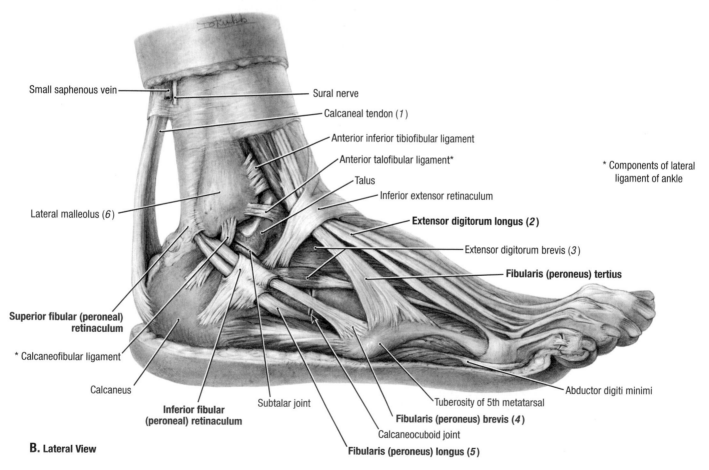

Small saphenous vein

Sural nerve

Calcaneal tendon (*1*)

Anterior inferior tibiofibular ligament

Anterior talofibular ligament*

Talus

Inferior extensor retinaculum

Extensor digitorum longus (*2*)

Lateral malleolus (*6*)

Extensor digitorum brevis (*3*)

Fibularis (peroneus) tertius

Superior fibular (peroneal) retinaculum

* Calcaneofibular ligament

Calcaneus

Abductor digiti minimi

Inferior fibular (peroneal) retinaculum

Subtalar joint

Tuberosity of 5th metatarsal

Fibularis (peroneus) brevis (*4*)

Calcaneocuboid joint

Fibularis (peroneus) longus (*5*)

* Components of lateral ligament of ankle

B. Lateral View

6.66 **Synovial Sheaths and Tendons at Ankle**

A. Surface anatomy. Numbers refer to structures labeled in *Part B*. **B.** Tendons at lateral aspect of ankle.

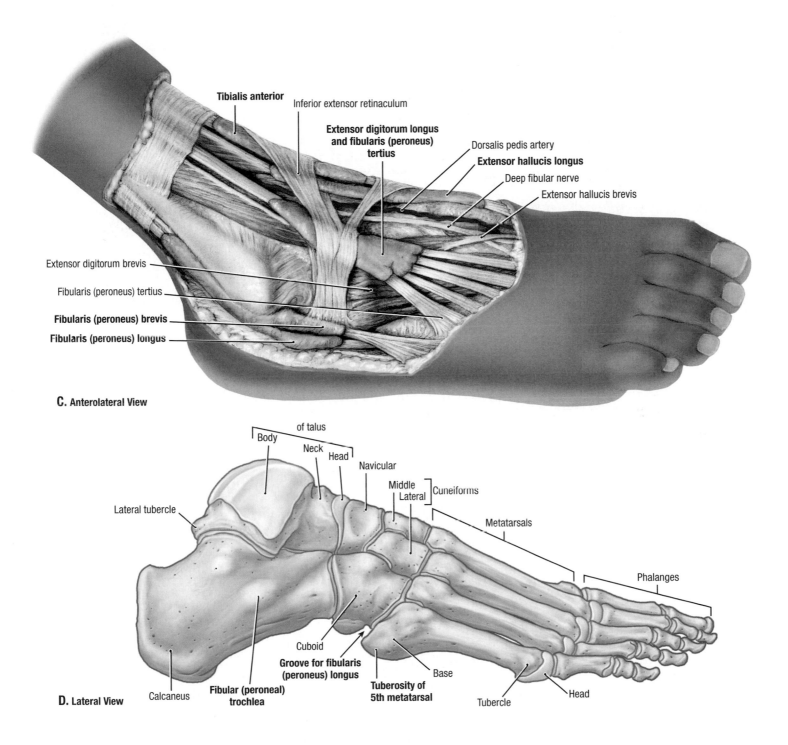

C. Anterolateral View

D. Lateral View

Synovial Sheaths and Tendons at Ankle (continued)

C. Synovial sheaths of tendons on anterolateral aspect of ankle. The tendons of the fibularis (peroneus) longus and fibularis (peroneus) brevis muscles are enclosed in a common synovial sheath posterior to the lateral malleolus. This sheath splits into two, one for each tendon, posterior to the fibular (peroneal) trochlea. **D. Lateral aspect of bones of foot.**

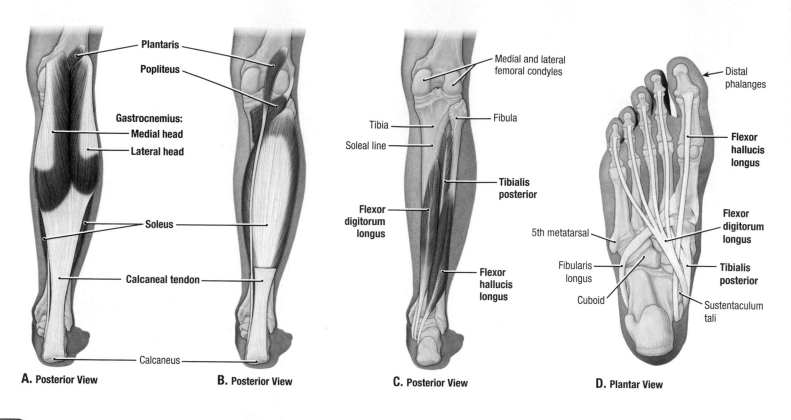

A. Posterior View   **B.** Posterior View   **C.** Posterior View   **D.** Plantar View

6.67   Posterior Leg: Muscles

A. and **B.** Muscles of superficial compartment. **C.** and **D.** Muscles of deep compartment.

TABLE 6.14   Muscles of Posterior Compartment of Leg

Muscle	Proximal Attachment		Distal Attachment	Innervation[a]	Main Actions
Superficial muscles					
Gastrocnemius	*Lateral head:* lateral aspect of lateral condyle of femur		Posterior surface of calcaneus via calcaneal tendon (tendocalcaneus)	Tibial nerve (S1 and S2)	Plantar flexes ankle joint when knee joint is extended; raises heel during walking, and flexes knee joint
	Medial head: popliteal surface of femur, superior to medial condyle				
Soleus	Posterior aspect of head of fibula, superior fourth of posterior surface of fibula, soleal line and medial border of tibia				Plantar flexes ankle joint (independent of knee position) and steadies leg on foot
Plantaris	Inferior end of lateral supracondylar line of femur and oblique popliteal ligament		Posterior surface of calcaneus		Weakly assists gastrocnemius in plantar flexing ankle joint and flexing knee joint
Deep muscles					
Popliteus	Lateral surface of lateral condyle of femur and lateral meniscus		Posterior surface of tibia, superior to soleal line	Tibial nerve (**L4**, **L5**, and **S1**)	Unlocks fully extended knee joint (laterally rotates femur 5 degrees on planted tibia); weakly flexes knee joint
Flexor hallucis longus	Inferior two thirds of posterior surface of fibula and inferior part of interosseous membrane		Base of distal phalanx of great toe (hallux)		Flexes great toe at all joints and plantar flexes ankle joint; supports medial longitudinal arch of foot
Flexor digitorum longus	Medial part of posterior surface of tibia inferior to soleal line, and by a broad tendon to fibula		Bases of distal phalanges of lateral four digits	Tibial nerve (**S2** and **S3**)	Flexes lateral four digits and plantar flexes ankle joint; supports longitudinal arches of foot
Tibialis posterior	Interosseous membrane, posterior surface of tibia inferior to soleal line and posterior surface of fibula		Tuberosity of navicular, cuneiform, and cuboid and bases of metatarsals 2–4	Tibial nerve (**L4** and **L5**)	Plantar flexes ankle joint and inverts foot

[a]Numbers indicate spinal cord segmental innervation of nerves (e.g., S2, and S3 indicate that the part of the tibial nerve supplying flexor digitorum longus is derived from two segments of the spinal cord; boldface type [**S2**] indicates main segmental innervation). Damage to one or more of these spinal cord segments or to motor nerve roots arising from these segments results in paralysis of the muscles concerned.

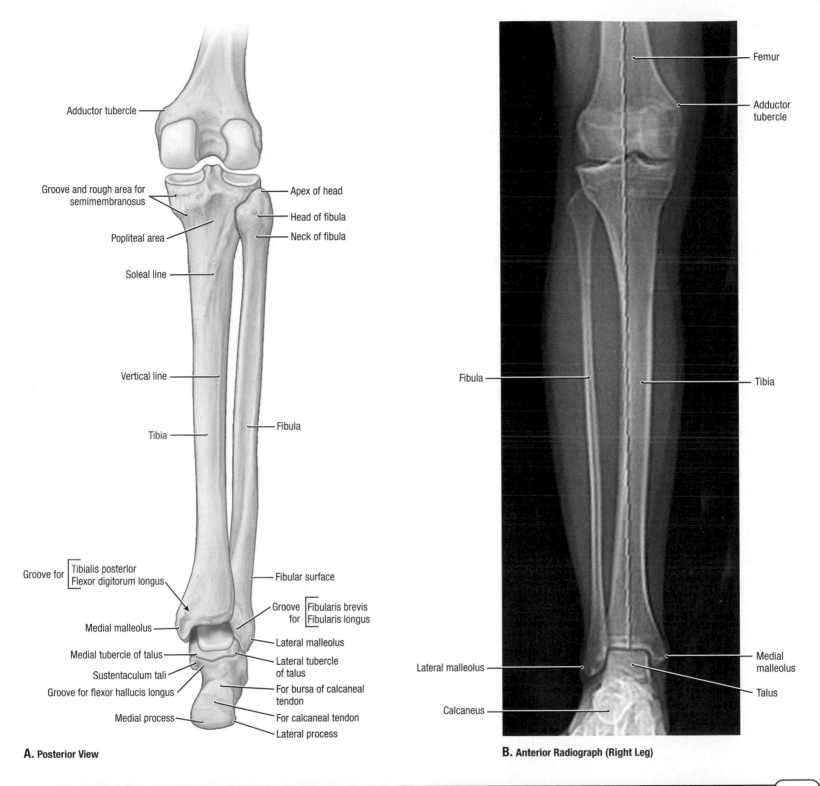

Adductor tubercle

Groove and rough area for
semimembranosus

Apex of head

Head of fibula

Popliteal area

Neck of fibula

Soleal line

Vertical line

Fibula

Tibia

Groove for ⎡ Tibialis posterior
        ⎣ Flexor digitorum longus

Fibular surface

Groove ⎡ Fibularis brevis
for   ⎣ Fibularis longus

Medial malleolus

Lateral malleolus

Medial tubercle of talus

Lateral tubercle
of talus

Sustentaculum tali

Groove for flexor hallucis longus

For bursa of calcaneal
tendon

Medial process

For calcaneal tendon

Lateral process

A. Posterior View

Femur

Adductor
tubercle

Fibula

Tibia

Lateral malleolus

Medial
malleolus

Calcaneus

Talus

B. Anterior Radiograph (Right Leg)

Posterior Leg: Bones

6.68

A. Features of bones. **B.** Radiograph.

Tibial fractures. The tibial shaft is narrowest at the junction of its middle and inferior thirds, which is the most frequent site of fracture. Unfortunately, this area of the bone also has the poorest blood supply.

Fibular fractures. These commonly occur 2 to 6 cm proximal to the distal end of the lateral malleolus and are often associated with fracture/dislocations of the ankle joint, which are combined with tibial fractures. When a person slips and the foot is forced into an excessively inverted position, the ankle ligaments tear, forcibly tilting the talus against the lateral malleolus and shearing it off.

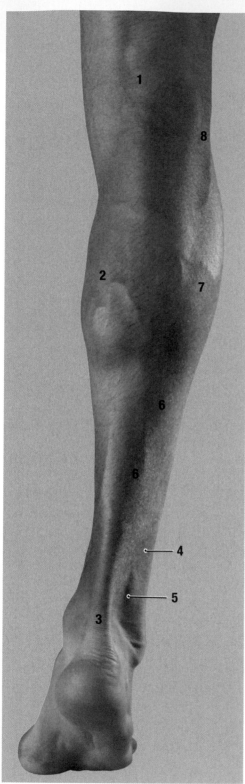

A. Posterior View

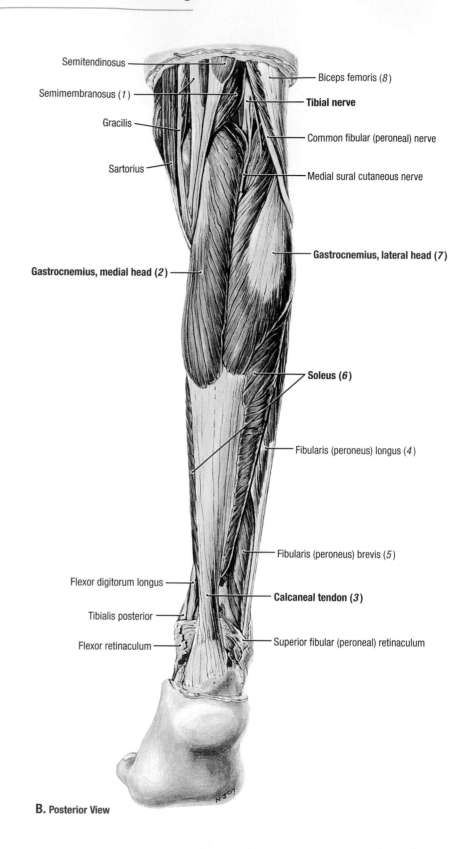

Semitendinosus

Semimembranosus (*1*)

Gracilis

Sartorius

Gastrocnemius, medial head (*2*)

Flexor digitorum longus

Tibialis posterior

Flexor retinaculum

Biceps femoris (*8*)

Tibial nerve

Common fibular (peroneal) nerve

Medial sural cutaneous nerve

Gastrocnemius, lateral head (*7*)

Soleus (*6*)

Fibularis (peroneus) longus (*4*)

Fibularis (peroneus) brevis (*5*)

Calcaneal tendon (*3*)

Superior fibular (peroneal) retinaculum

B. Posterior View

6.69 **Posterior Leg: Superficial Muscles of Posterior Compartment**

A. Surface anatomy. Numbers refer to structures labeled in *Part B*.
B. Dissection.
 Gastrocnemius strain (tennis leg) is a painful calf injury result-
ing from partial tearing of the medial belly of the muscle at or near

its musculotendinous junction. It is caused by overstretching the
muscle during simultaneous full extension of the knee joint and
dorsiflexion of the ankle joint.

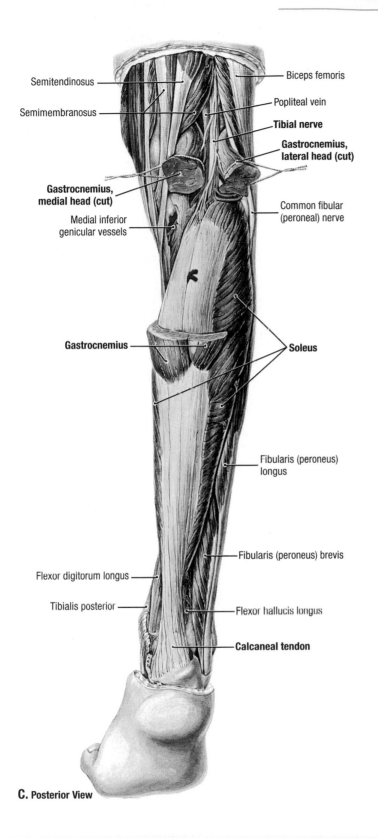

Semitendinosus

Semimembranosus

Gastrocnemius, medial head (cut)

Medial inferior genicular vessels

Gastrocnemius

Flexor digitorum longus

Tibialis posterior

Biceps femoris

Popliteal vein

Tibial nerve

Gastrocnemius, lateral head (cut)

Common fibular (peroneal) nerve

Soleus

Fibularis (peroneus) longus

Fibularis (peroneus) brevis

Flexor hallucis longus

Calcaneal tendon

C. Posterior View

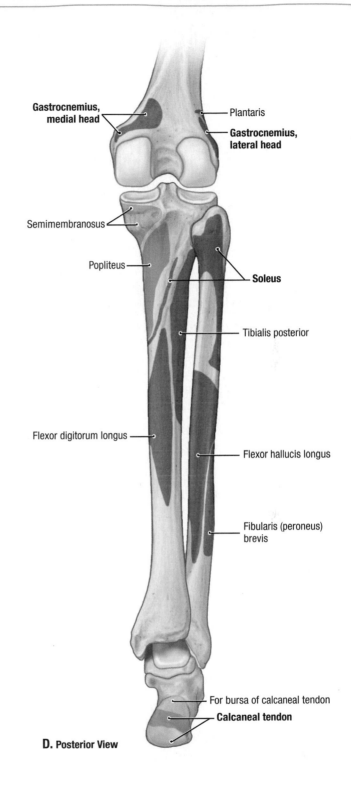

Gastrocnemius, medial head

Semimembranosus

Popliteus

Flexor digitorum longus

Plantaris

Gastrocnemius, lateral head

Soleus

Tibialis posterior

Flexor hallucis longus

Fibularis (peroneus) brevis

For bursa of calcaneal tendon

Calcaneal tendon

D. Posterior View

Posterior Leg: Superficial Muscles of Posterior Compartment *(continued)*

6.69

C. Dissection revealing soleus. **D.** Bones of leg showing muscle attachments.

Inflammation of the calcaneal tendon due to microscopic tears of collagen fibers in the tendon, particularly just superior to its attachment to the calcaneus, results in **calcaneal tendinitis**, which causes pain during walking. **Calcaneal tendon rupture** is probably the most severe acute muscular problem of the leg. Following complete rupture of the tendon, passive dorsiflexion is excessive, and the person cannot plantar flex against resistance.

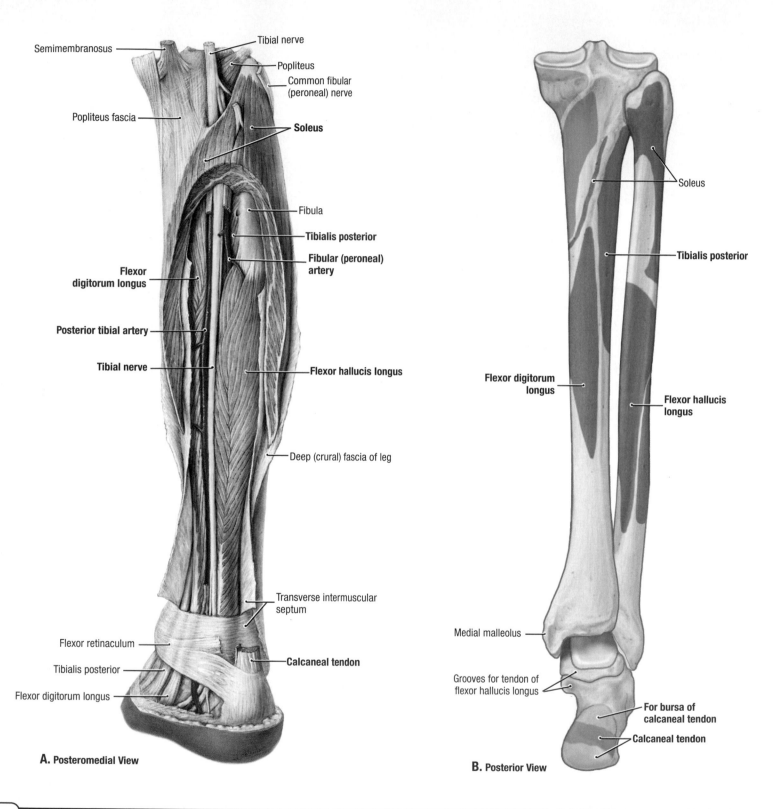

A. Posteromedial View

B. Posterior View

6.70   **Posterior Leg: Deep Muscles of Posterior Compartment**

A. Superficial dissection. The calcaneal (Achilles) tendon is cut, the gastrocnemius muscle is removed, and only a horseshoe-shaped proximal part of the soleus muscle remains in place.
B. Bones of leg showing muscle attachments. Tarsal tunnel syndrome, the entrapment and compression of the tibial nerve, occurs when there is edema and tightness in the ankle involving the synovial sheaths of the tendons of muscles in the posterior compartment of the leg. The area involved is from the medial malleolus to the calcaneus. The heel pain results from compression of the tibial nerve by the flexor retinaculum.

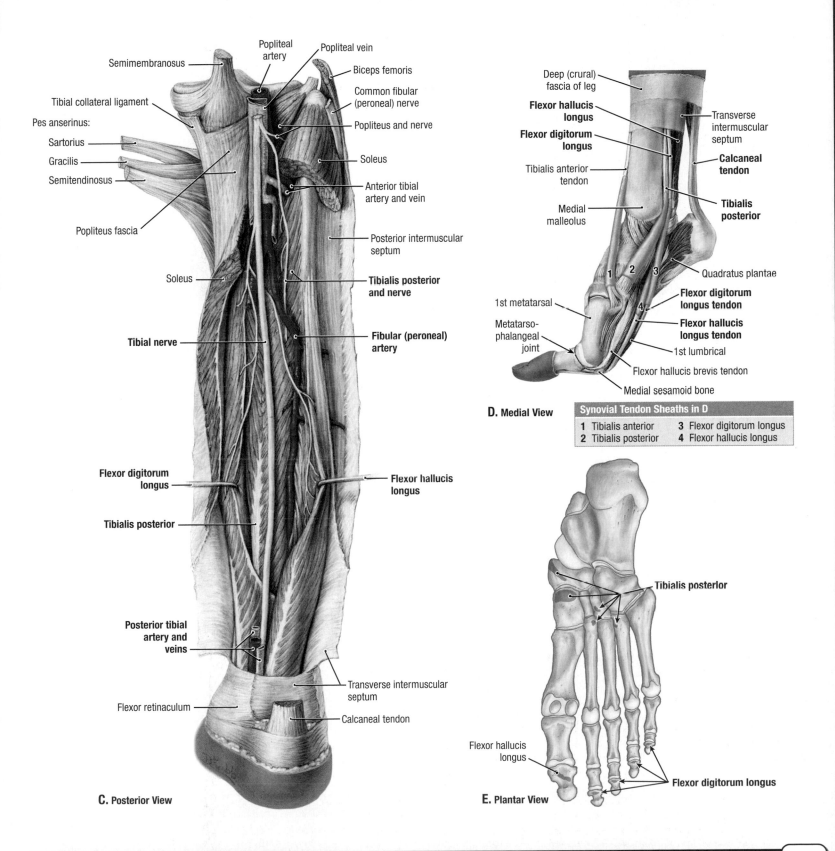

C. Posterior View

Semimembranosus

Popliteal artery

Popliteal vein

Biceps femoris

Tibial collateral ligament

Common fibular (peroneal) nerve

Popliteus and nerve

Pes anserinus:

Sartorius

Gracilis

Semitendinosus

Soleus

Anterior tibial artery and vein

Popliteus fascia

Posterior intermuscular septum

Soleus

Tibialis posterior and nerve

Tibial nerve

Fibular (peroneal) artery

Flexor digitorum longus

Flexor hallucis longus

Tibialis posterior

Posterior tibial artery and veins

Transverse intermuscular septum

Flexor retinaculum

Calcaneal tendon

D. Medial View

Deep (crural) fascia of leg

Flexor hallucis longus

Flexor digitorum longus

Transverse intermuscular septum

Tibialis anterior tendon

Calcaneal tendon

Medial malleolus

Tibialis posterior

1 2 3

Quadratus plantae

1st metatarsal

Flexor digitorum longus tendon

Metatarsophalangeal joint

4

Flexor hallucis longus tendon

1st lumbrical

Flexor hallucis brevis tendon

Medial sesamoid bone

Synovial Tendon Sheaths in D	
1 Tibialis anterior	**3** Flexor digitorum longus
2 Tibialis posterior	**4** Flexor hallucis longus

Tibialis posterior

Flexor hallucis longus

E. Plantar View

Flexor digitorum longus

Posterior Leg: Deep Muscles of Posterior Compartment *(continued)*   **6.70**

C. Deeper dissection. The flexor hallucis longus and flexor digitorum longus are pulled apart, and the posterior tibial artery is partly excised. The tibialis posterior lies deep to the two long digital flexors. **D. Structures passing posterior to medial malleolus.** Synovial sheaths of the tendons are purple; each is named in key. **E. Bones of foot showing muscle attachments.**

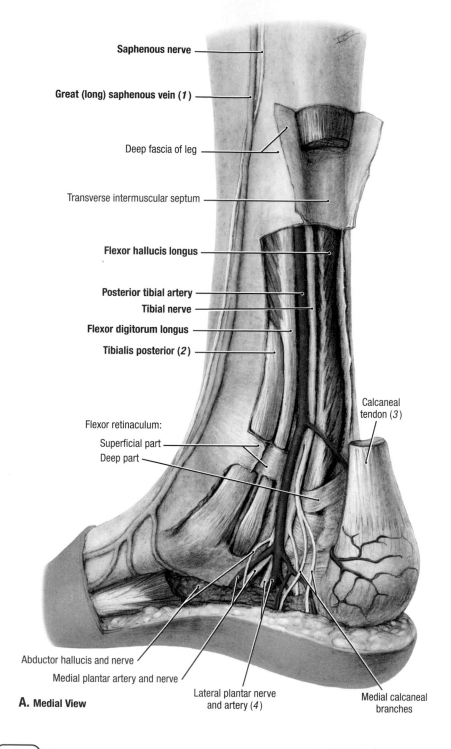

Saphenous nerve

Great (long) saphenous vein (*1*)

Deep fascia of leg

Transverse intermuscular septum

Flexor hallucis longus

Posterior tibial artery
Tibial nerve
Flexor digitorum longus
Tibialis posterior (*2*)

Flexor retinaculum:
  Superficial part
  Deep part

Calcaneal tendon (*3*)

Abductor hallucis and nerve
Medial plantar artery and nerve
Lateral plantar nerve and artery (*4*)
Medial calcaneal branches

A. Medial View

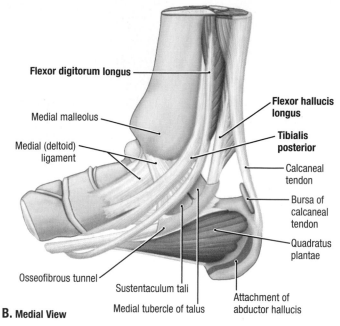

Flexor digitorum longus

Medial malleolus

Medial (deltoid) ligament

Osseofibrous tunnel

Sustentaculum tali
Medial tubercle of talus

Flexor hallucis longus

Tibialis posterior

Calcaneal tendon

Bursa of calcaneal tendon

Quadratus plantae

Attachment of abductor hallucis

B. Medial View

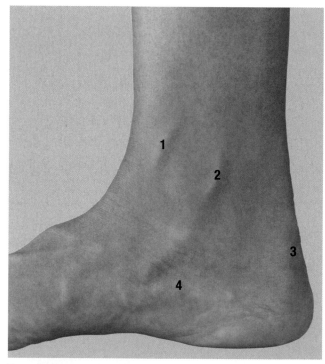

C. Medial View

6.71   Medial Ankle Region

A. Dissection. The calcaneal tendon and posterior part of the abductor hallucis were excised. **B. Schematic of tendons passing posterior to medial malleolus. C. Surface anatomy.** Numbers refer to structures labeled in *Part A*.
- The posterior tibial artery and the tibial nerve lie between the flexor digitorum longus and flexor hallucis longus muscles and divide into medial and lateral plantar branches.

- The tibialis posterior and flexor digitorum longus tendons occupy separate osseofibrous tunnels posterior to the medial malleolus.
- The **posterior tibial pulse** can usually be palpated between the posterior surface of the medial malleolus and the medial border of the calcaneal tendon.

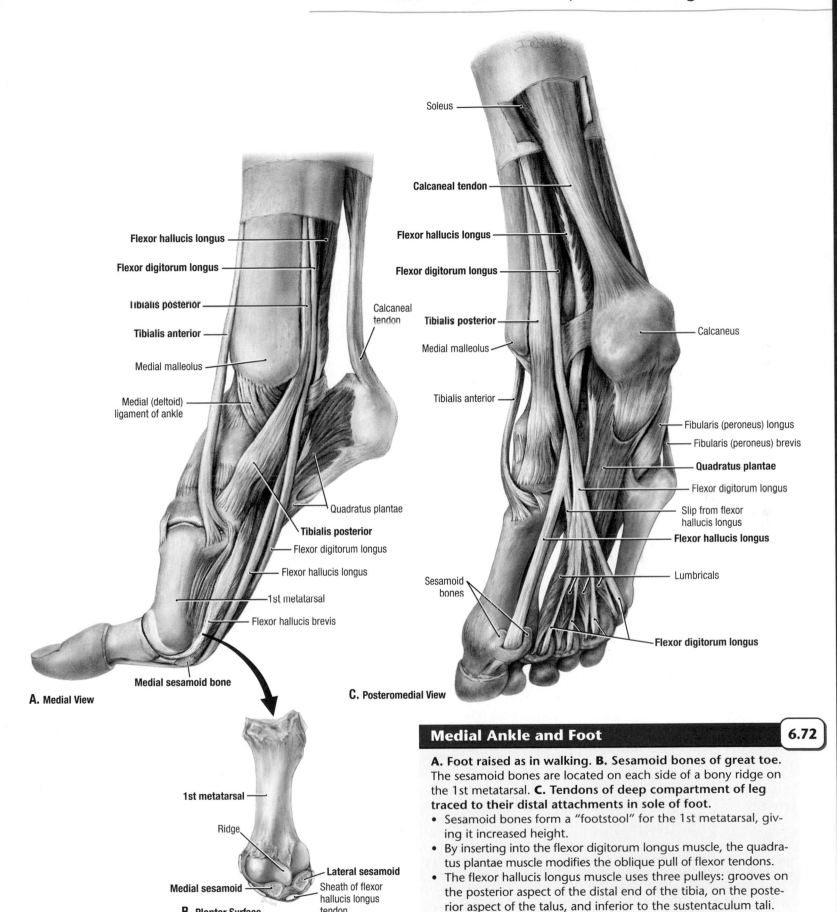

A. Medial View

Flexor hallucis longus
Flexor digitorum longus
Tibialis posterior
Tibialis anterior
Medial malleolus
Medial (deltoid) ligament of ankle
Calcaneal tendon
Quadratus plantae
Tibialis posterior
Flexor digitorum longus
Flexor hallucis longus
1st metatarsal
Flexor hallucis brevis
Medial sesamoid bone

B. Plantar Surface

1st metatarsal
Ridge
Lateral sesamoid
Medial sesamoid
Sheath of flexor hallucis longus tendon

C. Posteromedial View

Soleus
Calcaneal tendon
Flexor hallucis longus
Flexor digitorum longus
Tibialis posterior
Medial malleolus
Tibialis anterior
Calcaneus
Fibularis (peroneus) longus
Fibularis (peroneus) brevis
Quadratus plantae
Flexor digitorum longus
Slip from flexor hallucis longus
Flexor hallucis longus
Lumbricals
Sesamoid bones
Flexor digitorum longus

Medial Ankle and Foot

6.72

A. Foot raised as in walking. B. Sesamoid bones of great toe. The sesamoid bones are located on each side of a bony ridge on the 1st metatarsal. **C.** Tendons of deep compartment of leg traced to their distal attachments in sole of foot.

- Sesamoid bones form a "footstool" for the 1st metatarsal, giving it increased height.
- By inserting into the flexor digitorum longus muscle, the quadratus plantae muscle modifies the oblique pull of flexor tendons.
- The flexor hallucis longus muscle uses three pulleys: grooves on the posterior aspect of the distal end of the tibia, on the posterior aspect of the talus, and inferior to the sustentaculum tali.
- The flexor digitorum longus muscle crosses superficial to the tibialis posterior, superoposterior to the medial malleolus.

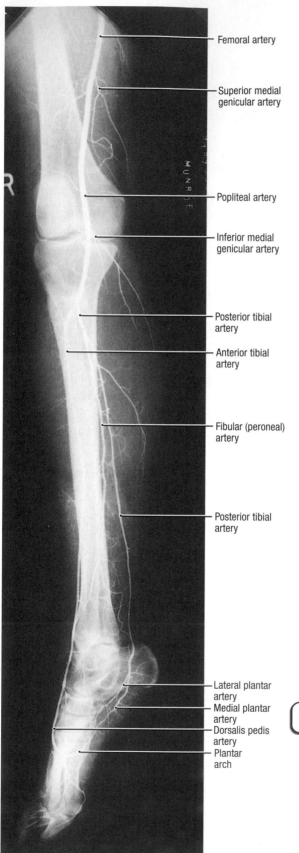

A. Medial Arteriogram

Femoral artery

Superior medial genicular artery

Popliteal artery

Inferior medial genicular artery

Posterior tibial artery

Anterior tibial artery

Fibular (peroneal) artery

Posterior tibial artery

Lateral plantar artery
Medial plantar artery
Dorsalis pedis artery
Plantar arch

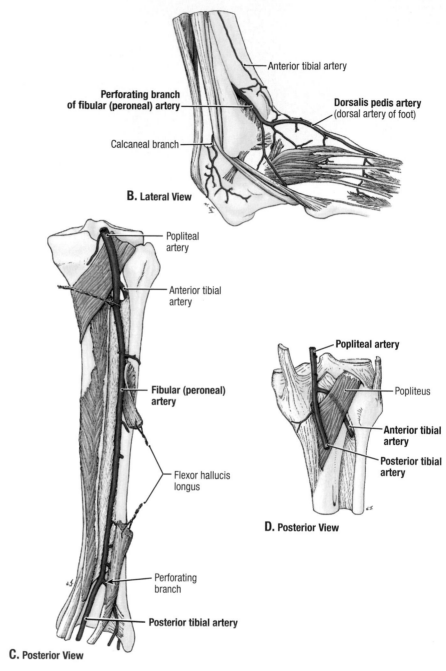

Anterior tibial artery

Perforating branch of fibular (peroneal) artery

Dorsalis pedis artery (dorsal artery of foot)

Calcaneal branch

B. Lateral View

Popliteal artery

Anterior tibial artery

Fibular (peroneal) artery

Flexor hallucis longus

Perforating branch

Posterior tibial artery

C. Posterior View

Popliteal artery

Popliteus

Anterior tibial artery

Posterior tibial artery

D. Posterior View

6.73   **Popliteal Arteriogram and Arterial Anomalies**

A. Popliteal arteriogram. The femoral artery becomes the popliteal artery at the adductor hiatus. The anterior tibial artery continues as the dorsalis pedis (dorsal artery of the foot). The posterior tibial artery terminates as the medial and lateral plantar arteries; its major branch is the fibular artery. **B. Anomalous dorsalis pedis artery.** The perforating branch of the fibular artery rarely continues as the dorsalis pedis artery, but when it does, the anterior tibial artery ends proximal to the ankle or is a slender vessel. **C. Absence of posterior tibial artery.** Compensatory enlargement of the fibular artery was found to occur in approximately 5% of limbs. **D. High division of popliteal artery.** Note that the anterior tibial artery descends anterior to the popliteus muscle. This anomaly was found to occur in approximately 2% of limbs.

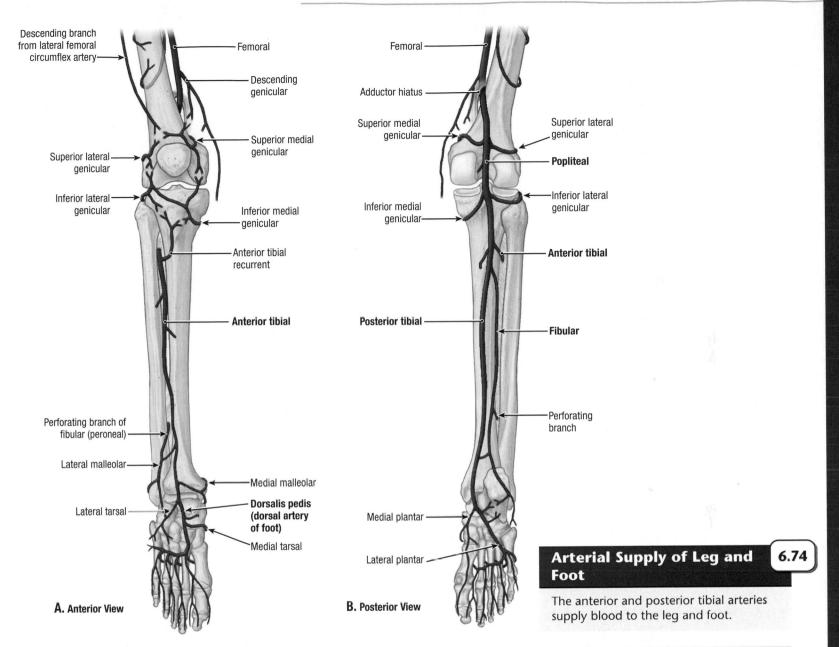

Descending branch from lateral femoral circumflex artery

Femoral

Descending genicular

Superior lateral genicular

Inferior lateral genicular

Superior medial genicular

Inferior medial genicular

Anterior tibial recurrent

Anterior tibial

Perforating branch of fibular (peroneal)

Lateral malleolar

Lateral tarsal

Medial malleolar

Dorsalis pedis (dorsal artery of foot)

Medial tarsal

A. Anterior View

Femoral

Adductor hiatus

Superior medial genicular

Inferior medial genicular

Superior lateral genicular

Popliteal

Inferior lateral genicular

Anterior tibial

Posterior tibial

Fibular

Perforating branch

Medial plantar

Lateral plantar

B. Posterior View

Arterial Supply of Leg and Foot   6.74

The anterior and posterior tibial arteries supply blood to the leg and foot.

TABLE 6.15   Arterial Supply of Leg and Foot

Artery	Origin	Course	Distribution in Leg
Popliteal	Continuation of femoral artery at adductor hiatus	Passes through popliteal fossa to leg; divides into anterior and posterior tibial arteries at lower border of popliteus	All aspects of knee via genicular arteries
Anterior tibial	From popliteal	Passes between tibia and fibula into anterior compartment through gap superior to interosseous membrane; descends between tibialis anterior and extensor digitorum longus muscles	Anterior compartment of leg
Dorsalis pedis (dorsal artery of foot)	Continuation of anterior tibial artery distal to talocrural joint	Descends to first interosseous space; pierces first dorsal interosseous muscle as deep plantar artery; joins deep plantar arch	Muscles on dorsum of foot
Posterior tibial	From popliteal	Passes through posterior compartment; divides into medial and lateral plantar arteries posterior to medial malleolus	Posterior and lateral compartments of leg, nutrient artery passes to tibia
Fibular (peroneal)		Descends in posterior compartment adjacent to posterior intermuscular septum	Posterior compartment: perforating branches supply lateral compartment
Medial plantar	From posterior tibial	In foot between abductor hallucis and flexor digitorum brevis muscles	Supplies mainly muscles of great toe and skin on medial side of sole of foot
Lateral plantar		Runs anterolaterally deep to abductor hallucis and flexor digitorum brevis and then arches medially to form deep plantar arch	Supplies lateral aspect of sole of foot

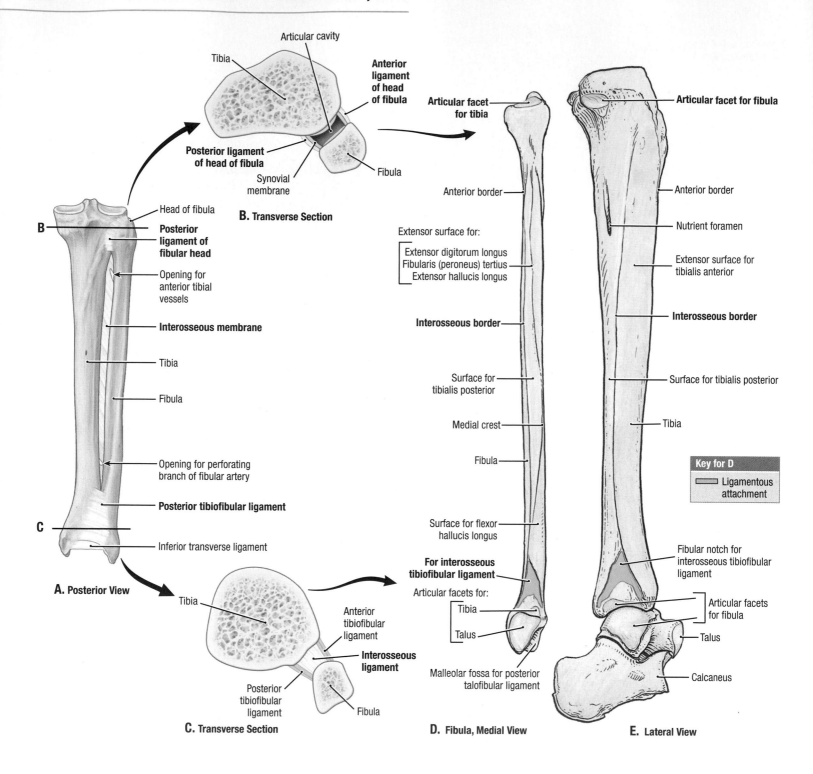

Articular cavity

Tibia

Anterior ligament of head of fibula

Articular facet for tibia

Articular facet for fibula

Posterior ligament of head of fibula

Synovial membrane

Fibula

B. Transverse Section

Head of fibula

Posterior ligament of fibular head

Opening for anterior tibial vessels

Interosseous membrane

Tibia

Fibula

Opening for perforating branch of fibular artery

Posterior tibiofibular ligament

Inferior transverse ligament

A. Posterior View

Anterior border

Nutrient foramen

Anterior border

Extensor surface for:
   Extensor digitorum longus
   Fibularis (peroneus) tertius
   Extensor hallucis longus

Extensor surface for tibialis anterior

Interosseous border

Interosseous border

Surface for tibialis posterior

Surface for tibialis posterior

Medial crest

Tibia

Fibula

Key for D

☐ Ligamentous attachment

Surface for flexor hallucis longus

For interosseous tibiofibular ligament

Fibular notch for interosseous tibiofibular ligament

Articular facets for:
   Tibia
   Talus

Articular facets for fibula

Talus

Malleolar fossa for posterior talofibular ligament

Calcaneus

D. Fibula, Medial View

E. Lateral View

Tibia

Anterior tibiofibular ligament

Interosseous ligament

Posterior tibiofibular ligament

Fibula

C. Transverse Section

6.75 Tibiofibular Joint and Tibiofibular Syndesmosis

A. Overview. **B.** Tibiofibular joint. **C.** Tibiofibular syndesmosis. **D.** and **E.** Tibia and fibula, disarticulated.

• The superior tibiofibular joint (proximal tibiofibular joint) is a plane type of synovial joint between the flat facet on the fibular head and a similar facet located posterolaterally on the lateral tibial condyle. The tense joint capsule surrounds the joint and attaches to the margins of the articular surfaces of the fibula and tibia.

• The tibiofibular syndesmosis is a fibrous joint. This articulation is essential for stability of the ankle joint because it keeps the lateral malleolus firmly against the lateral surface of the talus. The strong interosseous tibiofibular ligament is continuous superiorly with the interosseous membrane and forms the principal connection between the distal ends of the tibia and fibula.

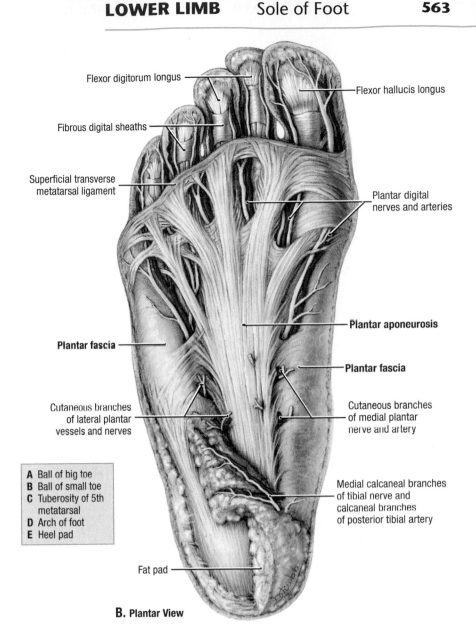

Flexor digitorum longus

Flexor hallucis longus

Fibrous digital sheaths

Superficial transverse metatarsal ligament

Plantar digital nerves and arteries

Plantar aponeurosis

Plantar fascia

Plantar fascia

Cutaneous branches of lateral plantar vessels and nerves

Cutaneous branches of medial plantar nerve and artery

Medial calcaneal branches of tibial nerve and calcaneal branches of posterior tibial artery

Fat pad

B. Plantar View

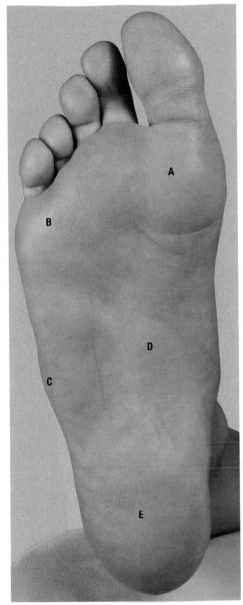

A Ball of big toe
B Ball of small toe
C Tuberosity of 5th metatarsal
D Arch of foot
E Heel pad

A. Plantar View

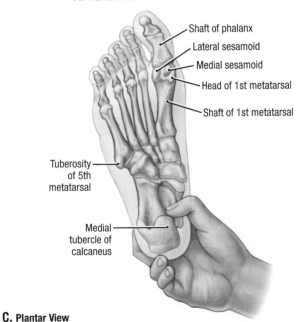

Shaft of phalanx

Lateral sesamoid

Medial sesamoid

Head of 1st metatarsal

Shaft of 1st metatarsal

Tuberosity of 5th metatarsal

Medial tubercle of calcaneus

C. Plantar View

Sole of Foot, Superficial

6.76

A. Surface anatomy. B. Dissection. Plantar aponeurosis and fascia, with neurovascular structures. **C. Palpation of medial tubercle of calcaneus.**

Plantar fasciitis, strain and inflammation of the plantar aponeurosis, may result from running and high-impact aerobics, especially when inappropriate footwear is worn. It causes pain on the plantar surface of the heel and on the medial aspect of the foot. Point tenderness is located at the proximal attachment of the plantar aponeurosis to the medial tubercle of the calcaneus and on the medial surface of this bone. The pain increases with passive extension of the great toe and may be further exacerbated by dorsiflexion of the ankle and/or weight bearing.

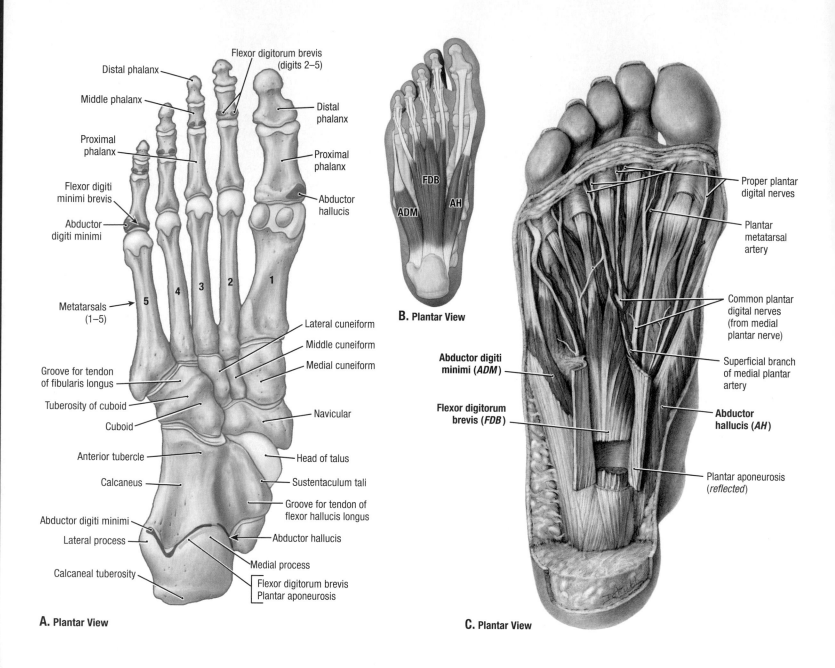

A. Plantar View

Distal phalanx

Middle phalanx

Proximal phalanx

Flexor digiti minimi brevis

Abductor digiti minimi

Metatarsals (1–5)

Groove for tendon of fibularis longus

Tuberosity of cuboid

Cuboid

Anterior tubercle

Calcaneus

Abductor digiti minimi

Lateral process

Calcaneal tuberosity

Flexor digitorum brevis (digits 2–5)

Distal phalanx

Proximal phalanx

Abductor hallucis

Lateral cuneiform

Middle cuneiform

Medial cuneiform

Navicular

Head of talus

Sustentaculum tali

Groove for tendon of flexor hallucis longus

Abductor hallucis

Medial process

Flexor digitorum brevis
Plantar aponeurosis

B. Plantar View

FDB

ADM

AH

C. Plantar View

Proper plantar digital nerves

Plantar metatarsal artery

Common plantar digital nerves (from medial plantar nerve)

Superficial branch of medial plantar artery

Abductor hallucis (AH)

Plantar aponeurosis (*reflected*)

Abductor digiti minimi (ADM)

Flexor digitorum brevis (FDB)

6.77   **First Layer of Muscles of Sole of Foot**

A. Bones. B. Overview. C. Dissection. Muscles and neurovascular structures.

TABLE 6.16	Muscles in Sole of Foot—First Layer			
Muscle	**Proximal Attachment**	**Distal Attachment**	**Innervation**	**Actions**[a]
Abductor hallucis	Medial process of tuberosity of calcaneus, flexor retinaculum, and plantar aponeurosis	Medial side of base of proximal phalanx of 1st digit	Medial plantar nerve (L5, S1)	Abducts and flexes 1st digit
Flexor digitorum brevis	Medial process of tuberosity of calcaneus, plantar aponeurosis, and intermuscular septa	Both sides of middle phalanges of lateral four digits		Flexes lateral four digits
Abductor digiti minimi	Medial and lateral processes of tuberosity of calcaneus, plantar aponeurosis, and intermuscular septa	Lateral side of base of proximal phalanx of 5th digit	Lateral plantar nerve (S1–S3)	Abducts and flexes 5th digit

[a]Although individual actions are described, the primary function of the intrinsic muscles of the foot is to act collectively to resist forces that stress (attempt to flatten) the arches of the foot.

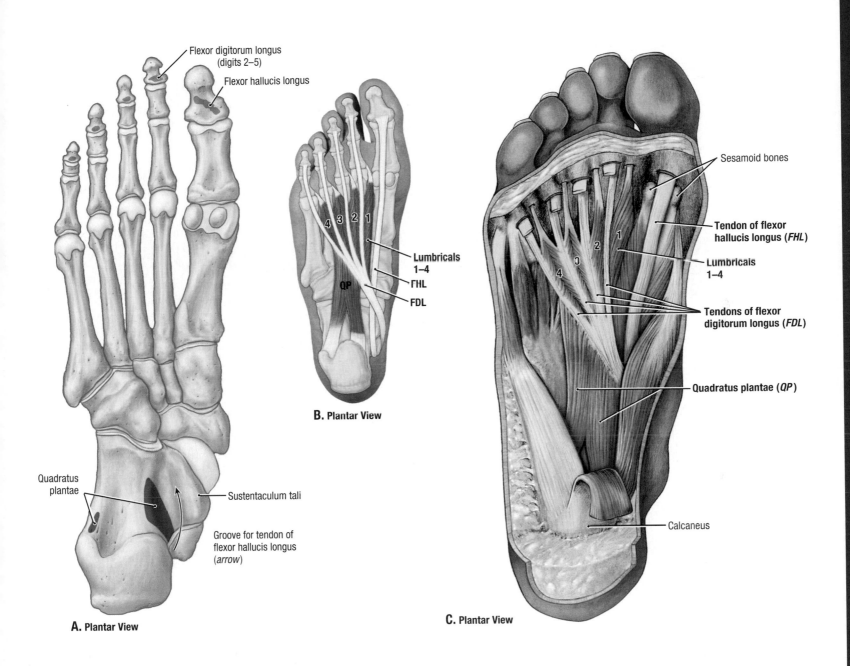

B. Plantar View

C. Plantar View

A. Plantar View

Second Layer of Muscles of Sole of Foot

6.78

A. Bony attachments. **B.** Overview. **C.** Dissection. Muscles as *in situ*.

TABLE 6.17	Muscles in Sole of Foot—Second Layer			
Muscle	**Proximal Attachment**	**Distal Attachment**	**Innervation**	**Actions[a]**
Quadratus plantae	Medial surface and lateral margin of plantar surface of calcaneus	Posterolateral margin of tendon of flexor digitorum longus	Lateral plantar nerve (S1–S3)	Assists flexor digitorum longus in flexing lateral four digits
Lumbricals	Tendons of flexor digitorum longus	Medial aspect of extensor expansion over lateral four digits	*Medial one:* medial plantar nerve (L5, S1) *Lateral three:* lateral plantar nerve (S1–S3)	Flex proximal phalanges and extend middle and distal phalanges of lateral four digits

[a]Although individual actions are described, the primary function of the intrinsic muscles of the foot is to act collectively to resist forces that stress (attempt to flatten) the arches of the foot.

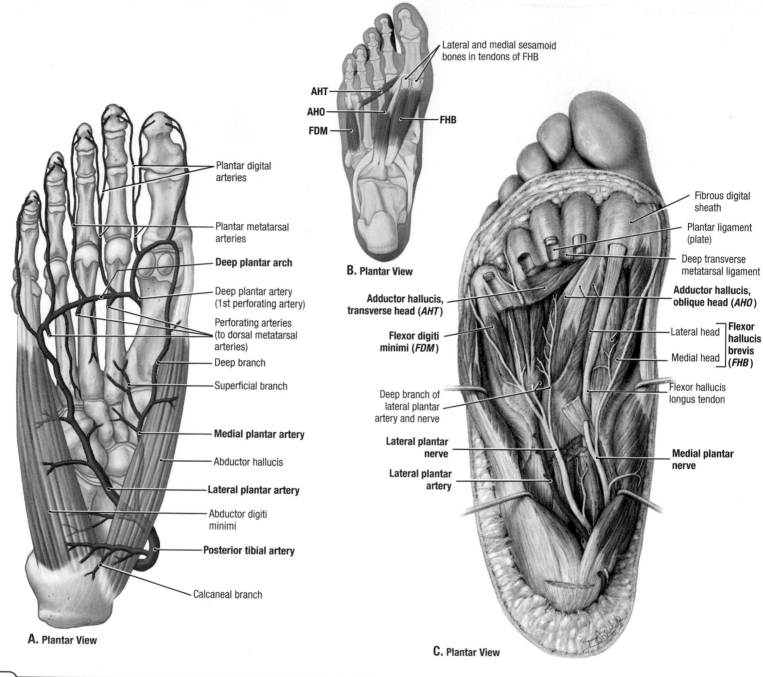

Plantar digital arteries

Plantar metatarsal arteries

Deep plantar arch

Deep plantar artery (1st perforating artery)

Perforating arteries (to dorsal metatarsal arteries)

Deep branch

Superficial branch

Medial plantar artery

Abductor hallucis

Lateral plantar artery

Abductor digiti minimi

Posterior tibial artery

Calcaneal branch

A. Plantar View

Lateral and medial sesamoid bones in tendons of FHB

AHT
AHO
FDM
FHB

B. Plantar View

Adductor hallucis, transverse head (*AHT*)

Flexor digiti minimi (*FDM*)

Deep branch of lateral plantar artery and nerve

Lateral plantar nerve

Lateral plantar artery

Fibrous digital sheath

Plantar ligament (plate)

Deep transverse metatarsal ligament

Adductor hallucis, oblique head (*AHO*)

Lateral head
Medial head
Flexor hallucis brevis (*FHB*)

Flexor hallucis longus tendon

Medial plantar nerve

C. Plantar View

6.79   **Third Layer of Muscles and Arterial Supply of Sole of Foot**

A. Arterial supply. **B.** Overview. **C.** Dissection. Muscles and neurovascular structures.

TABLE 6.18	Muscles in Sole of Foot—Third Layer			
Muscle	**Proximal Attachment**	**Distal Attachment**	**Innervation**	**Actions**[a]
Flexor hallucis brevis	Plantar surfaces of cuboid and lateral cuneiforms	Both sides of base of proximal phalanx of 1st digit	Medial plantar nerve (L5, S1)	Flexes proximal phalanx of 1st digit
Adductor hallucis	*Oblique head:* bases of metatarsals 2–4 *Transverse head:* plantar ligaments of metatarsophalangeal joints	Tendons of both heads attach to lateral side of base of proximal phalanx of 1st digit	Deep branch of lateral plantar nerve (S1–S3)	Adducts 1st digit; assists in maintaining transverse arch of foot
Flexor digiti minimi	Base of 5th metatarsal	Base of proximal phalanx of 5th digit	Superficial branch of lateral plantar nerve (S1–S3)	Flexes proximal phalanx of 5th digit, thereby assisting with its flexion

[a]Although individual actions are described, the primary function of the intrinsic muscles of the foot is to act collectively to resist forces that stress (attempt to flatten) the arches of the foot.

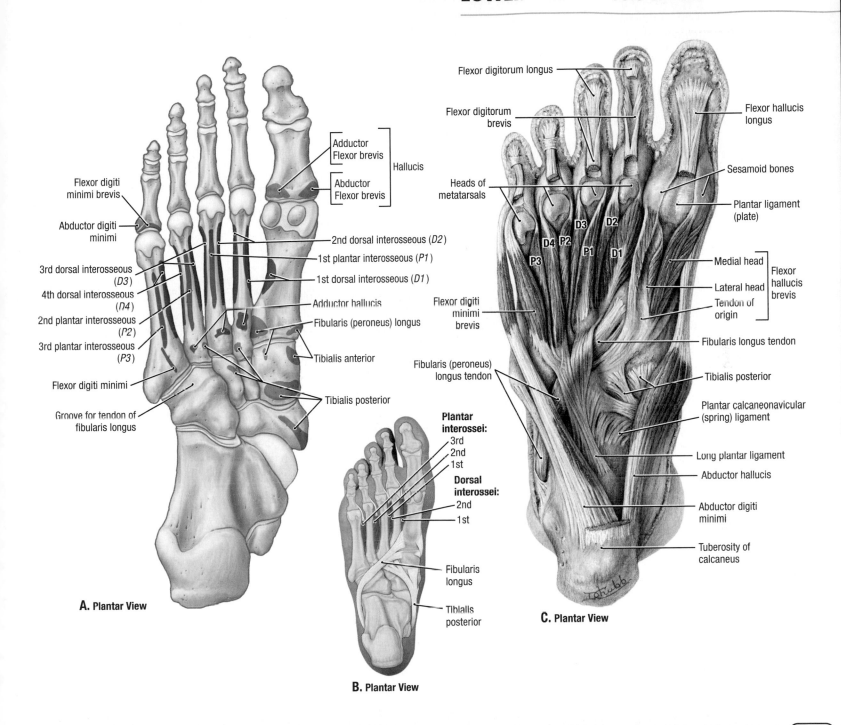

Flexor digitorum longus

Flexor digitorum brevis

Flexor digiti minimi brevis

Abductor digiti minimi

3rd dorsal interosseous (*D3*)

4th dorsal interosseous (*D4*)

2nd plantar interosseous (*P2*)

3rd plantar interosseous (*P3*)

Flexor digiti minimi

Groove for tendon of fibularis longus

Flexor digiti minimi brevis

Adductor Flexor brevis

Abductor Flexor brevis

Hallucis

2nd dorsal interosseous (*D2*)

1st plantar interosseous (*P1*)

1st dorsal interosseous (*D1*)

Adductor hallucis

Fibularis (peroneus) longus

Tibialis anterior

Tibialis posterior

A. Plantar View

Flexor hallucis longus

Flexor digitorum brevis

Heads of metatarsals

D4 P2

P3

D3 D2

P1 D1

Flexor hallucis longus

Sesamoid bones

Plantar ligament (plate)

Medial head

Lateral head

Flexor hallucis brevis

Tendon of origin

Flexor digiti minimi brevis

Fibularis (peroneus) longus tendon

Fibularis longus tendon

Tibialis posterior

Plantar calcaneonavicular (spring) ligament

Long plantar ligament

Abductor hallucis

Abductor digiti minimi

Tuberosity of calcaneus

C. Plantar View

Plantar interossei:
3rd
2nd
1st

Dorsal interossei:
2nd
1st

Fibularis longus

Tibialis posterior

B. Plantar View

Fourth Layer of Muscles of Sole of Foot

6.80

A. Bony attachments of muscles of third and fourth layers. **B.** Overview. **C.** Dissection. Muscles and ligaments.

TABLE 6.19	Muscles in Sole of Foot—Fourth Layer			
Muscle	**Proximal Attachment**	**Distal Attachment**	**Innervation**	**Actions**[a]
Plantar interossei (three muscles; P1–P3)	Plantar aspect of medial sides of shafts of metatarsals 3–5	Medial sides of bases of proximal phalanges of 3rd to 5th digits	Lateral plantar nerve (S1–S3)	Adduct digits 3–5 and flex metatarsophalangeal joints
Dorsal interossei (four muscles; D1–D4)	Adjacent sides of shafts of metatarsals 1–5	First: medial side of proximal phalanx of 2nd digit Second to fourth: lateral sides of 2nd to 4th digits		Abduct digits 2–4 and flex metatarsophalangeal joints

[a]Although individual actions are described, the primary function of the intrinsic muscles of the foot is to act collectively to resist forces that stress (attempt to flatten) the arches of the foot.

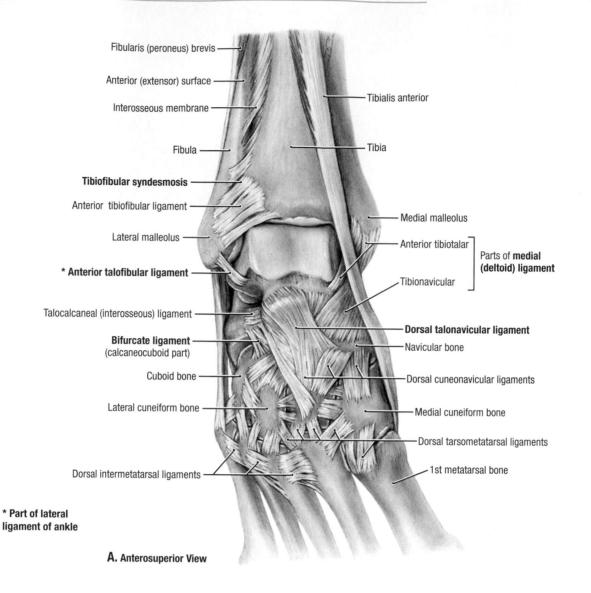

Fibularis (peroneus) brevis

Anterior (extensor) surface

Interosseous membrane

Fibula

Tibiofibular syndesmosis

Anterior tibiofibular ligament

Lateral malleolus

* Anterior talofibular ligament

Talocalcaneal (interosseous) ligament

Bifurcate ligament
(calcaneocuboid part)

Cuboid bone

Lateral cuneiform bone

Dorsal intermetatarsal ligaments

Tibialis anterior

Tibia

Medial malleolus

Anterior tibiotalar   Parts of **medial
(deltoid) ligament**

Tibionavicular

Dorsal talonavicular ligament

Navicular bone

Dorsal cuneonavicular ligaments

Medial cuneiform bone

Dorsal tarsometatarsal ligaments

1st metatarsal bone

*** Part of lateral
ligament of ankle**

A. Anterosuperior View

6.81 | **Ankle Joint and Ligaments of Dorsum of
Foot**

A. Dissection. The ankle joint is plantar flexed, and its anterior
capsular fibers are removed. Note that the bifurcate ligament, a
Y-shaped ligament consisting of calcaneocuboid and calcaneonavicular ligaments, and the dorsal talonavicular ligament are the
primary dorsal ligaments of the transverse tarsal joint. **B. Ankle
joint with joint cavity distended with injected latex.** Note the
relations of the tendons to the sustentaculum tali: the flexor hallucis longus inferior to it, flexor digitorum longus along its medial
aspect, and tibialis posterior superior to it and in contact with the
medial (deltoid) ligament.

A **Pott fracture-dislocation of the ankle** occurs when the
foot is forcibly everted. This action pulls on the extremely strong
medial (deltoid) ligament, often avulsing the medial malleolus and
compressing the lateral malleolus against the talus, shearing off
the malleolus or, more often, fracturing the fibula superior to the
tibiofibular syndesmosis.

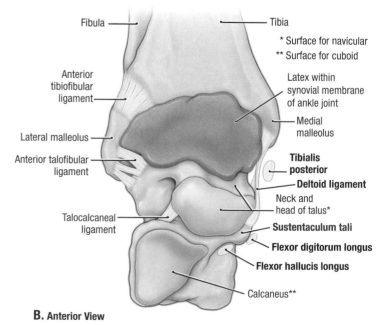

Fibula

Anterior
tibiofibular
ligament

Lateral malleolus

Anterior talofibular
ligament

Talocalcaneal
ligament

Tibia

* Surface for navicular
** Surface for cuboid

Latex within
synovial membrane
of ankle joint

Medial
malleolus

**Tibialis
posterior**

Deltoid ligament

Neck and
head of talus*

Sustentaculum tali

Flexor digitorum longus

Flexor hallucis longus

Calcaneus**

B. Anterior View

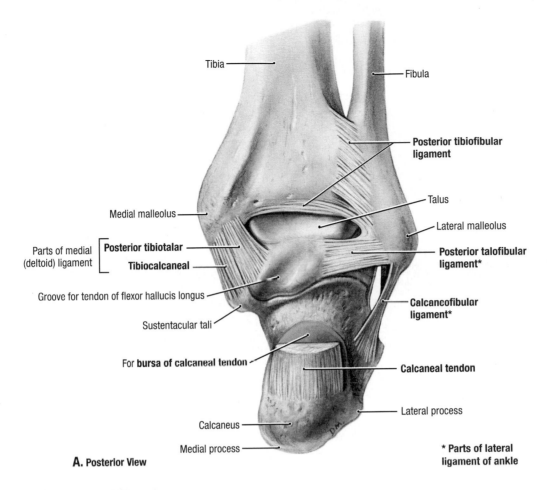

Tibia

Fibula

Posterior tibiofibular ligament

Talus

Medial malleolus

Lateral malleolus

Parts of medial (deltoid) ligament { **Posterior tibiotalar** **Tibiocalcaneal** }

Posterior talofibular ligament*

Groove for tendon of flexor hallucis longus

Calcaneofibular ligament*

Sustentacular tali

For **bursa of calcaneal tendon**

Calcaneal tendon

Lateral process

Calcaneus

Medial process

A. Posterior View

*** Parts of lateral ligament of ankle**

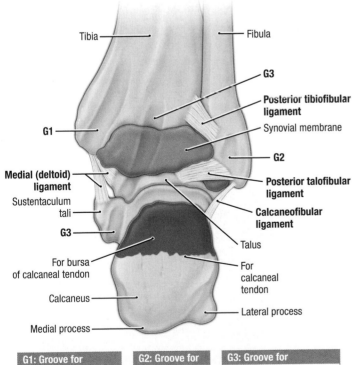

Tibia

Fibula

G3

Posterior tibiofibular ligament

Synovial membrane

G1

G2

Medial (deltoid) ligament

Posterior talofibular ligament

Sustentaculum tali

G3

Calcaneofibular ligament

For bursa of calcaneal tendon

Talus

For calcaneal tendon

Calcaneus

Lateral process

Medial process

G1: Groove for	G2: Groove for	G3: Groove for
Tibialis posterior Flexor digitorum longus	Fibularis brevis Fibularis longus	Flexor hallucis longus

B. Posterior View

Posterior Aspect of Ankle Joint   6.82

A. Dissection. B. Ankle joint with joint cavity distended with latex. Observe the grooves for the flexor hallucis longus muscle, which crosses the middle of the ankle joint posteriorly, the two tendons posterior to the medial malleolus, and the two tendons posterior to the lateral malleolus.

- The posterior aspect of the ankle joint is strengthened by the transversely oriented posterior tibiofibular and posterior talofibular ligaments.
- The calcaneofibular ligament stabilizes the joint laterally, and the posterior tibiotalar and tibiocalcanean parts of the medial (deltoid) ligament stabilize it medially.
- The groove for the flexor hallucis tendon is between the medial and lateral tubercles of the talus and continues inferior to the sustentaculum tali.

Calcaneal bursitis results from inflammation of the bursa of the calcaneal tendon located between the calcaneal tendon and the superior part of the posterior surface of the calcaneus. Calcaneal bursitis causes pain posterior to the heel and occurs commonly during long-distance running, basketball, and tennis. It is caused by excessive friction on the bursa as the calcaneal tendon continuously slides over it.

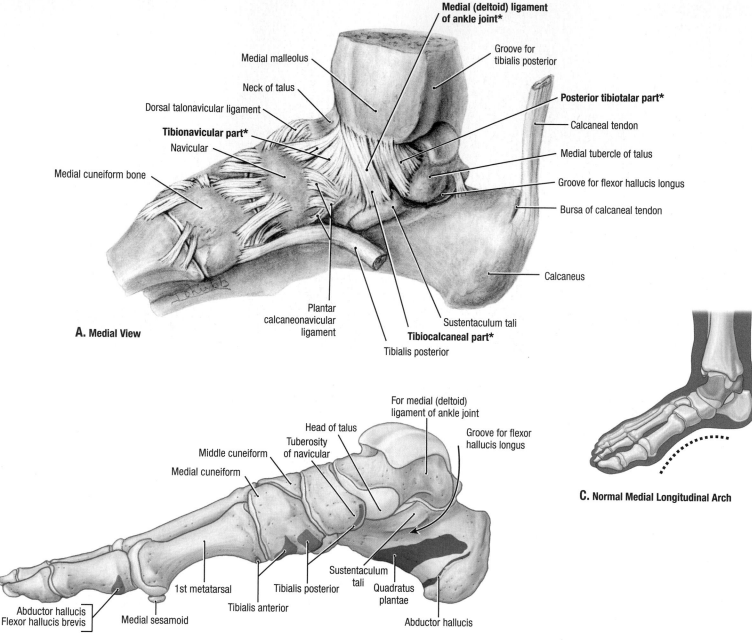

A. Medial View

Medial (deltoid) ligament of ankle joint*

Medial malleolus

Neck of talus

Dorsal talonavicular ligament

Tibionavicular part*

Navicular

Medial cuneiform bone

Groove for tibialis posterior

Posterior tibiotalar part*

Calcaneal tendon

Medial tubercle of talus

Groove for flexor hallucis longus

Bursa of calcaneal tendon

Calcaneus

Plantar calcaneonavicular ligament

Sustentaculum tali

Tibiocalcaneal part*

Tibialis posterior

B. Medial View

For medial (deltoid) ligament of ankle joint

Head of talus

Tuberosity of navicular

Groove for flexor hallucis longus

Middle cuneiform

Medial cuneiform

Sustentaculum tali

Quadratus plantae

Abductor hallucis

1st metatarsal

Tibialis posterior

Tibialis anterior

Abductor hallucis
Flexor hallucis brevis

Medial sesamoid

C. Normal Medial Longitudinal Arch

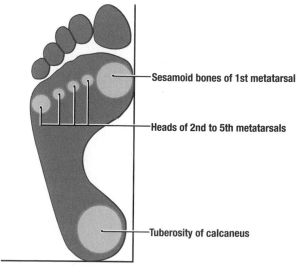

D. Plantar View

Sesamoid bones of 1st metatarsal

Heads of 2nd to 5th metatarsals

Tuberosity of calcaneus

6.83 Medial Ligaments of Ankle Region

A. Dissection. B. Bones. The joint capsule of the ankle joint is reinforced medially by the large, strong medial (deltoid) ligament that attaches proximally to the medial malleolus and fans out from it to attach distally to the talus, calcaneus, and navicular via four adjacent and continuous parts: the tibionavicular part, the tibiocalcaneal part, and the anterior and posterior tibiotalar parts. The medial ligament stabilizes the ankle joint during eversion of the foot and prevents subluxation (partial dislocation) of the ankle joint. **C. Normal medial longitudinal arch. D. Weight-bearing areas.** The weight of the body is transmitted to the talus from the tibia and fibula. It is then transmitted to the tuberosity of the calcaneus, the heads of the 2nd to 5th metatarsals, and the sesamoid bones of the 1st digit.

Key for A, B, and C

A	Calcaneal (Achilles) tendon
Ca	Calcaneus
Cb	Cuboid
Cu	Cuneiforms
F	Fat
L	Lateral malleolus
M	Medial malleolus
MT	Metatarsal
N	Navicular
S	Sustentaculum tali
Su	Superimposed tibia and fibula
T	Talus
TF	Tibiofibular syndesmosis
TH	Head of talus
TN	Neck of talus
TS	Tarsal sinus

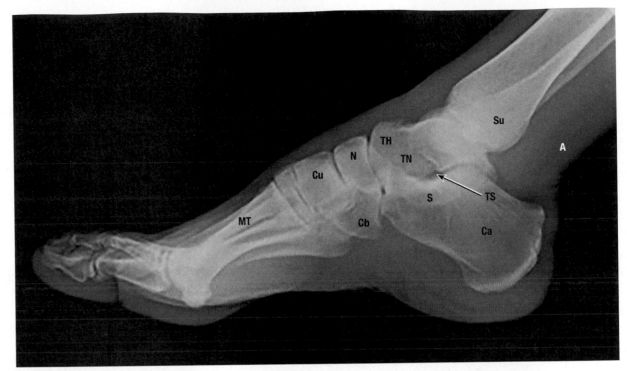

A. Medial Radiograph

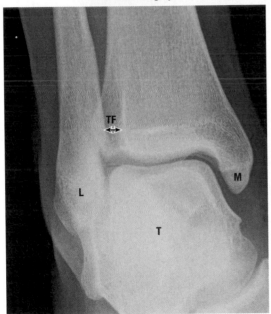

B. Anteroposterior Radiograph

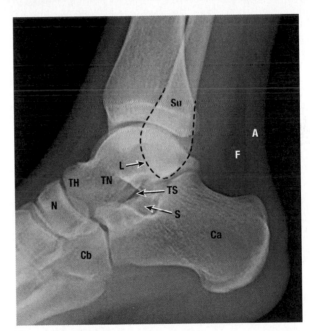

C. Lateral Radiograph

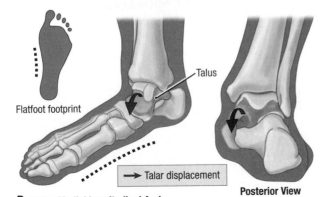

Flatfoot footprint

Talus

→ Talar displacement

D. Fallen Medial Longitudinal Arch

Posterior View

Radiographs of Ankle and Foot

6.84

A–C. Imaging of ankle region and tarsal bones. **D. Pes planus** (flatfeet). Acquired flatfeet ("fallen arches") are likely to be secondary to dysfunction of the tibialis posterior due to trauma, degeneration with age, or denervation. In the absence of normal passive or dynamic support, the plantar calcaneonavicular ligament fails to support the head of the talus. Consequently, the head of the talus displaces inferomedially. As a result, flattening of the medial longitudinal arch occurs along with lateral deviation of the forefoot. Flatfeet are common in older people, particularly if they undertake much unaccustomed standing or gain weight rapidly, adding stress on the muscles and increasing strain on the ligaments supporting the arches.

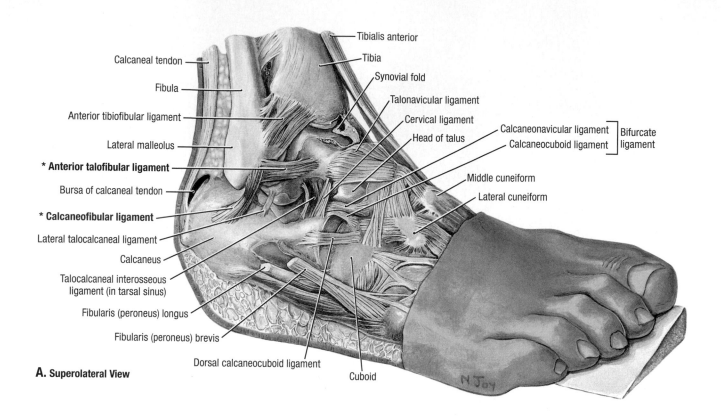

Tibialis anterior
Tibia
Synovial fold
Talonavicular ligament
Cervical ligament
Head of talus
Calcaneonavicular ligament ⎤
Calcaneocuboid ligament ⎦ Bifurcate ligament
Middle cuneiform
Lateral cuneiform

Calcaneal tendon
Fibula
Anterior tibiofibular ligament
Lateral malleolus
* **Anterior talofibular ligament**
Bursa of calcaneal tendon
* **Calcaneofibular ligament**
Lateral talocalcaneal ligament
Calcaneus
Talocalcaneal interosseous ligament (in tarsal sinus)
Fibularis (peroneus) longus
Fibularis (peroneus) brevis
Dorsal calcaneocuboid ligament
Cuboid

A. Superolateral View

* **Parts of lateral ligament of ankle**

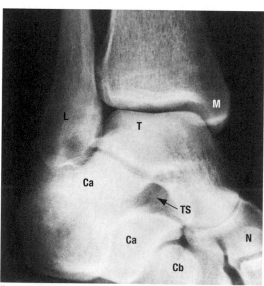

B. Lateral Radiograph

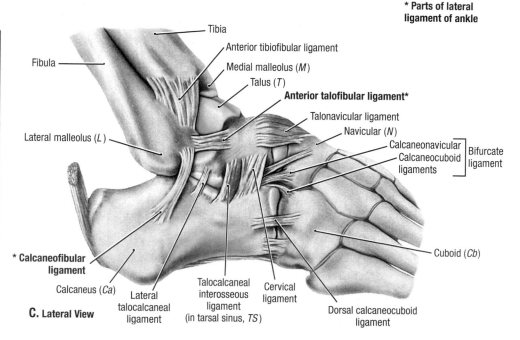

Tibia
Anterior tibiofibular ligament
Medial malleolus (*M*)
Talus (*T*)
Anterior talofibular ligament*
Talonavicular ligament
Navicular (*N*)
Calcaneonavicular ⎤
Calcaneocuboid ⎦ Bifurcate ligament
ligaments

Fibula
Lateral malleolus (*L*)
Cuboid (*Cb*)

* **Calcaneofibular ligament**
Calcaneus (*Ca*)
Lateral talocalcaneal ligament
Talocalcaneal interosseous ligament (in tarsal sinus, *TS*)
Cervical ligament
Dorsal calcaneocuboid ligament

C. Lateral View

6.85 | **Lateral Ligaments of Ankle Region**

A. Dissection with foot inverted by underlying wedge. B. Lateral radiograph. Abbreviations refer to structures labeled in *Part C.* **C. Dissection.**

The lateral ligament of the ankle consists of three separate ligaments: (1) anterior talofibular ligament, (2) calcaneofibular ligament, and (3) posterior talofibular ligament (see Fig. 6.82A).

Ankle sprains (partial or fully torn ligaments) are common injuries. Ankle sprains nearly always result from forceful inversion of the weight-bearing plantar flexed foot. The anterior talofibular ligament is most commonly injured, resulting in instability of the ankle. The calcaneofibular is also often torn.

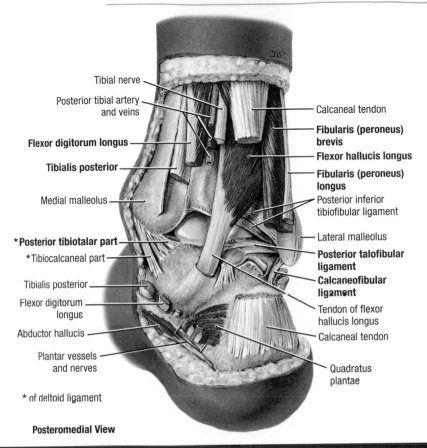

Tibial nerve

Posterior tibial artery and veins

Flexor digitorum longus

Tibialis posterior

Medial malleolus

*Posterior tibiotalar part

*Tibiocalcaneal part

Tibialis posterior

Flexor digitorum longus

Abductor hallucis

Plantar vessels and nerves

Calcaneal tendon

Fibularis (peroneus) brevis

Flexor hallucis longus

Fibularis (peroneus) longus

Posterior inferior tibiofibular ligament

Lateral malleolus

Posterior talofibular ligament

Calcaneofibular ligament

Tendon of flexor hallucis longus

Calcaneal tendon

Quadratus plantae

* of deltoid ligament

Posteromedial View

Relationship of Ankle Ligaments to Muscular and Neurovascular Structures

6.86

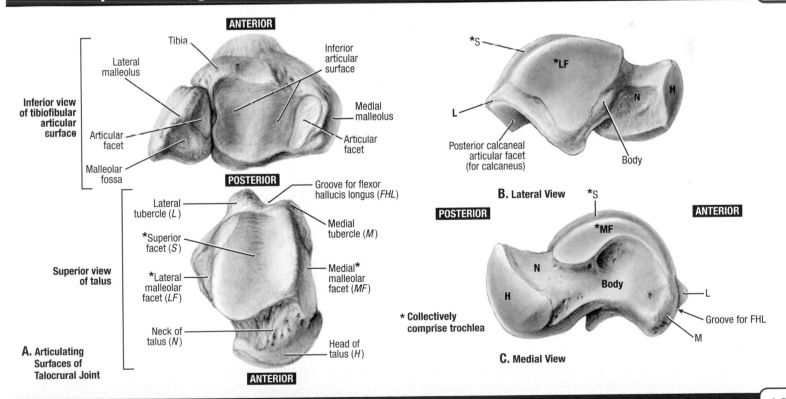

ANTERIOR

Tibia

Lateral malleolus

Inferior articular surface

Medial malleolus

Inferior view of tibiofibular articular surface

Articular facet

Articular facet

Malleolar fossa

POSTERIOR

Lateral tubercle (*L*)

Groove for flexor hallucis longus (*FHL*)

Medial tubercle (*M*)

*Superior facet (*S*)

*Lateral malleolar facet (*LF*)

Medial* malleolar facet (*MF*)

Superior view of talus

Neck of talus (*N*)

Head of talus (*H*)

A. Articulating Surfaces of Talocrural Joint

ANTERIOR

*S

*LF

N

H

L

Posterior calcaneal articular facet (for calcaneus)

Body

B. Lateral View

POSTERIOR

*S

*MF

N

Body

H

L

Groove for FHL

M

* Collectively comprise trochlea

ANTERIOR

C. Medial View

Articular Surfaces of Ankle Joint

6.87

A. Superior view of talus separated from distal ends of tibia and fibula. The superior articular surface of the talus is broader anteriorly than posteriorly. **B. Lateral view of talus.** The triangular lateral facet is for articulation with the lateral malleolus. **C. Medial view of talus.** The comma-shaped medial facet is for articulation with the medial malleolus.

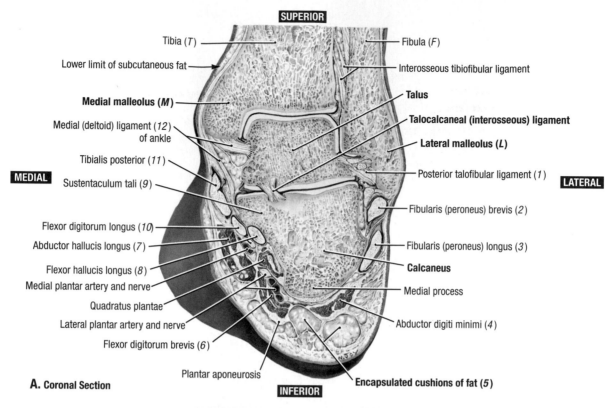

SUPERIOR

Tibia (T)

Fibula (F)

Lower limit of subcutaneous fat

Interosseous tibiofibular ligament

Medial malleolus (M)

Talus

Medial (deltoid) ligament (12) of ankle

Talocalcaneal (interosseous) ligament

Tibialis posterior (11)

Lateral malleolus (L)

MEDIAL

Sustentaculum tali (9)

Posterior talofibular ligament (1)

LATERAL

Fibularis (peroneus) brevis (2)

Flexor digitorum longus (10)

Abductor hallucis longus (7)

Fibularis (peroneus) longus (3)

Flexor hallucis longus (8)

Calcaneus

Medial plantar artery and nerve

Quadratus plantae

Medial process

Lateral plantar artery and nerve

Abductor digiti minimi (4)

Flexor digitorum brevis (6)

A. Coronal Section

Plantar aponeurosis

INFERIOR

Encapsulated cushions of fat (5)

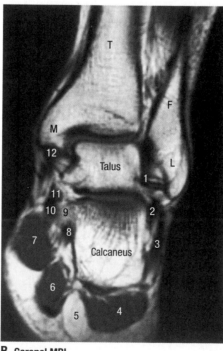

B. Coronal MRI

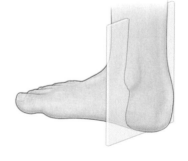

6.88   Coronal Section and MRI through Ankle

A. Coronal section. B. Coronal MRI. Numbers in *Part B* refer to labeled structures in *Part A*.

- The tibia rests on the talus, and the talus rests on the calcaneus; between the calcaneus and the skin are several encapsulated cushions of fat.

- The lateral malleolus descends farther inferiorly than the medial malleolus.

- The talocalcaneal (interosseous) ligament between the talus and calcaneus separates the subtalar, or posterior talocalcaneal joint from the talocalcaneonavicular joint.

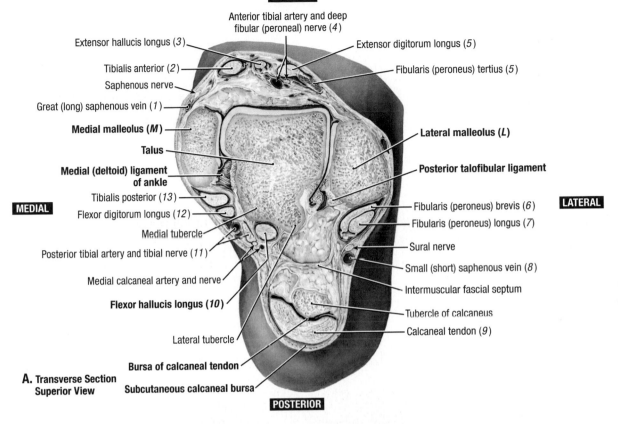

ANTERIOR

Anterior tibial artery and deep fibular (peroneal) nerve (4)

Extensor hallucis longus (3)

Extensor digitorum longus (5)

Tibialis anterior (2)

Fibularis (peroneus) tertius (5)

Saphenous nerve

Great (long) saphenous vein (1)

Medial malleolus (M)

Lateral malleolus (L)

Talus

Medial (deltoid) ligament of ankle

Posterior talofibular ligament

Tibialis posterior (13)

MEDIAL

LATERAL

Flexor digitorum longus (12)

Fibularis (peroneus) brevis (6)

Fibularis (peroneus) longus (7)

Medial tubercle

Posterior tibial artery and tibial nerve (11)

Sural nerve

Small (short) saphenous vein (8)

Medial calcaneal artery and nerve

Intermuscular fascial septum

Flexor hallucis longus (10)

Tubercle of calcaneus

Lateral tubercle

Calcaneal tendon (9)

Bursa of calcaneal tendon

A. Transverse Section Superior View

Subcutaneous calcaneal bursa

POSTERIOR

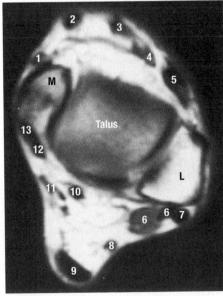

B. Transverse MRI

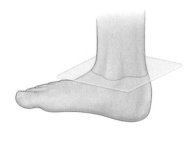

Transverse Section and MRI through Ankle

6.89

A. Transverse section. B. Transverse MRI. Numbers in *Part B* refer to labeled structures in *Part A*.
- The body of the talus is wedge shaped and positioned between the malleoli, which are bound to it by the medial (deltoid) and posterior talofibular ligaments.

- The flexor hallucis longus muscle lies within its osseofibrous sheath between the medial and lateral tubercles of the talus.
- There is a small, inconstant subcutaneous bursa superficial to the calcaneal tendon and a large, constant bursa of calcaneal tendon deep to it.

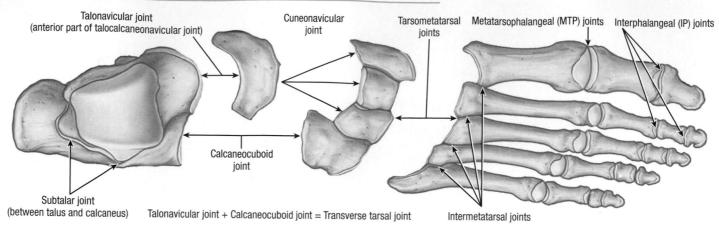

A. Superior View

Talonavicular joint (anterior part of talocalcaneonavicular joint)

Cuneonavicular joint

Tarsometatarsal joints

Metatarsophalangeal (MTP) joints

Interphalangeal (IP) joints

Calcaneocuboid joint

Subtalar joint (between talus and calcaneus)

Talonavicular joint + Calcaneocuboid joint = Transverse tarsal joint

Intermetatarsal joints

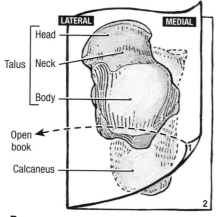

B. Superior (Dorsal) View

Talus — Head, Neck, Body

Open book

Calcaneus

Anterior facet for calcaneus

Facet for spring ligament

Middle facet for calcaneus

Sulcus tali for talocalcaneal (interosseous) ligament

Posterior calcaneal articular facet

Lateral tubercle

Groove for flexor hallucis longus

Medial tubercle

Plantar Surfaces of Talus

Anterior talar articular surface

Middle talar articular surface (on sustentaculum tali)

Calcaneal sulcus/ talocalcaneal interosseous ligament

Posterior talar articular surface

Dorsal Surface of Calcaneus

Talocalcaneal Joint

6.90   Joints of Foot

A. Overview. **B.** Talocalcaneal joint.

TABLE 6.20   Joints of Foot

Joint	Type	Articular Surface	Joint Capsule	Ligaments	Movements
Subtalar	Synovial (plane) joint	Inferior surface of body of talus articulates with superior surface of calcaneus	Attached to margins of articular surfaces	Medial, lateral, and posterior talocalcaneal ligaments support capsule; talocalcaneal (interosseous) ligament binds bones together	Inversion and eversion of foot
Talocalcaneonavicular	Synovial joint; talonavicular part is a pivot joint	Head of talus articulates with calcaneus and navicular bones	Incompletely encloses joint	Plantar calcaneonavicular ("spring") ligament supports head of talus	Gliding and rotary movements
Calcaneocuboid	Synovial (plane) joint	Anterior end of calcaneus articulates with posterior surface of cuboid	Encloses joint	Dorsal calcaneocuboid ligament, plantar calcaneocuboid ligament, and long plantar ligament support joint capsule	Inversion and eversion of foot
Cuneonavicular	Synovial (plane) joint	Anterior navicular articulates with posterior surface of cuneiforms	Common joint capsule	Dorsal and plantar ligaments	Limited gliding movement
Tarsometatarsal	Synovial (plane) joint	Anterior tarsal bones articulate with bases of metatarsal bones	Encloses joint	Dorsal, plantar, and interosseous ligaments	Gliding or sliding
Intermetatarsal	Synovial (plane) joint	Bases of metatarsal bones articulate with each other	Encloses each joint	Dorsal, plantar, and interosseous ligaments bind bones together	Little individual movement
Metatarsophalangeal	Synovial (condyloid) joint	Heads of metatarsal bones articulate with bases of proximal phalanges	Encloses each joint	Collateral ligaments support capsule on each side; plantar ligament supports plantar part of capsule	Flexion, extension, and some abduction, adduction and circumduction
Interphalangeal	Synovial (hinge) joint	Head of proximal or middle phalanx articulates with base of phalanx distal to it	Encloses each joint	Collateral and plantar ligaments support joints	Flexion and extension

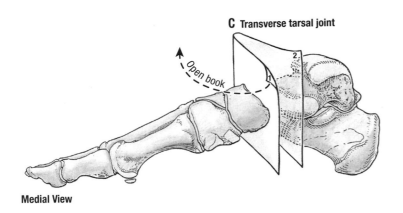

C Transverse tarsal joint

Medial View

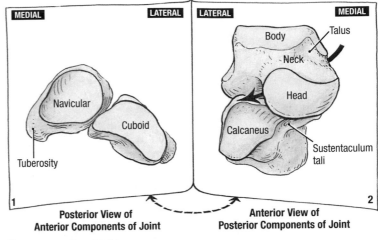

C. Transverse Tarsal Joint

Posterior View of Anterior Components of Joint

Anterior View of Posterior Components of Joint

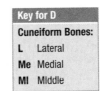

Key for D

Cuneiform Bones:

L   Lateral

Me   Medial

MI   Middle

D Cuneonavicular and cubonavicular joints

E Tarsometatarsal joint

Lateral View

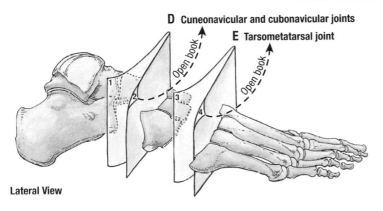

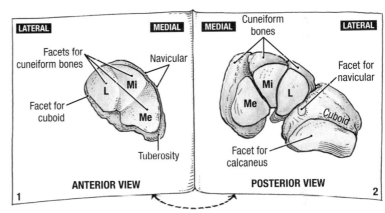

D. Cuneonavicular and Cubonavicular Joints

ANTERIOR VIEW

POSTERIOR VIEW

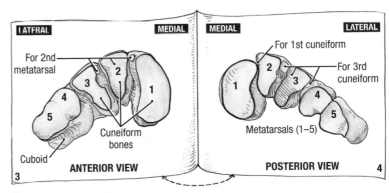

E. Tarsometatarsal Joints

ANTERIOR VIEW

POSTERIOR VIEW

Joints of Foot (continued)   6.90

C. Transverse tarsal joint. The *black arrow* traverses the tarsal sinus, in which the talocalcaneal (interosseous) ligament is located.
D. Cuneonavicular and cubonavicular joints. E. Tarsometatarsal joints.
- The joints of inversion and eversion are the subtalar (posterior talocalcaneal) joint, talocalcaneonavicular joint, and transverse tarsal (combined calcaneocuboid and talonavicular) joint.

- The talus participates in the ankle joint, of the posterior and anterior talocalcaneal joints, and of the talonavicular joint.
Metatarsal fractures (dancer's fracture) usually occur when the dancer loses balance, putting full body weight on the metatarsal. **Fatigue fractures of the metatarsals,** usually transverse, may result from prolonged walking with repeated stress on the metatarsals.

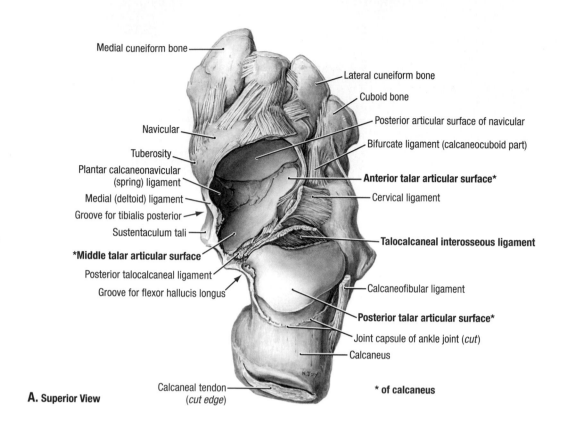

Medial cuneiform bone

Lateral cuneiform bone

Cuboid bone

Posterior articular surface of navicular

Navicular

Bifurcate ligament (calcaneocuboid part)

Tuberosity

Anterior talar articular surface*

Plantar calcaneonavicular (spring) ligament

Cervical ligament

Medial (deltoid) ligament

Groove for tibialis posterior

Sustentaculum tali

Talocalcaneal interosseous ligament

*Middle talar articular surface

Posterior talocalcaneal ligament

Calcaneofibular ligament

Groove for flexor hallucis longus

Posterior talar articular surface*

Joint capsule of ankle joint (*cut*)

Calcaneus

Calcaneal tendon (*cut edge*)

* of calcaneus

A. Superior View

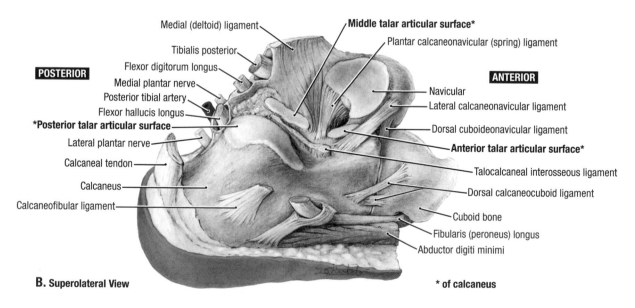

Medial (deltoid) ligament

Middle talar articular surface*

Plantar calcaneonavicular (spring) ligament

Tibialis posterior

Flexor digitorum longus

POSTERIOR

Medial plantar nerve

Posterior tibial artery

Flexor hallucis longus

*Posterior talar articular surface

Lateral plantar nerve

Calcaneal tendon

Calcaneus

Calcaneofibular ligament

ANTERIOR

Navicular

Lateral calcaneonavicular ligament

Dorsal cuboideonavicular ligament

Anterior talar articular surface*

Talocalcaneal interosseous ligament

Dorsal calcaneocuboid ligament

Cuboid bone

Fibularis (peroneus) longus

Abductor digiti minimi

B. Superolateral View

* of calcaneus

6.91 Joints of Inversion and Eversion

The joints of inversion and eversion are the subtalar (posterior talo-calcaneal), talocalcaneonavicular, and transverse tarsal (combined calcaneocuboid and talonavicular) joints. **A. Posterior and middle parts of foot with talus removed. B. Posterior part of foot with talus removed.** The convex posterior talar facet is separated from the concave middle, and anterior facets by the talocalcaneal (inter-osseous) ligament within the tarsal sinus. The posterior and anterior talocalcaneal joints are separated from each other by the sulcus tali and calcaneal sulcus, which, when the talus and calcaneus are in articulation, become the tarsal sinus.

Calcaneal fractures. A hard fall onto the heel (e.g., from a ladder) may fracture the calcaneus into several pieces, resulting in a comminuted fracture. A calcaneal fracture is usually disabling because it disrupts the subtalar (talocalcaneal) joint.

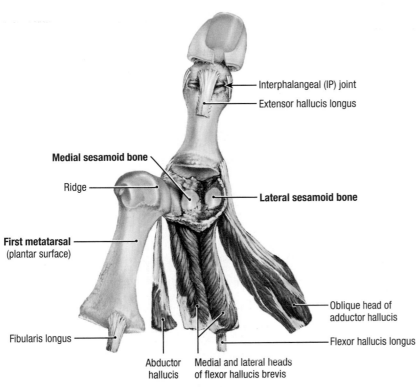
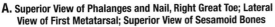

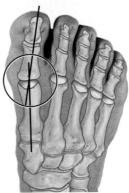

Interphalangeal (IP) joint

Extensor hallucis longus

Medial sesamoid bone

Ridge

Lateral sesamoid bone

First metatarsal
(plantar surface)

Oblique head of
adductor hallucis

Fibularis longus

Flexor hallucis longus

Abductor
hallucis

Medial and lateral heads
of flexor hallucis brevis

**A. Superior View of Phalanges and Nail, Right Great Toe; Lateral
View of First Metatarsal; Superior View of Sesamoid Bones**

Normal 1st metatarsophalangeal
joint (*circled*)

Bunion/hallux
valgus

B. Dorsal View

Metatarsophalangeal Joint of Great Toe   6.92

A. First metatarsal and sesamoid bones of right great toe. The
1st metatarsal has been reflected medially. **B. Hallux valgus.** This is
a foot deformity caused by pressure from footwear and degenerative
joint disease. It is characterized by lateral deviation of the base of
the 1st metatarsal and base of the proximal phalanx of the great toe
(L. *hallux*). In some people, the deviation is so great that the 1st toe

overlaps the 2nd toe. These individuals are unable to move their 1st
digit away from their 2nd digit because the sesamoid bones under
the head of the 1st metatarsal are displaced and lie in the space
between the heads of the 1st and 2nd metatarsals. In addition, a
subcutaneous bursa may form owing to pressure and friction against
the shoe. When tender and inflamed, the bursa is called a **bunion**.

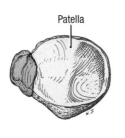

Patella

A. Posterior View

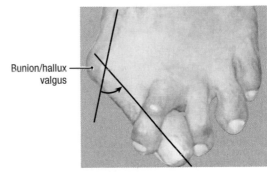

Talus

Os trigonum

B. Superior View

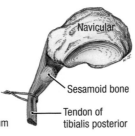

Navicular

Sesamoid bone

Tendon of
tibialis posterior

C. Posterior View

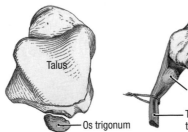

Cuboid

Sesamoid
bones

Tendon of fibularis
(peroneus) longus

D. Lateral View

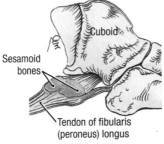

Femur

Tibia

Fibula

E. Lateral View (sesamoid bone circled)

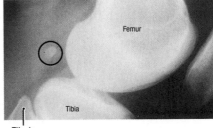

Bony Anomalies   6.93

A. Bipartite patella. Occasionally, the superolateral angle of the patella ossifies independently and remains discrete. **B. Os trigonum.**
The lateral (posterior) tubercle of the talus has a separate center of
ossification that appears from the ages of 7 to 13 years; when this
fails to fuse with the body of the talus, as in the left bone of this pair,
it is called an os trigonum. It was found in Dr. Grant's lab in 7.7% of
558 adult feet; 22 were paired, and 21 were unpaired. **C. Sesamoid**

bone in tendon of tibialis posterior. A sesamoid bone was found
in 23% of 348 adults. **D. Sesamoid bone in tendon of fibularis
(peroneus) longus.** A sesamoid bone was found in 26% of 92
specimens. In this specimen, it is bipartite, and the fibularis (peroneus) longus muscle has an additional attachment to the 5th metatarsal bone. **E. Fabella.** A sesamoid bone in the lateral head of the
gastrocnemius muscle was present in 21.6% of 116 limbs.

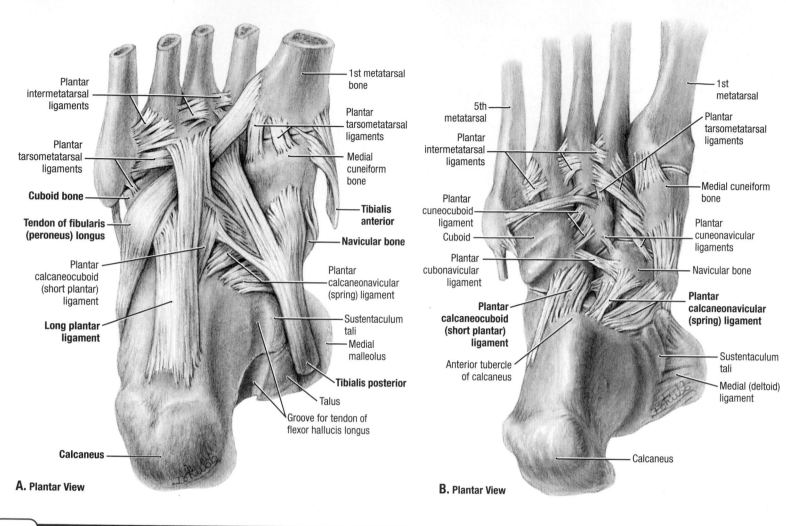

Plantar intermetatarsal ligaments

Plantar tarsometatarsal ligaments

Cuboid bone

Tendon of fibularis (peroneus) longus

Plantar calcaneocuboid (short plantar) ligament

Long plantar ligament

Calcaneus

A. Plantar View

1st metatarsal bone

Plantar tarsometatarsal ligaments

Medial cuneiform bone

Tibialis anterior

Navicular bone

Plantar calcaneonavicular (spring) ligament

Sustentaculum tali

Medial malleolus

Tibialis posterior

Talus

Groove for tendon of flexor hallucis longus

5th metatarsal

Plantar intermetatarsal ligaments

Plantar cuneocuboid ligament

Cuboid

Plantar cubonavicular ligament

Plantar calcaneocuboid (short plantar) ligament

Anterior tubercle of calcaneus

1st metatarsal

Plantar tarsometatarsal ligaments

Medial cuneiform bone

Plantar cuneonavicular ligaments

Navicular bone

Plantar calcaneonavicular (spring) ligament

Sustentaculum tali

Medial (deltoid) ligament

Calcaneus

B. Plantar View

6.94   Ligaments of Sole of Foot

A. Dissection of superficial ligaments. **B.** Dissection of deep ligaments. **C.** Bones lying deep to ligaments. The head of the talus is exposed between the sustentaculum tali of the calcaneus and the navicular.

In *Part A*:

- Note the insertions of three long tendons: fibularis (peroneus) longus, tibialis anterior, and tibialis posterior.
- The tendon of the fibularis (peroneus) longus muscle crosses the sole of the foot in the groove anterior to the tuberosity of the cuboid, is bridged by some fibers of the long plantar ligament, and inserts into the base of the 1st metatarsal.
- Observe the slips of the tibialis posterior tendon extending to the bones anterior to the transverse tarsal joint.

In *Part B*:

- The plantar calcaneocuboid (short plantar) and plantar calcaneonavicular (spring) ligaments are the primary plantar ligaments of the transverse tarsal joint.
- The ligaments of the anterior foot diverge laterally and posteriorly from each side of the long axis of the 3rd metatarsal and 3rd cuneiform; hence, a posterior thrust received by the 1st metatarsal, as when rising on the big toe while in walking, is transmitted directly to the navicular and talus by the first cuneiform and indirectly by the 2nd metatarsal, 2nd cuneiform, 3rd metatarsal, and 3rd cuneiform.
- A posterior thrust received by the 4th and 5th metatarsals is transmitted directly to the cuboid and calcaneus.

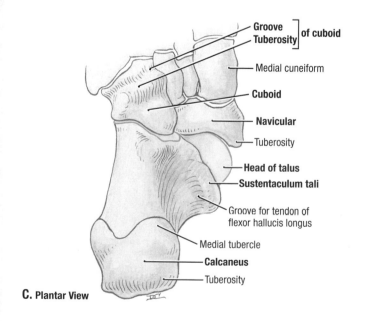

Groove
Tuberosity } of cuboid

Medial cuneiform

Cuboid

Navicular

Tuberosity

Head of talus

Sustentaculum tali

Groove for tendon of flexor hallucis longus

Medial tubercle

Calcaneus

Tuberosity

C. Plantar View

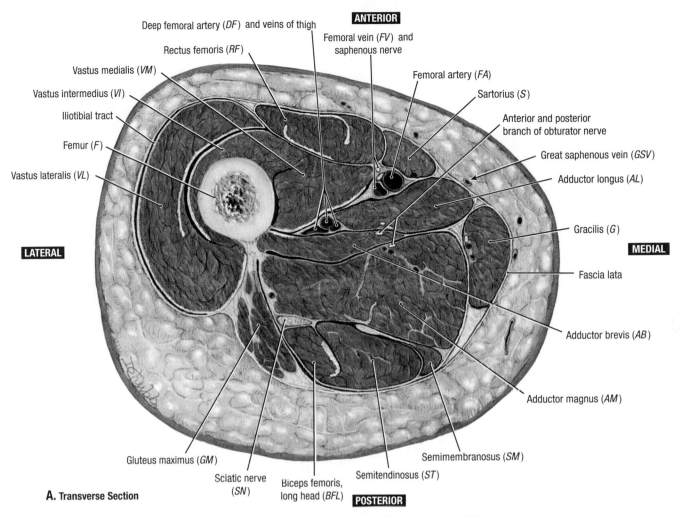

ANTERIOR

Deep femoral artery (*DF*) and veins of thigh

Femoral vein (*FV*) and saphenous nerve

Rectus femoris (*RF*)

Vastus medialis (*VM*)

Femoral artery (*FA*)

Vastus intermedius (*VI*)

Sartorius (*S*)

Iliotibial tract

Anterior and posterior branch of obturator nerve

Femur (*F*)

Great saphenous vein (*GSV*)

Vastus lateralis (*VL*)

Adductor longus (*AL*)

LATERAL

Gracilis (*G*)

MEDIAL

Fascia lata

Adductor brevis (*AB*)

Adductor magnus (*AM*)

Gluteus maximus (*GM*)

Semimembranosus (*SM*)

Sciatic nerve (*SN*)

Biceps femoris, long head (*BFL*)

Semitendinosus (*ST*)

POSTERIOR

A. Transverse Section

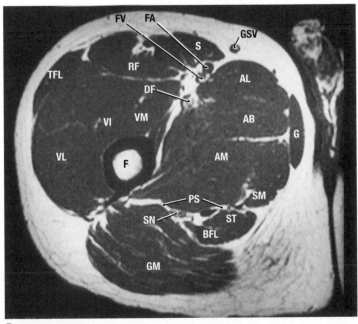

B. Transverse MRI

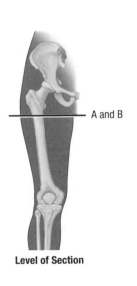

A and B

Level of Section

Transverse Sections and MRIs of Thigh

6.95

A. Anatomical section of proximal thigh. **B.** Transverse MRI of proximal thigh.

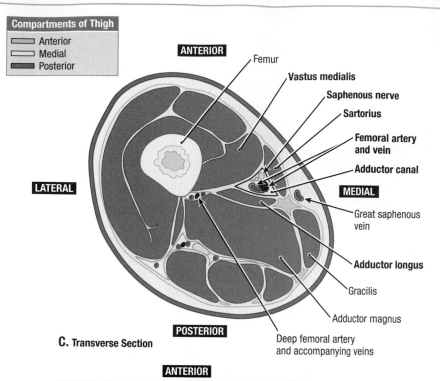

Compartments of Thigh
- Anterior
- Medial
- Posterior

ANTERIOR

Femur
Vastus medialis
Saphenous nerve
Sartorius
Femoral artery and vein
Adductor canal

LATERAL
MEDIAL

Great saphenous vein

Adductor longus

Gracilis

POSTERIOR
Adductor magnus

C. Transverse Section

Deep femoral artery and accompanying veins

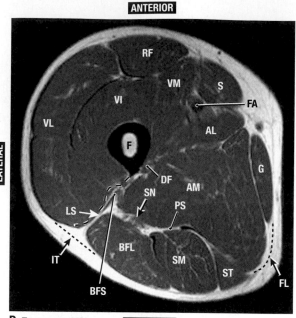

D. Transverse MRI

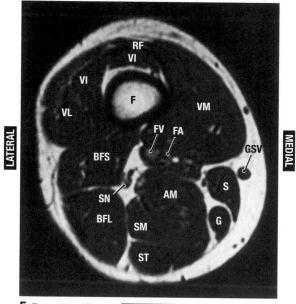

E. Transverse MRI

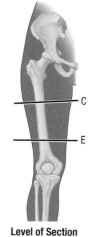

Level of Section

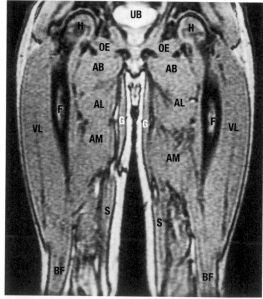

F. Coronal MRI

AB	Adductor brevis	IT	Iliotibial tract
AL	Adductor longus	LS	Lateral intermuscular septum
AM	Adductor magnus	OE	Obturator externus
BF	Biceps femoris	PS	Posteromedial intermuscular septum
BFL	Long head of biceps femoris		
BFS	Short head of biceps femoris	RF	Rectus femoris
DF	Deep femoral artery	S	Sartorius
F	Femur	SM	Semimembranosus
FA	Femoral artery	SN	Sciatic nerve
FL	Fascia lata	ST	Semitendinosus
FV	Femoral vein	TFL	Tensor fasciae latae
G	Gracilis	UB	Urinary bladder
GM	Gluteus maximus	VI	Vastus intermedius
GSV	Great saphenous vein	VL	Vastus lateralis
H	Head of femur	VM	Vastus medialis

6.95 **Transverse Sections and MRIs of Thigh** (continued)

C. Diagrammatic anatomical section. **D.** Transverse (axial) MRI of midthigh. **E.** Transverse (axial) MRI of distal thigh. **F.** Coronal MRI.

The thigh has three compartments, each with its own nerve supply and primary function: Anterior group extends the knee and is supplied by the femoral nerve, medial group adducts the hip and is supplied by the obturator nerve, and posterior group flexes the knee and is supplied by the sciatic nerve.

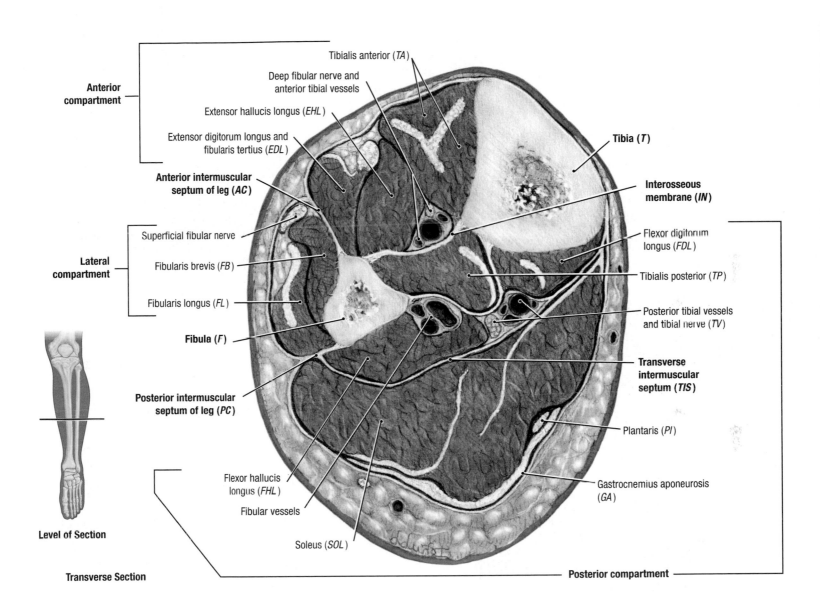

Anterior compartment

- Tibialis anterior (*TA*)
- Deep fibular nerve and anterior tibial vessels
- Extensor hallucis longus (*EHL*)
- Extensor digitorum longus and fibularis tertius (*EDL*)

Anterior intermuscular septum of leg (AC)

Lateral compartment

- Superficial fibular nerve
- Fibularis brevis (*FB*)
- Fibularis longus (*FL*)

Fibula (F)

Posterior intermuscular septum of leg (PC)

Flexor hallucis longus (*FHL*)

Fibular vessels

Soleus (*SOL*)

Tibia (T)

Interosseous membrane (IN)

Flexor digitorum longus (*FDL*)

Tibialis posterior (*TP*)

Posterior tibial vessels and tibial nerve (*TV*)

Transverse intermuscular septum (TIS)

Plantaris (*PI*)

Gastrocnemius aponeurosis (*GA*)

Level of Section

Transverse Section

Posterior compartment

Transverse Section of Leg

6.96

Boundaries of anterior, lateral, and posterior compartments of leg. Anterior compartment: tibia, interosseous membrane, fibula, anterior intermuscular septum, and crural fascia. Lateral compartment: fibula, anterior and posterior intermuscular septa, and the crural fascia. Posterior compartment: tibia, interosseous membrane, fibula, posterior intermuscular septum, and crural fascia. The posterior compartment is subdivided by the transverse intermuscular septum into superficial and deep subcompartments.

Compartmental infections in the leg. Because the septa and deep fascia forming the boundaries of the leg compartments

are strong, the increased volume consequent to infection with suppuration (formation of pus) increases intracompartmental pressure. Inflammation within the anterior and posterior compartments spreads chiefly in a distal direction; however, a purulent infection in the lateral compartment can ascend proximally into the popliteal fossa, presumably along the course of the fibular nerve. **Fasciotomy** may be necessary to relieve compartmental pressure and debride (remove by scraping) pockets of infection.

ANTERIOR

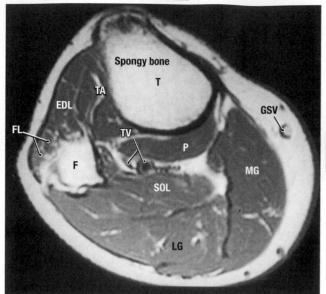

A. Transverse MRI

POSTERIOR

LATERAL

MEDIAL

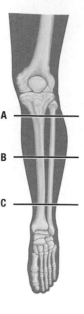

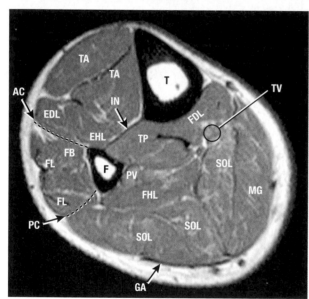

B. Transverse Section and MRI

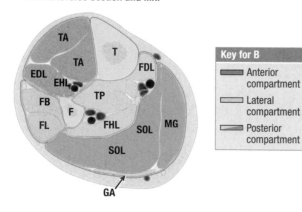

Key for B

	Anterior compartment
	Lateral compartment
	Posterior compartment

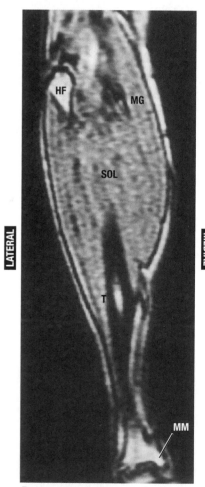

C. Transverse MRI

LATERAL   MEDIAL

D. Coronal MRI

AC	Anterior intermuscular septum
AV	Anterior tibial vessels and deep fibular nerve
EDL	Extensor digitorum longus
EHL	Extensor hallucis longus
F	Fibula
FB	Fibularis brevis
FDL	Flexor digitorum longus
FHL	Flexor hallucis longus
FL	Fibularis longus
GA	Gastrocnemius aponeurosis
GSV	Great saphenous vein
HF	Head of fibula
IN	Interosseous membrane
LG	Lateral head of gastrocnemius
MG	Medial head of gastrocnemius
MM	Medial malleolus
P	Popliteus
PC	Posterior intermuscular septum
PV	Peroneal vessels
SOL	Soleus
SSV	Small saphenous vein
T	Tibia
TA	Tibialis anterior
TC	Calcaneal tendon
TP	Tibialis posterior
TV	Tibial nerve and posterior tibial vessels

6.97   MRIs of Leg

A–C. Transverse (axial) MRIs. **D.** Coronal MRI.

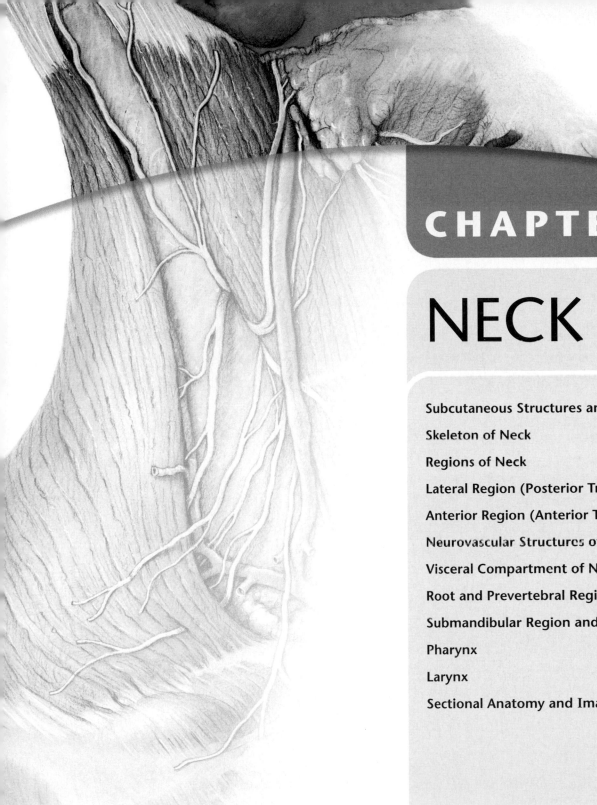

NECK

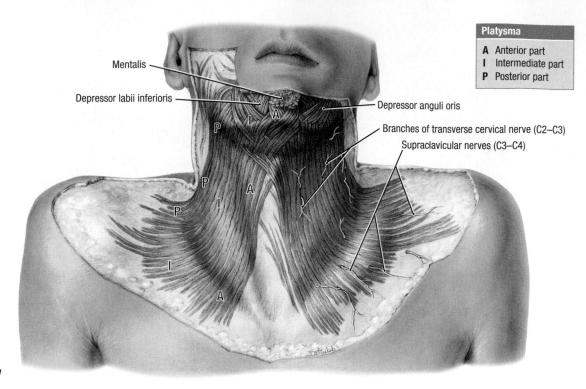

Mentalis

Depressor labii inferioris

Depressor anguli oris

Branches of transverse cervical nerve (C2–C3)

Supraclavicular nerves (C3–C4)

Platysma

A Anterior part
I Intermediate part
P Posterior part

A. Anterior View

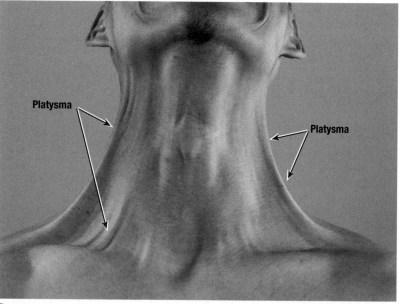

Platysma

Platysma

B. Anteroinferior View

7.1 Platysma

A. Parts of platysma. **B.** Surface anatomy.

TABLE 7.1	Platysma			
Muscle	**Superior Attachment**	**Inferior Attachment**	**Innervation**	**Main Action**
Platysma	*Anterior part:* Fibers interlace with contralateral muscle *Intermediate part:* Fibers pass deep to depressors anguli oris and labii inferioris to attach to inferior border of mandible *Posterior part:* Skin/subcutaneous tissue of lower face lateral to mouth	Subcutaneous tissue overlying superior parts of pectoralis major and sometimes deltoid muscles	Cervical branch of facial nerve (CN VII)	Draws corner of mouth inferiorly and widens it as in expressions of sadness and fright; draws the skin of the neck superiorly, forming tense vertical and oblique ridges over the anterior neck

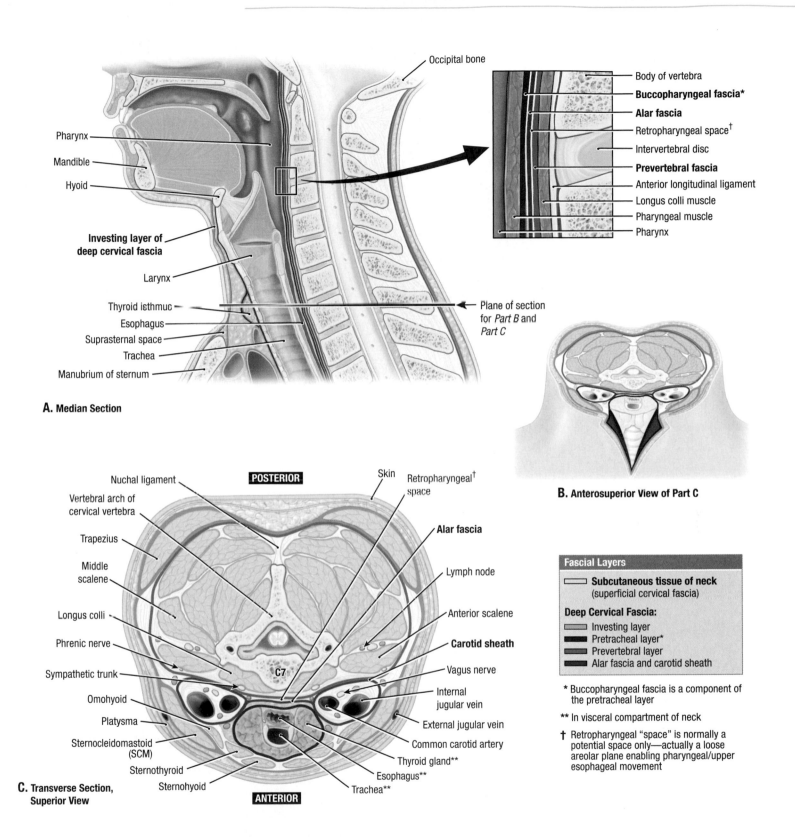

Occipital bone

Body of vertebra
Buccopharyngeal fascia*
Alar fascia
Retropharyngeal space†
Intervertebral disc
Prevertebral fascia
Anterior longitudinal ligament
Longus colli muscle
Pharyngeal muscle
Pharynx

Pharynx

Mandible

Hyoid

**Investing layer of
deep cervical fascia**

Larynx

Thyroid isthmus

Esophagus

Suprasternal space

Trachea

Manubrium of sternum

Plane of section
for *Part B* and
Part C

A. Median Section

B. Anterosuperior View of Part C

POSTERIOR

Nuchal ligament

Vertebral arch of
cervical vertebra

Trapezius

Middle
scalene

Longus colli

Phrenic nerve

Sympathetic trunk

Omohyoid

Platysma

Sternocleidomastoid
(SCM)

Sternothyroid

Sternohyoid

Skin

Retropharyngeal†
space

Alar fascia

Lymph node

Anterior scalene

Carotid sheath

Vagus nerve

Internal
jugular vein

External jugular vein

Common carotid artery

Thyroid gland**

Esophagus**

Trachea**

C7

ANTERIOR

**C. Transverse Section,
Superior View**

Fascial Layers

⬜ **Subcutaneous tissue of neck**
(superficial cervical fascia)

Deep Cervical Fascia:
◻ Investing layer
⬛ Pretracheal layer*
▦ Prevertebral layer
▣ Alar fascia and carotid sheath

* Buccopharyngeal fascia is a component of
the pretracheal layer

** In visceral compartment of neck

† Retropharyngeal "space" is normally a
potential space only—actually a loose
areolar plane enabling pharyngeal/upper
esophageal movement

Subcutaneous Tissue and Deep Fascia Neck

7.2

A. Median section. Fasciae of the neck are continuous inferiorly
and superiorly with thoracic and cranial fasciae. The *inset* illustrates
the fascia of the retropharyngeal region. **B.** and **C.** Transverse sections at **vertebral level C7**. Relationship of the main layers of deep
cervical fascia and the carotid sheath. Midline access to the cervical
viscera is possible with minimal disruption of tissues. The concentric
layers of fascia are apparent in this transverse section of neck at the
level indicated in *Part A*.

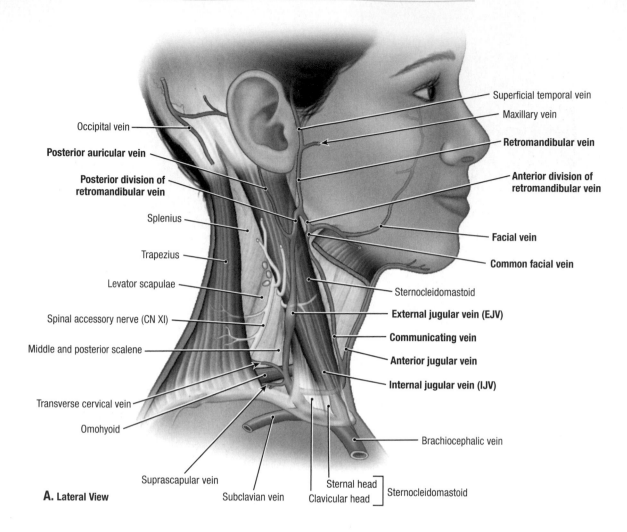

Superficial temporal vein
Maxillary vein
Retromandibular vein
Anterior division of retromandibular vein
Facial vein
Common facial vein
Sternocleidomastoid
External jugular vein (EJV)
Communicating vein
Anterior jugular vein
Internal jugular vein (IJV)
Brachiocephalic vein

Occipital vein
Posterior auricular vein
Posterior division of retromandibular vein
Splenius
Trapezius
Levator scapulae
Spinal accessory nerve (CN XI)
Middle and posterior scalene
Transverse cervical vein
Omohyoid
Suprascapular vein
Subclavian vein
Sternal head
Clavicular head
Sternocleidomastoid

A. Lateral View

7.3   Superficial Veins of Neck

A. Schematic of superficial veins of neck. The superficial temporal and maxillary veins merge to form the retromandibular vein. The posterior division of the retromandibular vein unites with the posterior auricular vein to form the external jugular vein. The facial vein receives the anterior division of the retromandibular vein, forming the common facial vein that empties into the internal jugular vein. Variations are common. **B. Surface anatomy of lateral cervical region (posterior triangle) of neck.** Note the external jugular vein and the muscles bounding this region.

External jugular vein (EJV). The EJV may serve as an "internal barometer." When venous pressure is in the normal range, the EJV is usually visible superior to the clavicle for only a short distance. However, when venous pressure rises (e.g., as in heart failure), the vein is prominent throughout its course along the side of the neck. Consequently, routine observation for distention of the EJVs during physical examinations may reveal diagnostic signs of heart failure, obstruction of the superior vena cava, enlarged supraclavicular lymph nodes, or increased intrathoracic pressure.

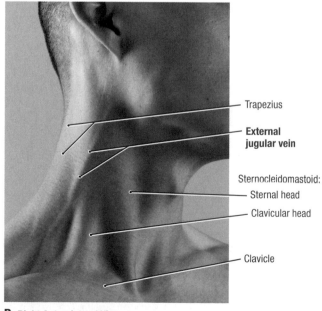

Trapezius
External jugular vein
Sternocleidomastoid:
Sternal head
Clavicular head
Clavicle

B. Right Anterolateral View

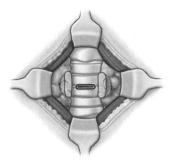

Incision in trachea after retracting infrahyoid muscles and incising isthmus of thyroid gland

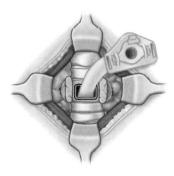

Tracheostomy tube inserted In tracheal opening

B. Tracheostomy

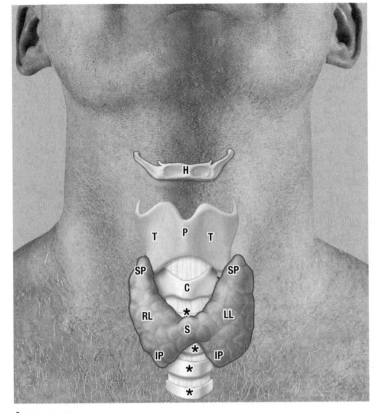

A. Anterior View

C	Cricoid cartilage
H	Hyoid bone
IP	Inferior pole of thyroid gland
LL	Left lobe of thyroid gland
P	Laryngeal prominence
RL	Right lobe of thyroid gland
S	Isthmus
SP	Superior pole of thyroid gland
T	Thyroid cartilage
＊	Tracheal rings

Surface Anatomy and Palpation of Cartilages and Hyoid of Anterior Neck 7.4

A. Surface anatomy and palpable structures. With the chin elevated, the subcutaneous laryngeal prominence, especially evident in males as the "Adam's apple," is readily apparent in the midline, produced by the junction of the laminae of the thyroid cartilage on each side of the prominence. The thyroid cartilage lies at the level of the C5 vertebra. The arch of the cricoid cartilage can be felt inferior to the laryngeal prominence, at the level of the C6 vertebra. The cartilaginous tracheal rings are palpable in the inferior part of the neck. The 2nd to 4th rings cannot be felt because the isthmus of the thyroid, connecting its right and left lobes, covers them. The 1st tracheal ring is immediately superior to the isthmus. The U-shaped hyoid bone lies superior to the thyroid cartilage at the level of the C3/C4 IV disc. The body and median tubercle lie subcutaneously in the midline, while the lesser and greater horns of both sides can be palpated by simultaneously passing the thumb and index finger along the sides of the hyoid, gently compressing while moving the hyoid from side to side.

B. Tracheostomy. A transverse incision through the skin of the neck and anterior wall of the trachea (*tracheostomy*) establishes an airway in patients with upper airway obstruction or respiratory failure. The infrahyoid muscles are retracted laterally, and the isthmus of the thyroid gland is either divided or retracted superiorly. An opening is made in the trachea between the 1st and 2nd tracheal rings or through the 2nd through 4th rings. A tracheostomy tube is then inserted into the trachea and secured. To avoid complications during a tracheostomy, the following anatomical relationships are important:

- The inferior thyroid veins arise from a venous plexus on the thyroid gland and descend anterior to the trachea (see Fig. 7.10).
- A small thyroid ima artery is present in approximately 10% of people; it ascends from the brachiocephalic trunk or the arch of the aorta to the isthmus of the thyroid gland (see Fig. 7.21).
- The left brachiocephalic vein, jugular venous arch, and pleurae may be encountered, particularly in infants and children.
- The thymus covers the inferior part of the trachea in infants and children.
- The trachea is small, mobile, and soft in infants, making it easy to cut through its posterior wall and damage the esophagus.

Cricothyrotomy. The incision is made through the cricothyroid membrane, and the tube inserted between the thyroid and cricoid cartilages.

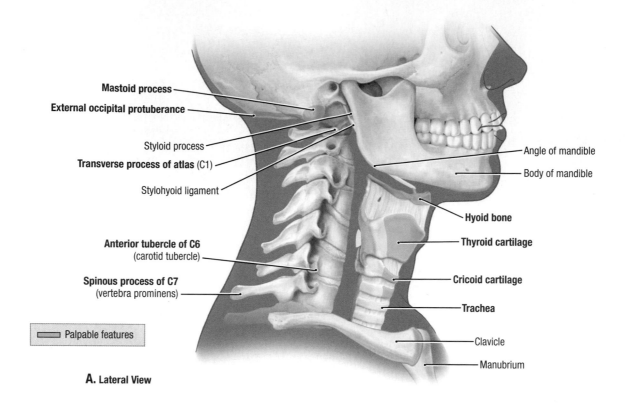

Mastoid process

External occipital protuberance

Styloid process

Transverse process of atlas (C1)

Stylohyoid ligament

Anterior tubercle of C6
(carotid tubercle)

Spinous process of C7
(vertebra prominens)

▭ Palpable features

Angle of mandible

Body of mandible

Hyoid bone

Thyroid cartilage

Cricoid cartilage

Trachea

Clavicle

Manubrium

A. Lateral View

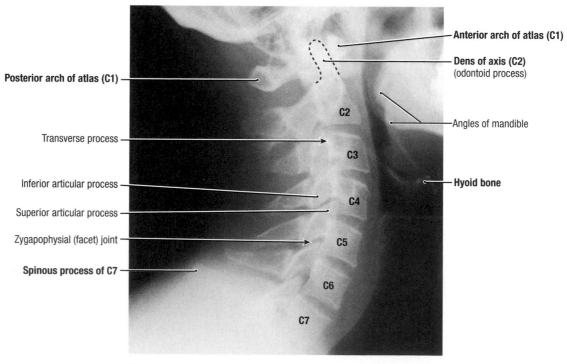

Posterior arch of atlas (C1)

Transverse process

Inferior articular process

Superior articular process

Zygapophysial (facet) joint

Spinous process of C7

Anterior arch of atlas (C1)

Dens of axis (C2)
(odontoid process)

Angles of mandible

Hyoid bone

C2

C3

C4

C5

C6

C7

B. Lateral Radiograph

| 7.5 | **Bones and Cartilages of Neck** |

A. Bony and cartilaginous landmarks of neck. B. Radiographic study of hyoid bone and cervical vertebrae (C1–C7). Because the upper cervical vertebrae lie posterior to the upper and lower jaws and teeth, they are best seen radiographically in lateral views, or in anterior views via the open mouth (see Fig. 1.9C in Chapter 1, Back).

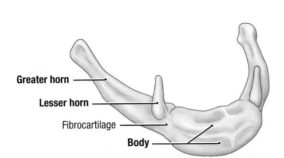

Greater horn

Lesser horn

Fibrocartilage

Body

Hyoid Bone

C. Right Anterolateral View

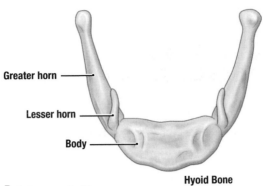

Greater horn

Lesser horn

Body

Hyoid Bone

D. Anterosuperior View

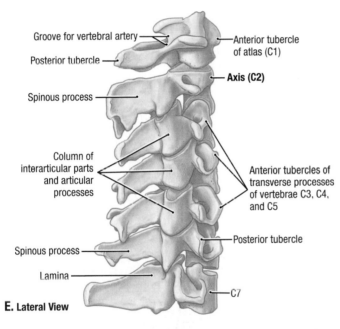

Groove for vertebral artery

Posterior tubercle

Spinous process

Column of interarticular parts and articular processes

Spinous process

Lamina

Anterior tubercle of atlas (C1)

Axis (C2)

Anterior tubercles of transverse processes of vertebrae C3, C4, and C5

Posterior tubercle

C7

E. Lateral View

Atlas { Anterior arch / Anterior tubercle }   C1

Dens (odontoid process) of axis (C2)

Uncovertebral joints

Space for intervertebral disc

Groove for spinal nerve

Anterior tubercle

Posterior tubercle

Carotid tubercle (anterior tubercle of C6)

C2

C3

C4

C5

C6

C7

F. Anterior View

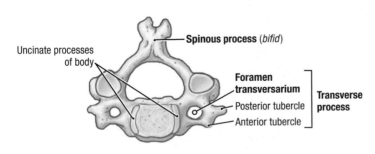

Uncinate processes of body

Spinous process (*bifid*)

Foramen transversarium

Posterior tubercle

Anterior tubercle

Transverse process

G. Superior View, Typical Cervical Vertebra (e.g., C4)

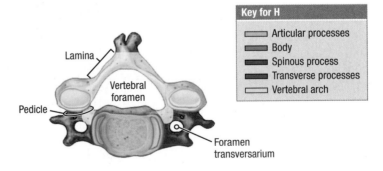

Lamina

Pedicle

Vertebral foramen

Foramen transversarium

Key for H

- Articular processes
- Body
- Spinous process
- Transverse processes
- Vertebral arch

H. Superior View

Bones and Cartilages of Neck (*continued*)   **7.5**

C. and **D.** Features of hyoid. **E.** and **F.** Articulated cervical vertebrae. **G.** and **H.** Features of typical cervical vertebrae.

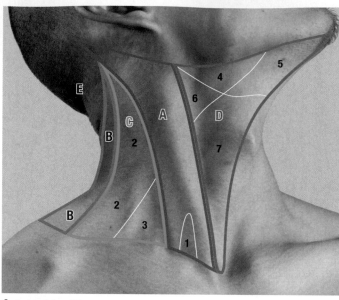

A. Anterolateral View

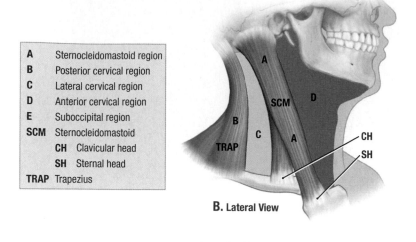

A	Sternocleidomastoid region
B	Posterior cervical region
C	Lateral cervical region
D	Anterior cervical region
E	Suboccipital region
SCM	Sternocleidomastoid
CH	Clavicular head
SH	Sternal head
TRAP	Trapezius

B. Lateral View

Parotid region

Digastric, posterior belly

Submandibular (digastric) triangle (4)

Digastric, anterior belly

Submental triangle (5)

Carotid triangle (6)

Superior belly of omohyoid

Muscular (omotracheal) triangle (7)

Lesser supraclavicular fossa (1)

Occipital triangle (2)

Spinal accessory nerve (CN XI)

Inferior belly of omohyoid

Omoclavicular (subclavian) triangle (3)

SCM

TRAP

C. Lateral View

7.6 Cervical Regions

A. Surface anatomy. **B.** and **C.** Regions and triangles of neck.

TABLE 7.2 Cervical Regions and Contents[a]

Region	Main Contents and Underlying Structures
Sternocleidomastoid region (A) Lesser supraclavicular fossa (1)	Sternocleidomastoid (SCM) muscle; superior part of the external jugular vein; greater auricular nerve; transverse cervical nerve
	Inferior part of internal jugular vein
Posterior cervical region (B)	Trapezius muscle; cutaneous branches of posterior rami of cervical spinal nerves; suboccipital region (E) lies deep to superior part of this region
Lateral cervical region (posterior triangle) (C) Occipital triangle (2) Omoclavicular triangle (3)	Part of external jugular vein; posterior branches of cervical plexus of nerves; spinal accessory nerve; transverse cervical artery; cervical lymph nodes
	Subclavian artery; part of subclavian vein (variable); suprascapular artery; supraclavicular lymph nodes; trunks of brachial plexus
Anterior cervical region (anterior triangle) (D) Submandibular (digastric) triangle (4) Submental triangle (5) Carotid triangle (6) Muscular (omotracheal) triangle (7)	Submandibular gland almost fills triangle; submandibular lymph nodes; hypoglossal nerve; mylohyoid nerve; parts of facial artery and vein
	Submental lymph nodes and small veins that unite to form anterior jugular vein
	Common carotid artery and its branches; internal jugular vein and its tributaries; vagus nerve; external carotid artery and some of its branches; hypoglossal nerve and superior root of ansa cervicalis; spinal accessory nerve; thyroid gland, larynx, and pharynx; deep cervical lymph nodes; branches of cervical plexus
	Sternothyroid and sternohyoid muscles; thyroid and parathyroid glands

[a]Letters and numbers in parentheses refer to *Part A, Part B,* and *Part C.*

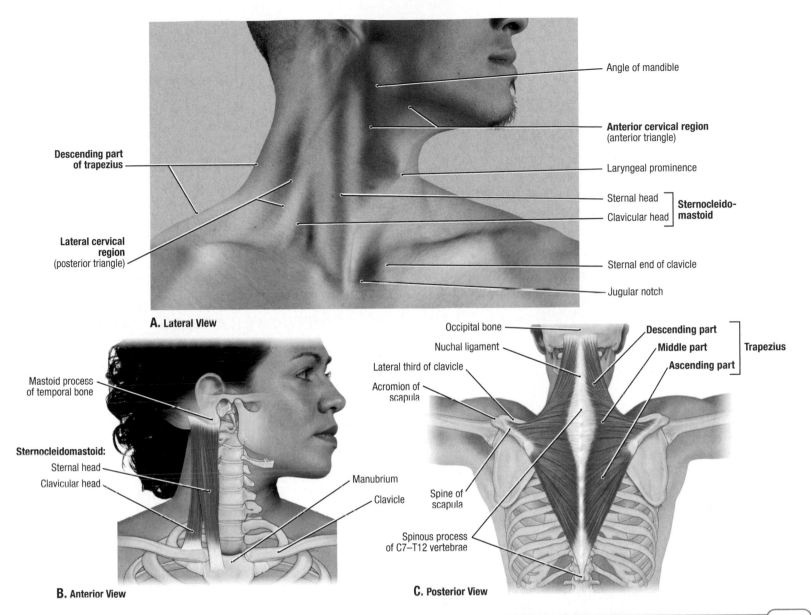

Descending part
of trapezius

Lateral cervical
region
(posterior triangle)

Angle of mandible

Anterior cervical region
(anterior triangle)

Laryngeal prominence

Sternal head
Clavicular head   } **Sternocleidomastoid**

Sternal end of clavicle

Jugular notch

A. Lateral View

Mastoid process
of temporal bone

Sternocleidomastoid:

Sternal head

Clavicular head

Manubrium

Clavicle

B. Anterior View

Occipital bone

Nuchal ligament

Lateral third of clavicle

Acromion of
scapula

Spine of
scapula

Spinous process
of C7–T12 vertebrae

Descending part

Middle part   **Trapezius**

Ascending part

C. Posterior View

7.7

Sternocleidomastoid and Trapezius

A. Surface anatomy. **B.** Sternocleidomastoid. **C.** Trapezius.

TABLE 7.3	Sternocleidomastoid and Trapezius			
Muscle	**Superior Attachment**	**Inferior Attachment**	**Innervation**	**Main Action**
Sternocleidomastoid	Lateral surface of mastoid process of temporal bone; lateral half of superior nuchal line	*Sternal head:* anterior surface of manubrium of sternum *Clavicular head:* superior surface of medial third of clavicle	Spinal accessory nerve (CN XI) [motor] and C2 and C3 nerves (pain and proprioception)	*Unilateral contraction:* laterally flexes neck; rotates neck so face is turned superiorly toward opposite side *Bilateral contraction:* (1) extends neck at atlantooccipital joints, (2) flexes cervical vertebrae so that chin approaches manubrium, or (3) extends superior cervical vertebrae while flexing inferior vertebrae, so chin is thrust forward with head kept level; with cervical vertebrae fixed, may elevate manubrium and medial end of clavicles, assisting deep respiration
Trapezius	Medial third of superior nuchal line, external occipital protuberance, nuchal ligament, spinous processes of C7–T12 vertebrae	Lateral third of clavicle, acromion, spine of scapula	Spinal accessory nerve (CN XI) [motor] and C2 and C3 nerves (pain and proprioception)	*Descending fibers* elevate pectoral girdle, maintain level of shoulders against gravity or resistance; *middle fibers* retract scapula; and *ascending fibers* depress shoulders; *superior* and *inferior fibers* work together to rotate scapula upward; *when shoulders are fixed,* bilateral contraction extends neck; unilateral contraction produces lateral flexion to same side

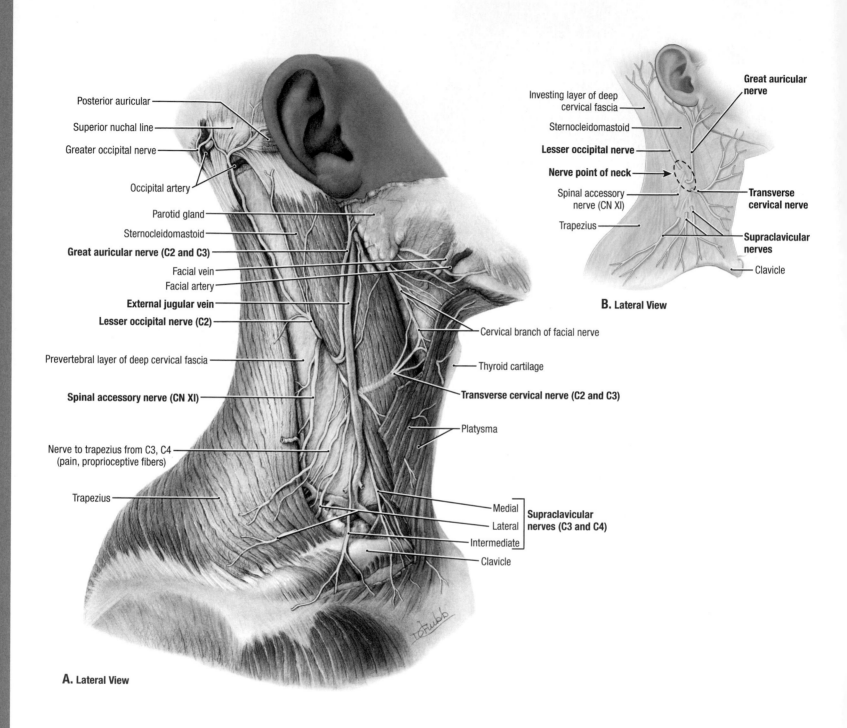

Posterior auricular

Superior nuchal line

Greater occipital nerve

Occipital artery

Parotid gland

Sternocleidomastoid

Great auricular nerve (C2 and C3)

Facial vein

Facial artery

External jugular vein

Lesser occipital nerve (C2)

Prevertebral layer of deep cervical fascia

Spinal accessory nerve (CN XI)

Nerve to trapezius from C3, C4
(pain, proprioceptive fibers)

Trapezius

Cervical branch of facial nerve

Thyroid cartilage

Transverse cervical nerve (C2 and C3)

Platysma

Medial
Lateral — **Supraclavicular
nerves (C3 and C4)**
Intermediate
Clavicle

A. Lateral View

Investing layer of deep
cervical fascia

Sternocleidomastoid

Lesser occipital nerve

Nerve point of neck

Spinal accessory
nerve (CN XI)

Trapezius

**Great auricular
nerve**

**Transverse
cervical nerve**

**Supraclavicular
nerves**

Clavicle

B. Lateral View

7.8 | Serial Dissections of Lateral Cervical Region (Posterior Triangle of Neck)

A. External jugular vein and cutaneous branches of cervical plexus. Subcutaneous fat, the part of the plasma overlying the inferior part of the lateral cervical region, and the investing layer of deep cervical fascia have all been removed. The external jugular vein descends vertically across the sternocleidomastoid and pierces the investing layer of deep cervical fascia superior to the clavicle to reach the subclavian vein.

• The spinal accessory nerve (CN XI) supplies the sternocleido-mastoid (SCM) and trapezius muscles; between them, it courses along the levator scapulae muscle but is separated from it by the prevertebral layer of deep cervical fascia.

B. Nerve point of neck. Cutaneous nerves of the neck emerge from the posterior border of the sternocleidomastoid in a small area about midway between the mastoid process and the clavicle (see Fig. 7.8E).

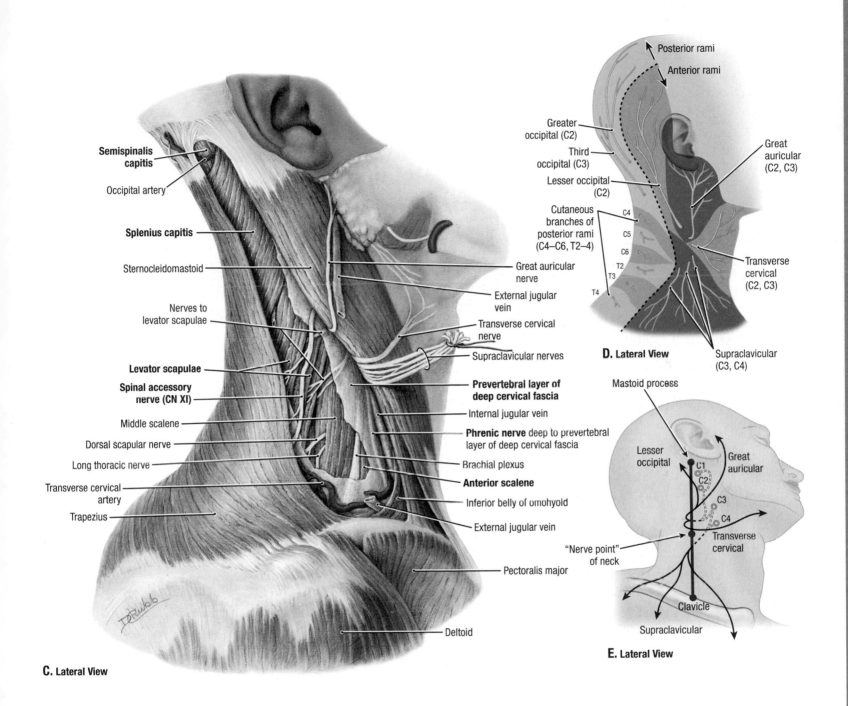

Posterior rami

Anterior rami

Greater occipital (C2)

Third occipital (C3)

Lesser occipital (C2)

Great auricular (C2, C3)

Cutaneous branches of posterior rami (C4–C6, T2–4)

C4
C5
C6
T2
T3
T4

Transverse cervical (C2, C3)

D. Lateral View

Supraclavicular (C3, C4)

Mastoid process

Lesser occipital

Great auricular

C1
C2
C3
C4

Transverse cervical

"Nerve point" of neck

Clavicle

Supraclavicular

E. Lateral View

Semispinalis capitis

Occipital artery

Splenius capitis

Sternocleidomastoid

Nerves to levator scapulae

Levator scapulae

Spinal accessory nerve (CN XI)

Middle scalene

Dorsal scapular nerve

Long thoracic nerve

Transverse cervical artery

Trapezius

Great auricular nerve

External jugular vein

Transverse cervical nerve

Supraclavicular nerves

Prevertebral layer of deep cervical fascia

Internal jugular vein

Phrenic nerve deep to prevertebral layer of deep cervical fascia

Brachial plexus

Anterior scalene

Inferior belly of omohyoid

External jugular vein

Pectoralis major

Deltoid

C. Lateral View

Serial Dissections of Lateral Cervical Region (Posterior Triangle of Neck) (continued) **7.8**

C. Muscles forming floor of lateral cervical region. The prevertebral layer of deep cervical fascia has been partially removed, and the motor nerves and most of the floor of the region are exposed.
- The phrenic nerve (C3, C4, C5) supplies the diaphragm and is located deep to the prevertebral layer of deep cervical fascia on the anterior surface of the anterior scalene muscle.

Severance of a phrenic nerve results in an ipsilateral paralysis of the diaphragm. A phrenic nerve block produces a short period of paralysis of the diaphragm on one side (e.g., for a lung operation). The anesthetic agent is injected around the nerve where it lies on the anterior surface of the anterior scalene muscle.

D. and **E. Sensory nerves of cervical plexus.** Branches arising from the nerve loop between the anterior rami of C2 and C3 are the lesser occipital, great auricular, and transverse cervical nerves. Branches arising from the loop formed between the anterior rami of C3 and C4 are the supraclavicular nerves, which emerge as a common trunk under cover of the SCM.

Regional anesthesia is often used for surgical procedures in the neck region or upper limb. In a **cervical plexus block**, an anesthetic agent is injected at several points along the posterior border of the SCM, mainly at its midpoint, the nerve point of the neck.

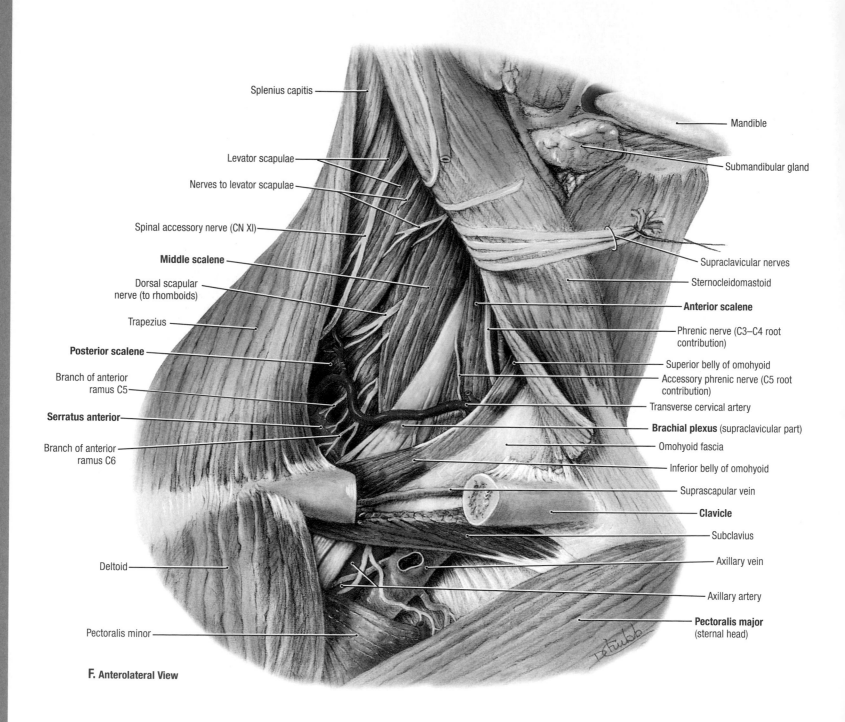

Splenius capitis

Levator scapulae

Nerves to levator scapulae

Spinal accessory nerve (CN XI)

Middle scalene

Dorsal scapular
nerve (to rhomboids)

Trapezius

Posterior scalene

Branch of anterior
ramus C5

Serratus anterior

Branch of anterior
ramus C6

Deltoid

Pectoralis minor

Mandible

Submandibular gland

Supraclavicular nerves

Sternocleidomastoid

Anterior scalene

Phrenic nerve (C3–C4 root
contribution)

Superior belly of omohyoid

Accessory phrenic nerve (C5 root
contribution)

Transverse cervical artery

Brachial plexus (supraclavicular part)

Omohyoid fascia

Inferior belly of omohyoid

Suprascapular vein

Clavicle

Subclavius

Axillary vein

Axillary artery

Pectoralis major
(sternal head)

F. Anterolateral View

7.8 | **Serial Dissections of Lateral Cervical Region (Posterior Triangle of Neck)** *(continued)*

F. Vessels and motor nerves of lateral cervical region. The clavicular head of the pectoralis major muscle and part of the clavicle
have been removed.

The muscles that form the floor of the region are the semispinalis capitis, splenius capitis, and levator scapulae superiorly and
the anterior, middle, and posterior scalenes and serratus anterior
inferiorly.

A **supraclavicular brachial plexus block** may be utilized for anesthesia of the upper limb. The anesthetic agent is injected around
the supraclavicular part of the brachial plexus. The main injection
site is superior to the midpoint of the clavicle.

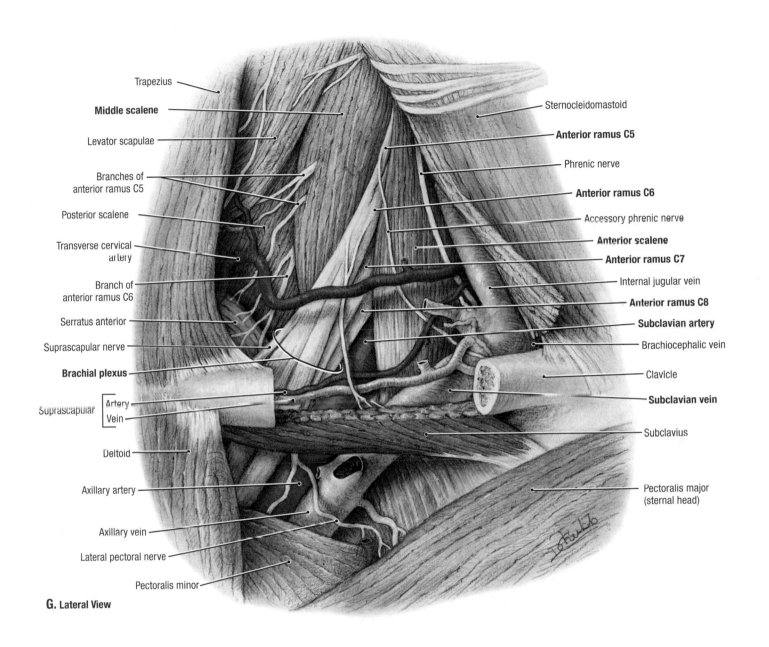

Trapezius

Middle scalene

Levator scapulae

Branches of anterior ramus C5

Posterior scalene

Transverse cervical artery

Branch of anterior ramus C6

Serratus anterior

Suprascapular nerve

Brachial plexus

Suprascapular {Artery / Vein}

Deltoid

Axillary artery

Axillary vein

Lateral pectoral nerve

Pectoralis minor

Sternocleidomastoid

Anterior ramus C5

Phrenic nerve

Anterior ramus C6

Accessory phrenic nerve

Anterior scalene

Anterior ramus C7

Internal jugular vein

Anterior ramus C8

Subclavian artery

Brachiocephalic vein

Clavicle

Subclavian vein

Subclavius

Pectoralis major (sternal head)

G. Lateral View

G. Structures of omoclavicular (subclavian) triangle. The omo-hyoid muscle and fascia have been removed, exposing the brachial plexus and subclavian vessels.

- The anterior rami of C5–T1 form the brachial plexus; the anterior ramus of T1 lies posterior to the subclavian artery.
- The brachial plexus and subclavian artery emerge between the middle and anterior scalene muscles.
- The anterior scalene muscle lies between the subclavian artery and vein.

The right or left subclavian vein is often the site of **placement for a central venous catheter**, used to insert intravenous tubes ("central venous lines") for the administration of parenteral nutritional fluids or medications, for testing blood chemistry or central venous pressure, or inserting electrode wires for heart pacemaker devices. The relationships of the subclavian vein to the sternocleidomastoid muscle, clavicle, sternoclavicular joint, and 1st rib are of clinical importance in line placement, and there is danger of puncture of the pleura or subclavian artery if the procedure is not performed correctly.

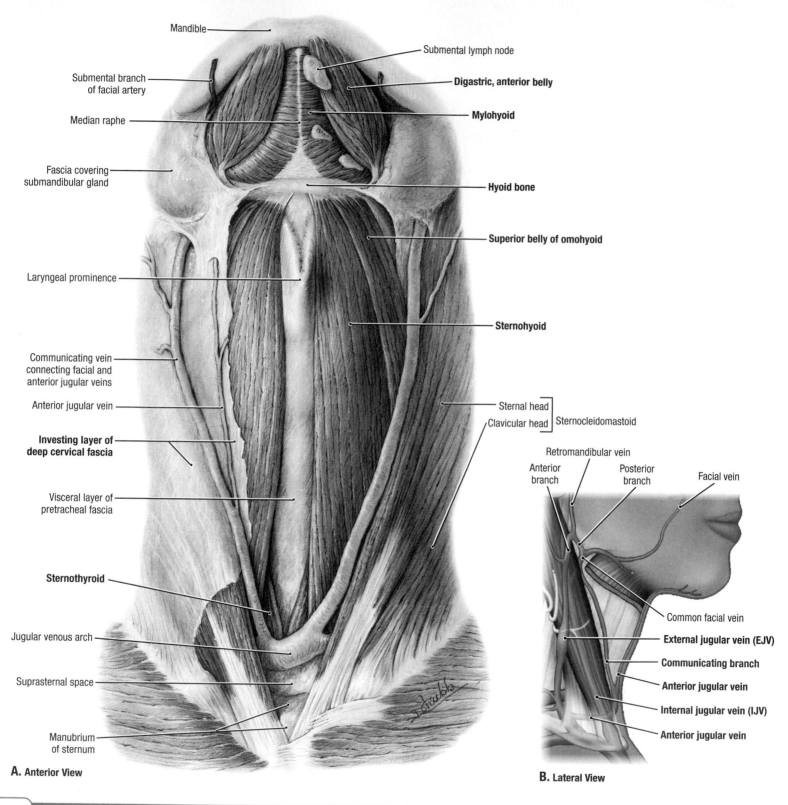

Mandible

Submental branch
of facial artery

Median raphe

Fascia covering
submandibular gland

Laryngeal prominence

Communicating vein
connecting facial and
anterior jugular veins

Anterior jugular vein

**Investing layer of
deep cervical fascia**

Visceral layer of
pretracheal fascia

Sternothyroid

Jugular venous arch

Suprasternal space

Manubrium
of sternum

Submental lymph node

Digastric, anterior belly

Mylohyoid

Hyoid bone

Superior belly of omohyoid

Sternohyoid

Sternal head ⎤
Clavicular head ⎦ Sternocleidomastoid

Retromandibular vein

Anterior   Posterior
branch   branch   Facial vein

Common facial vein

External jugular vein (EJV)

Communicating branch

Anterior jugular vein

Internal jugular vein (IJV)

Anterior jugular vein

A. Anterior View

B. Lateral View

7.9   Suprahyoid and Infrahyoid Muscles

A. Dissection. Much of the investing layer of deep cervical fascia
has been removed.
- The anterior bellies of the digastric muscles form the sides of the
  suprahyoid part of the anterior cervical region, or submental triangle (floor of mouth). The hyoid bone forms the triangle's base,
  and the mylohyoid muscles are its floor.

- The infrahyoid part of the anterior cervical region is shaped like
  an elongated diamond bounded by the sternohyoid muscle
  superiorly and sternothyroid muscle inferiorly.
- The longitudinal anterior jugular veins are absent.
B. Overview of superficial venous drainage.

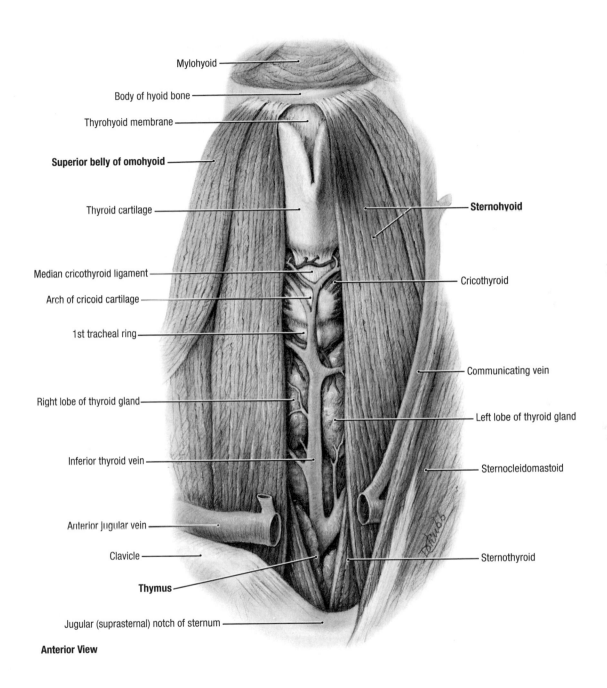

Mylohyoid

Body of hyoid bone

Thyrohyoid membrane

Superior belly of omohyoid

Thyroid cartilage

Median cricothyroid ligament

Arch of cricoid cartilage

1st tracheal ring

Right lobe of thyroid gland

Inferior thyroid vein

Anterior jugular vein

Clavicle

Thymus

Jugular (suprasternal) notch of sternum

Sternohyoid

Cricothyroid

Communicating vein

Left lobe of thyroid gland

Sternocleidomastoid

Sternothyroid

Anterior View

Infrahyoid Region, Superficial Muscular Layer

7.10

The pretracheal fascia, right anterior jugular vein, and jugular venous arch have been removed.
- A persistent thymus projects superiorly from the thorax.
- The two superficial depressors of the larynx ("strap muscles") are the omohyoid (only the superior belly of which is seen here) and sternohyoid.

Fracture of the hyoid. This results in depression of the body of the hyoid onto the thyroid cartilage. Inability to elevate the hyoid and move it anteriorly beneath the tongue makes swallowing and maintenance of the separation of the alimentary and respiratory tracts difficult and may result in **aspiration pneumonia.**

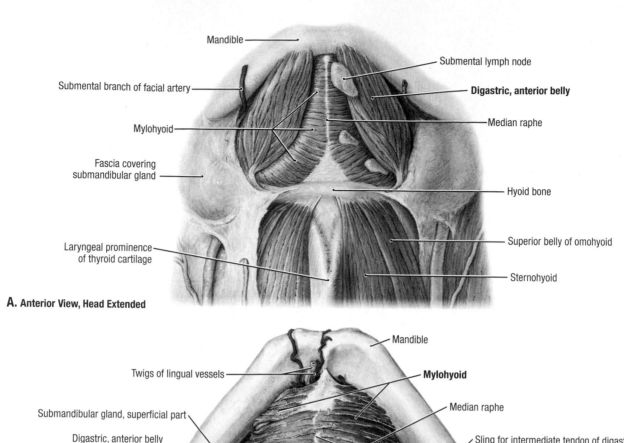

Mandible

Submental lymph node

Submental branch of facial artery

Digastric, anterior belly

Mylohyoid

Median raphe

Fascia covering submandibular gland

Hyoid bone

Superior belly of omohyoid

Laryngeal prominence of thyroid cartilage

Sternohyoid

A. Anterior View, Head Extended

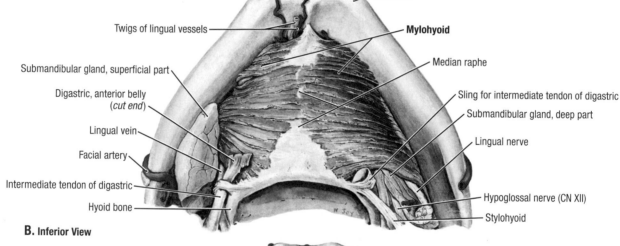

Mandible

Twigs of lingual vessels

Mylohyoid

Submandibular gland, superficial part

Median raphe

Digastric, anterior belly (*cut end*)

Sling for intermediate tendon of digastric

Lingual vein

Submandibular gland, deep part

Facial artery

Lingual nerve

Intermediate tendon of digastric

Hypoglossal nerve (CN XII)

Hyoid bone

Stylohyoid

B. Inferior View

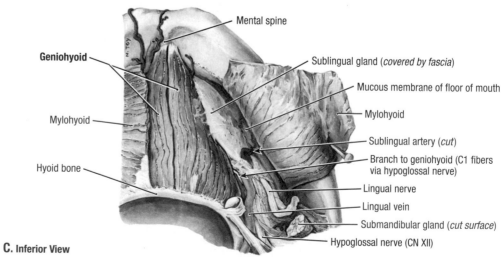

Mental spine

Geniohyoid

Sublingual gland (*covered by fascia*)

Mucous membrane of floor of mouth

Mylohyoid

Mylohyoid

Sublingual artery (*cut*)

Branch to geniohyoid (C1 fibers via hypoglossal nerve)

Hyoid bone

Lingual nerve

Lingual vein

Submandibular gland (*cut surface*)

Hypoglossal nerve (CN XII)

C. Inferior View

| 7.11 | **Suprahyoid Region (Submental Triangle)** |

A. Superficial layer—anterior belly of digastric. **B.** Intermediate layer—mylohyoid. **C.** Deep layer—geniohyoid.

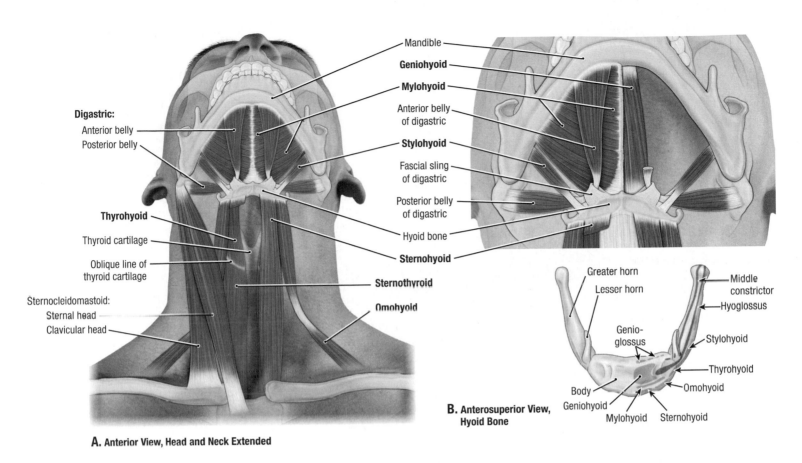

A. Anterior View, Head and Neck Extended

B. Anterosuperior View, Hyoid Bone

Suprahyoid and Infrahyoid Muscles

7.12

A. Overview. **B.** Muscular attachments onto hyoid bone.

TABLE 7.4	Muscles of Anterior Cervical Region			
Muscle	**Superior Attachment**	**Inferior Attachment**	**Innervation**	**Main Action**
Suprahyoid muscles				
Mylohyoid	Mylohyoid line of mandible	Raphe and body of hyoid bone	Nerve to mylohyoid, a branch of inferior alveolar nerve (CN V₃)	Elevates hyoid bone, floor of mouth and tongue during swallowing and speaking
Digastric	*Anterior belly:* digastric fossa of mandible *Posterior belly:* mastoid notch of temporal bone	Intermediate tendon to body and greater horn of hyoid bone	*Anterior belly:* nerve to mylohyoid, a branch of inferior alveolar nerve (CN V₃) *Posterior belly:* facial nerve (CN VII)	Elevates hyoid bone and steadies it during swallowing and speaking; depresses mandible against resistance
Geniohyoid	Inferior mental spine of mandible	Body of hyoid bone	Branch to geniohyoid (C1 fibers via the hypoglossal nerve [CN XII])	Pulls hyoid bone anterosuperiorly, shortens floor of mouth, and widens pharynx
Stylohyoid	Styloid process of temporal bone		Cervical branch of facial nerve (CN VII)	Elevates and retracts hyoid bone, thereby elongating floor of mouth
Infrahyoid muscles				
Sternohyoid	Body of hyoid bone	Manubrium of sternum and medial end of clavicle	C1–C3 by branches of ansa cervicalis	Depresses hyoid bone after it has been elevated during swallowing
Omohyoid	Inferior border of hyoid bone	Superior border of scapula near suprascapular notch		Depresses, retracts, and steadies hyoid bone
Sternothyroid	Oblique line of thyroid cartilage	Posterior surface of manubrium of sternum	C2 and C3 by a branch of ansa cervicalis	Depresses hyoid bone and larynx
Thyrohyoid	Inferior border of body and greater horn of hyoid bone	Oblique line of thyroid cartilage	Branch to thyrohyoid (C1 fibers via hypoglossal nerve [CN XII])	Depresses hyoid bone and elevates larynx

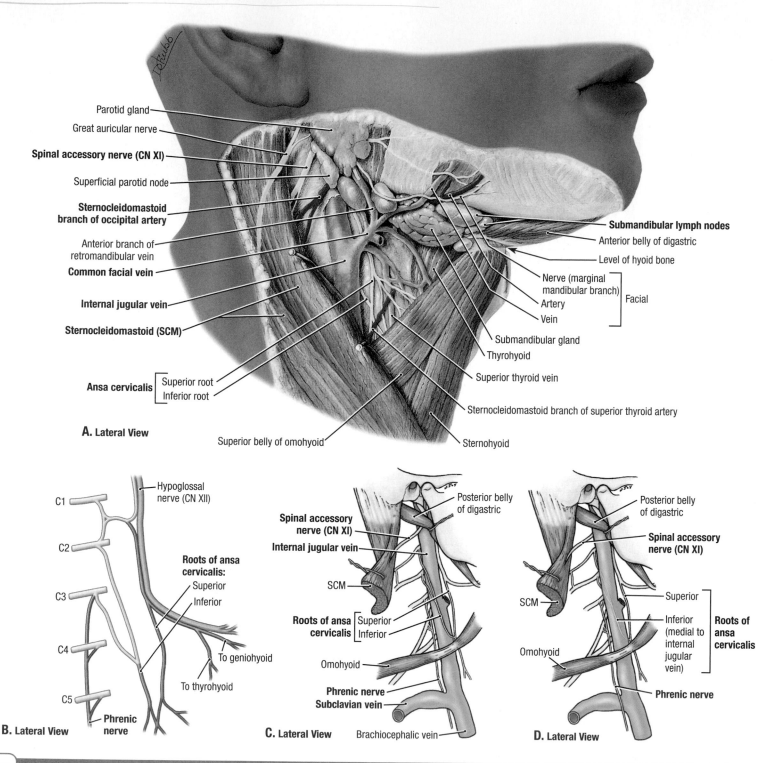

Parotid gland

Great auricular nerve

Spinal accessory nerve (CN XI)

Superficial parotid node

Sternocleidomastoid branch of occipital artery

Anterior branch of retromandibular vein

Common facial vein

Internal jugular vein

Sternocleidomastoid (SCM)

Ansa cervicalis [Superior root / Inferior root]

A. Lateral View

Superior belly of omohyoid

Submandibular lymph nodes

Anterior belly of digastric

Level of hyoid bone

Nerve (marginal mandibular branch)

Artery

Vein } Facial

Submandibular gland

Thyrohyoid

Superior thyroid vein

Sternocleidomastoid branch of superior thyroid artery

Sternohyoid

C1

C2

C3

C4

C5

Hypoglossal nerve (CN XII)

Roots of ansa cervicalis:

Superior

Inferior

To geniohyoid

To thyrohyoid

Phrenic nerve

B. Lateral View

Posterior belly of digastric

Spinal accessory nerve (CN XI)

Internal jugular vein

SCM

Roots of ansa cervicalis [Superior / Inferior]

Omohyoid

Phrenic nerve

Subclavian vein

C. Lateral View   Brachiocephalic vein

Posterior belly of digastric

Spinal accessory nerve (CN XI)

SCM

Superior

Inferior (medial to internal jugular vein) } **Roots of ansa cervicalis**

Omohyoid

Phrenic nerve

D. Lateral View

| 7.13 | **Superficial Dissection of Carotid Triangle** |

A. Lateral aspect of carotid triangle. The skin, subcutaneous tissue (with platysma), and the investing layer of deep cervical fascia, including the sheaths of the parotid and submandibular glands, have been removed.

- The spinal accessory nerve (CN XI) enters the deep surface of the sternocleidomastoid muscle and is joined along its anterior border by the sternocleidomastoid branch of the occipital artery.
- The (common) facial vein joins the internal jugular vein near the level of the hyoid bone; here, the facial vein is joined by several other veins.

- The submandibular lymph nodes lie deep to the investing layer of deep cervical fascia in the submandibular triangle; some of the nodes lie deep in the submandibular gland.

B. Diagram of motor branches of cervical plexus. C. Typical relationships of ansa cervicalis, spinal accessory nerve (CN XI), and phrenic nerve to internal jugular and subclavian veins. D. Atypical relationships.

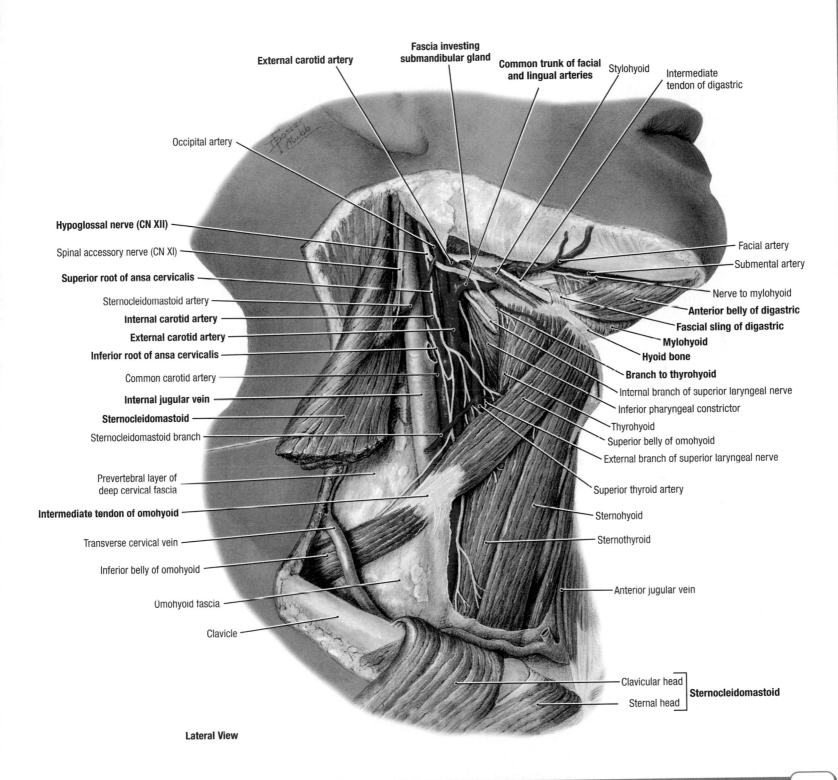

External carotid artery

Fascia investing
submandibular gland

Common trunk of facial
and lingual arteries

Stylohyoid

Intermediate
tendon of digastric

Occipital artery

Hypoglossal nerve (CN XII)

Spinal accessory nerve (CN XI)

Superior root of ansa cervicalis

Sternocleidomastoid artery

Internal carotid artery

External carotid artery

Inferior root of ansa cervicalis

Common carotid artery

Internal jugular vein

Sternocleidomastoid

Sternocleidomastoid branch

Prevertebral layer of
deep cervical fascia

Intermediate tendon of omohyoid

Transverse cervical vein

Inferior belly of omohyoid

Omohyoid fascia

Clavicle

Facial artery

Submental artery

Nerve to mylohyoid

Anterior belly of digastric

Fascial sling of digastric

Mylohyoid

Hyoid bone

Branch to thyrohyoid

Internal branch of superior laryngeal nerve

Inferior pharyngeal constrictor

Thyrohyoid

Superior belly of omohyoid

External branch of superior laryngeal nerve

Superior thyroid artery

Sternohyoid

Sternothyroid

Anterior jugular vein

Clavicular head

Sternal head

Sternocleidomastoid

Lateral View

Deep Dissection of Carotid Triangle

7.14

The sternocleidomastoid muscle has been severed; the inferior portion reflected inferiorly and superior portion posteriorly.

- The intermediate tendon of the digastric muscle is connected to the hyoid bone by a fascial sling derived from the muscular part of the pretracheal layer of deep cervical fascia; the tendon of the omohyoid muscle is similarly tethered to the clavicle.
- In this specimen, the facial and lingual arteries arise from a common trunk and pass deep to the stylohyoid and digastric muscles.

- The hypoglossal nerve (CN XII) crosses the internal and external carotid arteries and gives off two branches, the superior root of the ansa cervicalis and the nerve to the thyrohyoid, before passing anteriorly deep to the mylohyoid muscle. In this specimen, the inferior root of the ansa cervicalis lies deep to the internal jugular vein and emerges at its medial aspect.

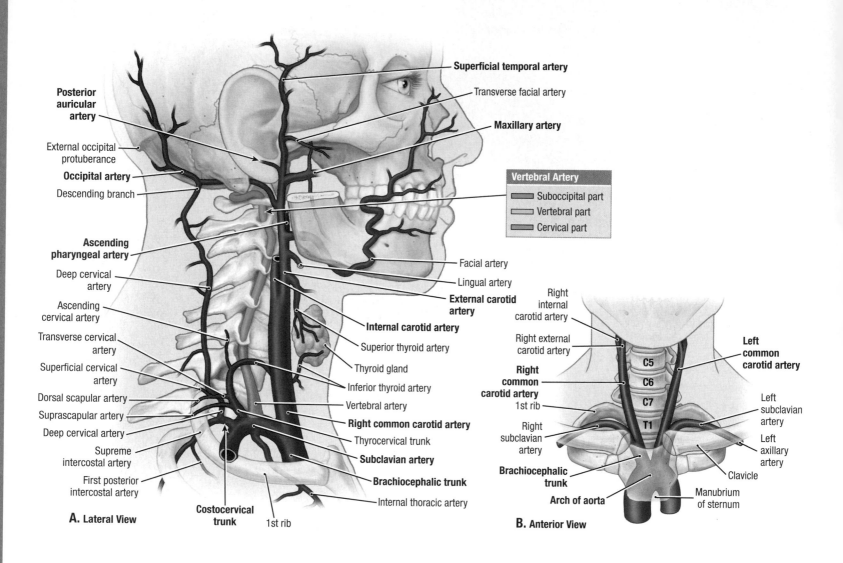

A. Lateral View

Superficial temporal artery

Transverse facial artery

Maxillary artery

Posterior auricular artery

External occipital protuberance

Occipital artery

Descending branch

Ascending pharyngeal artery

Deep cervical artery

Ascending cervical artery

Transverse cervical artery

Superficial cervical artery

Dorsal scapular artery

Suprascapular artery

Deep cervical artery

Supreme intercostal artery

First posterior intercostal artery

Costocervical trunk

1st rib

Vertebral Artery
- Suboccipital part
- Vertebral part
- Cervical part

Facial artery

Lingual artery

External carotid artery

Internal carotid artery

Superior thyroid artery

Thyroid gland

Inferior thyroid artery

Vertebral artery

Right common carotid artery

Thyrocervical trunk

Subclavian artery

Brachiocephalic trunk

Internal thoracic artery

B. Anterior View

Right internal carotid artery

Right external carotid artery

Right common carotid artery

1st rib

Right subclavian artery

Brachiocephalic trunk

Arch of aorta

C5 C6 C7 T1

Left common carotid artery

Left subclavian artery

Left axillary artery

Clavicle

Manubrium of sternum

7.15 Arteries of Neck

A. Overview. **B.** Common carotid and subclavian arteries.

TABLE 7.5	Arteries of Neck	
Artery	**Origin**	**Course and Distribution**
Right common carotid	Bifurcation of brachiocephalic trunk	Ascends in neck within carotid sheath with the internal jugular vein and vagus nerve (CN X). Terminates at superior border of thyroid cartilage (C4 vertebral level) by dividing into internal and external carotid arteries
Left common carotid	Arch of aorta	
Right and left internal carotid	Right and left common carotid	No branches in the neck. Enters cranium via carotid canal to supply brain and orbits. Proximal part location of carotid sinus, a baroreceptor that reacts to change in arterial blood pressure. The carotid body, a chemoreceptor that monitors oxygen level in blood, is located in bifurcation of common carotid
Right and left external carotid		Supplies most structures external to cranium; part of forehead, and scalp are supplied by ophthalmic artery from intracranial internal carotid artery
Ascending pharyngeal	External carotid	Ascends on pharynx to supply pharynx, prevertebral muscles, middle ear, and cranial meninges
Occipital		Passes posteriorly, medial and parallel to the posterior belly of digastric, ending in the posterior scalp
Posterior auricular		Ascends posteriorly between external acoustic meatus and mastoid process to supply adjacent muscles, parotid gland, facial nerve, auricle, and scalp

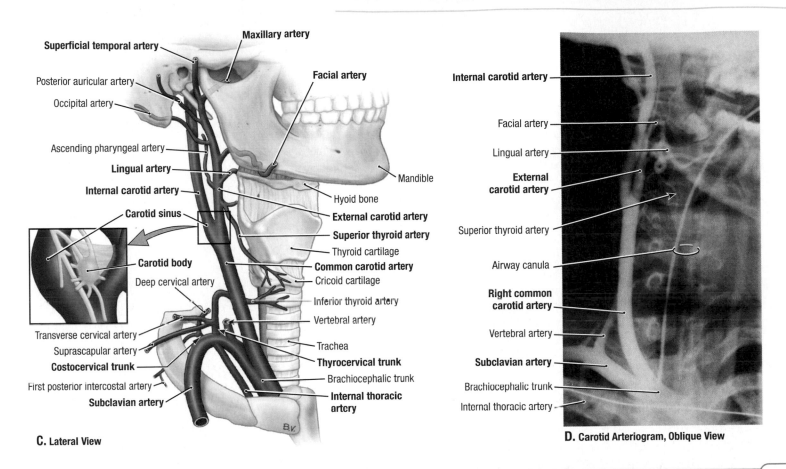

C. Lateral View

D. Carotid Arteriogram, Oblique View

Arteries of Neck *(continued)*

7.15

C. Branches of external carotid and subclavian arteries. The carotid sinus is a baroreceptor that reacts to changes in arterial blood pressure and is located in the dilatation of the proximal part of the internal carotid artery. The carotid body is an ovoid mass of tissue that lies at the bifurcation of the common carotid artery. It is a chemoreceptor that monitors the level of oxygen in the blood. **D.** Arteriogram of neck.

TABLE 7.5	**Arteries of Neck** *(continued)*	
Artery	**Origin**	**Course and Distribution**
Superior thyroid	External carotid	Runs anteroinferiorly deep to infrahyoid muscles to reach thyroid gland. Supplies thyroid gland, infrahyoid muscles, sternocleidomastoid (SCM), and larynx via *superior laryngeal artery*
Lingual		Lies on middle constrictor muscle of pharynx; arches superoanteriorly and passes deep to CN XII, stylohyoid muscle, and posterior belly of digastric then passes deep to hyoglossus, giving branches to the posterior tongue and bifurcating into *deep lingual* and *sublingual arteries*
Facial		After giving rise to *ascending palatine artery* and a tonsillar branch, it passes superiorly under cover of the angle of the mandible. It then loops anteriorly to supply the submandibular gland and give rise to the submental artery to the floor of the mouth before entering the face
Maxillary	Terminal branches of external carotid	Passes posterior to neck of mandible, enters infratemporal fossa then pterygopalatine fossa to supply teeth, nose, ear, and face
Superficial temporal		Ascends anterior to auricle to temporal region and ends in scalp
Vertebral	Subclavian	Passes through the foramina transversaria of the transverse processes of vertebrae C1–C6, runs in a groove on the posterior arch of the atlas, and enters the cranial cavity through the foramen magnum
Internal thoracic		No branches in neck; enters thorax
Thyrocervical trunk		Branches: the *inferior thyroid artery*, the main visceral artery of the neck; the transverse cervical and suprascapular arteries directly or via cervicodorsal trunk sending branches to the lateral cervical region, trapezius, and medial scapular arteries
Costocervical trunk		Trunk passes posterosuperiorly and divides into *superior intercostal* and *deep cervical arteries* to supply the 1st and 2nd intercostal spaces and posterior deep cervical muscles, respectively

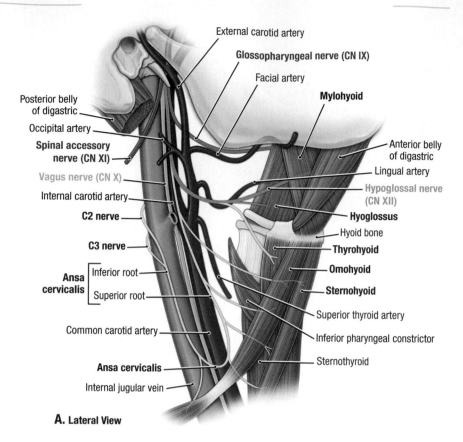

A. Lateral View

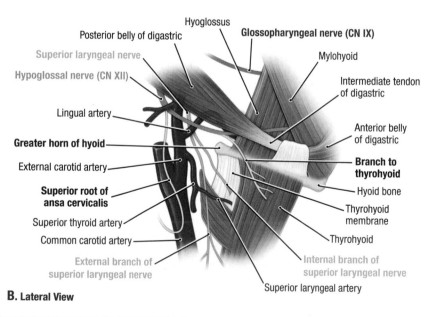

B. Lateral View

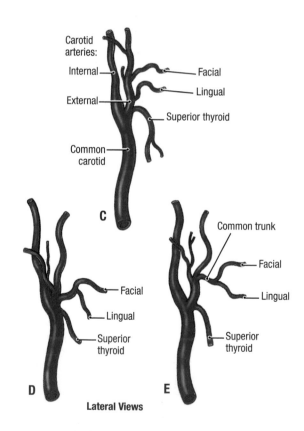

Lateral Views

Glossopharyngeal—CN IX	Vagus—CN X
Motor: stylopharyngeus, parotid gland **Sensory:** taste: posterior third of tongue; general sensation: pharynx, tonsillar sinus, pharyngotympanic tube, middle ear cavity	**Motor:** palate, pharynx, larynx, trachea, bronchial tree, heart, gastro-intestinal (GI) tract to left colic flexure **Sensory:** pharynx, larynx; reflex sensory from tracheo-bronchial tree, lungs, heart, GI tract to left colic flexure
Spinal accessory—CN XI	Hypoglossal—CN XII
Motor: sternocleidomastoid and trapezius	**Motor:** all intrinsic and extrinsic muscles of tongue (excluding palatoglossus—a palatine muscle)

7.16 **Relationships of Nerves and Vessels in Carotid Triangle of Neck**

A. Ansa cervicalis and strap muscles. B. Hypoglossal nerve (CN XII) and internal and external branches of superior laryngeal nerve (CN X). The palpable tip of the greater horn of the hyoid bone, indicated with a *circle*, is the reference point for many structures. **C–E. Variation in origin of lingual artery** (as studied by Dr. Grant in 211 specimens). In 80%, the superior thyroid, lingual, and facial arteries arose separately (*Part C*); in 20%, the lingual and facial arteries arose from a common stem inferiorly (*Part D*) or high on the external carotid artery (*Part E*). In one specimen, the superior thyroid and lingual arteries arose from a common stem.

Carotid occlusion, causing stenosis (narrowing), can be relieved by opening the artery at its origin and stripping off the atherosclerotic plaque with the artery's lining (intima). This procedure is called **carotid endarterectomy.** Because of the relationships of the internal carotid artery, there is a risk of cranial nerve injury during the procedure involving one or more of the following nerves: CN IX, CN X (or its branch, the superior laryngeal nerve), CN XI, or CN XII.

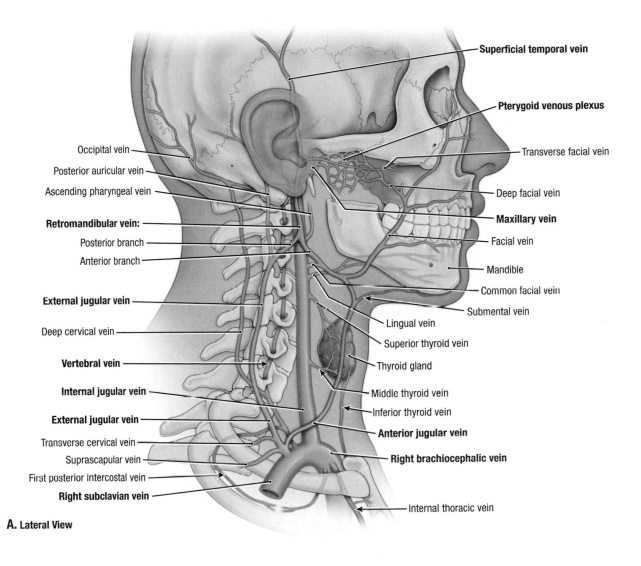

Superficial temporal vein

Pterygoid venous plexus

Occipital vein

Posterior auricular vein

Ascending pharyngeal vein

Transverse facial vein

Deep facial vein

Retromandibular vein:

Maxillary vein

Posterior branch

Facial vein

Anterior branch

Mandible

Common facial vein

External jugular vein

Submental vein

Deep cervical vein

Lingual vein

Superior thyroid vein

Vertebral vein

Thyroid gland

Internal jugular vein

Middle thyroid vein

External jugular vein

Inferior thyroid vein

Transverse cervical vein

Anterior jugular vein

Suprascapular vein

First posterior intercostal vein

Right brachiocephalic vein

Right subclavian vein

Internal thoracic vein

A. Lateral View

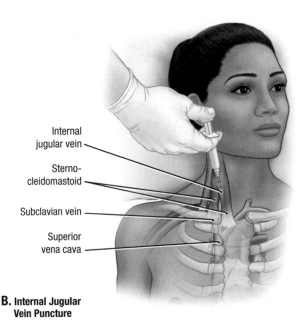

Internal jugular vein

Sterno-cleidomastoid

Subclavian vein

Superior vena cava

B. Internal Jugular Vein Puncture

Deep Veins of Neck 7.17

A. Overview. The internal jugular vein (IJV) begins at the jugular foramen as the continuation of the sigmoid sinus. From a dilated origin, the superior bulb of the IJV, the vein runs inferiorly through the neck in the carotid sheath. Posterior to the sternal end of the clavicle, the vein merges perpendicularly with the subclavian vein, forming the "venous angle" that marks the origin of the brachiocephalic vein. The inferior end of the IJV dilates superior to its terminal valve, forming the inferior bulb of the IJV. The valve permits blood to flow toward the heart while preventing backflow into the IJV. The external jugular vein drains blood from the occipital region and posterior neck to the subclavian vein, and the anterior jugular vein the anterior aspect of the neck.

B. Internal jugular vein puncture. A needle and catheter may be inserted into the IJV, using ultrasonic guidance, for diagnostic or therapeutic purposes. The right IJV is preferable to the left because it is usually larger and straighter. The clinician palpates the common carotid artery and inserts the needle into the IJV just lateral to it at a 30-degree angle, aiming at the apex of the triangle between the sternal and clavicular heads of the SCM. The needle is then directed inferolaterally toward the ipsilateral nipple. Venous access can also be achieved by other supra- and infraclavicular approaches.

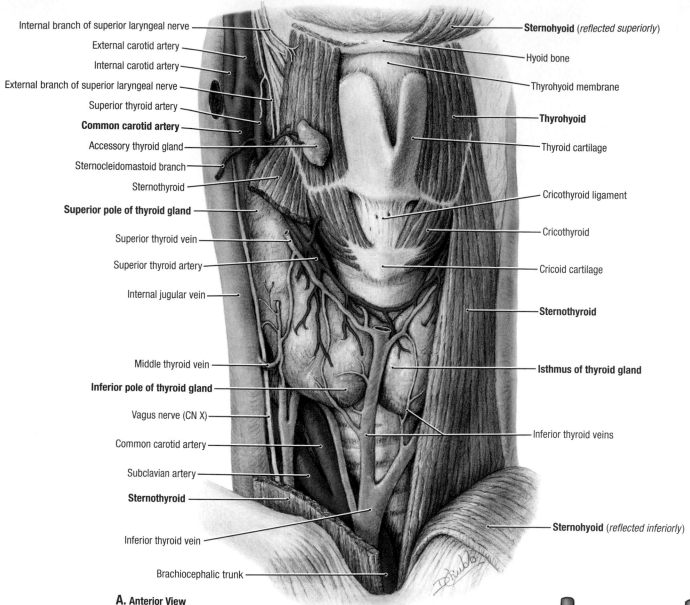

Internal branch of superior laryngeal nerve

External carotid artery

Internal carotid artery

External branch of superior laryngeal nerve

Superior thyroid artery

Common carotid artery

Accessory thyroid gland

Sternocleidomastoid branch

Sternothyroid

Superior pole of thyroid gland

Superior thyroid vein

Superior thyroid artery

Internal jugular vein

Middle thyroid vein

Inferior pole of thyroid gland

Vagus nerve (CN X)

Common carotid artery

Subclavian artery

Sternothyroid

Inferior thyroid vein

Brachiocephalic trunk

Sternohyoid (*reflected superiorly*)

Hyoid bone

Thyrohyoid membrane

Thyrohyoid

Thyroid cartilage

Cricothyroid ligament

Cricothyroid

Cricoid cartilage

Sternothyroid

Isthmus of thyroid gland

Inferior thyroid veins

Sternohyoid (*reflected inferiorly*)

A. Anterior View

| 7.18 | **Endocrine Layer of Visceral Compartment (I)** |

A. Dissection. On the left side of the specimen, the sternohyoid and omohyoid muscles are reflected or removed, exposing the sternothyroid and the thyrohyoid muscles; on the right side of the specimen, the sternothyroid muscle is largely excised. **B. Schematic of venous drainage of thyroid gland.** Except for the superior thyroid veins, the thyroid veins are not paired with arteries of corresponding names.

The **carotid pulse (neck pulse)** is easily felt by palpating the common carotid artery in the side of the neck, where it lies in a groove between the trachea and the infrahyoid muscles. It is usually easily palpated just deep to the anterior border of the SCM at the level of the superior border of the thyroid cartilage. It is routinely checked during **cardiopulmonary resuscitation** (CPR). **Absence of a carotid pulse** indicates cardiac arrest.

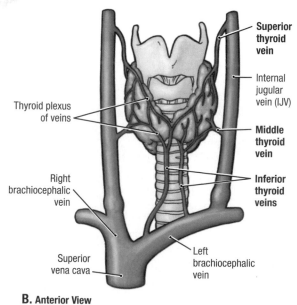

Superior thyroid vein

Internal jugular vein (IJV)

Middle thyroid vein

Inferior thyroid veins

Thyroid plexus of veins

Right brachiocephalic vein

Superior vena cava

Left brachiocephalic vein

B. Anterior View

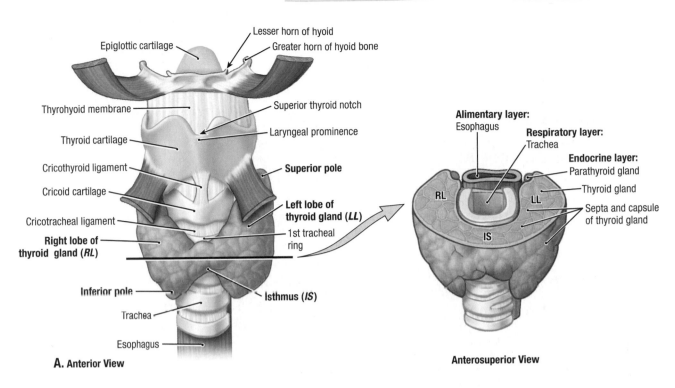

Epiglottic cartilage

Lesser horn of hyoid

Greater horn of hyoid bone

Thyrohyoid membrane

Superior thyroid notch

Laryngeal prominence

Thyroid cartilage

Cricothyroid ligament

Superior pole

Cricoid cartilage

Cricotracheal ligament

Left lobe of thyroid gland (LL)

1st tracheal ring

Right lobe of thyroid gland (RL)

Inferior pole

Isthmus (IS)

Trachea

Esophagus

A. Anterior View

Alimentary layer:
Esophagus

Respiratory layer:
Trachea

Endocrine layer:
Parathyroid gland

RL   LL

IS

Thyroid gland

Septa and capsule of thyroid gland

Anterosuperior View

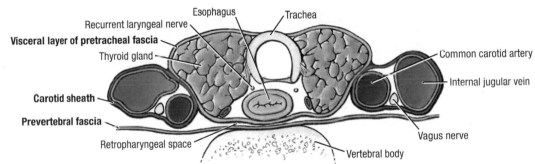

Esophagus   Trachea

Recurrent laryngeal nerve

Visceral layer of pretracheal fascia

Thyroid gland

Carotid sheath

Prevertebral fascia

Retropharyngeal space

Common carotid artery

Internal jugular vein

Vagus nerve

Vertebral body

B. Transverse Section, Inferior View

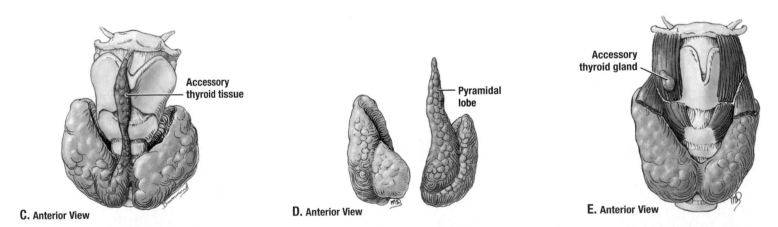

Accessory thyroid tissue

C. Anterior View

Pyramidal lobe

D. Anterior View

Accessory thyroid gland

E. Anterior View

Endocrine Layer of Visceral Compartment (II)

7.19

A. Relations of thyroid gland with transverse section showing alimentary, respiratory, and endocrine layers of visceral compartment. **B.** Fascial relationships. **C.** Accessory thyroid tissue. This tissue is located along the course of the thyroglossal duct, which was the path of migration of thyroid tissue from its embryonic site of development. **D.** Pyramidal lobe. Approximately

50% of glands have a pyramidal lobe that extends from near the isthmus to or toward the hyoid bone; the isthmus is occasionally absent, in which case the gland is in two parts. **E.** Accessory thyroid gland. An accessory gland can occur between the suprahyoid region and arch of the aorta (see Fig. 7.18A).

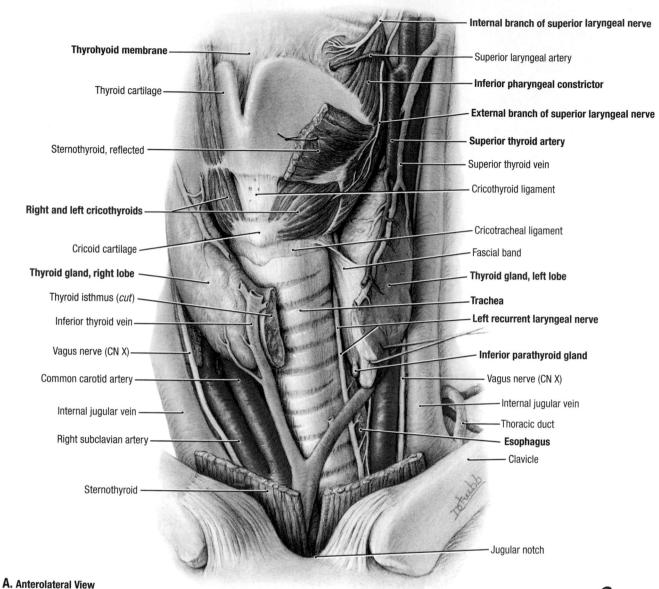

A. Anterolateral View

Internal branch of superior laryngeal nerve

Thyrohyoid membrane

Superior laryngeal artery

Thyroid cartilage

Inferior pharyngeal constrictor

External branch of superior laryngeal nerve

Sternothyroid, reflected

Superior thyroid artery

Superior thyroid vein

Cricothyroid ligament

Right and left cricothyroids

Cricotracheal ligament

Cricoid cartilage

Fascial band

Thyroid gland, right lobe

Thyroid gland, left lobe

Thyroid isthmus (cut)

Trachea

Inferior thyroid vein

Left recurrent laryngeal nerve

Vagus nerve (CN X)

Inferior parathyroid gland

Common carotid artery

Vagus nerve (CN X)

Internal jugular vein

Internal jugular vein

Right subclavian artery

Thoracic duct

Esophagus

Clavicle

Sternothyroid

Jugular notch

| 7.20 | **Respiratory Layer of Visceral Compartment** |

A. Dissection. The isthmus of the thyroid gland is divided, and the left lobe is retracted. The left recurrent laryngeal nerve ascends on the lateral aspect of the trachea between the trachea and esophagus. The internal branch of the superior laryngeal nerve runs along the superior border of the inferior pharyngeal constrictor muscle and pierces the thyrohyoid membrane. The external branch of the superior laryngeal nerve lies adjacent to the inferior pharyngeal constrictor muscle and supplies its lower portion; it continues to run along the anterior border of the superior thyroid artery, passing deep to the superior attachment of the sternothyroid muscle, and then supplies the cricothyroid muscle. **B. Blood supply of parathyroid glands and courses of left and right recurrent laryngeal nerves.**

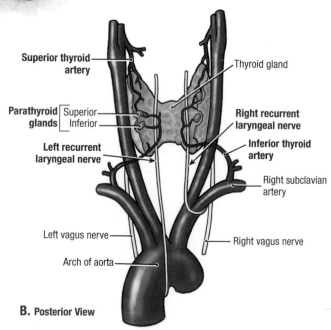

Superior thyroid artery

Thyroid gland

Parathyroid glands — Superior / Inferior

Right recurrent laryngeal nerve

Left recurrent laryngeal nerve

Inferior thyroid artery

Right subclavian artery

Left vagus nerve

Right vagus nerve

Arch of aorta

B. Posterior View

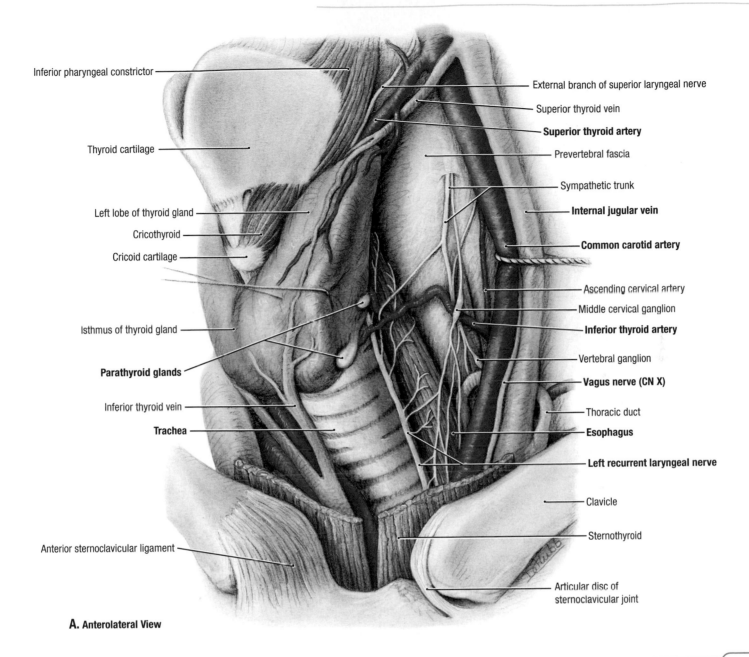

Inferior pharyngeal constrictor

External branch of superior laryngeal nerve

Superior thyroid vein

Superior thyroid artery

Thyroid cartilage

Prevertebral fascia

Sympathetic trunk

Left lobe of thyroid gland

Internal jugular vein

Cricothyroid

Common carotid artery

Cricoid cartilage

Ascending cervical artery

Middle cervical ganglion

Inferior thyroid artery

Isthmus of thyroid gland

Vertebral ganglion

Parathyroid glands

Vagus nerve (CN X)

Inferior thyroid vein

Thoracic duct

Trachea

Esophagus

Left recurrent laryngeal nerve

Clavicle

Sternothyroid

Anterior sternoclavicular ligament

Articular disc of sternoclavicular joint

A. Anterolateral View

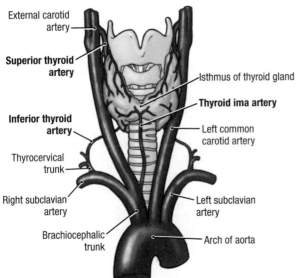

External carotid artery

Superior thyroid artery

Isthmus of thyroid gland

Thyroid ima artery

Inferior thyroid artery

Left common carotid artery

Thyrocervical trunk

Right subclavian artery

Left subclavian artery

Brachiocephalic trunk

Arch of aorta

B. Anterior View

Alimentary Layer of Visceral Compartment   7.21

A. Dissection of left side of root of neck. The three structures contained in the carotid sheath (internal jugular vein, common carotid artery, and vagus nerve) are retracted. The left recurrent laryngeal nerve ascends on the lateral aspect of the trachea, just anterior to the recess between the trachea and esophagus. **B. Arterial supply of thyroid gland.** The thyroid ima artery is infrequent (10%) and variable in its origin.

During a **total thyroidectomy** (e.g., excision of a malignant thyroid gland), the parathyroid glands are in danger of being inadvertently damaged or removed. These glands are safe during **subtotal thyroidectomy** because the most posterior part of the thyroid gland usually is preserved. Variability in the position of the parathyroid glands, especially the inferior ones, puts them in danger of being removed during surgery on the thyroid gland. If the parathyroid glands are inadvertently removed during surgery, the patient suffers from **tetany**, a severe convulsive disorder. The generalized convulsive muscle spasms result from a fall in blood calcium levels.

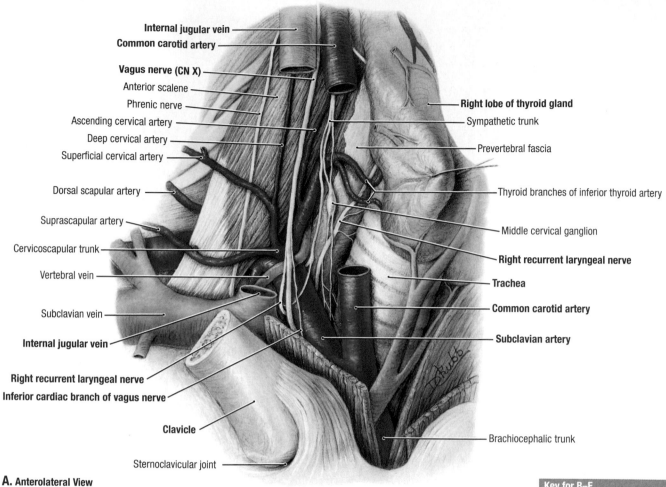

A. Anterolateral View

Internal jugular vein
Common carotid artery
Vagus nerve (CN X)
Anterior scalene
Phrenic nerve
Ascending cervical artery
Deep cervical artery
Superficial cervical artery
Dorsal scapular artery
Suprascapular artery
Cervicoscapular trunk
Vertebral vein
Subclavian vein
Internal jugular vein
Right recurrent laryngeal nerve
Inferior cardiac branch of vagus nerve
Clavicle
Sternoclavicular joint

Right lobe of thyroid gland
Sympathetic trunk
Prevertebral fascia
Thyroid branches of inferior thyroid artery
Middle cervical ganglion
Right recurrent laryngeal nerve
Trachea
Common carotid artery
Subclavian artery
Brachiocephalic trunk

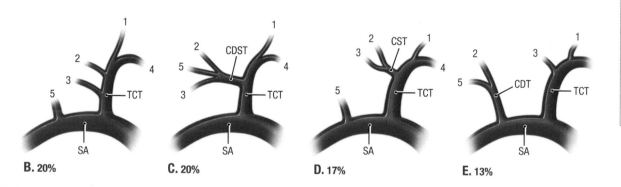

B. 20%   **C.** 20%   **D.** 17%   **E.** 13%

Key for B–E

1 Ascending cervical artery
2 Superficial cervical/ transverse cervical artery
3 Suprascapular artery
4 Inferior thyroid artery
5 Dorsal scapular artery
CDST Cervicodorsoscapular trunk
CDT Cervicodorsal trunk
CST Cervicoscapular trunk
SA Subclavian artery
TCT Thyrocervical trunk

7.22 Root of Neck

A. Dissection of right side of root of neck. The clavicle is cut, sections of the common carotid artery and internal jugular vein are removed, and the right lobe of the thyroid gland is retracted. The right vagus nerve crosses the first part of the subclavian artery and gives off an inferior cardiac branch and the right recurrent laryngeal nerve. The right recurrent laryngeal nerve loops inferior to the subclavian artery and passes posterior to the common carotid artery on its way to the posterolateral aspect of the trachea.

- **Recurrent laryngeal nerve injury** may occur during thyroidectomy and other surgeries in the anterior cervical region of the neck. Because the terminal branch of this nerve, the inferior

laryngeal nerve, innervates the muscles moving the vocal folds, injury to the nerve results in **paralysis of the vocal folds**.

- A non-neoplastic and noninflammatory enlargement of the thyroid gland, other than the variable enlargement that may occur during menstruation and pregnancy, is called a **goiter**. A goiter results from a lack of iodine.

B–E. Variations in arteries of posterior cervical region. B. Separate origin of *2* and *3* from thyrocervical trunk. **C.** Origin (*2, 3, 5*) from cervicodorsoscapular trunk from thyrocervical trunk. **D.** Origin (*2* and *3*) cervicoscapular trunk from thyrocervical trunk. **E.** Origin (*2* and *5*) from cervicodorsal trunk from subclavian artery.

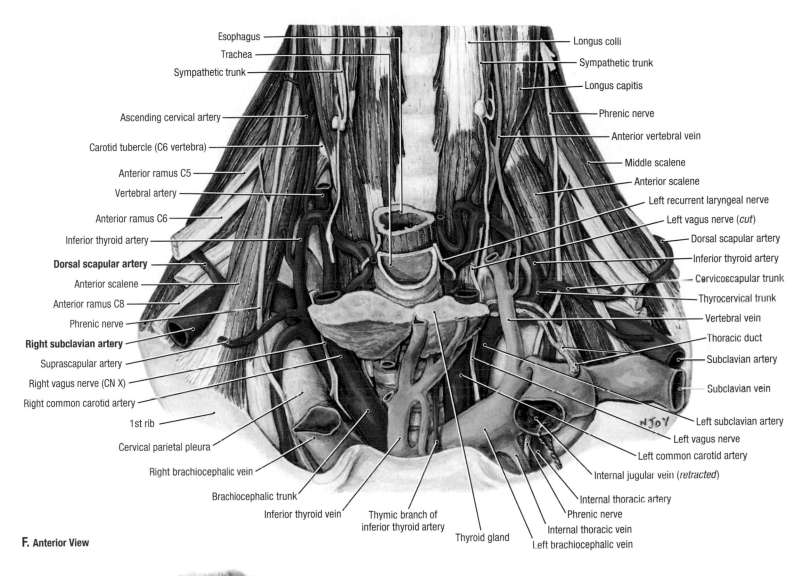

Esophagus
Trachea
Sympathetic trunk
Ascending cervical artery
Carotid tubercle (C6 vertebra)
Anterior ramus C5
Vertebral artery
Anterior ramus C6
Inferior thyroid artery
Dorsal scapular artery
Anterior scalene
Anterior ramus C8
Phrenic nerve
Right subclavian artery
Suprascapular artery
Right vagus nerve (CN X)
Right common carotid artery
1st rib
Cervical parietal pleura
Right brachiocephalic vein
Brachiocephalic trunk
Inferior thyroid vein
Thymic branch of inferior thyroid artery
Thyroid gland

Longus colli
Sympathetic trunk
Longus capitis
Phrenic nerve
Anterior vertebral vein
Middle scalene
Anterior scalene
Left recurrent laryngeal nerve
Left vagus nerve (cut)
Dorsal scapular artery
Inferior thyroid artery
Cervicoscapular trunk
Thyrocervical trunk
Vertebral vein
Thoracic duct
Subclavian artery
Subclavian vein
Left subclavian artery
Left vagus nerve
Left common carotid artery
Internal jugular vein (retracted)
Internal thoracic artery
Phrenic nerve
Internal thoracic vein
Left brachiocephalic vein

F. Anterior View

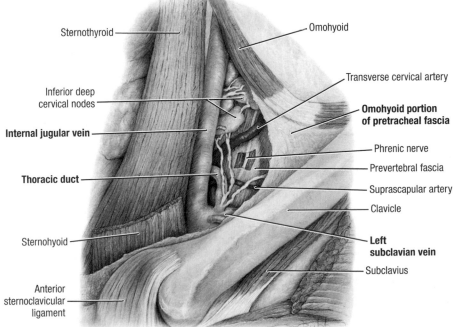

Sternothyroid
Inferior deep cervical nodes
Internal jugular vein
Thoracic duct
Sternohyoid
Anterior sternoclavicular ligament

Omohyoid
Transverse cervical artery
Omohyoid portion of pretracheal fascia
Phrenic nerve
Prevertebral fascia
Suprascapular artery
Clavicle
Left subclavian vein
Subclavius

G. Anterolateral View

Root of Neck (continued)   **7.22**

F. Deep anterior dissection. Note that the right dorsal scapular artery arises directly from the subclavian artery, a common variation.
G. Dissection of termination of thoracic duct. The sternocleidomastoid muscle is removed, the sternohyoid muscle is resected, and the omohyoid portion of the pretracheal fascia is partially removed. The thoracic duct arches laterally in the neck, passing posterior to the carotid sheath and anterior to the vertebral artery, thyrocervical trunk, and subclavian arteries; it enters the angle formed by the junction of the left subclavian and internal jugular veins to form the left brachiocephalic vein (the left venous angle).

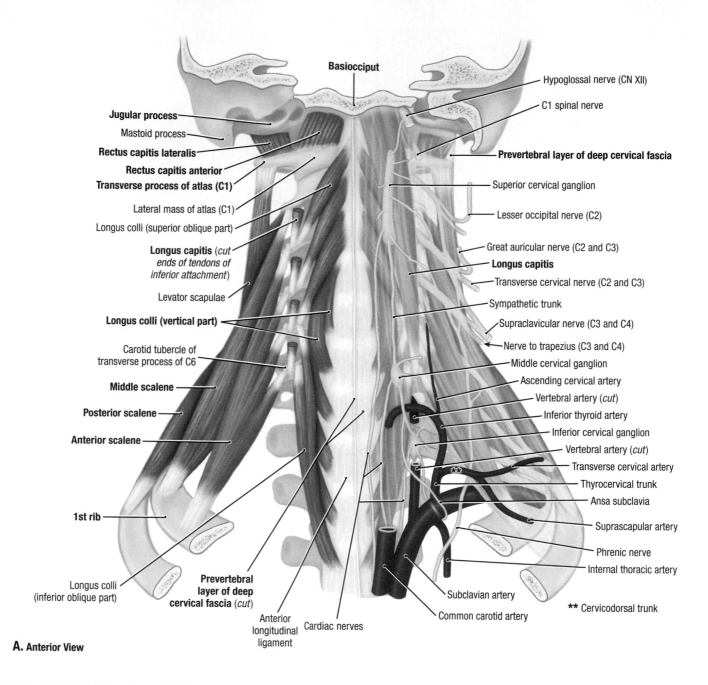

A. Anterior View

7.23   Prevertebral Region

A. and **B. Overview of muscles, nerves, and vessels.** In *Part A*, the prevertebral layer of deep cervical fascia is present on the left side of the specimen and has been removed from the right side.

TABLE 7.6   Prevertebral and Scalene Muscles

Muscle	Superior Attachment	Inferior Attachment	Innervation	Main Action
Longus colli				
Superior oblique part	Anterior tubercle of atlas (C1)	Anterior tubercles of TVP C3–C5	Anterior rami of C2–C6 spinal nerves (cervical plexus)	Rotation of cervical spine to opposite side (acting unilaterally)
Vertical part	Vertebral bodies of C2–C4	Vertebral bodies C5–T3		
Inferior oblique part	Anterior tubercles of TVP C5–C6	Vertebral bodies T1–T3		Flexion of cervical spine
Longus capitis	Basilar part of occipital bone	Anterior tubercles of TVP C3–C6	Anterior rami of C1–C3 spinal nerves (cervical plexus)	Flexion of head (atlantooccipital joints)

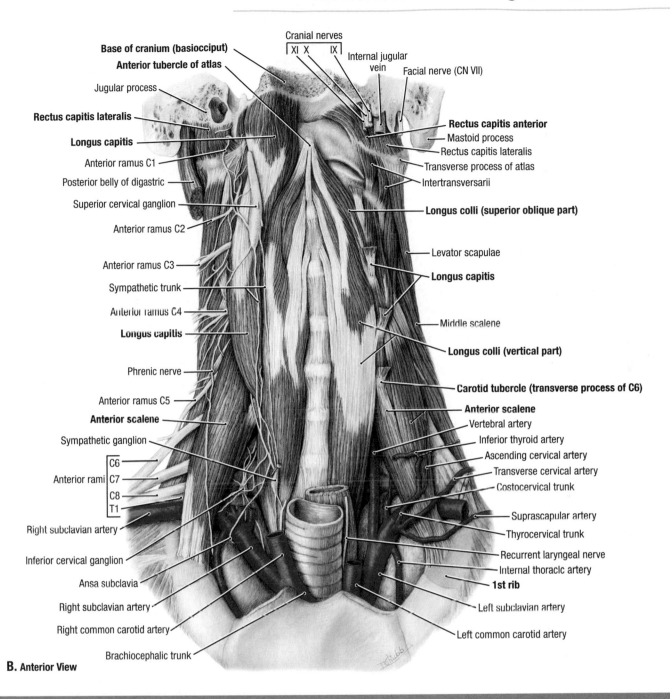

Cranial nerves
XI X IX

Base of cranium (basiocciput)
Anterior tubercle of atlas
Jugular process
Rectus capitis lateralis
Longus capitis
Anterior ramus C1
Posterior belly of digastric
Superior cervical ganglion
Anterior ramus C2
Anterior ramus C3
Sympathetic trunk
Anterior ramus C4
Longus capitis
Phrenic nerve
Anterior ramus C5
Anterior scalene
Sympathetic ganglion
Anterior rami C6 C7 C8 T1
Right subclavian artery
Inferior cervical ganglion
Ansa subclavia
Right subclavian artery
Right common carotid artery
Brachiocephalic trunk

Internal jugular vein
Facial nerve (CN VII)
Rectus capitis anterior
Mastoid process
Rectus capitis lateralis
Transverse process of atlas
Intertransversarii
Longus colli (superior oblique part)
Levator scapulae
Longus capitis
Middle scalene
Longus colli (vertical part)
Carotid tubercle (transverse process of C6)
Anterior scalene
Vertebral artery
Inferior thyroid artery
Ascending cervical artery
Transverse cervical artery
Costocervical trunk
Suprascapular artery
Thyrocervical trunk
Recurrent laryngeal nerve
Internal thoracic artery
1st rib
Left subclavian artery
Left common carotid artery

B. Anterior View

Prevertebral Region (continued)   **7.23**

TABLE 7.6   Prevertebral and Scalene Muscles (continued)

Muscle	Superior Attachment	Inferior Attachment	Innervation	Main Action
Rectus capitis anterior	Base of cranium, just anterior to occipital condyle	Anterior surface of lateral mass of atlas (C1)	Branches from loop between C1 and C2 spinal nerves	Lateral flexion at atlantooccipital joints (acting unilaterally)
Rectus capitis lateralis	Base of cranium just lateral to occipital condyle	TVP of atlas (C1)		Flexion at atlantooccipital joints (acting bilaterally)
Anterior scalene	Anterior tubercles of TVP C3–C6	Scalene tubercle of 1st rib	Anterior rami of C3–C8 (cervical and brachial plexus)	Forced inspiration: elevates 1st rib
Middle scalene	TVP C1–C2	Superior surface of 1st rib; posterior to groove for subclavian artery		
	Posterior tubercles of TVP C5–C7			Ribs fixed: lateral flexion of cervical spine (acting unilaterally) Flexes neck (acting bilaterally)
Posterior scalene	Posterior tubercles of TVP C3–C7	External border of 2nd rib		

TVP, transverse process.

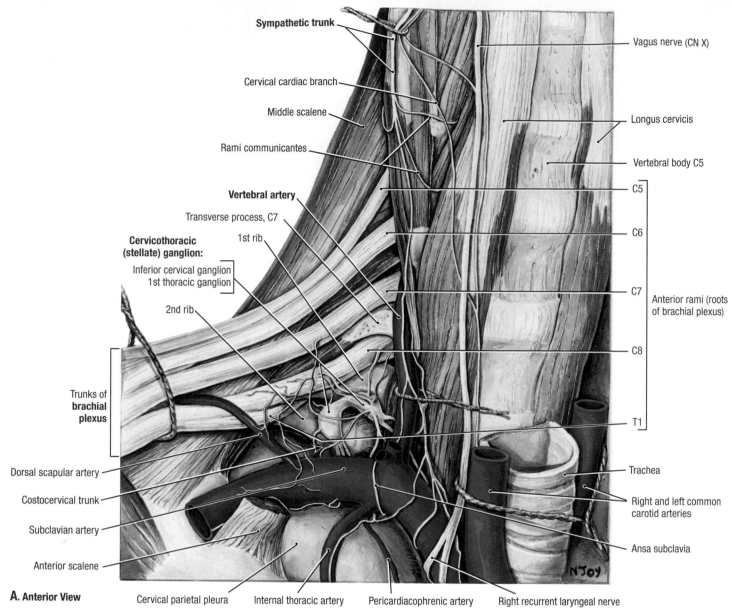

Sympathetic trunk

Cervical cardiac branch

Middle scalene

Rami communicantes

Vertebral artery

Transverse process, C7

Cervicothoracic (stellate) ganglion:

Inferior cervical ganglion
1st thoracic ganglion

1st rib

2nd rib

Trunks of **brachial plexus**

Dorsal scapular artery

Costocervical trunk

Subclavian artery

Anterior scalene

A. Anterior View

Cervical parietal pleura

Internal thoracic artery

Pericardiacophrenic artery

Right recurrent laryngeal nerve

Vagus nerve (CN X)

Longus cervicis

Vertebral body C5

C5

C6

C7

C8

T1

Anterior rami (roots of brachial plexus)

Trachea

Right and left common carotid arteries

Ansa subclavia

| 7.24 | **Brachial Plexus and Sympathetic Trunk in Root of Neck** |

A. Dissection of right side of specimen. The pleura has been depressed, the vertebral artery retracted medially, and the brachial plexus retracted superiorly to reveal the cervicothoracic (stellate) ganglion (the combined inferior cervical and 1st thoracic ganglia). Anesthetic injected around the cervicothoracic (stellate) ganglion blocks transmission of stimuli through the cervical and superior thoracic ganglia. This **stellate ganglion block** may relieve vascular spasms involving the brain and upper limb. It is also useful when deciding if surgical resection of the ganglion would be beneficial to a person with excess vasoconstriction of the ipsilateral limb.
B. Relation of brachial plexus and subclavian artery to anterior and middle scalene muscles.

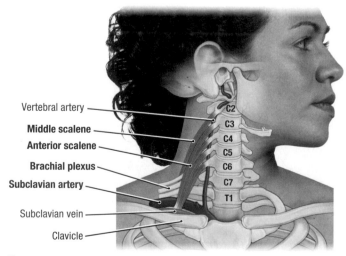

Vertebral artery

Middle scalene

Anterior scalene

Brachial plexus

Subclavian artery

Subclavian vein

Clavicle

C2
C3
C4
C5
C6
C7
T1

B. Anterolateral View

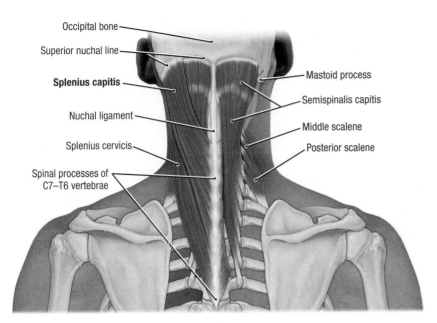

A. Posterior View

- Occipital bone
- Superior nuchal line
- **Splenius capitis**
- Nuchal ligament
- Splenius cervicis
- Spinal processes of C7–T6 vertebrae
- Mastoid process
- Semispinalis capitis
- Middle scalene
- Posterior scalene

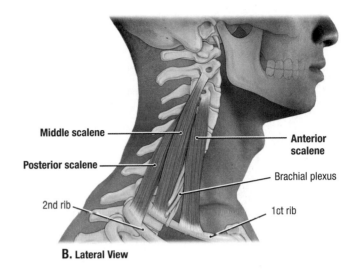

B. Lateral View

- **Middle scalene**
- **Posterior scalene**
- 2nd rib
- **Anterior scalene**
- Brachial plexus
- 1ct rib

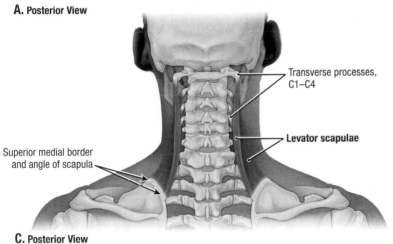

C. Posterior View

- Transverse processes, C1–C4
- **Levator scapulae**
- Superior medial border and angle of scapula

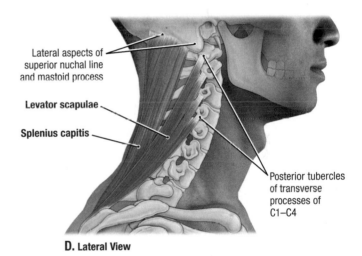

D. Lateral View

- Lateral aspects of superior nuchal line and mastoid process
- **Levator scapulae**
- **Splenius capitis**
- Posterior tubercles of transverse processes of C1–C4

Lateral Vertebral Muscles   7.25

A. Overview. **B.** Scalene muscles. **C.** Levator scapulae. **D.** Levator scapulae and splenius capitis.

TABLE 7.7 Lateral Vertebral Muscles[a]

Muscle	Superior Attachment	Inferior Attachment	Innervation	Main Action
Splenius capitis	Lateral aspect of mastoid process and lateral third of superior nuchal line	Inferior half of nuchal ligament and spinous processes of C7 and superior 3–4 thoracic vertebrae	Posterior rami of middle cervical spinal nerves	Laterally flexes and rotates head and neck to same side; acting bilaterally, extends head and neck[b]
Levator scapulae	Posterior tubercles of transverse processes of C1–C4 vertebrae	Superior part of medial border of scapula	Dorsal scapular nerve (C5) and cervical spinal nerves C3 and C4	Elevates scapula and tilts glenoid cavity inferiorly by rotating scapula

[a]Middle and posterior scalene; see Table 7.6.
[b]Rotation of head occurs at atlantoaxial joints.

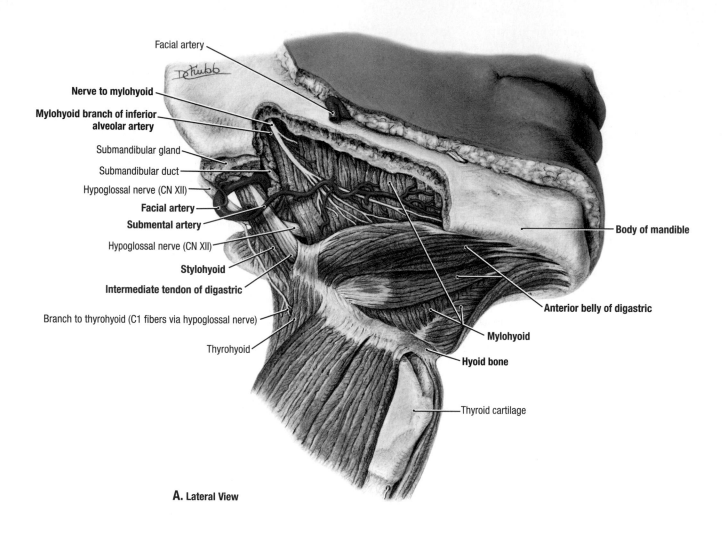

Facial artery

Nerve to mylohyoid

Mylohyoid branch of inferior alveolar artery

Submandibular gland

Submandibular duct

Hypoglossal nerve (CN XII)

Facial artery

Submental artery

Hypoglossal nerve (CN XII)

Stylohyoid

Intermediate tendon of digastric

Branch to thyrohyoid (C1 fibers via hypoglossal nerve)

Thyrohyoid

Body of mandible

Anterior belly of digastric

Mylohyoid

Hyoid bone

Thyroid cartilage

A. Lateral View

7.26 Serial Dissection of Submandibular Region and Floor of Mouth

A. Mylohyoid and digastric muscles. Structures overlying the mandible and a portion of the body of the mandible have been removed.

- The stylohyoid and posterior belly and intermediate tendon of the digastric muscle form the posterior border of the submandibular triangle; the facial artery passes superficial to these muscles.
- The anterior belly of the digastric muscle forms the anteromedial border of the submandibular triangle. In this specimen, the anterior belly has an additional origin from the hyoid. The mylohyoid muscle forms the floor of the triangle and has a thick, free posterior border.
- The nerve to mylohyoid, which supplies the mylohyoid muscle and anterior belly of the digastric muscle, is accompanied by the mylohyoid branch of the inferior alveolar artery posteriorly and the submental artery from the facial artery anteriorly.

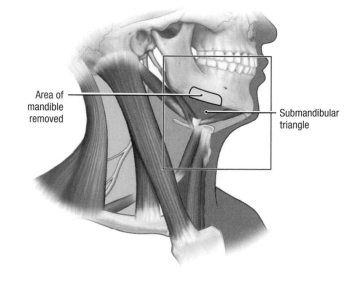

Area of mandible removed

Submandibular triangle

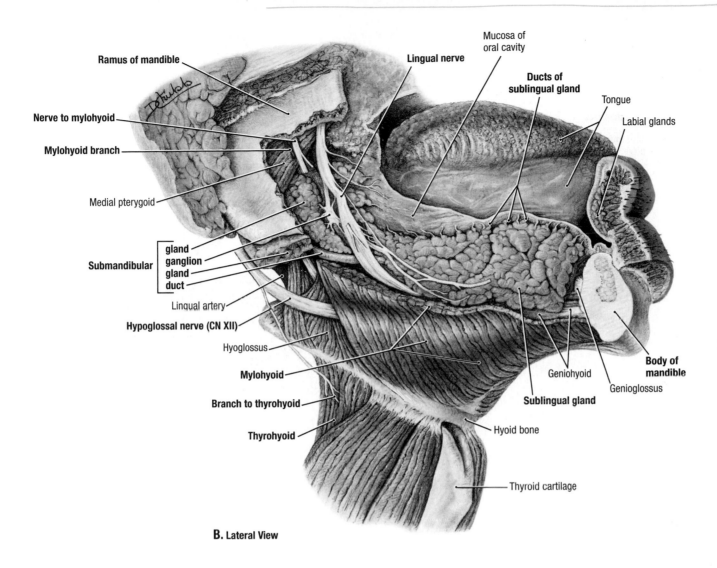

Ramus of mandible

Nerve to mylohyoid

Mylohyoid branch

Medial pterygoid

Submandibular
- gland
- ganglion
- gland
- duct

Linqual artery

Hypoglossal nerve (CN XII)

Hyoglossus

Mylohyoid

Branch to thyrohyoid

Thyrohyoid

Lingual nerve

Mucosa of
oral cavity

Ducts of
sublingual gland

Tongue

Labial glands

Geniohyoid

Genioglossus

Sublingual gland

Body of
mandible

Hyoid bone

Thyroid cartilage

B. Lateral View

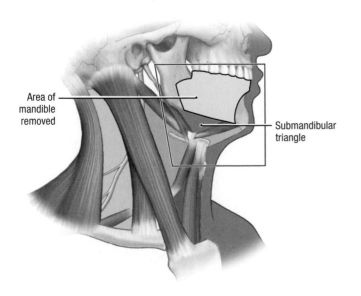

Area of
mandible
removed

Submandibular
triangle

**Serial Dissection of Submandibular Region
and Floor of Mouth** (continued)

7.26

B. Sublingual and submandibular glands. The body and adjacent portion of the ramus of the mandible have been removed.

- The sublingual salivary gland lies posterior to the mandible and is in contact with the deep part of the submandibular gland posteriorly.
- Numerous fine ducts pass from the superior border of the sublingual gland to open on the sublingual fold of the overlying mucosa.
- The lingual nerve lies between the sublingual gland and the deep part of the submandibular gland; the submandibular ganglion is suspended from this nerve.
- Spinal nerve C1 fibers, conveyed by the hypoglossal nerve (CN XII), pass to the thyrohyoid muscle before the hypoglossal nerve passes deep to the mylohyoid muscle.

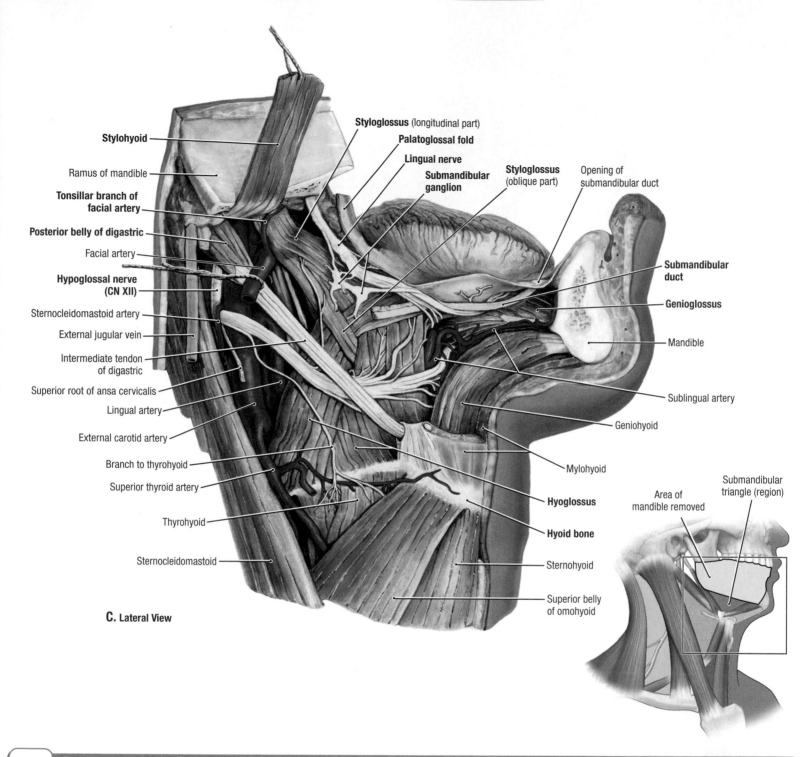

Stylohyoid

Ramus of mandible

Tonsillar branch of facial artery

Posterior belly of digastric

Facial artery

Hypoglossal nerve (CN XII)

Sternocleidomastoid artery

External jugular vein

Intermediate tendon of digastric

Superior root of ansa cervicalis

Lingual artery

External carotid artery

Branch to thyrohyoid

Superior thyroid artery

Thyrohyoid

Sternocleidomastoid

C. Lateral View

Styloglossus (longitudinal part)

Palatoglossal fold

Lingual nerve

Submandibular ganglion

Styloglossus (oblique part)

Opening of submandibular duct

Submandibular duct

Genioglossus

Mandible

Sublingual artery

Geniohyoid

Mylohyoid

Hyoglossus

Hyoid bone

Sternohyoid

Superior belly of omohyoid

Area of mandible removed

Submandibular triangle (region)

7.26   **Serial Dissection of Submandibular Region and Floor of Mouth** (continued)

C. Hyoglossus muscle, lingual (CN V₃) and hypoglossal (CN XII) nerves. All of the right half of the mandible, except the superior part of the ramus, has been removed. The stylohyoid muscle is reflected superiorly, and the posterior belly of the digastric muscle is left *in situ*.

- The hyoglossus muscle ascends from the greater horn and body of the hyoid bone to the side of the tongue.
- The styloglossus muscle is crossed by the tonsillar branch of the facial artery posterosuperiorly, and its oblique part interdigitates with bundles of the hyoglossus muscle inferiorly.

- The hypoglossal nerve (CN XII) supplies all of the muscles of the tongue, both extrinsic and intrinsic, except the palatoglossus (a palatine muscle, innervated by the vagus nerve, CN X).
- The submandibular duct runs anteriorly in contact with the hyoglossus and genioglossus muscles to its opening on the side of the frenulum of the tongue.
- The lingual nerve is in contact with the mandible posteriorly, looping inferior to the submandibular duct and ending in the tongue. The submandibular ganglion is suspended from the lingual nerve.

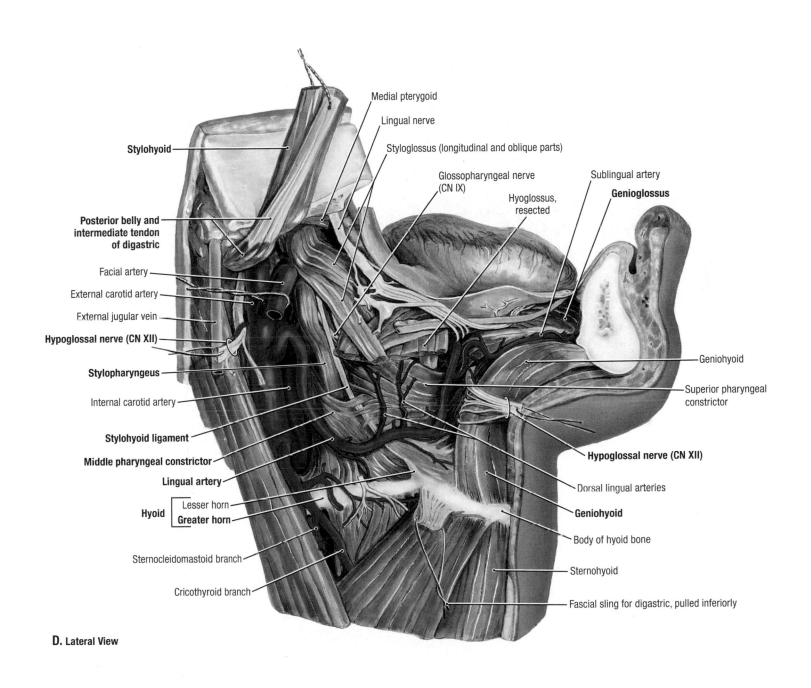

Medial pterygoid

Lingual nerve

Styloglossus (longitudinal and oblique parts)

Glossopharyngeal nerve
(CN IX)

Sublingual artery

Hyoglossus,
resected

Genioglossus

Stylohyoid

**Posterior belly and
intermediate tendon
of digastric**

Facial artery

External carotid artery

External jugular vein

Hypoglossal nerve (CN XII)

Stylopharyngeus

Internal carotid artery

Stylohyoid ligament

Middle pharyngeal constrictor

Lingual artery

Hyoid   Lesser horn
Greater horn

Sternocleidomastoid branch

Cricothyroid branch

Geniohyoid

Superior pharyngeal
constrictor

Hypoglossal nerve (CN XII)

Dorsal lingual arteries

Geniohyoid

Body of hyoid bone

Sternohyoid

Fascial sling for digastric, pulled inferiorly

D. Lateral View

Serial Dissection of Submandibular Region and Floor of Mouth *(continued)*   **7.26**

D. Genioglossus and geniohyoid muscles. The stylohyoid, posterior belly and intermediate tendon of the digastric muscle are reflected superiorly, the hypoglossal nerve (CN XII) is divided, and the hyoglossus muscle is mostly removed.

- The lingual artery passes deep to the hyoglossus muscle (resected here), close to the greater horn of the hyoid, and

then passes lateral to the middle pharyngeal constrictor muscle, stylohyoid ligament, and genioglossus muscle and turns into the tongue as the deep lingual arteries.

- In this specimen, the glossopharyngeal nerve does not make the usual spiral descent lateral to the stylopharyngeus muscle but descends medial to it.

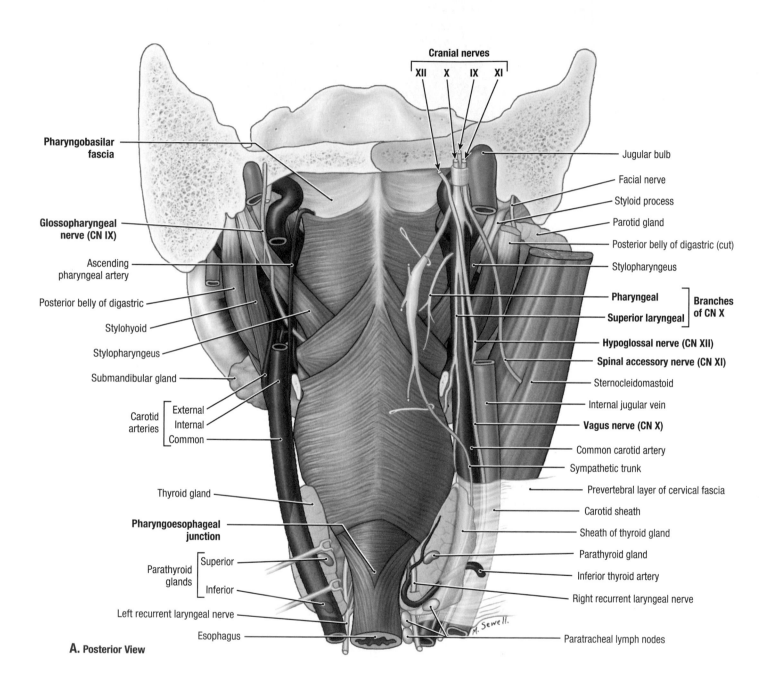

Cranial nerves

XII   X   IX   XI

Pharyngobasilar fascia

Glossopharyngeal nerve (CN IX)

Ascending pharyngeal artery

Posterior belly of digastric

Stylohyoid

Stylopharyngeus

Submandibular gland

Carotid arteries
- External
- Internal
- Common

Thyroid gland

Pharyngoesophageal junction

Parathyroid glands
- Superior
- Inferior

Left recurrent laryngeal nerve

Esophagus

Jugular bulb

Facial nerve

Styloid process

Parotid gland

Posterior belly of digastric (cut)

Stylopharyngeus

Pharyngeal
Superior laryngeal
} Branches of CN X

Hypoglossal nerve (CN XII)

Spinal accessory nerve (CN XI)

Sternocleidomastoid

Internal jugular vein

Vagus nerve (CN X)

Common carotid artery

Sympathetic trunk

Prevertebral layer of cervical fascia

Carotid sheath

Sheath of thyroid gland

Parathyroid gland

Inferior thyroid artery

Right recurrent laryngeal nerve

Paratracheal lymph nodes

M. Sewell.

A. Posterior View

7.27 **External Pharynx, Posterior Views**

A. Illustration. The sympathetic trunk (including the superior cervical ganglion), which normally lies posterior to the internal carotid artery, has been retracted medially.

- The pharyngobasilar fascia, between the superior pharyngeal constrictor muscle and the base of the skull, attaches the pharynx to the occipital bone and forms the wall of the pharyngeal recesses.

- As they exit the jugular foramen, CN IX lies anterior to CN X, and CN XI; CN XII, exiting the hypoglossal canal, lies medially.

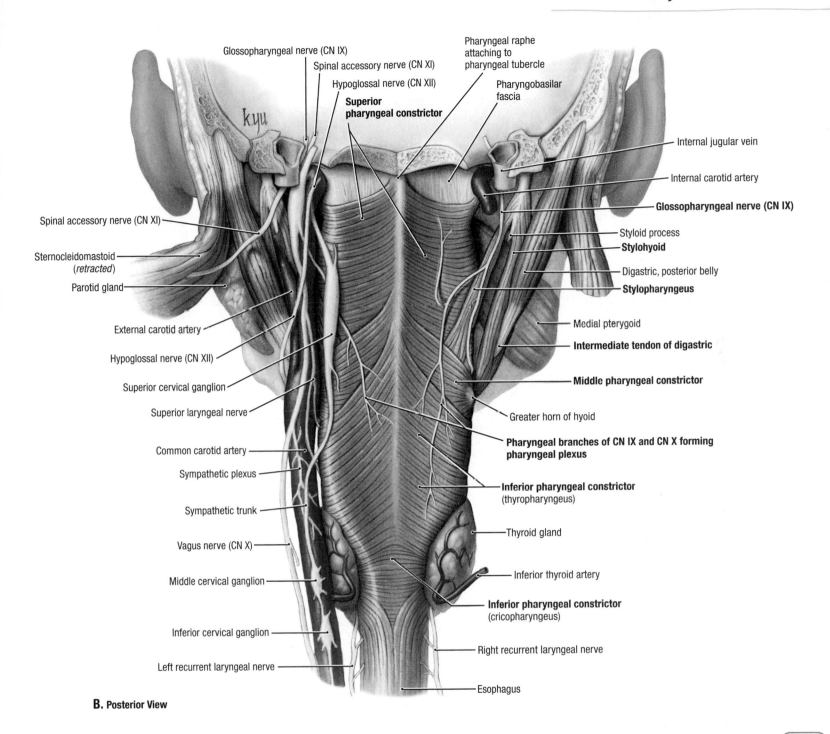

Glossopharyngeal nerve (CN IX)
Spinal accessory nerve (CN XI)
Hypoglossal nerve (CN XII)
Superior pharyngeal constrictor
Pharyngeal raphe attaching to pharyngeal tubercle
Pharyngobasilar fascia

Internal jugular vein
Internal carotid artery
Glossopharyngeal nerve (CN IX)
Styloid process
Stylohyoid
Digastric, posterior belly
Stylopharyngeus
Medial pterygoid
Intermediate tendon of digastric
Middle pharyngeal constrictor
Greater horn of hyoid
Pharyngeal branches of CN IX and CN X forming pharyngeal plexus
Inferior pharyngeal constrictor (thyropharyngeus)
Thyroid gland
Inferior thyroid artery
Inferior pharyngeal constrictor (cricopharyngeus)
Right recurrent laryngeal nerve
Esophagus

Spinal accessory nerve (CN XI)
Sternocleidomastoid (*retracted*)
Parotid gland
External carotid artery
Hypoglossal nerve (CN XII)
Superior cervical ganglion
Superior laryngeal nerve
Common carotid artery
Sympathetic plexus
Sympathetic trunk
Vagus nerve (CN X)
Middle cervical ganglion
Inferior cervical ganglion
Left recurrent laryngeal nerve

B. Posterior View

External Pharynx, Posterior Views (*continued*)   **7.27**

B. Dissection. A large wedge of occipital bone (including the foramen magnum) and the articulated cervical vertebrae have been separated from the remainder (anterior portion) of the head and cervical viscera at the retropharyngeal space and removed.

- The pharynx is a unique portion of the alimentary tract, having a circular layer of muscle externally and a longitudinal layer internally.
- The circular layer of the pharynx consists of the three pharyngeal constrictor muscles (superior, middle, and inferior), which overlap one another.
- On the right side of the specimen, the stylopharyngeus muscle and glossopharyngeal nerve (CN IX) pass from the medial

side of the styloid process anteromedially through the interval between the superior and middle pharyngeal constrictor muscles to become part of the internal longitudinal layer. The stylohyoid muscle passes from the lateral side of the styloid process anterolaterally and splits on its way to the hyoid bone to accommodate passage of the intermediate tendon of the digastric.

Pharyngeal branches of the glossopharyngeal nerve (CN IX) and the vagus nerve (CN X) form the pharyngeal plexus, which provides most of the pharyngeal innervation. The glossopharyngeal nerve supplies the sensory component, plus motor innervation to the stylopharyngeus, while the vagus nerve supplies motor innervation to the remainder.

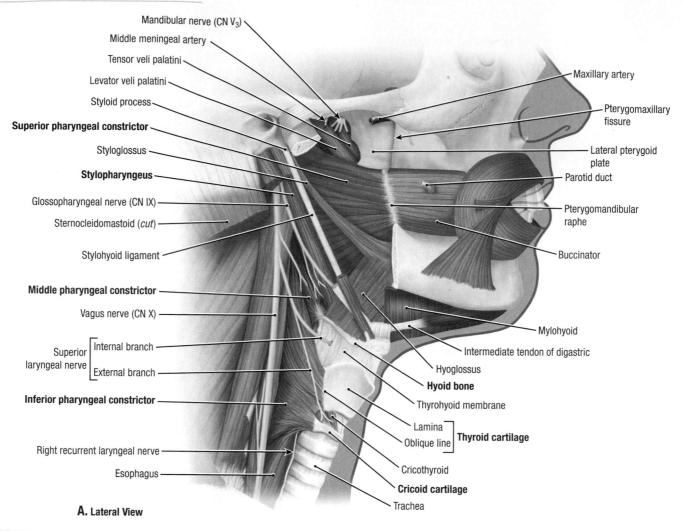

Mandibular nerve (CN V₃)
Middle meningeal artery
Tensor veli palatini
Levator veli palatini
Styloid process
Superior pharyngeal constrictor
Styloglossus
Stylopharyngeus
Glossopharyngeal nerve (CN IX)
Sternocleidomastoid (*cut*)
Stylohyoid ligament
Middle pharyngeal constrictor
Vagus nerve (CN X)
Superior laryngeal nerve — Internal branch / External branch
Inferior pharyngeal constrictor
Right recurrent laryngeal nerve
Esophagus

Maxillary artery
Pterygomaxillary fissure
Lateral pterygoid plate
Parotid duct
Pterygomandibular raphe
Buccinator
Mylohyoid
Intermediate tendon of digastric
Hyoglossus
Hyoid bone
Thyrohyoid membrane
Lamina / Oblique line **Thyroid cartilage**
Cricothyroid
Cricoid cartilage
Trachea

A. Lateral View

7.28 **External Pharynx, Lateral Views**

A. Illustration showing relationships of nerves and muscles.

TABLE 7.8 Muscles of Pharynx

Muscle	Origin	Insertion	Innervation	Main Action(s)
Superior pharyngeal constrictor	Pterygoid hamulus, pterygomandibular raphe, posterior end of mylohyoid line of mandible, and side of tongue	Pharyngeal raphe	Pharyngeal and superior laryngeal branches of vagus (CN X) through pharyngeal plexus	Constrict wall of pharynx during swallowing
Middle pharyngeal constrictor	Stylohyoid ligament and superior (greater) and inferior (lesser) horns of hyoid bone			
Inferior pharyngeal constrictor: Thyropharyngeus	Oblique line of thyroid cartilage			
Cricopharyngeus	Side of cricoid cartilage	Contralateral side of cricoid cartilage	Pharyngeal and superior laryngeal branches of vagus (CN X) through pharyngeal plexus + external laryngeal plexus	Serves as superior esophageal sphincter
Palatopharyngeus (see Fig. 7.29B)	Hard palate and palatine aponeurosis	Posterior border of lamina of thyroid cartilage and side of pharynx and esophagus	Pharyngeal and superior laryngeal branches of vagus (CN X) through pharyngeal plexus	Elevate pharynx and larynx during swallowing and speaking
Salpingopharyngeus (see Fig. 7.29B)	Cartilaginous part of pharyngotympanic tube	Blends with palatopharyngeus		
Stylopharyngeus	Styloid process of temporal bone	Posterior and superior borders of thyroid cartilage with palatopharyngeus	Glossopharyngeal nerve (CN IX)	

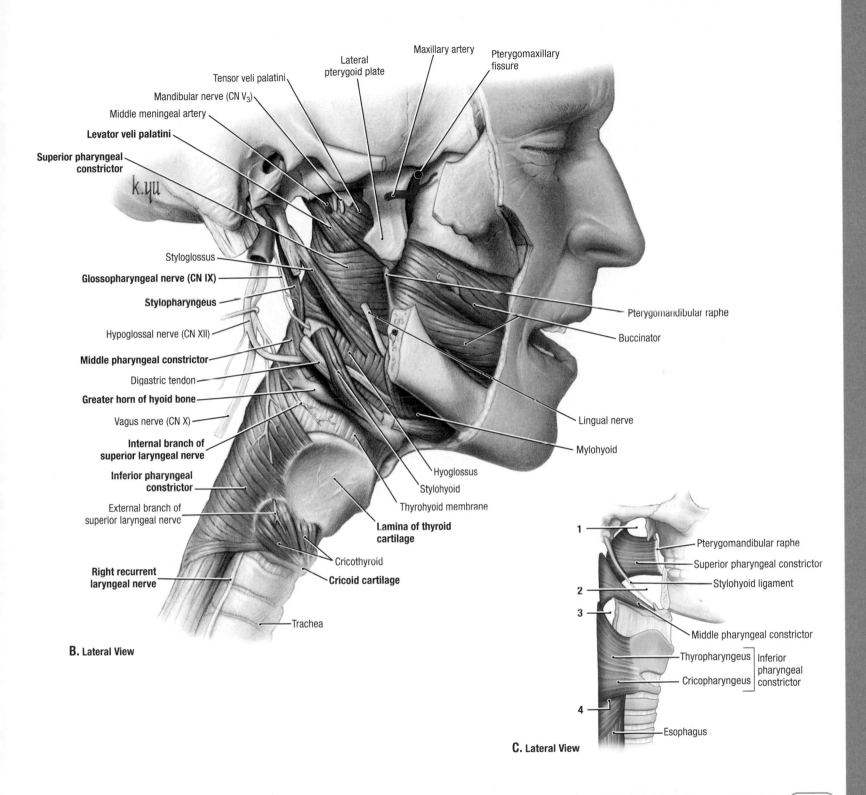

Maxillary artery

Pterygomaxillary fissure

Lateral pterygoid plate

Tensor veli palatini

Mandibular nerve (CN V₃)

Middle meningeal artery

Levator veli palatini

Superior pharyngeal constrictor

Styloglossus

Glossopharyngeal nerve (CN IX)

Stylopharyngeus

Hypoglossal nerve (CN XII)

Middle pharyngeal constrictor

Digastric tendon

Greater horn of hyoid bone

Vagus nerve (CN X)

Internal branch of superior laryngeal nerve

Inferior pharyngeal constrictor

External branch of superior laryngeal nerve

Right recurrent laryngeal nerve

Trachea

Pterygomandibular raphe

Buccinator

Lingual nerve

Mylohyoid

Hyoglossus

Stylohyoid

Thyrohyoid membrane

Lamina of thyroid cartilage

Cricothyroid

Cricoid cartilage

B. Lateral View

Pterygomandibular raphe

Superior pharyngeal constrictor

Stylohyoid ligament

Middle pharyngeal constrictor

Thyropharyngeus | Inferior pharyngeal constrictor

Cricopharyngeus |

Esophagus

C. Lateral View

External Pharynx, Lateral Views (*continued*)

7.28

B. Dissection. C. Relationships of pharyngeal constrictor muscles.
Observe that there are gaps in the pharyngeal musculature
(*1 to 4* in *Part C*) allowing the entry of structures:
1. Superior to the superior constrictor muscle: levator veli palatini muscle and pharyngotympanic (auditory) tube.
2. Between the superior and middle constrictors: stylopharyngeus muscle, CN IX, and stylohyoid ligament.

3. Between the middle and inferior constrictors: internal branch of superior laryngeal nerve and superior laryngeal artery.
4. Inferior to the inferior constrictor muscle: recurrent laryngeal nerve.

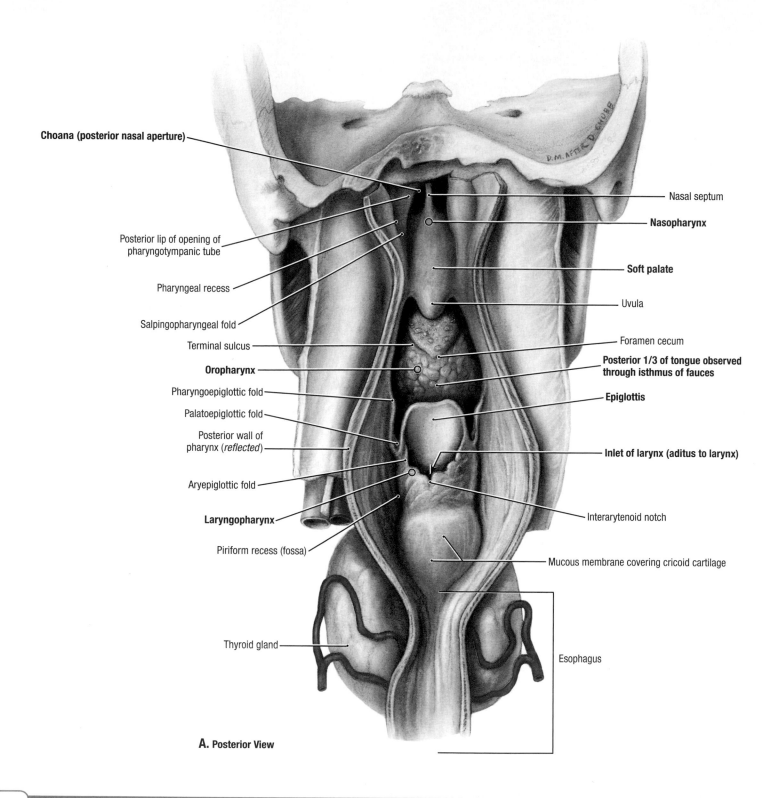

Choana (posterior nasal aperture)

Posterior lip of opening of
pharyngotympanic tube

Pharyngeal recess

Salpingopharyngeal fold

Terminal sulcus

Oropharynx

Pharyngoepiglottic fold

Palatoepiglottic fold

Posterior wall of
pharynx (*reflected*)

Aryepiglottic fold

Laryngopharynx

Piriform recess (fossa)

Thyroid gland

Nasal septum

Nasopharynx

Soft palate

Uvula

Foramen cecum

**Posterior 1/3 of tongue observed
through isthmus of fauces**

Epiglottis

Inlet of larynx (aditus to larynx)

Interarytenoid notch

Mucous membrane covering cricoid cartilage

Esophagus

A. Posterior View

7.29 | **Internal Pharynx**

A. Dissection. The posterior wall of the pharynx has been split in
the midline and the halves retracted laterally to reveal the internal
aspect of the anterior wall of the pharynx. The pharynx consists of
three continuous parts: (1) The nasal part (nasopharynx), superior
to the level of the soft palate, communicates anteriorly through
the choanae with the nasal cavities; (2) the oral part (oropharynx),
between the soft palate and the epiglottis, communicates anteriorly
through the isthmus of the fauces with the oral cavity; and (3) the
laryngeal part (laryngopharynx), posterior to the larynx, communicates with the vestibule of the larynx through the inlet of (aditus
to) the larynx. The pharynx extends from the cranial base to the
inferior border of the cricoid cartilage.

Vagus nerve (CN X)

Nasal septum

Cartilaginous part of pharyngotympanic tube

Internal carotid artery

Internal jugular vein

Pharyngobasilar fascia (wall of pharyngeal recess)

Salpingopharyngeus

Spinal accessory nerve (CN XI)

Superior pharyngeal constrictor

Stylopharyngeus

Posterior belly of digastric

Sternocleidomastoid

Musculus uvulae

Levator veli palatini

Palatopharyngeus

Vallate papilla

Uvula

Hypoglossal nerve (CN XII)

Palatine tonsil

Root of tongue

Pharyngoepiglottic fold

Epiglottis

Aryepiglottic muscle

Fibers from stylopharyngeus

Oblique
Transverse } Arytenoid

Palatopharyngeus

Posterior cricoarytenoid

Common carotid artery

Circular } Muscle of
Longitudinal } esophagus

Thyroid gland

Inferior thyroid artery

Vagus nerve (CN X)

Right recurrent laryngeal nerve

B. Posterior View

Internal Pharynx (continued)

7.29

B. Illustration. The posterior wall of the pharynx has been split in the midline and reflected laterally as in *Part A* and then the mucous membrane was removed to expose the underlying musculature. The muscles of the soft palate, pharynx, and larynx work together during swallowing, elevating the soft palate, narrowing the pharyngeal isthmus (passageway between the nasal and oral parts of the pharynx) and laryngeal inlet, retracting the epiglottis, and closing the glottis, to keep food and drink out of the nasopharynx and larynx as they pass from oral cavity to esophagus. At other times, as when blowing one's nose, the palatopharyngeus muscles, partially encircling the opening to the oral cavity, constrict this opening and depress the soft palate, working with placement and expansion of the posterior tongue to direct expired air through the nasal cavity.

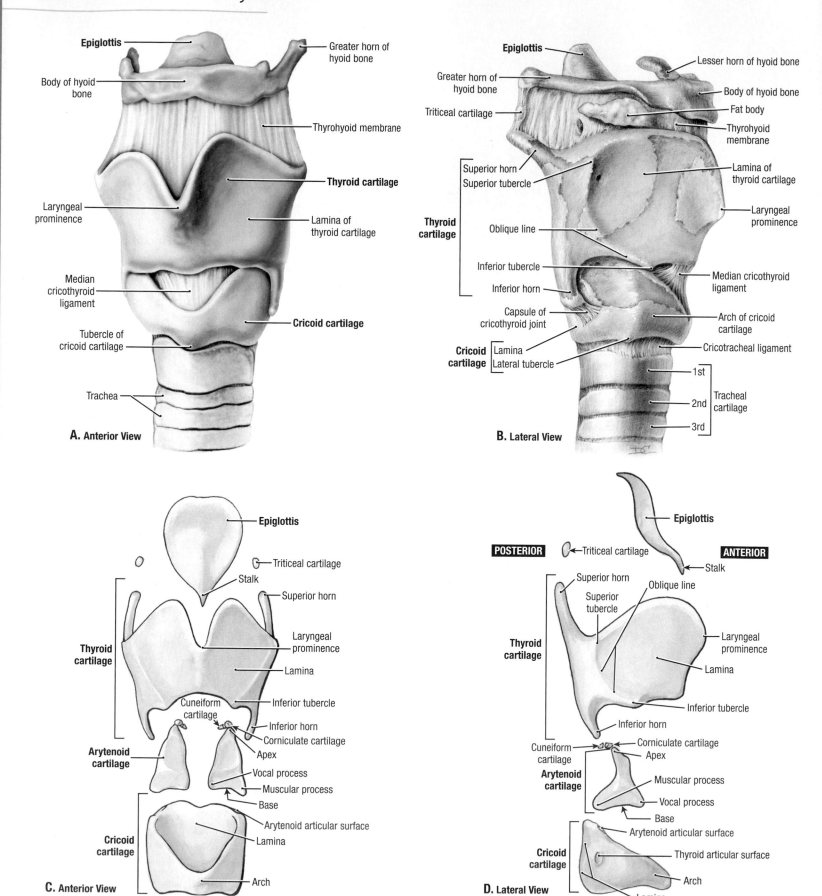

Epiglottis
Body of hyoid bone
Laryngeal prominence
Median cricothyroid ligament
Tubercle of cricoid cartilage
Trachea

Greater horn of hyoid bone
Thyrohyoid membrane
Thyroid cartilage
Lamina of thyroid cartilage
Cricoid cartilage

A. Anterior View

Epiglottis
Greater horn of hyoid bone
Triticeal cartilage
Thyroid cartilage
Superior horn
Superior tubercle
Oblique line
Inferior tubercle
Inferior horn
Capsule of cricothyroid joint
Cricoid cartilage Lamina
Lateral tubercle

Lesser horn of hyoid bone
Body of hyoid bone
Fat body
Thyrohyoid membrane
Lamina of thyroid cartilage
Laryngeal prominence
Median cricothyroid ligament
Arch of cricoid cartilage
Cricotracheal ligament
1st
2nd Tracheal cartilage
3rd

B. Lateral View

Epiglottis
Triticeal cartilage
Stalk
Superior horn
Thyroid cartilage
Laryngeal prominence
Lamina
Cuneiform cartilage
Inferior tubercle
Inferior horn
Corniculate cartilage
Apex
Arytenoid cartilage
Vocal process
Muscular process
Base
Arytenoid articular surface
Cricoid cartilage
Lamina
Arch

C. Anterior View

Epiglottis
POSTERIOR Triticeal cartilage ANTERIOR
Stalk
Superior horn
Oblique line
Superior tubercle
Thyroid cartilage
Laryngeal prominence
Lamina
Inferior tubercle
Inferior horn
Cuneiform cartilage
Corniculate cartilage
Apex
Arytenoid cartilage
Muscular process
Vocal process
Base
Arytenoid articular surface
Cricoid cartilage
Thyroid articular surface
Arch
Lamina

D. Lateral View

7.30 **Cartilages of Laryngeal Skeleton**

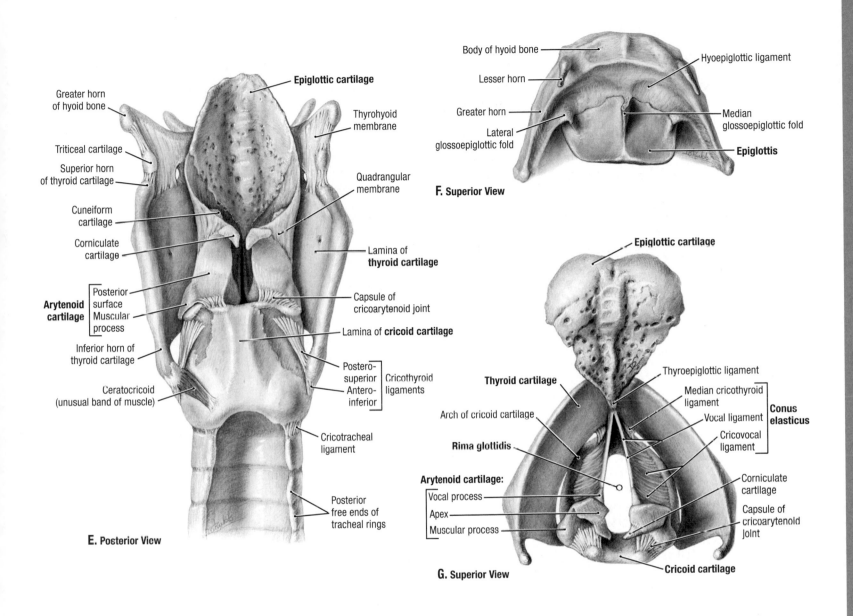

Epiglottic cartilage

Greater horn
of hyoid bone

Thyrohyoid
membrane

Triticeal cartilage

Superior horn
of thyroid cartilage

Cuneiform
cartilage

Corniculate
cartilage

Quadrangular
membrane

Lamina of
thyroid cartilage

**Arytenoid
cartilage**
Posterior
surface
Muscular
process

Inferior horn of
thyroid cartilage

Ceratocricoid
(unusual band of muscle)

Capsule of
cricoarytenoid joint

Lamina of **cricoid cartilage**

Postero-
superior
Antero-
inferior
Cricothyroid
ligaments

Cricotracheal
ligament

Posterior
free ends of
tracheal rings

E. Posterior View

Body of hyoid bone

Hyoepiglottic ligament

Lesser horn

Greater horn

Lateral
glossoepiglottic fold

Median
glossoepiglottic fold

Epiglottis

F. Superior View

Epiglottic cartilage

Thyroid cartilage

Thyroepiglottic ligament

Median cricothyroid
ligament

**Conus
elasticus**

Arch of cricoid cartilage

Vocal ligament

Cricovocal
ligament

Rima glottidis

Arytenoid cartilage:

Vocal process

Apex

Muscular process

Corniculate
cartilage

Capsule of
cricoarytenoid
joint

Cricoid cartilage

G. Superior View

Cartilages of Laryngeal Skeleton *(continued)*

7.30

A, **B**, and **E**. Articulated laryngeal skeleton. **C**. and **D**. Cartilages disarticulated and separated. **F.** Epiglottis and hyoepiglottic ligament. **G.** Conus elasticus and rima glottidis.

- The larynx extends vertically from the tip of the epiglottis to the inferior border of the cricoid cartilage. The hyoid bone is generally not regarded as part of the larynx.
- The cricoid cartilage is the only cartilage that totally encircles the airway.
- The rima glottidis is the aperture between the vocal folds. During normal respiration, it is narrow and wedge shaped; during forced respiration, it is wide. Variations in the tension and length

of the vocal folds, in the width of the rima glottidis, and in the intensity of the expiratory effort produce changes in the pitch of the voice.

- Laryngeal fractures may result from blows received in sports such as kickboxing and hockey or from compression by a shoulder strap during an automobile accident. Laryngeal fractures produce submucous hemorrhage and edema, respiratory obstruction, hoarseness, and sometimes a temporary inability to speak. The thyroid, cricoid, and most of the arytenoid cartilages often ossify as age advances, commencing at approximately 25 years of age in the thyroid cartilage.

Greater horn of hyoid bone

Thyrohyoid membrane

Epiglottis

Median raphe of pharynx

Thyropharyngeus

Inferior pharyngeal constrictor

Cricopharyngeus

Parathyroid glands — Superior / Inferior

Inferior laryngeal nerve, posterior branch

Esophagus

Submucous coat of esophagus

Internal branch ⎤ **Superior laryngeal nerve**
External branch ⎦ **(CN X)**

Sheath of thyroid gland

Right lobe of thyroid gland

Parathyroid glands

Inferior thyroid artery

Inferior laryngeal nerve, anterior branch

Right recurrent laryngeal nerve (CN X)

Paratracheal lymph nodes

Incision to open posterior wall of larynx and trachea (Fig. 7.33A)

A. Posterior View

| 7.31 | **External Larynx and Laryngeal Nerves** |

A. Posterior aspect.
- The internal branch of the superior laryngeal nerve innervates the mucous membrane superior to the vocal folds, and the external laryngeal branch supplies the inferior pharyngeal constrictor and cricothyroid muscles.
- The recurrent laryngeal nerve supplies the esophagus, trachea, and inferior pharyngeal constrictor muscle. It supplies sensory innervation inferior to the vocal folds and motor innervation to the intrinsic muscles of the larynx, except the cricothyroid.

B. Laryngocele. A laryngocele (enlarged laryngeal saccule) projects through the thyrohyoid membrane and communicates with the larynx through the ventricle. This air sac can form a bulge in the neck, especially on coughing. The inferior laryngeal nerves are vulnerable to injury during operations in the anterior triangles of the neck. **Injury of the recurrent laryngeal nerve** results in paralysis of the vocal fold. The voice is initially poor because the paralyzed fold cannot adduct to meet the normal vocal fold. In a bilateral paralysis, the voice is almost absent. **Injury to the external branch of the superior laryngeal nerve** results in a voice that is monotonous in character because the cricothyroid muscle is unable to vary the tension of the vocal fold. Hoarseness is the most common symptom of serious disorders of the larynx.

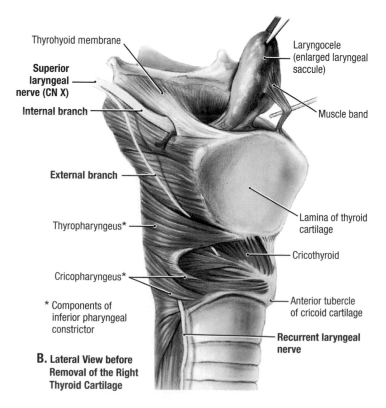

Thyrohyoid membrane

Superior laryngeal nerve (CN X)

Internal branch

External branch

Thyropharyngeus*

Cricopharyngeus*

* Components of inferior pharyngeal constrictor

Laryngocele (enlarged laryngeal saccule)

Muscle band

Lamina of thyroid cartilage

Cricothyroid

Anterior tubercle of cricoid cartilage

Recurrent laryngeal nerve

B. Lateral View before Removal of the Right Thyroid Cartilage

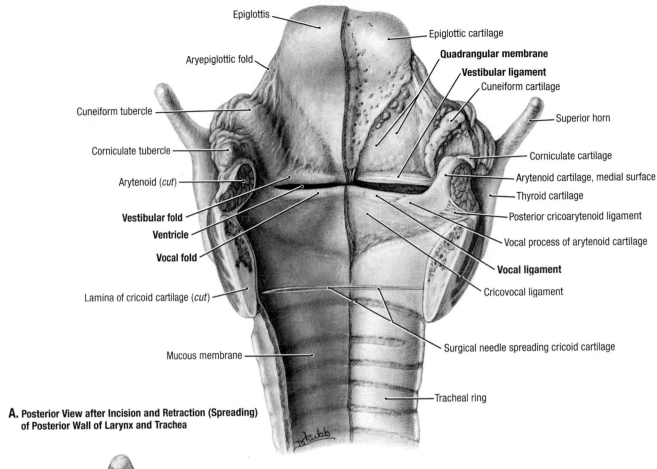

Epiglottis

Aryepiglottic fold

Cuneiform tubercle

Corniculate tubercle

Arytenoid (*cut*)

Vestibular fold

Ventricle

Vocal fold

Lamina of cricoid cartilage (*cut*)

Mucous membrane

Epiglottic cartilage

Quadrangular membrane

Vestibular ligament

Cuneiform cartilage

Superior horn

Corniculate cartilage

Arytenoid cartilage, medial surface

Thyroid cartilage

Posterior cricoarytenoid ligament

Vocal process of arytenoid cartilage

Vocal ligament

Cricovocal ligament

Surgical needle spreading cricoid cartilage

Tracheal ring

A. Posterior View after Incision and Retraction (Spreading) of Posterior Wall of Larynx and Trachea

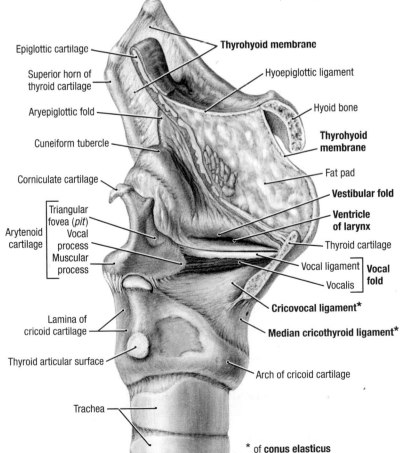

Epiglottic cartilage

Superior horn of thyroid cartilage

Aryepiglottic fold

Cuneiform tubercle

Corniculate cartilage

Arytenoid cartilage

Triangular fovea (*pit*)

Vocal process

Muscular process

Lamina of cricoid cartilage

Thyroid articular surface

Trachea

Thyrohyoid membrane

Hyoepiglottic ligament

Hyoid bone

Thyrohyoid membrane

Fat pad

Vestibular fold

Ventricle of larynx

Thyroid cartilage

Vocal ligament / Vocalis — **Vocal fold**

Cricovocal ligament*

Median cricothyroid ligament*

Arch of cricoid cartilage

* of **conus elasticus**

B. Lateral View after Removal of the Right Thyroid Cartilage

Internal Larynx   7.32

A. Dissection. The posterior wall of the larynx is split in the median plane (see Fig. 7.31A), and the two sides held apart. On the left side of the specimen, the mucous membrane is intact; on the right side, the mucous and submucous coats are peeled off revealing the cartilages, ligaments, and fibroelastic membrane. **B. Interior of larynx superior to vocal folds.** The larynx is sectioned near the median plane to reveal the interior of its left side. Inferior to this level, the right side of the intact larynx is dissected.

- The three compartments of the larynx are (1) the superior compartment of the vestibule, superior to the level of the vestibular folds (false cords); (2) the middle, between the levels of the vestibular and vocal folds; and (3) the inferior, or infraglottic, cavity, inferior to the level of the vocal folds.
- The quadrangular membrane underlies the aryepiglottic fold superiorly and is thickened inferiorly to form the vestibular ligament. The cricothyroid ligament (conus elasticus) begins inferiorly as the strong median cricothyroid ligament and is thickened superiorly as the vocal ligament. The lateral recess between the vocal and vestibular ligaments is the ventricle.

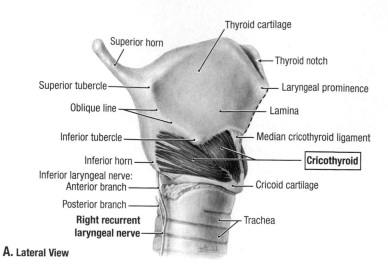

A. Lateral View

Thyroid cartilage
Superior horn
Superior tubercle
Oblique line
Inferior tubercle
Inferior horn
Inferior laryngeal nerve:
Anterior branch
Posterior branch
Right recurrent laryngeal nerve
Thyroid notch
Laryngeal prominence
Lamina
Median cricothyroid ligament
Cricothyroid
Cricoid cartilage
Trachea

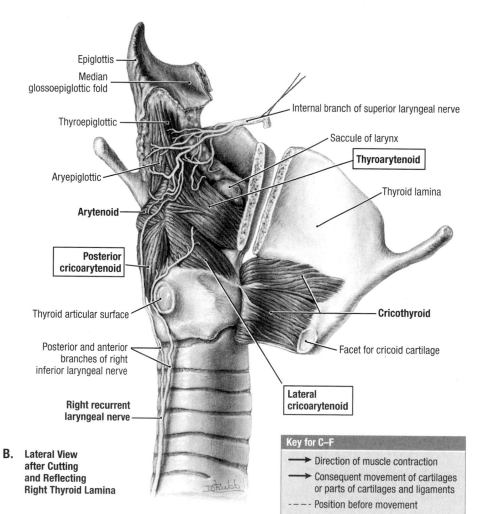

Epiglottis
Median glossoepiglottic fold
Thyroepiglottic
Aryepiglottic
Arytenoid
Posterior cricoarytenoid
Thyroid articular surface
Posterior and anterior branches of right inferior laryngeal nerve
Right recurrent laryngeal nerve
Internal branch of superior laryngeal nerve
Saccule of larynx
Thyroarytenoid
Thyroid lamina
Cricothyroid
Facet for cricoid cartilage
Lateral cricoarytenoid

B.   Lateral View after Cutting and Reflecting Right Thyroid Lamina

Key for C–F

→ Direction of muscle contraction
→ Consequent movement of cartilages or parts of cartilages and ligaments
- - - Position before movement

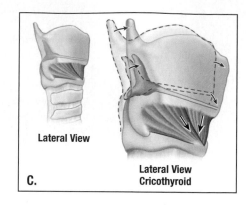

C.

Lateral View

Lateral View Cricothyroid

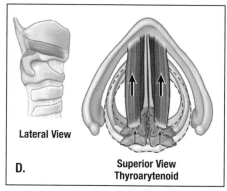

Lateral View

D.

Superior View Thyroarytenoid

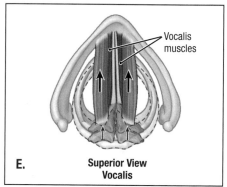

Vocalis muscles

Lateral View

E.

Superior View Vocalis

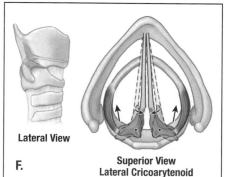

Lateral View

F.

Superior View Lateral Cricoarytenoid

7.33   **Muscles of Larynx**

A. Cricothyroid dissection. B. Laryngeal musculature deep to thyroid cartilage. The thyroid cartilage has been cut along *dashed line (Part A)* and the right thyroid lamina reflected anteriorly. **C.** Cricothyroid. **D.** Thyroarytenoid. **E.** Vocalis. **F.** Lateral cricoarytenoid.

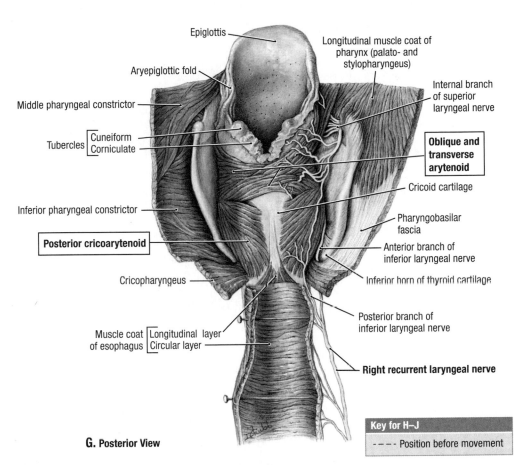

Epiglottis

Longitudinal muscle coat of pharynx (palato- and stylopharyngeus)

Aryepiglottic fold

Internal branch of superior laryngeal nerve

Middle pharyngeal constrictor

Tubercles { Cuneiform / Corniculate }

Oblique and transverse arytenoid

Cricoid cartilage

Inferior pharyngeal constrictor

Pharyngobasilar fascia

Posterior cricoarytenoid

Anterior branch of inferior laryngeal nerve

Cricopharyngeus

Inferior horn of thyroid cartilage

Muscle coat { Longitudinal layer / Circular layer } of esophagus

Posterior branch of inferior laryngeal nerve

Right recurrent laryngeal nerve

G. Posterior View

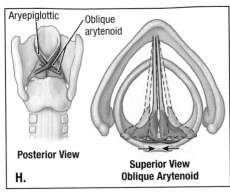

Aryepiglottic   Oblique arytenoid

Posterior View

Superior View Oblique Arytenoid

H.

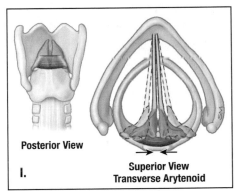

Posterior View

Superior View Transverse Arytenoid

I.

Key for H–J

– – – Position before movement

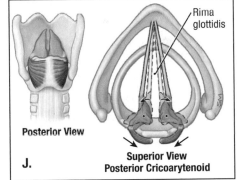

Rima glottidis

Posterior View

Superior View Posterior Cricoarytenoid

J.

Muscles of Larynx *(continued)*   7.33

G. Posterior view of muscles of larynx. **H.** Oblique arytenoid. **I.** Transverse arytenoid. **J.** Posterior cricoarytenoid.

   The intrinsic laryngeal muscles move the laryngeal cartilages, making alterations in the length and tension of the vocal folds and in the size and shape of the rima glottidis. All but one of the intrinsic muscles of the larynx are supplied by the inferior laryngeal nerves, terminal branches of the recurrent laryngeal nerve (CN X). The cricothyroid muscle (*Part A* and *Part B*) is supplied by the external laryngeal nerve, one of the two terminal branches of the superior laryngeal nerve.

TABLE 7.9	**Muscles of Larynx**			
Muscle	**Origin**	**Insertion**	**Innervation**	**Main Action(s)**
Cricothyroid	Anterolateral part of cricoid cartilage	Inferior margin and inferior horn of thyroid cartilage	External branch of superior laryngeal nerve (CN X)	Tenses vocal fold
Posterior cricoarytenoid	Posterior surface of laminae of cricoid cartilage	Muscular process of arytenoid cartilage	Inferior laryngeal nerves (terminal part of recurrent laryngeal nerve—CN X)	Abducts vocal fold
Lateral cricoarytenoid	Arch of cricoid cartilage			Adducts vocal fold
Thyroarytenoid[a]	Posterior surface of thyroid cartilage			Relaxes vocal fold
Transverse and oblique arytenoids[b]	One arytenoid cartilage	Opposite arytenoid cartilage		Close inlet of larynx by approximating arytenoid cartilages
Vocalis[c]	Angle between laminae of thyroid cartilage	Vocal ligament, between origin and vocal process of arytenoid cartilage		Alters vocal fold during phonation

[a]Superior fibers of the thyroarytenoid muscle pass into the aryepiglottic fold, and some of them reach the epiglottic cartilage. These fibers constitute the thyroepiglottic muscle, which widens the inlet of the larynx.
[b]Some fibers of the oblique arytenoid muscle continue as the aryepiglottic muscle.
[c]This slender muscular slip is derived from inferior deeper fibers of the thyroarytenoid muscle.

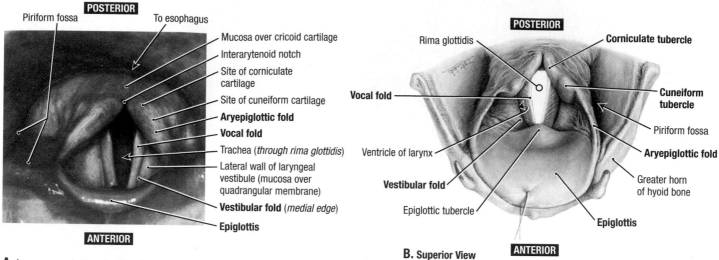

A. Laryngoscopic Examination, Superior View

B. Superior View

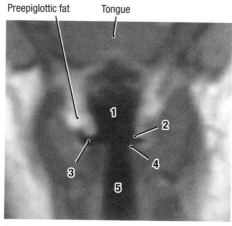

C. Coronal MRI

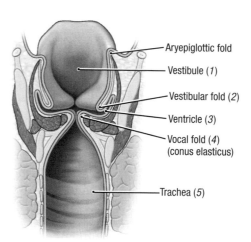

D. Coronal Section, Posterior View

7.34 | Laryngoscopic Examination and MRI of Larynx

A. Laryngoscopic examination. Laryngoscopy is the procedure used to examine the interior of the larynx. The larynx may be examined visually by indirect laryngoscopy using a laryngeal mirror or it may be viewed by direct laryngoscopy using a tubular and endoscopic instrument, a laryngoscope. The vestibular and vocal folds can be observed. **B. Vocal folds and rima glottidis.** The inlet, or aditus, to the larynx is bounded anteriorly by the epiglottis; posteriorly by the arytenoid cartilages, the corniculate cartilages that cap them, and the interarytenoid fold that unites them; and on each side by the aryepiglottic fold, which contains the superior end of the cuneiform cartilage. The vocal apparatus of the larynx, the glottis, includes the vocal folds, vocal processes of the arytenoid cartilages, and the rima glottidis, the aperture between the vocal folds. **C. Coronal MRI. D. Coronal section.** Numbers in parentheses on diagram refer to numbered structures on MRI.

A **foreign body** such as a piece of steak may accidentally aspirate through the laryngeal inlet into the vestibule of the larynx, where it becomes trapped superior to the vestibular folds. When a foreign body enters the vestibule, the laryngeal muscles go into spasm, tensing the vocal folds. The rima glottidis closes and no air enters the trachea. **Asphyxiation** occurs, and the person will die in approximately 5 minutes from lack of oxygen if the obstruction is not removed. Emergency therapy must be given to open the airway. The procedure used depends on the condition of the patient, the facilities available, and the experience of the person giving first aid. Because the lungs still contain air, sudden compression of the abdomen (**Heimlich maneuver**) causes the diaphragm to elevate and compress the lungs, expelling air from the trachea into the larynx. This maneuver may dislodge the food or other material from the larynx.

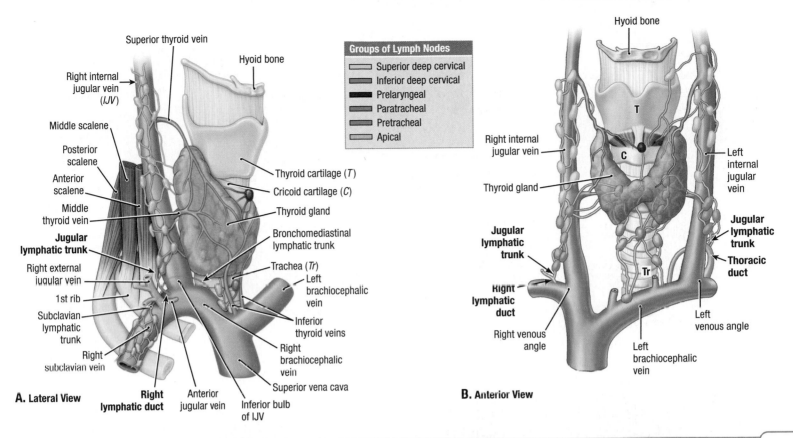

Groups of Lymph Nodes

- Superior deep cervical
- Inferior deep cervical
- Prelaryngeal
- Paratracheal
- Pretracheal
- Apical

A. Lateral View

B. Anterior View

| Lymphatic Drainage of Thyroid Gland, Larynx, and Trachea | 7.35 |

Radical neck dissections are performed when cancer invades the lymphatics. During the procedure, the deep cervical lymph nodes and the tissues around them are removed as completely as possible. Although major arteries, the brachial plexus, CN X, and the phrenic nerve are preserved, most cutaneous branches of the cervical plexus are removed. The aim of the dissection is to remove all tissue that contains lymph nodes in one piece.

Lateral View

| Sympathetic Trunk and Sympathetic Periarterial Plexus | 7.36 |

A **lesion of a sympathetic trunk** in the neck results in a sympathetic disturbance called **Horner syndrome**, which is characterized by the following:

- **Pupillary constriction** resulting from paralysis of the dilator pupillae muscle.
- **Ptosis** (drooping of the superior eyelid), resulting from paralysis of the smooth (tarsal) muscle intermingled with striated muscle of the levator palpebrae superioris.
- Sinking in of the eyeball (**enophthalmos**), possibly caused by paralysis of smooth (orbitalis) muscle in the floor of the orbit.
- Vasodilation and absence of sweating on the face and neck (**anhydrosis**), caused by a lack of sympathetic (vasoconstrictive) nerve supply to the blood vessels and sweat glands.

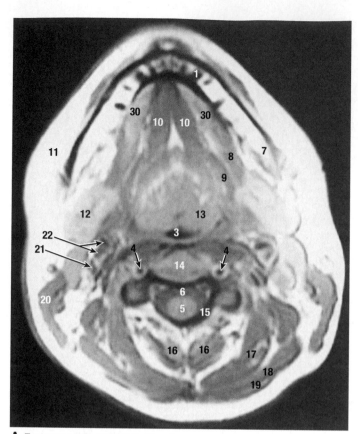

A. Transverse MRI, C3 Vertebral Level

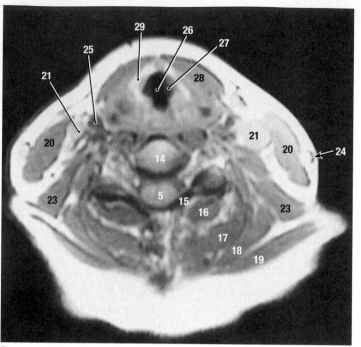

B. Transverse MRI, Upper C6 Vertebral Level

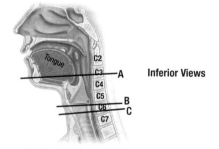

Median Section   **Inferior Views**

1	Tooth	16	Semispinalis cervicis
2	Cricoid cartilage	17	Semispinalis capitis
3	Pharynx	18	Splenius capitis
4	Vertebral artery	19	Trapezius
5	Spinal cord	20	Sternocleidomastoid
6	Cerebrospinal fluid in subarachnoid space	21	Internal jugular vein
		22	Bifurcation of common carotid artery
7	Body of mandible	23	Levator scapulae
8	Mylohyoid	24	External jugular vein
9	Hyoglossus	25	Common carotid artery
10	Genioglossus	26	Rima glottidis
11	Buccal fat pad	27	Vocal fold
12	Submandibular gland	28	Strap muscles
13	Intrinsic muscles of tongue	29	Thyroid cartilage
14	Vertebral body	30	Sublingual gland
15	Lamina of vertebra	31	Inferior pharyngeal constrictor

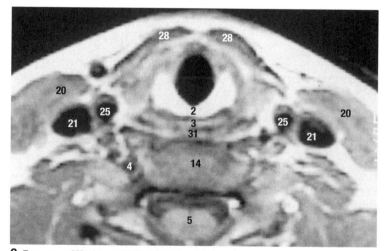

C. Transverse MRI, Lower C6 Vertebral Level

7.37   Transverse MRIs of Neck

The orientation figure indicates the vertebral level of the MRI sections.

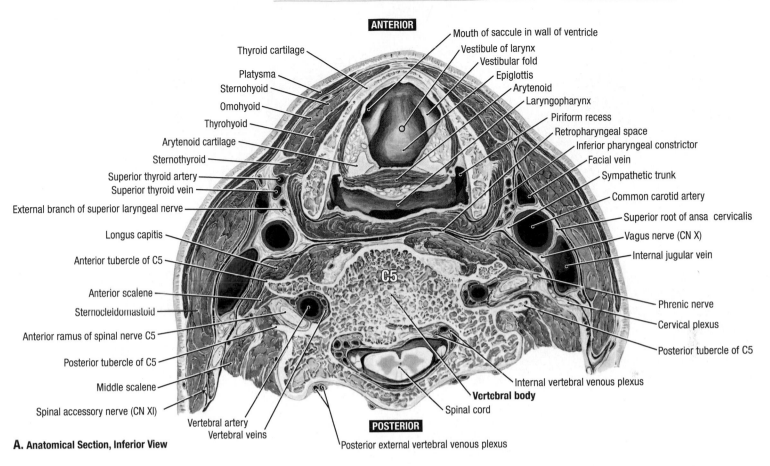

ANTERIOR

Thyroid cartilage
Platysma
Sternohyoid
Omohyoid
Thyrohyoid
Arytenoid cartilage
Sternothyroid
Superior thyroid artery
Superior thyroid vein
External branch of superior laryngeal nerve
Longus capitis
Anterior tubercle of C5
Anterior scalene
Sternocleidomastoid
Anterior ramus of spinal nerve C5
Posterior tubercle of C5
Middle scalene
Spinal accessory nerve (CN XI)

Mouth of saccule in wall of ventricle
Vestibule of larynx
Vestibular fold
Epiglottis
Arytenoid
Laryngopharynx
Piriform recess
Retropharyngeal space
Inferior pharyngeal constrictor
Facial vein
Sympathetic trunk
Common carotid artery
Superior root of ansa cervicalis
Vagus nerve (CN X)
Internal jugular vein
Phrenic nerve
Cervical plexus
Posterior tubercle of C5
Internal vertebral venous plexus
Vertebral body
Spinal cord

C5

Vertebral artery
Vertebral veins
Posterior external vertebral venous plexus

POSTERIOR

A. Anatomical Section, Inferior View

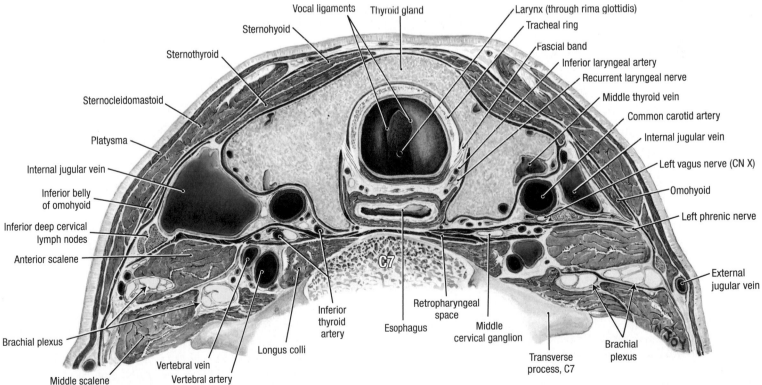

Vocal ligaments
Thyroid gland
Sternohyoid
Sternothyroid
Sternocleidomastoid
Platysma
Internal jugular vein
Inferior belly of omohyoid
Inferior deep cervical lymph nodes
Anterior scalene
Brachial plexus
Middle scalene
Vertebral vein
Vertebral artery
Longus colli
Inferior thyroid artery
Esophagus

Larynx (through rima glottidis)
Tracheal ring
Fascial band
Inferior laryngeal artery
Recurrent laryngeal nerve
Middle thyroid vein
Common carotid artery
Internal jugular vein
Left vagus nerve (CN X)
Omohyoid
Left phrenic nerve
External jugular vein
Brachial plexus
Transverse process, C7
Middle cervical ganglion
Retropharyngeal space

C7

B. Anatomical Section, Inferior View

Transverse Anatomical Sections of Neck

7.38

A. At level of laryngopharynx. **B.** At level of trachea.

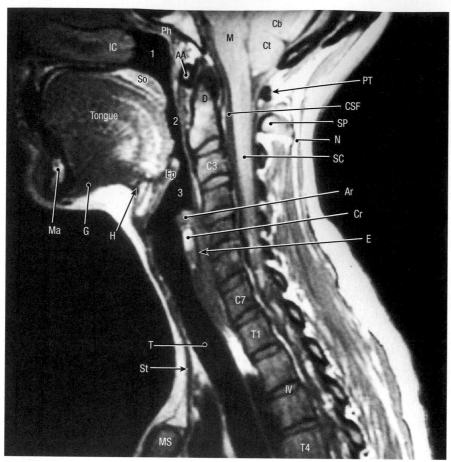

A. Median MRI

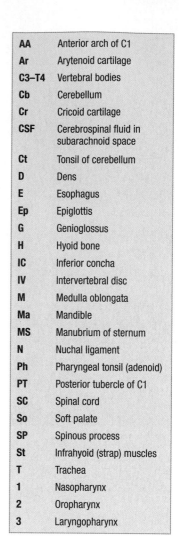

AA	Anterior arch of C1
Ar	Arytenoid cartilage
C3–T4	Vertebral bodies
Cb	Cerebellum
Cr	Cricoid cartilage
CSF	Cerebrospinal fluid in subarachnoid space
Ct	Tonsil of cerebellum
D	Dens
E	Esophagus
Ep	Epiglottis
G	Genioglossus
H	Hyoid bone
IC	Inferior concha
IV	Intervertebral disc
M	Medulla oblongata
Ma	Mandible
MS	Manubrium of sternum
N	Nuchal ligament
Ph	Pharyngeal tonsil (adenoid)
PT	Posterior tubercle of C1
SC	Spinal cord
So	Soft palate
SP	Spinous process
St	Infrahyoid (strap) muscles
T	Trachea
1	Nasopharynx
2	Oropharynx
3	Laryngopharynx

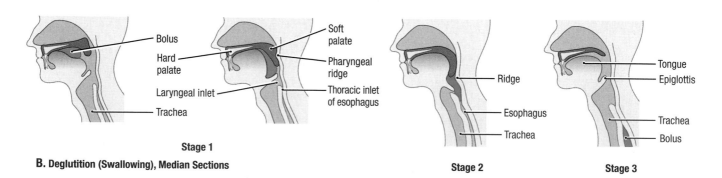

B. Deglutition (Swallowing), Median Sections

Stage 1   **Stage 2**   **Stage 3**

7.39   **Relationship and Function of Air and Food Passages in Breathing and Swallowing**

A. Study revealing normal relationships of structures in median plane during breathing. B. Swallowing. There are three main stages of swallowing:
- Stage 1: Voluntary; the bolus is compressed against the palate and pushed from the mouth into the oropharynx, mainly by coordinated movements of the muscles of the tongue and soft palate.
- Stage 2: Involuntary and rapid; the soft palate is elevated, sealing off the nasopharynx from the oropharynx and laryngopharynx.

The pharynx widens and shortens to receive the bolus of food as the suprahyoid and longitudinal pharyngeal muscles contract, elevating the larynx.
- Stage 3: Involuntary; sequential contraction of all three pharyngeal constrictor muscles forces the food bolus inferiorly into the esophagus.

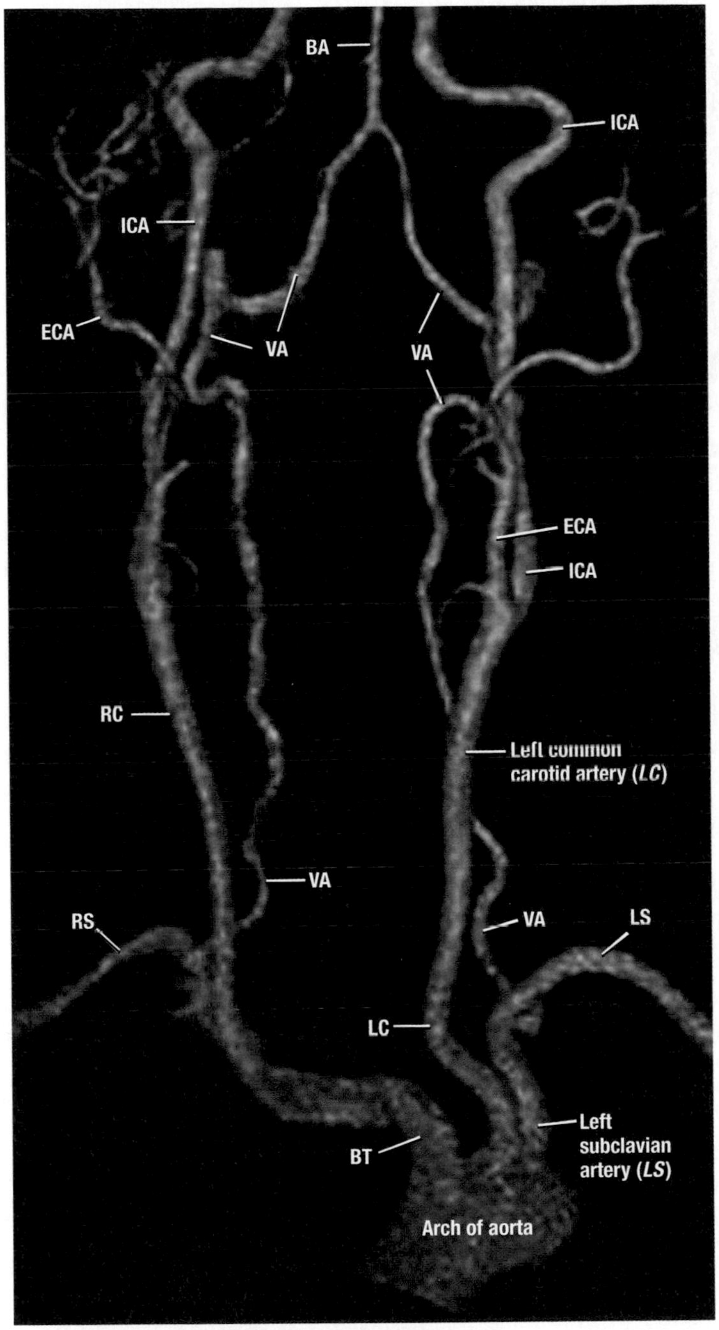
BA
ICA
ICA
ECA
VA
VA
ECA
ICA
RC
Left common carotid artery (LC)
VA
RS
VA
LS
LC
BT
Left subclavian artery (LS)
Arch of aorta

A. Reconstructed CT Angiogram, Anterior View

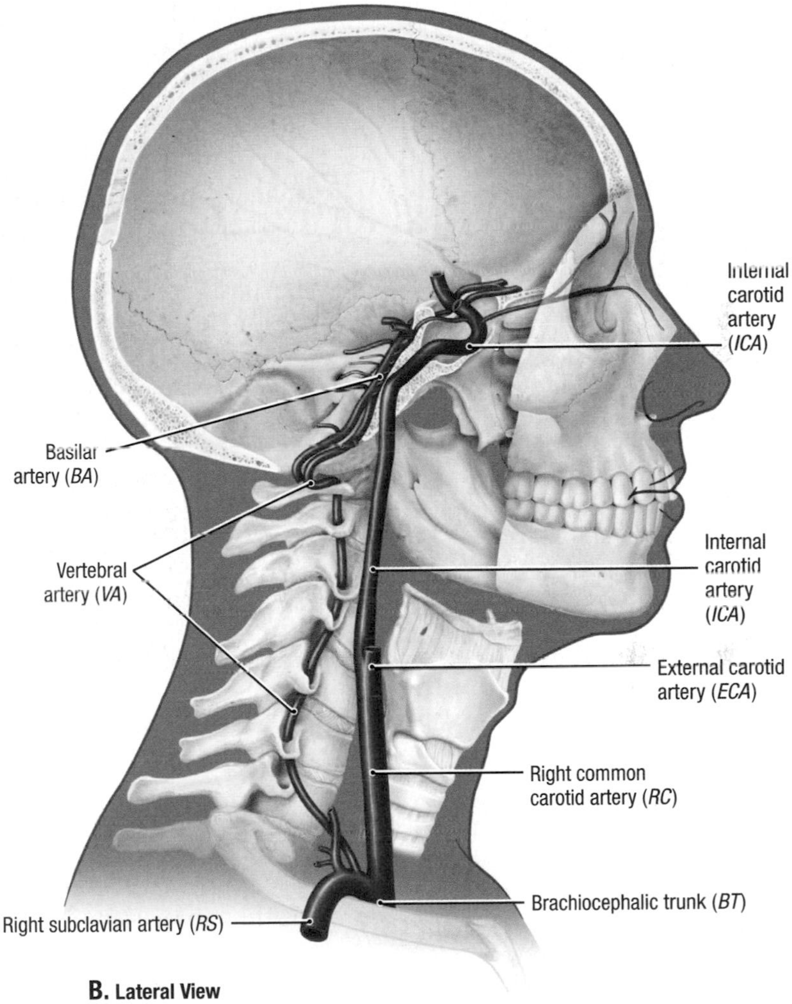
Internal carotid artery (ICA)
Basilar artery (BA)
Vertebral artery (VA)
Internal carotid artery (ICA)
External carotid artery (ECA)
Right common carotid artery (RC)
Right subclavian artery (RS)
Brachiocephalic trunk (BT)

B. Lateral View

Imaging of Blood Supply of Head and Neck

7.40

A. Arteries of neck and cranial base. Letters refer to labels in *Part B*. **B. Schematic of arteries in relation to skeletal structures.** Posterior cranium has been resected to midline.

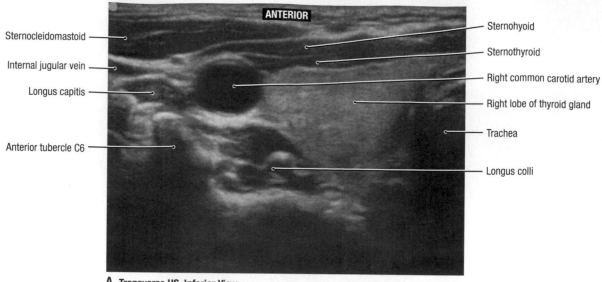

ANTERIOR

Sternocleidomastoid

Internal jugular vein

Longus capitis

Anterior tubercle C6

Sternohyoid

Sternothyroid

Right common carotid artery

Right lobe of thyroid gland

Trachea

Longus colli

A. Transverse US, Inferior View

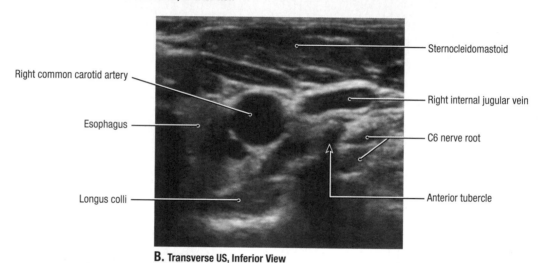

Right common carotid artery

Esophagus

Longus colli

Sternocleidomastoid

Right internal jugular vein

C6 nerve root

Anterior tubercle

B. Transverse US, Inferior View

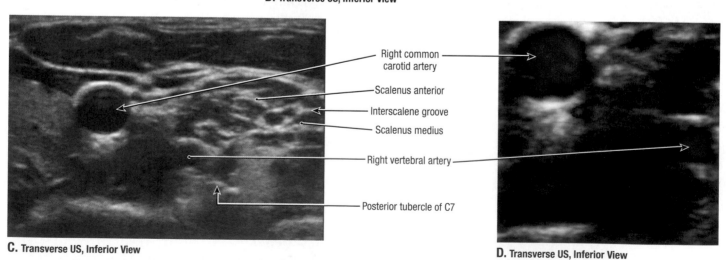

Right common carotid artery

Scalenus anterior

Interscalene groove

Scalenus medius

Right vertebral artery

Posterior tubercle of C7

C. Transverse US, Inferior View

D. Transverse US, Inferior View

| 7.41 | **Ultrasound Imaging of Head and Neck** |

Ultrasonography is a useful diagnostic imaging technique for studying soft tissues of the neck. Ultrasound (US) provides images of many abnormal conditions noninvasively, at relatively low cost, and with minimal discomfort. US is useful for distinguishing solid from cystic masses, for example, which may be difficult to determine during physical examination. Vascular imaging of arteries and veins of the neck is possible using intravascular US. The images are produced by placing the transducer over the blood vessel. Doppler US techniques help evaluate blood flow through a vessel (e.g., for detecting stenosis [narrowing] of a carotid artery).

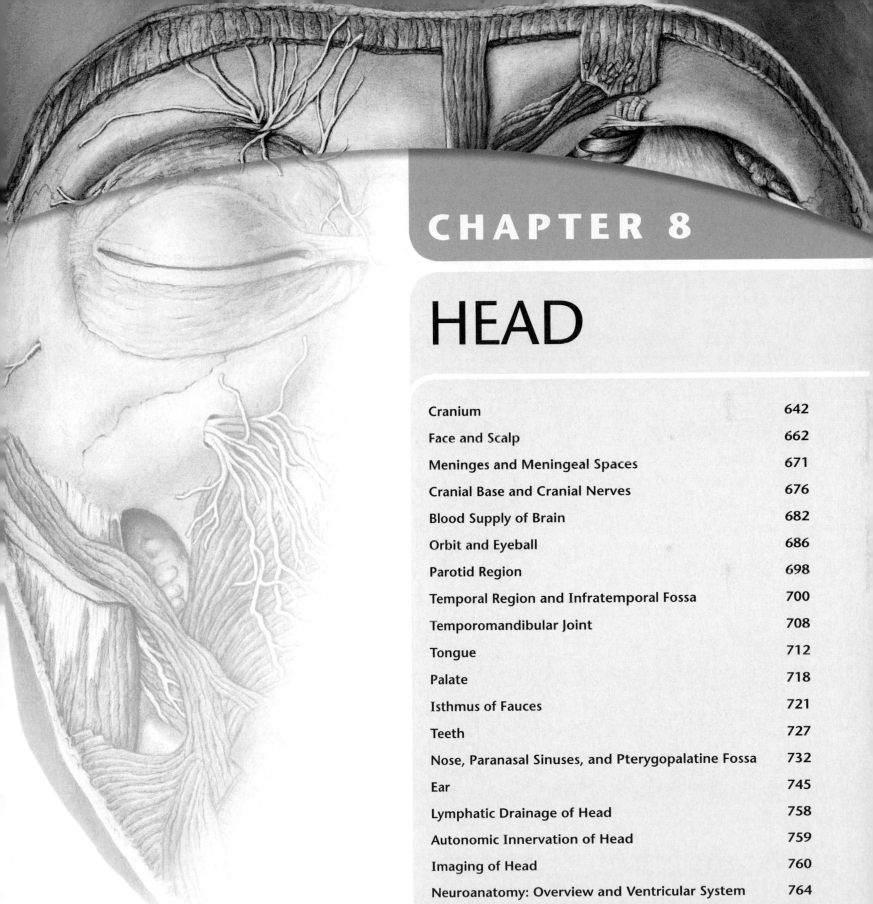

CHAPTER 8

HEAD

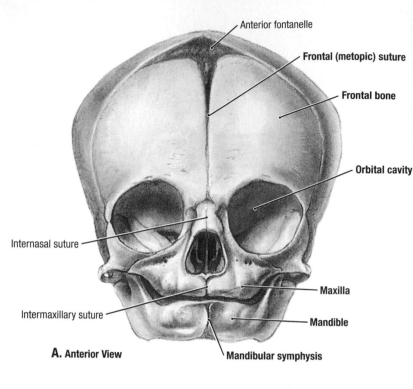

Anterior fontanelle

Frontal (metopic) suture

Frontal bone

Orbital cavity

Internasal suture

Intermaxillary suture

Maxilla

Mandible

A. Anterior View

Mandibular symphysis

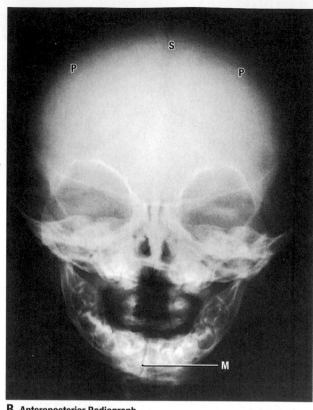

S

P   P

M

B. Anteroposterior Radiograph

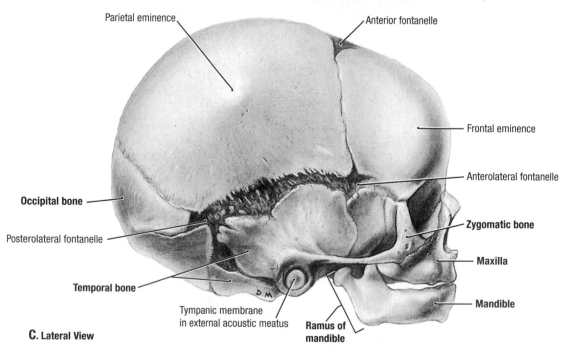

Parietal eminence

Anterior fontanelle

Frontal eminence

Anterolateral fontanelle

Occipital bone

Zygomatic bone

Posterolateral fontanelle

Maxilla

Temporal bone

Mandible

Tympanic membrane
in external acoustic meatus

Ramus of
mandible

C. Lateral View

8.1   Cranium at Birth and in Early Childhood

A. Cranium at birth, anterior aspect. **B.** Radiograph of 6½-month-old child. **C.** Cranium at birth, lateral aspect.
   Compared with the adult skull (see Figs. 8.2, 8.3, & 8.4):
- The maxilla and mandible are proportionately small.
- The mandibular symphysis, which closes during the second year, and the frontal suture, which closes during the sixth year, are still open (unfused).

- The orbital cavities are proportionately large, but the face is small; the facial skeleton forming only one eighth of the whole cranium, while in the adult, it forms one third.
- The increase in size is largely due to the development of primary and secondary dentition. The lateral view of *Part C* makes it appear that the tympanic membrane is vertical, but it is actually obliquely disposed in the neonate, closer to horizontal than vertical, requiring downward traction on the external ear to examine with an otoscope.

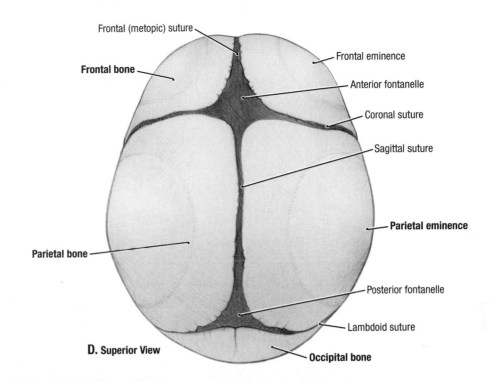

Frontal (metopic) suture

Frontal eminence

Frontal bone

Anterior fontanelle

Coronal suture

Sagittal suture

Parietal eminence

Parietal bone

Posterior fontanelle

Lambdoid suture

D. Superior View

Occipital bone

Key for B, E, and F	
A	Angles of mandible
B	Body of mandible
C	Coronal suture
F	Frontal bone
L	Lambdoid suture
M	Mandibular symphysis
O	Occipital bone
P	Parietal eminence
S	Sagittal suture
SP	Sphenoid
T	Temporal bone
X	Maxilla
Y	Mastoid process
Z	Zygomatic bone
➤	Outline of cartilaginous portion of developing parietal bone.

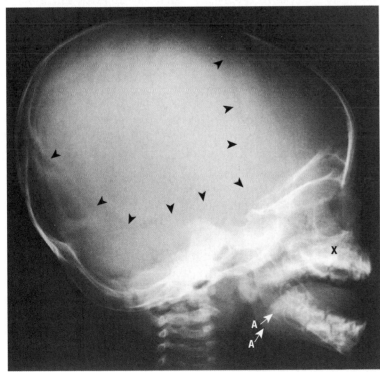

E. Lateral Radiograph

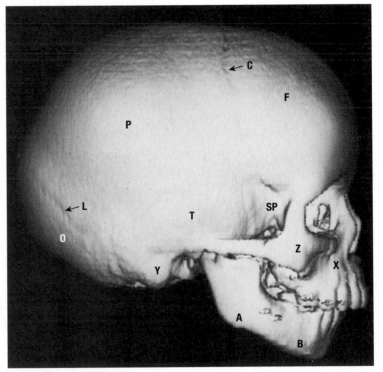

F. Lateral Reconstructed CT

Cranium at Birth and in Early Childhood *(continued)*

8.1

D. Cranium at birth, superior aspect. **E.** Radiograph of 6½-month-old child. **F.** Three-dimensional computer-generated image of 3-year-old child's cranium.

• The parietal eminence is a shallow, rounded cone. Ossification, which starts at the eminences, has not yet reached the ultimate

four angles of the parietal bone; accordingly, these regions are membranous, and the membrane is blended with the pericranium externally and the dura mater internally to form the fontanelles. The fontanelles are usually closed by the second year. There is no mastoid process until the second year.

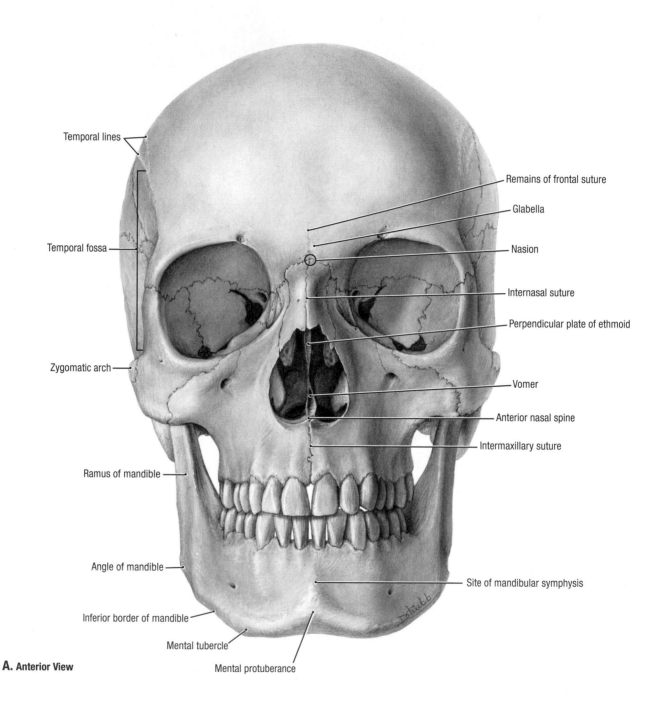

Temporal lines

Temporal fossa

Zygomatic arch

Ramus of mandible

Angle of mandible

Inferior border of mandible

Mental tubercle

Remains of frontal suture

Glabella

Nasion

Internasal suture

Perpendicular plate of ethmoid

Vomer

Anterior nasal spine

Intermaxillary suture

Site of mandibular symphysis

A. Anterior View

Mental protuberance

8.2 **Cranium, Facial (Front) Aspect**

A. Formations of bony cranium. B. Bones of cranium and their features. The individual bones forming the cranium are color coded. (For orbital cavity, see Fig. 8.36A.)

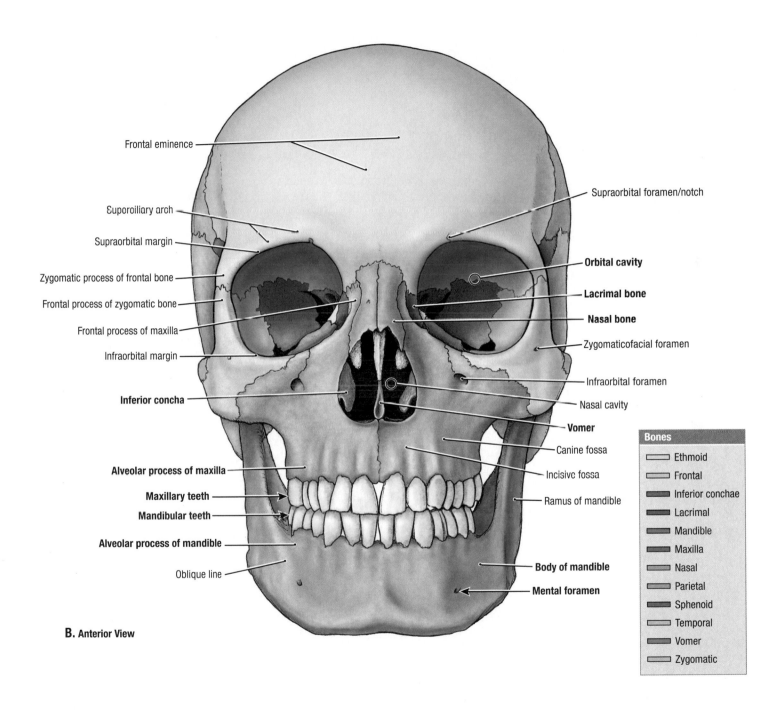

Frontal eminence

Superciliary arch

Supraorbital margin

Zygomatic process of frontal bone

Frontal process of zygomatic bone

Frontal process of maxilla

Infraorbital margin

Inferior concha

Alveolar process of maxilla

Maxillary teeth

Mandibular teeth

Alveolar process of mandible

Oblique line

Supraorbital foramen/notch

Orbital cavity

Lacrimal bone

Nasal bone

Zygomaticofacial foramen

Infraorbital foramen

Nasal cavity

Vomer

Canine fossa

Incisive fossa

Ramus of mandible

Body of mandible

Mental foramen

B. Anterior View

Bones

▭	Ethmoid
▭	Frontal
▭	Inferior conchae
▭	Lacrimal
▭	Mandible
▭	Maxilla
▭	Nasal
▭	Parietal
▭	Sphenoid
▭	Temporal
▭	Vomer
▭	Zygomatic

Cranium, Facial (Front) Aspect *(continued)*   **8.2**

Extraction of teeth causes the alveolar bone to resorb in the affected region(s). Following complete loss or extraction of teeth, the sockets begin to fill in with bone, and the alveolar processes begin to resorb.

The mental foramen may eventually lie near the superior border of the body of the mandible. In some cases, mental foramina resorption may extend to the mental nerves, exposing them to injury.

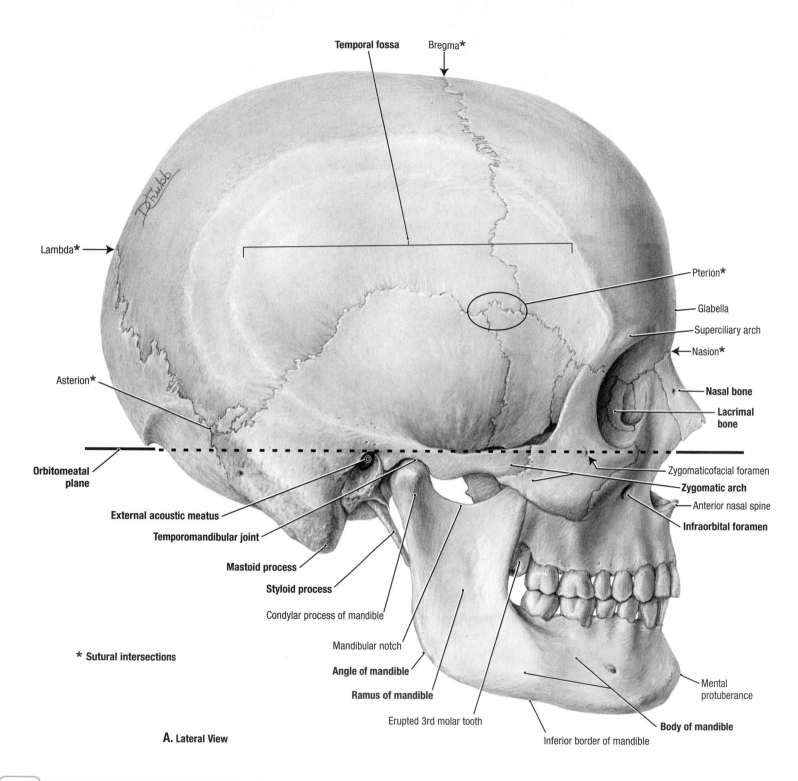

Temporal fossa   Bregma*

Lambda*

Pterion*

Glabella

Superciliary arch

Nasion*

Nasal bone

Lacrimal bone

Asterion*

Orbitomeatal plane

Zygomaticofacial foramen

Zygomatic arch

Anterior nasal spine

Infraorbital foramen

External acoustic meatus

Temporomandibular joint

Mastoid process

Styloid process

Condylar process of mandible

Mandibular notch

Angle of mandible

Ramus of mandible

Erupted 3rd molar tooth

Mental protuberance

Body of mandible

Inferior border of mandible

* Sutural intersections

A. Lateral View

| 8.3 | **Cranium, Lateral Aspect** |

A. Bony cranium. B. Cranium with bones color coded. The cranium is in the anatomical position when the orbitomeatal plane is horizontal. **C. Buttresses of cranium.** The buttresses are thicker portions of cranial bones that transfer forces around the weaker regions of the orbits and nasal cavity.

The convexity of the neurocranium (braincase) distributes and thereby minimizes the effects of a blow to it. However, hard blows to the head in thin areas of the cranium (e.g., in the temporal fossa) are likely to produce **depressed fractures**, in which a fragment of bone is depressed inward, compressing and/or injuring the brain. In **comminuted fractures**, the bone is broken into several pieces. **Linear fractures**, the most frequent type, usually occur at the point of impact, but fracture lines often radiate away from it in two or more directions.

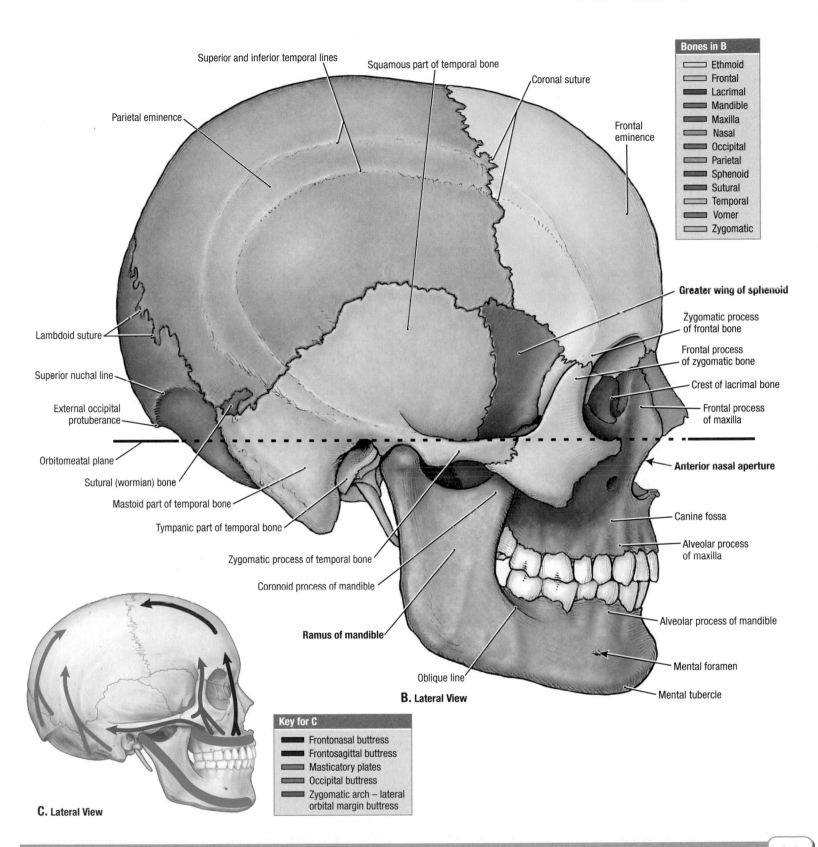

Superior and inferior temporal lines

Squamous part of temporal bone

Coronal suture

Parietal eminence

Frontal eminence

Bones in B

- Ethmoid
- Frontal
- Lacrimal
- Mandible
- Maxilla
- Nasal
- Occipital
- Parietal
- Sphenoid
- Sutural
- Temporal
- Vomer
- Zygomatic

Lambdoid suture

Superior nuchal line

External occipital protuberance

Orbitomeatal plane

Sutural (wormian) bone

Mastoid part of temporal bone

Tympanic part of temporal bone

Zygomatic process of temporal bone

Coronoid process of mandible

Ramus of mandible

Oblique line

Greater wing of sphenoid

Zygomatic process of frontal bone

Frontal process of zygomatic bone

Crest of lacrimal bone

Frontal process of maxilla

Anterior nasal aperture

Canine fossa

Alveolar process of maxilla

Alveolar process of mandible

Mental foramen

Mental tubercle

B. Lateral View

Key for C

- Frontonasal buttress
- Frontosagittal buttress
- Masticatory plates
- Occipital buttress
- Zygomatic arch – lateral orbital margin buttress

C. Lateral View

Cranium, Lateral Aspect *(continued)*

8.3

If the area of the neurocranium is thick at the site of impact, the bone usually bends inward without fracturing; however, a fracture may occur some distance from the site of direct trauma where the calvaria is thinner. In a **contrecoup (counterblow) fracture**, the fracture occurs on the opposite side of the cranium rather than at the point of impact. One or more sutural (accessory) bones may be located along the lambdoid suture or near the mastoid process.

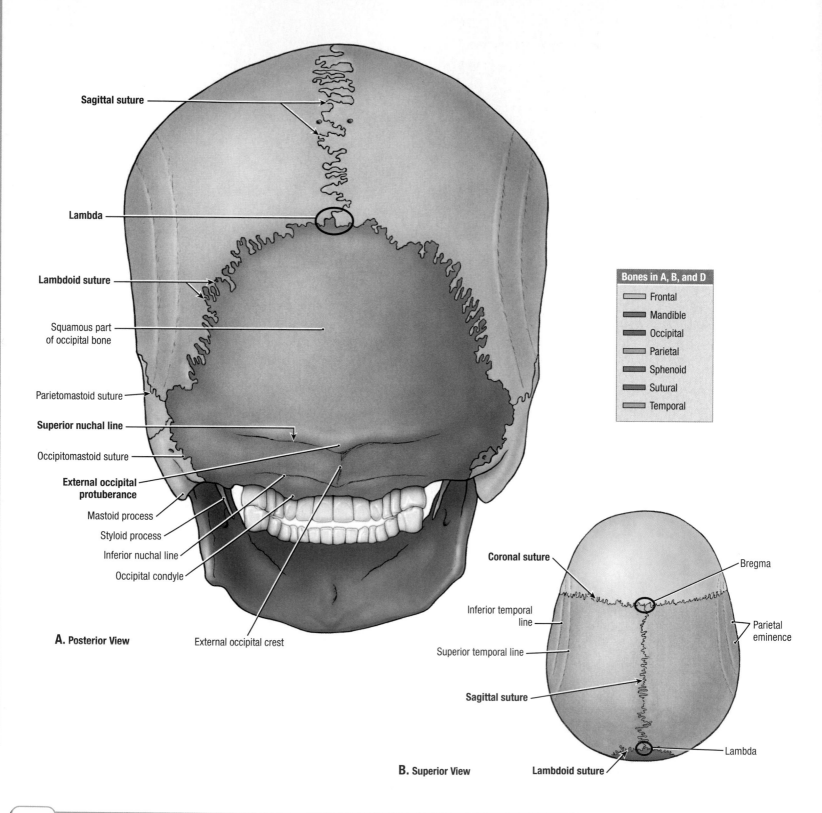

Sagittal suture

Lambda

Lambdoid suture

Squamous part
of occipital bone

Parietomastoid suture

Superior nuchal line

Occipitomastoid suture

**External occipital
protuberance**

Mastoid process

Styloid process

Inferior nuchal line

Occipital condyle

A. Posterior View

External occipital crest

Bones in A, B, and D

- Frontal
- Mandible
- Occipital
- Parietal
- Sphenoid
- Sutural
- Temporal

Coronal suture

Bregma

Inferior temporal
line

Parietal
eminence

Superior temporal line

Sagittal suture

Lambda

B. Superior View

Lambdoid suture

| **8.4** | **Cranium, Occipital Aspect, Calvaria, and Anterior Part of Posterior Cranial Fossa** |

A. Cranium, posterior aspect. The lambda, near the center of this convex surface, is located at the junction of the sagittal and lambdoid sutures. **B. Cranium, superior aspect.** The roof of the neurocranium, or calvaria (skullcap), is formed primarily by the paired parietal bones, the frontal bone, and the occipital bone.

Premature closure of the coronal suture results in a high, towerlike cranium, called **oxycephaly** or **turricephaly**. Premature closure of sutures usually does not affect brain development. When premature closure occurs on one side only, the cranium is asymmetrical, a condition known as **plagiocephaly**.

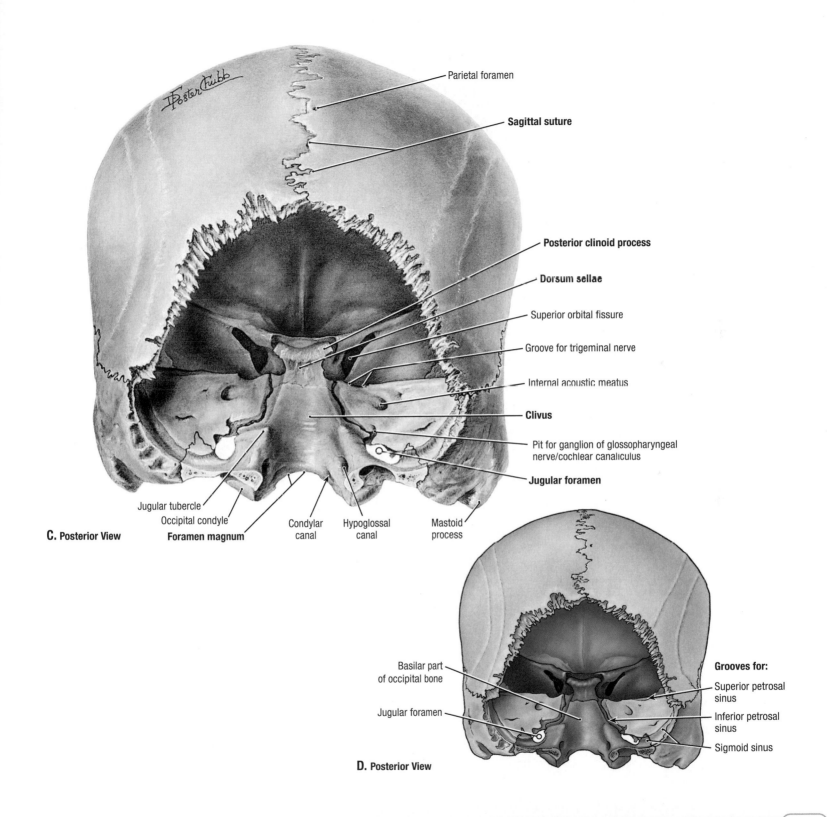

Parietal foramen

Sagittal suture

Posterior clinoid process

Dorsum sellae

Superior orbital fissure

Groove for trigeminal nerve

Internal acoustic meatus

Clivus

Pit for ganglion of glossopharyngeal nerve/cochlear canaliculus

Jugular foramen

Jugular tubercle
Occipital condyle
Foramen magnum
Condylar canal
Hypoglossal canal
Mastoid process

C. Posterior View

Basilar part of occipital bone

Jugular foramen

Grooves for:

Superior petrosal sinus

Inferior petrosal sinus

Sigmoid sinus

D. Posterior View

Cranium, Occipital Aspect, Calvaria, and Anterior Part of Posterior Cranial Fossa *(continued)*   **8.4**

C. and **D.** Cranium after removal of squamous part of occipital bone.
- The dorsum sellae projects from the body of the sphenoid; the posterior clinoid processes form its superolateral corners.
- The clivus is the slope descending from the dorsum sellae to the foramen magnum.

- The grooves for the sigmoid sinus and inferior petrosal sinus lead inferiorly to the jugular foramen.

Premature closure of the sagittal suture, in which the anterior fontanelle is small or absent, results in a long, narrow, wedge-shaped cranium, a condition called **scaphocephaly.**

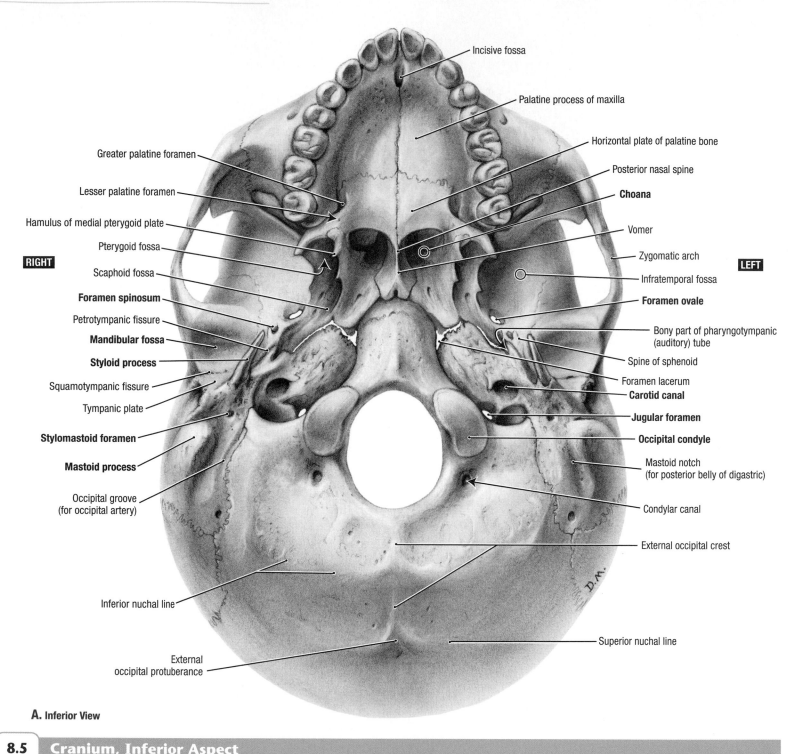

A. Inferior View

8.5   Cranium, Inferior Aspect

A. Bony cranium. **B.** Diagram of cranium with bones color coded.

TABLE 8.1	Foramina and Other Apertures of Neurocranium and Contents
Foramen cecum: Nasal emissary vein (1% of population)	**Optic canals:** Optic nerve (CN II) and ophthalmic arteries
Cribriform plate: Olfactory nerves (CN I)	**Superior orbital fissure:** Ophthalmic veins; ophthalmic nerve (CN V_1); CN III, IV, and VI; and sympathetic fibers
Anterior and posterior ethmoidal foramina: Vessels and nerves with same names	**Foramen rotundum:** Maxillary nerve (CN V_2)
Foramen ovale: Mandibular nerve (CN V_3) and accessory meningeal artery	**Jugular foramen:** CN IX, X, and XI; superior bulb of internal jugular vein; inferior petrosal and sigmoid sinuses; meningeal branches of ascending pharyngeal and occipital arteries

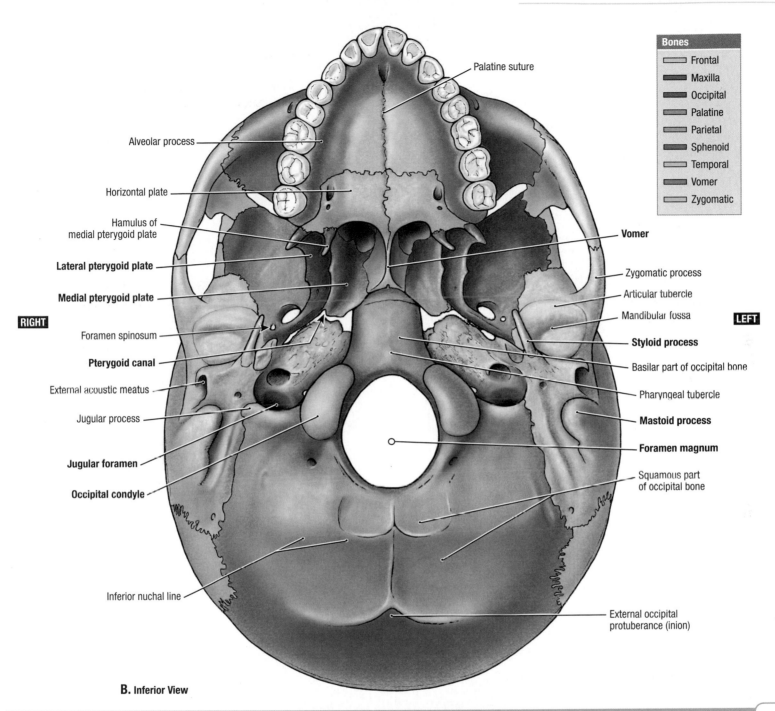

Bones
- Frontal
- Maxilla
- Occipital
- Palatine
- Parietal
- Sphenoid
- Temporal
- Vomer
- Zygomatic

Palatine suture

Alveolar process

Horizontal plate

Hamulus of medial pterygoid plate

Lateral pterygoid plate

Medial pterygoid plate

RIGHT

Foramen spinosum

Pterygoid canal

External acoustic meatus

Jugular process

Jugular foramen

Occipital condyle

Inferior nuchal line

Vomer

Zygomatic process

Articular tubercle

Mandibular fossa

Styloid process

Basilar part of occipital bone

Pharyngeal tubercle

Mastoid process

Foramen magnum

Squamous part of occipital bone

LEFT

External occipital protuberance (inion)

B. Inferior View

Cranium, Inferior Aspect (continued)

8.5

TABLE 8.1   Foramina and Other Apertures of Neurocranium and Contents (continued)

Foramen spinosum: Middle meningeal artery/vein and meningeal branch of CN V₃	**Hypoglossal canal:** Hypoglossal nerve (CN XII)
Foramen lacerum[a]: Deep petrosal nerve, some meningeal arterial branches, and small veins	**Foramen magnum:** Spinal cord; spinal accessory nerve (CN XI); vertebral arteries; internal vertebral venous plexus
Groove of greater petrosal nerve: Greater petrosal nerve and petrosal branch of middle meningeal artery	**Condylar canal:** Condyloid emissary vein (passes from sigmoid sinus to vertebral veins in neck)
Carotid canal: Internal carotid artery and accompanying sympathetic and venous plexuses	**Stylomastoid foramen:** Facial nerve (CN VII)
Internal acoustic meatus: Facial nerve/intermediate nerve (CN VII); vestibulocochlear nerve (CN VIII); labyrinthine artery	**Mastoid foramina:** Mastoid emissary vein from sigmoid sinus and meningeal branch of occipital artery

[a]The internal carotid artery and its accompanying sympathetic and venous plexuses actually pass horizontally across (rather than vertically through) the area of the foramen lacerum, an artifact of dry crania, which is closed by cartilage in life.

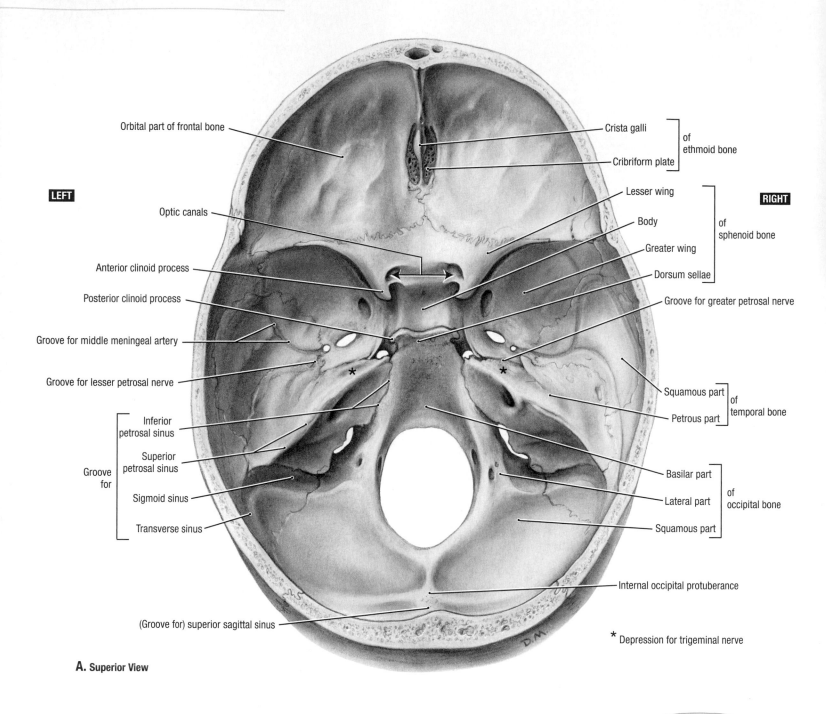

Orbital part of frontal bone

Crista galli ⎤ of
                ⎦ ethmoid bone

Cribriform plate

LEFT

Optic canals

Lesser wing ⎤
Body   ⎥ of
Greater wing ⎥ sphenoid bone

RIGHT

Anterior clinoid process

Dorsum sellae

Posterior clinoid process

Groove for greater petrosal nerve

Groove for middle meningeal artery

Groove for lesser petrosal nerve

Squamous part ⎤ of
Petrous part ⎦ temporal bone

Inferior petrosal sinus

Groove for ⎱ Superior petrosal sinus
             ⎰ Sigmoid sinus
               Transverse sinus

Basilar part ⎤
Lateral part ⎥ of
             ⎥ occipital bone
Squamous part ⎦

Internal occipital protuberance

(Groove for) superior sagittal sinus

* Depression for trigeminal nerve

A. **Superior View**

Sphenoidal crest

Superior border of petrous part of temporal bone

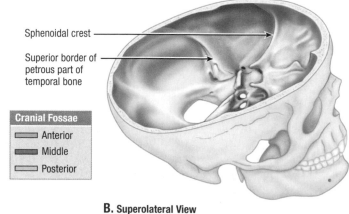

Cranial Fossae
— Anterior
— Middle
— Posterior

B. **Superolateral View**

8.6   Interior of Cranial Base

A. Bony cranial base. **B.** Anterior, middle, and posterior cranial fossae. **C.** Diagrammatic cranial base with bones color coded.

- **Fractures in the floor of the anterior cranial fossa** may involve the cribriform plate of the ethmoid, resulting in leakage of cerebrospinal fluid (CSF) through the nose (CSF rhinorrhea). **CSF rhinorrhea** may be a primary indication of a cranial base fracture which increases the risk of meningitis because an infection could spread to the meninges from the ear or nose.

Frontal crest

Foramen cecum

Crista galli

Cribriform plate

Ethmoidal foramina [Anterior / Posterior]

Cribriform foramina

Optic canal

Ethmoidal spine

Superior orbital fissure

Prechiasmatic groove

LEFT

RIGHT

Anterior clinoid process

Tuberculum sellae

Foramen rotundum

Carotid groove

Hypophysial fossa

Foramen ovale

Posterior clinoid process

Foramen spinosum

Groove for greater petrosal nerve

Dorsum sellae

Foramen lacerum

Arcuate eminence

Clivus

Internal acoustic meatus

Jugular foramen

Hypoglossal canal

Groove for sigmoid sinus

Jugular tubercle

Foramen magnum

Cerebellar fossa

Inner table of bone

Diploë

Groove for transverse sinus

Outer table of bone

C. Superior View

Internal occipital protuberance

Internal occipital crest

Bones	
▭	Ethmoid
▭	Frontal
▭	Occipital
▭	Parietal
▭	Sphenoid
▭	Temporal

Interior of Cranial Base *(continued)*

8.6

In *Part B* and *Part C*, note the following midline features:

- In the anterior cranial fossa, the frontal crest and crista galli for anterior attachment of the falx cerebri have between them the foramen cecum, which, during development, transmits a vein connecting the superior sagittal sinus with the veins of the frontal sinus and root of the nose.
- In the middle cranial fossa, the tuberculum sellae, hypophysial fossa, dorsum sellae, and posterior clinoid processes constitute the sella turcica (L., *Turkish saddle*).

- In the posterior cranial fossa, note the clivus, foramen magnum, internal occipital crest for attachment of the falx cerebelli, and the internal occipital protuberance, from which the grooves for the transverse sinuses course laterally.
- The jugular foramen is at the base of the petrous temporal bone. It transmits three cranial nerves and the sigmoid sinus that exits the skull as the internal jugular vein. The hypoglossal canal lies superior to the anterolateral margins of the foramen magnum.

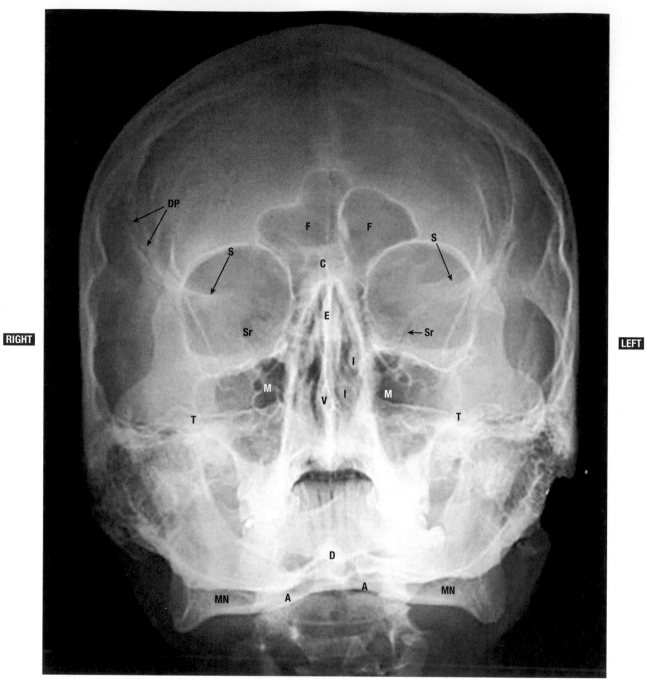

A. Posteroanterior Radiograph

A	Lateral masses of atlas	**M**	Maxillary sinus
C	Crista galli	**MN**	Mandible
D	Dens	**S**	Lesser wing of the sphenoid
DP	Diploic veins	**Sr**	Superior orbital fissure
E	Perpendicular plate of ethmoid	**T**	Superior surface of petrous part
F	Frontal sinus		of temporal bone
I	Inferior and middle conchae	**V**	Vomer

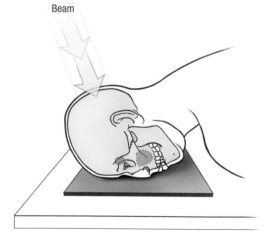

8.7   Radiographs of Cranium

A. Posteroanterior (*Caldwell*) radiograph. This view places the orbits centrally in the head and is used to examine the orbits and paranasal sinuses.

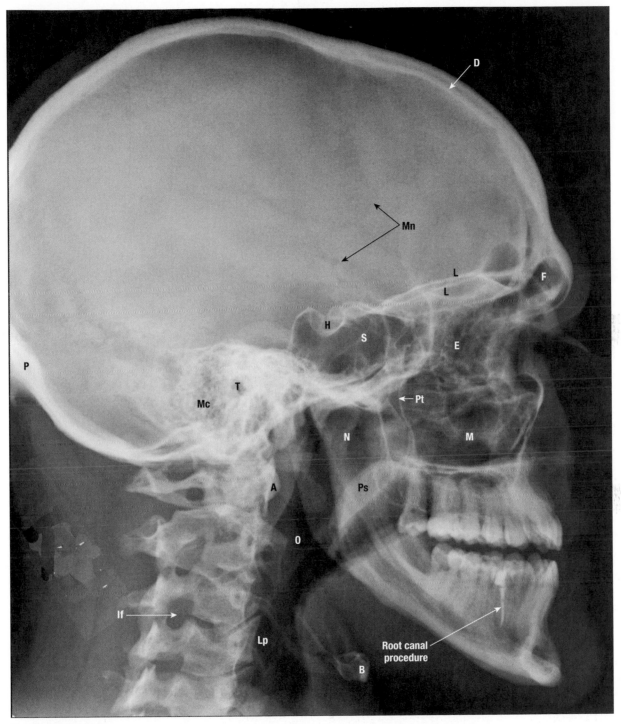

B. Lateral Radiograph

A	Anterior tubercle of atlas	**Lp**	Laryngopharynx	**O**	Oropharynx
B	Hyoid	**M**	Maxillary sinuses	**P**	Internal occipital protuberance
D	Diploë	**Mc**	Mastoid cells	**Ps**	Soft palate
E	Ethmoidal cells	**Mn**	Grooves for branches of	**Pt**	Pterygopalatine fossa
F	Frontal		middle meningeal vessels	**S**	Sphenoidal
H	Hypophysial fossa	**N**	Nasopharynx	**T**	Petrous part of temporal bone
If	Intervertebral foramen				

Radiographs of Cranium (continued)

B. Lateral radiograph of cranium. Most of the relatively thin bone of the facial skeleton (viscerocranium) is radiolucent (appears *black*). The right and left orbital plates of the frontal bone are not superimposed; thus, the floor of the anterior cranial fossa appears as two lines (*L*).

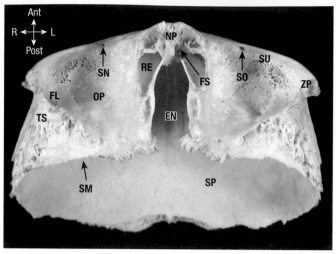

A. Inferior View

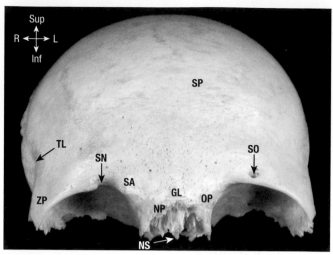

B. Anterior View

Key for A and B: Frontal Bone

EN	Ethmoidal notch	**NP**	Nasal part	**SA**	Superciliary arch	**SU**	Supraorbital margin
FL	Fossa for lacrimal gland	**NS**	Nasal spine	**SM**	Sphenoidal margin	**TL**	Temporal line
FS	Opening of frontal sinus	**OP**	Orbital part	**SN**	Supraorbital notch	**TS**	Temporal surface
GL	Glabella	**RE**	Root of ethmoid cells	**SO**	Supraorbital foramen	**ZP**	Zygomatic process
				SP	Squamous part		

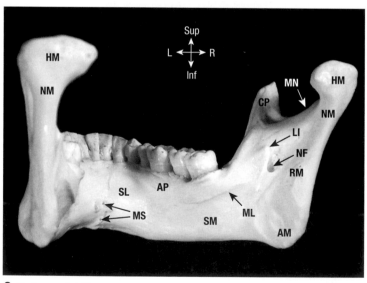

C. Posteromedial View

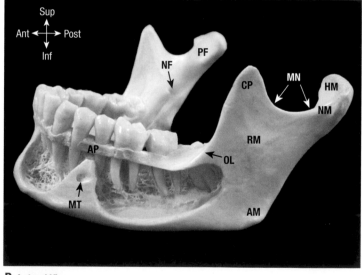

D. Lateral View

Key for C and D: Mandible

AM	Angle of mandible (Gonion)	**LI**	Lingula	**MT**	Mental foramen	**PF**	Pterygoid fovea
AP	Alveolar part	**ML**	Mylohyoid groove	**NF**	Mandibular foramen	**RM**	Ramus of mandible
CP	Coronoid process	**MN**	Mandibular notch	**NM**	Neck of mandible	**SL**	Sublingual fossa
HM	Head of mandible	**MS**	Mental (genial) spines	**OL**	Oblique line	**SM**	Submandibular fossa

8.8 **Mandible and Maxilla and Ethmoid, Frontal, Nasal, and Palatine Bones**

A. and **B.** Frontal bone. **C.** and **D.** Mandible.

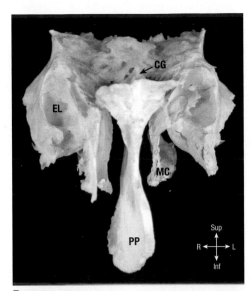

E. Anterior View

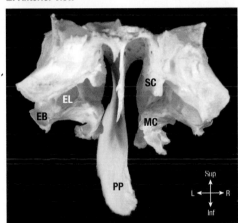

F. Posterior View

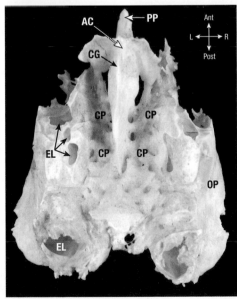

G. Superior View

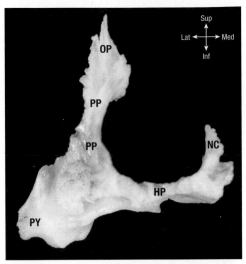

H. Anterior View

Key for H: Palatine Bone			
HP	Horizontal plate	**PP**	Perpendicular plate
NC	Nasal crest	**PY**	Pyramidal process
OP	Orbital process		

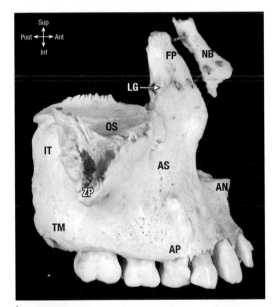

I. Lateral View

Key for I: Maxilla and Nasal Bone			
AN	Anterior nasal spine	**LG**	Lacrimal groove
AP	Alveolar process	**NB**	Nasal bone
AS	Anterior surface	**OS**	Orbital surface
FP	Frontal process	**TM**	Maxillary tuberosity
IT	Infratemporal surface	**ZP**	Zygomatic process

Mandible and Maxilla and Ethmoid, Frontal, Nasal, and Palatine Bones *(continued)*

8.8

Key for E–G: Ethmoid Bone					
AC	Ala of crista galli	**EB**	Ethmoidal bulla	**OP**	Orbital plate
CG	Crista galli	**EL**	Ethmoidal labyrinth (cells)	**PP**	Perpendicular plate
CP	Cribriform plate	**MC**	Bony middle nasal concha	**SC**	Bony superior nasal concha

E–G. Ethmoid bone. **H.** Palatine bone. **I.** Maxilla.

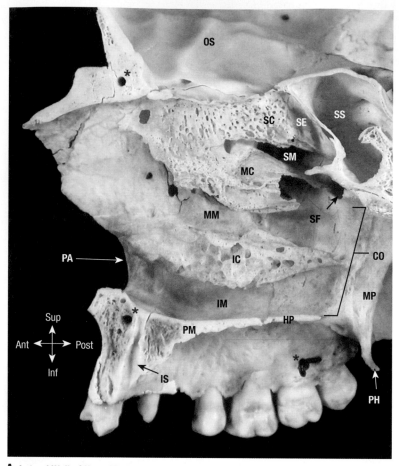

A. Lateral Wall of Nose, Medial View

Key for A: Lateral Wall of Nose	
CO	Choana (posterior nasal aperture)
HP	Horizontal plate of palatine bone
IC	Inferior nasal concha
IM	Inferior nasal meatus
IS	Incisive canal
MC	Bony middle nasal concha
MM	Middle nasal meatus
MP	Medial pterygoid plate
OS	Orbital surface of frontal bone
PA	Piriform aperture
PH	Pterygoid hamulus
PM	Palatine process of maxilla
SC	Bony superior nasal concha
SE	Sphenoethmoidal recess
SF	Sphenopalatine foramen
SM	Superior nasal meatus
SS	Sphenoidal sinus

* Artifact (drilled holes and wire)

B. Infratemporal Region, Inferolateral View

Key for B: Infratemporal Region	
AT	Articular tubercle
EM	External acoustic meatus
FL	Foramen lacerum
FO	Foramen ovale
FS	Foramen spinosum
GW	Greater wing of sphenoid
IOF	Inferior orbital fissure
LP	Lateral pterygoid plate
MF	Mandibular fossa
MP	Medial pterygoid plate
MX	Maxilla
PF	Pterygopalatine fossa
PMF	Pterygomaxillary fissure
PQ	Petrosquamous fissure
TG	Tegmen tympani
TS	Temporal bone (squamous part)
TT	Temporal bone (tympanic part)
ZB	Zygomatic bone
ZF	Zygomaticofacial foramen
ZPM	Zygomatic process of maxilla
ZPT	Zygomatic process of temporal bone

8.9 **Lateral Wall of Nose and Infratemporal Region**

A. Lateral wall of nose. **B.** Infratemporal region.

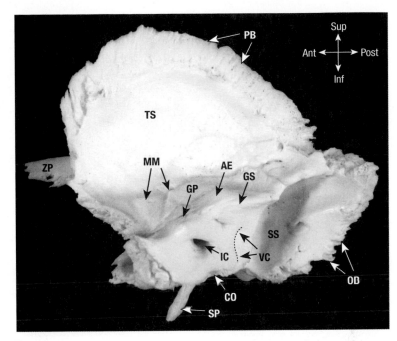

A. Lateral View

B. Medial View

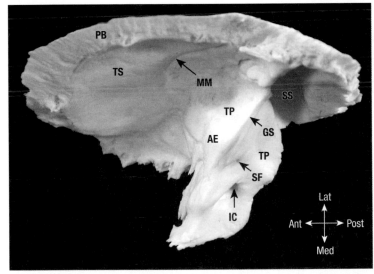

C. Superior View

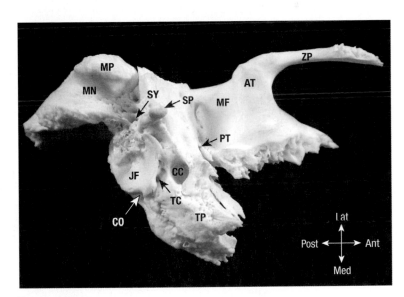

D. Inferior View

Key for A–D: Temporal Bone					
AE	Arcuate eminence	**MF**	Mandibular fossa	**SM**	Sphenoid margin
AT	Articular tubercle	**MM**	Groove for middle meningeal artery	**SP**	Styloid process
CC	Carotid canal	**MN**	Mastoid notch	**SS**	Groove for sigmoid sinus
CO	Cochlear canaliculus	**MP**	Mastoid process	**SY**	Stylomastoid foramen
EM	External acoustic meatus	**OB**	Occipital border	**TC**	Tympanic canaliculus
GP	Hiatus for greater petrosal nerve	**PB**	Parietal border	**TP**	Temporal bone (petrous part)
GS	Groove for superior petrosal sinus	**PN**	Parietal notch	**TS**	Temporal bone (squamous part)
IC	Internal acoustic meatus	**PT**	Petrotympanic fissure	**TT**	Temporal bone (tympanic part)
JF	Jugular fossa	**SC**	Supramastoid crest	**VC**	Vestibular canaliculus
		SF	Subarcuate fossa	**ZP**	Zygomatic process

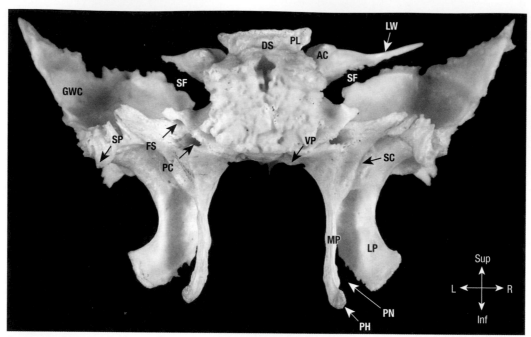

A. Posterior View

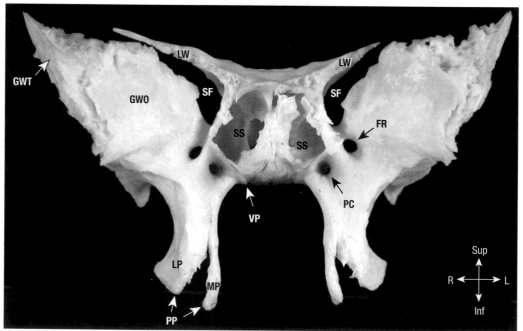

B. Anterior View

Key for A–D: Sphenoid Bone					
AC	Anterior clinoid process	**FO**	Foramen ovale	**GWO**	Greater wing (orbital surface)
CG	Carotid sulcus	**FR**	Foramen rotundum	**GWT**	Greater wing (temporal surface)
CS	Chiasmatic sulcus	**FS**	Foramen spinosum	**H**	Hypophysial fossa
DS	Dorsum sellae	**GWC**	Greater wing (cerebral surface)	**LP**	Lateral pterygoid plate
ES	Ethmoidal spine	**GWI**	Greater wing (infratemporal surface)	**LW**	Lesser wing

8.11 Sphenoid Bone

A. Posterior aspect. B. Anterior aspect. The sphenoid is an irregular unpaired bone that is wedged between the frontal, temporal, and occipital bones.

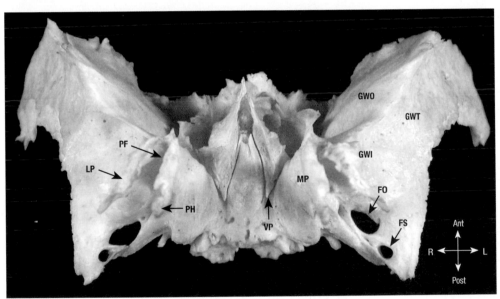

C. Superior View

D. Inferior View

Key for A–D: Sphenoid Bone (*continued*)					
MP	Medial pterygoid plate	**PL**	Posterior clinoid process	**SP**	Spine of sphenoid bone
OC	Optic canal	**PN**	Pterygoid notch	**SS**	Sphenoidal sinus (in body of sphenoid)
PC	Pterygoid canal	**PP**	Pterygoid process	**TS**	Tuberculum sellae
PF	Pterygoid fossa	**SC**	Scaphoid fossa	**VP**	Vaginal process
PH	Pterygoid hamulus	**SF**	Superior orbital fissure		

Sphenoid Bone (*continued*)   **8.11**

C. Superior aspect. D. Inferior aspect. It consists of a body and three pairs of processes: greater wings, lesser wings, and pterygoid processes.

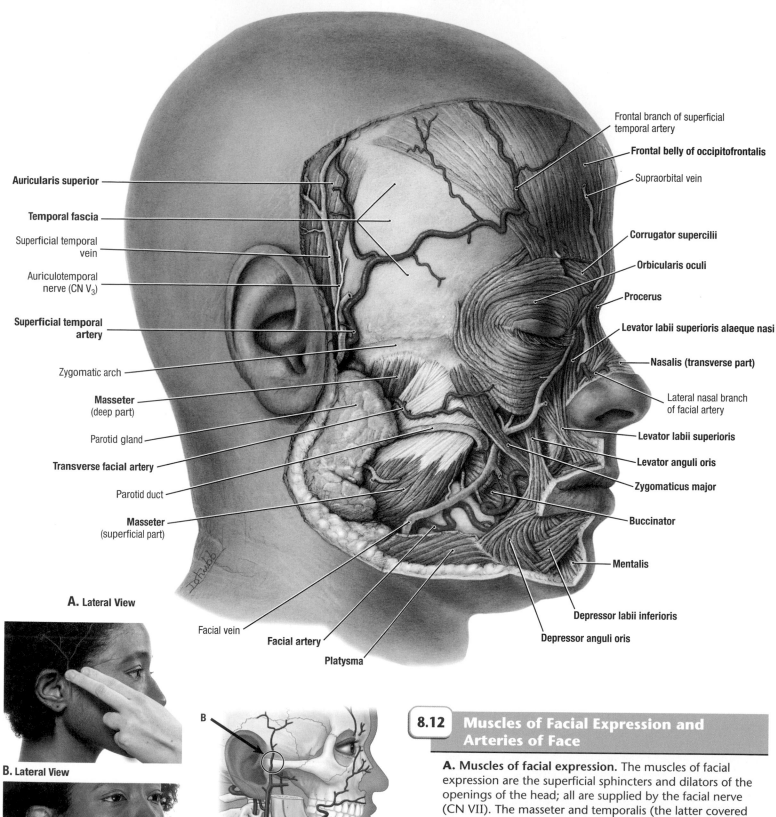

A. Lateral View

Auricularis superior

Temporal fascia

Superficial temporal vein

Auriculotemporal nerve (CN V₃)

Superficial temporal artery

Zygomatic arch

Masseter (deep part)

Parotid gland

Transverse facial artery

Parotid duct

Masseter (superficial part)

Facial vein

Facial artery

Platysma

Frontal branch of superficial temporal artery

Frontal belly of occipitofrontalis

Supraorbital vein

Corrugator supercilii

Orbicularis oculi

Procerus

Levator labii superioris alaeque nasi

Nasalis (transverse part)

Lateral nasal branch of facial artery

Levator labii superioris

Levator anguli oris

Zygomaticus major

Buccinator

Mentalis

Depressor labii inferioris

Depressor anguli oris

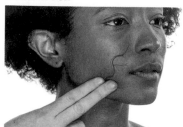

B. Lateral View

C. Anterolateral View

D. Lateral View

B

C

8.12 Muscles of Facial Expression and Arteries of Face

A. Muscles of facial expression. The muscles of facial expression are the superficial sphincters and dilators of the openings of the head; all are supplied by the facial nerve (CN VII). The masseter and temporalis (the latter covered here by temporal fascia) are muscles of mastication that are innervated by the trigeminal nerve (CN V). **B. Superficial temporal pulse.** The pulse is palpated anterior to the auricle as the artery crosses the zygomatic arch. **C. Facial pulse.** The pulse is palpated where the facial artery crosses the inferior border of the mandible immediately anterior to the masseter. **D. Superficial arteries of face.**

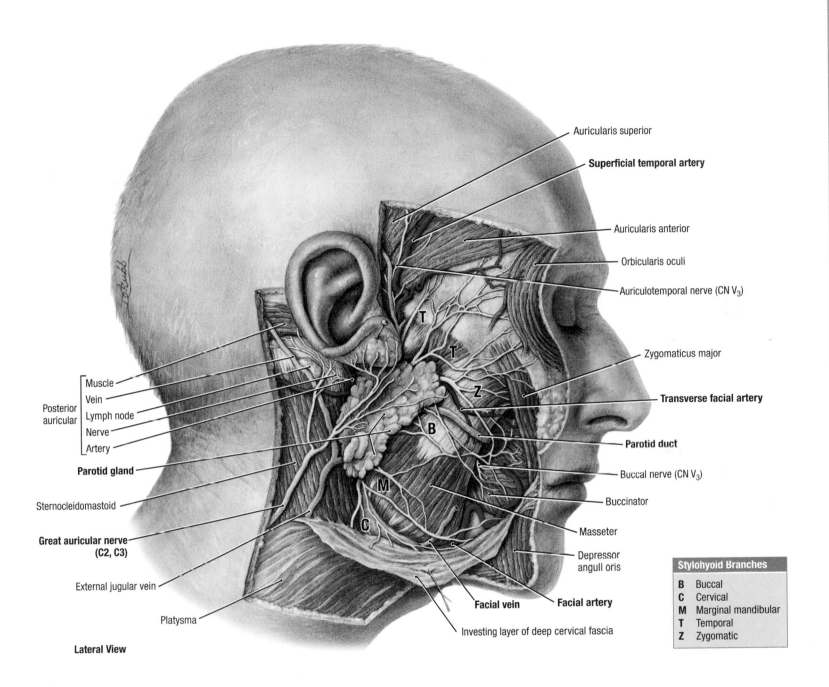

Auricularis superior

Superficial temporal artery

Auricularis anterior

Orbicularis oculi

Auriculotemporal nerve (CN V$_3$)

Zygomaticus major

Transverse facial artery

Parotid duct

Buccal nerve (CN V$_3$)

Buccinator

Masseter

Depressor
anguli oris

Muscle
Vein
Posterior   Lymph node
auricular   Nerve
Artery

Parotid gland

Sternocleidomastoid

**Great auricular nerve
(C2, C3)**

External jugular vein

Platysma

Lateral View

Facial vein   **Facial artery**

Investing layer of deep cervical fascia

Stylohyoid Branches	
B	Buccal
C	Cervical
M	Marginal mandibular
T	Temporal
Z	Zygomatic

Relationships of Branches of Facial Nerve and Vessels to Parotid Gland and Duct   8.13

- The parotid duct extends across the masseter muscle just inferior to the zygomatic arch; the duct turns medially to pierce the buccinator and opens into the oral vestibule.
- The facial nerve (CN VII) innervates the muscles of facial expression. After emerging from the stylomastoid foramen, the main stem of the facial nerve has posterior auricular, digastric, and stylohyoid branches; the parotid plexus gives rise to the temporal, zygomatic, buccal, marginal mandibular, cervical, and posterior auricular branches. These branches form a plexus within the parotid gland, the branches of which radiate over the face, anastomosing with each other and the branches of the trigeminal nerve.

- During **parotidectomy** (surgical excision of the parotid gland), identification, dissection, and preservation of the branches of the facial nerve are critical.
- The parotid gland may become infected by infectious agents that pass through the bloodstream, as occurs in mumps, an acute communicable viral disease. Infection of the gland causes inflammation, parotiditis, and swelling of the gland. Severe pain occurs because the parotid sheath, innervated by the great auricular nerve, is distended by swelling.

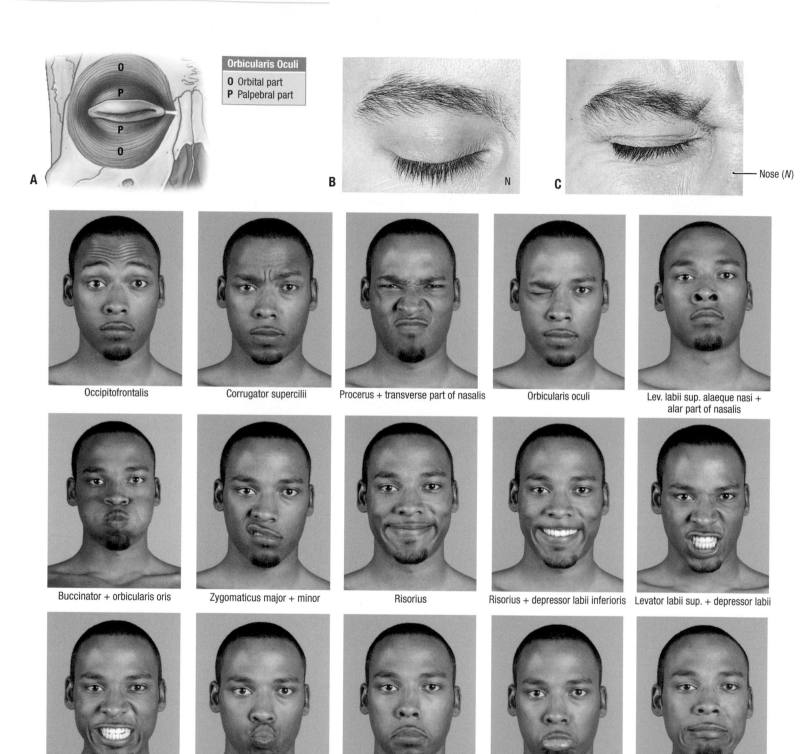

Orbicularis Oculi
O Orbital part
P Palpebral part

Nose (*N*)

Occipitofrontalis

Corrugator supercilii

Procerus + transverse part of nasalis

Orbicularis oculi

Lev. labii sup. alaeque nasi + alar part of nasalis

Buccinator + orbicularis oris

Zygomaticus major + minor

Risorius

Risorius + depressor labii inferioris

Levator labii sup. + depressor labii

Dilators of mouth:
Risorius plus levator labii superioris + depressor labii inferioris

D. Anterior Views

Orbicularis oris

Depressor anguli oris

Mentalis

Platysma

| 8.14 | **Muscles of Facial Expression** |

A. Orbicularis oculi: palpebral and orbital parts. Eyelids close from lateral to medial washing lacrimal fluid across the cornea. **B. Gentle** closure of eyelid (palpebral part). **C. Tight closure of eyelid** (orbital part). **D. Actions of selected muscles of facial expression.**

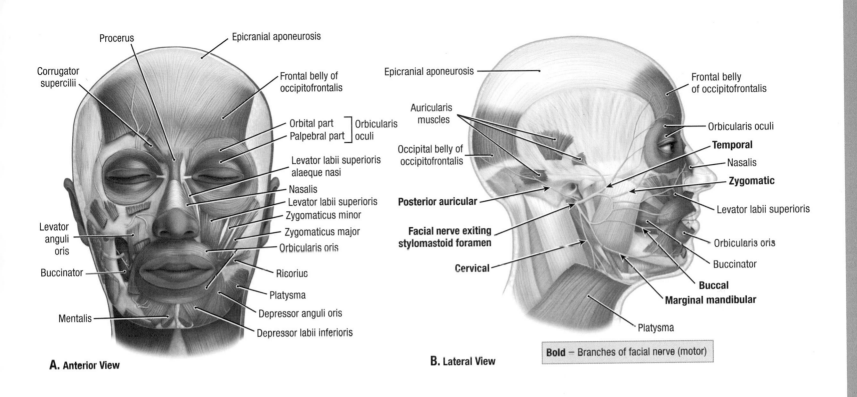

A. Anterior View

B. Lateral View

Bold – Branches of facial nerve (motor)

Branches of Facial Nerve and Muscles of Facial Expression

8.15

A. Muscles. **B.** Branches of facial nerve.

TABLE 8.2	Main Muscles of Facial Expression		
Muscle[a,b]	**Origin**	**Insertion**	**Action**
Occipitofrontalis, frontal belly	Epicranial aponeurosis	Skin of and subcutaneous tissue of eyebrows and forehead	Elevates eyebrows and wrinkles skin of forehead; protracts scalp (indicating surprise or curiosity)
Occipitofrontalis, occipital belly	Lateral two thirds of superior nuchal line	Epicranial aponeurosis	Retracts scalp, increasing effectiveness of frontal belly
Orbicularis oculi	Medial orbital margin, medial palpebral ligament; lacrimal bone	Skin around margin of orbit; superior and inferior tarsal plates	Closes eyelids; palpebral part does so gently; orbital part tightly (winking)
Orbicularis oris	Medial maxilla and mandible; deep surface of perioral skin; angle of mouth (modiolus)	Mucous membrane of lips	Tonus closes oral fissure; phasic contraction compresses and protrudes lips (kissing) or resists distension (when blowing)
Levator labii superioris	Infraorbital margin (maxilla)	Skin of upper lip	Part of dilators of mouth; retract (elevate) and/or evert upper lip; deepen nasolabial sulcus (showing sadness)
Zygomaticus minor	Anterior aspect, zygomatic bone		
Buccinator	Mandible, alveolar processes of maxilla and mandible; pterygomandibular raphe	Angle of mouth (modiolus); orbicularis oris	Presses cheek against molar teeth; works with tongue to keep food between occlusal surfaces and out of oral vestibule; resists distension (when blowing)
Zygomaticus major	Lateral aspect of zygomatic bone	Angle of mouth (modiolus)	Part of dilators of mouth; elevate labial commissure—bilaterally to smile (happiness); unilaterally to sneer (disdain)
Risorius	Parotid fascia and buccal skin (highly variable)		Part of dilators of mouth; widens oral fissure
Platysma	Subcutaneous tissue of infraclavicular and supraclavicular regions	Base of mandible; skin of cheek and lower lip; angle of mouth (modiolus); orbicularis oris	Depresses mandible (against resistance); tenses skin of inferior face and neck (conveying tension and stress)

[a]All of these muscles are supplied by the facial nerve (CN VII).
[b]Muscles of nose (procerus, nasalis, levator labii superioris alaeque nasi) not included.

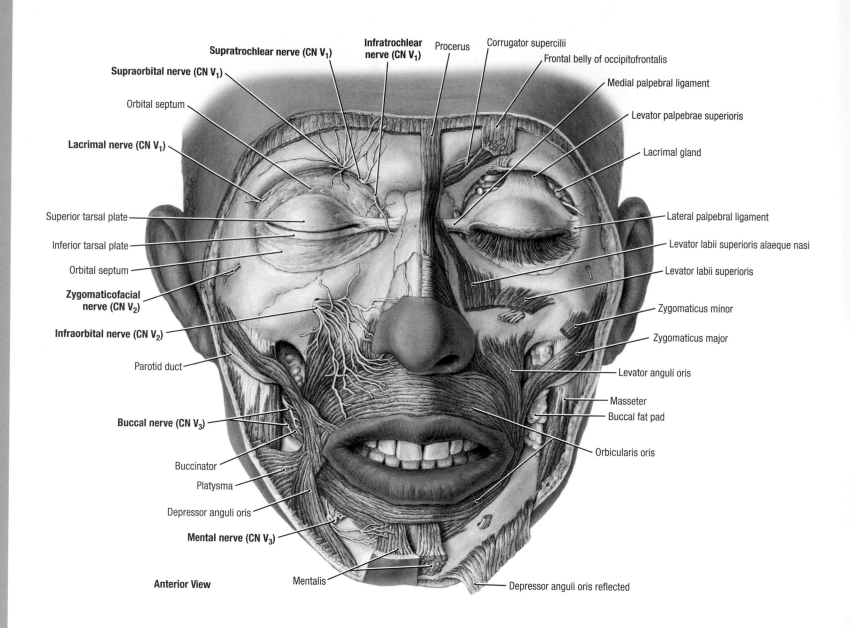

Supratrochlear nerve (CN V₁)

Supraorbital nerve (CN V₁)

Orbital septum

Lacrimal nerve (CN V₁)

Superior tarsal plate

Inferior tarsal plate

Orbital septum

Zygomaticofacial nerve (CN V₂)

Infraorbital nerve (CN V₂)

Parotid duct

Buccal nerve (CN V₃)

Buccinator

Platysma

Depressor anguli oris

Mental nerve (CN V₃)

Anterior View

Mentalis

Infratrochlear nerve (CN V₁)

Procerus

Corrugator supercilii

Frontal belly of occipitofrontalis

Medial palpebral ligament

Levator palpebrae superioris

Lacrimal gland

Lateral palpebral ligament

Levator labii superioris alaeque nasi

Levator labii superioris

Zygomaticus minor

Zygomaticus major

Levator anguli oris

Masseter

Buccal fat pad

Orbicularis oris

Depressor anguli oris reflected

8.16 **Cutaneous Branches of Trigeminal Nerve, Muscles of Facial Expression, and Eyelid**

Injury to the facial nerve (CN VII) or its branches produces paralysis of some or all of the facial muscles on the affected side (Bell facial palsy). The affected area sags, and facial expression is distorted. The loss of tonus causes the inferior lid to evert (fall away from the surface of the eyeball). As a result, the lacrimal fluid is not spread over the cornea, preventing adequate lubrication, hydration, and flushing of the cornea. This makes the cornea vulnerable to ulceration. If the injury weakens or paralyzes the buccinator and orbicularis oris, food will accumulate in the oral vestibule during chewing, usually requiring continual removal with a finger. When the sphincters or dilators of the mouth are affected, displacement of the mouth (drooping of the corner) is produced by gravity and contraction of unopposed contralateral facial muscles, resulting in food and saliva dribbling out of the side of the mouth. Weakened lip muscles affect speech. Affected people cannot whistle or blow a wind instrument effectively. They frequently dab their eyes and mouth with a handkerchief to wipe the fluid (tears and saliva) that runs from the drooping lid and mouth.

Because the face does not have a distinct layer of deep fascia and the subcutaneous tissue is loose between the attachments of facial muscles, **facial lacerations** tend to gap (part widely). Consequently, the skin must be sutured carefully to prevent scarring. The looseness of the subcutaneous tissue also enables fluid and blood to accumulate in the loose connective tissue causing **bruising of the face**.

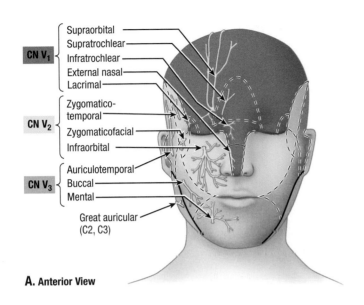

A. Anterior View

CN V₁
- Supraorbital
- Supratrochlear
- Infratrochlear
- External nasal
- Lacrimal

CN V₂
- Zygomatico-temporal
- Zygomaticofacial
- Infraorbital

CN V₃
- Auriculotemporal
- Buccal
- Mental

Great auricular (C2, C3)

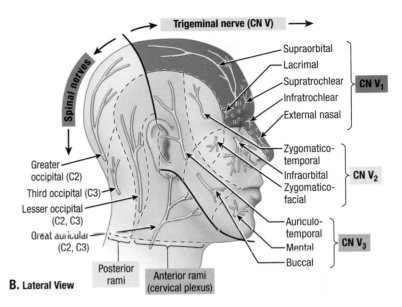

B. Lateral View

Trigeminal nerve (CN V)

Spinal nerves

- Supraorbital
- Lacrimal
- Supratrochlear
- Infratrochlear
- External nasal
CN V₁

- Zygomatico-temporal
- Infraorbital
- Zygomatico-facial
CN V₂

- Auriculo-temporal
- Mental
- Buccal
CN V₃

Greater occipital (C2)
Third occipital (C3)
Lesser occipital (C2, C3)
Great auricular (C2, C3)

Posterior rami   Anterior rami (cervical plexus)

Cutaneous Nerves of Face and Scalp

8.17

Cutaneous (sensory) innervation of the face and anterosuperior part of the scalp is primarily from the trigeminal nerve (CN V).

TABLE 8.3 Cutaneous Nerves of Face and Scalp

Nerve	Origin	Course	Distribution
Frontal	Ophthalmic nerve (CN V₁)	Crosses orbit on superior aspect of levator palpebrae superioris; divides into supraorbital and supratrochlear branches	Skin of forehead, scalp, superior eyelid; conjunctiva of superior lid and mucosa of frontal sinus
Supraorbital	Continuation of frontal nerve (CN V₁)	Emerges through supraorbital notch, or foramen, and breaks up into small branches	Mucous membrane of frontal sinus and conjunctiva (lining) of superior eyelid; skin of forehead as far as vertex
Supratrochlear	Frontal nerve (CN V₁)	Continues anteromedially along roof of orbit, passing lateral to trochlea	Skin in middle of forehead to hairline
Infratrochlear	Nasociliary nerve (CN V₁)	Follows medial wall of orbit passing inferior to trochlea to superior eyelid	Skin and conjunctiva (lining) of superior eyelid and nose
Lacrimal	Ophthalmic nerve (CN V₁)	Passes through palpebral fascia of superior eyelid near lateral angle (canthus) of eye	Lacrimal gland and small area of skin and conjunctiva of lateral part of superior eyelid
External nasal	Anterior ethmoidal nerve (CN V₁)	Runs in nasal cavity and emerges on face between nasal bone and lateral nasal cartilage	Skin on dorsum of nose, including tip of nose
Zygomatic	Maxillary nerve (CN V₂)	Arises in floor of orbit, divides into zygomaticofacial and zygomaticotemporal nerves, which traverse foramina of same name	Skin over zygomatic arch and anterior temporal region
Infraorbital	Terminal branch of maxillary nerve (CN V₂)	Runs in floor of orbit and emerges at infraorbital foramen	Skin of cheek, inferior lid, lateral side of nose and inferior septum and superior lip, upper premolar incisors and canine teeth; mucosa of maxillary sinus and superior lip
Auriculotemporal	Mandibular nerve (CN V₃)	From posterior division of CN V₃, it passes between neck of mandible and external acoustic meatus to accompany superficial temporal artery	Skin anterior to ear and posterior temporal region, tragus and part of helix of auricle, and roof of external acoustic meatus and upper tympanic membrane
Buccal	Mandibular nerve (CN V₃)	From the anterior division of CN V₃ in infratemporal fossa, it passes anteriorly to reach cheek	Skin and mucosa of cheek, buccal gingiva adjacent to 2nd and 3rd molar teeth
Mental	Terminal branch of inferior alveolar nerve (CN V₃)	Emerges from mandibular canal at mental foramen	Skin of chin and inferior lip and mucosa of lower lip

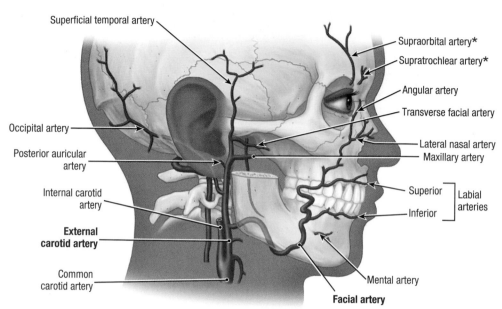

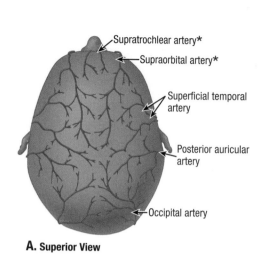

A. Superior View

B. Lateral View

* Source = internal carotid artery (ophthalmic artery); all other labeled arteries are from external carotid

8.18 Arteries of Face and Scalp

Most superficial arteries of the face are branches or derivatives of the external carotid artery. The facial artery, a branch of the external carotid artery, provides the major arterial supply to the face. The facial artery winds its way to the inferior border of the mandible, just anterior to the masseter, and then courses over the face to the medial angle (canthus) of the eye, where the superior and inferior eyelids meet.

TABLE 8.4 Arteries of Superficial Face and Scalp

Artery	Origin	Course	Distribution
Facial	External carotid artery	Ascends deep to submandibular gland, winds around inferior border of mandible and enters face	Most muscles of facial expression and centrolateral aspects of face
Inferior labial	Facial artery near angle of mouth	Runs medially in lower lip	Lower lip and chin
Superior labial		Runs medially in upper lip	Upper lip and ala (side) and septum of nose
Lateral nasal	Facial artery as it ascends alongside nose	Passes to ala of nose	Skin on ala and dorsum of nose
Angular	Terminal branch of facial artery	Passes to medial angle (canthus) of eye	Superior part of cheek and lower eyelid
Occipital	External carotid artery	Passes medial to posterior belly of digastric and mastoid process; accompanies occipital nerve in occipital region	Scalp of back of head, as far as vertex
Posterior auricular		Passes posteriorly, deep to parotid, along styloid process between mastoid and ear	Scalp posterior to auricle and auricle
Superficial temporal	Smaller terminal branch of external carotid artery	Ascends anterior to ear to temporal region and ends in scalp	Facial muscles and skin of frontal and temporal regions
Transverse facial	Superficial temporal artery within parotid gland	Crosses face superficial to masseter and inferior to zygomatic arch	Parotid gland and duct, muscles and skin of face
Mental	Terminal branch of inferior alveolar artery	Emerges from mental foramen and passes to chin	Facial muscles and skin of chin
Supraorbital	Terminal branch of ophthalmic artery, a branch of internal carotid	Passes superiorly from supraorbital foramen	Muscles and skin of forehead and scalp
Supratrochlear		Passes superiorly from supratrochlear notch	Muscles and skin of scalp

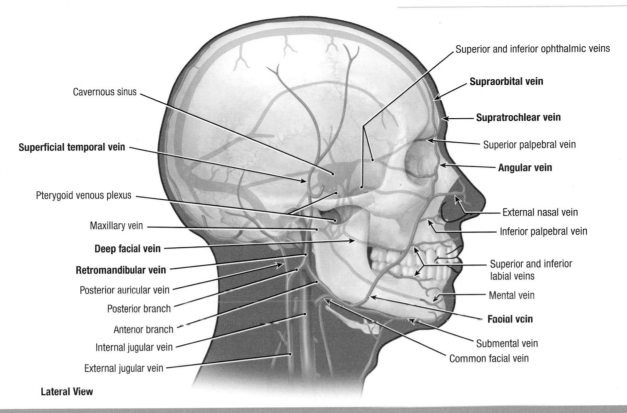

Superior and inferior ophthalmic veins

Supraorbital vein

Supratrochlear vein

Superior palpebral vein

Angular vein

External nasal vein

Inferior palpebral vein

Superior and inferior labial veins

Mental vein

Facial vein

Submental vein

Common facial vein

Cavernous sinus

Superficial temporal vein

Pterygoid venous plexus

Maxillary vein

Deep facial vein

Retromandibular vein

Posterior auricular vein

Posterior branch

Anterior branch

Internal jugular vein

External jugular vein

Lateral View

Veins of Face   8.19

TABLE 8.5	Veins of Face			
Vein	**Origin**	**Course**	**Termination**	**Area Drained**
Supratrochlear	Begins from a venous plexus on the forehead and scalp, through which it communicates with the frontal branch of the superficial temporal vein, its contralateral partner, and the supraorbital vein	Descends near the midline of the forehead to the root of the nose where it joins the supraorbital vein	Angular vein at the root of the nose	Anterior part of scalp and forehead
Supraorbital	Begins in the forehead by anastomosing with a frontal tributary of the superficial temporal vein	Passes medially superior to the orbit and joins the supratrochlear vein; a branch passes through the supraorbital notch and joins with the superior ophthalmic vein		
Angular	Begins at root of nose by union of supratrochlear and supraorbital veins	Descends obliquely along the root and side of the nose to the inferior margin of the orbit	Becomes the facial vein at the inferior margin of the orbit	In addition to above, drains upper and lower lids and conjunctiva; may receive drainage from cavernous sinus
Facial	Continuation of angular vein past inferior margin of orbit	Descends along lateral border of the nose, receiving external nasal and inferior palpebral veins, then obliquely across face to mandible; receives anterior division of retromandibular vein, after which it is sometimes called the common facial vein	Internal jugular vein at or inferior to the level of the hyoid bone	Anterior scalp and forehead, eyelids, external nose, and anterior cheek, lips, chin, and submandibular gland
Deep facial	Pterygoid venous plexus	Runs anteriorly on maxilla above buccinator and deep to masseter, emerging medial to anterior border of masseter onto face	Enters posterior aspect of facial vein	Infratemporal fossa (most areas supplied by maxillary artery)
Superficial temporal	Begins from a widespread plexus of veins on the side of the scalp and along the zygomatic arch	Its frontal and parietal tributaries unite anterior to the auricle; it crosses the temporal root of the zygomatic arch to pass from the temporal region and enters the substance of the parotid gland	Joins the maxillary vein posterior to the neck of the mandible to form the retromandibular vein	Side of the scalp, superficial aspect of the temporal muscle, and external ear
Retromandibular	Formed anterior to the ear by the union of the superficial temporal and maxillary veins	Runs posterior and deep to the ramus of the mandible through the substance of the parotid gland; communicates at its inferior end with the facial vein	*Anterior branch* unites with facial vein to form common facial vein; *posterior branch* unites with the posterior auricular vein to form the external jugular vein	Parotid gland and masseter muscle

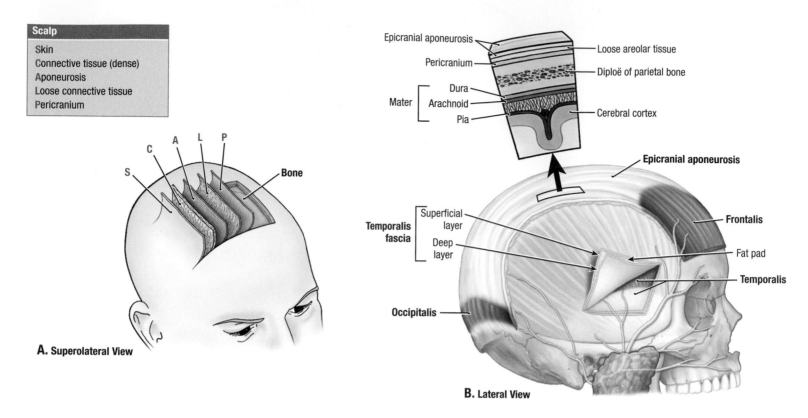

Scalp

Skin
Connective tissue (dense)
Aponeurosis
Loose connective tissue
Pericranium

Epicranial aponeurosis
Pericranium

Mater
Dura
Arachnoid
Pia

Loose areolar tissue
Diploë of parietal bone
Cerebral cortex

A. Superolateral View

Bone

Epicranial aponeurosis

Temporalis fascia
Superficial layer
Deep layer

Frontalis
Fat pad
Temporalis

Occipitalis

B. Lateral View

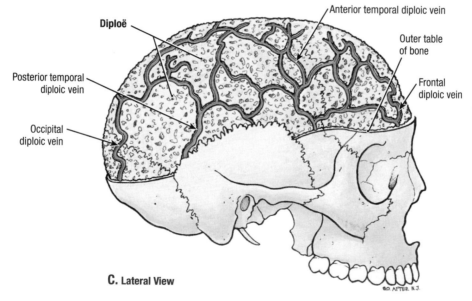

Diploë

Anterior temporal diploic vein

Posterior temporal diploic vein

Outer table of bone

Frontal diploic vein

Occipital diploic vein

C. Lateral View

8.20 **Scalp**

A. Layers of scalp. B. Epicranial aponeurosis. C. Diploic veins. The outer layer of the compact bone of the cranium has been filed away, exposing the channels for the diploic veins in the cancellous bone that composes the diploë.

Scalp injuries and infections. The loose areolar tissue layer is the danger area of the scalp because pus or blood spreads easily in it. Infection in this layer can pass into the cranial cavity through emissary veins, which pass through parietal foramina in the calvaria and reach intracranial structures such as the meninges. An infection cannot pass into the neck because the occipital belly of the occipitofrontalis attaches to the occipital bone and mastoid parts of the temporal bones. Neither can a scalp infection spread laterally beyond the zygomatic arches because the epicranial aponeurosis is continuous with the temporalis fascia that attaches to these arches. An infection or fluid (e.g., pus or blood) can enter the eyelids and the root of the nose because the frontal belly of the occipitofrontalis inserts into the skin and dense subcutaneous tissue and does not attach to the bone. **Ecchymoses**, or purple patches, develop as a result of extravasation of blood into the subcutaneous tissue, skin of the eyelids, and surrounding regions.

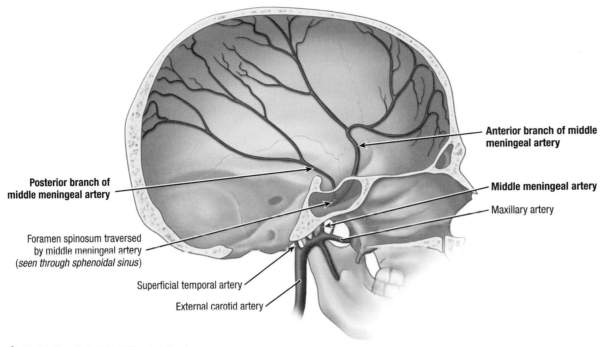

A. Medial View, Left Half of Bisected Cranium

Anterior branch of middle meningeal artery

Posterior branch of middle meningeal artery

Middle meningeal artery

Maxillary artery

Foramen spinosum traversed by middle meningeal artery (*seen through sphenoidal sinus*)

Superficial temporal artery

External carotid artery

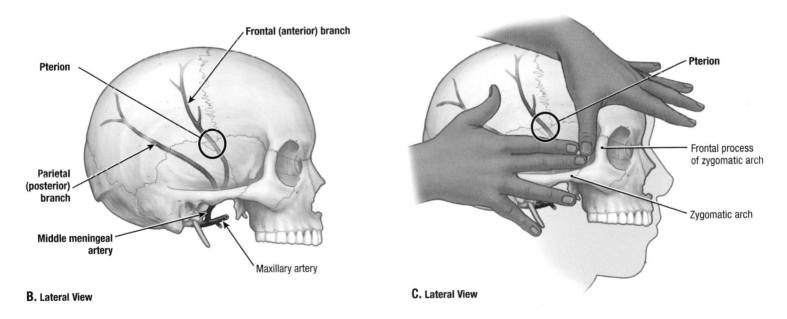

Frontal (anterior) branch

Pterion

Pterion

Parietal (posterior) branch

Middle meningeal artery

Maxillary artery

Frontal process of zygomatic arch

Zygomatic arch

B. Lateral View

C. Lateral View

Middle Meningeal Artery and Pterion

8.21

A. Course of middle meningeal artery in cranium. B. Surface projections of middle meningeal artery. C. Locating pterion.
The pterion is located two fingers breadth superior to the zygomatic arch and one thumb breadth posterior to the frontal process of the zygomatic bone (approximately 4 cm superior to the midpoint of the zygomatic arch); the anterior branch of the middle meningeal artery crosses the pterion.

A hard blow to the side of the head may fracture the thin bones forming the pterion, rupturing the anterior branch of the middle meningeal artery crossing the pterion. The resulting **extradural (epidural) hematoma** exerts pressure on the underlying cerebral cortex. Untreated middle meningeal artery hemorrhage may cause death in a few hours.

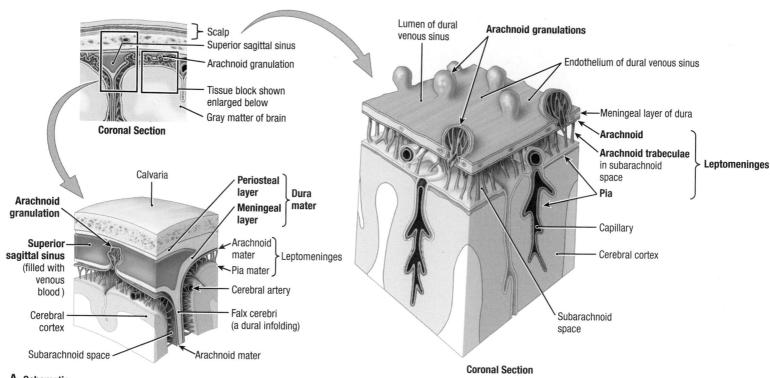

Coronal Section

Coronal Section

A. **Schematic**

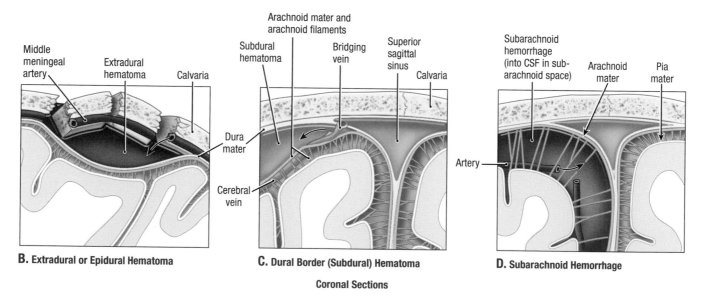

B. **Extradural or Epidural Hematoma**

C. **Dural Border (Subdural) Hematoma**

D. **Subarachnoid Hemorrhage**

Coronal Sections

8.22 Meninges

A. Cranium and meninges. The three meningeal spaces include the extradural (epidural) space between the cranial bones and dura, which is a potential space normally (it becomes a real space pathologically if blood accumulates in it); the similarly potential subdural space between the dura and arachnoid; and the subarachnoid space, the normal realized space between the arachnoid and pia, which contains cerebrospinal fluid (CSF).

B. Extradural (epidural) hematoma. These hematomas result from bleeding from a torn middle meningeal artery. **C. Dural border (subdural) hematoma.** These hematomas commonly result from tearing of a cerebral vein as it enters the superior sagittal sinus. **D. Subarachnoid hemorrhage.** This hemorrhage results from bleeding within the subarachnoid space (e.g., from rupture of an aneurysm).

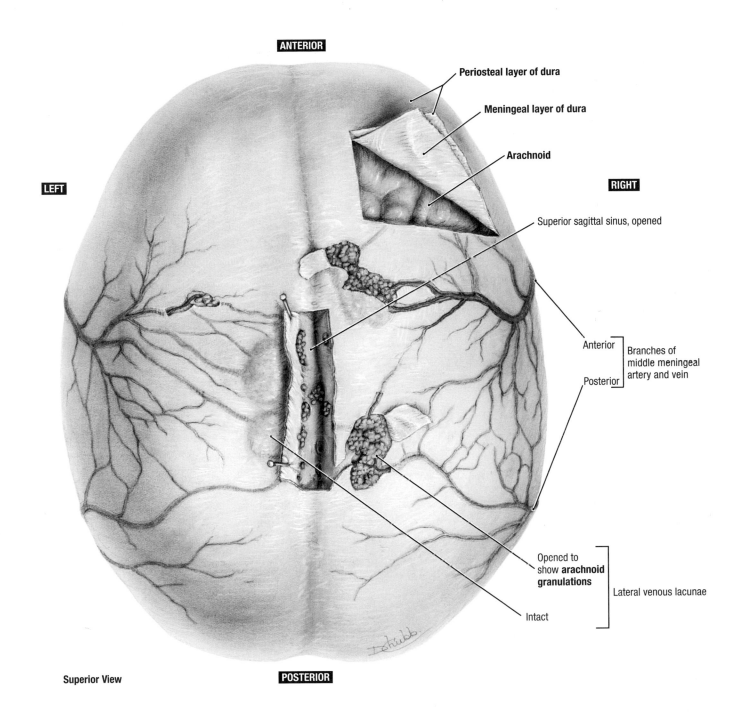

ANTERIOR

Periosteal layer of dura

Meningeal layer of dura

Arachnoid

LEFT

RIGHT

Superior sagittal sinus, opened

Anterior   Branches of
            middle meningeal
Posterior   artery and vein

Opened to
show **arachnoid
granulations**

Lateral venous lacunae

Intact

Superior View

POSTERIOR

Dura Mater and Arachnoid Granulations

8.23

- The calvaria is removed. In the median plane, the thick roof of the superior sagittal sinus is partly pinned aside, and laterally, the thin roofs of two lateral lacunae are reflected.
- The middle meningeal artery courses with the middle meningeal veins, which enlarge superiorly and drain into a lateral lacunae. Other channels drain the lateral lacunae into the superior sagittal sinus.
- Arachnoid granulations in the lacunae are responsible for absorption of CSF from the subarachnoid space into the venous system.

- The dura is sensitive to pain, especially where it is related to the dural venous sinuses and meningeal arteries. Although the causes of **headache** are numerous, distention of the scalp or meningeal vessels (or both) is believed to be one cause of headache. Many headaches appear to be dural in origin, such as the headache occurring after a lumbar spinal puncture for removal of CSF. These headaches are thought to result from stimulation of sensory nerve endings in the dura.

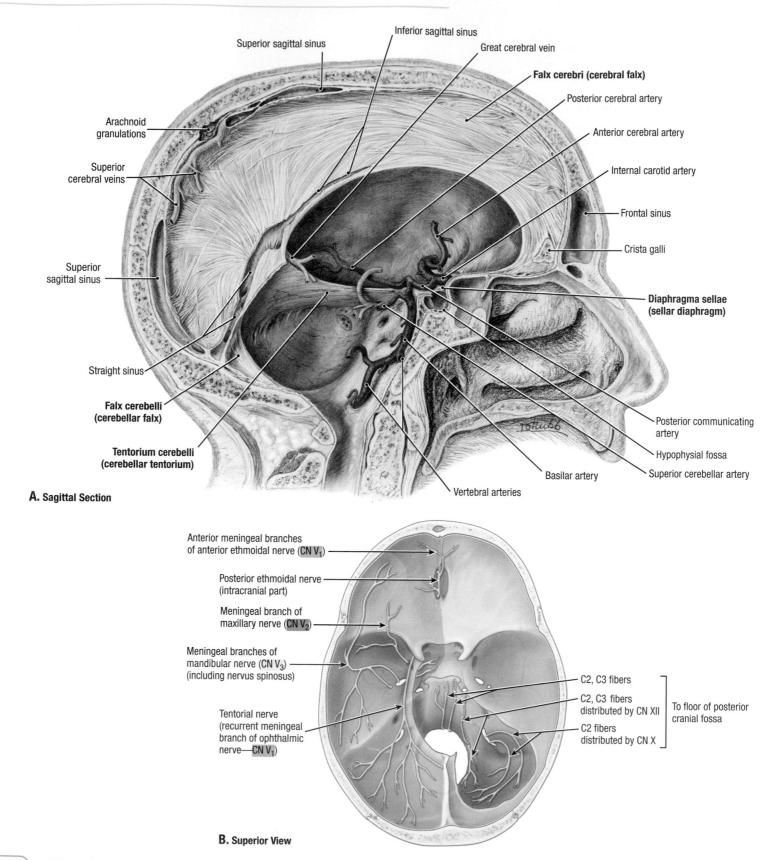

Superior sagittal sinus

Inferior sagittal sinus

Great cerebral vein

Falx cerebri (cerebral falx)

Posterior cerebral artery

Anterior cerebral artery

Internal carotid artery

Frontal sinus

Crista galli

Diaphragma sellae (sellar diaphragm)

Arachnoid granulations

Superior cerebral veins

Superior sagittal sinus

Straight sinus

Falx cerebelli (cerebellar falx)

Tentorium cerebelli (cerebellar tentorium)

Posterior communicating artery

Hypophysial fossa

Superior cerebellar artery

Basilar artery

Vertebral arteries

A. Sagittal Section

Anterior meningeal branches of anterior ethmoidal nerve (CN V₁)

Posterior ethmoidal nerve (intracranial part)

Meningeal branch of maxillary nerve (CN V₂)

Meningeal branches of mandibular nerve (CN V₃) (including nervus spinosus)

Tentorial nerve (recurrent meningeal branch of ophthalmic nerve—CN V₁)

C2, C3 fibers

C2, C3 fibers distributed by CN XII

C2 fibers distributed by CN X

To floor of posterior cranial fossa

B. Superior View

8.24 **Dura Mater**

A. Reflections of dura mater. B. Innervation of dura of cranial base. The dura of the cranial base is innervated by branches of the trigeminal nerve and sensory fibers of cervical spinal nerves (C2, C3) passing directly from those nerves or via meningeal branches of the vagus (CN X) and hypoglossal (CN XII) nerves.

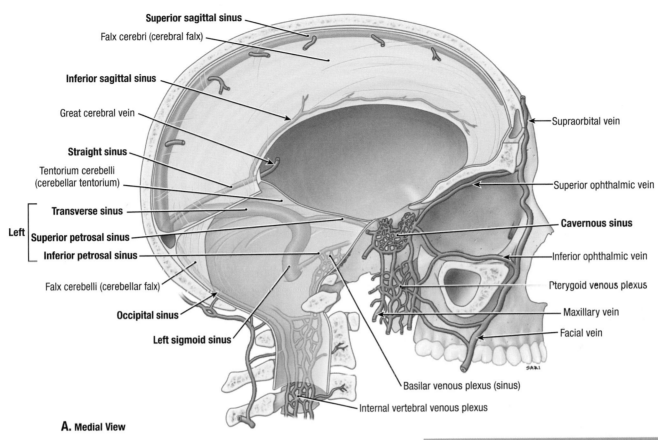

A. Medial View

Superior sagittal sinus
Falx cerebri (cerebral falx)
Inferior sagittal sinus
Great cerebral vein
Straight sinus
Tentorium cerebelli (cerebellar tentorium)
Transverse sinus
Left
Superior petrosal sinus
Inferior petrosal sinus
Falx cerebelli (cerebellar falx)
Occipital sinus
Left sigmoid sinus
Supraorbital vein
Superior ophthalmic vein
Cavernous sinus
Inferior ophthalmic vein
Pterygoid venous plexus
Maxillary vein
Facial vein
Basilar venous plexus (sinus)
Internal vertebral venous plexus

ANTERIOR

Superior ophthalmic vein
Sphenoparietal sinus
Cavernous sinus
Superior petrosal sinus
Inferior petrosal sinus
LEFT
Sigmoid sinus
Straight sinus
B. Superior View
POSTERIOR

Intercavernous sinus
Basilar venous plexus (sinus)
Great cerebral vein
Transition of sigmoid sinus into internal jugular vein
RIGHT
Tentorial notch
Tentorium cerebelli
Right transverse sinus
Inferior sagittal sinus
Superior sagittal sinus

Venous Sinuses of Dura Mater   8.25

A. Schematic of left half of cranial cavity and right facial skeleton. **B.** Venous sinuses of cranial base.

- The superior sagittal sinus is at the superior border of the falx cerebri, and the inferior sagittal sinus is in its free border. The great cerebral vein joins the inferior sagittal sinus to form the straight sinus.
- The superior sagittal sinus usually becomes the right transverse sinus, which drains into the right sigmoid sinus, and next into the right internal jugular vein; the straight sinus similarly drains through the left transverse sinus, left sigmoid sinus, and left internal jugular vein.
- The cavernous sinus communicates with the veins of the face through the ophthalmic veins and pterygoid plexus of veins and with the sigmoid sinus through the superior and inferior petrosal sinuses.
- **Metastasis of tumor cells to dural sinuses.** The basilar and occipital sinuses communicate through the foramen magnum with the internal vertebral venous plexuses. Because these venous channels are valveless, increased intra-abdominopelvic or intrathoracic pressure, as occurs during heavy coughing and straining, may force venous blood from these regions into the internal vertebral venous system and from it into the dural venous sinuses. As a result, pus in abscesses and tumor cells in these regions may spread to the vertebrae and brain.

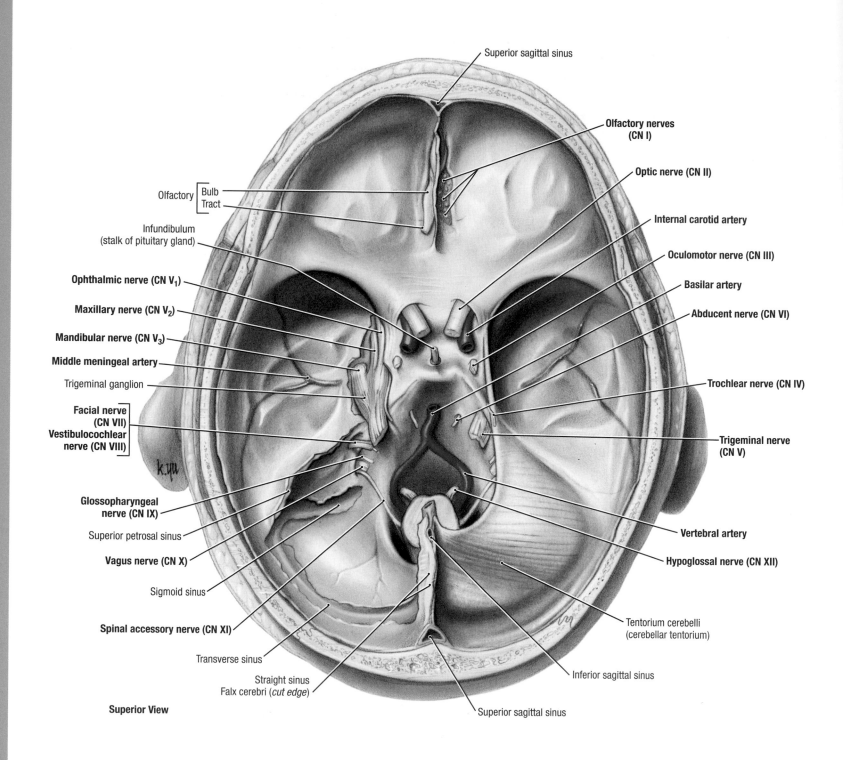

Superior sagittal sinus

Olfactory nerves (CN I)

Optic nerve (CN II)

Internal carotid artery

Oculomotor nerve (CN III)

Basilar artery

Abducent nerve (CN VI)

Trochlear nerve (CN IV)

Trigeminal nerve (CN V)

Vertebral artery

Hypoglossal nerve (CN XII)

Tentorium cerebelli (cerebellar tentorium)

Inferior sagittal sinus

Superior sagittal sinus

Olfactory [Bulb / Tract]

Infundibulum (stalk of pituitary gland)

Ophthalmic nerve (CN V₁)

Maxillary nerve (CN V₂)

Mandibular nerve (CN V₃)

Middle meningeal artery

Trigeminal ganglion

Facial nerve (CN VII)
Vestibulocochlear nerve (CN VIII)

Glossopharyngeal nerve (CN IX)

Superior petrosal sinus

Vagus nerve (CN X)

Sigmoid sinus

Spinal accessory nerve (CN XI)

Transverse sinus

Straight sinus
Falx cerebri (*cut edge*)

Superior View

| 8.26 | **Nerves and Vessels of Interior of Base of Cranium** |

- On the left of the specimen, the dura mater forming the roof of the trigeminal cave is cut away to expose the trigeminal ganglion and its three branches. The tentorium cerebelli is removed to reveal the transverse and superior petrosal sinuses.
- The frontal lobes of the cerebrum are located in the anterior cranial fossa, the temporal lobes in the middle cranial fossa, and

the brainstem and cerebellum in the posterior cranial fossa; the occipital lobes rest on the tentorium cerebelli.
- The sites where the 12 cranial nerves and the internal carotid, vertebral, and basilar, arteries penetrate the dura mater are shown.

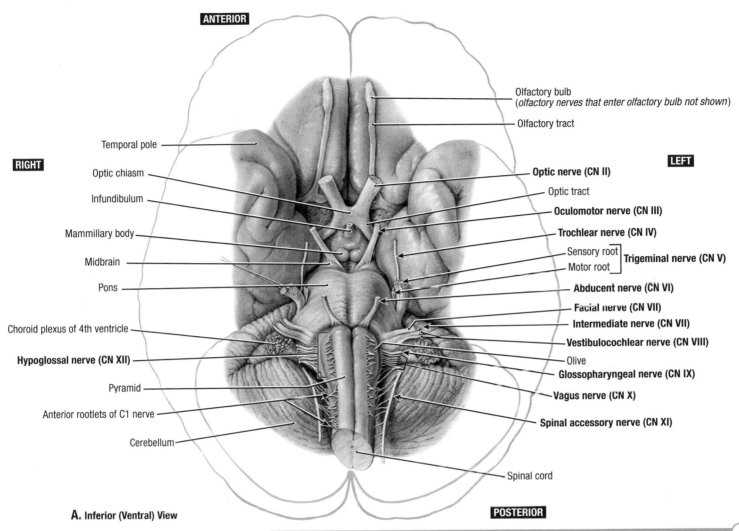

A. Inferior (Ventral) View

Labels (top to bottom, right side):
ANTERIOR

RIGHT — LEFT

Temporal pole

Olfactory bulb (*olfactory nerves that enter olfactory bulb not shown*)

Olfactory tract

Optic chiasm

Optic nerve (CN II)

Infundibulum

Optic tract

Oculomotor nerve (CN III)

Mammillary body

Trochlear nerve (CN IV)

Midbrain

Sensory root ⎤
Motor root ⎦ **Trigeminal nerve (CN V)**

Pons

Abducent nerve (CN VI)

Facial nerve (CN VII)

Choroid plexus of 4th ventricle

Intermediate nerve (CN VII)

Vestibulocochlear nerve (CN VIII)

Hypoglossal nerve (CN XII)

Olive

Glossopharyngeal nerve (CN IX)

Pyramid

Vagus nerve (CN X)

Anterior rootlets of C1 nerve

Spinal accessory nerve (CN XI)

Cerebellum

Spinal cord

POSTERIOR

Base of Brain and Superficial Origins of Cranial Nerves | 8.27

A. Cranial nerves in relation to base of brain. B. Cranial fossae. Foramina of skull and their associated cranial nerve(s) are listed below.

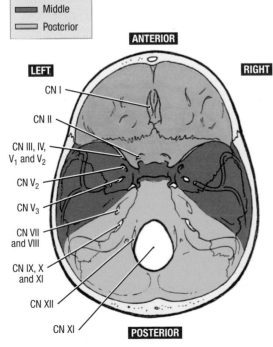

Cranial Fossae
- ▢ Anterior
- ▣ Middle
- ▢ Posterior

ANTERIOR

LEFT — RIGHT

CN I
CN II
CN III, IV, V₁ and V₂
CN V₂
CN V₃
CN VII and VIII
CN IX, X and XI
CN XII
CN XI

POSTERIOR

B. Superior View

TABLE 8.6	Openings by Which Cranial Nerves Traverse Cranial Base
Foramina/Apertures	**Cranial Nerve(s)**
Anterior cranial fossa	
Cribriform foramina in cribriform plate	Axons of olfactory cells in olfactory epithelium form olfactory nerves (CN I)
Middle cranial fossa	
Optic canal	Optic nerve (CN II)
Superior orbital fissure	Ophthalmic nerve (CN V₁) and branches, oculomotor nerve (CN III), trochlear nerve (CN IV), and abducent nerve (CN VI)
Foramen rotundum	Maxillary nerve (CN V₂)
Foramen ovale	Mandibular nerve (CN V₃)
Posterior cranial fossa	
Internal auditory meatus	Facial nerve (CN VII), vestibulocochlear nerve (CN VIII)
Foramen magnum	Spinal accessory nerve (CN XI)
Jugular foramen	Glossopharyngeal nerve (CN IX), vagus nerve (CN X), and spinal accessory nerve (CN XI)
Hypoglossal canal	Hypoglossal nerve (CN XII)

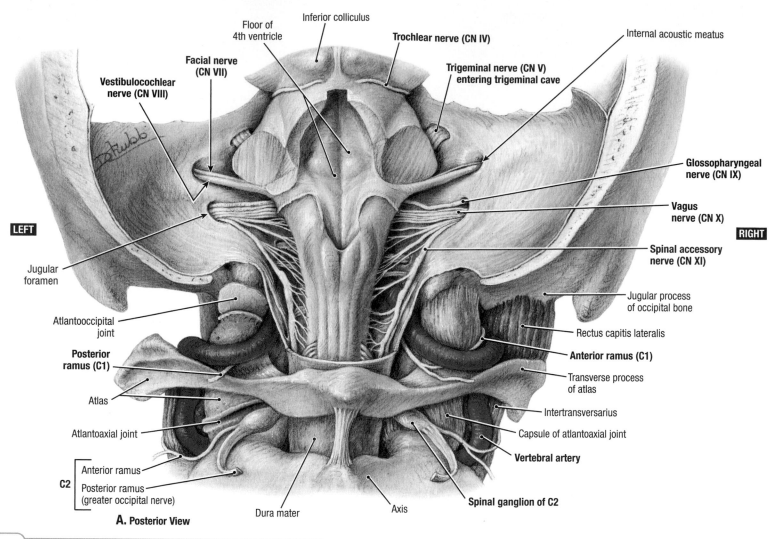

Inferior colliculus

Floor of
4th ventricle

Trochlear nerve (CN IV)

Internal acoustic meatus

Facial nerve
(CN VII)

Trigeminal nerve (CN V)
entering trigeminal cave

Vestibulocochlear
nerve (CN VIII)

Glossopharyngeal
nerve (CN IX)

Vagus
nerve (CN X)

LEFT

RIGHT

Spinal accessory
nerve (CN XI)

Jugular
foramen

Jugular process
of occipital bone

Atlantooccipital
joint

Rectus capitis lateralis

**Posterior
ramus (C1)**

Anterior ramus (C1)

Transverse process
of atlas

Atlas

Intertransversarius

Atlantoaxial joint

Capsule of atlantoaxial joint

Anterior ramus

Vertebral artery

C2

Posterior ramus
(greater occipital nerve)

Spinal ganglion of C2

Dura mater

Axis

A. Posterior View

8.28 Posterior Exposures of Cranial Nerves

A. Brainstem *in situ*. Squamous part of occipital bone has been removed posterior to foramen magnum to reveal dural cavity of posterior cranial fossa.
B. Brainstem removed (*right side*). The trochlear nerves (CN IV) arise from the dorsal aspect of the midbrain, just inferior to the inferior colliculi.

- The sensory and motor roots of the trigeminal nerves (CN V) pass anterolaterally to enter the mouth of the trigeminal cave.
- The facial (CN VII) and vestibulocochlear (CN VIII) nerves course laterally to enter the internal acoustic meatus.
- The glossopharyngeal nerve (CN IX) pierces the dura mater separately but passes with the vagus (CN X) and spinal accessory (CN XI) nerves through the jugular foramen.
- An **acoustic neuroma** (neurofibroma) is a slow-growing benign tumor of the neurolemma (Schwann) cells. The tumor begins in the vestibulocochlear nerve (CN VIII) while it is in the internal acoustic meatus. The early symptom of an acoustic neuroma is usually loss of hearing. Dysequilibrium and tinnitus also may occur.

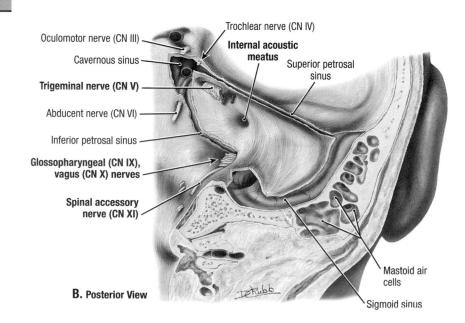

Oculomotor nerve (CN III)

Trochlear nerve (CN IV)

**Internal acoustic
meatus**

Cavernous sinus

Superior petrosal
sinus

Trigeminal nerve (CN V)

Abducent nerve (CN VI)

Inferior petrosal sinus

**Glossopharyngeal (CN IX),
vagus (CN X) nerves**

**Spinal accessory
nerve (CN XI)**

Mastoid air
cells

B. Posterior View

Sigmoid sinus

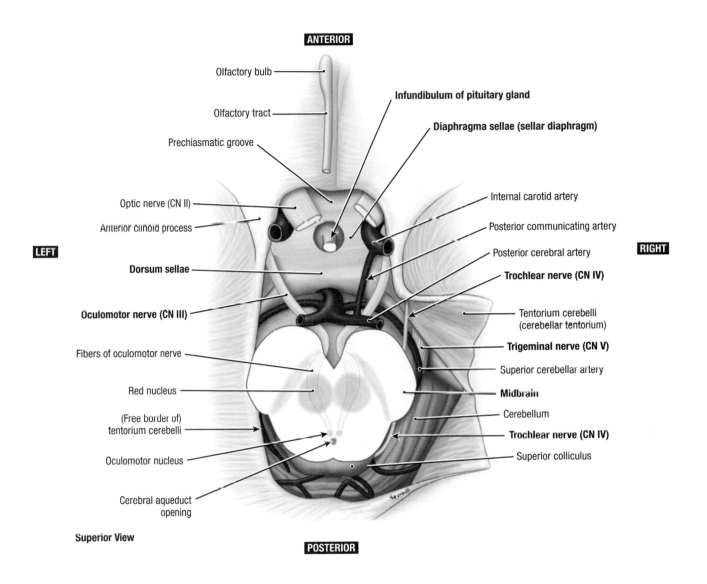

ANTERIOR

Olfactory bulb

Olfactory tract

Prechiasmatic groove

Infundibulum of pituitary gland

Diaphragma sellae (sellar diaphragm)

Optic nerve (CN II)

Anterior clinoid process

LEFT

RIGHT

Internal carotid artery

Posterior communicating artery

Posterior cerebral artery

Dorsum sellae

Trochlear nerve (CN IV)

Oculomotor nerve (CN III)

Tentorium cerebelli
(cerebellar tentorium)

Trigeminal nerve (CN V)

Fibers of oculomotor nerve

Superior cerebellar artery

Red nucleus

Midbrain

Cerebellum

(Free border of)
tentorium cerebelli

Trochlear nerve (CN IV)

Oculomotor nucleus

Superior colliculus

Cerebral aqueduct
opening

Superior View

POSTERIOR

Tentorial Notch   **8.29**

- The brain has been removed by cutting through the midbrain, revealing the tentorial notch through which the brainstem extends from the posterior into the middle cranial fossa.
- On the right side of the specimen, the tentorium cerebelli is divided and reflected. The trochlear nerve (CN IV) passes around the midbrain under the free edge of the tentorium cerebelli; the roots of the trigeminal nerve (CN V) enter the mouth of the trigeminal cave.
- There is a circular opening in the diaphragma sellae for the infundibulum, the stalk of the pituitary gland.
- The oculomotor nerve (CN III) passes between the posterior cerebral and superior cerebellar arteries and then laterally around the posterior clinoid process.

- The tentorial notch is the opening in the tentorium cerebelli for the brainstem, which is slightly larger than is necessary to accommodate the midbrain. Hence, space-occupying lesions, such as tumors in the supratentorial compartment, produce increased intracranial pressure that may cause part of the adjacent temporal lobe of the brain to herniate through the tentorial notch. During **tentorial herniation**, the temporal lobe may be lacerated by the tough tentorium cerebelli, and the oculomotor nerve (CN III) may be stretched, compressed, or both. Oculomotor lesions may produce paralysis of the extrinsic eye muscles supplied by CN III.

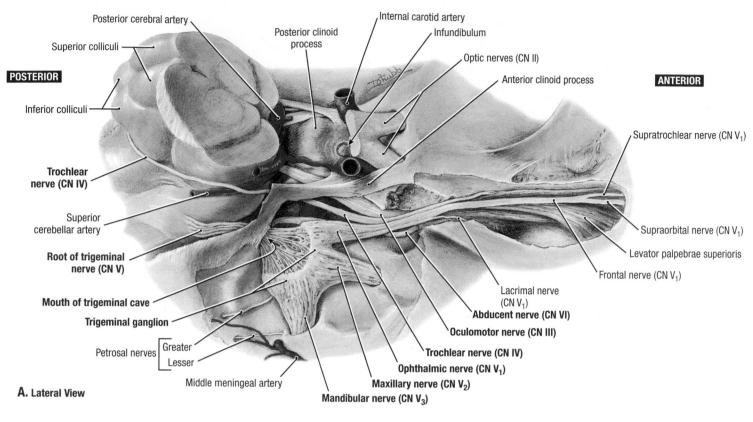

Posterior cerebral artery

Superior colliculi

POSTERIOR

Inferior colliculi

Trochlear nerve (CN IV)

Superior cerebellar artery

Root of trigeminal nerve (CN V)

Mouth of trigeminal cave

Trigeminal ganglion

Petrosal nerves [Greater / Lesser]

Middle meningeal artery

A. Lateral View

Posterior clinoid process

Internal carotid artery

Infundibulum

Optic nerves (CN II)

Anterior clinoid process

ANTERIOR

Supratrochlear nerve (CN V₁)

Supraorbital nerve (CN V₁)

Levator palpebrae superioris

Frontal nerve (CN V₁)

Lacrimal nerve (CN V₁)

Abducent nerve (CN VI)

Oculomotor nerve (CN III)

Trochlear nerve (CN IV)

Ophthalmic nerve (CN V₁)

Maxillary nerve (CN V₂)

Mandibular nerve (CN V₃)

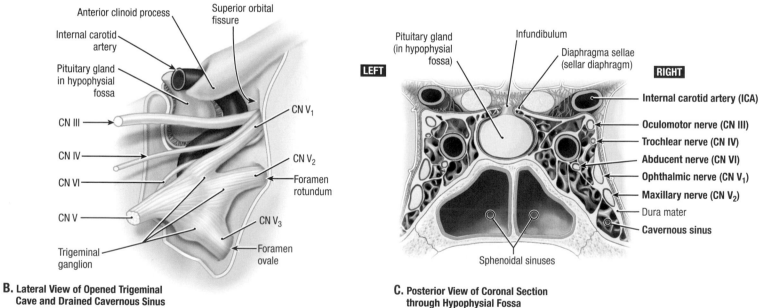

Anterior clinoid process

Superior orbital fissure

Internal carotid artery

Pituitary gland in hypophysial fossa

CN III

CN IV

CN VI

CN V

Trigeminal ganglion

CN V₁

CN V₂

Foramen rotundum

CN V₃

Foramen ovale

B. Lateral View of Opened Trigeminal Cave and Drained Cavernous Sinus

Pituitary gland (in hypophysial fossa)

Infundibulum

Diaphragma sellae (sellar diaphragm)

LEFT

RIGHT

Internal carotid artery (ICA)

Oculomotor nerve (CN III)

Trochlear nerve (CN IV)

Abducent nerve (CN VI)

Ophthalmic nerve (CN V₁)

Maxillary nerve (CN V₂)

Dura mater

Cavernous sinus

Sphenoidal sinuses

C. Posterior View of Coronal Section through Hypophysial Fossa

8.30 **Nerves and Vessels of Middle Cranial Fossa (I)**

A. Superficial dissection. The tentorium cerebelli is cut away. The dura mater is largely removed from the middle cranial fossa. The roof of the orbit is partly removed. **B. Relationship of oculomotor, trochlear, trigeminal, and abducent nerves to internal carotid artery. C. Coronal section through hypophysial fossa and cavernous sinuses.**

In fractures of the cranial base, the internal carotid artery may be torn, producing an arteriovenous fistula within the cavernous sinus. Arterial blood rushes into the sinus, enlarging it and forcing retrograde blood flow into its venous tributaries, especially the ophthalmic veins. As a result, the eyeball protrudes (exophthalmos) and the conjunctiva becomes engorged (chemosis). Because CN III, CN IV, CN VI, CN V₁, and CN V₂ lie in or close to the lateral wall of the cavernous sinus, these nerves may also be affected.

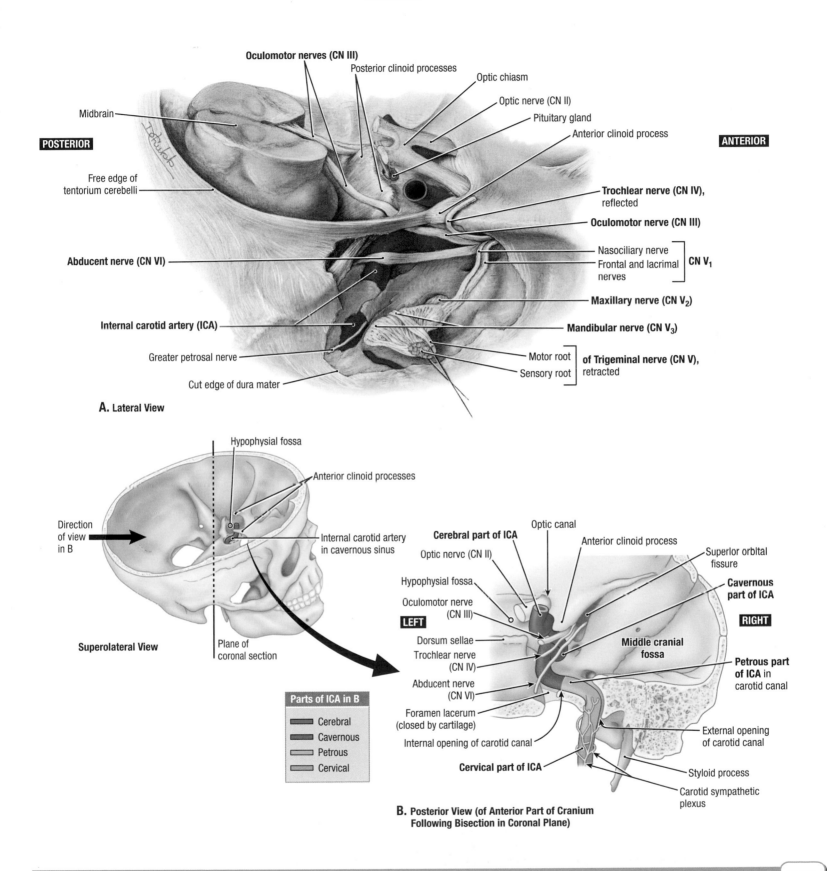

A. Lateral View

Oculomotor nerves (CN III)
Posterior clinoid processes
Optic chiasm
Optic nerve (CN II)
Pituitary gland
Anterior clinoid process
Midbrain
POSTERIOR
ANTERIOR
Free edge of tentorium cerebelli
Trochlear nerve (CN IV), reflected
Oculomotor nerve (CN III)
Nasociliary nerve
Frontal and lacrimal nerves
CN V₁
Abducent nerve (CN VI)
Maxillary nerve (CN V₂)
Internal carotid artery (ICA)
Mandibular nerve (CN V₃)
Greater petrosal nerve
Motor root
Sensory root
of Trigeminal nerve (CN V), retracted
Cut edge of dura mater

Hypophysial fossa
Anterior clinoid processes
Direction of view in B
Internal carotid artery in cavernous sinus
Superolateral View
Plane of coronal section

Parts of ICA in B
Cerebral
Cavernous
Petrous
Cervical

Optic canal
Cerebral part of ICA
Anterior clinoid process
Optic nerve (CN II)
Superior orbital fissure
Hypophysial fossa
Cavernous part of ICA
Oculomotor nerve (CN III)
LEFT
RIGHT
Dorsum sellae
Trochlear nerve (CN IV)
Middle cranial fossa
Petrous part of ICA in carotid canal
Abducent nerve (CN VI)
Foramen lacerum (closed by cartilage)
Internal opening of carotid canal
External opening of carotid canal
Cervical part of ICA
Styloid process
Carotid sympathetic plexus

B. Posterior View (of Anterior Part of Cranium Following Bisection in Coronal Plane)

Nerves and Vessels of Middle Cranial Fossa (II)

8.31

A. Deep dissection. The roots of the trigeminal nerve are divided, withdrawn from the mouth of the trigeminal cave, and turned anteriorly. The trochlear nerve is reflected anteriorly. **B. Course of internal carotid artery.**

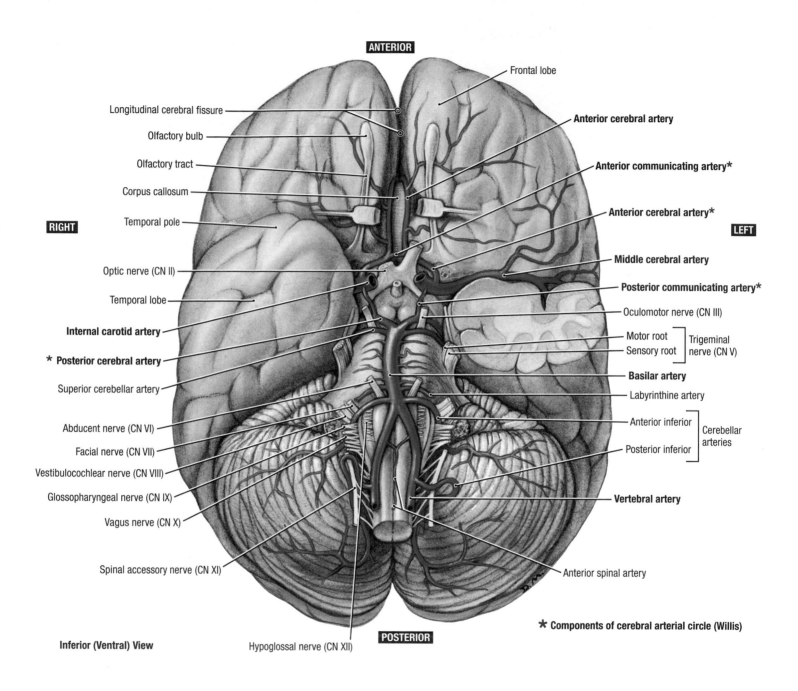

ANTERIOR

Frontal lobe

Longitudinal cerebral fissure

Olfactory bulb

Olfactory tract

Corpus callosum

RIGHT

Temporal pole

Optic nerve (CN II)

Temporal lobe

Internal carotid artery

* Posterior cerebral artery

Superior cerebellar artery

Abducent nerve (CN VI)

Facial nerve (CN VII)

Vestibulocochlear nerve (CN VIII)

Glossopharyngeal nerve (CN IX)

Vagus nerve (CN X)

Spinal accessory nerve (CN XI)

Anterior cerebral artery

Anterior communicating artery*

Anterior cerebral artery*

LEFT

Middle cerebral artery

Posterior communicating artery*

Oculomotor nerve (CN III)

Motor root ⎤ Trigeminal
Sensory root ⎦ nerve (CN V)

Basilar artery

Labyrinthine artery

Anterior inferior ⎤ Cerebellar
Posterior inferior ⎦ arteries

Vertebral artery

Anterior spinal artery

* Components of cerebral arterial circle (Willis)

Inferior (Ventral) View   Hypoglossal nerve (CN XII)   POSTERIOR

8.32   **Base of Brain and Cerebral Arterial Circle**

The anterior part of the left temporal lobe is removed to enable visualization of the middle cerebral artery in the lateral fissure. The frontal lobes are separated to expose the anterior cerebral arteries and corpus callosum.

An **ischemic stroke** denotes the sudden development of neurological deficits that are consequences of impaired cerebral blood flow. The most common causes of strokes are spontaneous cerebrovascular accidents such as cerebral embolism, thrombosis, or hemorrhage, and subarachnoid hemorrhage. The cerebral arterial circle is an important means of collateral circulation in the event of gradual obstruction of one of the major arteries forming the circle. Sudden

occlusion, even if only partial, results in neurological deficits. In elderly persons, the anastomoses are often inadequate when a large artery (e.g., internal carotid) is occluded, even if the occlusion is gradual. In such cases, function is impaired at least to some degree.

Hemorrhagic stroke follows the rupture of an artery or a saccular aneurysm, a saclike dilation on a weak part of the arterial wall. The most common type of saccular aneurysm is a berry aneurysm, occurring in the vessels of or near the cerebral arterial circle. In time, especially in people with hypertension (high blood pressure), the weak part of the arterial wall expands and may rupture, allowing blood to enter the subarachnoid space.

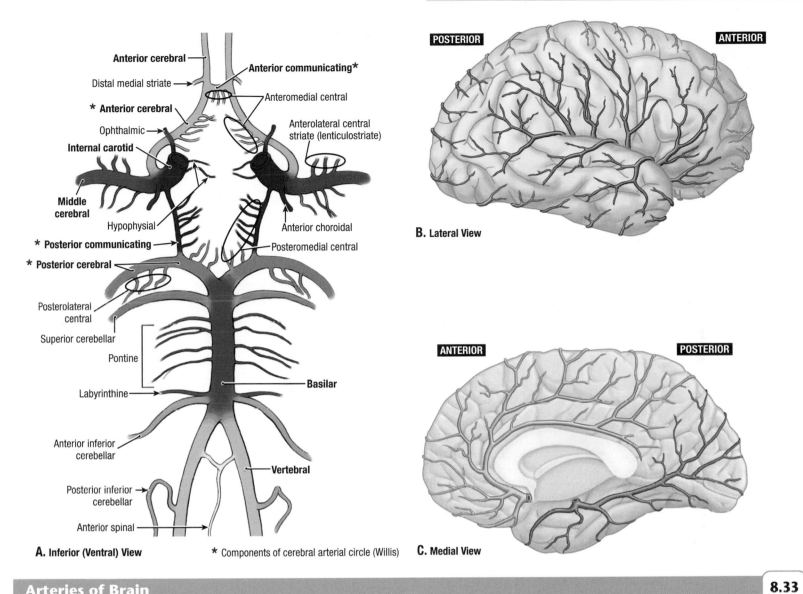

A. Inferior (Ventral) View

* Components of cerebral arterial circle (Willis)

B. Lateral View

C. Medial View

Arteries of Brain

8.33

A. Schematic overview. **B.** and **C.** Distribution of anterior, middle, and posterior cerebral arteries.

TABLE 8.7	Arterial Supply to Brain	
Artery	**Origin**	**Distribution**
Vertebral	Subclavian artery	Cranial meninges and cerebellum
Posterior inferior cerebellar	Vertebral artery	Extraocular aspect of cerebellum
Basilar	Formed by junction of vertebral arteries	Brainstem, cerebellum, and cerebrum
Pontine		Numerous branches to brainstem
Anterior inferior cerebellar	Basilar artery	Inferior aspect of cerebellum
Superior cerebellar		Superior aspect of cerebellum
Internal carotid	Common carotid artery at superior border of thyroid cartilage	Gives branches in cavernous sinus and provides supply to brain
Anterior cerebral	Internal carotid artery	Cerebral hemispheres, except for occipital lobes
Middle cerebral	Continuation of the internal carotid artery distal to anterior cerebral artery	Most of lateral surface of cerebral hemispheres
Posterior cerebral	Terminal branch of basilar artery	Inferior aspect of cerebral hemisphere and occipital lobe
Anterior communicating	Anterior cerebral artery	Cerebral arterial circle
Posterior communicating	Internal carotid artery	

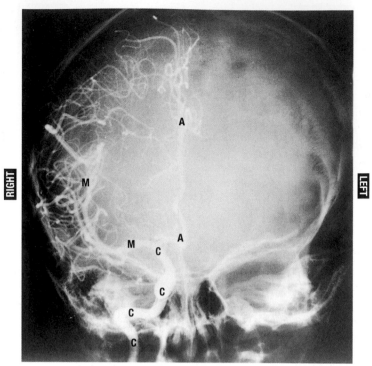

A. Posteroanterior Angiogram

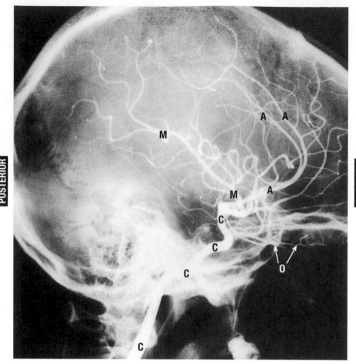

B. Lateral Angiogram

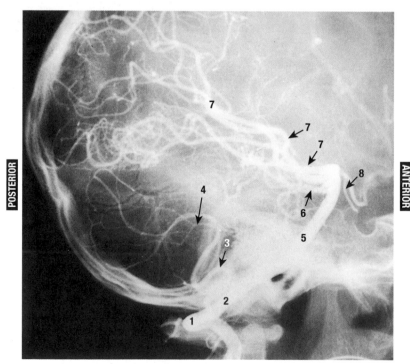

C. Lateral Angiogram

A	Anterior cerebral artery
C	Internal carotid artery
M	Middle cerebral artery
O	Ophthalmic artery
1	Vertebral artery on posterior arch of atlas
2	Vertebral artery entering skull through foramen magnum
3	Posterior inferior cerebellar artery
4	Anterior inferior cerebellar artery
5	Basilar artery
6	Superior cerebellar artery
7	Posterior cerebral artery
8	Posterior communicating artery

8.34   **Cerebral Angiograms**

A. and **B. Carotid angiogram.** The four Cs indicate the parts of the internal carotid artery: cervical, before entering the cranium; petrous, within the temporal bone; cavernous, within the sinus; and cerebral, within the cranial subarachnoid space. **C. Vertebral angiogram.**

Transient ischemic attacks (TIAs) refer to neurological symptoms resulting from ischemia (deficient blood supply) of the brain.

The symptoms of a TIA may be ambiguous: staggering, dizziness, light-headedness, fainting, and paresthesias (e.g., tingling in a limb). Most TIAs last a few minutes, but some persist longer. Individuals with TIAs are at increased risk for myocardial infarction and *ischemic stroke.*

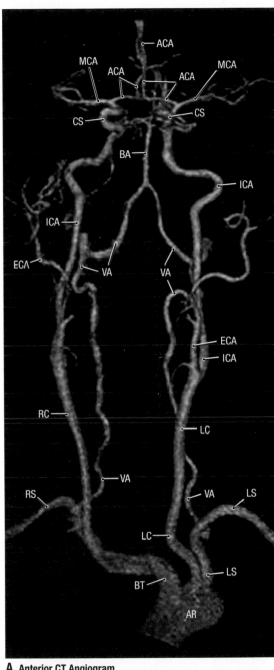

A. Anterior CT Angiogram

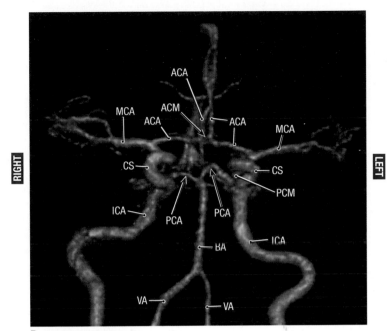

B. Anterior CT Angiogram

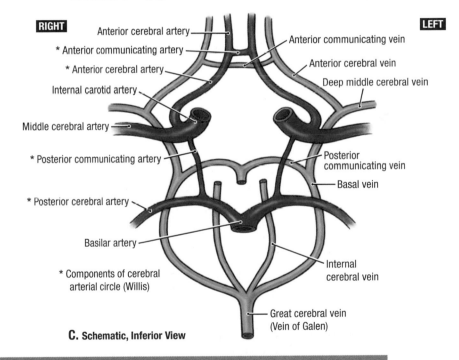

C. Schematic, Inferior View

Anterior cerebral artery

* Anterior communicating artery

* Anterior cerebral artery

Internal carotid artery

Middle cerebral artery

* Posterior communicating artery

* Posterior cerebral artery

Basilar artery

* Components of cerebral arterial circle (Willis)

Anterior communicating vein

Anterior cerebral vein

Deep middle cerebral vein

Posterior communicating vein

Basal vein

Internal cerebral vein

Great cerebral vein (Vein of Galen)

Key for A and B							
ACA	Anterior cerebral artery	**BT**	Brachiocephalic trunk	**LC**	Left common carotid artery	**PCM**	Posterior communicating artery
ACM	Anterior communicating artery	**CS**	Carotid siphon	**LS**	Left subclavian artery	**RC**	Right common carotid artery
AR	Arch of aorta	**ECA**	External carotid artery	**MCA**	Middle cerebral artery	**RS**	Right subclavian artery
BA	Basilar artery	**ICA**	Internal carotid artery	**PCA**	Posterior cerebral artery	**VA**	Vertebral artery

Blood Supply of Head and Neck

A. CT angiogram of arteries of head and neck. **B.** CT angiogram of cerebral arterial circle (circle of Willis). **C.** Schematic of cerebral arterial circle and veins of cerebral base.

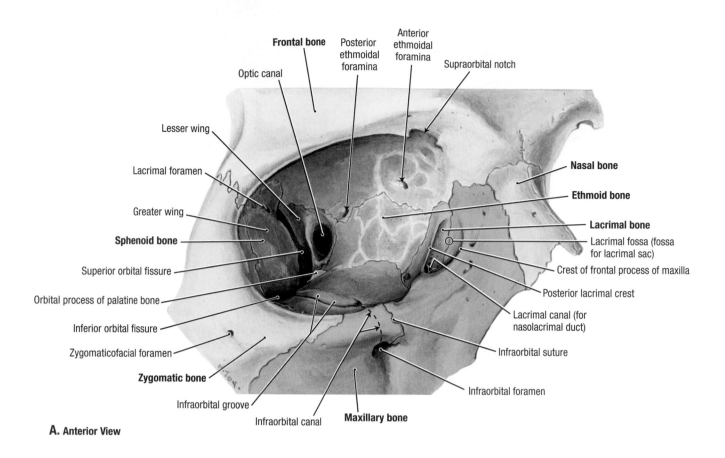

Frontal bone
Posterior ethmoidal foramina
Anterior ethmoidal foramina
Supraorbital notch
Optic canal
Lesser wing
Nasal bone
Lacrimal foramen
Ethmoid bone
Greater wing
Lacrimal bone
Sphenoid bone
Lacrimal fossa (fossa for lacrimal sac)
Superior orbital fissure
Crest of frontal process of maxilla
Orbital process of palatine bone
Posterior lacrimal crest
Inferior orbital fissure
Lacrimal canal (for nasolacrimal duct)
Zygomaticofacial foramen
Infraorbital suture
Zygomatic bone
Infraorbital foramen
Infraorbital groove
Infraorbital canal
Maxillary bone

A. Anterior View

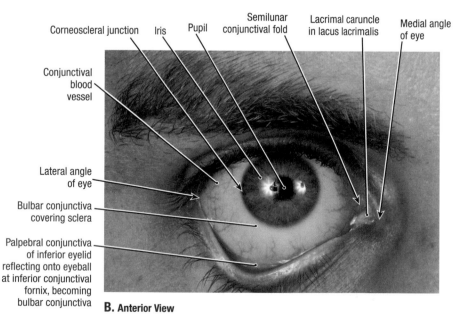

Corneoscleral junction
Iris
Pupil
Semilunar conjunctival fold
Lacrimal caruncle in lacus lacrimalis
Medial angle of eye
Conjunctival blood vessel
Lateral angle of eye
Bulbar conjunctiva covering sclera
Palpebral conjunctiva of inferior eyelid reflecting onto eyeball at inferior conjunctival fornix, becoming bulbar conjunctiva

B. Anterior View

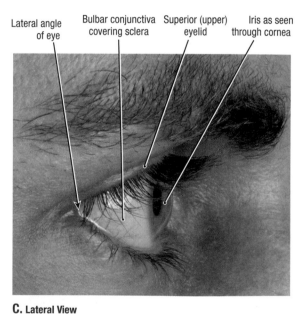

Lateral angle of eye
Bulbar conjunctiva covering sclera
Superior (upper) eyelid
Iris as seen through cornea

C. Lateral View

8.36 **Orbital Cavity and Surface Anatomy of Eye**

A. Bones and features of orbital cavity. B. and C. Surface anatomy of eye. The inferior eyelid is everted to demonstrate the palpebral conjunctiva (*Part B*). When powerful blows impact directly on the bony rim of the orbit, the resulting orbital fractures usually occur at the sutures between the bones forming the orbital margin. Fractures of the inferior wall may involve the maxillary sinus; fractures of the medial wall are less common and may involve the ethmoidal and sphenoidal sinuses. Although the superior wall is stronger, it is thin enough to be translucent and may be readily penetrated. Thus, a sharp object may pass through it into the frontal lobe of the brain. Orbital fractures often result in intraorbital bleeding, which exerts pressure on the eyeball, causing **exophthalmos** (protrusion of the eyeball).

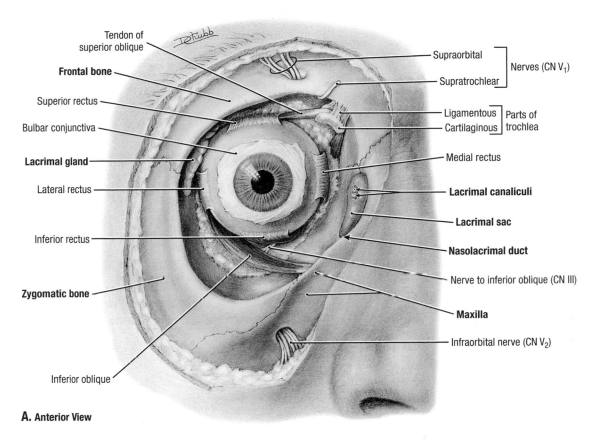

Tendon of superior oblique

Supraorbital ⎤
Supratrochlear ⎦ Nerves (CN V₁)

Frontal bone

Superior rectus

Ligamentous ⎤ Parts of
Cartilaginous ⎦ trochlea

Bulbar conjunctiva

Lacrimal gland

Medial rectus

Lateral rectus

Lacrimal canaliculi

Lacrimal sac

Inferior rectus

Nasolacrimal duct

Nerve to inferior oblique (CN III)

Zygomatic bone

Maxilla

Infraorbital nerve (CN V₂)

Inferior oblique

A. Anterior View

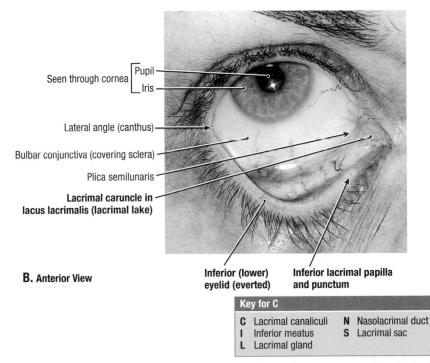

Seen through cornea ⎡ Pupil
⎣ Iris

Lateral angle (canthus)

Bulbar conjunctiva (covering sclera)

Plica semilunaris

**Lacrimal caruncle in
lacus lacrimalis (lacrimal lake)**

B. Anterior View

**Inferior (lower)
eyelid (everted)**

**Inferior lacrimal papilla
and punctum**

Key for C			
C	Lacrimal canaliculi	**N**	Nasolacrimal duct
I	Inferior meatus	**S**	Lacrimal sac
L	Lacrimal gland		

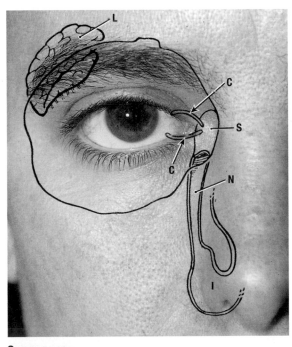

C. Anterior View

Eye and Lacrimal Apparatus

8.37

A. Anterior dissection of orbital cavity. The eyelids, orbital septum, levator palpebrae superioris, and some fats are removed. **B. Surface features, with inferior eyelid everted. C. Surface projection of lacrimal apparatus.** Tears, secreted by the lacrimal gland in the superolateral angle of the bony orbit, pass across the eyeball and enter the lacus lacrimalis (lacrimal lake) at the medial angle of the eye; from here they drain through the lacrimal puncta and lacrimal canaliculi to the lacrimal sac. The lacrimal sac drains into the nasolacrimal duct, which empties into the inferior meatus of the nasal cavity.

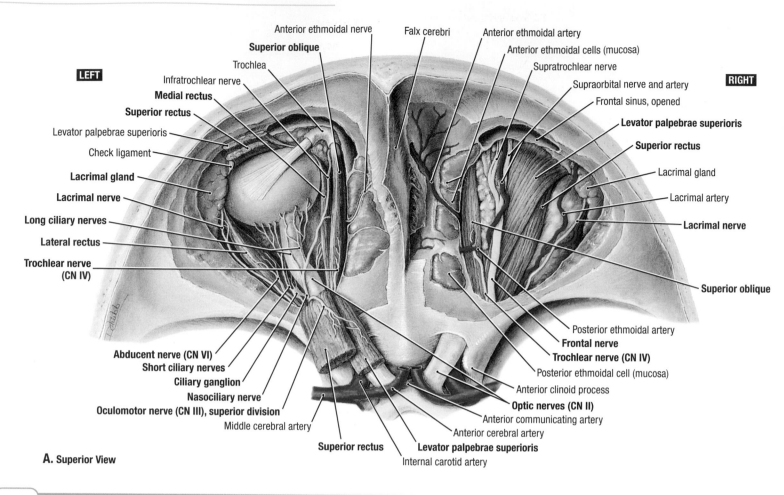

Anterior ethmoidal nerve

Superior oblique

Trochlea

Infratrochlear nerve

Medial rectus

Superior rectus

Levator palpebrae superioris

Check ligament

Lacrimal gland

Lacrimal nerve

Long ciliary nerves

Lateral rectus

Trochlear nerve (CN IV)

Abducent nerve (CN VI)

Short ciliary nerves

Ciliary ganglion

Nasociliary nerve

Oculomotor nerve (CN III), superior division

Middle cerebral artery

Falx cerebri

Anterior ethmoidal artery

Anterior ethmoidal cells (mucosa)

Supratrochlear nerve

Supraorbital nerve and artery

Frontal sinus, opened

Levator palpebrae superioris

Superior rectus

Lacrimal gland

Lacrimal artery

Lacrimal nerve

Superior oblique

Posterior ethmoidal artery

Frontal nerve

Trochlear nerve (CN IV)

Posterior ethmoidal cell (mucosa)

Anterior clinoid process

Optic nerves (CN II)

Anterior communicating artery

Anterior cerebral artery

Superior rectus

Levator palpebrae superioris

Internal carotid artery

A. Superior View

LEFT

RIGHT

8.38 Orbital Cavity, Superior Approach

A. Superficial dissection. On the right side, the orbital plate of the frontal bone is removed. On the left side, the levator palpebrae and superior rectus muscles are reflected.

- The trochlear nerve (CN IV) lies on the medial side of the superior oblique muscle, and the abducent nerve (CN VI) on the medial side of the lateral rectus muscle.
- The lacrimal nerve runs superior to the lateral rectus muscle supplying sensory fibers to the conjunctiva and skin of the superior eyelid; it receives a communicating branch of the zygomaticotemporal nerve carrying secretory motor fibers from the pterygopalatine ganglion prior to entering or within the lacrimal gland.
- The parasympathetic ciliary ganglion, placed between the lateral rectus muscle and the optic nerve (CN II), gives rise to many short ciliary nerves; the nasociliary nerve gives rise to two long ciliary nerves that anastomose with each other and the short ciliary nerves.

B. Distribution of nerve fibers to ciliary ganglion and eyeball.

Horner syndrome results from interruption of a cervical sympathetic trunk and is manifest by the absence of sympathetically stimulated functions on the ipsilateral side of the head. The syndrome includes the following signs: constriction of the pupil (**miosis**), drooping of the superior eyelid (**ptosis**), redness and increased temperature of the skin (**vasodilatation**), and absence of sweating (**anhidrosis**).

- The ciliary ganglion receives sensory fibers from the nasociliary branches of CN VI, postsynaptic sympathetic fibers from the continuation of the internal carotid plexus extending along the ophthalmic artery, and presynaptic parasympathetic fibers from the inferior branch of the oculomotor nerve; only the latter synapse in the ganglion.

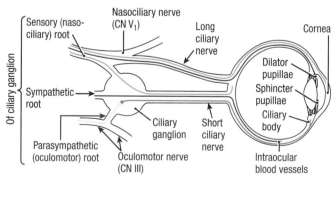

Sensory (naso-ciliary) root

Nasociliary nerve (CN V$_1$)

Long ciliary nerve

Cornea

Dilator pupillae

Sphincter pupillae

Ciliary body

Of ciliary ganglion

Sympathetic root

Ciliary ganglion

Short ciliary nerve

Parasympathetic (oculomotor) root

Oculomotor nerve (CN III)

Intraocular blood vessels

B. Schematic, Distribution of Nerve Fibers to Ciliary Ganglion and Eyeball

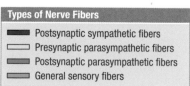

Types of Nerve Fibers

- Postsynaptic sympathetic fibers
- Presynaptic parasympathetic fibers
- Postsynaptic parasympathetic fibers
- General sensory fibers

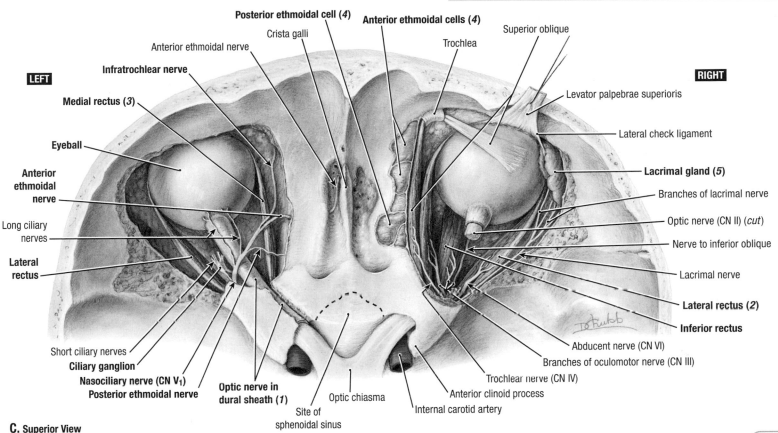

Posterior ethmoidal cell (*4*)

Anterior ethmoidal nerve

Crista galli

Anterior ethmoidal cells (*4*)

Superior oblique

Trochlea

Infratrochlear nerve

LEFT

RIGHT

Levator palpebrae superioris

Medial rectus (*3*)

Eyeball

Lateral check ligament

Anterior ethmoidal nerve

Lacrimal gland (*5*)

Branches of lacrimal nerve

Long ciliary nerves

Optic nerve (CN II) (*cut*)

Nerve to inferior oblique

Lateral rectus

Lacrimal nerve

Lateral rectus (*2*)

Inferior rectus

Short ciliary nerves

Abducent nerve (CN VI)

Ciliary ganglion

Branches of oculomotor nerve (CN III)

Nasociliary nerve (CN V₁)

Trochlear nerve (CN IV)

Posterior ethmoidal nerve

Optic nerve in dural sheath (*1*)

Anterior clinoid process

Optic chiasma

Internal carotid artery

Site of sphenoidal sinus

C. Superior View

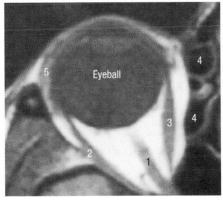

Eyeball

D. Transverse MRI of Orbit

Orbital Cavity, Superior Approach (*continued*)   **8.38**

C. Deep dissection. On the left side of the specimen, the optic nerve (CN II) is intact; on the right side the optic nerve (CN II) is sectioned. **D. Transverse (axial) MRI of orbital cavity.** The numbers refer to structures labeled in *Part C*.

Observe on the right side of *Part C*:

• The eyeball occupies the anterior half of the orbital cavity.

Observe on the left of *Part C*:

• The parasympathetic ciliary ganglion lies posteriorly between the lateral rectus muscle and the sheath of the optic nerve.

• The nasociliary nerve (CN V₁) sends a branch to the ciliary ganglion and crosses the optic nerve (CN II), where it gives off two long ciliary nerves (sensory to the eyeball and cornea) and the posterior ethmoidal nerve (to the sphenoidal sinus and posterior ethmoidal cells). The nasociliary nerve then divides into the anterior ethmoidal and infratrochlear nerves.

TABLE 8.8	**Muscles of Orbit**			
Muscle	**Origin**	**Insertion**	**Innervation**	**Main Action(s)**[a]
Levator palpebrae superioris	Lesser wing of sphenoid bone, superior and anterior to optic canal	Superior tarsus and skin of superior eyelid	Oculomotor nerve; deep layer (superior tarsal muscle) supplied by sympathetic fibers	Elevates superior eyelid
Superior oblique (SO)	Body of sphenoid bone	Tendon passes through trochlea to insert into sclera, deep to SR	Trochlear nerve (CN IV)	Rotates eyeball medially (intorsion) and abducts and depresses eyeball
Inferior oblique (IO)	Anterior part of floor of orbit	Sclera deep to lateral rectus muscle	Oculomotor nerve (CN III)	Rotates eyeball laterally (extorsion) and abducts and elevates eyeball
Superior rectus (SR)	Common tendinous ring	Sclera just posterior to corneoscleral junction		Rotates eyeball medially (intorsion) and elevates and adducts eyeball
Inferior rectus (IR)				Rotates eyeball laterally (extorsion) and depresses and adducts eyeball
Medial rectus (MR)				Adducts eyeball
Lateral rectus (LR)			Abducent nerve (CN VI)	Abducts eyeball

[a]It is essential to appreciate that all muscles are continuously involved in eyeball movements; thus, the individual actions are not usually tested clinically.

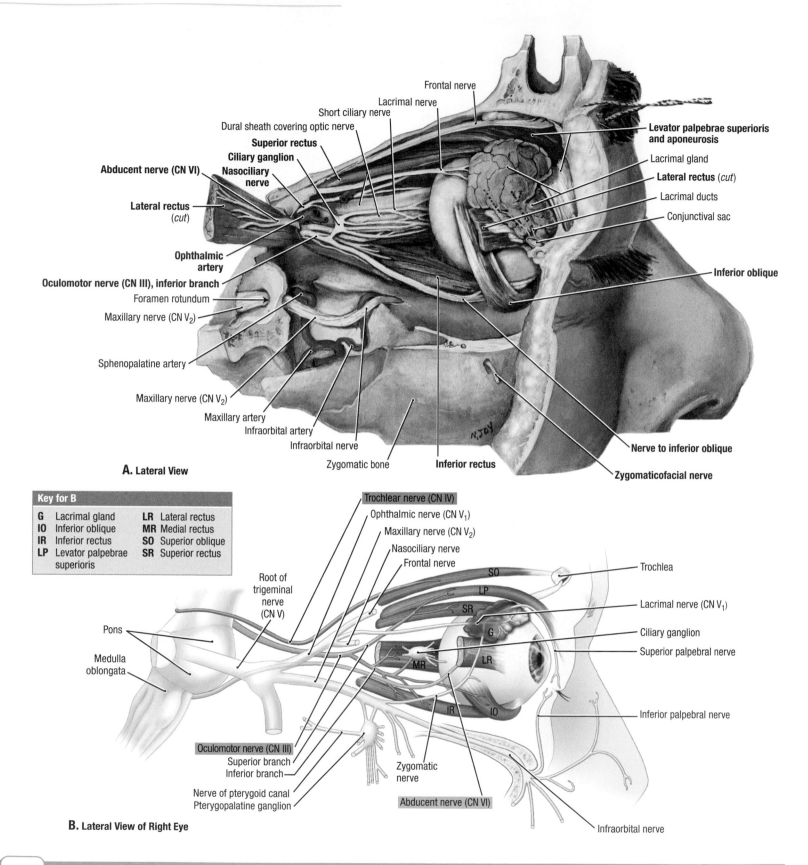

Frontal nerve
Lacrimal nerve
Short ciliary nerve
Dural sheath covering optic nerve
Superior rectus
Ciliary ganglion
Abducent nerve (CN VI) **Nasociliary nerve**
Lateral rectus (cut)
Ophthalmic artery
Oculomotor nerve (CN III), inferior branch
Foramen rotundum
Maxillary nerve (CN V₂)
Sphenopalatine artery
Maxillary nerve (CN V₂)
Maxillary artery
Infraorbital artery
Infraorbital nerve
Zygomatic bone
Inferior rectus

Levator palpebrae superioris and aponeurosis
Lacrimal gland
Lateral rectus (cut)
Lacrimal ducts
Conjunctival sac
Inferior oblique
Nerve to inferior oblique
Zygomaticofacial nerve

A. Lateral View

Key for B

G	Lacrimal gland	**LR**	Lateral rectus
IO	Inferior oblique	**MR**	Medial rectus
IR	Inferior rectus	**SO**	Superior oblique
LP	Levator palpebrae superioris	**SR**	Superior rectus

Trochlear nerve (CN IV)
Ophthalmic nerve (CN V₁)
Maxillary nerve (CN V₂)
Nasociliary nerve
Frontal nerve
Root of trigeminal nerve (CN V)
Pons
Medulla oblongata
Oculomotor nerve (CN III)
Superior branch
Inferior branch
Nerve of pterygoid canal
Pterygopalatine ganglion
Zygomatic nerve
Abducent nerve (CN VI)

SO
LP
SR
G
MR
LR
IR
IO

Trochlea
Lacrimal nerve (CN V₁)
Ciliary ganglion
Superior palpebral nerve
Inferior palpebral nerve
Infraorbital nerve

B. Lateral View of Right Eye

8.39 **Lateral Aspect of Orbit and Structure of Eyelid**

A. Dissection. B. Nerves. C. Sagittal and cross section through optic nerve. The subarachnoid space around the optic nerve is continuous with the subarachnoid space around the brain.

D. Sagittal MRI. The numbers refer to structures labeled in *Part C.* *Circled area,* optic foramen; *M,* maxillary sinus; *S,* superior ophthalmic vein. **E. Structure of eyelid.**

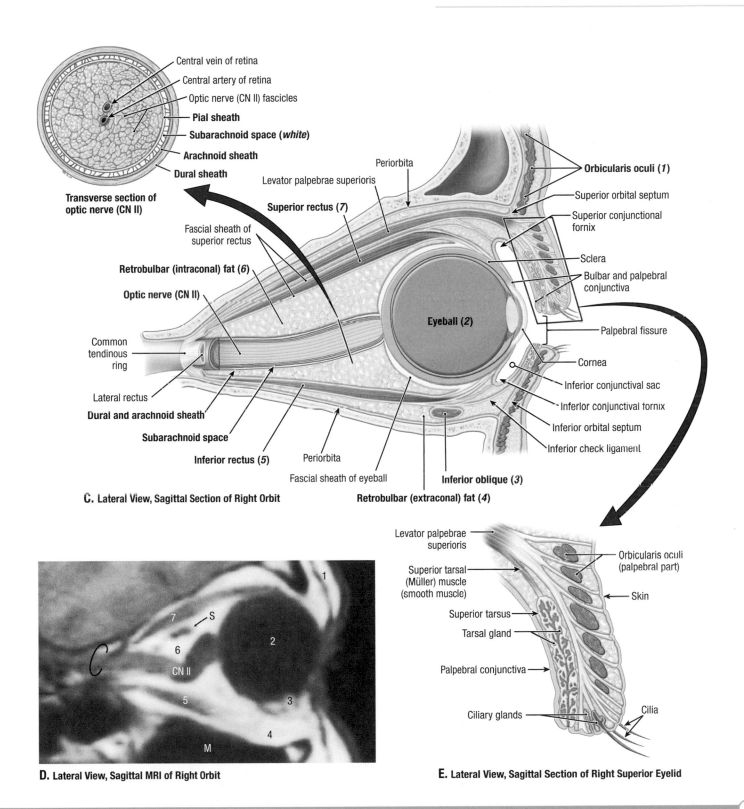

Central vein of retina
Central artery of retina
Optic nerve (CN II) fascicles
Pial sheath
Subarachnoid space (*white*)
Arachnoid sheath
Dural sheath

Transverse section of optic nerve (CN II)

Periorbita
Levator palpebrae superioris

Orbicularis oculi (*1*)
Superior orbital septum
Superior conjunctional fornix

Fascial sheath of superior rectus
Superior rectus (*7*)

Sclera
Bulbar and palpebral conjunctiva

Retrobulbar (intraconal) fat (*6*)

Optic nerve (CN II)

Eyeball (*2*)

Palpebral fissure

Common tendinous ring

Cornea

Lateral rectus
Dural and arachnoid sheath
Subarachnoid space

Inferior conjunctival sac
Inferior conjunctival fornix
Inferior orbital septum
Inferior check ligament

Inferior rectus (*5*)   Periorbita
Fascial sheath of eyeball   **Inferior oblique** (*3*)
Retrobulbar (extraconal) fat (*4*)

C. Lateral View, Sagittal Section of Right Orbit

D. Lateral View, Sagittal MRI of Right Orbit

Levator palpebrae superioris

Orbicularis oculi (palpebral part)

Superior tarsal (Müller) muscle (smooth muscle)

Skin

Superior tarsus
Tarsal gland

Palpebral conjunctiva

Ciliary glands

Cilia

E. Lateral View, Sagittal Section of Right Superior Eyelid

Lateral Aspect of Orbit and Structure of Eyelid (*continued*)   **8.39**

- Foreign objects, such as sand or metal filings, produce **corneal abrasions** that cause sudden, stabbing eye pain and tears. Opening and closing the eyelids is also painful. **Corneal lacerations** are caused by sharp objects such as fingernails or the corner of a page of a book.
- Any of the glands in the eyelid may become inflamed and swollen from infection or obstruction of their ducts. If the ducts of

the ciliary glands are obstructed, a painful red suppurative (pus-producing) swelling, a stye (**hordeolum**), develops on the eyelid. **Obstruction of a tarsal gland** produces inflammation, a **tarsal chalazion**, that protrudes toward the eyeball and rubs against it as the eyelids blink.

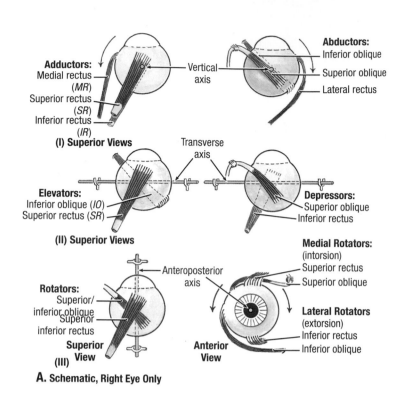

Adductors:
Medial rectus (*MR*)
Superior rectus (*SR*)
Inferior rectus (*IR*)

Vertical axis

Abductors:
Inferior oblique
Superior oblique
Lateral rectus

(I) Superior Views

Transverse axis

Elevators:
Inferior oblique (*IO*)
Superior rectus (*SR*)

Depressors:
Superior oblique
Inferior rectus

(II) Superior Views

Anteroposterior axis

Rotators:
Superior/inferior oblique
Superior inferior rectus

Superior View (III)

Medial Rotators: (intorsion)
Superior rectus
Superior oblique

Lateral Rotators: (extorsion)
Inferior rectus
Inferior oblique

Anterior View

A. Schematic, Right Eye Only

TABLE 8.9 Actions of Muscles of Orbit Starting from Primary Position[a]

Muscle	Main Action		
	Horizontal Axis (I)	Vertical Axis (II)	Anteroposterior Axis (III)
Superior rectus (SR)	Elevates	Adducts	Rotates medially (intorsion)
Inferior rectus (IR)	Depresses	Adducts	Rotates laterally (extorsion)
Superior oblique (SO)	Depresses	Abducts	Rotates medially (intorsion)
Inferior oblique (IO)	Elevates	Abducts	Rotates laterally (extorsion)
Medial rectus (MR)	N/A	Adducts	N/A
Lateral rectus (LR)	N/A	Abducts	N/A

[a]Primary position, gaze directed anteriorly.

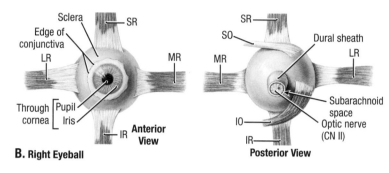

Sclera — SR
Edge of conjunctiva
LR
MR
Through cornea [Pupil / Iris]
IR **Anterior View**

SR
SO
MR
Dural sheath
LR
Subarachnoid space
Optic nerve (CN II)
IO
IR

B. Right Eyeball / **Posterior View**

8.40 **Extraocular Muscles and Their Movements**

A. Axes, muscle direction, and movements of right eye. The line of pull of the muscles relative to the eyeball and the axes around which movements occur. The orientation of the orbit is important in understanding the actions of the extraocular muscles. The common tendinous ring (origin of the recti), the origin of the inferior oblique, and the trochlea of the superior oblique all lie medial to the eyeball and to the anteroposterior (A-P) and vertical axes. (I) The medial and lateral recti are the primary adductors and abductors of the eyeball. However, when movements begin from the primary position (gaze directed anteriorly along the A-P axis): (1) the line of pull of the superior and inferior rectus muscles passes medial and anterior to the vertical axis, resulting in secondary actions of adduction; and (2) the line of pull of the superior and inferior oblique muscles passes medial and posterior to the vertical axis, resulting in secondary actions of abduction. (II) Pulling in opposite directions relative to the transverse axis, the superior rectus and inferior oblique muscles are synergistic elevators, and the inferior rectus and superior oblique are synergistic depressors. (III) Medial pull produced by the muscles attaching to the superior eyeball (superior rectus and oblique) produces secondary actions of medial rotation (intorsion), and that produced by muscles attaching to the inferior eyeball (inferior rectus and oblique) produces lateral rotation (extorsion). **B. Muscles of eyeball.**

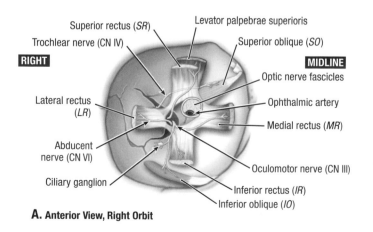

Superior rectus (*SR*)
Trochlear nerve (CN IV)
RIGHT
Lateral rectus (*LR*)
Abducent nerve (CN VI)
Ciliary ganglion
Levator palpebrae superioris
Superior oblique (*SO*)
MIDLINE
Optic nerve fascicles
Ophthalmic artery
Medial rectus (*MR*)
Oculomotor nerve (CN III)
Inferior rectus (*IR*)
Inferior oblique (*IO*)

A. Anterior View, Right Orbit

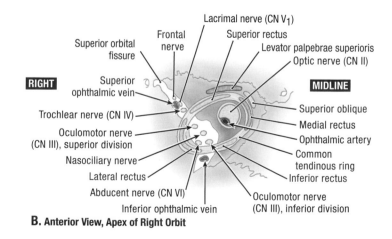

Lacrimal nerve (CN V₁)
Frontal nerve
Superior rectus
Levator palpebrae superioris
Optic nerve (CN II)
Superior orbital fissure
Superior ophthalmic vein
RIGHT
Trochlear nerve (CN IV)
Oculomotor nerve (CN III), superior division
Nasociliary nerve
Lateral rectus
Abducent nerve (CN VI)
Inferior ophthalmic vein
Superior oblique
MIDLINE
Medial rectus
Ophthalmic artery
Common tendinous ring
Inferior rectus
Oculomotor nerve (CN III), inferior division

B. Anterior View, Apex of Right Orbit

8.41 **Relationship of Nerves and Muscles at Apex of Orbit**

A. Eyeball enucleated. **B.** Tendinous ring and superior and inferior orbital fissures.

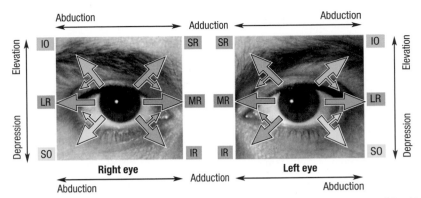

A. Anterior View, Single Movements Starting from Primary Position (*smaller arrows*, medial and lateral rotation)

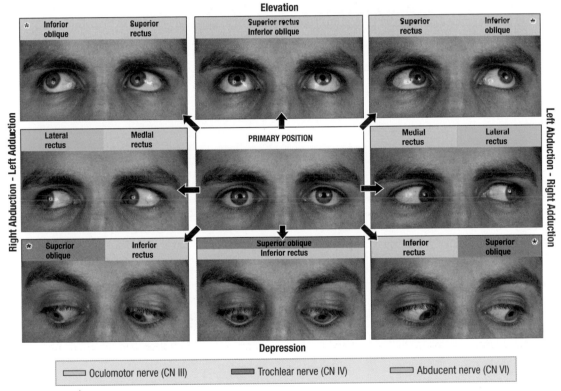

B. Anterior View, Single Movements Starting from Primary Position

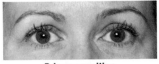

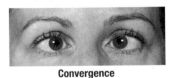

C. Anterior Views   **Primary position**   **Convergence**

Single Movements of Eye Starting from Primary Position

8.42

A. Movements produced by isolated contraction of four rectus and two oblique muscles, starting from primary position. *Large arrows* indicate prime movers for the six cardinal movements. Movements in directions between *large arrows* (e.g., vertical elevation or depression) require synergistic actions of adjacent muscles. Contralaterally paired muscles that work synergistically to direct parallel binocular gaze are called yoke muscles. For example, the right lateral rectus and left medial rectus act as yoke muscles in directing gaze to the right. **B. Anatomical movements of extraocular muscles** (single movements directly from primary position). **C. Convergence.**

Angle of gaze coinciding
with angle of muscle
ELEVATION ONLY

Angle of gaze coinciding
with angle of muscle
DEPRESSION ONLY

Angle of gaze coinciding
with angle of muscle
DEPRESSION ONLY

Angle of gaze coinciding
with angle of muscle
ELEVATION ONLY

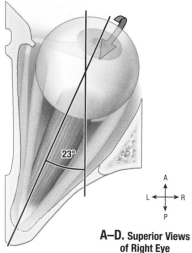

23°

23°

51°

51°

A
L ✛ R
P

A–D. Superior Views
of Right Eye

A. Superior Rectus

B. Inferior Rectus

C. Superior Oblique

D. Inferior Oblique

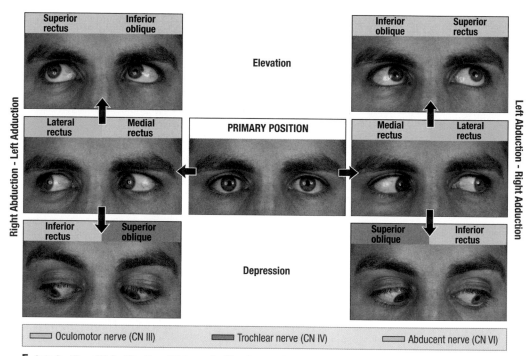

E. Anterior View, Clinical Testing of Extraocular Muscles and Cranial Nerves by Sequential Movements

---

8.43 **Clinical Testing of Extraocular Muscles and Motor Nerves (CN III, IV, and VI)**

A. and **B.** When eye is initially abducted by lateral rectus (LR), only rectus muscles can produce elevation and depression. **C.** and **D.** When eye is adducted by medial rectus (MR), only oblique muscles can produce these movements. **E.** Clinical testing of extraocular muscles using two-movement sequences (elevation or depression following left or right gaze). Following movements of the examiner's finger, the pupil is moved in an extended H pattern to isolate and test individual extraocular muscles and the integrity of their nerves.

• Complete **oculomotor nerve palsy** affects four of the six ocular muscles, the levator palpebrae superioris, and the sphincter

pupillae. The superior eyelid droops (**ptosis**) and cannot be raised voluntarily because of the unopposed activity of the orbicularis oculi (supplied by the facial nerve). The pupil is also fully dilated and nonreactive because of the unopposed dilator pupillae. The pupil is fully abducted and depressed ("down and out") because of the unopposed activity of the lateral rectus and superior oblique, respectively.

• A **lesion of the abducent nerve** results in loss of lateral gaze to the ipsilateral side because of paralysis of the lateral rectus muscle. On forward gaze, the eye is diverted medially because of the absence of normal resting tone in the lateral rectus, resulting in diplopia (double vision).

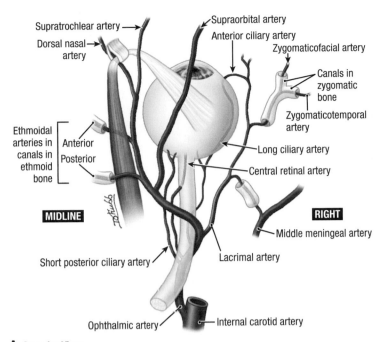

A. Superior View

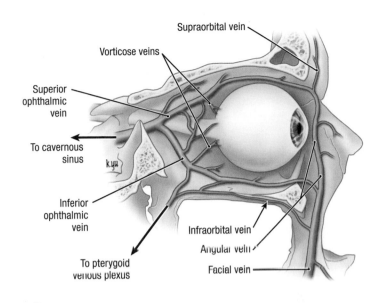

B. Lateral View

Arteries and Veins of Orbit

8.44

A. Arteries.

Blockage of central retinal artery. The terminal branches of the central retinal artery are end arteries. Obstruction of the artery by an embolus results in instant and total blindness. Blockage of the artery is usually unilateral and occurs in older people. **B. Veins.** The superior and inferior ophthalmic veins receive the vorticose veins from the eyeball and drain into the cavernous sinus posteriorly and the pterygoid plexus inferiorly. They communicate with the facial and supraorbital veins anteriorly.

- The facial veins make clinically important connections with the cavernous sinus through the superior ophthalmic veins. **Cavernous sinus thrombosis** usually results from infections in the orbit, nasal sinuses, and superior part of the face (the danger triangle). In persons with thrombophlebitis of the facial vein, pieces of an infected thrombus may extend into the cavernous sinus, producing **thrombophlebitis of the cavernous sinus**. The infection usually involves only one sinus initially but may spread to the opposite side through the intercavernous sinuses.

- **Blockade of central retinal vein.** The central retinal vein enters the cavernous sinus. Thrombophlebitis of this sinus may result in passage of a thrombus to the central retinal vein and produce a blockage in one of the small retinal veins. Occlusion of a branch of the central vein of the retina usually results in slow, painless loss of vision.

TABLE 8.10   Arteries of Orbit

Artery	Origin	Course and Distribution
Ophthalmic	Internal carotid artery	Traverses optic foramen to reach orbital cavity
Central retinal	Ophthalmic artery	Runs in dural sheath of optic nerve, entering nerve near eyeball; appears at center of optic disc; supplies optic retina (except cones and rods)
Supraorbital		Passes superiorly and posteriorly from supraorbital foramen to supply forehead and scalp
Supratrochlear		Passes from supraorbital margin to forehead and scalp
Lacrimal		Passes along superior border of lateral rectus muscle to supply lacrimal gland, conjunctiva, and eyelids
Dorsal nasal		Courses along dorsal aspect of nose and supplies its surface
Short posterior ciliary		Pierces sclera at periphery of optic nerve to supply choroid, which, in turn, supplies cones and rods of optic retina
Long posterior ciliary		Pierces sclera to supply ciliary body and iris
Posterior ethmoidal		Passes through posterior ethmoidal foramen to posterior ethmoidal cells
Anterior ethmoidal		Passes through anterior ethmoidal foramen to anterior cranial fossa; supplies anterior and middle ethmoidal cells, frontal sinus, nasal cavity, and skin on dorsum of nose
Anterior ciliary	Muscular rami of the ophthalmic and infraorbital arteries	Pierces sclera at attachments of rectus muscles and forms network in iris and ciliary body
Infraorbital	Third part of maxillary artery	Passes along infraorbital groove and exits through infraorbital foramen to face

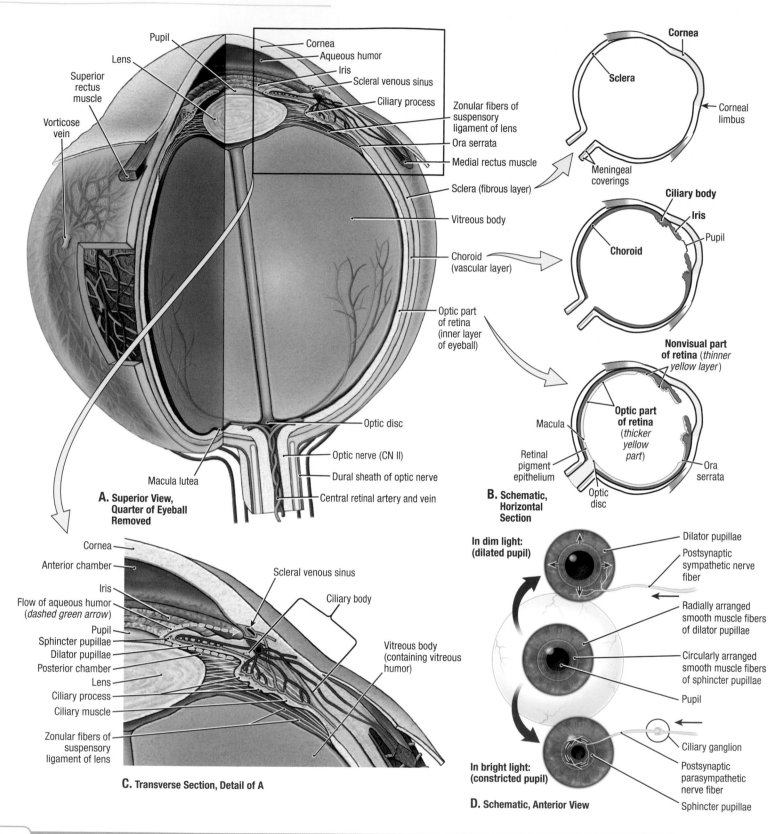

Pupil
Lens
Superior rectus muscle
Vorticose vein

Cornea
Aqueous humor
Iris
Scleral venous sinus
Ciliary process
Zonular fibers of suspensory ligament of lens
Ora serrata
Medial rectus muscle
Sclera (fibrous layer)
Vitreous body
Choroid (vascular layer)
Optic part of retina (inner layer of eyeball)
Optic disc
Optic nerve (CN II)
Dural sheath of optic nerve
Central retinal artery and vein
Macula lutea

A. Superior View, Quarter of Eyeball Removed

Cornea
Sclera
Corneal limbus
Meningeal coverings

Ciliary body
Iris
Pupil
Choroid

B. Schematic, Horizontal Section

Nonvisual part of retina (*thinner yellow layer*)
Optic part of retina (*thicker yellow part*)
Macula
Retinal pigment epithelium
Ora serrata
Optic disc

Cornea
Anterior chamber
Iris
Flow of aqueous humor (*dashed green arrow*)
Pupil
Sphincter pupillae
Dilator pupillae
Posterior chamber
Lens
Ciliary process
Ciliary muscle
Zonular fibers of suspensory ligament of lens
Scleral venous sinus
Ciliary body
Vitreous body (containing vitreous humor)

C. Transverse Section, Detail of A

In dim light: (dilated pupil)
Dilator pupillae
Postsynaptic sympathetic nerve fiber
Radially arranged smooth muscle fibers of dilator pupillae
Circularly arranged smooth muscle fibers of sphincter pupillae
Pupil
Ciliary ganglion
Postsynaptic parasympathetic nerve fiber
Sphincter pupillae
In bright light: (constricted pupil)

D. Schematic, Anterior View

8.45 **Illustration of a Dissected Eyeball**

A. Parts of eyeball. B. Layers (coats) of eyeball. C. Anterior segment. D. Structure and function of iris. The aqueous humor is produced by the ciliary processes and provides nutrients for the avascular cornea and lens; the aqueous humor drains into the scleral venous sinus (also called the sinus venosus sclerae or canal of Schlemm). **Glaucoma.** If drainage of the aqueous humor is reduced significantly, pressure builds up in the chambers of the eye (glaucoma). Blindness can result from compression of the inner layer of the retina and retinal arteries if aqueous humor production is not reduced to maintain normal intraocular pressure.

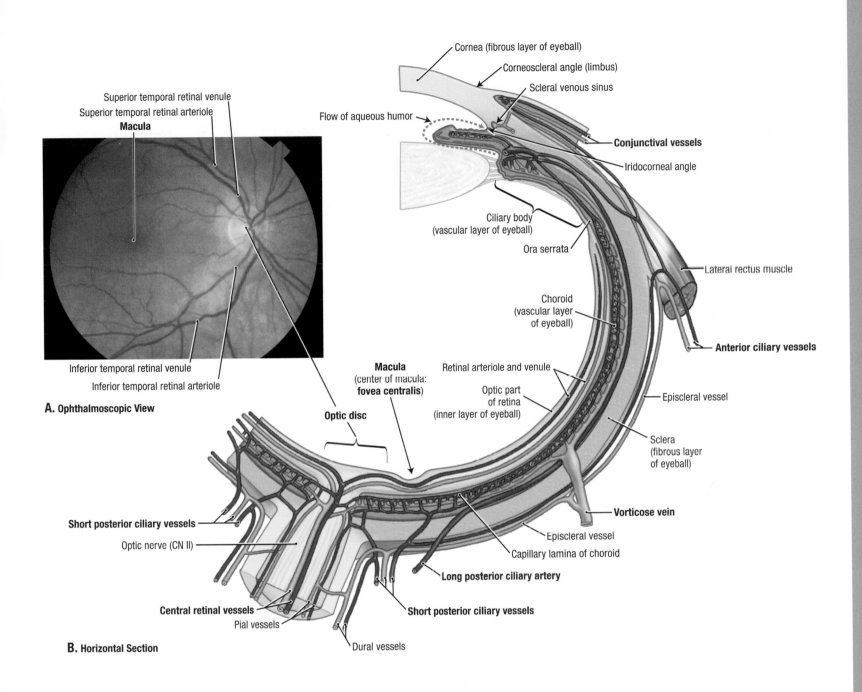

A. Ophthalmoscopic View

B. Horizontal Section

Ocular Fundus and Blood Supply to Eyeball   8.46

A. Right ocular fundus, ophthalmoscopic view. Retinal venules (wider) and retinal arterioles (narrower) radiate from the center of the oval optic disc, formed in relation to the entry of the optic nerve into the eyeball. The round, dark area lateral to the disc is the macula; branches of vessels extend to this area but do not reach its center, the fovea centralis, a depressed spot that is the area of most acute vision. It is avascular but, like the rest of the outermost (cones and rods) layer of the retina, is nourished by the adjacent choriocapillaris. Increased intracranial pressure is transmitted through the CSF in the subarachnoid space surrounding the optic nerve, causing the optic disc to protrude. The protrusion, called **papilledema**, is apparent during ophthalmoscopy. **B. Blood supply to eyeball.** The

eyeball has three layers: (1) the external, fibrous layer is the sclera and cornea; (2) the middle, vascular layer is the choroid, ciliary body, and iris; and (3) the internal, neural layer or retina consists of a pigment cell layer and a neural layer. The central artery of the retina, a branch of the ophthalmic artery, is an end artery. Of the eight posterior ciliary arteries, six are short posterior ciliary arteries and supply the choroid, which in turn nourishes the outer, non-vascular layer of the retina. Two long posterior ciliary arteries, one on each side of the eyeball, run between the sclera and choroid to anastomose with the anterior ciliary arteries, which are derived from muscular branches. The choroid is drained by posterior ciliary veins, and four to five vorticose veins that drain into the ophthalmic veins.

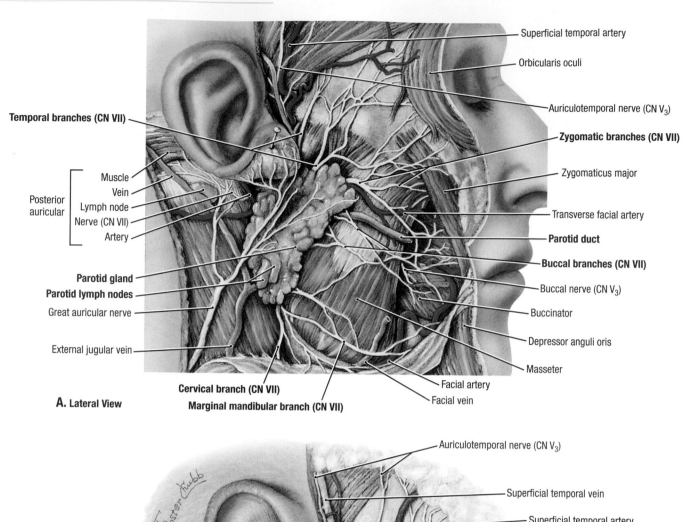

Superficial temporal artery

Orbicularis oculi

Auriculotemporal nerve (CN V₃)

Zygomatic branches (CN VII)

Zygomaticus major

Transverse facial artery

Parotid duct

Buccal branches (CN VII)

Buccal nerve (CN V₃)

Buccinator

Depressor anguli oris

Masseter

Facial artery

Facial vein

Temporal branches (CN VII)

Posterior auricular {
Muscle
Vein
Lymph node
Nerve (CN VII)
Artery
}

Parotid gland
Parotid lymph nodes

Great auricular nerve

External jugular vein

Cervical branch (CN VII)
Marginal mandibular branch (CN VII)

A. Lateral View

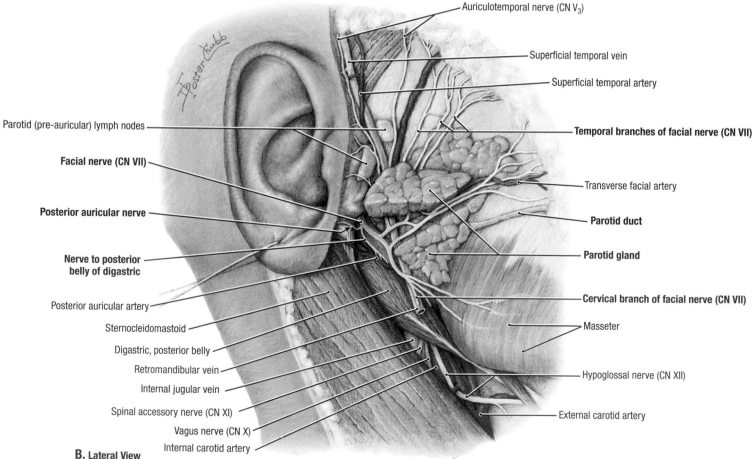

Auriculotemporal nerve (CN V₃)

Superficial temporal vein

Superficial temporal artery

Temporal branches of facial nerve (CN VII)

Transverse facial artery

Parotid duct

Parotid gland

Cervical branch of facial nerve (CN VII)

Masseter

Hypoglossal nerve (CN XII)

External carotid artery

Parotid (pre-auricular) lymph nodes

Facial nerve (CN VII)

Posterior auricular nerve

Nerve to posterior belly of digastric

Posterior auricular artery

Sternocleidomastoid

Digastric, posterior belly

Retromandibular vein

Internal jugular vein

Spinal accessory nerve (CN XI)

Vagus nerve (CN X)

Internal carotid artery

B. Lateral View

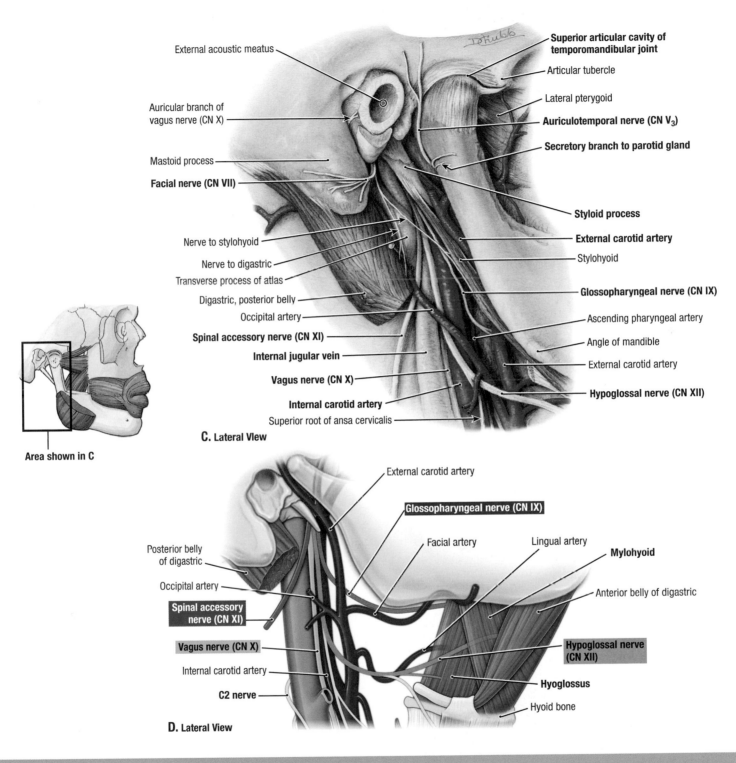

External acoustic meatus

Auricular branch of
vagus nerve (CN X)

Mastoid process

Facial nerve (CN VII)

Nerve to stylohyoid

Nerve to digastric

Transverse process of atlas

Digastric, posterior belly

Occipital artery

Spinal accessory nerve (CN XI)

Internal jugular vein

Vagus nerve (CN X)

Internal carotid artery

Superior root of ansa cervicalis

Superior articular cavity of
temporomandibular joint

Articular tubercle

Lateral pterygoid

Auriculotemporal nerve (CN V₃)

Secretory branch to parotid gland

Styloid process

External carotid artery

Stylohyoid

Glossopharyngeal nerve (CN IX)

Ascending pharyngeal artery

Angle of mandible

External carotid artery

Hypoglossal nerve (CN XII)

C. Lateral View

Area shown in C

External carotid artery

Glossopharyngeal nerve (CN IX)

Posterior belly
of digastric

Occipital artery

**Spinal accessory
nerve (CN XI)**

Vagus nerve (CN X)

Internal carotid artery

C2 nerve

Facial artery

Lingual artery

Mylohyoid

Anterior belly of digastric

**Hypoglossal nerve
(CN XII)**

Hyoglossus

Hyoid bone

D. Lateral View

8.47

Parotid Region *(continued)*

**A. Superficial dissection. B. Deep dissection with part of gland
removed.** During **parotidectomy** (surgical excision of the parotid
gland), identification, dissection, and preservation of the facial
nerve are critical. The parotid gland has superficial and deep parts.
In parotidectomy the superficial part is removed, then the plexus
may be retracted to remove the deep part. **C. Deep dissection
following removal of parotid gland and auricle.** The facial nerve,
posterior belly of the digastric muscle, and its nerve are retracted;
the external carotid artery, stylohyoid muscle, and the nerve to the

stylohyoid remain *in situ*. The internal jugular vein, internal carotid
artery, and glossopharyngeal (CN IX), vagus (CN X), spinal accessory (CN XI), and hypoglossal (CN XII) nerves cross anterior to
the transverse process of the atlas and deep to the styloid process.
D. Relationship of nerves and vessels.

Hypoglossal nerve palsy. Trauma, such as a fractured mandible,
may injure the hypoglossal nerve (CN XII), resulting in paralysis
and eventual atrophy of one side of the tongue. The tongue
deviates to the paralyzed side during protrusion.

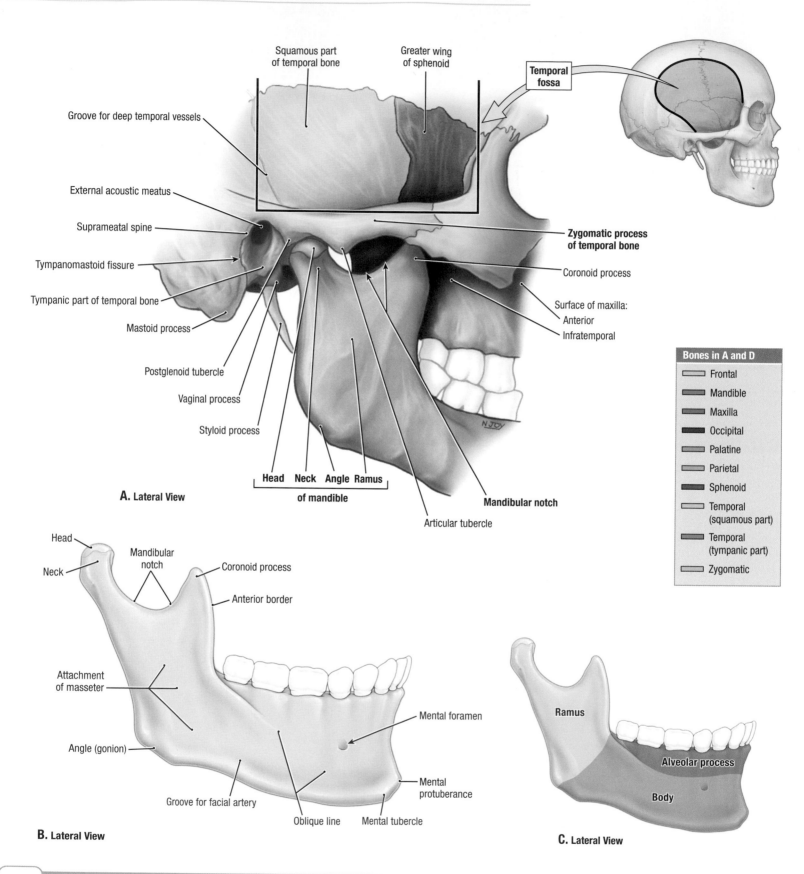

Squamous part
of temporal bone

Greater wing
of sphenoid

Temporal
fossa

Groove for deep temporal vessels

External acoustic meatus

Suprameatal spine

Tympanomastoid fissure

Tympanic part of temporal bone

Mastoid process

Postglenoid tubercle

Vaginal process

Styloid process

**Zygomatic process
of temporal bone**

Coronoid process

Surface of maxilla:
Anterior
Infratemporal

Head   Neck   Angle Ramus
of mandible

A. Lateral View

Mandibular notch

Articular tubercle

Head

Neck

Mandibular
notch

Coronoid process

Anterior border

Attachment
of masseter

Mental foramen

Angle (gonion)

Groove for facial artery

Mental
protuberance

Oblique line   Mental tubercle

B. Lateral View

Ramus

Alveolar process

Body

C. Lateral View

Bones in A and D

- Frontal
- Mandible
- Maxilla
- Occipital
- Palatine
- Parietal
- Sphenoid
- Temporal
  (squamous part)
- Temporal
  (tympanic part)
- Zygomatic

8.48   **Temporal and Infratemporal Fossae and Mandible**

A. Bones and bony features. Note that superficially, the zygomatic process of the temporal bone is the boundary between the

temporal fossa superiorly and the infratemporal fossa inferiorly.
B. External surface of mandible. C. Parts of mandible.

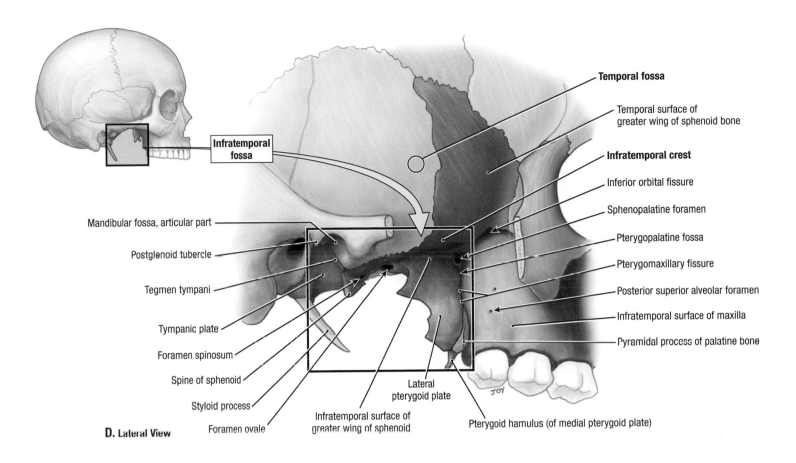

Temporal fossa

Temporal surface of greater wing of sphenoid bone

Infratemporal crest

Inferior orbital fissure

Sphenopalatine foramen

Pterygopalatine fossa

Pterygomaxillary fissure

Posterior superior alveolar foramen

Infratemporal surface of maxilla

Pyramidal process of palatine bone

Infratemporal fossa

Mandibular fossa, articular part

Postglenoid tubercle

Tegmen tympani

Tympanic plate

Foramen spinosum

Spine of sphenoid

Styloid process

Foramen ovale

Infratemporal surface of greater wing of sphenoid

Lateral pterygoid plate

Pterygoid hamulus (of medial pterygoid plate)

D. Lateral View

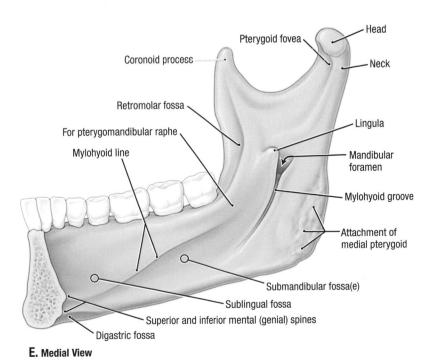

Pterygoid fovea

Head

Coronoid process

Neck

Retromolar fossa

For pterygomandibular raphe

Mylohyoid line

Lingula

Mandibular foramen

Mylohyoid groove

Attachment of medial pterygoid

Submandibular fossa(e)

Sublingual fossa

Superior and inferior mental (genial) spines

Digastric fossa

E. Medial View

Temporal and Infratemporal Fossae and Mandible (continued)   8.48

D. Bones and bony features of infratemporal fossa. The mandible and part of the zygomatic arch have been removed. Deeply, the infratemporal crest separates the temporal and infratemporal fossae. **E. Internal surface of mandible.**

- The temporal region is the region of the head that includes the lateral area of the scalp and the deeper soft tissues overlying the temporal fossa of the cranium, superior to the zygomatic arch. The temporal fossa, occupied primarily by the upper portion of the temporalis muscle, is bounded by the inferior temporal lines (see Fig. 8.3B).
- The infratemporal fossa is an irregularly shaped space deep and inferior to the zygomatic arch, deep to the ramus of the mandible and posterior to the maxilla. It communicates with the temporal fossa through the interval between the zygomatic arch and the cranial bones.

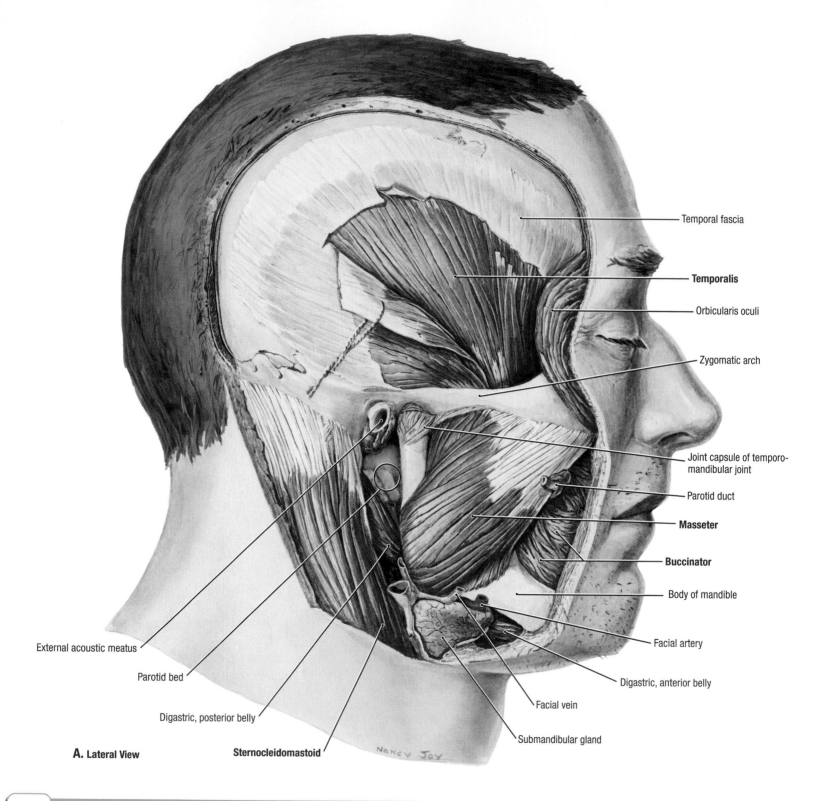

Temporal fascia

Temporalis

Orbicularis oculi

Zygomatic arch

Joint capsule of temporo-mandibular joint

Parotid duct

Masseter

Buccinator

Body of mandible

Facial artery

Digastric, anterior belly

Facial vein

Submandibular gland

External acoustic meatus

Parotid bed

Digastric, posterior belly

Sternocleidomastoid

NANCY JOY

A. Lateral View

8.49 **Temporalis and Masseter**

A. Superficial dissection.
- The temporalis and masseter muscles are supplied by the mandibular nerve (CN V₃), and both elevate the mandible. The buccinator muscle, supplied by the facial nerve (CN VII), functions during chewing to keep food between the teeth but does not act on the mandible.
- The sternocleidomastoid muscle, supplied by the spinal accessory nerve (CN XI), is the chief flexor of the head and neck; it forms the lateral part of the posterior boundary of the parotid region/parotid bed.

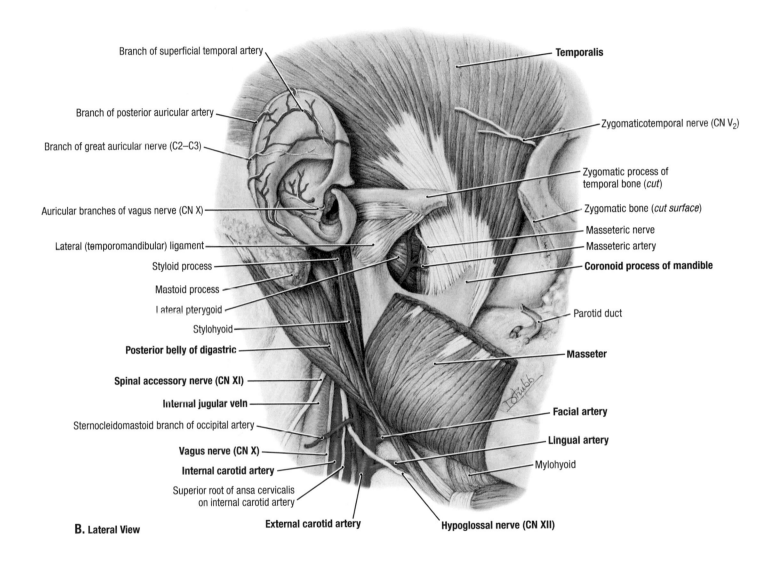

Branch of superficial temporal artery

Branch of posterior auricular artery

Branch of great auricular nerve (C2–C3)

Auricular branches of vagus nerve (CN X)

Lateral (temporomandibular) ligament

Styloid process

Mastoid process

Lateral pterygoid

Stylohyoid

Posterior belly of digastric

Spinal accessory nerve (CN XI)

Internal jugular vein

Sternocleidomastoid branch of occipital artery

Vagus nerve (CN X)

Internal carotid artery

Superior root of ansa cervicalis
on internal carotid artery

B. **Lateral View**

External carotid artery

Temporalis

Zygomaticotemporal nerve (CN V₂)

Zygomatic process of
temporal bone (cut)

Zygomatic bone (cut surface)

Masseteric nerve

Masseteric artery

Coronoid process of mandible

Parotid duct

Masseter

Facial artery

Lingual artery

Mylohyoid

Hypoglossal nerve (CN XII)

Temporalis and Masseter (continued)

B. Deep dissection.
- Parts of the zygomatic arch and masseter muscle have been removed to expose the attachment of the temporalis muscle to the coronoid process of the mandible.
- The carotid sheath surrounding the internal jugular vein, internal carotid artery, and the vagus nerve (CN X) has been removed.

The external carotid artery and its lingual, facial, and occipital branches, and the spinal accessory (CN XI) and hypoglossal (CN XII) nerves pass medial to the posterior belly of the digastric muscle.

8.49

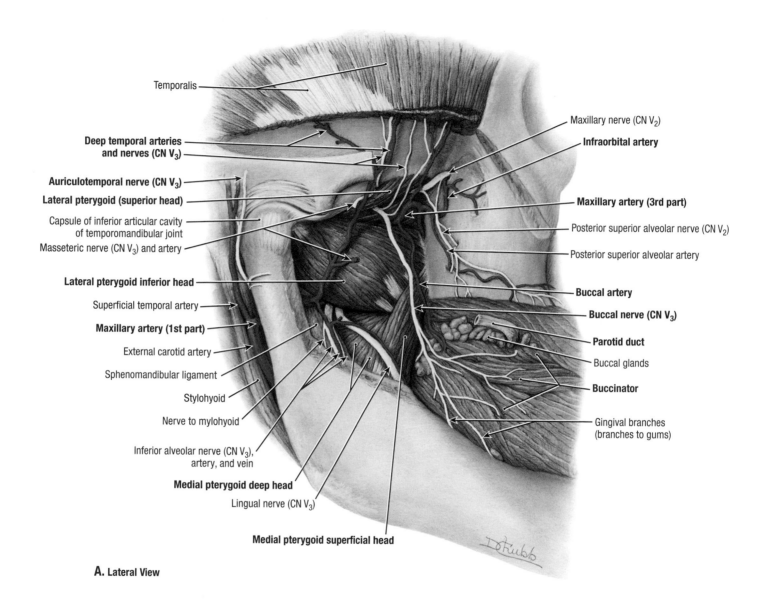

Temporalis

Deep temporal arteries
and nerves (CN V₃)

Auriculotemporal nerve (CN V₃)

Lateral pterygoid (superior head)

Capsule of inferior articular cavity
of temporomandibular joint

Masseteric nerve (CN V₃) and artery

Lateral pterygoid inferior head

Superficial temporal artery

Maxillary artery (1st part)

External carotid artery

Sphenomandibular ligament

Stylohyoid

Nerve to mylohyoid

Inferior alveolar nerve (CN V₃),
artery, and vein

Medial pterygoid deep head

Lingual nerve (CN V₃)

Medial pterygoid superficial head

Maxillary nerve (CN V₂)

Infraorbital artery

Maxillary artery (3rd part)

Posterior superior alveolar nerve (CN V₂)

Posterior superior alveolar artery

Buccal artery

Buccal nerve (CN V₃)

Parotid duct

Buccal glands

Buccinator

Gingival branches
(branches to gums)

A. Lateral View

8.50 Infratemporal Region

A. Superficial dissection.
- The maxillary artery, the larger of two terminal branches of the external carotid, is divided into three parts relative to the lateral pterygoid muscle.
- The buccinator is pierced by the parotid duct, the ducts of the buccal glands, and the sensory branches of the buccal nerve.
- The lateral pterygoid muscle arises by two heads, one head from the roof, and the other head from the lateral surface of the lateral pterygoid plate; both heads insert in relation to the temporomandibular joint (TMJ)—the superior head attaching primarily to the articular disc of the joint and the inferior head

primarily to the anterior aspect of the neck of the mandible (pterygoid fovea).
- Because of the close relationship of the facial and auriculotemporal nerves to the temporomandibular joint (TMJ), care must be taken during **surgical procedures on the temporomandibular joint** to preserve both the branches of the facial nerve overlying it and the articular branches of the auriculotemporal nerve that enter the posterior part of the joint. Injury to articular branches of the auriculotemporal nerve supplying the TMJ—associated with traumatic dislocation and rupture of the joint capsule and lateral ligament—leads to laxity and instability of the TMJ.

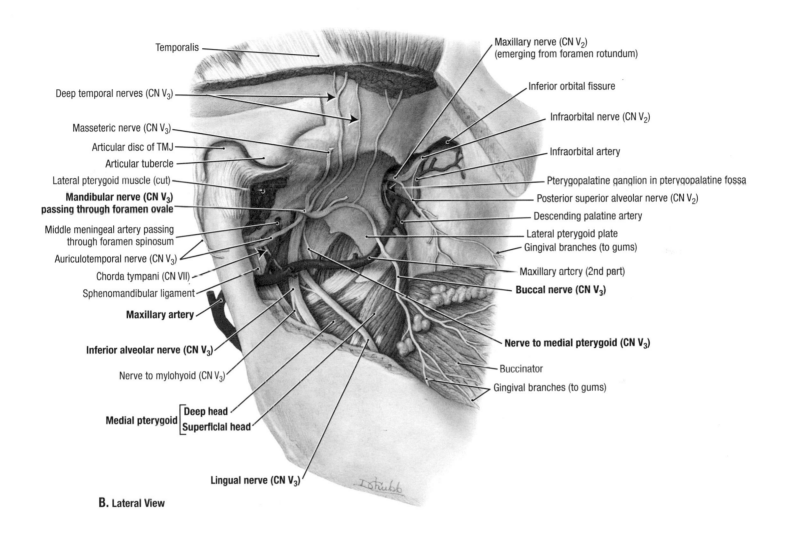

Temporalis

Deep temporal nerves (CN V₃)

Masseteric nerve (CN V₃)

Articular disc of TMJ

Articular tubercle

Lateral pterygoid muscle (cut)

**Mandibular nerve (CN V₃)
passing through foramen ovale**

Middle meningeal artery passing
through foramen spinosum

Auriculotemporal nerve (CN V₃)

Chorda tympani (CN VII)

Sphenomandibular ligament

Maxillary artery

Inferior alveolar nerve (CN V₃)

Nerve to mylohyoid (CN V₃)

Medial pterygoid — [Deep head / Superficial head]

Lingual nerve (CN V₃)

B. Lateral View

Maxillary nerve (CN V₂)
(emerging from foramen rotundum)

Inferior orbital fissure

Infraorbital nerve (CN V₂)

Infraorbital artery

Pterygopalatine ganglion in pterygopalatine fossa

Posterior superior alveolar nerve (CN V₂)

Descending palatine artery

Lateral pterygoid plate

Gingival branches (to gums)

Maxillary artery (2nd part)

Buccal nerve (CN V₃)

Nerve to medial pterygoid (CN V₃)

Buccinator

Gingival branches (to gums)

Infratemporal Region (continued) 8.50

B. Deeper dissection.
- The lateral pterygoid muscle and most of the branches of the maxillary artery have been removed to expose the mandibular nerve (CN V₃) entering the infratemporal fossa through the foramen ovale and the middle meningeal artery passing through the foramen spinosum.
- The deep head of the medial pterygoid muscle arises from the medial surface of the lateral pterygoid plate and the pyramidal process of the palatine bone. It has a small, superficial head that arises from the tuberosity of the maxilla.
- The inferior alveolar and lingual nerves descend on the medial pterygoid muscle. The inferior alveolar nerve gives off the nerve

to mylohyoid and nerve to anterior belly of the digastric muscle, and the lingual nerve receives the chorda tympani, which carries secretory parasympathetic fibers and fibers of taste.
- Motor nerves arising from CN V₃ supply the four muscles of mastication: the masseter, temporalis, and lateral and medial pterygoids. The buccal nerve from the mandibular nerve is sensory; the buccal branch of the facial nerve is the motor supply to the buccinator muscle.
- To perform a **mandibular nerve block,** an anesthetic agent is injected near the mandibular nerve where it enters the infratemporal fossa. This block usually anesthetizes the auriculotemporal, inferior alveolar, lingual, and buccal branches of the mandibular nerve.

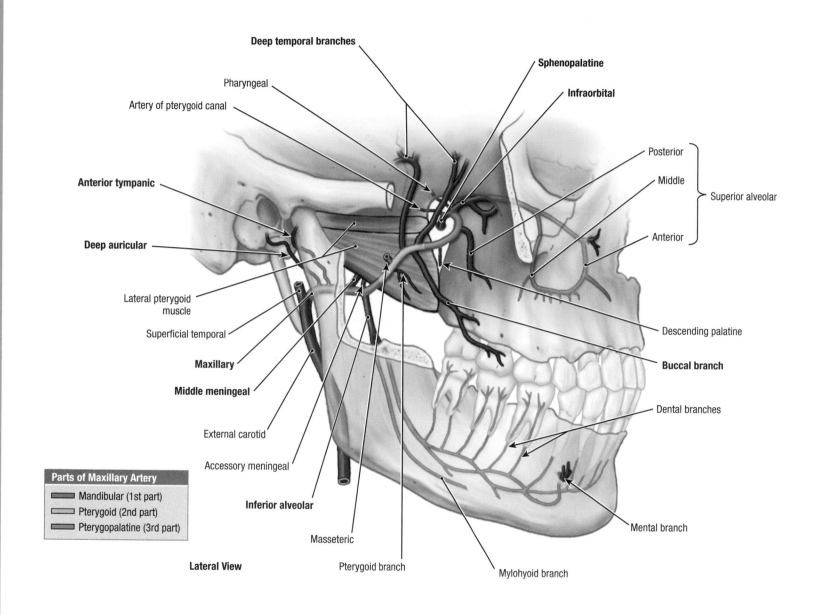

Deep temporal branches

Sphenopalatine

Pharyngeal

Infraorbital

Artery of pterygoid canal

Posterior

Middle

Superior alveolar

Anterior tympanic

Anterior

Deep auricular

Descending palatine

Lateral pterygoid muscle

Superficial temporal

Buccal branch

Maxillary

Middle meningeal

Dental branches

External carotid

Accessory meningeal

Parts of Maxillary Artery

Mandibular (1st part)
Pterygoid (2nd part)
Pterygopalatine (3rd part)

Inferior alveolar

Mental branch

Lateral View

Masseteric

Pterygoid branch

Mylohyoid branch

8.51 Branches of Maxillary Artery

- The maxillary artery arises at the neck of the mandible and is divided into three parts (mandibular, pterygoid, and pterygopalatine) by the lateral pterygoid muscle; it can pass medial or lateral to the lateral pterygoid.
- The branches of the *first (mandibular) part* pass through foramina or canals: the deep auricular to the external acoustic meatus, the anterior tympanic to the tympanic cavity, the middle and accessory meningeal to the cranial cavity, and the inferior alveolar to the mandible and teeth.

- The branches of the *second (pterygoid) part*, directly related to the lateral pterygoid muscle, supply muscles via the masseteric, deep temporal, pterygoid, and buccal branches.
- The branches of the *third (pterygopalatine) part* (posterior superior alveolar, infraorbital, descending palatine, and sphenopalatine arteries) arise immediately proximal to and within the pterygopalatine fossa.

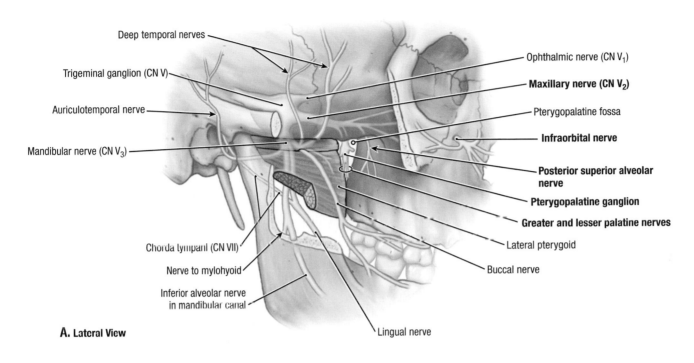

Deep temporal nerves

Trigeminal ganglion (CN V)

Auriculotemporal nerve

Mandibular nerve (CN V₃)

Chorda tympani (CN VII)

Nerve to mylohyoid

Inferior alveolar nerve in mandibular canal

Ophthalmic nerve (CN V₁)

Maxillary nerve (CN V₂)

Pterygopalatine fossa

Infraorbital nerve

Posterior superior alveolar nerve

Pterygopalatine ganglion

Greater and lesser palatine nerves

Lateral pterygoid

Buccal nerve

Lingual nerve

A. Lateral View

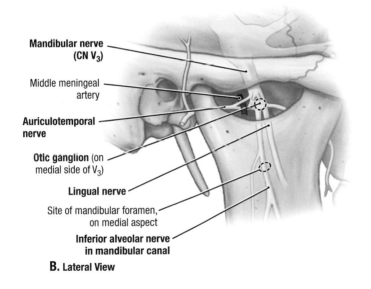

Mandibular nerve (CN V₃)

Middle meningeal artery

Auriculotemporal nerve

Otic ganglion (on medial side of V₃)

Lingual nerve

Site of mandibular foramen, on medial aspect

Inferior alveolar nerve in mandibular canal

B. Lateral View

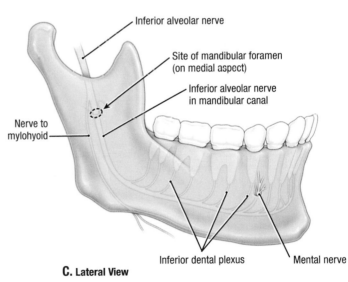

Inferior alveolar nerve

Site of mandibular foramen (on medial aspect)

Inferior alveolar nerve in mandibular canal

Nerve to mylohyoid

Inferior dental plexus

Mental nerve

C. Lateral View

Branches of Maxillary and Mandibular Nerves

8.52

A. Infratemporal region and pterygopalatine fossa. Branches of the maxillary (CN V₂) and mandibular (CN V₃) nerves accompany branches from the three parts of the maxillary artery. **B. Nerves of infratemporal fossa and otic ganglion. C. Mandible and inferior alveolar nerve.**

An **alveolar nerve block**—commonly used by dentists when repairing mandibular teeth—anesthetizes the inferior alveolar nerve, a branch of CN V₃. The anesthetic agent is injected around the

mandibular foramen, the opening into the mandibular canal on the medial aspect of the ramus of the mandible. This canal gives passage to the inferior alveolar nerve, artery, and vein. When this nerve block is successful, all mandibular teeth are anesthetized to the median plane. The skin and mucous membrane of the lower lip, the labial alveolar mucosa and gingiva, and the skin of the chin are also anesthetized because they are supplied by the mental branch of this nerve.

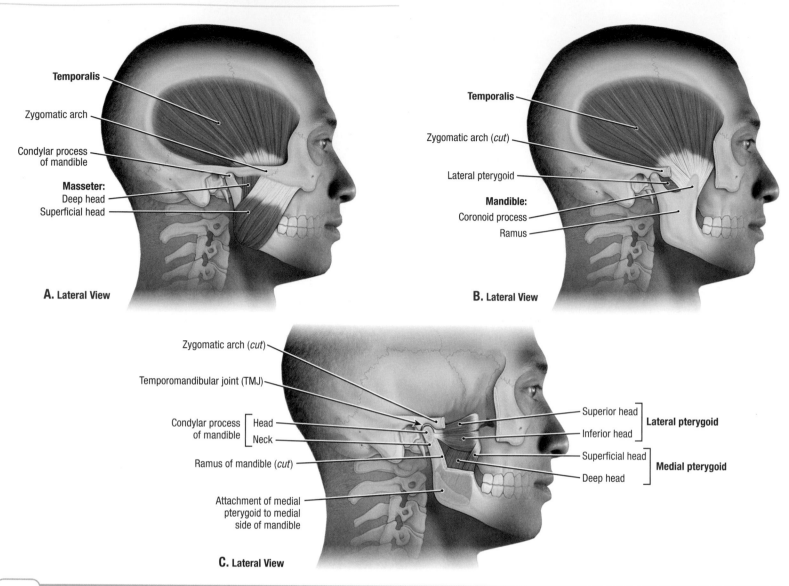

Temporalis
Zygomatic arch
Condylar process
of mandible
Masseter:
Deep head
Superficial head

A. Lateral View

Temporalis
Zygomatic arch (*cut*)
Lateral pterygoid
Mandible:
Coronoid process
Ramus

B. Lateral View

Zygomatic arch (*cut*)
Temporomandibular joint (TMJ)
Condylar process | Head
of mandible | Neck
Ramus of mandible (*cut*)
Attachment of medial
pterygoid to medial
side of mandible
Superior head } **Lateral pterygoid**
Inferior head
Superficial head } **Medial pterygoid**
Deep head

C. Lateral View

8.53 Muscles of Mastication

A. Temporalis and masseter. **B.** Temporalis. Zygomatic arch has been removed. **C.** Medial and lateral pterygoid.

TABLE 8.11	Muscles of Mastication (Acting on Temporomandibular Joint)			
Muscle	**Origin**	**Insertion**	**Innervation**	**Main Action**
Temporalis	Floor of temporal fossa and deep surface of temporal fascia	Tip and medial surface of coronoid process and anterior border of ramus of mandible	Deep temporal branches of mandibular nerve (CN V_3)	Elevates mandible, closing jaws; posterior fibers retrude mandible after protrusion
Masseter	Inferior border and medial surface of zygomatic arch	Lateral surface of ramus of mandible and coronoid process	Mandibular nerve (CN V_3) through masseteric nerve that enters deep surface of the muscle	Elevates and protrudes mandible, thus closing jaws; deep fibers retrude it
Lateral pterygoid	*Superior head*: infratemporal surface and infratemporal crest of greater wing of sphenoid bone *Inferior head*: lateral surface of lateral pterygoid plate	Neck of mandible, articular disc, and capsule of temporomandibular joint	Mandibular nerve (CN V_3) through lateral pterygoid nerve which enters its deep surface	*Acting bilaterally*, protrude mandible and depress chin; *acting unilaterally* alternately, they produce side-to-side movements of mandible
Medial pterygoid	*Deep head*: medial surface of lateral pterygoid plate and pyramidal process of palatine bone *Superficial head*: tuberosity of maxilla	Medial surface of ramus of mandible, inferior to mandibular foramen	Mandibular nerve (CN V_3) through medial pterygoid nerve	Helps elevate mandible, closing jaws; *acting bilaterally* protrude mandible; *acting unilaterally*, protrudes side of jaw; acting alternately, they produce a grinding motion

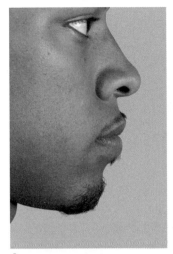

A. Elevation of mandible

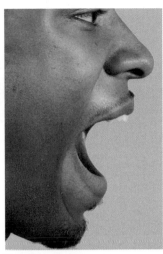

B. Depression of mandible

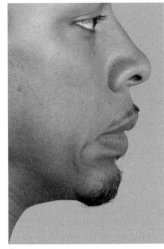

C. Retrusion

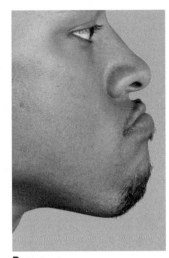

D. Protrusion

Lateral Views

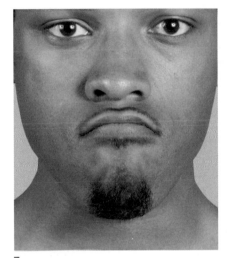

E. Protrusion

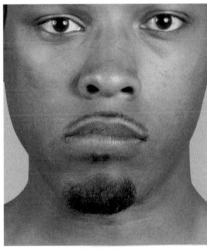

F. Lateral movement to right side

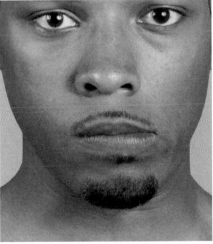

G. Lateral movement to left side

Anterior Views

Movements of Temporomandibular Joint

8.54

Temporomandibular joint movements are produced chiefly by the muscles of mastication. These four muscles (temporalis, masseter, and medial and lateral pterygoid muscles) develop from the mesoderm of the first pharyngeal arch; consequently, they are innervated by the nerve of that arch, the motor root of the mandibular nerve (CN V₃).

TABLE 8.12 Movements of Temporomandibular Joint

Movements	Muscles
Elevation (close mouth) (*Part A*)	Temporalis, masseter, and medial pterygoid
Depression (open mouth) (*Part B*)	Lateral pterygoid; suprahyoid and infrahyoid muscles; gravity
Retrusion (retrude chin) (*Part C*)	Temporalis (posterior oblique and near horizontal fibers) and masseter
Protrusion (protrude chin) (*Part D* and *Part E*)	Lateral pterygoid, masseter, and medial pterygoid
Lateral movements (grinding and chewing) (*Part F* and *Part G*)	Temporalis of same side, pterygoids of opposite side, and masseter

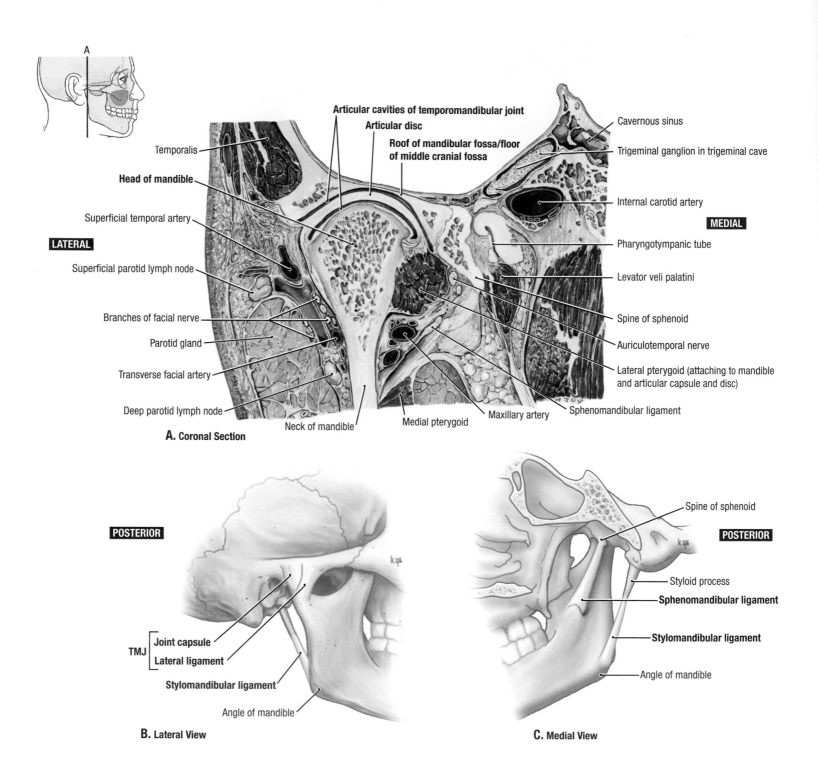

A. Coronal Section

Temporalis

Head of mandible

Superficial temporal artery

LATERAL

Superficial parotid lymph node

Branches of facial nerve

Parotid gland

Transverse facial artery

Deep parotid lymph node

Neck of mandible

Articular cavities of temporomandibular joint

Articular disc

Roof of mandibular fossa/floor of middle cranial fossa

Cavernous sinus

Trigeminal ganglion in trigeminal cave

Internal carotid artery

MEDIAL

Pharyngotympanic tube

Levator veli palatini

Spine of sphenoid

Auriculotemporal nerve

Lateral pterygoid (attaching to mandible and articular capsule and disc)

Sphenomandibular ligament

Maxillary artery

Medial pterygoid

B. Lateral View

POSTERIOR

TMJ

Joint capsule

Lateral ligament

Stylomandibular ligament

Angle of mandible

C. Medial View

Spine of sphenoid

POSTERIOR

Styloid process

Sphenomandibular ligament

Stylomandibular ligament

Angle of mandible

8.55 | **Temporomandibular Joint**

A. Coronal section. B. Temporomandibular joint (TMJ) and stylomandibular ligament. The joint capsule of the temporomandibular joint attaches to the margins of the mandibular fossa and articular tubercle of the temporal bone and around the neck of the mandible; the lateral (temporomandibular) ligament strengthens the lateral aspect of the joint. **C. Stylomandibular**

and sphenomandibular ligaments. The strong sphenomandibular ligament descends from near the spine of the sphenoid to the lingula of the mandible and is the "swinging hinge" by which the mandible is suspended; the weaker stylomandibular ligament is a thickened part of the parotid sheath that joins the styloid process to the angle of the mandible.

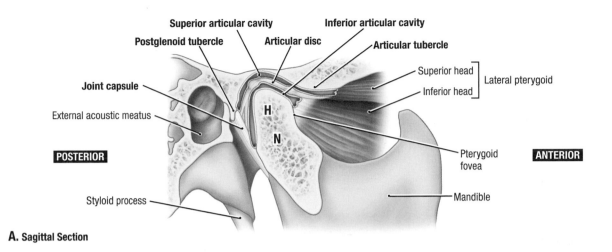

Superior articular cavity

Postglenoid tubercle

Articular disc

Inferior articular cavity

Articular tubercle

Joint capsule

Superior head ⎱
Inferior head ⎰ Lateral pterygoid

External acoustic meatus

H

N

POSTERIOR

ANTERIOR

Pterygoid fovea

Styloid process

Mandible

A. Sagittal Section

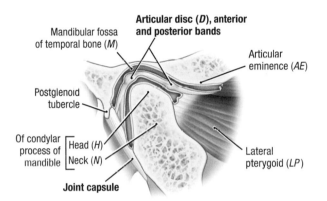

Mandibular fossa of temporal bone (*M*)

Articular disc (*D*), anterior and posterior bands

Articular eminence (*AE*)

Postglenoid tubercle

Of condylar process of mandible ⎱ Head (*H*) / Neck (*N*)

Lateral pterygoid (*LP*)

Joint capsule

B. Closed Mouth, Sagittal Section

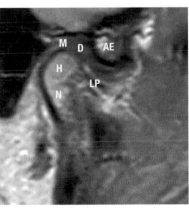

D. Sagittal MRI, Closed Mouth

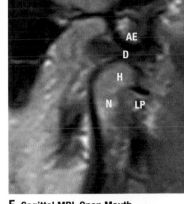

E. Sagittal MRI, Open Mouth

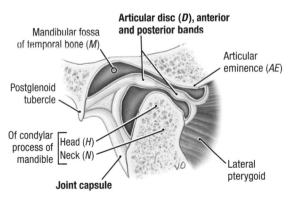

Mandibular fossa of temporal bone (*M*)

Articular disc (*D*), anterior and posterior bands

Articular eminence (*AE*)

Postglenoid tubercle

Of condylar process of mandible ⎱ Head (*H*) / Neck (*N*)

Lateral pterygoid

Joint capsule

C. Open Mouth, Sagittal Section

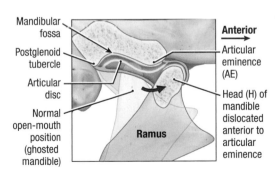

Mandibular fossa

Postglenoid tubercle

Articular disc

Normal open-mouth position (ghosted mandible)

Anterior →

Articular eminence (AE)

Head (H) of mandible dislocated anterior to articular eminence

Ramus

F. Lateral View

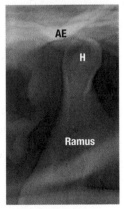

AE

H

Ramus

Lateral Radiograph

Sectional Anatomy of Temporomandibular Joint

8.56

A. Temporomandibular joint and related structures, sagittal section. **B.** Sagittal section through temporomandibular joint, closed mouth. **C.** Sagittal section through temporomandibular joint, open mouth. **D.** MRI, closed mouth. **E.** MRI, open mouth. **F.** Dislocation of mandible.

Dislocation of mandible. During yawning or taking large bites, excessive contraction of the lateral pterygoids can cause the head of the mandible to dislocate (pass anterior to the articular tubercle). In this position, the mouth remains wide open, and the person cannot close it without manual distraction.

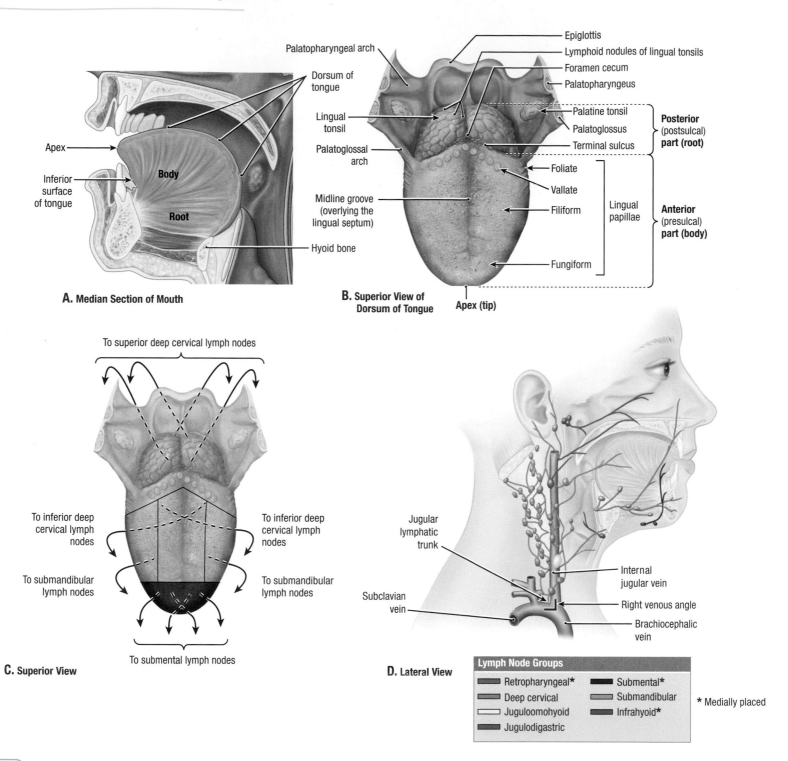

A. **Median Section of Mouth**

B. **Superior View of Dorsum of Tongue**

C. **Superior View**

D. **Lateral View**

Lymph Node Groups

Retropharyngeal*		Submental*	
Deep cervical		Submandibular	
Juguloomohyoid		Infrahyoid*	
Jugulodigastric			

* Medially placed

8.57 Parts and Lymphatic Drainage of Tongue

A. Parts of tongue. B. Features of dorsum of tongue. The foramen cecum is the upper end of the primitive thyroglossal duct; the arms of the V-shaped terminal sulcus diverge from the foramen, demarcating the posterior third of the tongue from the anterior two thirds. **C. Lymphatic drainage of dorsum of tongue. D. Lymphatic drainage of tongue, mouth, nasal cavity, and nose.**

Carcinoma of tongue. Malignant tumors in the posterior part of the tongue metastasize to the superior deep cervical lymph nodes on both sides. In contrast, tumors in the apex and anterolateral parts usually do not metastasize to the inferior deep cervical nodes

until late in the disease. Because the deep nodes are closely related to the internal jugular vein (IJV), metastases from the carcinoma may spread to the submental and submandibular regions and along the IJV into the neck.

Gag reflex. One may touch the anterior part of the tongue without feeling discomfort; however, when the posterior part is touched, one usually gags. CN IX and CN X are responsible for the muscular contraction of each side of the pharynx. Glossopharyngeal branches (CN IX) provide the afferent limb of the gag reflex.

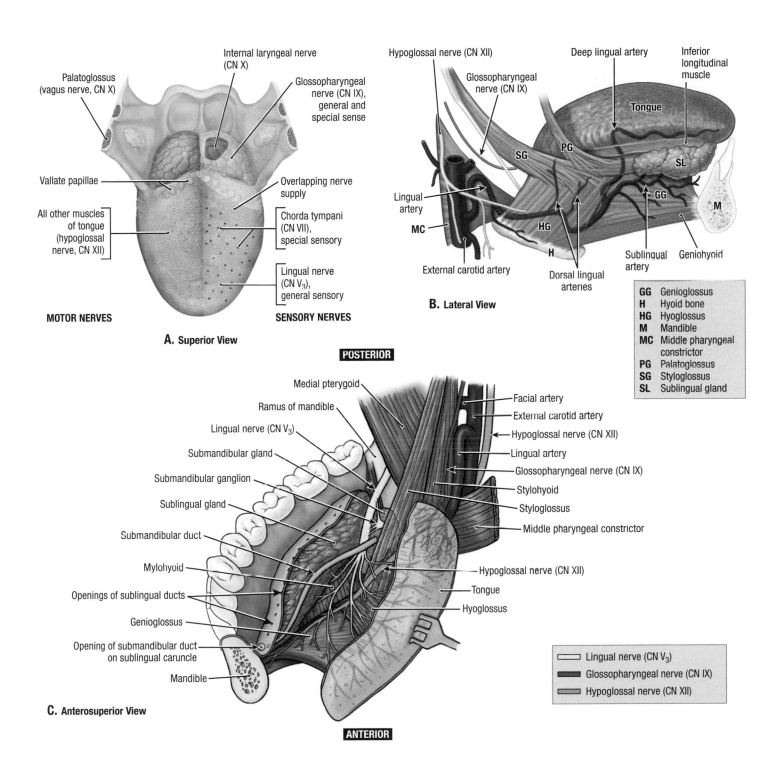

A. Superior View

Palatoglossus (vagus nerve, CN X)

Internal laryngeal nerve (CN X)

Glossopharyngeal nerve (CN IX), general and special sense

Vallate papillae

Overlapping nerve supply

All other muscles of tongue (hypoglossal nerve, CN XII)

Chorda tympani (CN VII), special sensory

Lingual nerve (CN V₃), general sensory

MOTOR NERVES

SENSORY NERVES

B. Lateral View

Hypoglossal nerve (CN XII)

Deep lingual artery

Inferior longitudinal muscle

Glossopharyngeal nerve (CN IX)

Tongue

SG   PG

SL

Lingual artery

GG

MC

M

External carotid artery

HG

H

Dorsal lingual arteries

Sublingual artery

Geniohyoid

GG	Genioglossus
H	Hyoid bone
HG	Hyoglossus
M	Mandible
MC	Middle pharyngeal constrictor
PG	Palatoglossus
SG	Styloglossus
SL	Sublingual gland

POSTERIOR

Medial pterygoid

Ramus of mandible

Lingual nerve (CN V₃)

Submandibular gland

Submandibular ganglion

Sublingual gland

Submandibular duct

Mylohyoid

Openings of sublingual ducts

Genioglossus

Opening of submandibular duct on sublingual caruncle

Mandible

Facial artery

External carotid artery

Hypoglossal nerve (CN XII)

Lingual artery

Glossopharyngeal nerve (CN IX)

Stylohyoid

Styloglossus

Middle pharyngeal constrictor

Hypoglossal nerve (CN XII)

Tongue

Hyoglossus

C. Anterosuperior View

	Lingual nerve (CN V₃)
	Glossopharyngeal nerve (CN IX)
	Hypoglossal nerve (CN XII)

ANTERIOR

Arteries and Nerves of Tongue

8.58

A. General sensory, special sensory (taste), and motor innervation of tongue. **B.** Course and distribution of lingual artery. **C.** Dissection of right side of floor of mouth.

Sialography. The parotid and submandibular salivary glands may be examined radiographically after the injection of a contrast medium into their ducts. This special type of radiograph (sialogram) demonstrates the salivary ducts and some secretory units. Because of the small size and number of sublingual ducts of the sublingual glands, one cannot usually inject contrast medium into them.

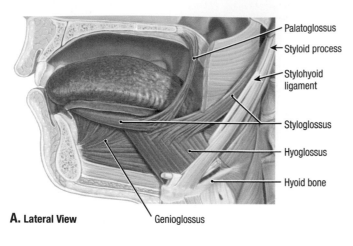

A. Lateral View

Palatoglossus
Styloid process
Stylohyoid ligament
Styloglossus
Hyoglossus
Hyoid bone
Genioglossus

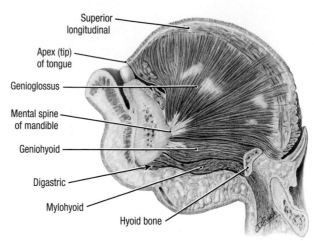

Superior longitudinal
Apex (tip) of tongue
Genioglossus
Mental spine of mandible
Geniohyoid
Digastric
Mylohyoid
Hyoid bone

B. Medial View of Right Half of Bisected Tongue

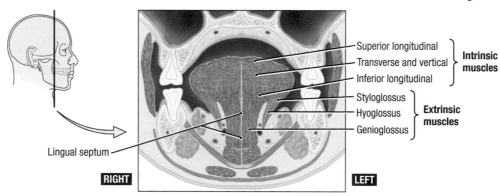

Superior longitudinal
Transverse and vertical — **Intrinsic muscles**
Inferior longitudinal
Styloglossus
Hyoglossus — **Extrinsic muscles**
Genioglossus
Lingual septum

RIGHT   LEFT

C. Anterior View of Coronal Section of Mouth

8.59 **Muscles of Tongue**

A. Extrinsic muscles. B. Median section. C. Coronal section. The extrinsic muscles of the tongue originate outside the tongue and attach to it, whereas the intrinsic muscles have their attachments entirely within the tongue and are not attached to bone.

TABLE 8.13   Muscles of Tongue

Extrinsic Muscles

Muscle	Origin	Insertion	Innervation	Main Action
Genioglossus	Superior part of mental spine of mandible	Dorsum of tongue and body of hyoid bone	Hypoglossal nerve (CN XII)	Depresses tongue; its posterior part pulls tongue anteriorly for protrusion[a]
Hyoglossus	Body and greater horn of hyoid bone	Side and inferior aspect of tongue		Depresses and retracts tongue
Styloglossus	Styloid process of temporal bone and stylohyoid ligament	Side and inferior aspect of tongue		Retracts tongue and draws it up to create a trough for swallowing
Palatoglossus	Palatine aponeurosis of soft palate	Side of tongue	CN X and pharyngeal plexus	Elevates posterolateral part of tongue

Intrinsic Muscles

Muscle	Origin	Insertion	Innervation	Main Action
Superior longitudinal	Submucous fibrous layer and lingual septum	Margins and mucous membrane of tongue	Hypoglossal nerve (CN XII)	Curls tip and sides of tongue superiorly and shortens tongue
Inferior longitudinal	Root of tongue and body of hyoid bone	Apex of tongue		Curls tip of tongue inferiorly and shortens tongue
Transverse	Lingual septum	Fibrous tissue at margins of tongue		Narrows and elongates the tongue[a]
Vertical	Superior surface of borders of tongue	Inferior surface of borders of tongue		Flattens and broadens the tongue[a]

[a]Act simultaneously to protrude tongue.

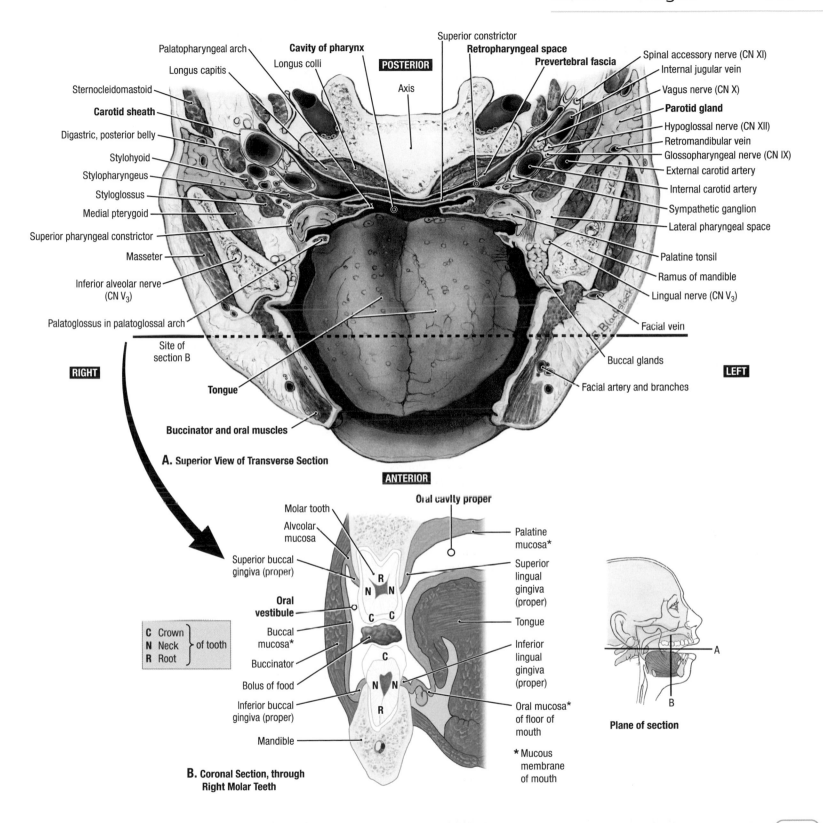

Palatopharyngeal arch
Longus capitis
Sternocleidomastoid
Carotid sheath
Digastric, posterior belly
Stylohyoid
Stylopharyngeus
Styloglossus
Medial pterygoid
Superior pharyngeal constrictor
Masseter
Inferior alveolar nerve (CN V₃)
Palatoglossus in palatoglossal arch

Cavity of pharynx
Longus colli
POSTERIOR
Axis

Superior constrictor
Retropharyngeal space
Prevertebral fascia

Spinal accessory nerve (CN XI)
Internal jugular vein
Vagus nerve (CN X)
Parotid gland
Hypoglossal nerve (CN XII)
Retromandibular vein
Glossopharyngeal nerve (CN IX)
External carotid artery
Internal carotid artery
Sympathetic ganglion
Lateral pharyngeal space
Palatine tonsil
Ramus of mandible
Lingual nerve (CN V₃)

Site of section B
RIGHT
Tongue
Buccinator and oral muscles
A. Superior View of Transverse Section
ANTERIOR
Facial vein
Buccal glands
Facial artery and branches
LEFT

Molar tooth
Alveolar mucosa
Superior buccal gingiva (proper)
Oral vestibule
Buccal mucosa*
Buccinator
Bolus of food
Inferior buccal gingiva (proper)
Mandible

Oral cavity proper
Palatine mucosa*
Superior lingual gingiva (proper)
Tongue
Inferior lingual gingiva (proper)
Oral mucosa* of floor of mouth

C	Crown	
N	Neck	} of tooth
R	Root	

B. Coronal Section, through Right Molar Teeth

* Mucous membrane of mouth

Plane of section

Sections through Mouth **8.60**

A. Coronal section of viscerocranium at C2 vertebral level. The plane of section passes through the oral fissure anteriorly. The retropharyngeal space (opened up in this specimen) allows the pharynx to contract and relax during swallowing; the retropharyngeal space is closed laterally at the carotid sheath and limited posteriorly by the prevertebral fascia. The beds of the parotid glands are also demonstrated. **B. Buccinator.** Schematic coronal section demonstrating how the tongue and buccinator (or, anteriorly, the orbicularis oris) work together to retain food between the teeth when chewing. The buccinator and superior part of the orbicularis oris are innervated by the buccal branch of the facial nerve (CN VII).

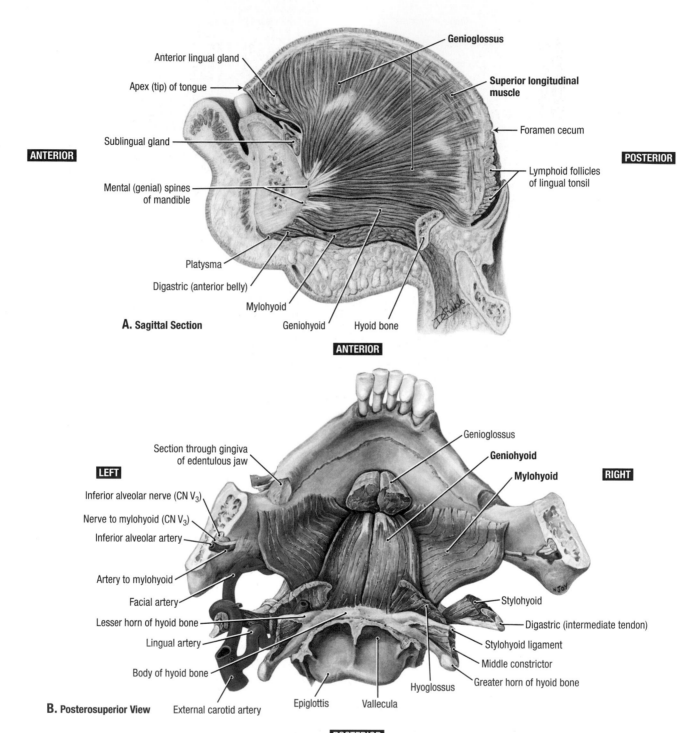

Anterior lingual gland

Apex (tip) of tongue

ANTERIOR

Sublingual gland

Mental (genial) spines
of mandible

Platysma

Digastric (anterior belly)

Mylohyoid

Geniohyoid

Hyoid bone

Genioglossus

**Superior longitudinal
muscle**

Foramen cecum

Lymphoid follicles
of lingual tonsil

POSTERIOR

A. Sagittal Section

ANTERIOR

Section through gingiva
of edentulous jaw

LEFT

Inferior alveolar nerve (CN V₃)

Nerve to mylohyoid (CN V₃)

Inferior alveolar artery

Artery to mylohyoid

Facial artery

Lesser horn of hyoid bone

Lingual artery

Body of hyoid bone

B. Posterosuperior View

External carotid artery

Epiglottis

Vallecula

Genioglossus

Geniohyoid

Mylohyoid

RIGHT

Stylohyoid

Digastric (intermediate tendon)

Stylohyoid ligament

Middle constrictor

Greater horn of hyoid bone

Hyoglossus

POSTERIOR

8.61 | **Tongue and Floor of Mouth**

A. Median section through tongue and lower jaw. The tongue is composed mainly of muscle; extrinsic muscles alter the position of the tongue, and intrinsic muscles alter its shape. The genioglossus is the extrinsic muscle apparent in this plane, and the superior longitudinal muscle is the intrinsic muscle. **B. Muscles of floor of mouth viewed posterosuperiorly.** The mylohyoid muscle extends between the two mylohyoid lines of the mandible. It has a thick, free posterior border and becomes thinner anteriorly.

Genioglossus paralysis. When the genioglossus is paralyzed, the tongue mass has a tendency to shift posteriorly, obstructing the airway and presenting the risk of suffocation. Total relaxation of the genioglossus muscles occurs during general anesthesia; therefore, the tongue of an anesthetized patient must be prevented from relapsing by inserting an airway.

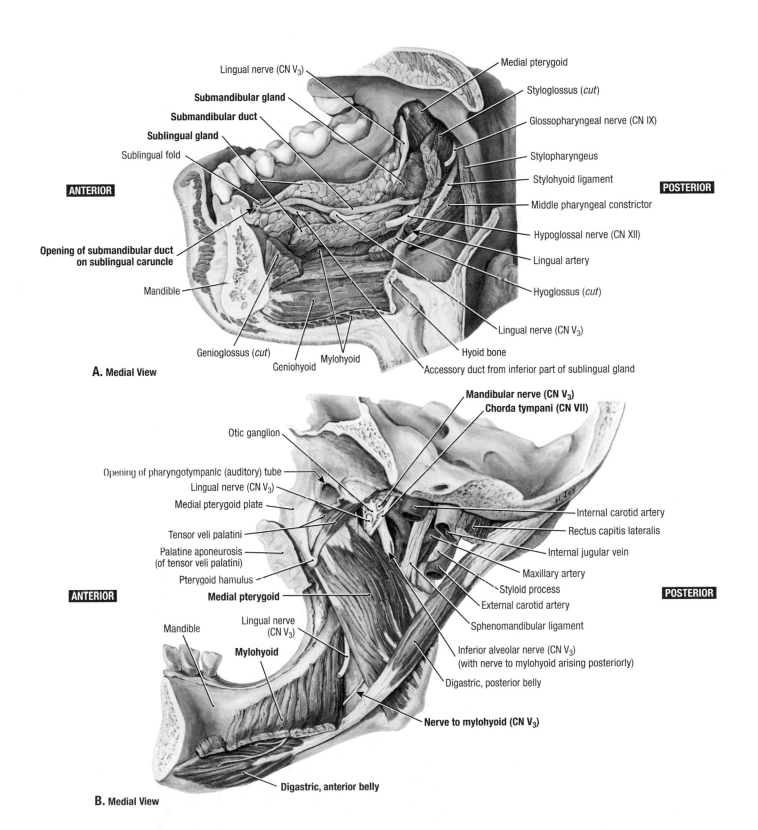

Lingual nerve (CN V₃)

Submandibular gland

Submandibular duct

Sublingual gland

Sublingual fold

ANTERIOR

Opening of submandibular duct on sublingual caruncle

Mandible

Genioglossus (*cut*)

Geniohyoid

Mylohyoid

A. Medial View

Medial pterygoid

Styloglossus (*cut*)

Glossopharyngeal nerve (CN IX)

Stylopharyngeus

Stylohyoid ligament

POSTERIOR

Middle pharyngeal constrictor

Hypoglossal nerve (CN XII)

Lingual artery

Hyoglossus (*cut*)

Lingual nerve (CN V₃)

Hyoid bone

Accessory duct from inferior part of sublingual gland

Mandibular nerve (CN V₃)

Chorda tympani (CN VII)

Otic ganglion

Opening of pharyngotympanic (auditory) tube

Lingual nerve (CN V₃)

Medial pterygoid plate

Tensor veli palatini

Palatine aponeurosis (of tensor veli palatini)

Pterygoid hamulus

ANTERIOR

Medial pterygoid

Mandible

Lingual nerve (CN V₃)

Mylohyoid

Internal carotid artery

Rectus capitis lateralis

Internal jugular vein

Maxillary artery

Styloid process

External carotid artery

Sphenomandibular ligament

Inferior alveolar nerve (CN V₃) (with nerve to mylohyoid arising posteriorly)

Digastric, posterior belly

POSTERIOR

Nerve to mylohyoid (CN V₃)

Digastric, anterior belly

B. Medial View

Muscles, Glands, and Vessels of Floor of Mouth and Medial Aspect of Mandible   **8.62**

A. Sublingual and submandibular glands. The tongue has been excised. **B. Structures related to medial surface of mandible.** The otic ganglion lies medial to the mandibular nerve (CN V₃) and between the foramen ovale superiorly and the medial pterygoid muscle inferiorly.

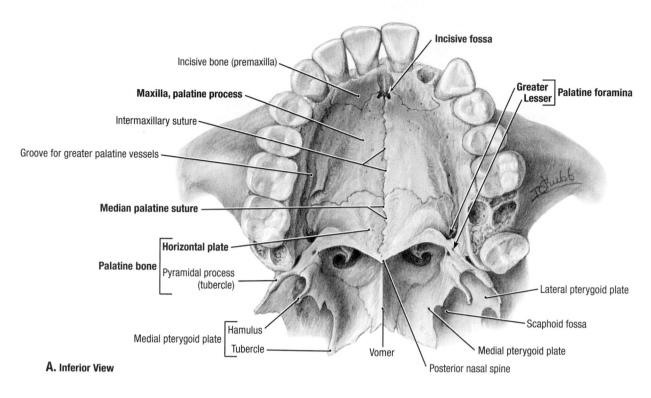

Incisive fossa

Incisive bone (premaxilla)

Maxilla, palatine process

Intermaxillary suture

Groove for greater palatine vessels

Greater | **Palatine foramina**
Lesser

Median palatine suture

Horizontal plate

Palatine bone

Pyramidal process (tubercle)

Lateral pterygoid plate

Scaphoid fossa

Medial pterygoid plate

Hamulus

Medial pterygoid plate

Tubercle

Vomer

Medial pterygoid plate

Posterior nasal spine

A. Inferior View

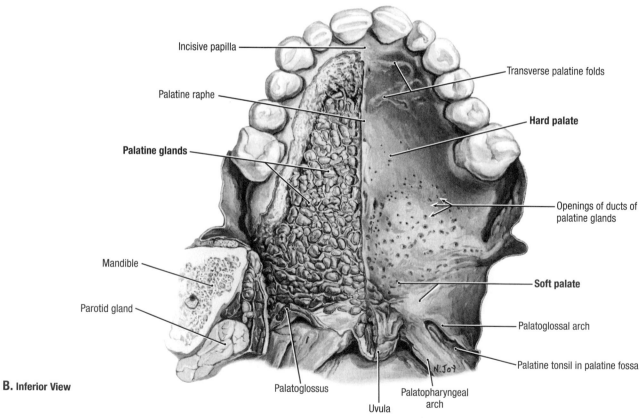

Incisive papilla

Transverse palatine folds

Palatine raphe

Hard palate

Palatine glands

Openings of ducts of palatine glands

Mandible

Parotid gland

Soft palate

Palatoglossal arch

Palatine tonsil in palatine fossa

Palatoglossus

Uvula

Palatopharyngeal arch

B. Inferior View

8.63   **Palate**

A. Bones of hard palate and nasopharynx. The palatine aponeurosis (*Part C* and *Part D*), which forms the fibrous "skeleton" of the soft palate, stretches between the hamuli of the medial pterygoid plates. **B. Mucous membrane and glands of palate.**

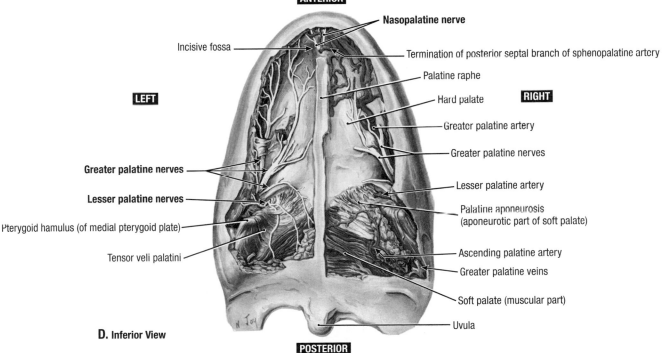

Inferior concha

Middle concha

Superior concha

Pterygopalatine ganglion

Medial pterygoid plate

Greater and lesser palatine nerves

Pharyngobasilar fascia

Levator veli palatini

Palatine aponeurosis

Palatine muscles

Musculus uvulae

Palatine glands

Lesser palatine arteries and nerves

Greater palatine arteries and nerves

Mucous membrane, separated from palate by blunt dissection

C. Lateral View

ANTERIOR

Nasopalatine nerve

Incisive fossa

Termination of posterior septal branch of sphenopalatine artery

Palatine raphe

LEFT

Hard palate

RIGHT

Greater palatine artery

Greater palatine nerves

Greater palatine nerves

Lesser palatine nerves

Lesser palatine artery

Pterygoid hamulus (of medial pterygoid plate)

Palatine aponeurosis (aponeurotic part of soft palate)

Tensor veli palatini

Ascending palatine artery

Greater palatine veins

Soft palate (muscular part)

Uvula

D. Inferior View

POSTERIOR

Palate (continued)

8.63

C. Nerves and vessels of palatine canal. The lateral wall of the nasal cavity is shown. The posterior ends of the middle and inferior conchae are excised along with the mucoperiosteum; the thin, perpendicular plate of the palatine bone is removed to expose the palatine nerves and arteries. **D. Dissection of an edentulous palate.** The greater palatine nerve supplies the gingivae and hard palate, the nasopalatine nerves the incisive region, and the lesser palatine nerves the soft palate. **Anesthesia of palatine nerves.** The nasopalatine nerves can be anesthetized by injecting anesthetic into the mouth of the incisive fossa in the hard palate. The anesthetized tissues are the palatal mucosa, the lingual gingivae, the six anterior maxillary teeth, and associated alveolar bone. The greater palatine nerve can be anesthetized by injecting anesthetic into the greater palatine foramen. The nerve emerges between the second and third maxillary molar teeth. This nerve block anesthetizes the palatal mucosa and lingual gingivae posterior to the maxillary canine teeth, and the underlying bone of the palate.

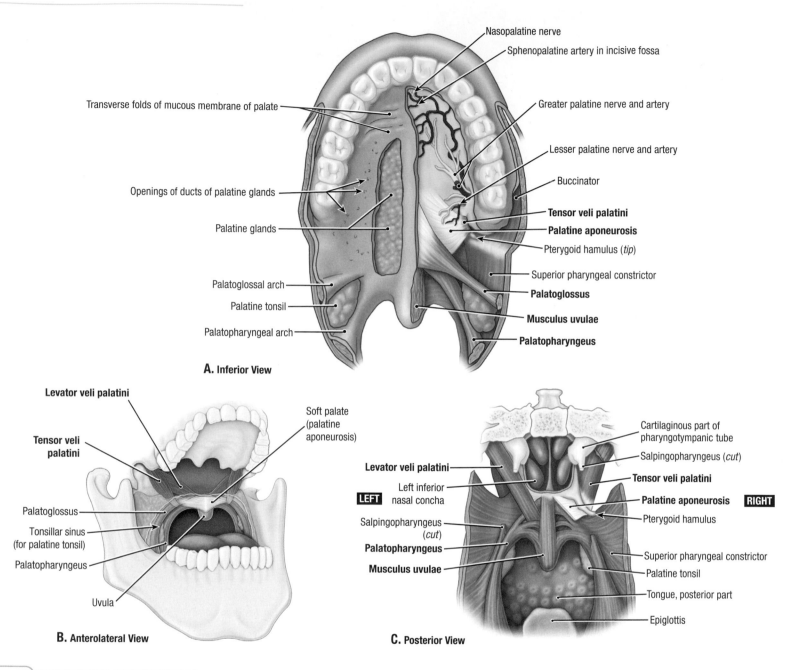

A. Inferior View

Nasopalatine nerve

Sphenopalatine artery in incisive fossa

Transverse folds of mucous membrane of palate

Greater palatine nerve and artery

Lesser palatine nerve and artery

Buccinator

Openings of ducts of palatine glands

Tensor veli palatini

Palatine aponeurosis

Pterygoid hamulus (*tip*)

Palatine glands

Superior pharyngeal constrictor

Palatoglossal arch

Palatoglossus

Palatine tonsil

Musculus uvulae

Palatopharyngeal arch

Palatopharyngeus

B. Anterolateral View

Levator veli palatini

Soft palate (palatine aponeurosis)

Tensor veli palatini

Palatoglossus

Tonsillar sinus (for palatine tonsil)

Palatopharyngeus

Uvula

C. Posterior View

Cartilaginous part of pharyngotympanic tube

Salpingopharyngeus (*cut*)

Levator veli palatini

Left inferior nasal concha

LEFT

Tensor veli palatini

Palatine aponeurosis   **RIGHT**

Pterygoid hamulus

Salpingopharyngeus (*cut*)

Palatopharyngeus

Superior pharyngeal constrictor

Musculus uvulae

Palatine tonsil

Tongue, posterior part

Epiglottis

8.64   Muscles of Soft Palate

TABLE 8.14	Muscles of Soft Palate			
Muscle	**Superior Attachment**	**Inferior Attachment**	**Innervation**	**Main Action(s)**
Levator veli palatini	Cartilage of pharyngotympanic tube and petrous part of temporal bone	Palatine aponeurosis	Pharyngeal branch of vagus nerve through pharyngeal plexus	Elevates soft palate during swallowing and yawning
Tensor veli palatini	Scaphoid fossa of medial pterygoid plate, spine of sphenoid bone, and cartilage of pharyngotympanic tube		Medial pterygoid nerve (CN V_3) through otic ganglion	Tenses soft palate and opens mouth of pharyngotympanic tube during swallowing and yawning
Palatoglossus	Palatine aponeurosis	Side of tongue		Elevates posterior part of tongue and draws soft palate onto tongue
Palatopharyngeus	Hard palate and palatine aponeurosis	Lateral wall of pharynx	Pharyngeal branch of vagus nerve (CN X) via pharyngeal plexus	Tenses soft palate and pulls walls of pharynx superiorly, anteriorly, and medially during swallowing
Musculus uvulae	Posterior nasal spine and palatine aponeurosis	Mucosa of uvula		Shortens uvula and pulls it superiorly

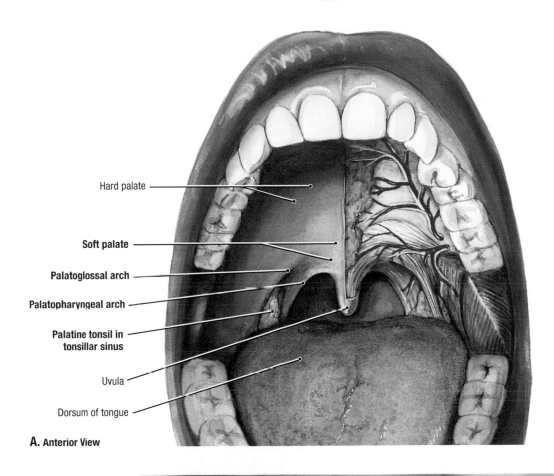

Hard palate

Soft palate

Palatoglossal arch

Palatopharyngeal arch

Palatine tonsil in tonsillar sinus

Uvula

Dorsum of tongue

A. Anterior View

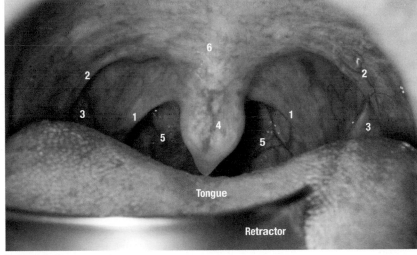

Key for B

1 Palatopharyngeal arch
2 Palatoglossal arch
3 Palatine tonsil
4 Uvula
5 Oropharynx (posterior wall)
6 Soft palate

Tongue

Retractor

B. Anterior View

Surface Anatomy of Isthmus of Fauces (Oropharyngeal Isthmus)   8.65

A. Oral cavity and isthmus demonstrating sinus (bed) of tonsils.
B. Tonsillar sinuses with palatine tonsils *in situ* and oropharynx in adult.

- The fauces (throat), the passage from the mouth to the pharynx, is bounded superiorly by the soft palate, inferiorly by the root (base) of the tongue, and laterally by the palatoglossal and palatopharyngeal arches (folds).
- The palatine tonsils are located between the palatoglossal and palatopharyngeal arches, formed by mucosa overlying the similarly

named muscles; the arches form the boundaries, and the superior pharyngeal constrictor the floor, of the tonsillar sinuses.

- Normal palatine tonsils. In the adult, the palatine tonsils are normally involuted, with little glandular tissue in the tonsillar sinuses (*Part B*). In contrast in young children, the palatine tonsils are large relative to the adult since most of the development of the lymphoid system occurs prior to puberty. Despite their large size, as long as the tonsils are not inflamed and not interfering with swallowing/breathing, they are considered normal.

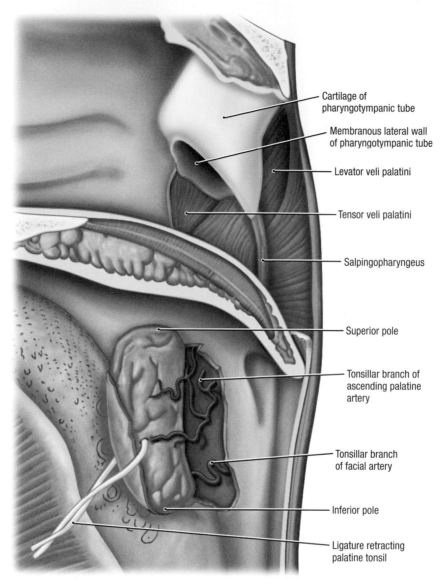

Cartilage of
pharyngotympanic tube

Membranous lateral wall
of pharyngotympanic tube

Levator veli palatini

Tensor veli palatini

Salpingopharyngeus

Superior pole

Tonsillar branch of
ascending palatine
artery

Tonsillar branch
of facial artery

Inferior pole

Ligature retracting
palatine tonsil

A. Medial View of Right Half of Head

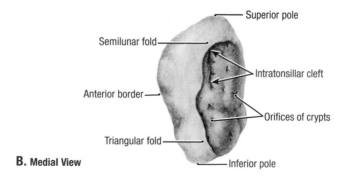

Superior pole

Semilunar fold

Intratonsillar cleft

Anterior border

Orifices of crypts

Triangular fold

B. Medial View

Inferior pole

8.66 **Palatine Tonsil**

A. Isolated palatine tonsil. B. Tonsillectomy. The procedure
involves removal of the tonsil and the fascial sheet covering the
tonsillar fossa. Because of the rich blood supply of the tonsil,
bleeding commonly arises from the large external palatine vein
or less commonly from the tonsillar artery or other arterial twigs.

The glossopharyngeal nerve accompanies the tonsillar artery
on the lateral wall of the pharynx and is vulnerable to injury
because this wall is thin. The internal carotid artery is especially
vulnerable when it is tortuous, as it lies directly lateral to the
tonsil.

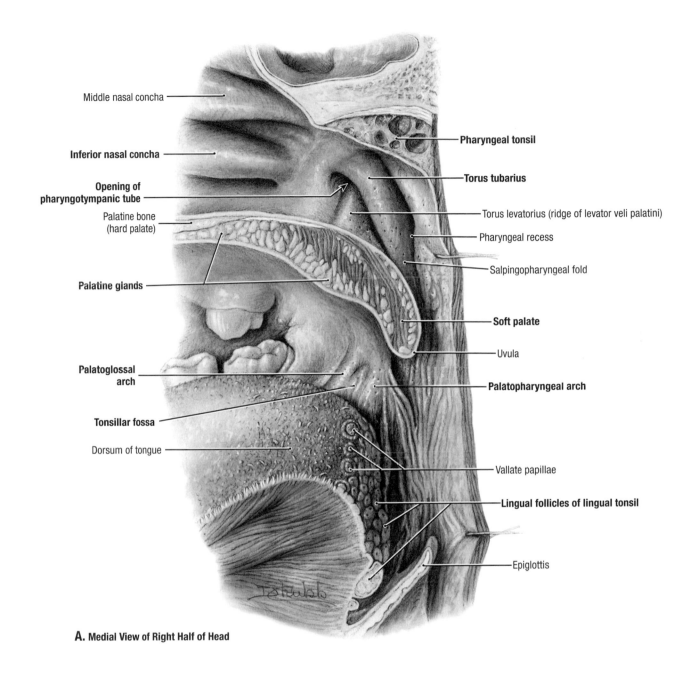

Middle nasal concha

Inferior nasal concha

Opening of pharyngotympanic tube

Palatine bone (hard palate)

Palatine glands

Palatoglossal arch

Tonsillar fossa

Dorsum of tongue

Pharyngeal tonsil

Torus tubarius

Torus levatorius (ridge of levator veli palatini)

Pharyngeal recess

Salpingopharyngeal fold

Soft palate

Uvula

Palatopharyngeal arch

Vallate papillae

Lingual follicles of lingual tonsil

Epiglottis

A. **Medial View of Right Half of Head**

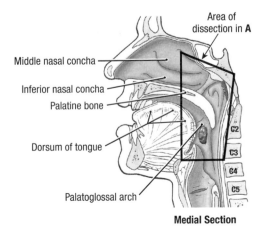

Area of dissection in **A**

Middle nasal concha

Inferior nasal concha

Palatine bone

Dorsum of tongue

Palatoglossal arch

C2

C3

C4

C5

Medial Section

Serial Dissection of Isthmus of Fauces and Lateral Wall of Nasopharynx

8.67

- The pharyngeal opening of the pharyngotympanic tube is located approximately 1 cm posterior to the inferior concha.
- The pharyngeal tonsil lies in the mucous membrane of the roof and posterior wall of the nasopharynx.
- The palatine glands lie in the soft palate.
- The palatine tonsil lies in the tonsillar fossa between the palatoglossal and palatopharyngeal arches.
- Each lingual follicle has the duct of a mucous gland opening onto its surface; collectively, the follicles are known as the lingual tonsil.

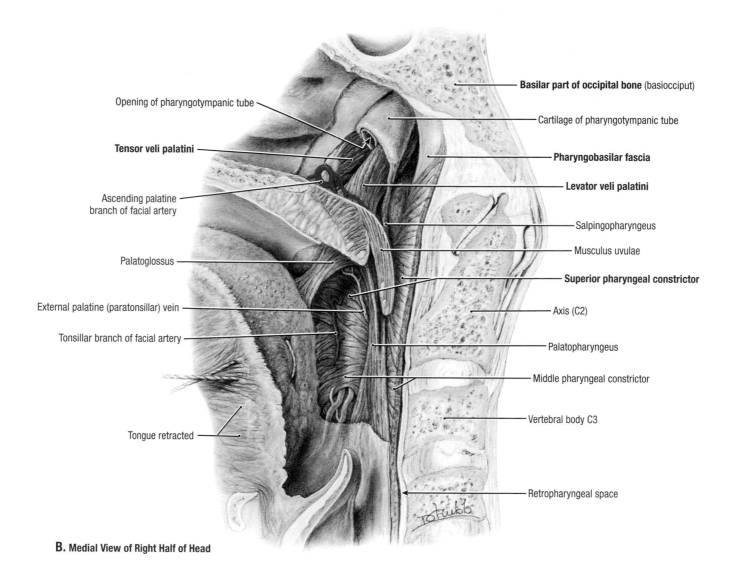

Opening of pharyngotympanic tube

Tensor veli palatini

Ascending palatine branch of facial artery

Palatoglossus

External palatine (paratonsillar) vein

Tonsillar branch of facial artery

Tongue retracted

Basilar part of occipital bone (basiocciput)

Cartilage of pharyngotympanic tube

Pharyngobasilar fascia

Levator veli palatini

Salpingopharyngeus

Musculus uvulae

Superior pharyngeal constrictor

Axis (C2)

Palatopharyngeus

Middle pharyngeal constrictor

Vertebral body C3

Retropharyngeal space

B. Medial View of Right Half of Head

8.67 Serial Dissection of Isthmus of Fauces and Lateral Wall of Nasopharynx *(continued)*

Muscles underlying tonsillar fossa and wall of nasopharynx. The palatine and pharyngeal tonsils and mucous membrane have been removed. The pharyngobasilar fascia, which attaches the pharynx to the basilar part of the occipital bone, was also removed, except at the superior, arched border of the superior pharyngeal constrictor.

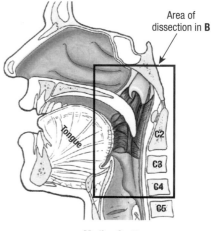

Area of dissection in **B**

Tongue

C2

C3

C4

C5

Median Section

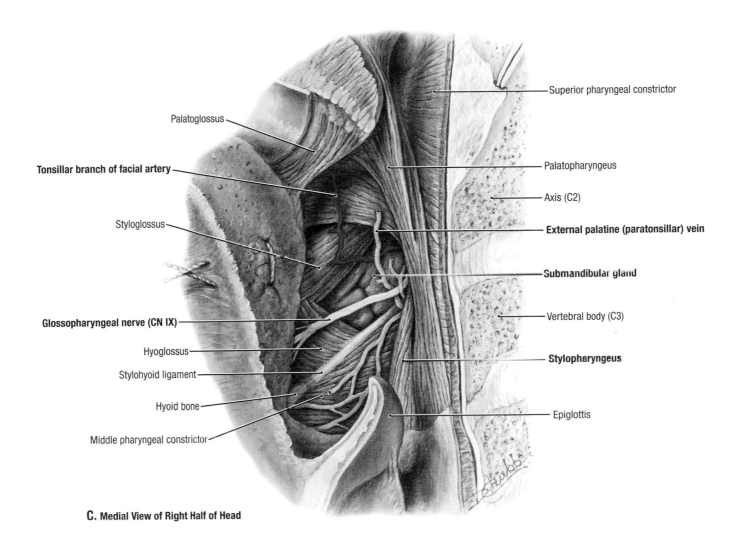

Palatoglossus

Tonsillar branch of facial artery

Styloglossus

Glossopharyngeal nerve (CN IX)

Hyoglossus

Stylohyoid ligament

Hyoid bone

Middle pharyngeal constrictor

Superior pharyngeal constrictor

Palatopharyngeus

Axis (C2)

External palatine (paratonsillar) vein

Submandibular gland

Vertebral body (C3)

Stylopharyngeus

Epiglottis

C. Medial View of Right Half of Head

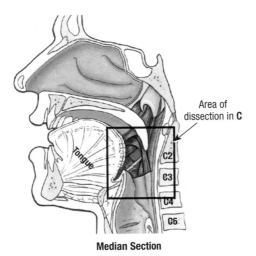

Area of
dissection in **C**

Median Section

**Serial Dissection of Isthmus of Fauces and
Lateral Wall of Nasopharynx** *(continued)*   8.67

Neurovascular structures of tonsillar sinus and longitudinal
muscles of the pharynx are shown.

- In this deeper dissection, the tongue was pulled anteriorly,
  and the inferior part of the origin of the superior pharyngeal
  constrictor muscle was cut away.
- The glossopharyngeal nerve passes to the posterior one third
  of the tongue and lies anterior to the stylopharyngeus muscle.
- The tonsillar branch of the facial artery sends a branch (cut
  short here) to accompany the glossopharyngeal nerve to the
  tongue; the submandibular gland is seen lateral to the artery
  and external palatine (paratonsillar) vein.

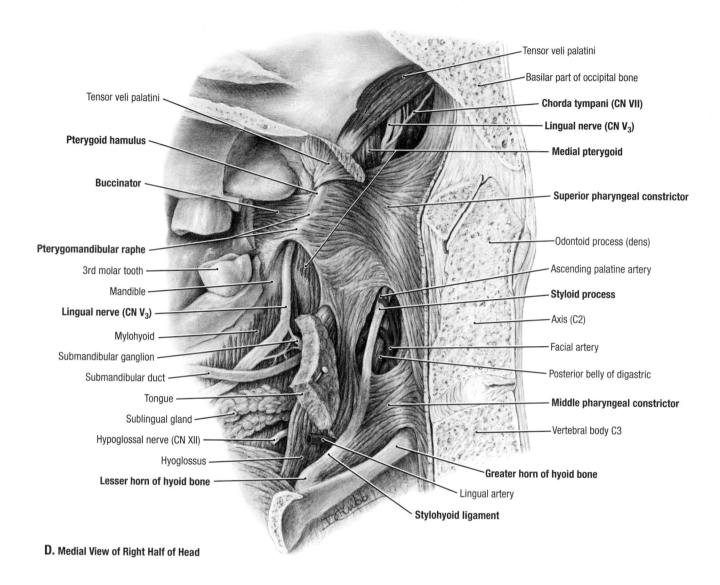

Tensor veli palatini

Basilar part of occipital bone

Chorda tympani (CN VII)

Lingual nerve (CN V₃)

Medial pterygoid

Superior pharyngeal constrictor

Odontoid process (dens)

Ascending palatine artery

Styloid process

Axis (C2)

Facial artery

Posterior belly of digastric

Middle pharyngeal constrictor

Vertebral body C3

Greater horn of hyoid bone

Lingual artery

Tensor veli palatini

Pterygoid hamulus

Buccinator

Pterygomandibular raphe

3rd molar tooth

Mandible

Lingual nerve (CN V₃)

Mylohyoid

Submandibular ganglion

Submandibular duct

Tongue

Sublingual gland

Hypoglossal nerve (CN XII)

Hyoglossus

Lesser horn of hyoid bone

Stylohyoid ligament

D. Medial View of Right Half of Head

| 8.67 | **Serial Dissection of Isthmus of Fauces and Lateral Wall of Nasopharynx** (continued) |

- The superior pharyngeal constrictor muscle arises from (1) the pterygomandibular raphe, which unites it to the buccinator muscle; (2) the bones at each end of the raphe, the hamulus of the medial pterygoid plate superiorly and the mandible inferiorly; and (3) the root (posterior part) of the tongue.
- The middle pharyngeal constrictor muscle arises from the angle formed by the greater and lesser horns of the hyoid bone and from the stylohyoid ligament; in this specimen, the styloid process is long and, therefore, a lateral relation of the tonsil.
- The lingual nerve is joined by the chorda tympani, disappears at the posterior border of the medial pterygoid muscle, and reappears at the anterior border to follow the mandible.

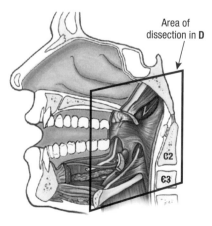

Area of dissection in **D**

C2

C3

Median Section

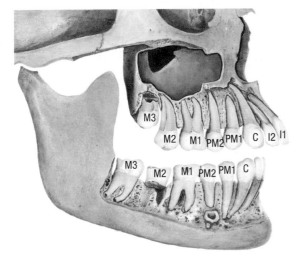

A. Lateral View

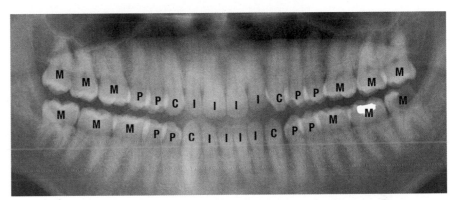

B. Panoramic Radiograph

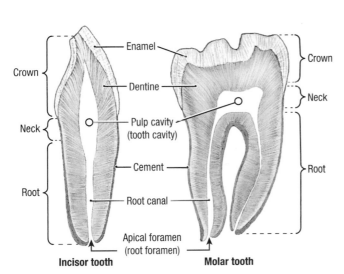

Incisor tooth   **Molar tooth**

C. Longitudinal Section

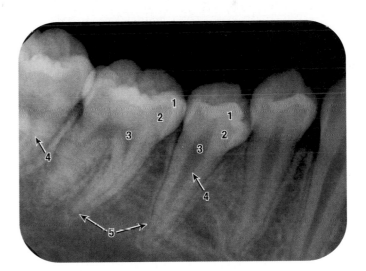

D. Lateral Radiograph

Key for D		
1 Enamel	**3** Pulp cavity	**5** Root apex
2 Dentin	**4** Root canal	

Permanent Teeth (I)   8.68

A. Teeth *in situ* with roots exposed. Incisors (*I1*, *I2*), canine (*C*), premolars (*PM1*, *PM2*), and molars (*M1*, *M2*, *M3*). The roots of the 2nd lower molar have been removed. **B. Pantomographic radiograph of mandible and maxilla.** The left lower third molar is not present. **C. Longitudinal sections of an incisor and a molar tooth. D. Lateral radiograph.**

Decay of the hard tissues of a tooth results in the formation of **dental caries** (cavities). Invasion of the pulp of the tooth by a carious lesion (cavity) results in infection and irritation of the tissues in the pulp cavity. This condition causes an inflammatory process (pulpitis). Because the pulp cavity is a rigid space, the swollen pulpal tissues cause pain (toothache).

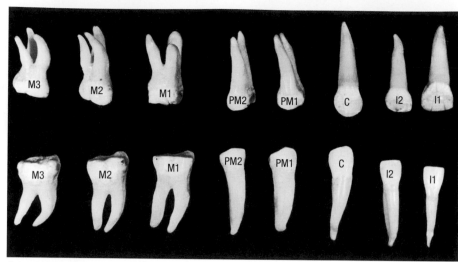

A. Vestibular View

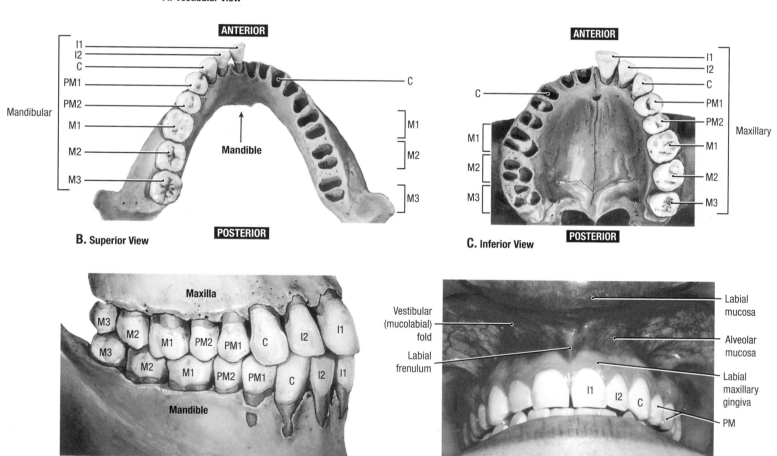

B. Superior View

C. Inferior View

D. Anterolateral View

E. Anterior View

8.69   Permanent Teeth (II)

A. Removed teeth, displaying roots. There are 32 permanent teeth; 8 are on each side of each dental arch on the top (maxillary teeth) and bottom (mandibular teeth): 2 incisors (*I1*, *I2*), 1 canine (C), 2 premolars (*PM1*, *PM2*), and 3 molars (*M1* to *M3*).

B. Permanent mandibular teeth and their dental alveoli (sockets). **C. Permanent maxillary teeth and their dental alveoli. D. Teeth in occlusion. E. Vestibule and gingivae of maxilla.**

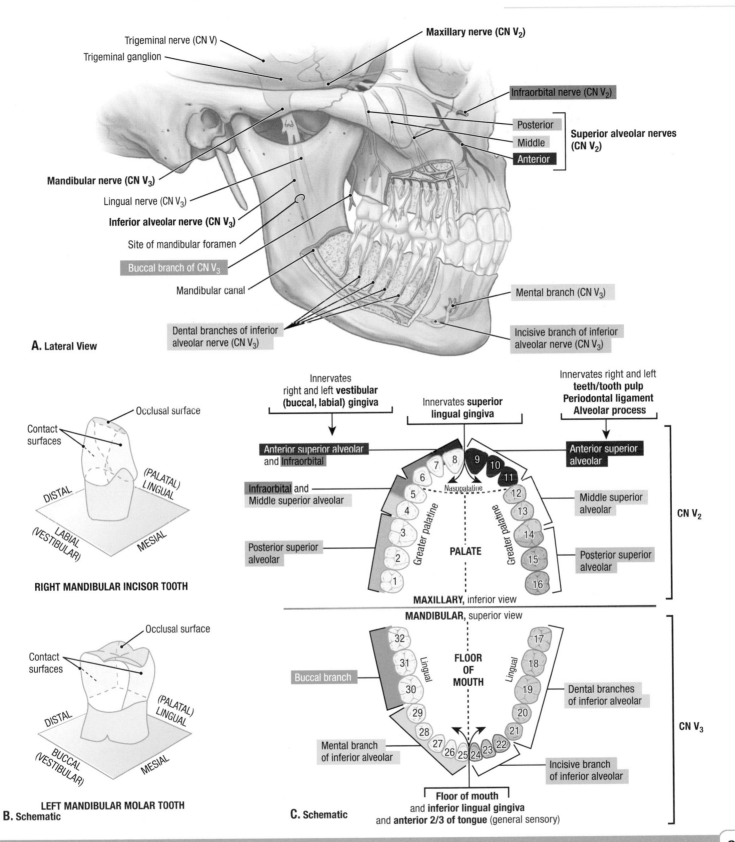

Trigeminal nerve (CN V)
Trigeminal ganglion
Maxillary nerve (CN V₂)
Infraorbital nerve (CN V₂)
Posterior
Middle
Anterior
Superior alveolar nerves (CN V₂)
Mandibular nerve (CN V₃)
Lingual nerve (CN V₃)
Inferior alveolar nerve (CN V₃)
Site of mandibular foramen
Buccal branch of CN V₃
Mandibular canal
Mental branch (CN V₃)
Dental branches of inferior alveolar nerve (CN V₃)
Incisive branch of inferior alveolar nerve (CN V₃)

A. Lateral View

Occlusal surface
Contact surfaces
(PALATAL) LINGUAL
DISTAL
LABIAL (VESTIBULAR)
MESIAL

RIGHT MANDIBULAR INCISOR TOOTH

Occlusal surface
Contact surfaces
(PALATAL) LINGUAL
DISTAL
BUCCAL (VESTIBULAR)
MESIAL

LEFT MANDIBULAR MOLAR TOOTH
B. Schematic

Innervates right and left **vestibular (buccal, labial) gingiva**
Innervates **superior lingual gingiva**
Innervates right and left **teeth/tooth pulp Periodontal ligament Alveolar process**

Anterior superior alveolar and Infraorbital
Infraorbital and Middle superior alveolar
Posterior superior alveolar

Anterior superior alveolar
Middle superior alveolar
Posterior superior alveolar

Nasopalatine
Greater palatine
PALATE
Greater palatine

MAXILLARY, inferior view

CN V₂

MANDIBULAR, superior view

FLOOR OF MOUTH
Lingual
Buccal branch
Mental branch of inferior alveolar

Lingual
Dental branches of inferior alveolar
Incisive branch of inferior alveolar

Floor of mouth and **inferior lingual gingiva** and **anterior 2/3 of tongue** (general sensory)

CN V₃

C. Schematic

Innervation of Teeth

8.70

A. Superior and inferior alveolar nerves. **B.** Surfaces of an incisor and molar tooth. **C.** Innervation of mouth and teeth.

Improper oral hygiene results in food deposits in tooth and gingival crevices, which may cause inflammation of the gingivae, gingivitis. If untreated, the disease spreads to other supporting structures (including the alveolar bone), producing **periodontitis**. Periodontitis results in inflammation of the gingivae and may result in absorption of alveolar bone and gingival recession. Gingival recession exposes the sensitive cement of the teeth.

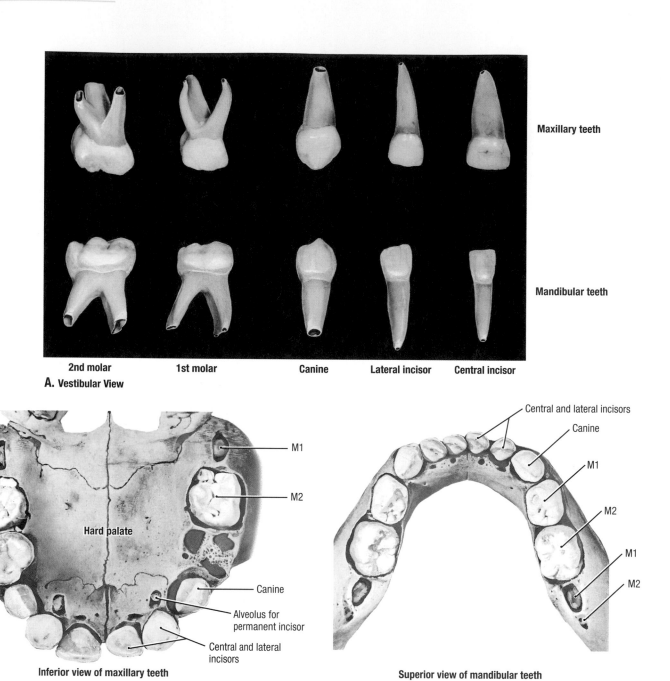

A. Vestibular View

2nd molar   1st molar   Canine   Lateral incisor   Central incisor

Maxillary teeth

Mandibular teeth

B. Teeth *in Situ*

M1
M2
Hard palate
Canine
Alveolus for permanent incisor
Central and lateral incisors

Inferior view of maxillary teeth

Central and lateral incisors
Canine
M1
M2
M1
M2

Superior view of mandibular teeth

8.71   Primary Teeth

A. Removed teeth. There are 20 primary (deciduous) teeth, 5 in each half of the mandible and 5 in each maxilla. They are named central incisor, lateral incisor, canine, 1st molar (*M1*), and 2nd molar (*M2*). Primary teeth differ from permanent teeth in that the primary teeth are smaller and whiter; the molars also have more bulbous crowns and more divergent roots. **B. Teeth *in situ*, younger than 2 years of age.** Permanent teeth are colored orange; the crowns of the unerupted 1st and 2nd permanent molars are partly visible.

TABLE 8.15   Primary (Deciduous) Teeth

Deciduous Teeth	Central Incisor	Lateral Incisor	Canine	First Molar	Second Molar
Eruption (months)[a]	6–8	8–10	16–20	12–16	20–24
Shedding (years)	6–7	7–8	10–12	9–11	10–12

[a]In some normal infants, the first teeth (medial incisors) may not erupt until 12 to 13 months of age.

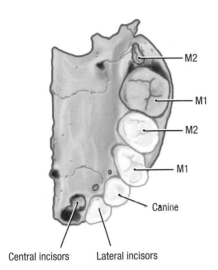

M2

M1

M2

M1

Canine

Central incisors   Lateral incisors

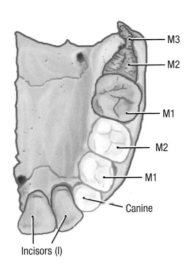

M3

M2

M1

M2

M1

Canine

Incisors (I)

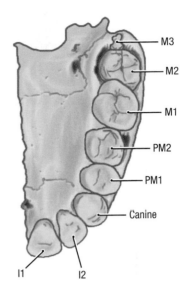

M3

M2

M1

PM2

PM1

Canine

I1   I2

Inferior Views

Central incisors   Lateral incisors

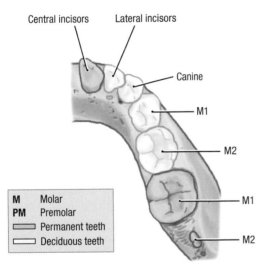

Canine

M1

M2

M1

M2

M	Molar
PM	Premolar
	Permanent teeth
	Deciduous teeth

A. Age: 6–7 years

Incisors

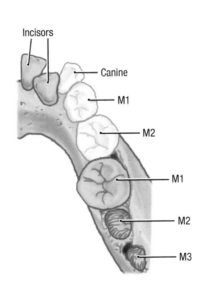

Canine

M1

M2

M1

M2

M3

B. Age: 8 years

I1   I2

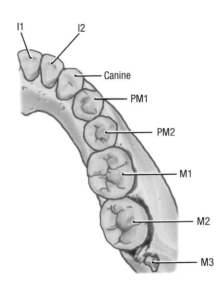

Canine

PM1

PM2

M1

M2

M3

C. Age: 12 years

Superior Views

Permanent (Secondary) Teeth

8.72

TABLE 8.16	Permanent (Secondary) Teeth							
Permanent Teeth	**Central Incisor**	**Lateral Incisor**	**Canine**	**First Premolar**	**Second Premolar**	**First Molar**	**Second Molar**	**Third Molar**
Eruption (years)	7–8	8–9	10–12	10–11	11–12	6–7	12	13–25

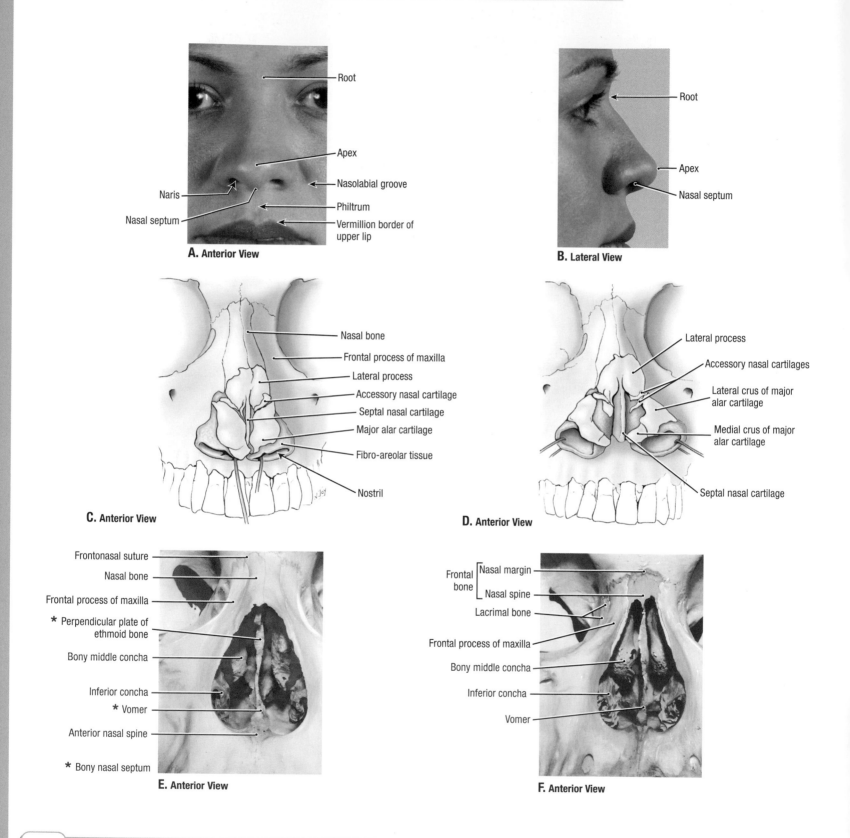

A. Anterior View

Root
Apex
Nasolabial groove
Naris
Philtrum
Nasal septum
Vermillion border of upper lip

B. Lateral View

Root
Apex
Nasal septum

C. Anterior View

Nasal bone
Frontal process of maxilla
Lateral process
Accessory nasal cartilage
Septal nasal cartilage
Major alar cartilage
Fibro-areolar tissue
Nostril

D. Anterior View

Lateral process
Accessory nasal cartilages
Lateral crus of major alar cartilage
Medial crus of major alar cartilage
Septal nasal cartilage

E. Anterior View

Frontonasal suture
Nasal bone
Frontal process of maxilla
* Perpendicular plate of ethmoid bone
Bony middle concha
Inferior concha
* Vomer
Anterior nasal spine
* Bony nasal septum

F. Anterior View

Frontal bone [Nasal margin
Nasal spine]
Lacrimal bone
Frontal process of maxilla
Bony middle concha
Inferior concha
Vomer

8.73   **Surface Anatomy, Cartilages, and Bones of Nose**

A. Surface features of anterior aspect of nose. **B.** Surface features of lateral aspect of nose. **C.** Nasal cartilages, with septum pulled inferiorly. **D.** Nasal cartilages, separated and retracted laterally. **E.** Lower conchae and bony septum seen through

piriform aperture. The margin of the piriform aperture is sharp and formed by the maxillae and nasal bones. **F.** Nasal bones removed. The areas of the frontal processes of the maxillae (*yellow*) and of the frontal bone (*blue*) that articulate with the nasal bones can be seen.

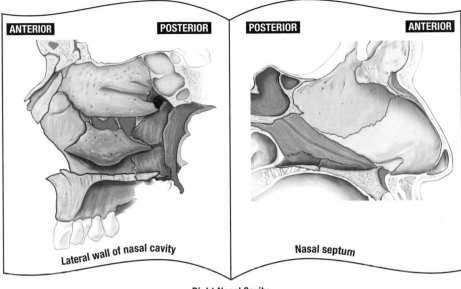

ANTERIOR   POSTERIOR   POSTERIOR   ANTERIOR

Lateral wall of nasal cavity   Nasal septum

Right Nasal Cavity

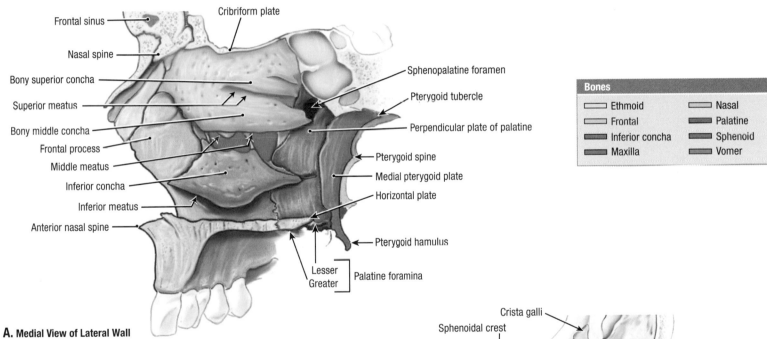

Frontal sinus

Nasal spine

Bony superior concha

Superior meatus

Bony middle concha

Frontal process

Middle meatus

Inferior concha

Inferior meatus

Anterior nasal spine

Cribriform plate

Sphenopalatine foramen

Pterygoid tubercle

Perpendicular plate of palatine

Pterygoid spine

Medial pterygoid plate

Horizontal plate

Pterygoid hamulus

Lesser
Greater   Palatine foramina

A. Medial View of Lateral Wall

Bones	
▭ Ethmoid	▭ Nasal
▭ Frontal	▭ Palatine
▭ Inferior concha	▭ Sphenoid
▭ Maxilla	▭ Vomer

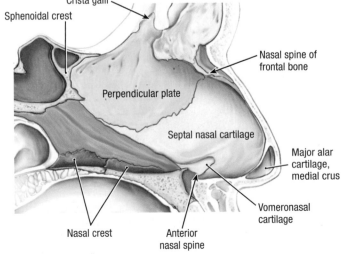

Crista galli

Sphenoidal crest

Nasal spine of
frontal bone

Perpendicular plate

Septal nasal cartilage

Major alar
cartilage,
medial crus

Nasal crest   Anterior
nasal spine

Vomeronasal
cartilage

B. Lateral View of Nasal Septum

Bones of Nasal Wall and Septum   8.74

A. Lateral wall of nose. The superior and middle bony conchae are parts of the ethmoid bone, whereas the inferior concha is itself a bone. **B. Nasal septum.**

Deformity of the external nose usually is present with a fracture, particularly when a lateral force is applied by someone's elbow, for example. When the injury results from a direct blow (e.g., from a hockey stick), the cribriform plate of the ethmoid bone may fracture, resulting in CSF rhinorrhea.

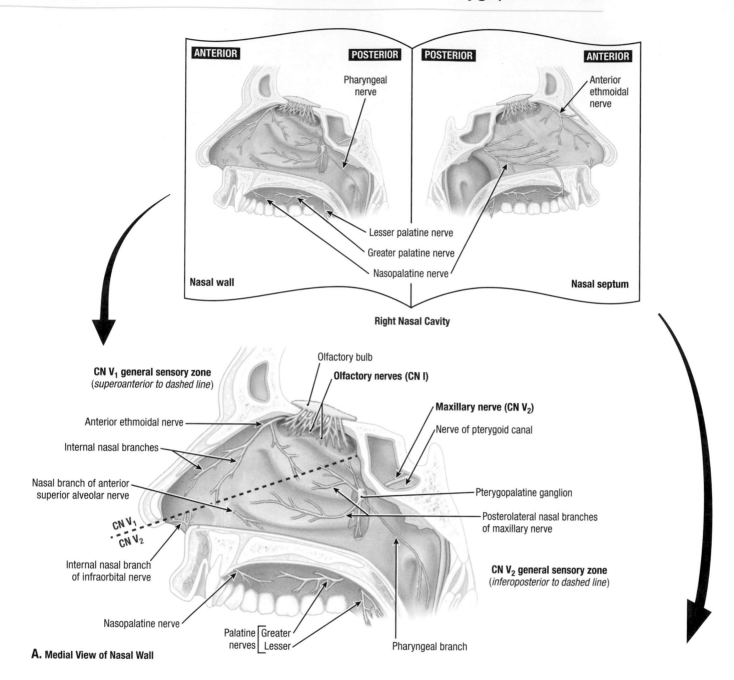

ANTERIOR | **POSTERIOR**

Pharyngeal nerve

POSTERIOR | **ANTERIOR**

Anterior ethmoidal nerve

Lesser palatine nerve

Greater palatine nerve

Nasopalatine nerve

Nasal wall

Nasal septum

Right Nasal Cavity

CN V₁ general sensory zone (*superoanterior to dashed line*)

Olfactory bulb

Olfactory nerves (CN I)

Maxillary nerve (CN V₂)

Anterior ethmoidal nerve

Nerve of pterygoid canal

Internal nasal branches

Nasal branch of anterior superior alveolar nerve

CN V₁

CN V₂

Pterygopalatine ganglion

Posterolateral nasal branches of maxillary nerve

Internal nasal branch of infraorbital nerve

CN V₂ general sensory zone (*inferoposterior to dashed line*)

Nasopalatine nerve

Palatine nerves [Greater / Lesser]

Pharyngeal branch

A. Medial View of Nasal Wall

| 8.75 | **Innervation of Nasal Wall and Septum** |

A. Lateral wall of nose. *Dashed diagonal lines* demarcate CN V₁ and CN V₂ general sensory zones. The olfactory neuroepithelium is in the superior part of the lateral and septal walls of the nasal cavity. The central processes of the olfactory neurosensory cells of each side form approximately 20 bundles that together form an olfactory nerve (CN I). **B. Nasal septum.** The nasopalatine nerve from the pterygopalatine ganglion supplies the extraocular septum, and the anterior ethmoidal nerve (branch of CN V₁) supplies the anterosuperior septum.

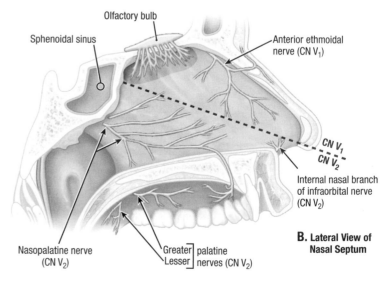

Olfactory bulb

Sphenoidal sinus

Anterior ethmoidal nerve (CN V₁)

CN V₁

CN V₂

Internal nasal branch of infraorbital nerve (CN V₂)

Nasopalatine nerve (CN V₂)

Greater / Lesser] palatine nerves (CN V₂)

B. Lateral View of Nasal Septum

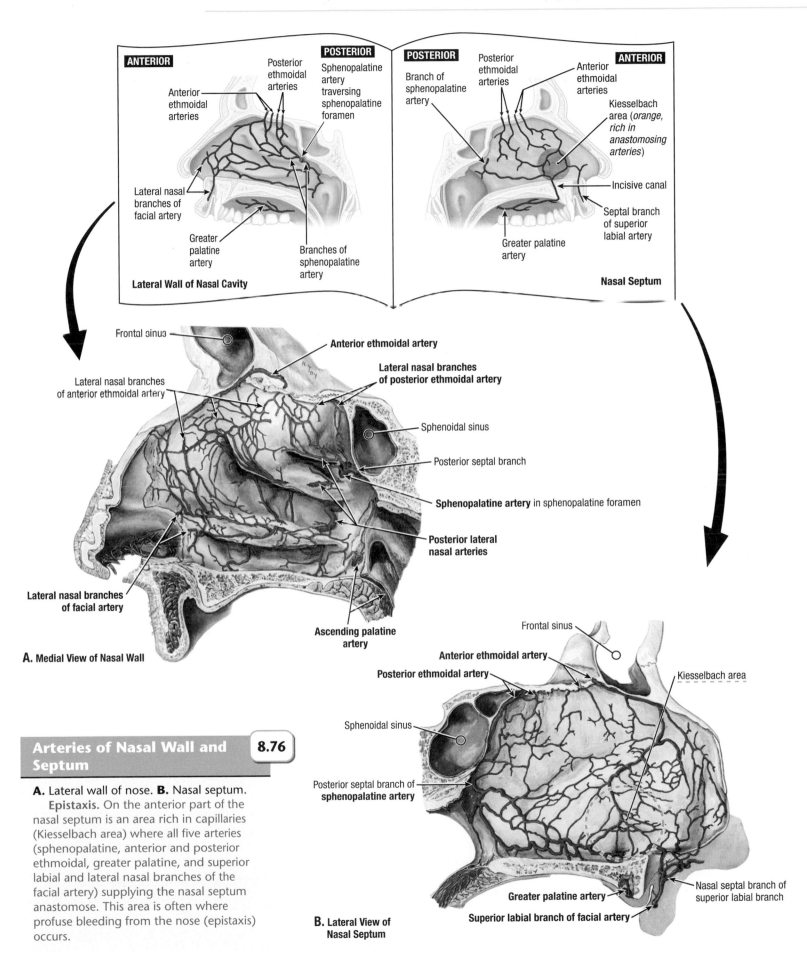

ANTERIOR

Anterior ethmoidal arteries

Posterior ethmoidal arteries

Sphenopalatine artery traversing sphenopalatine foramen

POSTERIOR

Lateral nasal branches of facial artery

Greater palatine artery

Branches of sphenopalatine artery

Lateral Wall of Nasal Cavity

POSTERIOR

Branch of sphenopalatine artery

Posterior ethmoidal arteries

Anterior ethmoidal arteries

Kiesselbach area (*orange, rich in anastomosing arteries*)

ANTERIOR

Incisive canal

Septal branch of superior labial artery

Greater palatine artery

Nasal Septum

Frontal sinus

Lateral nasal branches of anterior ethmoidal artery

Anterior ethmoidal artery

Lateral nasal branches of posterior ethmoidal artery

Sphenoidal sinus

Posterior septal branch

Sphenopalatine artery in sphenopalatine foramen

Posterior lateral nasal arteries

Lateral nasal branches of facial artery

Ascending palatine artery

A. Medial View of Nasal Wall

Frontal sinus

Anterior ethmoidal artery

Posterior ethmoidal artery

Kiesselbach area

Sphenoidal sinus

Posterior septal branch of **sphenopalatine artery**

Nasal septal branch of superior labial branch

Greater palatine artery

Superior labial branch of facial artery

B. Lateral View of Nasal Septum

Arteries of Nasal Wall and Septum   **8.76**

A. Lateral wall of nose. **B.** Nasal septum.
Epistaxis. On the anterior part of the nasal septum is an area rich in capillaries (Kiesselbach area) where all five arteries (sphenopalatine, anterior and posterior ethmoidal, greater palatine, and superior labial and lateral nasal branches of the facial artery) supplying the nasal septum anastomose. This area is often where profuse bleeding from the nose (epistaxis) occurs.

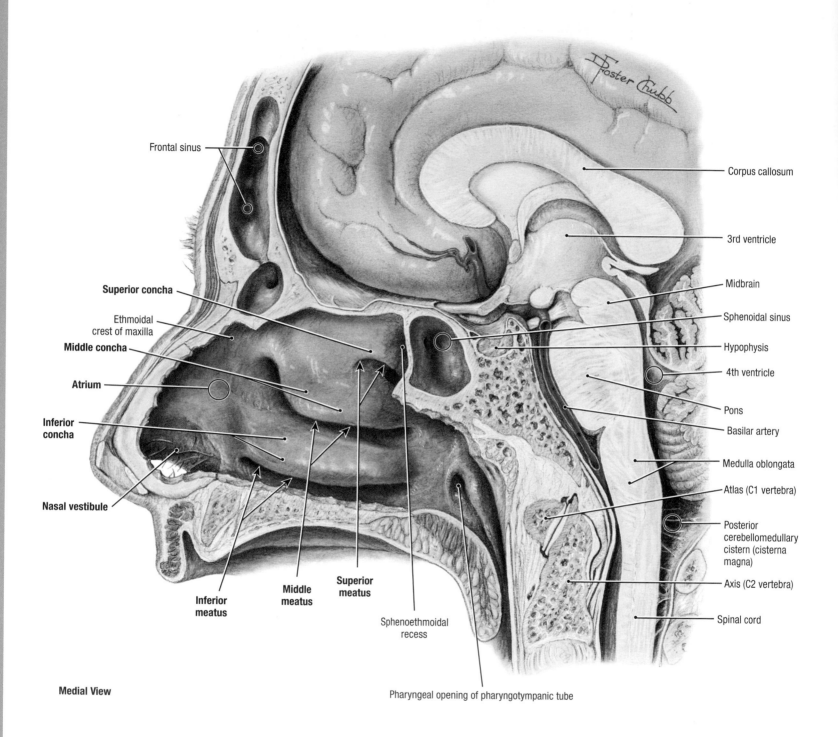

Frontal sinus

Corpus callosum

3rd ventricle

Superior concha

Midbrain

Ethmoidal crest of maxilla

Sphenoidal sinus

Middle concha

Hypophysis

4th ventricle

Atrium

Pons

Basilar artery

Inferior concha

Medulla oblongata

Atlas (C1 vertebra)

Nasal vestibule

Posterior cerebellomedullary cistern (cisterna magna)

Axis (C2 vertebra)

Spinal cord

Inferior meatus

Middle meatus

Superior meatus

Sphenoethmoidal recess

Medial View

Pharyngeal opening of pharyngotympanic tube

8.77 **Right Half of Hemisected Head Demonstrating Upper Respiratory Tract**

- The vestibule is superior to the nostril and anterior to the inferior meatus; hairs grow from its skin-lined surface. The atrium is superior to the vestibule and anterior to the middle meatus.
- The inferior and middle bony conchae curve inferiorly and medially from the lateral wall, dividing it into three nearly equal parts and covering the inferior and middle meatuses, respectively. The bony middle concha ends inferior to the sphenoidal sinus, and

the inferior concha ends inferior to the bony middle concha, just anterior to the orifice of the auditory tube. The bony superior concha is small and anterior to the sphenoidal sinus.
- The roof comprises an anterior sloping part corresponding to the bridge of the nose; an intermediate horizontal part; a perpendicular part anterior to the sphenoidal sinus; and a curved part, inferior to the sinus, that is continuous with the roof of the nasopharynx.

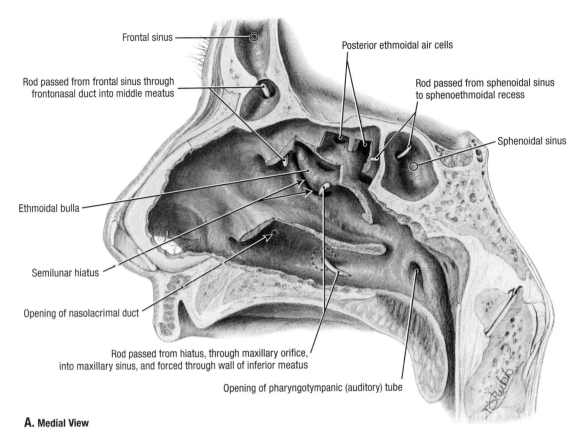

Frontal sinus

Rod passed from frontal sinus through frontonasal duct into middle meatus

Posterior ethmoidal air cells

Rod passed from sphenoidal sinus to sphenoethmoidal recess

Sphenoidal sinus

Ethmoidal bulla

Semilunar hiatus

Opening of nasolacrimal duct

Rod passed from hiatus, through maxillary orifice, into maxillary sinus, and forced through wall of inferior meatus

Opening of pharyngotympanic (auditory) tube

A. Medial View

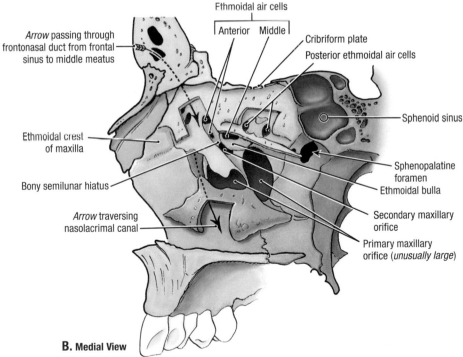

Ethmoidal air cells

Anterior   Middle

Cribriform plate

Posterior ethmoidal air cells

Arrow passing through frontonasal duct from frontal sinus to middle meatus

Sphenoid sinus

Ethmoidal crest of maxilla

Bony semilunar hiatus

Sphenopalatine foramen

Ethmoidal bulla

Arrow traversing nasolacrimal canal

Secondary maxillary orifice

Primary maxillary orifice (unusually large)

B. Medial View

Bones in B		Openings
☐ Ethmoid	☐ Maxilla	■ Openings of adjacent spaces in nasal wall
☐ Frontal	☐ Nasal	
■ Inferior concha	☐ Palatine	
■ Lacrimal	☐ Sphenoid	

Communications through Nasal Wall

8.78

A. Dissection. Parts of the superior, middle, and inferior conchae are cut away to reveal the openings of the air sinuses. **B. Diagram of bones and openings of lateral wall of nasal cavity following dissection.** Note one *arrow* passing from the frontal sinus through the frontonasal duct into the middle meatus and another *arrow* coming from the anteromedial orbit via the nasolacrimal canal.

Rhinitis. The nasal mucosa becomes swollen and inflamed (rhinitis) during upper respiratory infections and allergic reactions (e.g., hay fever). Swelling of this mucous membrane occurs readily because of its vascularity and abundant mucosal glands. Infections of the nasal cavities may spread to the anterior cranial fossa through the cribriform plate, nasopharynx and retropharyngeal soft tissues, middle ear through the pharyngotympanic (auditory) tube, paranasal sinuses, lacrimal apparatus, and conjunctiva.

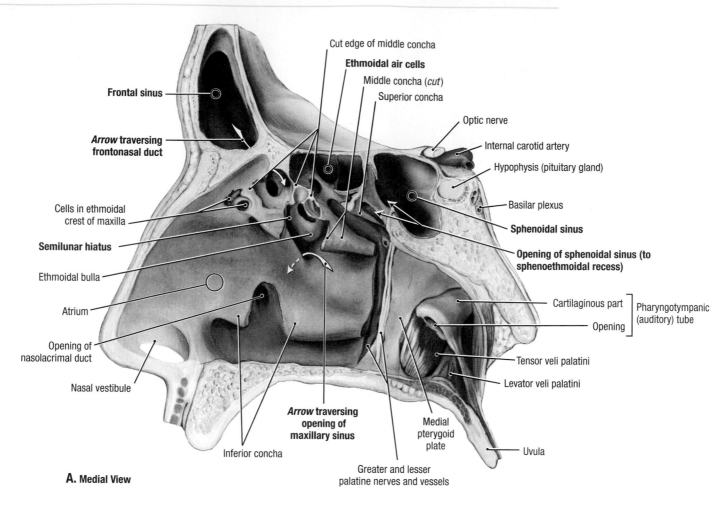

Cut edge of middle concha

Ethmoidal air cells

Middle concha (*cut*)

Superior concha

Frontal sinus

Optic nerve

Internal carotid artery

***Arrow* traversing frontonasal duct**

Hypophysis (pituitary gland)

Basilar plexus

Cells in ethmoidal crest of maxilla

Sphenoidal sinus

Semilunar hiatus

Opening of sphenoidal sinus (to sphenoethmoidal recess)

Ethmoidal bulla

Cartilaginous part — Pharyngotympanic (auditory) tube

Atrium

Opening

Opening of nasolacrimal duct

Tensor veli palatini

Levator veli palatini

Nasal vestibule

***Arrow* traversing opening of maxillary sinus**

Medial pterygoid plate

Uvula

Inferior concha

Greater and lesser palatine nerves and vessels

A. Medial View

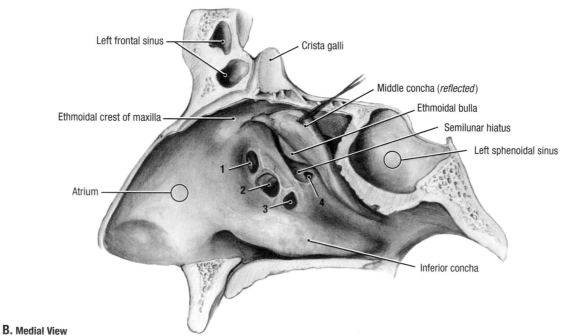

Left frontal sinus

Crista galli

Middle concha (*reflected*)

Ethmoidal bulla

Ethmoidal crest of maxilla

Semilunar hiatus

Left sphenoidal sinus

Atrium

1

2

3

4

Inferior concha

B. Medial View

8.79 **Paranasal Sinuses, Openings, and Palatine Muscles in Nasal Wall**

A. Dissection. Parts of the middle and inferior conchae and lateral wall of the nasal cavity are cut away to expose the nerves and vessels in the palatine canal and the extrinsic palatine muscles.

B. Accessory maxillary orifices. In addition to the primary, or normal, ostium (not shown), there are four secondary, or acquired, ostia (numbered *1* to *4*).

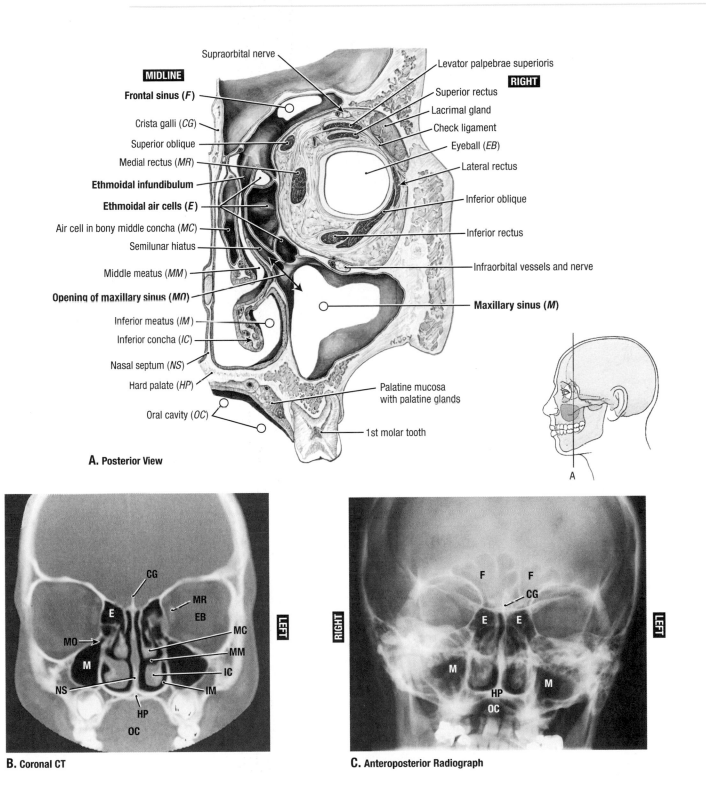

Supraorbital nerve

MIDLINE

Frontal sinus (F)

Crista galli (*CG*)

Superior oblique

Medial rectus (*MR*)

Ethmoidal infundibulum

Ethmoidal air cells (E)

Air cell in bony middle concha (*MC*)

Semilunar hiatus

Middle meatus (*MM*)

Opening of maxillary sinus (MO)

Inferior meatus (*IM*)

Inferior concha (*IC*)

Nasal septum (*NS*)

Hard palate (*HP*)

Oral cavity (*OC*)

Levator palpebrae superioris

RIGHT

Superior rectus

Lacrimal gland

Check ligament

Eyeball (*EB*)

Lateral rectus

Inferior oblique

Inferior rectus

Infraorbital vessels and nerve

Maxillary sinus (M)

N.JOY

Palatine mucosa with palatine glands

1st molar tooth

A. Posterior View

A

B. Coronal CT

RIGHT — CG, MR, E, EB, MC, MO, MM, M, IC, NS, IM, HP, OC — LEFT

C. Anteroposterior Radiograph

RIGHT — F, F, CG, E, E, M, M, HP, OC — LEFT

Paranasal Sinuses and Nasal Cavity

8.80

A. Coronal section of right side of head. B. CT image. C. Radiograph of cranium. Letters in *Part B* and *Part C* refer to structures labeled in *Part A*.

If nasal drainage is blocked, **infections of the ethmoidal cells** of the ethmoidal sinuses may break through the fragile medial wall of the orbit. Severe infections from this source may cause blindness but could also affect the dural sheath of the optic nerve, causing **optic neuritis**.

During removal of a maxillary molar tooth, a **fracture of a tooth root** may occur. If proper retrieval methods are not used, a piece of the root may be driven superiorly into the maxillary sinus.

Radiographs/CT images of the frontal sinuses may be used for **forensic identification of unknown individuals**. The frontal sinuses are unique to each person, much like fingerprints.

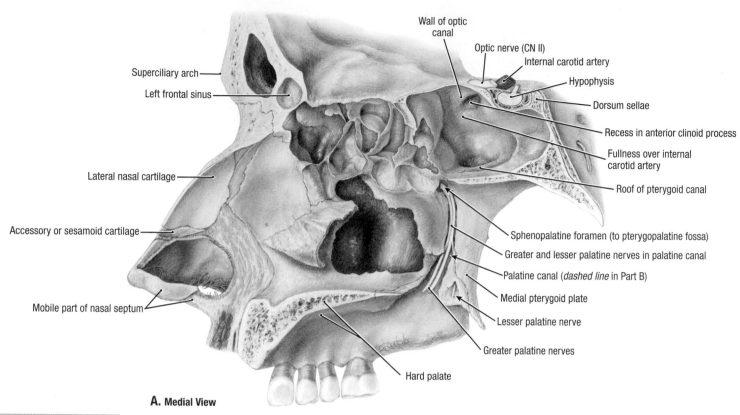

Superciliary arch

Left frontal sinus

Lateral nasal cartilage

Accessory or sesamoid cartilage

Mobile part of nasal septum

Wall of optic canal

Optic nerve (CN II)

Internal carotid artery

Hypophysis

Dorsum sellae

Recess in anterior clinoid process

Fullness over internal carotid artery

Roof of pterygoid canal

Sphenopalatine foramen (to pterygopalatine fossa)

Greater and lesser palatine nerves in palatine canal

Palatine canal (*dashed line* in Part B)

Medial pterygoid plate

Lesser palatine nerve

Greater palatine nerves

Hard palate

A. Medial View

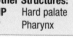

Sinuses:
Ethmoidal air cells (*E*)
Frontal sinus (*F*)
Maxillary sinus (*M*)
Sphenoidal sinus (*S*)

Other Structures:
HP Hard palate
P Pharynx

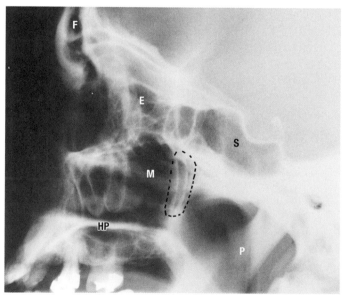

B. Lateral Radiograph

8.81 Paranasal Sinuses

A. Opened sinuses. Sinuses are color coded. **B. Radiograph of cranium.** The maxillary sinuses are the most commonly infected, as their ostia are small and located high on their superomedial walls, a poor location for natural drainage of the sinus. When the mucous membrane of the sinus is congested, the maxillary openings (ostia) often are obstructed. The **maxillary sinusitis** is treated with antibiotics; the sinus can also be cannulated and drained. For chronic maxillary sinusitis, **sinuplasty** or **maxillary antrostomy** is used to improve the drainage of the maxillary sinus by enlarging the opening of the ostia of one or more sinuses.

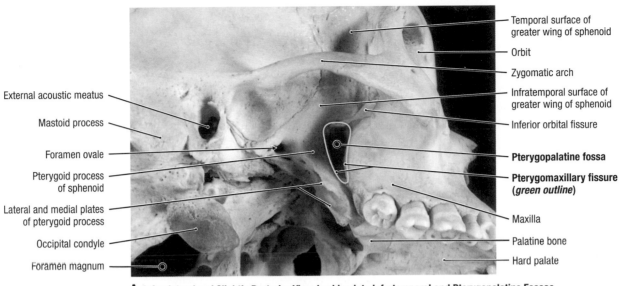

Temporal surface of
greater wing of sphenoid

Orbit

Zygomatic arch

Infratemporal surface of
greater wing of sphenoid

Inferior orbital fissure

Pterygopalatine fossa

Pterygomaxillary fissure
(*green outline*)

Maxilla

Palatine bone

Hard plate

External acoustic meatus

Mastoid process

Foramen ovale

Pterygoid process
of sphenoid

Lateral and medial plates
of pterygoid process

Occipital condyle

Foramen magnum

A. Inferolateral and Slightly Posterior View, Looking into Infratemporal and Pterygopalatine Fossae

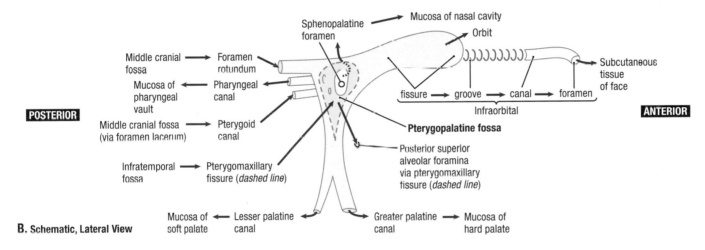

Sphenopalatine
foramen

Mucosa of nasal cavity

Orbit

Middle cranial → Foramen
fossa   rotundum

Mucosa of ← Pharyngeal
pharyngeal   canal
vault

Middle cranial → Pterygoid
fossa (via foramen lacerum) canal

fissure → groove → canal → foramen

Subcutaneous
tissue
of face

Infraorbital

POSTERIOR

ANTERIOR

Pterygopalatine fossa

Infratemporal → Pterygomaxillary
fossa   fissure (*dashed line*)

Posterior superior
alveolar foramina
via pterygomaxillary
fissure (*dashed line*)

Mucosa of ← Lesser palatine
soft palate   canal

Greater palatine → Mucosa of
canal   hard palate

B. Schematic, Lateral View

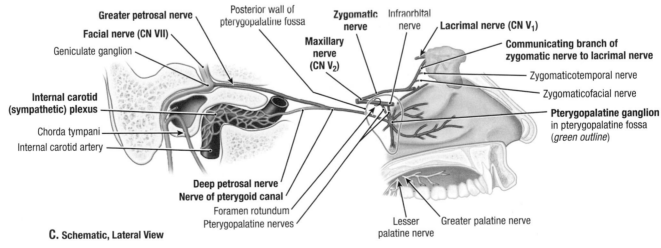

Greater petrosal nerve

Posterior wall of
pterygopalatine fossa

Zygomatic
nerve

Infraorbital
nerve

Lacrimal nerve (CN V₁)

Facial nerve (CN VII)

Geniculate ganglion

Maxillary
nerve
(CN V₂)

Communicating branch of
zygomatic nerve to lacrimal nerve

Zygomaticotemporal nerve

Zygomaticofacial nerve

Internal carotid
(sympathetic) plexus

Pterygopalatine ganglion
in pterygopalatine fossa
(*green outline*)

Chorda tympani

Internal carotid artery

Deep petrosal nerve
Nerve of pterygoid canal

Foramen rotundum
Pterygopalatine nerves

Lesser
palatine nerve

Greater palatine nerve

C. Schematic, Lateral View

Pterygopalatine Fossa   **8.82**

A. Bony relationships. The pterygopalatine fossa is a small pyramidal space inferior to the apex of the orbit. It lies between the pterygoid process of the sphenoid and the posterior aspect of the maxilla anteriorly. **B. Schematic. C.** Pterygopalatine ganglion and related nerves.

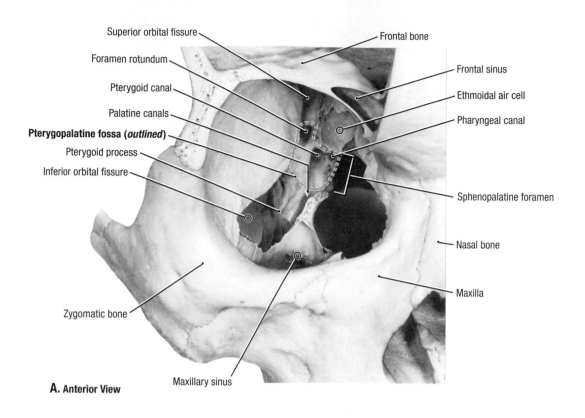

Superior orbital fissure

Foramen rotundum

Pterygoid canal

Palatine canals

Pterygopalatine fossa (*outlined*)

Pterygoid process

Inferior orbital fissure

Zygomatic bone

Maxillary sinus

Frontal bone

Frontal sinus

Ethmoidal air cell

Pharyngeal canal

Sphenopalatine foramen

Nasal bone

Maxilla

A. Anterior View

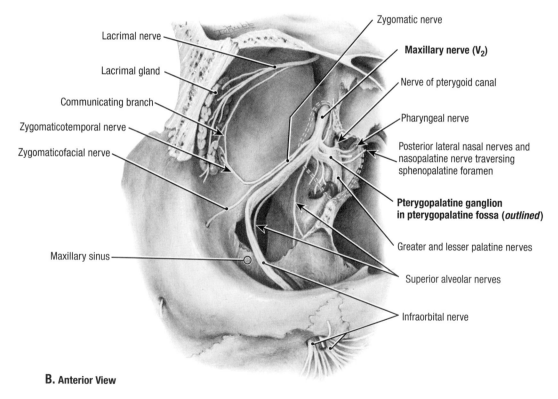

Lacrimal nerve

Lacrimal gland

Communicating branch

Zygomaticotemporal nerve

Zygomaticofacial nerve

Maxillary sinus

Zygomatic nerve

Maxillary nerve (V₂)

Nerve of pterygoid canal

Pharyngeal nerve

Posterior lateral nasal nerves and
nasopalatine nerve traversing
sphenopalatine foramen

**Pterygopalatine ganglion
in pterygopalatine fossa (*outlined*)**

Greater and lesser palatine nerves

Superior alveolar nerves

Infraorbital nerve

B. Anterior View

8.83   **Nerves of Pterygopalatine Fossa**

**A. Bones and foramina, orbital approach. B. Vessels and nerves,
orbital approach.** In *Part A* and *Part B*, the pterygopalatine fossa
has been exposed through the maxillary sinus after removal of the
floor of the orbit.

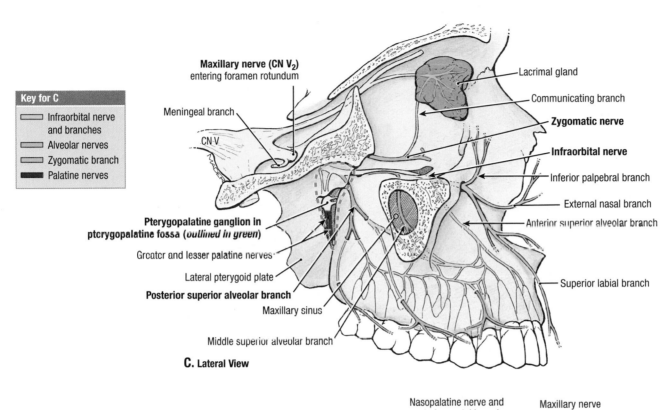

Key for C

- Infraorbital nerve and branches
- Alveolar nerves
- Zygomatic branch
- Palatine nerves

Maxillary nerve (CN V₂) entering foramen rotundum

Meningeal branch

CN V

Pterygopalatine ganglion in pterygopalatine fossa (outlined in green)

Greater and lesser palatine nerves

Lateral pterygoid plate

Posterior superior alveolar branch

Maxillary sinus

Middle superior alveolar branch

Lacrimal gland

Communicating branch

Zygomatic nerve

Infraorbital nerve

Inferior palpebral branch

External nasal branch

Anterior superior alveolar branch

Superior labial branch

C. Lateral View

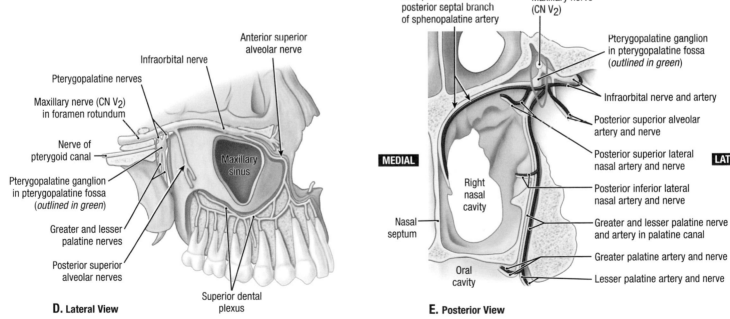

Anterior superior alveolar nerve

Infraorbital nerve

Pterygopalatine nerves

Maxillary nerve (CN V₂) in foramen rotundum

Nerve of pterygoid canal

Pterygopalatine ganglion in pterygopalatine fossa (outlined in green)

Greater and lesser palatine nerves

Posterior superior alveolar nerves

Maxillary sinus

Superior dental plexus

D. Lateral View

Nasopalatine nerve and posterior septal branch of sphenopalatine artery

Maxillary nerve (CN V₂)

MEDIAL

Right nasal cavity

Nasal septum

Oral cavity

Pterygopalatine ganglion in pterygopalatine fossa (outlined in green)

Infraorbital nerve and artery

Posterior superior alveolar artery and nerve

Posterior superior lateral nasal artery and nerve

LATERAL

Posterior inferior lateral nasal artery and nerve

Greater and lesser palatine nerve and artery in palatine canal

Greater palatine artery and nerve

Lesser palatine artery and nerve

E. Posterior View

C. Maxillary nerve (CN V₂) and branches. D. Pterygopalatine fossa, viewed laterally. Part of the wall of the maxillary sinus has been removed. **E. Nasopalatine and greater and lesser palatine nerves.**

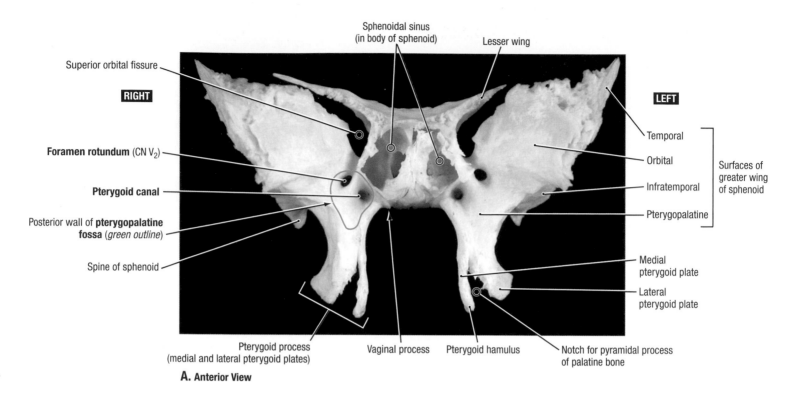

Sphenoidal sinus
(in body of sphenoid)

Lesser wing

Superior orbital fissure

RIGHT

Foramen rotundum (CN V₂)

Pterygoid canal

Posterior wall of **pterygopalatine fossa** (*green outline*)

Spine of sphenoid

LEFT

Temporal

Orbital

Infratemporal

Pterygopalatine

Surfaces of greater wing of sphenoid

Medial pterygoid plate

Lateral pterygoid plate

Pterygoid process
(medial and lateral pterygoid plates)

Vaginal process

Pterygoid hamulus

Notch for pyramidal process of palatine bone

A. Anterior View

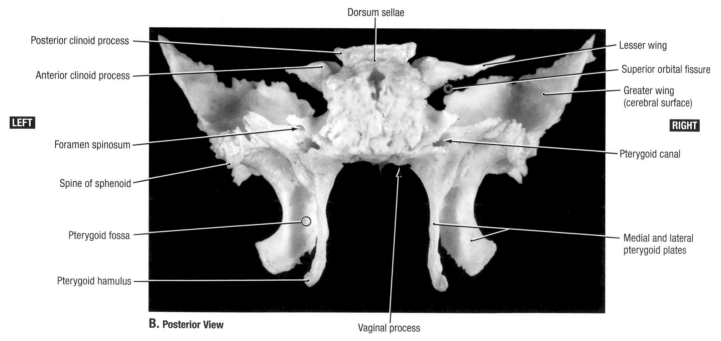

Dorsum sellae

Posterior clinoid process

Anterior clinoid process

LEFT

Foramen spinosum

Spine of sphenoid

Pterygoid fossa

Pterygoid hamulus

Lesser wing

Superior orbital fissure

Greater wing
(cerebral surface)

RIGHT

Pterygoid canal

Medial and lateral pterygoid plates

B. Posterior View

Vaginal process

8.84   **Sphenoid Bone: Features and Relationship to Pterygopalatine Fossa**

A. and **B. Bony features.** The pterygopalatine fossa communicates posterosuperiorly with the middle cranial fossa through the foramen rotundum and pterygoid canal.

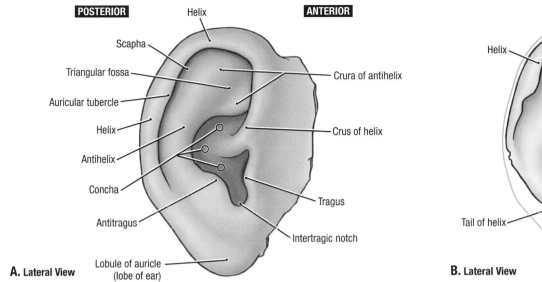

POSTERIOR

Helix

Scapha

Triangular fossa

Auricular tubercle

Helix

Antihelix

Concha

Antitragus

Lobule of auricle
(lobe of ear)

A. Lateral View

ANTERIOR

Crura of antihelix

Crus of helix

Tragus

Intertragic notch

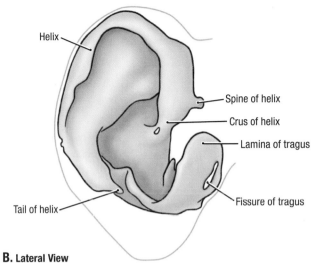

Helix

Spine of helix

Crus of helix

Lamina of tragus

Tail of helix

Fissure of tragus

B. Lateral View

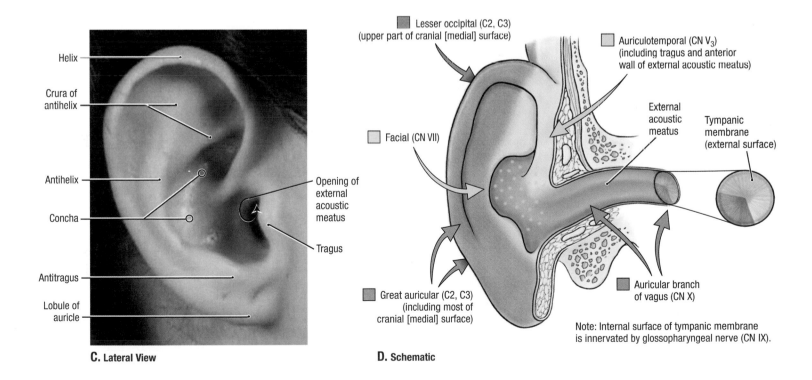

Helix

Crura of
antihelix

Antihelix

Concha

Antitragus

Lobule of
auricle

Opening of
external
acoustic
meatus

Tragus

C. Lateral View

Lesser occipital (C2, C3)
(upper part of cranial [medial] surface)

Auriculotemporal (CN V₃)
(including tragus and anterior
wall of external acoustic meatus)

Facial (CN VII)

External
acoustic
meatus

Tympanic
membrane
(external surface)

Great auricular (C2, C3)
(including most of
cranial [medial] surface)

Auricular branch
of vagus (CN X)

Note: Internal surface of tympanic membrane
is innervated by glossopharyngeal nerve (CN IX).

D. Schematic

A. Features of auricle. **B.** Cartilage of auricle. **C.** Surface anatomy of auricle. **D.** Sensory innervation.

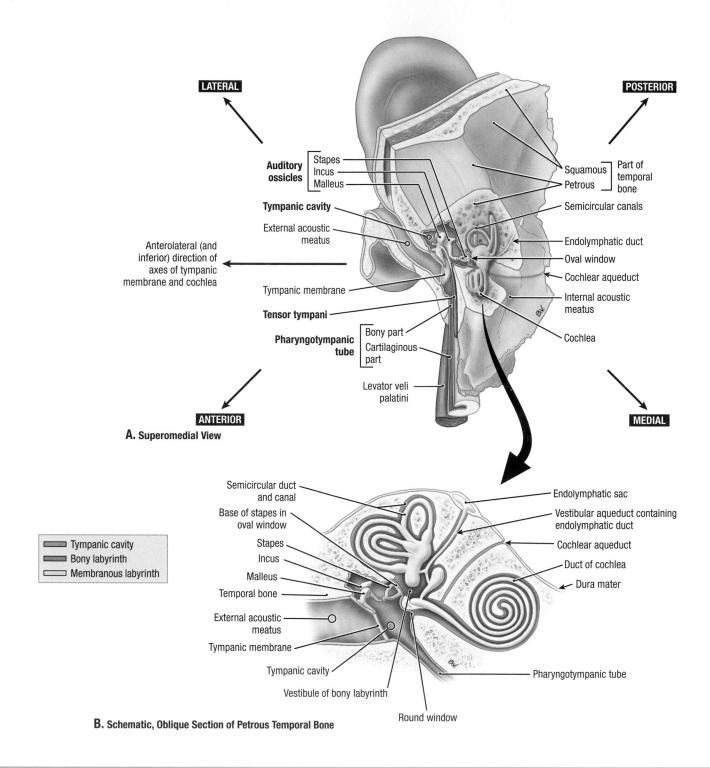

LATERAL

Auditory ossicles { Stapes / Incus / Malleus

Tympanic cavity

External acoustic meatus

Anterolateral (and inferior) direction of axes of tympanic membrane and cochlea

Tympanic membrane

Tensor tympani

Pharyngotympanic tube { Bony part / Cartilaginous part

Levator veli palatini

ANTERIOR

A. Superomedial View

POSTERIOR

Squamous } Part of temporal bone
Petrous

Semicircular canals

Endolymphatic duct

Oval window

Cochlear aqueduct

Internal acoustic meatus

Cochlea

MEDIAL

Tympanic cavity
Bony labyrinth
Membranous labyrinth

Semicircular duct and canal

Base of stapes in oval window

Stapes

Incus

Malleus

Temporal bone

External acoustic meatus

Tympanic membrane

Tympanic cavity

Vestibule of bony labyrinth

Round window

Endolymphatic sac

Vestibular aqueduct containing endolymphatic duct

Cochlear aqueduct

Duct of cochlea

Dura mater

Pharyngotympanic tube

B. Schematic, Oblique Section of Petrous Temporal Bone

8.86 **External, Middle, and Internal Ear (I): Overviews**

A. Right temporal bone and auricle, sectioned in planes of externa acoustic meatus and pharyngotympanic tube. **B.** Schematic section of petrous temporal bone.

- The external ear comprises the auricle and external acoustic (auditory) meatus.
- The middle ear (tympanum) lies between the tympanic membrane and internal ear. Three ossicles extend from the lateral to the medial walls of the tympanum. Of these, the malleus is attached to the tympanic membrane. The stapes is attached by

the annular ligament to the oval window, and the incus connects to the malleus and stapes. The pharyngotympanic tube, extending from the nasopharynx, opens into the anterior wall of the tympanic cavity.

- The membranous labyrinth comprises a closed system of membranous tubes and bulbs filled with fluid, endolymph and bathed in surrounding fluid, called perilymph; both membranous labyrinth and perilymph are contained within the bony labyrinth.

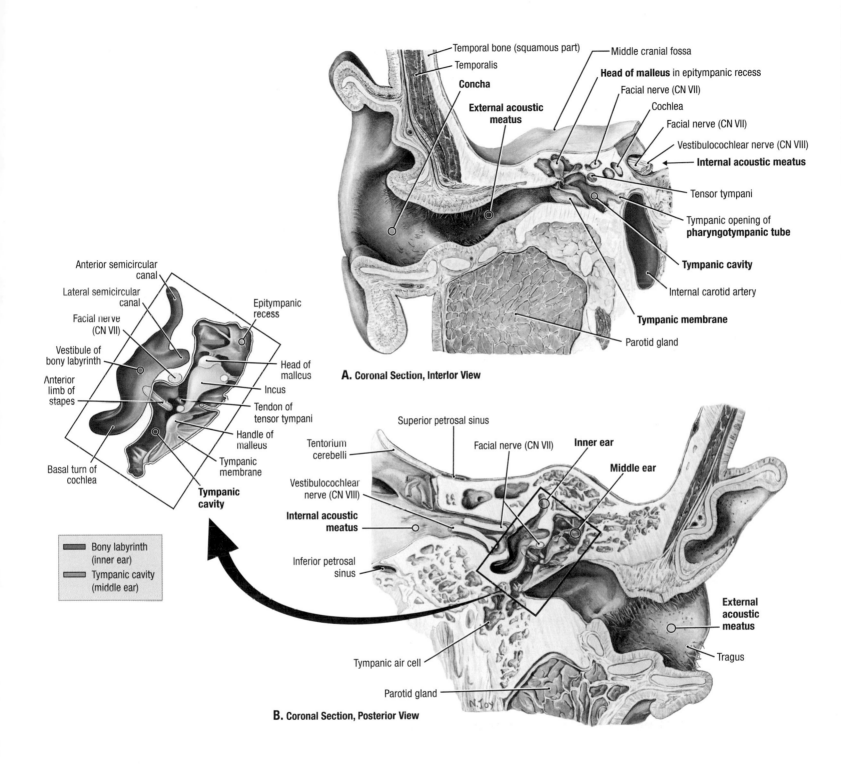

Temporal bone (squamous part)

Middle cranial fossa

Temporalis

Head of malleus in epitympanic recess

Concha

Facial nerve (CN VII)

Cochlea

External acoustic meatus

Facial nerve (CN VII)

Vestibulocochlear nerve (CN VIII)

Internal acoustic meatus

Tensor tympani

Tympanic opening of **pharyngotympanic tube**

Tympanic cavity

Internal carotid artery

Tympanic membrane

Parotid gland

A. Coronal Section, Interior View

Anterior semicircular canal

Lateral semicircular canal

Facial nerve (CN VII)

Epitympanic recess

Vestibule of bony labyrinth

Head of malleus

Anterior limb of stapes

Incus

Tendon of tensor tympani

Handle of malleus

Basal turn of cochlea

Tympanic membrane

Tympanic cavity

Bony labyrinth (inner ear)

Tympanic cavity (middle ear)

Superior petrosal sinus

Tentorium cerebelli

Facial nerve (CN VII)

Inner ear

Middle ear

Vestibulocochlear nerve (CN VIII)

Internal acoustic meatus

Inferior petrosal sinus

External acoustic meatus

Tympanic air cell

Tragus

Parotid gland

B. Coronal Section, Posterior View

External, Middle, and Internal Ear (II): Coronally Sectioned

8.87

A. Anterior portion. B. Posterior portion. The inset (*outlined by the box*) is an enlargement of the structures of the middle and internal ear as they appear in *Part B*.

- The external acoustic meatus is about 3 cm long; half is cartilaginous and half is bony. It is narrowest at the isthmus, near the junction of the cartilaginous and bony parts.
- The external acoustic meatus is innervated by the auriculotemporal branch of the mandibular nerve (CN V_3) and the auricular branches of the vagus nerve (CN X); the middle ear is innervated by the glossopharyngeal nerve (CN IX).
- The cartilaginous part of the external acoustic meatus is lined with thick skin; the bony part is lined with thin skin that adheres to the periosteum and forms the outermost layer of the tympanic membrane.

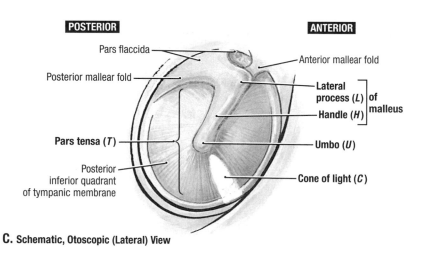

POSTERIOR   ANTERIOR

Posterior mallear fold

Pars flaccida

Anterior mallear fold

Lateral process of malleus

Handle of malleus

Umbo

Cone of light

A. Lateral View

POSTERIOR   ANTERIOR

Lateral ligament of malleus

Lateral process of malleus

Anterior mallear fold

Posterior mallear fold

Tensor tympani tendon

Long limb of incus (*I*)

Pyramidal eminence

Processus cochleariformis

Handle of malleus

Stapedius tendon

Promontory

Posterior limb of stapes (*S*)

Tympanic nerve (branch of CN IX)

Tympanic cells

B. Lateral View   Fossa of round window

POSTERIOR   ANTERIOR

Pars flaccida

Anterior mallear fold

Posterior mallear fold

Lateral process (*L*) of malleus

Handle (*H*)

Pars tensa (*T*)

Posterior inferior quadrant of tympanic membrane

Umbo (*U*)

Cone of light (*C*)

C. Schematic, Otoscopic (Lateral) View

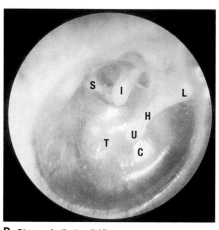

D. Otoscopic (Lateral) View

8.88   Tympanic Membrane

A. External (lateral) surface of tympanic membrane. B. Tympanic membrane removed, demonstrating structures that lie medially. C. Diagram of otoscopic view of tympanic membrane. D. Otoscopic view of tympanic membrane. Letter labels are identified in *Part B* and *Part C*.

- The oval tympanic membrane is a shallow cone deepest at the central apex, the umbo, where the membrane is attached to the tip of the handle of the malleus. The handle of the malleus is attached to the membrane along its entire length as it extends anterosuperiorly toward the periphery of the membrane.
- Superior to the lateral process of the malleus, the membrane is thin (pars flaccida); the flaccid part lacks the radial and circular fibers present in the remainder of the membrane (pars tensa).

The junction between the two parts is marked by anterior and posterior mallear folds.

- The lateral surface of the tympanic membrane is innervated by the auricular branch of the auriculotemporal nerve (CN V₃) and the auricular branch of the vagus nerve (CN X); the medial surface is innervated by tympanic branches of CN IX.

Examination of the external acoustic meatus and tympanic membrane begins by straightening the meatus. In adults, the helix is grasped and pulled posterosuperiorly (up, out, and back). These movements reduce the curvature of the external acoustic meatus, facilitating insertion of the otoscope. The external acoustic meatus is relatively short in infants; therefore, extra care must be taken to prevent damage to the tympanic membrane.

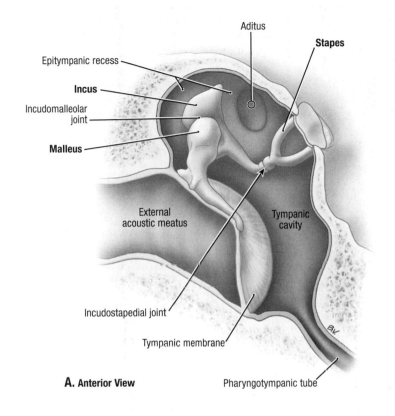

Aditus

Stapes

Epitympanic recess

Incus

Incudomalleolar joint

Malleus

External acoustic meatus

Tympanic cavity

Incudostapedial joint

Tympanic membrane

Pharyngotympanic tube

A. Anterior View

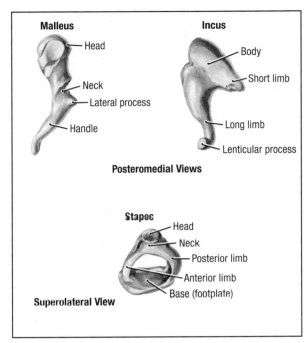

Malleus
- Head
- Neck
- Lateral process
- Handle

Incus
- Body
- Short limb
- Long limb
- Lenticular process

Posteromedial Views

Stapoc
- Head
- Neck
- Posterior limb
- Anterior limb
- Base (footplate)

Superolateral View

B. Ossicles

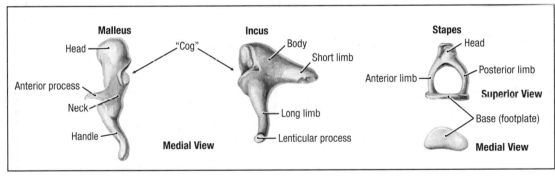

Malleus
- Head
- "Cog"
- Anterior process
- Neck
- Handle

Medial View

Incus
- Body
- Short limb
- Long limb
- Lenticular process

Stapes
- Head
- Anterior limb
- Posterior limb

Superior View

- Base (footplate)

Medial View

C. Ossicles

Ossicles of Middle Ear

8.89

A. Ossicles *in situ*, as revealed by a coronal section of temporal bone. **B.** and **C.** Isolated ossicles.
- The head of the malleus and body and short process of the incus lie in the epitympanic recess, and the handle of the malleus is embedded in the tympanic membrane.
- The saddle-shaped articular surface of the head of the malleus and the reciprocally shaped articular surface of the body of the incus form the incudomalleolar synovial joint.
- A convex articular facet at the end of the long process of the incus articulates with the head of the stapes to compose the incudostapedial synovial joint.

- An earache and bulging red tympanic membrane may indicate pus or fluid in the middle ear, a sign of **otitis media**. Infection of the middle ear often is secondary to upper respiratory infections. Inflammation and swelling of the mucous membrane lining the tympanic cavity may cause partial or complete blockage of the pharyngotympanic tube. The tympanic membrane becomes red and bulges and the person may complain of "ear popping." If untreated, otitis media may produce impaired hearing as the result of scarring of the auditory ossicles, limiting the ability of these bones to move in response to sound.

Aditus to mastoid antrum (forming posterior wall)

Prominence of lateral semicircular canal

Epitympanic recess

Lesser petrosal nerve

Malleus

Incus

Stapes

LATERAL

Chorda tympani nerve

Tensor tympani

Facial nerve (CN VII)

Prominence of canal for facial nerve

MEDIAL

Tympanic membrane

Tympanic plexus on **promontory** of labyrinthine wall

Stapedius tendon
Pyramidal eminence

Tympanic nerve (from CN IX)

A. Anterior View

Facial nerve

Walls of Tympanic Cavity

Tegmental wall (roof)
Jugular wall (floor)
Membranous (lateral) wall
Labyrinthine (medial) wall
Mastoid (posterior) wall

Carotid (anterior) wall was removed to provide this view.

SUPERIOR

Epitympanic recess

Neck of malleus

Head
Anterior process

Malleus

Anterior ligament of malleus

Lateral ligament of malleus

Superior recess of tympanic membrane

ANTERIOR

POSTERIOR

Tensor tympani

Tympanic opening of pharyngotympanic tube

Tubal cells

Chorda tympani

Facial nerve in its sheath within facial canal

Anterior recess of tympanic membrane

Posterior recess of tympanic membrane

Tendon of tensor tympani

N.Joy

Tympanic membrane

Tympanic cells

Margin of tympanic membrane

Handle of malleus

B. Medial View of Lateral Wall

8.90   Structures of Tympanic Cavity

A. Schematic of tympanic cavity with anterior wall removed. B. Lateral wall of tympanic cavity. The facial nerve lies within the facial canal surrounded by a tough periosteal tube; the chorda tympani leaves the facial nerve and lies within two crescentic folds of mucous membrane, crossing the neck of the malleus superior to the tendon of tensor tympani.

Perforation of the tympanic membrane (ruptured eardrum) may result from otitis media. Perforation may also result from foreign bodies in the external acoustic meatus, trauma, or excessive pressure. Because the superior half of the tympanic membrane is much more vascular than the inferior half, incisions are made extraocularly through the membrane. This incision also avoids injury to the chorda tympani nerve and auditory ossicles.

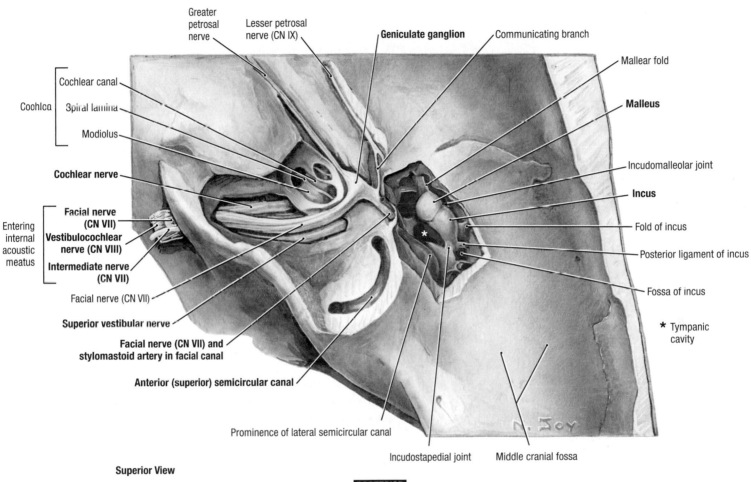

ANTERIOR

Greater petrosal nerve

Lesser petrosal nerve (CN IX)

Geniculate ganglion

Communicating branch

Mallear fold

Cochlear canal

Coohlca

Spiral lamina

Modiolus

Malleus

Cochlear nerve

Incudomalleolar joint

Incus

Entering internal acoustic meatus

Facial nerve (CN VII)

Vestibulocochlear nerve (CN VIII)

Intermediate nerve (CN VII)

Fold of incus

Posterior ligament of incus

Facial nerve (CN VII)

Fossa of incus

Superior vestibular nerve

* Tympanic cavity

Facial nerve (CN VII) and stylomastoid artery in facial canal

Anterior (superior) semicircular canal

Prominence of lateral semicircular canal

Incudostapedial joint

Middle cranial fossa

Superior View

POSTERIOR

Middle and Inner Ear *In Situ*

8.91

The tegmen tympani has been removed to expose the middle ear. In addition, the arcuate eminence has been removed to reveal the anterior semicircular canal and the course of the facial and vestibulocochlear nerves through the internal acoustic meatus and internal ear. At the geniculate ganglion, the facial nerve executes a sharp bend, called the genu, and then curves extraocularly within the bony facial canal; the thin lateral wall of the facial canal separates the facial nerve from the tympanic cavity of the middle ear.

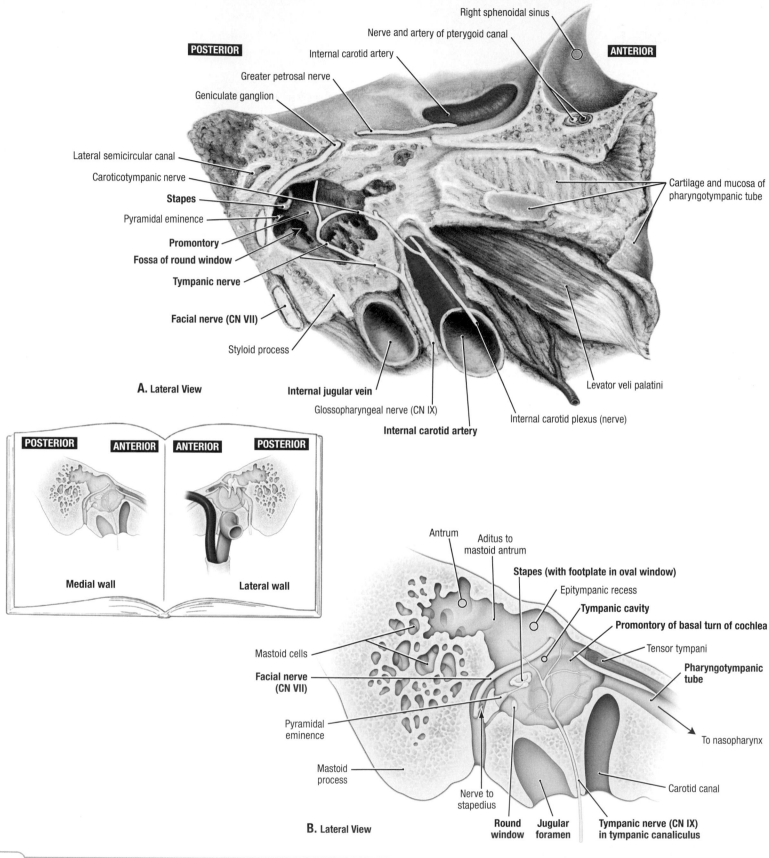

A. Lateral View

Right sphenoidal sinus

Nerve and artery of pterygoid canal

Internal carotid artery

POSTERIOR

Greater petrosal nerve

Geniculate ganglion

ANTERIOR

Lateral semicircular canal

Caroticotympanic nerve

Stapes

Pyramidal eminence

Promontory

Fossa of round window

Tympanic nerve

Facial nerve (CN VII)

Styloid process

Cartilage and mucosa of
pharyngotympanic tube

Internal jugular vein

Glossopharyngeal nerve (CN IX)

Internal carotid artery

Levator veli palatini

Internal carotid plexus (nerve)

POSTERIOR   ANTERIOR   ANTERIOR   POSTERIOR

Medial wall

Lateral wall

B. Lateral View

Antrum

Aditus to
mastoid antrum

Stapes (with footplate in oval window)

Epitympanic recess

Tympanic cavity

Promontory of basal turn of cochlea

Tensor tympani

**Pharyngotympanic
tube**

Mastoid cells

**Facial nerve
(CN VII)**

Pyramidal
eminence

Mastoid
process

Nerve to
stapedius

**Round
window**

**Jugular
foramen**

**Tympanic nerve (CN IX)
in tympanic canaliculus**

To nasopharynx

Carotid canal

8.92   **Right Tympanic Cavity and Pharyngotympanic Tube (I)**

A. Dissection of medial wall. B. Schematic of medial wall. The cut surfaces of this longitudinally sectioned specimen are displayed as pages in a book.

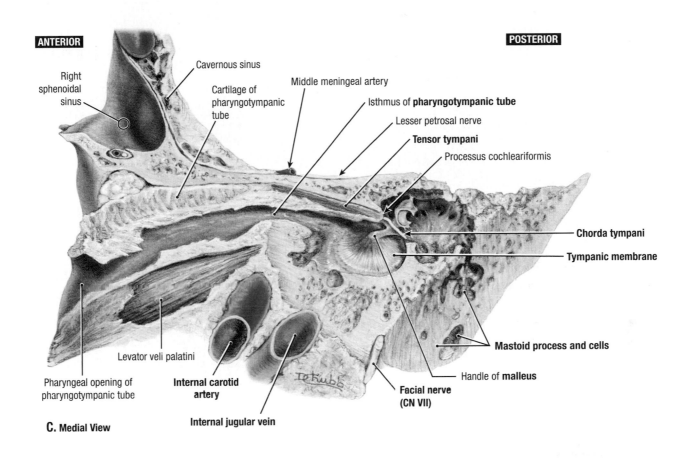

ANTERIOR

POSTERIOR

Right sphenoidal sinus

Cavernous sinus

Cartilage of pharyngotympanic tube

Middle meningeal artery

Isthmus of **pharyngotympanic tube**

Lesser petrosal nerve

Tensor tympani

Processus cochleariformis

Chorda tympani

Tympanic membrane

Mastoid process and cells

Handle of **malleus**

Levator veli palatini

Pharyngeal opening of pharyngotympanic tube

Internal carotid artery

Internal jugular vein

Facial nerve (CN VII)

C. Medial View

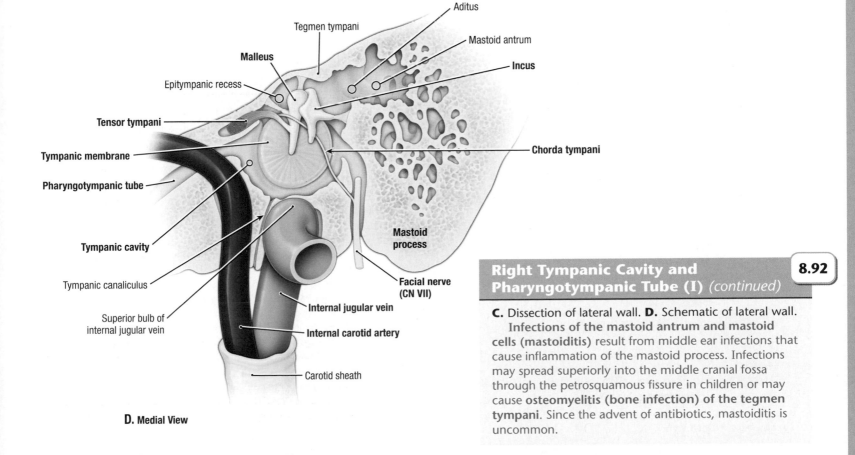

Tegmen tympani

Aditus

Mastoid antrum

Incus

Malleus

Epitympanic recess

Tensor tympani

Tympanic membrane

Pharyngotympanic tube

Chorda tympani

Tympanic cavity

Tympanic canaliculus

Superior bulb of internal jugular vein

Mastoid process

Facial nerve (CN VII)

Internal jugular vein

Internal carotid artery

Carotid sheath

D. Medial View

Right Tympanic Cavity and Pharyngotympanic Tube (I) *(continued)*

8.92

C. Dissection of lateral wall. **D.** Schematic of lateral wall. Infections of the mastoid antrum and mastoid cells (mastoiditis) result from middle ear infections that cause inflammation of the mastoid process. Infections may spread superiorly into the middle cranial fossa through the petrosquamous fissure in children or may cause **osteomyelitis (bone infection) of the tegmen tympani**. Since the advent of antibiotics, mastoiditis is uncommon.

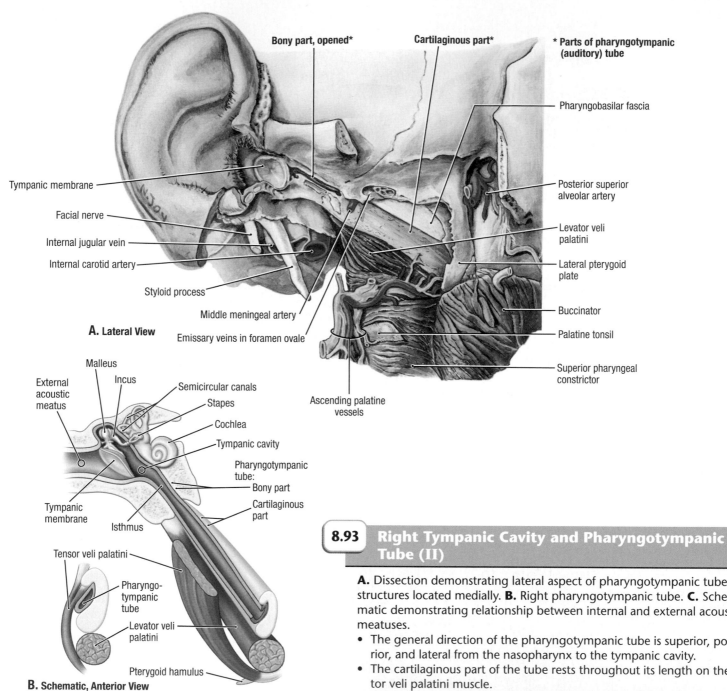

Bony part, opened*

Cartilaginous part*

* Parts of pharyngotympanic (auditory) tube

Pharyngobasilar fascia

Tympanic membrane

Facial nerve

Internal jugular vein

Internal carotid artery

Styloid process

Middle meningeal artery

Emissary veins in foramen ovale

A. Lateral View

Posterior superior alveolar artery

Levator veli palatini

Lateral pterygoid plate

Buccinator

Palatine tonsil

Superior pharyngeal constrictor

Ascending palatine vessels

Malleus

Incus

External acoustic meatus

Semicircular canals

Stapes

Cochlea

Tympanic cavity

Pharyngotympanic tube:

Bony part

Cartilaginous part

Tympanic membrane

Isthmus

Tensor veli palatini

Pharyngo-tympanic tube

Levator veli palatini

Pterygoid hamulus

B. Schematic, Anterior View

Cells

Antrum Mastoid

Aditus

Cochlea

Cranial cavity

Internal acoustic meatus

External acoustic meatus

Membrane

Cavity

Tympanic

Pharyngotympanic tube

Nasopharynx

C. Schematic, Superior View

8.93 **Right Tympanic Cavity and Pharyngotympanic Tube (II)**

A. Dissection demonstrating lateral aspect of pharyngotympanic tube and structures located medially. **B.** Right pharyngotympanic tube. **C.** Schematic demonstrating relationship between internal and external acoustic meatuses.

- The general direction of the pharyngotympanic tube is superior, posterior, and lateral from the nasopharynx to the tympanic cavity.
- The cartilaginous part of the tube rests throughout its length on the levator veli palatini muscle.
- The line of the meatuses and the line of the airway, from nasopharynx to mastoid cells, intersect at the tympanic cavity.
- The tegmen tympani forms the roof of the tympanic cavity and mastoid antrum.

The function of the pharyngotympanic tube is **equalizing pressure in the middle ear** with the atmospheric pressure, thereby allowing free movement of the tympanic membrane. By allowing air to enter and leave the tympanic cavity, this tube balances the pressure on both sides of the membrane. Because the walls of the cartilaginous part of the tube are normally in apposition, the tube must be actively opened. The tube is opened by the expanding girth of the belly of the levator veli palatini as it contracts longitudinally, pushing against one wall while the tensor veli palatini pulls on the other. Because these are muscles of the soft palate, equalizing pressure (popping the eardrums) is commonly associated with activities such as yawning and swallowing.

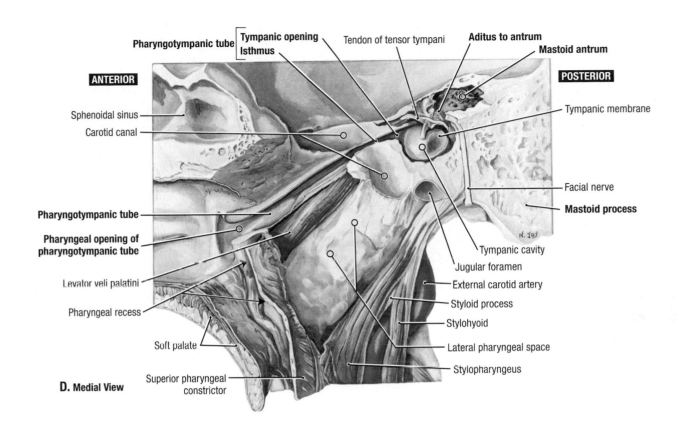

Pharyngotympanic tube | **Tympanic opening** | Tendon of tensor tympani | **Aditus to antrum**
Pharyngotympanic tube | **Isthmus** | | **Mastoid antrum**

ANTERIOR

POSTERIOR

Sphenoidal sinus

Carotid canal

Tympanic membrane

Facial nerve

Mastoid process

Pharyngotympanic tube

**Pharyngeal opening of
pharyngotympanic tube**

Tympanic cavity

Jugular foramen

Levator veli palatini

External carotid artery

Pharyngeal recess

Styloid process

Stylohyoid

Soft palate

Lateral pharyngeal space

Stylopharyngeus

D. Medial View

Superior pharyngeal
constrictor

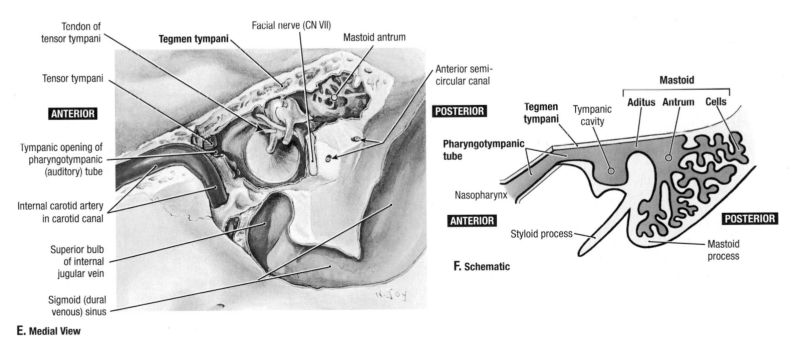

Tendon of
tensor tympani

Facial nerve (CN VII)

Tegmen tympani

Mastoid antrum

Tensor tympani

Anterior semi-
circular canal

ANTERIOR

POSTERIOR

Tympanic opening of
pharyngotympanic
(auditory) tube

**Tegmen
tympani**

Tympanic
cavity

Mastoid

Aditus **Antrum** **Cells**

Internal carotid artery
in carotid canal

**Pharyngotympanic
tube**

Superior bulb
of internal
jugular vein

Nasopharynx

ANTERIOR

POSTERIOR

Sigmoid (dural
venous) sinus

Styloid process

Mastoid
process

F. Schematic

E. Medial View

Right Tympanic Cavity and Pharyngotympanic Tube (II) *(continued)*

D. Spaces of tympanic bone. **E.** Relationship of tympanic cavity
to internal carotid artery, sigmoid sinus, and middle cranial fossa.
F. Diagram of tegmen tympani.

• The internal carotid artery is the primary relationship of the anterior
wall, the internal jugular vein is the primary relationship of the floor,
and the facial nerve is the primary relationship of the posterior wall.

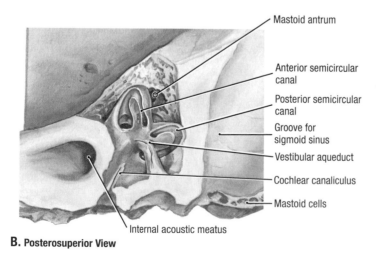

A. Superior View

Dorsum sellae
Foramen lacerum
Foramen ovale
Squamous part of temporal bone
Petrosquamous fissure
Cochlea
Anterior
Lateral
Posterior
Semicircular canals
Vestibular aqueduct
Petrous part of temporal bone
Internal acoustic meatus
Groove for sigmoid sinus
Mastoid part of temporal bone
Groove for inferior petrosal sinus
Foramen magnum

B. Posterosuperior View

Mastoid antrum
Anterior semicircular canal
Posterior semicircular canal
Groove for sigmoid sinus
Vestibular aqueduct
Cochlear canaliculus
Mastoid cells
Internal acoustic meatus

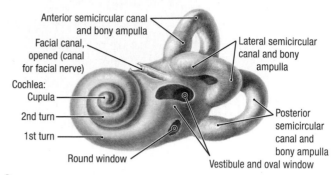

Anterior semicircular canal and bony ampulla
Facial canal, opened (canal for facial nerve)
Cochlea:
Cupula
2nd turn
1st turn
Round window
Lateral semicircular canal and bony ampulla
Posterior semicircular canal and bony ampulla
Vestibule and oval window

C. Anterolateral View of Left Otic Capsule

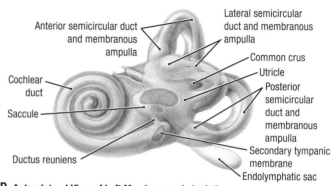

Anterior semicircular duct and membranous ampulla
Lateral semicircular duct and membranous ampulla
Common crus
Utricle
Posterior semicircular duct and membranous ampulla
Secondary tympanic membrane
Endolymphatic sac
Cochlear duct
Saccule
Ductus reuniens

D. Anterolateral View of Left Membranous Labyrinth (through Transparent Otic Capsule)

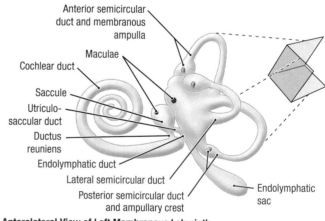

Anterior semicircular duct and membranous ampulla
Maculae
Cochlear duct
Saccule
Utriculo-saccular duct
Ductus reuniens
Endolymphatic duct
Lateral semicircular duct
Posterior semicircular duct and ampullary crest
Endolymphatic sac

E. Anterolateral View of Left Membranous Labyrinth

8.94   Bony and Membranous Labyrinths

A. Location and orientation of bony labyrinth within petrous temporal bone. B. Semicircular canals and aqueducts *in situ*. The tegmen tympani has been excised, and the softer bone surrounding the harder bone of the otic capsule has been drilled away.

C. Walls of left bony labyrinth (otic capsule). The bony labyrinth is the fluid-filled space contained within this formation. **D. Membranous labyrinth within surrounding bony labyrinth. E. Isolated left membranous labyrinth.**

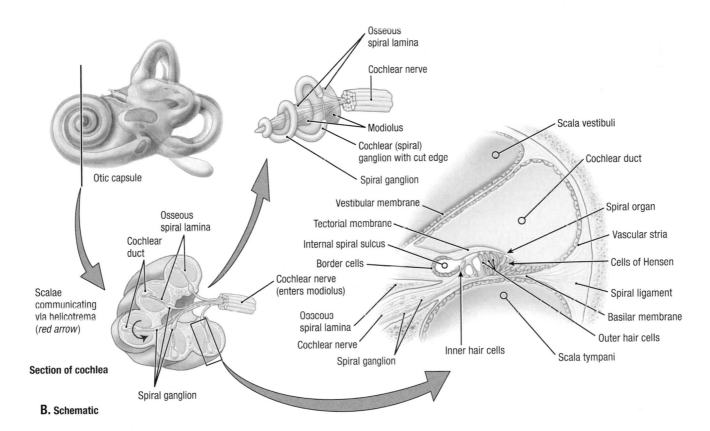

A. Schematic

Section of cochlea

B. Schematic

Vestibulocochlear Nerve (CN VIII) and Structure of Cochlea

A. Distribution of vestibulocochlear nerve (schematic). **B. Structure of cochlea.** The cochlea has been sectioned along the bony core of the cochlea (modiolus), the axis about which the cochlea winds. An isolated modiolus is shown after the turns of the cochlea are removed, leaving only the spiral lamina winding around it. The large drawing shows the details of the area enclosed in the rectangle, including a cross section of the cochlear duct of the membranous labyrinth.

- The maculae of the membranous labyrinth are primarily static organs, which have small dense particles (otoliths) embedded among the hair cells. Under the influence of gravity, the otoliths cause bending of the hair cells, which stimulate the vestibular nerve and provide awareness of the position of the head in space; the hairs also respond to quick tilting movements and to linear acceleration and deceleration. **Motion sickness** results mainly from discordance between vestibular and visual stimuli.

- Persistent exposure to excessively loud sound causes degenerative changes in the spiral organ, resulting in **high-tone deafness**. This type of hearing loss commonly occurs in workers who are exposed to loud noises and do not wear protective earmuffs.

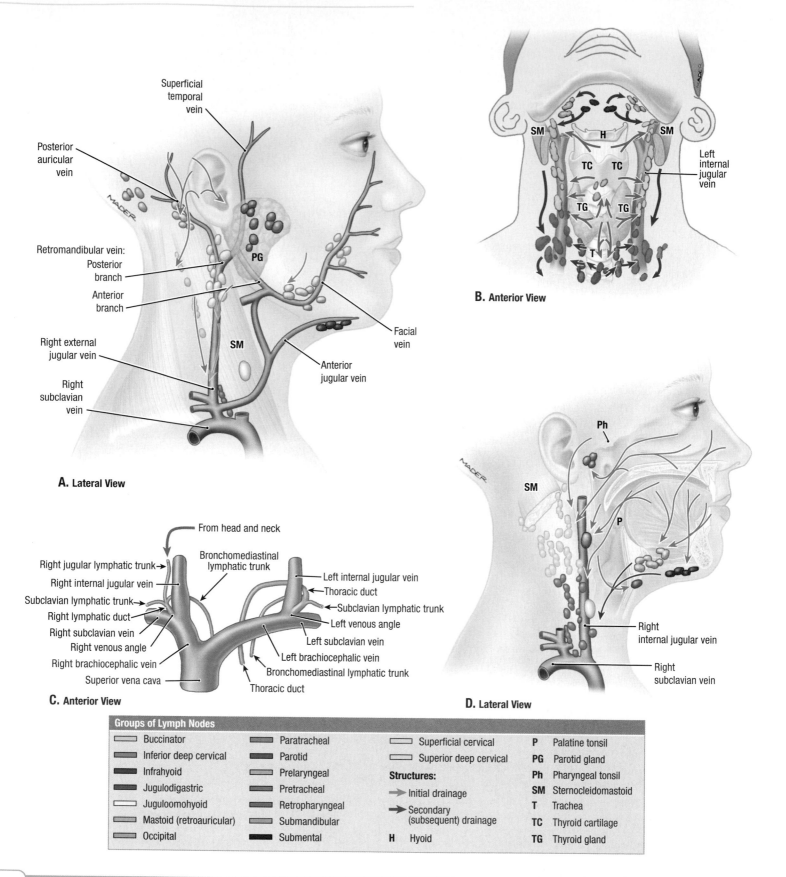

Superficial
temporal
vein

Posterior
auricular
vein

Retromandibular vein:
Posterior
branch

Anterior
branch

Right external
jugular vein

Right
subclavian
vein

PG

SM

Facial
vein

Anterior
jugular vein

A. Lateral View

SM   H   SM

Left
internal
jugular
vein

TC   TC

TG   TG

T

B. Anterior View

From head and neck

Right jugular lymphatic trunk →
Right internal jugular vein
Subclavian lymphatic trunk →
Right lymphatic duct
Right subclavian vein
Right venous angle
Right brachiocephalic vein
Superior vena cava

Bronchomediastinal
lymphatic trunk

← Thoracic duct
← Subclavian lymphatic trunk
← Left venous angle
Left subclavian vein
Left brachiocephalic vein
Bronchomediastinal lymphatic trunk
Thoracic duct

Left internal jugular vein

C. Anterior View

Ph

SM

P

Right
internal jugular vein

Right
subclavian vein

D. Lateral View

Groups of Lymph Nodes			
Buccinator	Paratracheal	Superficial cervical	**P** Palatine tonsil
Inferior deep cervical	Parotid	Superior deep cervical	**PG** Parotid gland
Infrahyoid	Prelaryngeal	**Structures:**	**Ph** Pharyngeal tonsil
Jugulodigastric	Pretracheal	→ Initial drainage	**SM** Sternocleidomastoid
Juguloomohyoid	Retropharyngeal	→ Secondary	**T** Trachea
Mastoid (retroauricular)	Submandibular	(subsequent) drainage	**TC** Thyroid cartilage
Occipital	Submental	**H** Hyoid	**TG** Thyroid gland

8.96   **Lymphatic and Venous Drainage of Head and Neck**

A. Superficial drainage. **B.** Drainage of trachea, thyroid gland, larynx, and floor of mouth. **C.** Termination of right and left jugular lymphatic trunks. **D.** Deep drainage.

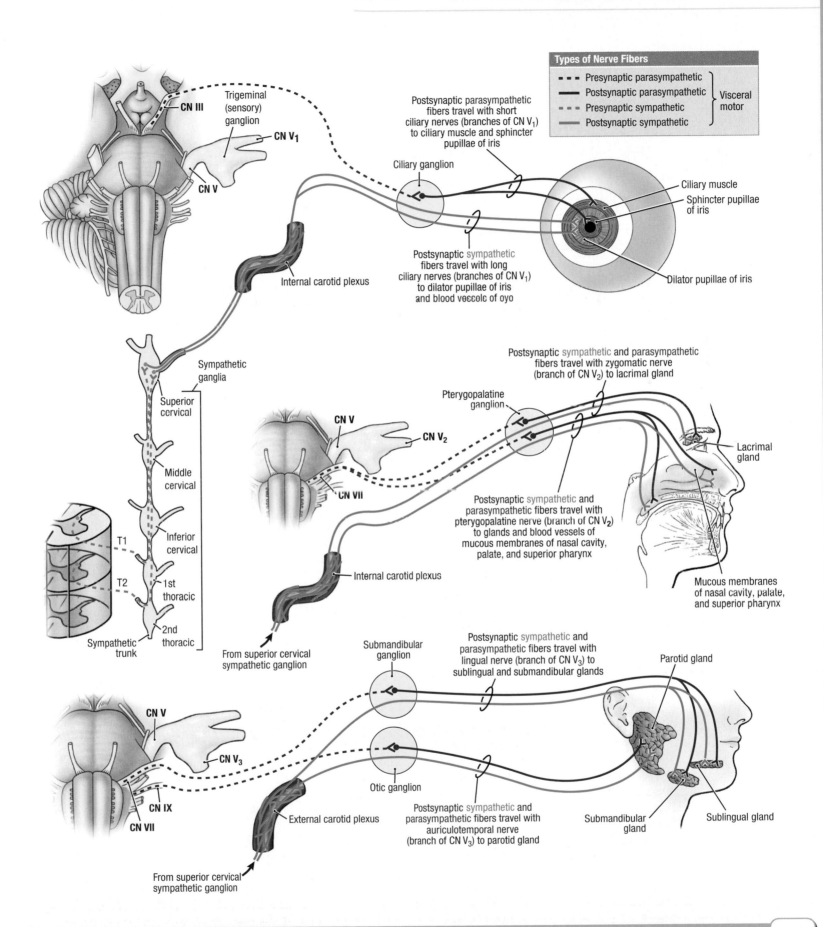

Trigeminal (sensory) ganglion

CN III

CN V₁

CN V

Internal carotid plexus

Sympathetic ganglia

Superior cervical

Middle cervical

Inferior cervical

1st thoracic

2nd thoracic

Sympathetic trunk

T1

T2

Types of Nerve Fibers
- - - Presynaptic parasympathetic
—— Postsynaptic parasympathetic } Visceral motor
- - - Presynaptic sympathetic
—— Postsynaptic sympathetic

Postsynaptic parasympathetic fibers travel with short ciliary nerves (branches of CN V₁) to ciliary muscle and sphincter pupillae of iris

Ciliary ganglion

Ciliary muscle

Sphincter pupillae of iris

Postsynaptic sympathetic fibers travel with long ciliary nerves (branches of CN V₁) to dilator pupillae of iris and blood vessels of eye

Dilator pupillae of iris

Postsynaptic sympathetic and parasympathetic fibers travel with zygomatic nerve (branch of CN V₂) to lacrimal gland

CN V

CN V₂

Pterygopalatine ganglion

Lacrimal gland

CN VII

Postsynaptic sympathetic and parasympathetic fibers travel with pterygopalatine nerve (branch of CN V₂) to glands and blood vessels of mucous membranes of nasal cavity, palate, and superior pharynx

Internal carotid plexus

Mucous membranes of nasal cavity, palate, and superior pharynx

From superior cervical sympathetic ganglion

Submandibular ganglion

Postsynaptic sympathetic and parasympathetic fibers travel with lingual nerve (branch of CN V₃) to sublingual and submandibular glands

Parotid gland

CN V

CN V₃

Otic ganglion

Postsynaptic sympathetic and parasympathetic fibers travel with auriculotemporal nerve (branch of CN V₃) to parotid gland

Submandibular gland

Sublingual gland

CN IX

CN VII

External carotid plexus

From superior cervical sympathetic ganglion

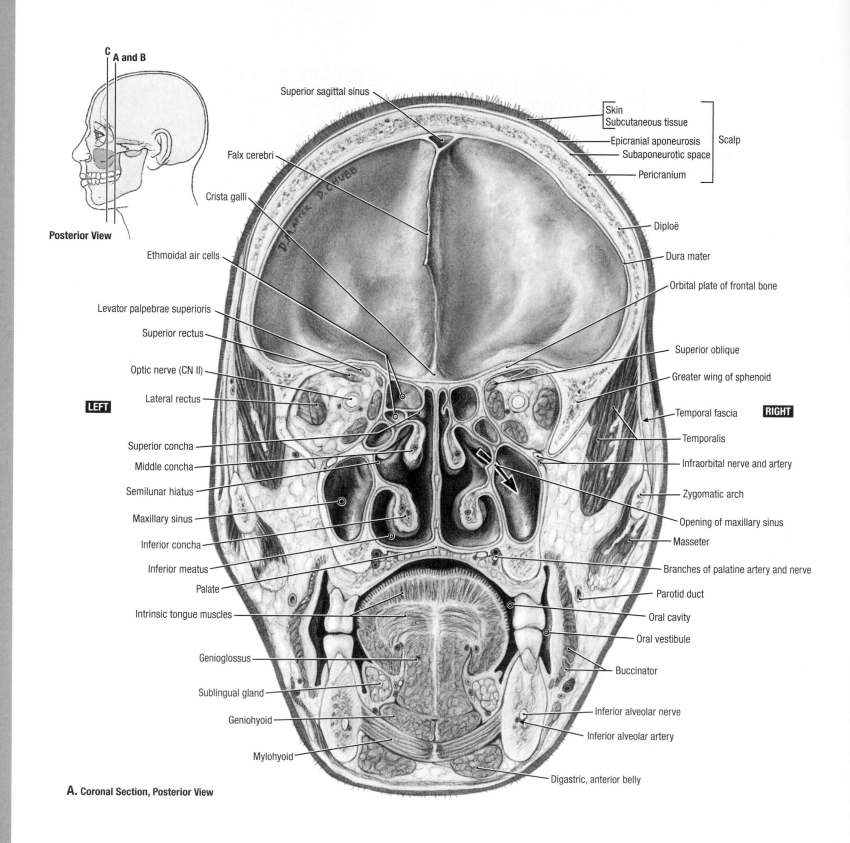

Posterior View

C | A and B

Superior sagittal sinus

Falx cerebri

Crista galli

Ethmoidal air cells

Levator palpebrae superioris

Superior rectus

Optic nerve (CN II)

Lateral rectus

Superior concha

Middle concha

Semilunar hiatus

Maxillary sinus

Inferior concha

Inferior meatus

Palate

Intrinsic tongue muscles

Genioglossus

Sublingual gland

Geniohyoid

Mylohyoid

LEFT

Skin
Subcutaneous tissue
Epicranial aponeurosis
Subaponeurotic space
Pericranium
Scalp

Diploë

Dura mater

Orbital plate of frontal bone

Superior oblique

Greater wing of sphenoid

Temporal fascia

Temporalis

Infraorbital nerve and artery

Zygomatic arch

Opening of maxillary sinus

Masseter

Branches of palatine artery and nerve

Parotid duct

Oral cavity

Oral vestibule

Buccinator

Inferior alveolar nerve

Inferior alveolar artery

Digastric, anterior belly

RIGHT

A. Coronal Section, Posterior View

8.98 **Coronal Section and MRIs of Nasopharynx and Oral Cavity**

A. Coronal section.

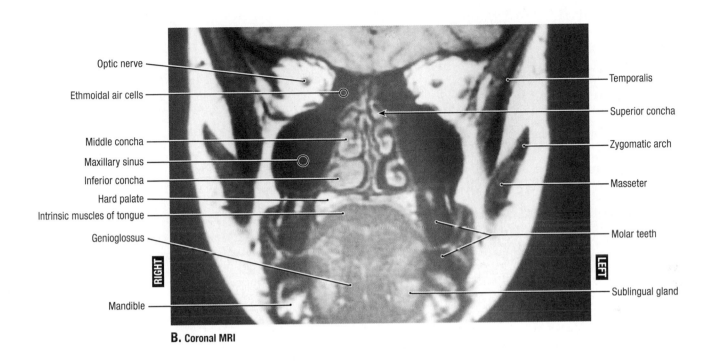

Optic nerve

Ethmoidal air cells

Middle concha

Maxillary sinus

Inferior concha

Hard palate

Intrinsic muscles of tongue

Genioglossus

Mandible

Temporalis

Superior concha

Zygomatic arch

Masseter

Molar teeth

Sublingual gland

RIGHT   **LEFT**

B. Coronal MRI

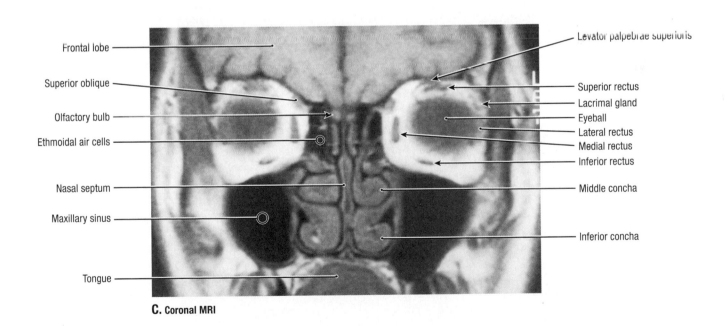

Frontal lobe

Superior oblique

Olfactory bulb

Ethmoidal air cells

Nasal septum

Maxillary sinus

Tongue

Levator palpebrae superioris

Superior rectus

Lacrimal gland

Eyeball

Lateral rectus

Medial rectus

Inferior rectus

Middle concha

Inferior concha

C. Coronal MRI

Coronal Section and MRIs of Nasopharynx and Oral Cavity *(continued)*

8.98

B. and **C.** Coronal MRIs.

   Deviation of nasal septum. The nasal septum is usually deviated to one side or the other. This could be the result of a birth injury, but more often, the deviation occurs during adolescence and adulthood from trauma. Sometimes, the deviation is so severe that the nasal septum is in contact with the lateral wall of the nasal cavity and often obstructs breathing or exacerbates snoring. The deviation can be corrected surgically.

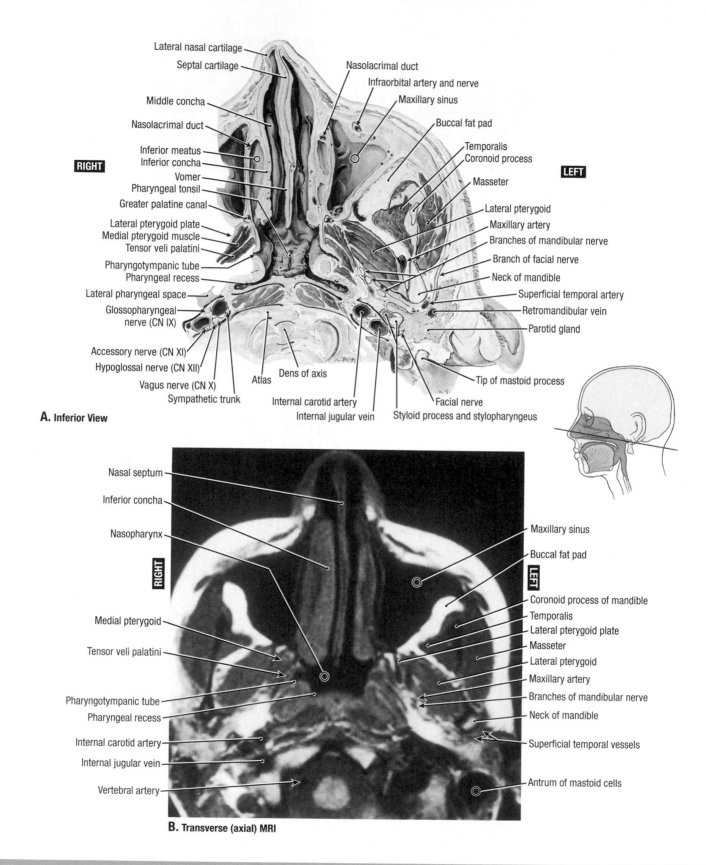

Lateral nasal cartilage
Septal cartilage
Nasolacrimal duct
Infraorbital artery and nerve
Maxillary sinus
Middle concha
Nasolacrimal duct
Buccal fat pad
Temporalis
Coronoid process
RIGHT
Inferior meatus
Inferior concha
Masseter
LEFT
Vomer
Pharyngeal tonsil
Lateral pterygoid
Greater palatine canal
Maxillary artery
Lateral pterygoid plate
Branches of mandibular nerve
Medial pterygoid muscle
Branch of facial nerve
Tensor veli palatini
Pharyngotympanic tube
Neck of mandible
Pharyngeal recess
Superficial temporal artery
Lateral pharyngeal space
Retromandibular vein
Glossopharyngeal
nerve (CN IX)
Parotid gland
Accessory nerve (CN XI)
Hypoglossal nerve (CN XII)
Atlas   Dens of axis
Tip of mastoid process
Vagus nerve (CN X)
Sympathetic trunk
Internal carotid artery
Facial nerve
Internal jugular vein   Styloid process and stylopharyngeus

A. Inferior View

Nasal septum
Inferior concha
Nasopharynx
Maxillary sinus
Buccal fat pad
RIGHT
LEFT
Coronoid process of mandible
Temporalis
Medial pterygoid
Lateral pterygoid plate
Masseter
Tensor veli palatini
Lateral pterygoid
Maxillary artery
Branches of mandibular nerve
Pharyngotympanic tube
Neck of mandible
Pharyngeal recess
Internal carotid artery
Superficial temporal vessels
Internal jugular vein
Vertebral artery
Antrum of mastoid cells

B. Transverse (axial) MRI

8.99 **Transverse Section and MRI of Nasal Cavity and Nasopharynx**

A. Transverse section of left side of head. B. Transverse (axial) MRI. The maxillary artery can course either superficial (as in *Part A*) or deep to the lateral pterygoid (as in *Part B*).

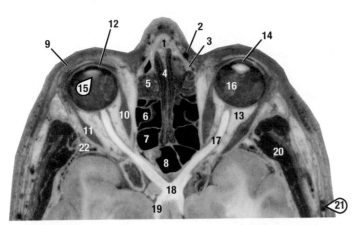

A. Transverse Section

B. Transverse (Axial) MRI Scan

1	Nasal bones	7	Posterior ethmoidal air cell	13	Retrobulbar fat
2	Angular artery	8	Sphenoid sinus	14	Anterior chamber
3	Frontal process of maxilla	9	Orbicularis oculi muscle	15	Lens
4	Nasal septum	10	Medial rectus muscle	16	Vitreous body
5	Anterior ethmoidal cell	11	Lateral rectus muscle	17	Optic nerve
6	Middle ethmoidal cell	12	Cornea	18	Optic chiasm

19	Optic tract
20	Temporalis muscle
21	Superficial temporal vessels
22	Greater wing of sphenoid
23	Squamous part of temporal bone

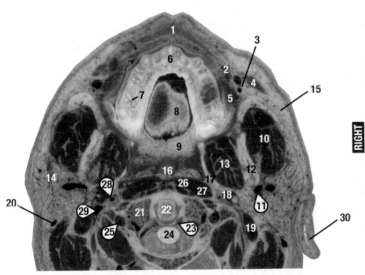

C. Transverse Section

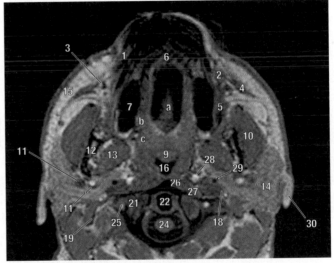

D. Transverse (Axial) MRI Scan

1	Orbicularis oris muscle	12	Ramus of mandible	23	Transverse ligament of atlas
2	Levator anguli oris muscle	13	Lateral pterygoid muscle	24	Spinal cord
3	Facial artery and vein	14	Parotid gland	25	Vertebral artery in foramina transversaria
4	Zygomaticus major muscle	15	Subcutaneous tissue	26	Longus colli muscle
5	Buccinator muscle	16	Region of pharyngeal tubercle	27	Longus capitis muscle
6	Maxilla	17	Sphenoid bone	28	Internal carotid artery
7	Alveolar process of maxilla	18	Stylohyoid ligament and muscle	29	Internal jugular vein
8	Dorsum of tongue	19	Posterior belly of digastric muscle	30	Inferior portion of helix of auricle
9	Soft palate (uvula apparent in image)	20	Occipital artery	a	Hard palate
10	Masseter muscle	21	First cervical vertebrae (atlas)	b	Palatoglossus muscle
11	Retromandibular vein	22	Dens (axis)	c	Palatopharyngeus muscle

A. and **B.** Transverse section and MRI through plane of optic nerve. **C.** and **D.** Transverse section and MRI at level of atlas/dens.

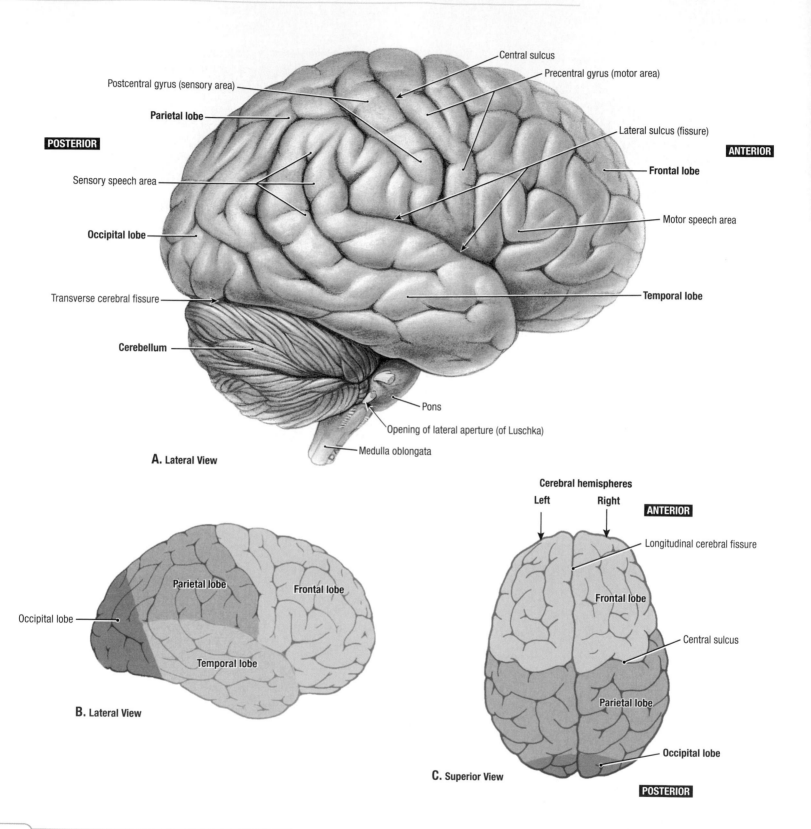

Central sulcus

Precentral gyrus (motor area)

Postcentral gyrus (sensory area)

Parietal lobe

POSTERIOR

Lateral sulcus (fissure)

ANTERIOR

Sensory speech area

Frontal lobe

Occipital lobe

Motor speech area

Transverse cerebral fissure

Temporal lobe

Cerebellum

Pons

Opening of lateral aperture (of Luschka)

Medulla oblongata

A. Lateral View

Cerebral hemispheres

Left   **Right**   **ANTERIOR**

Parietal lobe   **Frontal lobe**

Longitudinal cerebral fissure

Occipital lobe

Frontal lobe

Central sulcus

Temporal lobe

Parietal lobe

B. Lateral View

C. Superior View

Occipital lobe

POSTERIOR

8.101 **Brain**

A. Cerebrum, cerebellum, and brainstem, lateral aspect. **B.** Lobes of cerebral hemispheres, lateral aspect. **C.** Lobes of cerebral hemispheres, superior aspect.

Cerebral contusion (bruising) results from brain trauma in which the pia is stripped from the injured surface of the brain and may be torn, allowing blood to enter the subarachnoid space. The bruising results from the sudden impact of the moving brain against the stationary cranium or from the suddenly moving cranium against the stationary brain. Cerebral contusion may result in an extended loss of consciousness.

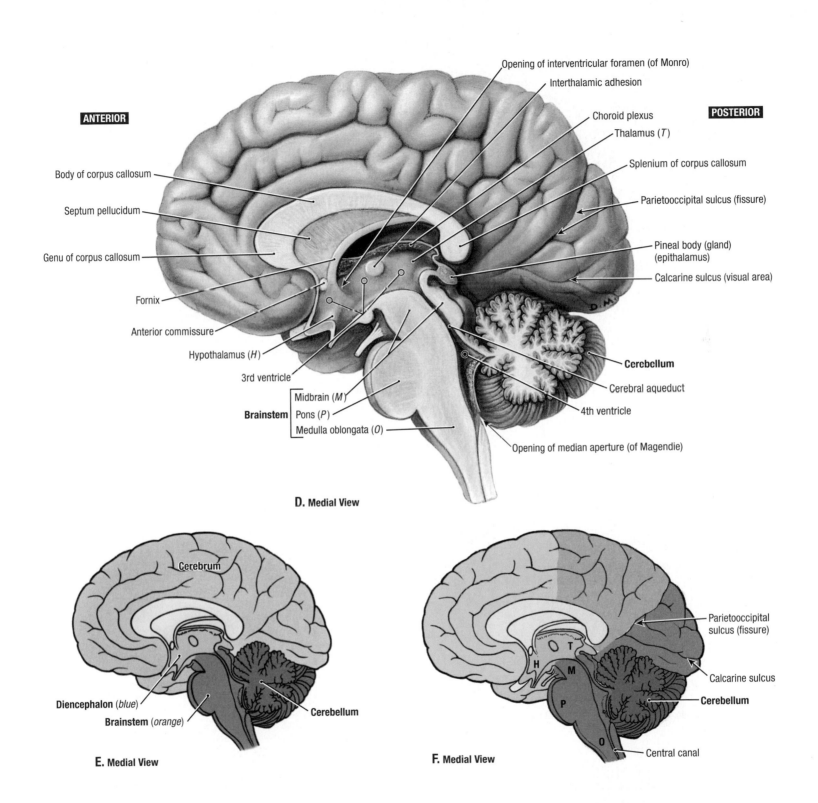

Opening of interventricular foramen (of Monro)

Interthalamic adhesion

ANTERIOR

POSTERIOR

Choroid plexus

Thalamus (*T*)

Body of corpus callosum

Splenium of corpus callosum

Septum pellucidum

Parietooccipital sulcus (fissure)

Genu of corpus callosum

Pineal body (gland) (epithalamus)

Calcarine sulcus (visual area)

Fornix

Anterior commissure

Hypothalamus (*H*)

Cerebellum

3rd ventricle

Cerebral aqueduct

Brainstem { Midbrain (*M*)
Pons (*P*)
Medulla oblongata (*O*) }

4th ventricle

Opening of median aperture (of Magendie)

D. Medial View

Cerebrum

Parietooccipital sulcus (fissure)

Calcarine sulcus

Diencephalon (*blue*)

Cerebellum

Brainstem (*orange*)

Cerebellum

Central canal

E. Medial View

F. Medial View

D. Cerebrum, cerebellum, and brainstem, median section.
E. Parts of brain, median section. **F.** Lobes of cerebral hemisphere, median section. See *Part D* for labeling key.

   Cerebral compression may be produced by intracranial collections of blood, obstruction of CSF circulation or absorption, intracranial tumors or abscesses, and brain swelling caused by brain edema, an increase in brain volume resulting from an increase in water and sodium content.

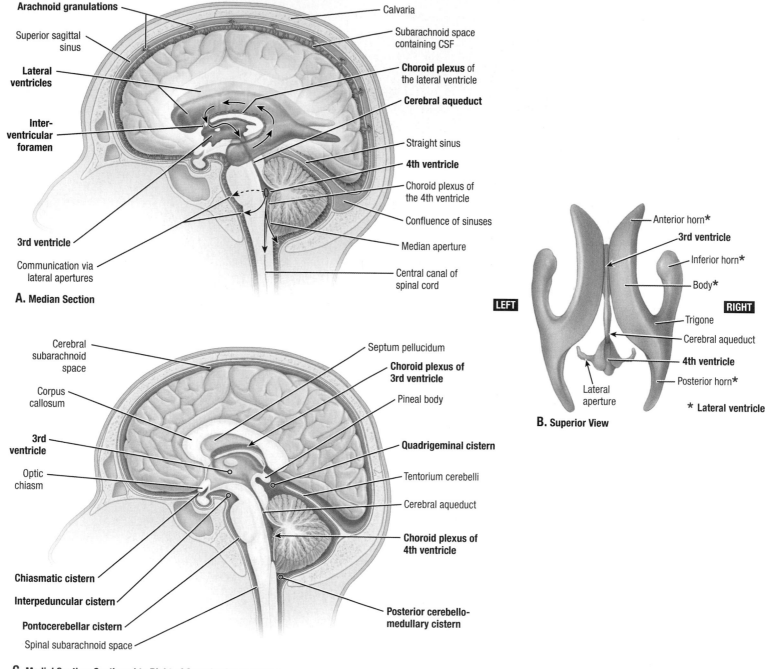

A. Median Section

- Arachnoid granulations
- Superior sagittal sinus
- **Lateral ventricles**
- **Interventricular foramen**
- **3rd ventricle**
- Communication via lateral apertures
- Calvaria
- Subarachnoid space containing CSF
- **Choroid plexus** of the lateral ventricle
- **Cerebral aqueduct**
- Straight sinus
- **4th ventricle**
- Choroid plexus of the 4th ventricle
- Confluence of sinuses
- Median aperture
- Central canal of spinal cord

B. Superior View

LEFT   RIGHT

- Anterior horn*
- **3rd ventricle**
- Inferior horn*
- Body*
- Trigone
- Cerebral aqueduct
- **4th ventricle**
- Posterior horn*
- Lateral aperture
- *** Lateral ventricle**

C. Medial Section, Sectioned to Right of Superior Sagittal Sinus

- Cerebral subarachnoid space
- Corpus callosum
- **3rd ventricle**
- Optic chiasm
- **Chiasmatic cistern**
- **Interpeduncular cistern**
- **Pontocerebellar cistern**
- Spinal subarachnoid space
- Septum pellucidum
- **Choroid plexus of 3rd ventricle**
- Pineal body
- **Quadrigeminal cistern**
- Tentorium cerebelli
- Cerebral aqueduct
- **Choroid plexus of 4th ventricle**
- **Posterior cerebello-medullary cistern**

8.102   Ventricular System

A. Circulation of cerebrospinal fluid (*CSF*). **B.** Ventricles: lateral, third, and fourth. **C.** Subarachnoid cisterns.

- The ventricular system consists of two lateral ventricles located in the cerebral hemispheres, a 3rd ventricle located between the right and left halves of the diencephalon, and a 4th ventricle located in the posterior parts of the pons and medulla.
- CSF secreted by choroid plexus in the ventricles drains via the interventricular foramen from the lateral to the 3rd ventricle, via the cerebral aqueduct from the 3rd to the 4th ventricle, and via

the median and lateral apertures into the subarachnoid space. CSF is absorbed by arachnoid granulations into the venous sinuses (especially the superior sagittal sinus).

- **Hydrocephalus.** Overproduction of CSF, obstruction of its flow, or interference with its absorption results in an excess of CSF in the ventricles and enlargement of the head, a condition known as hydrocephalus. Excess CSF dilates the ventricles; thins the brain; and, in infants, separates the bones of the calvaria because the sutures and fontanelles are still open.

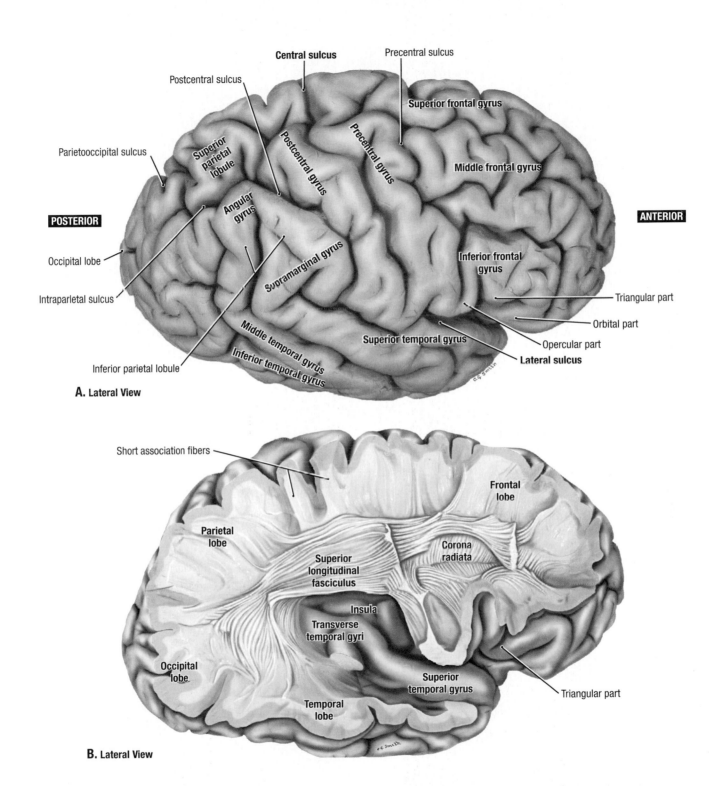

Central sulcus

Precentral sulcus

Postcentral sulcus

Superior frontal gyrus

Parietooccipital sulcus

Superior parietal lobule

Postcentral gyrus

Precentral gyrus

Middle frontal gyrus

POSTERIOR

ANTERIOR

Angular gyrus

Occipital lobe

Supramarginal gyrus

Inferior frontal gyrus

Intraparietal sulcus

Triangular part

Orbital part

Middle temporal gyrus

Superior temporal gyrus

Opercular part

Inferior parietal lobule

Inferior temporal gyrus

Lateral sulcus

A. Lateral View

Short association fibers

Frontal lobe

Parietal lobe

Corona radiata

Superior longitudinal fasciculus

Insula

Transverse temporal gyri

Occipital lobe

Superior temporal gyrus

Triangular part

Temporal lobe

B. Lateral View

Serial Dissections of Lateral Aspect of Cerebral Hemisphere

8.103

The dissections begin from the lateral surface of the cerebral hemisphere (*Part A*) and proceed sequentially medially (*Part B* to *Part F*).

A. Sulci and gyri of lateral surface of right cerebral hemisphere. Each gyrus is a fold of cerebral cortex with a core of white matter. The furrows are called sulci. The pattern of sulci and gyri, formed shortly before birth, is recognizable in some adult brains, as shown in this specimen. Usually, the expanding cortex acquires secondary foldings, which make identification of this basic pattern more difficult. **B. Superior longitudinal fasciculus, transverse temporal gyri, and insula.** The cortex and short association fiber bundles around the lateral fissure have been removed.

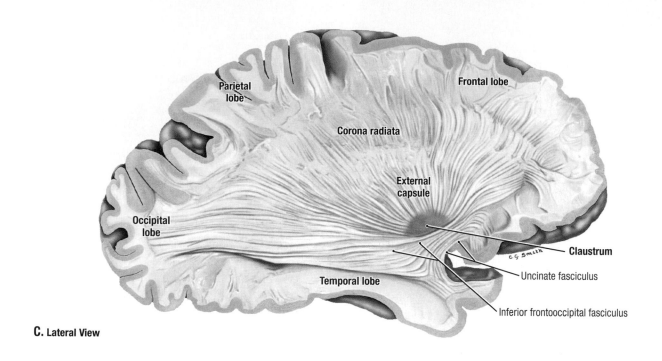

C. Lateral View

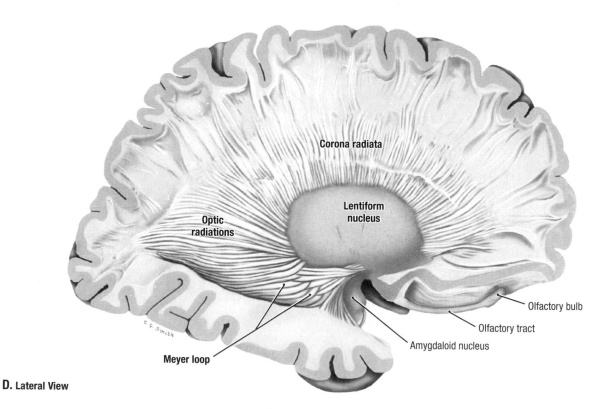

D. Lateral View

8.103 **Serial Dissections of Lateral Aspect of Cerebral Hemisphere** *(continued)*

C. Uncinate and inferior frontooccipital fasciculi and external capsule. The external capsule consists of projection fibers that pass between the claustrum laterally and the lentiform nucleus medially. **D. Lentiform nucleus and corona radiata.** The inferior longitudinal and uncinate fasciculi, claustrum, and external capsule have been removed. The fibers of these right hemisphere optic radiations convey impulses from the right half of the retina of each eye; the fibers extending closest to the temporal pole (Meyer loop) carry impulses from the lower portion of each retina.

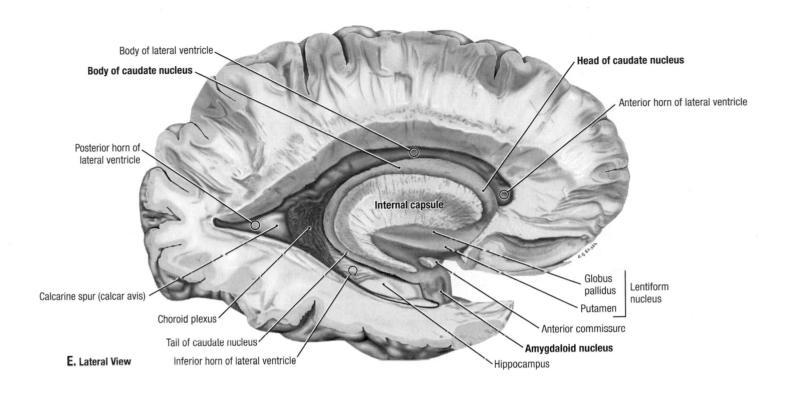

Body of lateral ventricle

Body of caudate nucleus

Head of caudate nucleus

Anterior horn of lateral ventricle

Posterior horn of lateral ventricle

Internal capsule

Calcarine spur (calcar avis)

Globus pallidus

Putamen

Lentiform nucleus

Choroid plexus

Anterior commissure

Tail of caudate nucleus

Amygdaloid nucleus

E. Lateral View

Inferior horn of lateral ventricle

Hippocampus

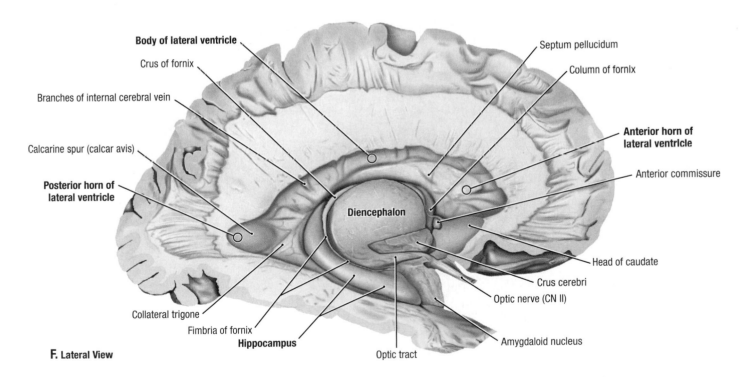

Body of lateral ventricle

Septum pellucidum

Crus of fornix

Column of fornix

Branches of internal cerebral vein

Anterior horn of lateral ventricle

Calcarine spur (calcar avis)

Anterior commissure

Posterior horn of lateral ventricle

Diencephalon

Head of caudate

Crus cerebri

Optic nerve (CN II)

Collateral trigone

Fimbria of fornix

Hippocampus

Optic tract

Amygdaloid nucleus

F. Lateral View

Serial Dissections of Lateral Aspect of Cerebral Hemisphere *(continued)*

8.103

E. Caudate and amygdaloid nuclei and internal capsule. The lateral wall of the lateral ventricle, the marginal part of the internal capsule, the anterior commissure, and the superior part of the lentiform nucleus have been removed. **F. Lateral ventricle, hippocampus, and diencephalon.** The inferior parts of the lentiform nucleus, internal capsule, and caudate nucleus have been removed.

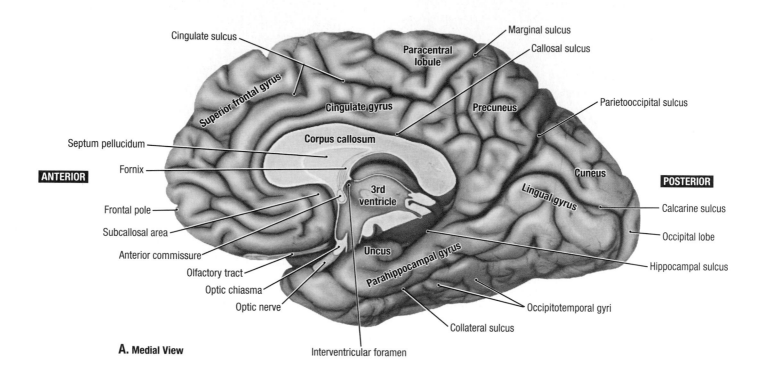

Cingulate sulcus

Marginal sulcus

Paracentral lobule

Callosal sulcus

Superior frontal gyrus

Cingulate gyrus

Precuneus

Parietooccipital sulcus

Septum pellucidum

Corpus callosum

Fornix

Cuneus

ANTERIOR

3rd ventricle

Lingual gyrus

POSTERIOR

Frontal pole

Calcarine sulcus

Subcallosal area

Occipital lobe

Anterior commissure

Uncus

Parahippocampal gyrus

Hippocampal sulcus

Olfactory tract

Optic chiasma

Occipitotemporal gyri

Optic nerve

Collateral sulcus

A. Medial View

Interventricular foramen

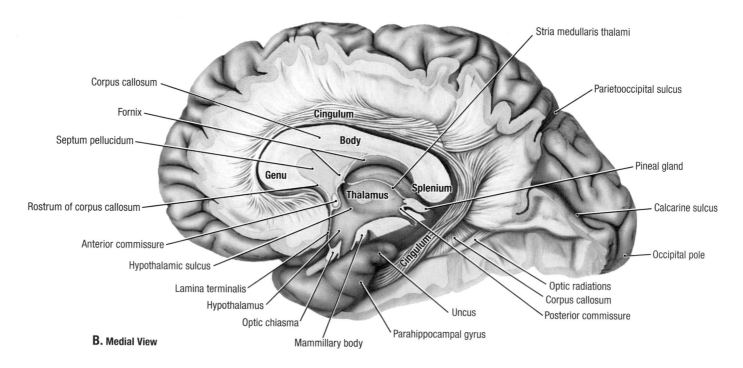

Stria medullaris thalami

Corpus callosum

Parietooccipital sulcus

Fornix

Cingulum

Septum pellucidum

Body

Pineal gland

Genu

Thalamus

Splenium

Rostrum of corpus callosum

Calcarine sulcus

Anterior commissure

Cingulum

Occipital pole

Hypothalamic sulcus

Lamina terminalis

Optic radiations

Hypothalamus

Corpus callosum

Optic chiasma

Uncus

Posterior commissure

B. Medial View

Mammillary body

Parahippocampal gyrus

8.104   Serial Dissections of Medial Aspect of Cerebral Hemisphere

The dissections begin from the medial surface of the cerebral hemisphere (*Part A*) and proceed sequentially laterally (*Part B* to *Part D*).

    A. Sulci and gyri of medial surface of cerebral hemisphere. The corpus callosum consists of the rostrum, genu, body, and

splenium; the cingulate and parahippocampal gyri form the limbic lobe. **B. Cingulum.** The cortex and short association fibers were removed from the medial aspect of the hemisphere. The cingulum is a long association fiber bundle that lies in the core of the cingulate and parahippocampal gyri.

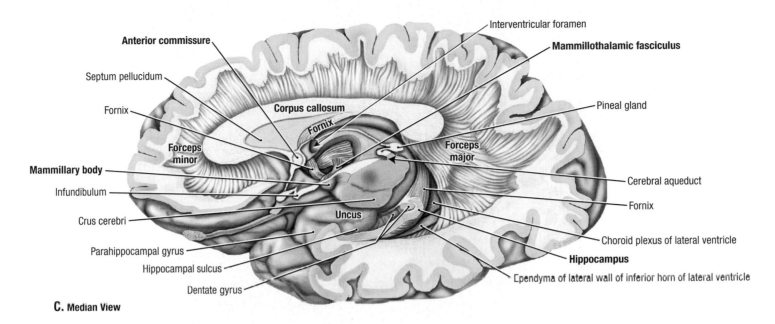

Anterior commissure

Septum pellucidum

Fornix

Corpus callosum

Interventricular foramen

Mammillothalamic fasciculus

Pineal gland

Forceps minor

Fornix

Forceps major

Mammillary body

Infundibulum

Crus cerebri

Uncus

Cerebral aqueduct

Fornix

Parahippocampal gyrus

Hippocampal sulcus

Dentate gyrus

Choroid plexus of lateral ventricle

Hippocampus

Ependyma of lateral wall of inferior horn of lateral ventricle

C. Median View

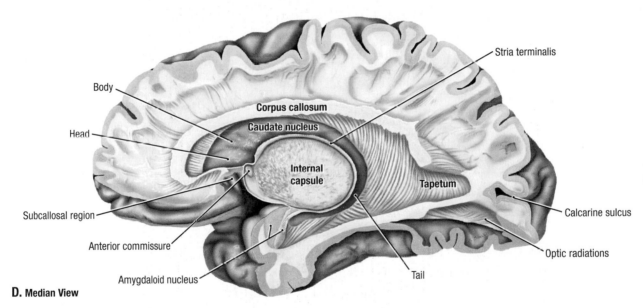

Body

Head

Subcallosal region

Anterior commissure

Amygdaloid nucleus

Corpus callosum

Caudate nucleus

Internal capsule

Stria terminalis

Tapetum

Tail

Calcarine sulcus

Optic radiations

D. Median View

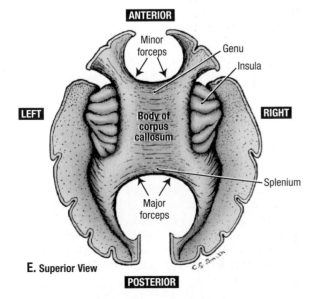

ANTERIOR

Minor forceps

Genu

Insula

LEFT

Body of corpus callosum

RIGHT

Splenium

Major forceps

E. Superior View

POSTERIOR

Serial Dissections of Medial Aspect of Cerebral Hemisphere *(continued)*   8.104

C. Fornix, mammillothalamic fasciculus, and forceps major and minor. The cingulum and a portion of the wall of the 3rd ventricle have been removed. The fornix begins at the hippocampus and terminates in the mammillary body by passing anterior to the interventricular foramen and posterior to the anterior commissure. The mammillothalamic fasciculus emerges from the mammillary body and terminates in the anterior nucleus of the thalamus. **D. Caudate nucleus and internal capsule.** The diencephalon was removed, along with the ependyma of the lateral ventricle, except where it covers the caudate and amygdaloid nuclei. **E. Corpus callosum.** The body of the corpus callosum connects the two cerebral hemispheres; the minor (frontal) forceps (at the genu of corpus callosum) connects the frontal lobes, and the major (occipital) forceps (at splenium) connects the occipital lobes.

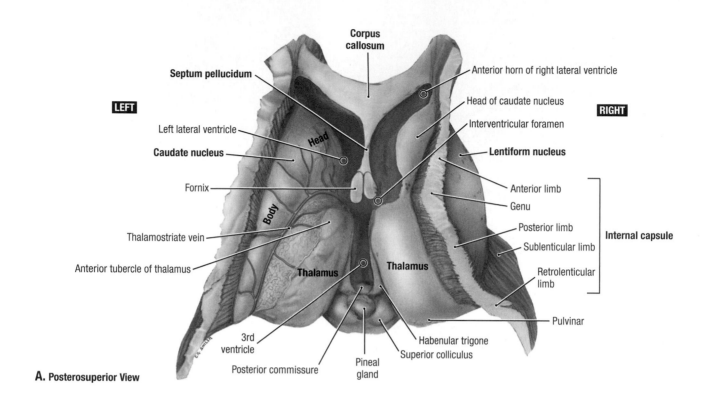

A. Posterosuperior View

Corpus callosum

Septum pellucidum

LEFT

Left lateral ventricle

Caudate nucleus

Fornix

Thalamostriate vein

Anterior tubercle of thalamus

Head

Body

Thalamus

3rd ventricle

Posterior commissure

Pineal gland

Anterior horn of right lateral ventricle

Head of caudate nucleus

Interventricular foramen

Lentiform nucleus

RIGHT

Anterior limb

Genu

Posterior limb

Sublenticular limb

Retrolenticular limb

Internal capsule

Thalamus

Pulvinar

Habenular trigone

Superior colliculus

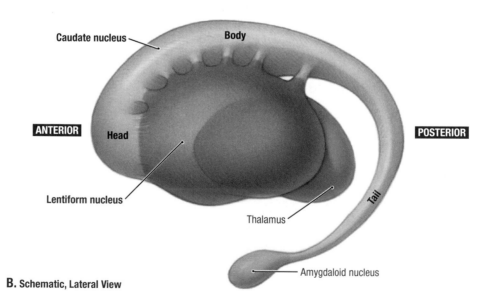

B. Schematic, Lateral View

Caudate nucleus

Body

ANTERIOR

Head

Lentiform nucleus

Thalamus

Tail

Amygdaloid nucleus

POSTERIOR

8.105 **Caudate and Lentiform Nuclei**

A. Relationship to lateral ventricles and internal capsule. The dorsal surface of the diencephalon has been exposed by dissecting away the two cerebral hemispheres, except the anterior part of the corpus callosum, the inferior part of the septum pellucidum, the internal capsule, and the caudate and lentiform nuclei.

On the right side of the specimen, the thalamus, caudate, and lentiform nuclei have been cut horizontally at the level of the interventricular foramen. The parts of the internal capsule include the anterior, posterior, retrolenticular and sublenticular limbs, and genu. **B. Schematic of nuclei.**

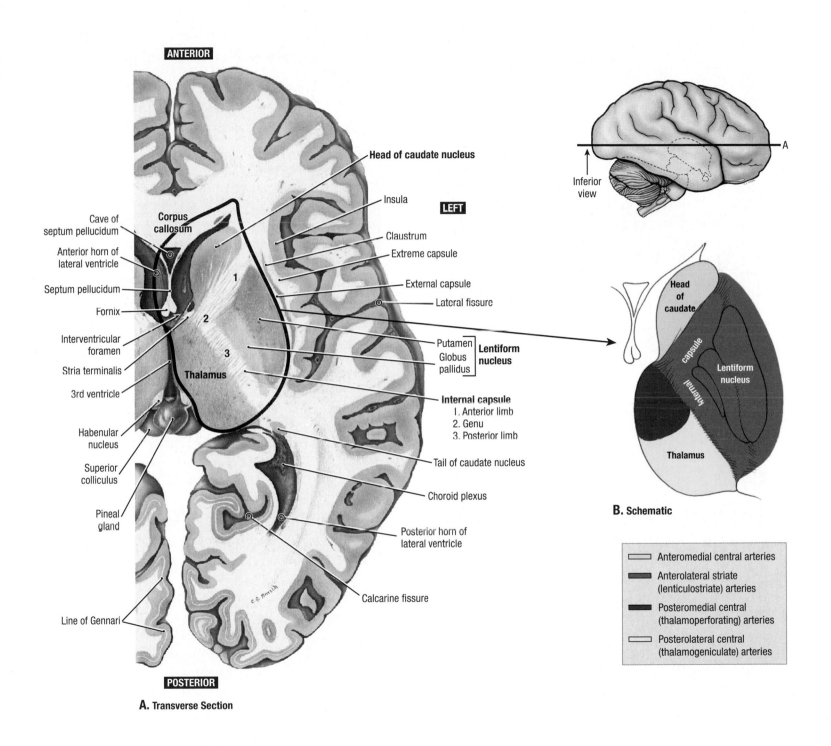

A. Transverse Section

ANTERIOR

Head of caudate nucleus

Cave of
septum pellucidum

Corpus
callosum

Insula

LEFT

Claustrum

Anterior horn of
lateral ventricle

Extreme capsule

Septum pellucidum

External capsule

Lateral fissure

Fornix

Interventricular
foramen

Putamen
Globus
pallidus

Lentiform
nucleus

Stria terminalis

Thalamus

3rd ventricle

Internal capsule
1. Anterior limb
2. Genu
3. Posterior limb

Habenular
nucleus

Tail of caudate nucleus

Superior
colliculus

Choroid plexus

Pineal
gland

Posterior horn of
lateral ventricle

Line of Gennari

Calcarine fissure

POSTERIOR

Inferior
view

A

Head
of
caudate

Internal capsule

Lentiform
nucleus

Thalamus

B. Schematic

Anteromedial central arteries

Anterolateral striate
(lenticulostriate) arteries

Posteromedial central
(thalamoperforating) arteries

Posterolateral central
(thalamogeniculate) arteries

A. Relationships of internal capsule. **B.** Blood supply of region.

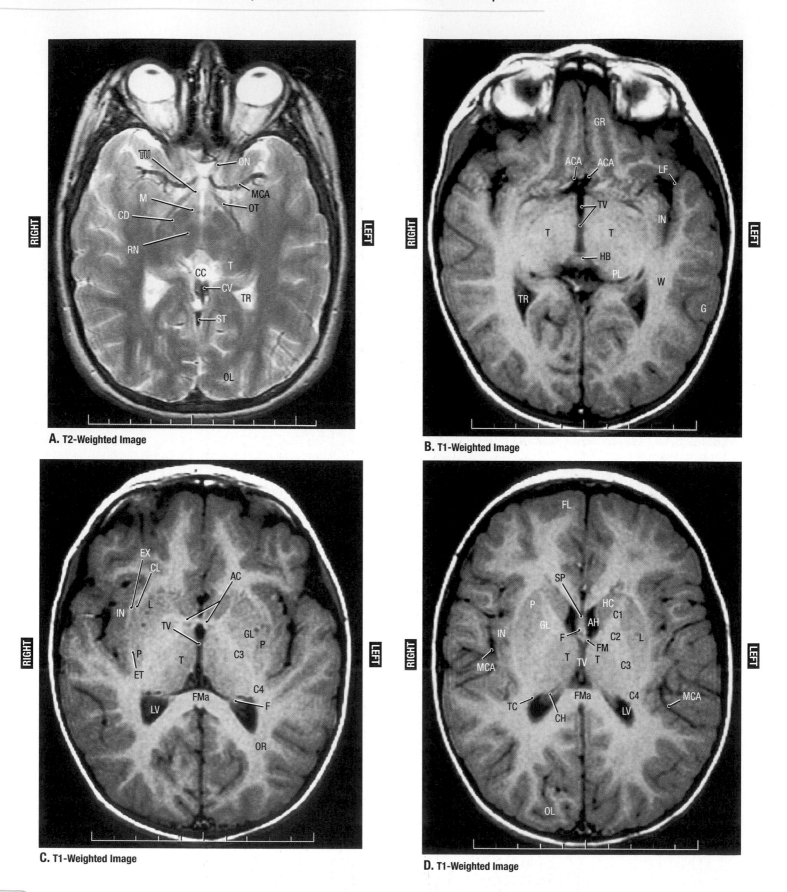

A. T2-Weighted Image

B. T1-Weighted Image

C. T1-Weighted Image

D. T1-Weighted Image

8.107 **Axial (Transverse) MRIs through Cerebral Hemispheres**

See orientation drawing for sites of scans (*Part A* to *Part F*).

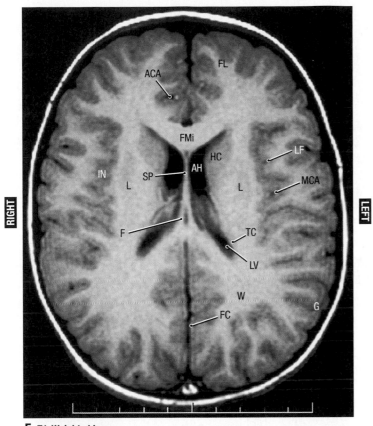

E. T1-Weighted Image

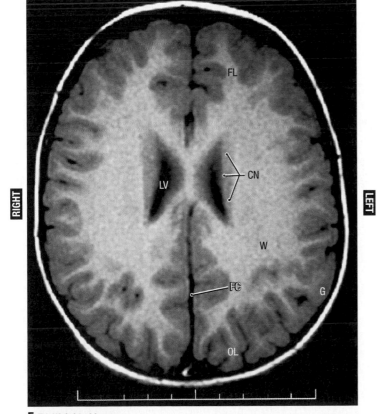

F. T1-Weighted Image

AC	Anterior commissure	**GL**	Globus pallidus
ACA	Anterior cerebral artery	**GR**	Gyrus rectus
AH	Anterior horn of lateral ventricle	**HB**	Habenular commissure
		HC	Head of caudate nucleus
C1	Anterior limb of internal capsule	**IN**	Insular cortex
		L	Lentiform nucleus
C2	Genu of internal capsule	**LF**	Lateral fissure
C3	Posterior limb of internal capsule	**LV**	Lateral ventricle
		M	Mammillary body
C4	Retrolenticular limb of internal capsule	**MCA**	Middle cerebral artery
		OL	Occipital lobe
CC	Collicular cistern	**ON**	Optic nerve
CD	Cerebral peduncle	**OR**	Optic radiations
CH	Choroid plexus	**OT**	Optic tract
CL	Claustrum	**P**	Putamen
CN	Caudate nucleus	**PL**	Pulvinar
CV	Great cerebral vein	**RN**	Red nucleus
ET	External capsule	**SP**	Septum pellucidum
EX	Extreme capsule	**ST**	Straight sinus
F	Fornix	**T**	Thalamus
FC	Falx cerebri	**TC**	Tail of caudate nucleus
FL	Frontal lobe	**TR**	Trigone of lateral ventricle
FM	Interventricular foramen	**TU**	Tuber cinereum
FMa	Forceps major	**TV**	Third ventricle
FMi	Forceps minor	**W**	White matter
G	Gray matter		

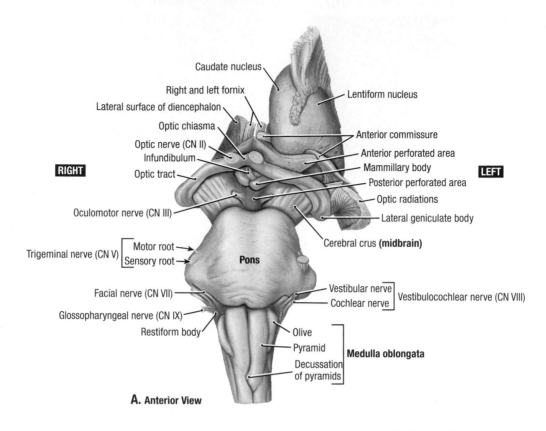

Caudate nucleus
Right and left fornix
Lateral surface of diencephalon
Optic chiasma
Optic nerve (CN II)
Infundibulum
Optic tract
Lentiform nucleus
Anterior commissure
Anterior perforated area
Mammillary body
Posterior perforated area
Optic radiations
Lateral geniculate body
Cerebral crus **(midbrain)**

RIGHT   **LEFT**

Oculomotor nerve (CN III)

Trigeminal nerve (CN V) { Motor root → / Sensory root → }   **Pons**

Facial nerve (CN VII)
Glossopharyngeal nerve (CN IX)
Restiform body
Vestibular nerve / Cochlear nerve } Vestibulocochlear nerve (CN VIII)
Olive
Pyramid
Decussation of pyramids
Medulla oblongata

A. Anterior View

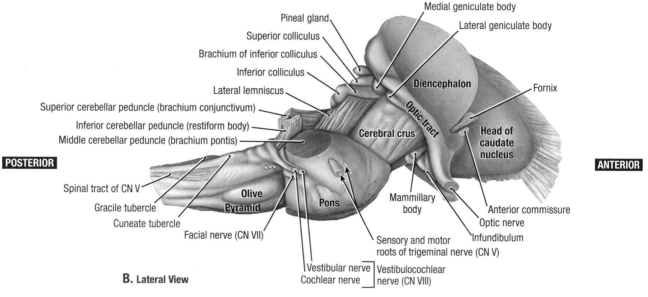

Pineal gland
Superior colliculus
Brachium of inferior colliculus
Inferior colliculus
Lateral lemniscus
Superior cerebellar peduncle (brachium conjunctivum)
Inferior cerebellar peduncle (restiform body)
Middle cerebellar peduncle (brachium pontis)
Medial geniculate body
Lateral geniculate body
Diencephalon
Fornix
Optic tract
Cerebral crus
Head of caudate nucleus

POSTERIOR   **ANTERIOR**

Spinal tract of CN V
Gracile tubercle
Cuneate tubercle
Facial nerve (CN VII)
Olive
Pyramid
Pons
Mammillary body
Anterior commissure
Optic nerve
Infundibulum
Sensory and motor roots of trigeminal nerve (CN V)
Vestibular nerve / Cochlear nerve } Vestibulocochlear nerve (CN VIII)

B. Lateral View

8.108   **Brainstem**

The brainstem has been exposed by removing the cerebellum, all of the right cerebral hemisphere, and the major portion of the left hemisphere.
   A. Ventral aspect.
- The brainstem consists of the medulla oblongata, pons, and midbrain.
- The pyramid is on the ventral surface of the medulla; the decussation of the pyramids is formed by the decussating (crossing) lateral corticospinal tract.
- The trigeminal nerve (CN V) emerges as sensory and motor roots.

- The crus cerebri are part of the midbrain.
- The oculomotor nerve emerges from the interpeduncular fossa.
B. Lateral aspect.
- The vestibulocochlear nerve (CN VIII) consists of two nerves, the vestibular and cochlear nerves.
- The spinal tract of the trigeminal nerve is exposed where it comes to the surface of the medulla to form the tuber cinereum.
- The three are cerebellar peduncles: superior, middle, and inferior.
- The medial and lateral lemnisci are on the lateral aspect of the midbrain

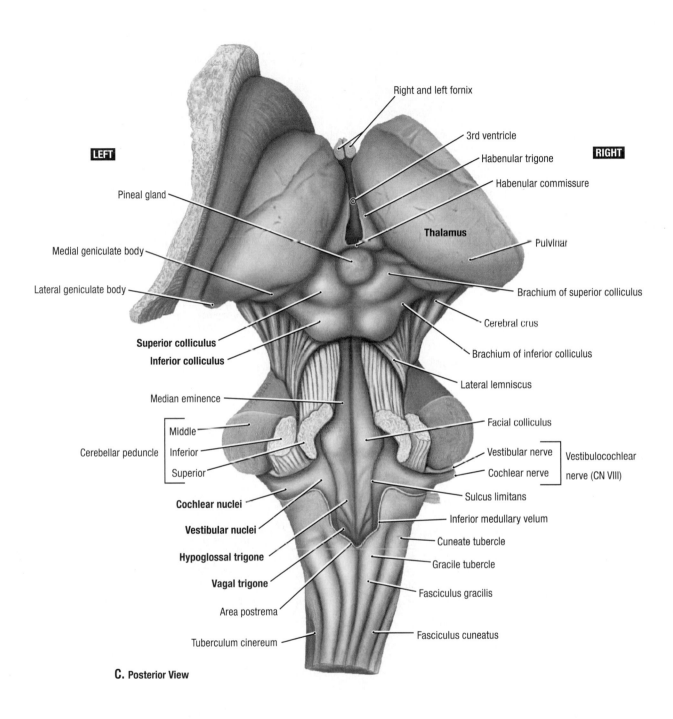

Right and left fornix

3rd ventricle

Habenular trigone

Habenular commissure

LEFT

RIGHT

Pineal gland

Thalamus

Pulvinar

Medial geniculate body

Brachium of superior colliculus

Lateral geniculate body

Cerebral crus

Superior colliculus

Brachium of inferior colliculus

Inferior colliculus

Lateral lemniscus

Median eminence

Facial colliculus

Middle

Inferior

Cerebellar peduncle

Superior

Vestibular nerve   Vestibulocochlear
nerve (CN VIII)

Cochlear nerve

Sulcus limitans

Cochlear nuclei

Inferior medullary velum

Vestibular nuclei

Cuneate tubercle

Hypoglossal trigone

Gracile tubercle

Vagal trigone

Fasciculus gracilis

Area postrema

Fasciculus cuneatus

Tuberculum cinereum

C. Posterior View

Brainstem (continued)

8.108

C. Dorsal aspect.
- Ridges are formed by the fasciculus gracilis and cuneatus.
- The gracile and cuneate tubercles are the sites of the nucleus gracilis and nucleus cuneatus.
- The diamond-shaped floor of the 4th ventricle; lateral to the sulcus limitans are the vestibular and cochlear nuclei and

medially are the hypoglossal and vagal trigones and the facial colliculus.
- The superior and inferior colliculi form the dorsal surface of the midbrain.

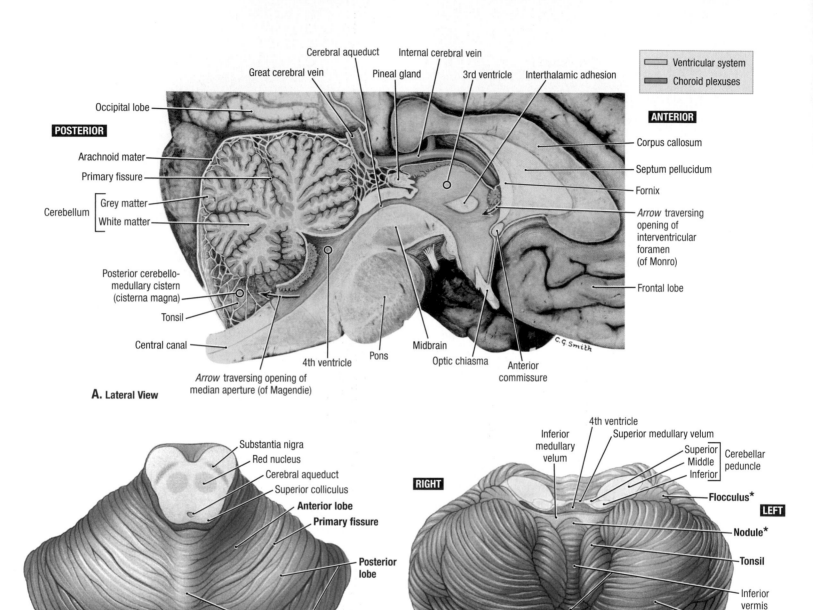

A. Lateral View

Occipital lobe
POSTERIOR
Arachnoid mater
Primary fissure
Cerebellum { Grey matter / White matter }
Posterior cerebello-medullary cistern (cisterna magna)
Tonsil
Central canal
Arrow traversing opening of median aperture (of Magendie)
4th ventricle
Pons
Midbrain
Optic chiasma
Anterior commissure

Cerebral aqueduct
Great cerebral vein
Pineal gland
Internal cerebral vein
3rd ventricle
Interthalamic adhesion
ANTERIOR
Corpus callosum
Septum pellucidum
Fornix
Arrow traversing opening of interventricular foramen (of Monro)
Frontal lobe

Ventricular system
Choroid plexuses

B. Superior View

Substantia nigra
Red nucleus
Cerebral aqueduct
Superior colliculus
Anterior lobe
Primary fissure
Posterior lobe
RIGHT
LEFT
Superior vermis

C. Inferior View

Inferior medullary velum
4th ventricle
Superior medullary velum
Superior / Middle / Inferior } Cerebellar peduncle
Flocculus*
RIGHT
LEFT
Nodule*
Tonsil
Inferior vermis
Posterior lobe
Horizontal fissure

*** Flocculonodular lobe**

8.109   **Cerebellum**

A. Median section. The arachnoid mater was removed except where it covered the cerebellum and the occipital lobe. **Cisternal puncture.** CSF may be obtained, for diagnostic purposes, from the posterior cerebellomedullary cistern, using a procedure known as cisternal puncture. The subarachnoid space or the ventricular system may also be entered for measuring or monitoring CSF pressure, injecting antibiotics, or administering contrast media for radiography. **B. Superior view of cerebellum.** The right and left cerebellar hemispheres are united by the superior vermis; the anterior and posterior lobes are separated by the primary fissure. **C. Inferior view of cerebellum.** The flocculonodular lobe, the oldest part of the cerebellum, consists of the flocculus and nodule; the cerebellar tonsils typically extend into the foramen magnum.

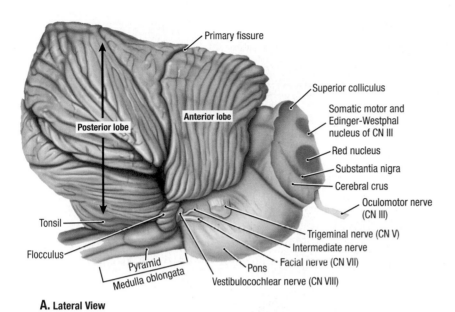

A. Lateral View

Labels for A:
Primary fissure
Superior colliculus
Somatic motor and Edinger-Westphal nucleus of CN III
Red nucleus
Substantia nigra
Cerebral crus
Oculomotor nerve (CN III)
Trigeminal nerve (CN V)
Intermediate nerve
Facial nerve (CN VII)
Vestibulocochlear nerve (CN VIII)
Anterior lobe
Posterior lobe
Tonsil
Flocculus
Pyramid
Medulla oblongata
Pons

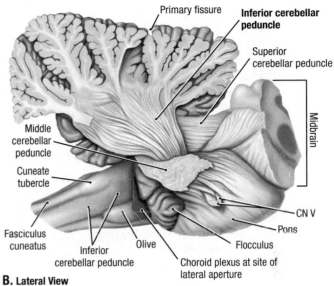

B. Lateral View

Labels for B:
Primary fissure
Inferior cerebellar peduncle
Superior cerebellar peduncle
Midbrain
Middle cerebellar peduncle
Cuneate tubercle
Fasciculus cuneatus
Inferior cerebellar peduncle
Olive
CN V
Pons
Flocculus
Choroid plexus at site of lateral aperture

C. Lateral View

Labels for C:
Primary fissure
Middle cerebellar peduncle
Superior cerebellar peduncle
Inferior colliculus
Superior colliculus
Lateral lemniscus
Cerebral crus
Motor root
Sensory root
Trigeminal nerve CN V
Pons
Facial nerve (CN VII)
Pyramid
Olive
Flocculus
Vestibulocochlear nerve (CN VIII)

D. Lateral View

Labels for D:
Inferior cerebellar peduncle
Primary fissure
Fastigiobulbar tract
Superior cerebellar peduncle
Dentate nucleus
Red nucleus
Substantia nigra
Cerebral crus
Pons
Middle cerebellar peduncle
Flocculus
Choroid plexus at the site of the lateral aperture (of Luschka)

Serial Dissections of Cerebellum

8.110

The series begins with the lateral surface of the cerebellar hemispheres (*Part A*) and proceeds medially in sequence (*Part B* to *Part D*).
 A. Cerebellum and brainstem. B. Inferior cerebellar peduncle. The fibers of the middle cerebellar peduncle were cut dorsal to the trigeminal nerve and peeled away to expose the fibers of the inferior cerebellar peduncle. **C. Middle cerebellar peduncle.**

The fibers of the middle cerebellar peduncle were exposed by peeling away the lateral portion of the lobules of the cerebellar hemisphere. **D. Superior cerebellar peduncle and dentate nucleus.** The fibers of the inferior cerebellar peduncle were cut just dorsal to the previously sectioned middle cerebellar peduncle and peeled away until the gray matter of the dentate nucleus could be seen.

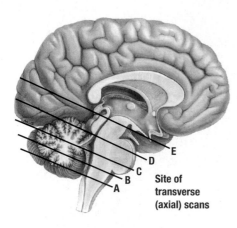

Site of transverse (axial) scans

Blood Supply

- Posterior cerebral
- Superior cerebellar
- Anterior inferior cerebellar
- Posterior inferior cerebellar
- Vertebral
- Anterior spinal
- Posterior spinal

Basilar:
- Long circumferential branches
- Short circumferential branches
- Paramedian branches

AICA	Anterior inferior cerebellar artery
AM	Internal acoustic meatus
BA	Basilar artery
C	Cerebral crus
CA	Cerebral aqueduct
CB	Ciliary body
CC	Common carotid artery
CI	Colliculi
CL	Left cerebellar hemisphere
CP	Cochlear perilymph
CR	Right cerebellar hemisphere
CSF	CSF in subarachnoid space
DS	Dorsum sellae
EB	Eyeball
F	CN VII and CN VIII
FC	Facial colliculus
FI	Fat in infratemporal fossa
FL	Flocculus
FV	Fourth ventricle
G	Gray matter
HF	Hypophysial fossa
HP	Hippocampus
IC	Interpeduncular cistern
ICA	Internal carotid artery
ICP	Inferior cerebellar peduncle
IF	Inferior concha
IH	Inferior horn (lateral ventricle)
IJV	Internal jugular vein
IN	Infundibulum
IP	Interpeduncular fossa
IV	Inferior vermis
L	Lens
LP	Lateral pterygoid
MA	Mastoid air cells
MB	Mandible
MC	Middle concha
MCP	Middle cerebellar peduncle
MD	Midbrain
MO	Medulla oblongata
MS	Maxillary sinus
MT	Masseter
MX	Maxilla
ND	Nodule of cerebellum
NS	Nasal septum
OB	Occipital bone
OC	Optic chiasm

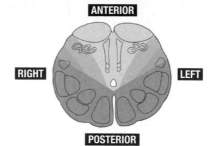

Transverse section through lower medulla oblongata (*Part A*)

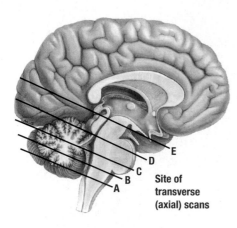

A. T1-Weighted Image

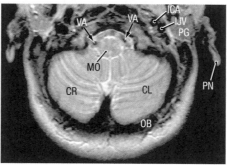

T2-Weighted Image

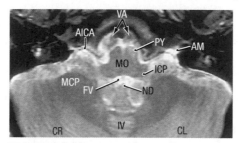

Transverse section through upper medulla oblongata (*Part B*)

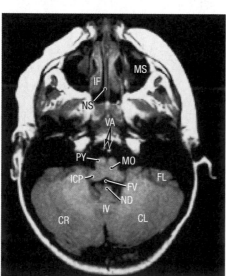

B. T1-Weighted Image

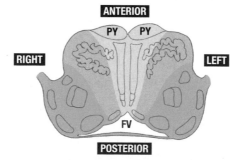

T2-Weighted Image

8.111 **Axial (Transverse) MRIs through Brainstem, Inferior Views**

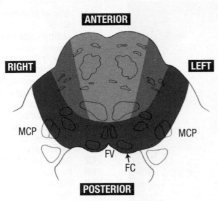

Transverse section through pons (*Parts C & D*)

OL	Occipital lobe
ON	Optic nerve (CN II)
P	Pons
PA	Pharynx
PCA	Posterior cerebral artery
PF	Parapharyngeal fat
PG	Parotid gland
PH	Posterior horn (lateral ventricle)
PN	Pinna
PY	Pyramid
RN	Red nucleus
SC	Semicircular canal
SCP	Superior cerebellar peduncle
SE	Suprasellar cistern
SH	Superior concha
SN	Substantia nigra
SS	Superior sagittal sinus
ST	Straight sinus
SV	Superior vermis
TG	Tongue
TL	Temporal lobe
TP	Temporalis
UN	Uncus
VA	Vertebral artery
VP	Vestibular perilymph
VT	Vitreous body
W	White matter

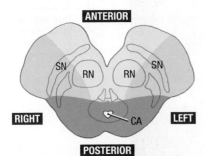

Transverse section through midbrain (*Part E*)

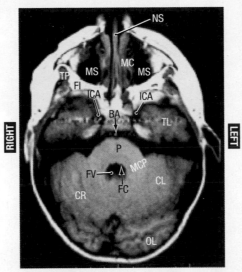

C. T1-Weighted Image

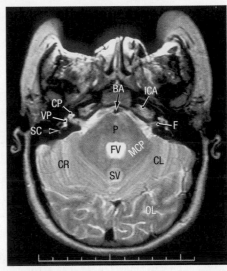

T2-Weighted Image

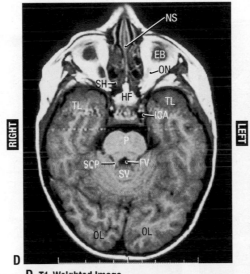

D. T1-Weighted Image

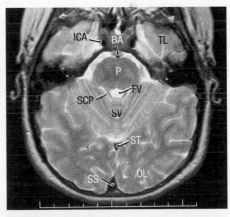

T2-Weighted Image

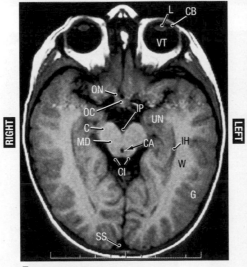

E. T1-Weighted Image

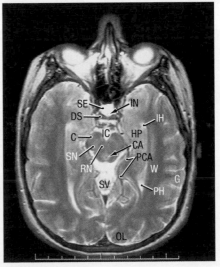

T2-Weighted Image

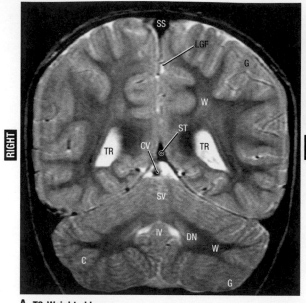

A. T2-Weighted Image

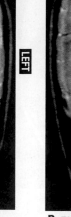

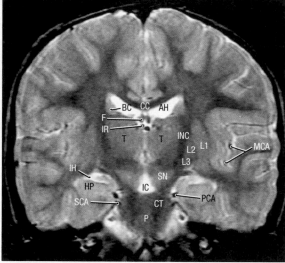

B. T2-Weighted Image

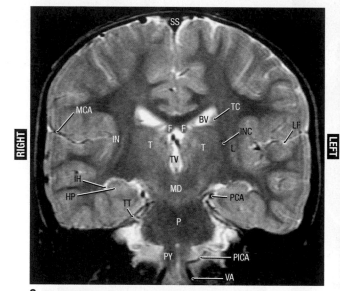

C. T2-Weighted Image

D. T2-Weighted Image

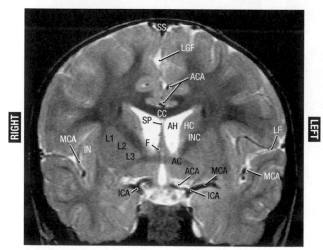

E. T2-Weighted Image

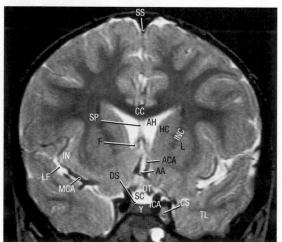

F. T2-Weighted Image

AA	Anterior communicating artery
AC	Anterior commissure
ACA	Anterior cerebral artery
AH	Anterior horn of lateral ventricle
BC	Body of caudate nucleus
BV	Body of lateral ventricle
C	Cerebellum
CC	Corpus callosum
CH	Choroid plexus
CS	Cavernous sinus
CT	Corticospinal tract
CV	Great cerebral vein
DN	Dentate nucleus
DS	Diaphragma sellae
F	Fornix
G	Gray matter
HC	Head of caudate nucleus
HP	Hippocampus
IC	Interpeduncular cistern
ICA	Internal carotid artery
IH	Interior horn of lateral ventricle
IN	Insular cortex
INC	Internal capsule
IR	Intervertebral vein
IV	Inferior vermis
L	Lentiform nucleus
L1	Putamen
L2	External (lateral) segment of globus pallidus
L3	Internal (medial) segment of globus pallidus
LF	Lateral fissure
LGF	Longitudinal fissure
MCA	Middle cerebral artery
MD	Midbrain
OT	Optic tract
P	Pons
PCA	Posterior cerebral artery
PH	Posterior horn of lateral ventricle
PICA	Posterior inferior cerebellar artery
PY	Pyramid
SC	Supracerebellar cistern
SCA	Superior cerebellar artery
SN	Substantia nigra
SP	Septum pellucidum
SS	Superior sagittal sinus
ST	Straight sinus
SV	Superior vermis
T	Thalamus
TC	Tail of caudate nucleus
TL	Temporal lobe
To	Cerebellar tonsil
TR	Trigone of lateral ventricle
TT	Tentorium cerebelli
TV	Third ventricle
VA	Vertebral artery
W	White matter
Y	Hypophysis

8.112 **Coronal MRIs (T2-Weighted) and Sections of Brain**

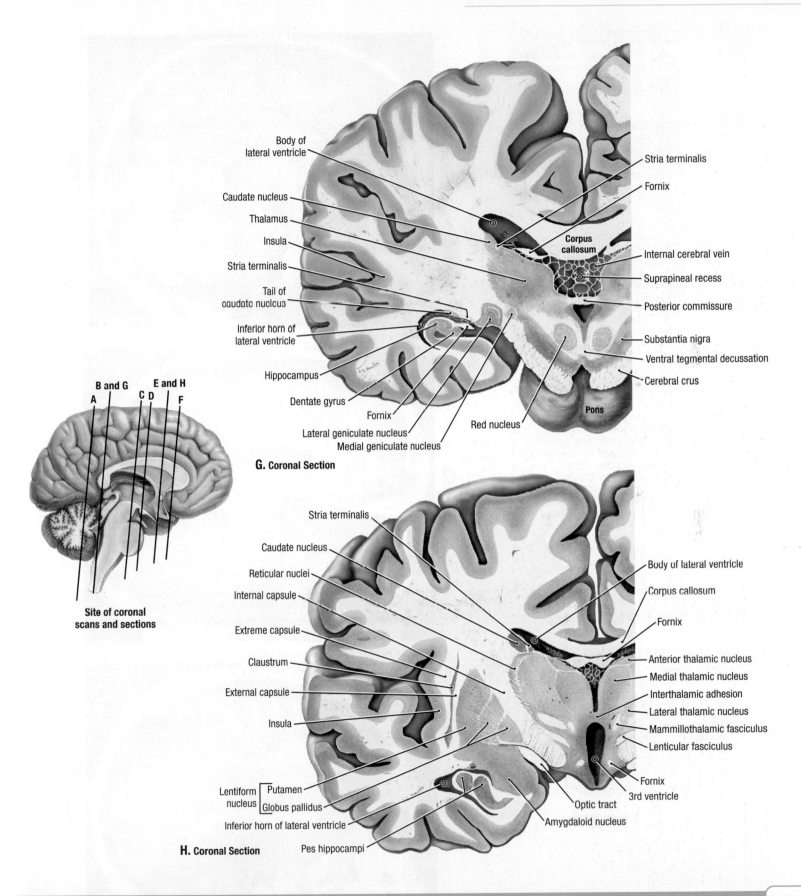

Body of
lateral ventricle

Caudate nucleus

Thalamus

Insula

Stria terminalis

Tail of
caudate nucleus

Inferior horn of
lateral ventricle

Hippocampus

Dentate gyrus

Fornix

Lateral geniculate nucleus

Medial geniculate nucleus

Stria terminalis

Fornix

**Corpus
callosum**

Internal cerebral vein

Suprapineal recess

Posterior commissure

Substantia nigra

Ventral tegmental decussation

Cerebral crus

Pons

Red nucleus

G. Coronal Section

B and G

E and H

A

C D

F

**Site of coronal
scans and sections**

Stria terminalis

Caudate nucleus

Reticular nuclei

Internal capsule

Extreme capsule

Claustrum

External capsule

Insula

Lentiform { Putamen
nucleus { Globus pallidus

Inferior horn of lateral ventricle

Pes hippocampi

Body of lateral ventricle

Corpus callosum

Fornix

Anterior thalamic nucleus

Medial thalamic nucleus

Interthalamic adhesion

Lateral thalamic nucleus

Mammillothalamic fasciculus

Lenticular fasciculus

Fornix

3rd ventricle

Optic tract

Amygdaloid nucleus

H. Coronal Section

G. and **H.** Coronal sections, posterior views.

ACA	Anterior cerebral artery
AH	Anterior horn of lateral ventricle
B	Body of corpus callosum
BA	Basilar artery
BV	Body of lateral ventricle
C	Colliculi
C1	Anterior tubercle of atlas
Cal	Calcarine sulcus
Cb	Cerebellum
CG	Cingulate nucleus
CQ	Cerebral aqueduct
CS	Cingulate sulcus
D	Dens (odontoid process)
F	Fornix
FM	Foramen magnum
FP	Frontal pole
FV	Fourth ventricle
G	Cerebral cortex (gray matter)
GC	Genus of corpus callosum
H	Hypothalamus
HC	Head of caudate nucleus
I	Infundibulum
IN	Insular cortex
M	Mammillary body
MCA	Middle cerebral artery
MD	Midbrain
MO	Medulla oblongata
OP	Occipital pole
P	Pons
PA	Pharynx
PD	Cerebral peduncle
PI	Pineal
PO	Parietooccipital fissure
R	Rostrum of corpus callosum
S	Splenium of corpus callosum
SC	Spinal cord
SF	Superior frontal sulcus
ST	Straight sinus
STS	Superior temporal sulcus
SV	Superior medullary vellum
T	Thalamus
To	Cerebellar tonsil
TP	Temporal pole
TS	Transverse sinus
W	White matter
Y	Hypophysis

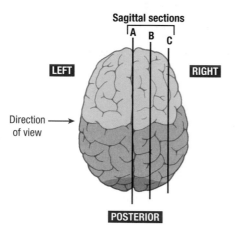

Sagittal sections

LEFT   **RIGHT**

Direction of view →

POSTERIOR

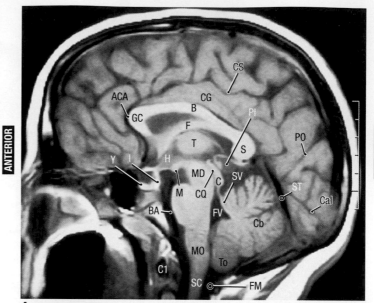

A. T1-Weighted Image

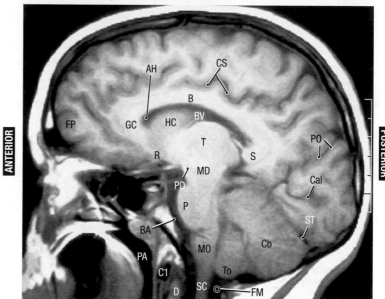

B. T1-Weighted Image

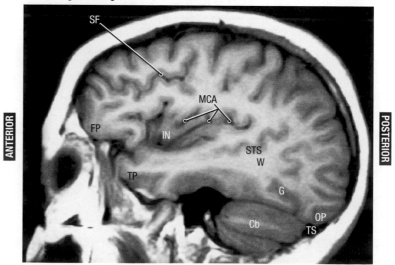

C. T1-Weighted Image

8.113   **Sagittal MRIs (T1-Weighted) and Median Section of Brain**

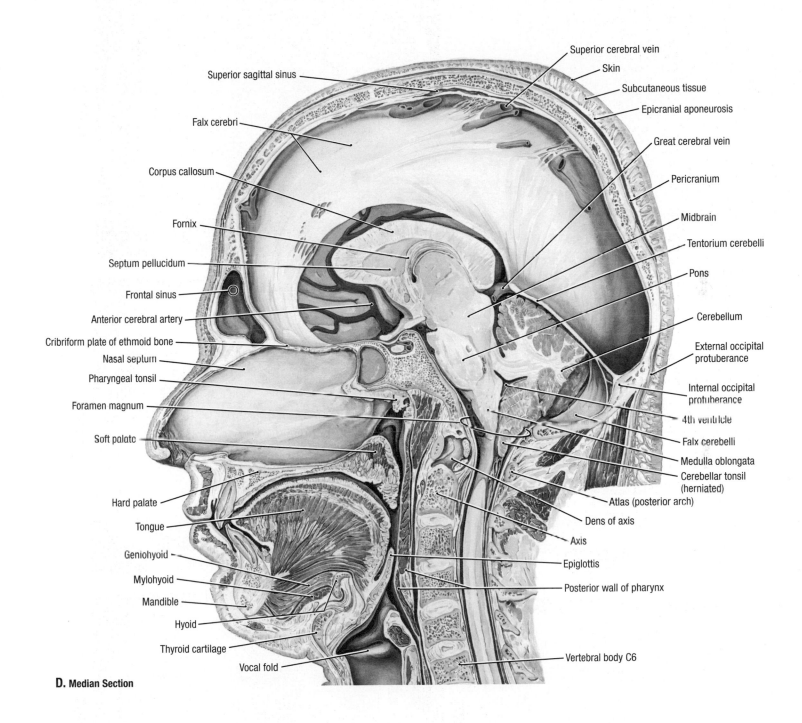

Superior cerebral vein

Skin

Subcutaneous tissue

Epicranial aponeurosis

Great cerebral vein

Pericranium

Midbrain

Tentorium cerebelli

Pons

Cerebellum

External occipital protuberance

Internal occipital protuberance

4th ventricle

Falx cerebelli

Medulla oblongata

Cerebellar tonsil (herniated)

Atlas (posterior arch)

Dens of axis

Axis

Epiglottis

Posterior wall of pharynx

Vertebral body C6

Superior sagittal sinus

Falx cerebri

Corpus callosum

Fornix

Septum pellucidum

Frontal sinus

Anterior cerebral artery

Cribriform plate of ethmoid bone

Nasal septum

Pharyngeal tonsil

Foramen magnum

Soft palate

Hard palate

Tongue

Geniohyoid

Mylohyoid

Mandible

Hyoid

Thyroid cartilage

Vocal fold

D. Median Section

Sagittal MRIs (T1-Weighted) and Median Section of Brain *(continued)*   **8.113**

See orientation drawing for sites of scans (*Part A* to *Part C*).
  Increased intracranial pressure (e.g., due to a tumor) may cause displacement of the cerebellar tonsils through the foramen magnum, resulting in a foraminal (tonsillar) herniation. Compression of the brainstem, if severe, may result in respiratory and cardiac arrest.

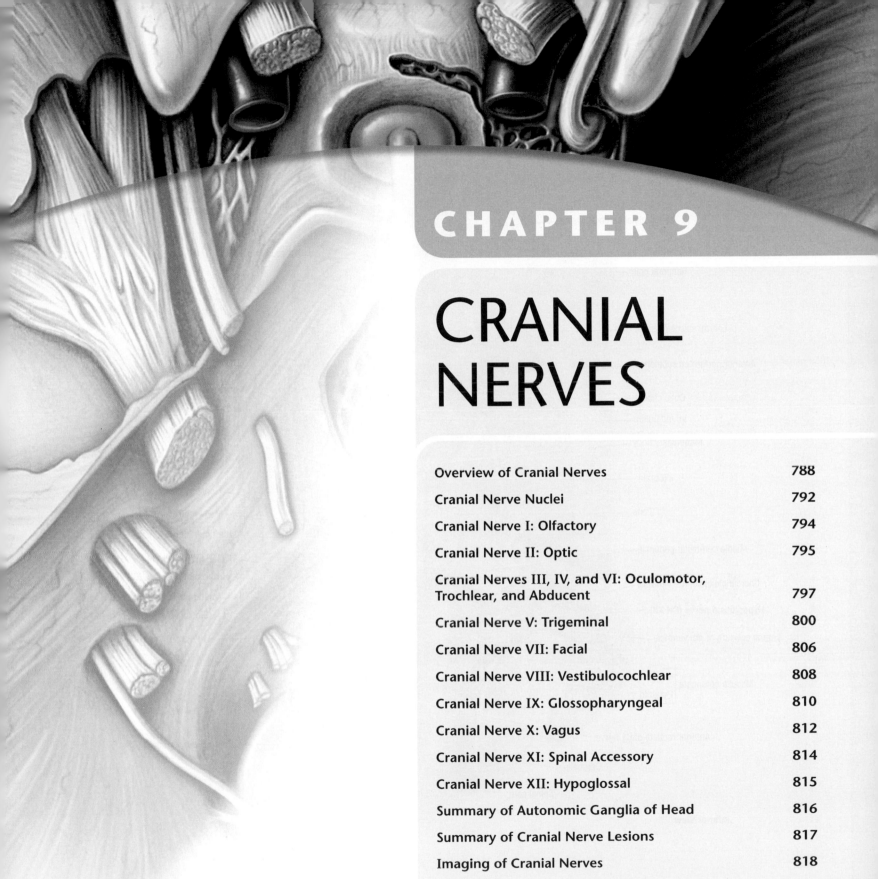

CHAPTER 9

CRANIAL NERVES

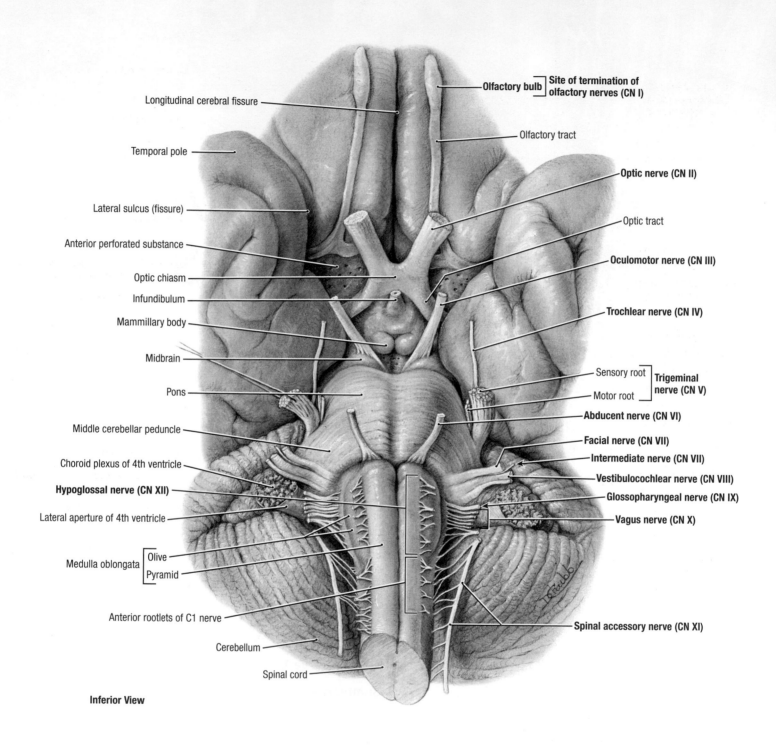

Longitudinal cerebral fissure

Temporal pole

Lateral sulcus (fissure)

Anterior perforated substance

Optic chiasm

Infundibulum

Mammillary body

Midbrain

Pons

Middle cerebellar peduncle

Choroid plexus of 4th ventricle

Hypoglossal nerve (CN XII)

Lateral aperture of 4th ventricle

Medulla oblongata [Olive / Pyramid]

Anterior rootlets of C1 nerve

Cerebellum

Spinal cord

Inferior View

Olfactory bulb] **Site of termination of olfactory nerves (CN I)**

Olfactory tract

Optic nerve (CN II)

Optic tract

Oculomotor nerve (CN III)

Trochlear nerve (CN IV)

Sensory root] **Trigeminal**
Motor root] **nerve (CN V)**

Abducent nerve (CN VI)

Facial nerve (CN VII)

Intermediate nerve (CN VII)

Vestibulocochlear nerve (CN VIII)

Glossopharyngeal nerve (CN IX)

Vagus nerve (CN X)

Spinal accessory nerve (CN XI)

9.1 **Cranial Nerves in Relation to Base of Brain**

Cranial nerves are nerves that exit from the cranial cavity through openings in the cranium. There are 12 pairs of cranial nerves that are named and numbered in rostrocaudal sequence of their superficial origins from the brain, brainstem, and superior spinal cord.

The olfactory nerves (CN I, *not shown*) end in the olfactory bulb. The entire origin of the spinal accessory nerve (CN XI) from the spinal cord is not included here; it extends inferiorly as far as the C6 spinal cord segment.

ANTERIOR

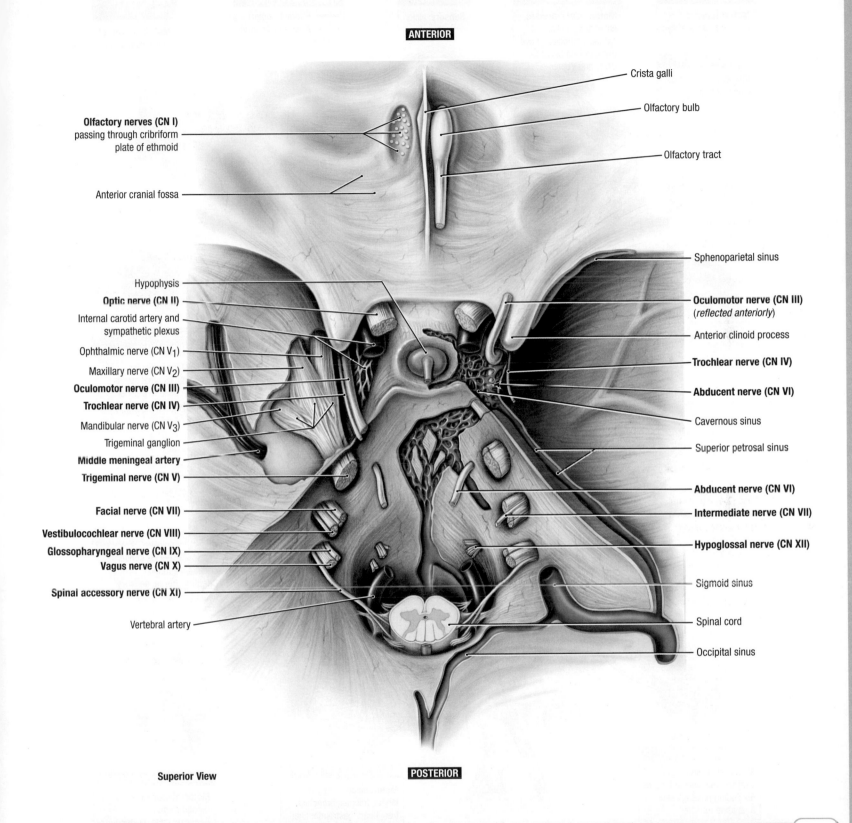

Crista galli

Olfactory bulb

Olfactory nerves (CN I)
passing through cribriform
plate of ethmoid

Olfactory tract

Anterior cranial fossa

Sphenoparietal sinus

Hypophysis

Optic nerve (CN II)

Oculomotor nerve (CN III)
(*reflected anteriorly*)

Internal carotid artery and
sympathetic plexus

Anterior clinoid process

Ophthalmic nerve (CN V$_1$)

Trochlear nerve (CN IV)

Maxillary nerve (CN V$_2$)

Oculomotor nerve (CN III)

Abducent nerve (CN VI)

Trochlear nerve (CN IV)

Cavernous sinus

Mandibular nerve (CN V$_3$)

Trigeminal ganglion

Superior petrosal sinus

Middle meningeal artery

Trigeminal nerve (CN V)

Abducent nerve (CN VI)

Facial nerve (CN VII)

Intermediate nerve (CN VII)

Vestibulocochlear nerve (CN VIII)

Glossopharyngeal nerve (CN IX)

Hypoglossal nerve (CN XII)

Vagus nerve (CN X)

Spinal accessory nerve (CN XI)

Sigmoid sinus

Vertebral artery

Spinal cord

Occipital sinus

Superior View

POSTERIOR

Cranial Nerves in Relation to Internal Aspect of Cranial Base

9.2

The venous sinuses have been opened on the right side. The ophthalmic division of the trigeminal nerve (CN V$_1$) and the trochlear (CN IV) and oculomotor (CN III) nerves have been dissected from the lateral wall of the cavernous sinus. Although there are no sympathetic fibers in cranial nerves as they leave the brain, postsynaptic sympathetic nerve fibers "hitchhike" onto branches of cranial nerves having traveled to the region via major blood vessels.

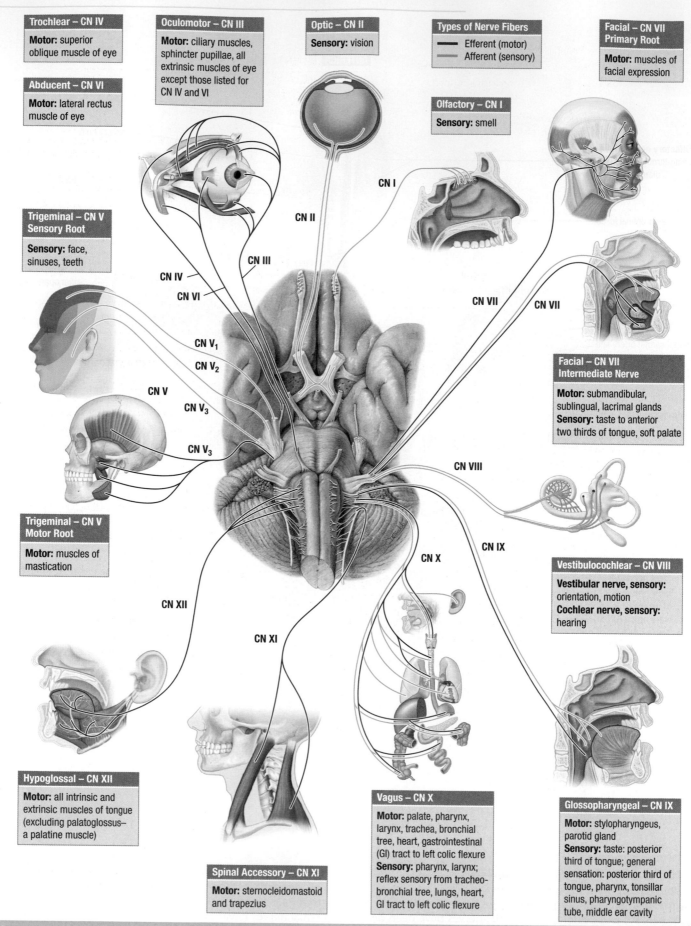

Trochlear – CN IV

Motor: superior oblique muscle of eye

Abducent – CN VI

Motor: lateral rectus muscle of eye

Oculomotor – CN III

Motor: ciliary muscles, sphincter pupillae, all extrinsic muscles of eye except those listed for CN IV and VI

Optic – CN II

Sensory: vision

Types of Nerve Fibers

— Efferent (motor)
— Afferent (sensory)

Facial – CN VII Primary Root

Motor: muscles of facial expression

Olfactory – CN I

Sensory: smell

Trigeminal – CN V Sensory Root

Sensory: face, sinuses, teeth

Facial – CN VII Intermediate Nerve

Motor: submandibular, sublingual, lacrimal glands
Sensory: taste to anterior two thirds of tongue, soft palate

Trigeminal – CN V Motor Root

Motor: muscles of mastication

Vestibulocochlear – CN VIII

Vestibular nerve, sensory: orientation, motion
Cochlear nerve, sensory: hearing

Hypoglossal – CN XII

Motor: all intrinsic and extrinsic muscles of tongue (excluding palatoglossus– a palatine muscle)

Vagus – CN X

Motor: palate, pharynx, larynx, trachea, bronchial tree, heart, gastrointestinal (GI) tract to left colic flexure
Sensory: pharynx, larynx; reflex sensory from tracheobronchial tree, lungs, heart, GI tract to left colic flexure

Spinal Accessory – CN XI

Motor: sternocleidomastoid and trapezius

Glossopharyngeal – CN IX

Motor: stylopharyngeus, parotid gland
Sensory: taste: posterior third of tongue; general sensation: posterior third of tongue, pharynx, tonsillar sinus, pharyngotympanic tube, middle ear cavity

CN I
CN II
CN III
CN IV
CN VI
CN V₁
CN V₂
CN V
CN V₃
CN V₃
CN VII
CN VII
CN VIII
CN IX
CN X
CN XI
CN XII

9.3   Summary of Cranial Nerves

TABLE 9.1 Summary of Cranial Nerves

Nerve	Components	Location of Nerve Cell Bodies	Cranial Exit	Function
Olfactory (CN I)	Special sensory	Olfactory epithelium (olfactory cells)	Foramina in cribriform plate of ethmoid bone	Smell from nasal mucosa of roof of each nasal cavity, superior sides of nasal septum and superior concha
Optic (CN II)	Special sensory	Retina (ganglion cells)	Optic canal	Vision from retina
Oculomotor (CN III)	Somatic motor	Midbrain (nucleus of CN III)	Superior orbital fissure	Motor to levator palpebrae superioris, inferior oblique, and superior, inferior and medial rectus muscles that raise upper eyelid and direct gaze superiorly, inferiorly, and medially
	Visceral motor	Presynaptic: midbrain (Edinger-Westphal nucleus) Postsynaptic: ciliary ganglion		Parasympathetic innervation to sphincter pupillae and ciliary muscles that constrict pupil and accommodate lens of eye
Trochlear (CN IV)	Somatic motor	Midbrain (nucleus of CN IV)		Motor to superior oblique that assists in directing gaze inferolaterally
Trigeminal (CN V) Ophthalmic division (CN V$_1$)	Somatic (general) sensory	Trigeminal ganglion Synapse: sensory nucleus of CN V		Sensation from: cornea, skin of forehead, scalp, eyelids and nose; mucosa of nasal cavity and paranasal sinuses; cranial dura
Maxillary division (CN V$_2$)			Foramen rotundum	Sensation from skin of face over maxilla including upper lip, maxillary teeth, mucosa of nose, maxillary sinuses, palate, and cranial dura
Mandibular division (CN V$_3$)			Foramen ovale	Sensation from: skin over mandible, including lower lip, side of head, mandibular teeth and temporomandibular joint; mucosa of mouth; anterior two thirds of tongue; cranial dura
	Somatic (branchial) motor	Pons (motor nucleus of CN V)		Motor to muscles of mastication, mylohyoid, anterior belly of digastric, tensor veli palatini, and tensor tympani
Abducent (CN VI)	Somatic motor	Pons (nucleus of CN VI)	Superior orbital fissure	Motor to lateral rectus to direct gaze laterally
Facial (CN VII)	Somatic (branchial) motor	Pons (motor nucleus of CN VII)	Internal acoustic meatus, facial canal, and stylomastoid foramen	Motor to muscles of facial expression and scalp; also supplies stapedius of middle ear, stylohyoid, and posterior belly of digastric
	Special sensory	Geniculate ganglion Synapse: nuclei of solitary tract		Taste from anterior two thirds of tongue and soft palate
	General sensory	Geniculate ganglion Synapse: sensory nucleus of CN V		Sensation from skin of external acoustic meatus
	Visceral motor	Presynaptic: pons (superior salivatory nucleus) Postsynaptic: pterygopalatine ganglion and submandibular ganglion		Parasympathetic innervation to submandibular and sublingual salivary glands, lacrimal gland, and glands of nose and palate
Vestibulocochlear (CN VIII) Vestibular cochlear	Special sensory	Vestibular ganglion Synapse: vestibular nuclei	Internal acoustic meatus	Vestibular sensation from semicircular ducts, utricle, and saccule related to position and movement of head
	Special sensory	Spiral ganglion Synapse: cochlear nuclei		Hearing from spiral organ
Glossopharyngeal (CN IX)	Somatic (br.) motor	Medulla (nucleus ambiguus)	Jugular foramen	Motor to stylopharyngeus that assists with swallowing
	Visceral motor	Presynaptic: medulla (inferior salivatory nucleus) Postsynaptic: otic ganglion		Parasympathetic innervation to parotid gland
	Visceral sensory	Inferior ganglion		Visceral sensation from carotid body and sinus
	Special sensory	Inferior ganglion Synapse: nuclei of solitary tract		Taste from posterior third of tongue and pharynx
	General sensory	Superior and inferior ganglia Synapse: sensory nucleus of CN V		Sensation from external ear, tympanic cavity membrane, mastoid air cells, pharyngotympanic tube, pharynx, posterior third of tongue
Vagus (CN X)	Somatic (branchial) motor	Medulla (nucleus ambiguus)		Motor to constrictor muscles of pharynx, intrinsic muscles of larynx, muscles of palate (except tensor veli palatini), and striated muscle in superior two thirds of esophagus
	Visceral motor	Presynaptic: medulla Postsynaptic: neurons in, on, or near viscera		Smooth muscle of trachea, bronchi, and digestive tract, and cardiac muscle
	Visceral sensory	Inferior ganglion Synapse: nuclei of solitary tract		Visceral sensation from base of tongue, pharynx, larynx, trachea, bronchi, heart, esophagus, stomach, and intestine
	Special sensory	Inferior ganglion Synapse: nuclei of solitary tract		Taste from epiglottis and palate
	Somatic (general) sensory	Superior ganglion Synapse: sensory nucleus of trigeminal nerve		Sensation from posterior auricle, tragus, external acoustic meatus, and dura mater of posterior cranial fossa
Spinal accessory nerve (CN XI)	Somatic motor	Cervical spinal cord		Motor to sternocleidomastoid and trapezius
Hypoglossal (CN XII)	Somatic motor	Medulla (nucleus of CN XII)	Hypoglossal canal	Motor to muscles of tongue (except palatoglossus)

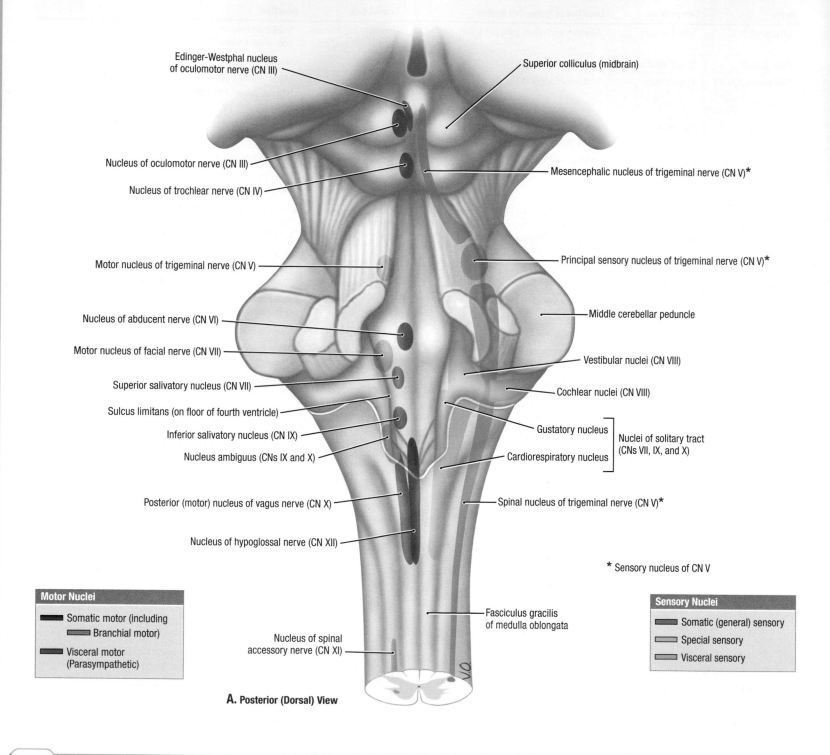

Edinger-Westphal nucleus
of oculomotor nerve (CN III)

Superior colliculus (midbrain)

Nucleus of oculomotor nerve (CN III)

Mesencephalic nucleus of trigeminal nerve (CN V)*

Nucleus of trochlear nerve (CN IV)

Motor nucleus of trigeminal nerve (CN V)

Principal sensory nucleus of trigeminal nerve (CN V)*

Nucleus of abducent nerve (CN VI)

Middle cerebellar peduncle

Motor nucleus of facial nerve (CN VII)

Vestibular nuclei (CN VIII)

Superior salivatory nucleus (CN VII)

Cochlear nuclei (CN VIII)

Sulcus limitans (on floor of fourth ventricle)

Gustatory nucleus

Inferior salivatory nucleus (CN IX)

Nuclei of solitary tract
(CNs VII, IX, and X)

Nucleus ambiguus (CNs IX and X)

Cardiorespiratory nucleus

Posterior (motor) nucleus of vagus nerve (CN X)

Spinal nucleus of trigeminal nerve (CN V)*

Nucleus of hypoglossal nerve (CN XII)

* Sensory nucleus of CN V

Motor Nuclei

■ Somatic motor (including
▬ Branchial motor)
▬ Visceral motor
(Parasympathetic)

Nucleus of spinal
accessory nerve (CN XI)

Fasciculus gracilis
of medulla oblongata

Sensory Nuclei

▬ Somatic (general) sensory
▬ Special sensory
▬ Visceral sensory

A. Posterior (Dorsal) View

| 9.4 | **Cranial Nerve Nuclei** |

The fibers of the cranial nerves are connected to nuclei (groups of nerve cell bodies in the central nervous system), in which afferent (sensory) fibers terminate and from which efferent (motor) fibers originate. Nuclei of common functional types (motor, sensory, parasympathetic, and special sensory nuclei) have a generally columnar placement within the brainstem, with the sulcus limitans demarcating motor and sensory columns.

Somatic motor: Motor fibers innervating voluntary (striated muscle). For the muscles derived from the embryonic pharyngeal arches, their somatic motor innervation can be referred to more specifically as **branchial motor**.

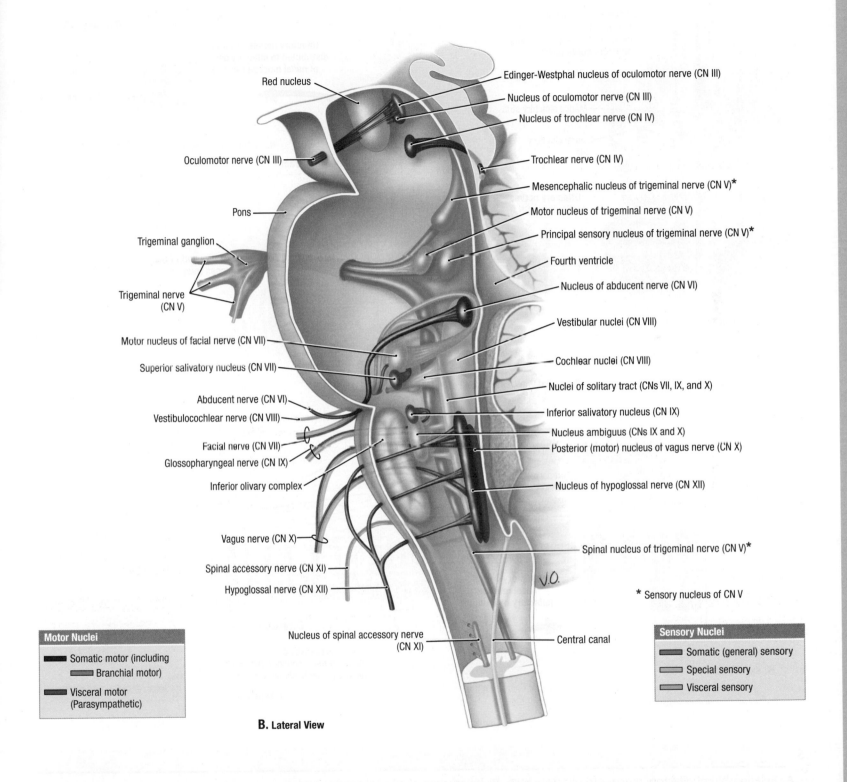

Red nucleus

Edinger-Westphal nucleus of oculomotor nerve (CN III)

Nucleus of oculomotor nerve (CN III)

Nucleus of trochlear nerve (CN IV)

Oculomotor nerve (CN III)

Trochlear nerve (CN IV)

Mesencephalic nucleus of trigeminal nerve (CN V)*

Pons

Motor nucleus of trigeminal nerve (CN V)

Principal sensory nucleus of trigeminal nerve (CN V)*

Trigeminal ganglion

Fourth ventricle

Trigeminal nerve (CN V)

Nucleus of abducent nerve (CN VI)

Vestibular nuclei (CN VIII)

Motor nucleus of facial nerve (CN VII)

Cochlear nuclei (CN VIII)

Superior salivatory nucleus (CN VII)

Nuclei of solitary tract (CNs VII, IX, and X)

Abducent nerve (CN VI)

Inferior salivatory nucleus (CN IX)

Vestibulocochlear nerve (CN VIII)

Nucleus ambiguus (CNs IX and X)

Facial nerve (CN VII)

Posterior (motor) nucleus of vagus nerve (CN X)

Glossopharyngeal nerve (CN IX)

Inferior olivary complex

Nucleus of hypoglossal nerve (CN XII)

Vagus nerve (CN X)

Spinal nucleus of trigeminal nerve (CN V)*

Spinal accessory nerve (CN XI)

V.O.

Hypoglossal nerve (CN XII)

* Sensory nucleus of CN V

Motor Nuclei

Somatic motor (including
Branchial motor)

Visceral motor
(Parasympathetic)

Nucleus of spinal accessory nerve
(CN XI)

Central canal

Sensory Nuclei

Somatic (general) sensory

Special sensory

Visceral sensory

B. Lateral View

Cranial Nerve Nuclei (continued)

9.4

Visceral motor: parasympathetic innervation to glands and involuntary (smooth) muscle.

Somatic (general) sensory: fibers transmitting general sensation from skin and membranes (e.g., touch, pressure, heat, cold).

Visceral sensory: fibers conveying sensation from viscera (organs) and mucous membranes.

Special sensory: taste, smell, vision, hearing, and balance.

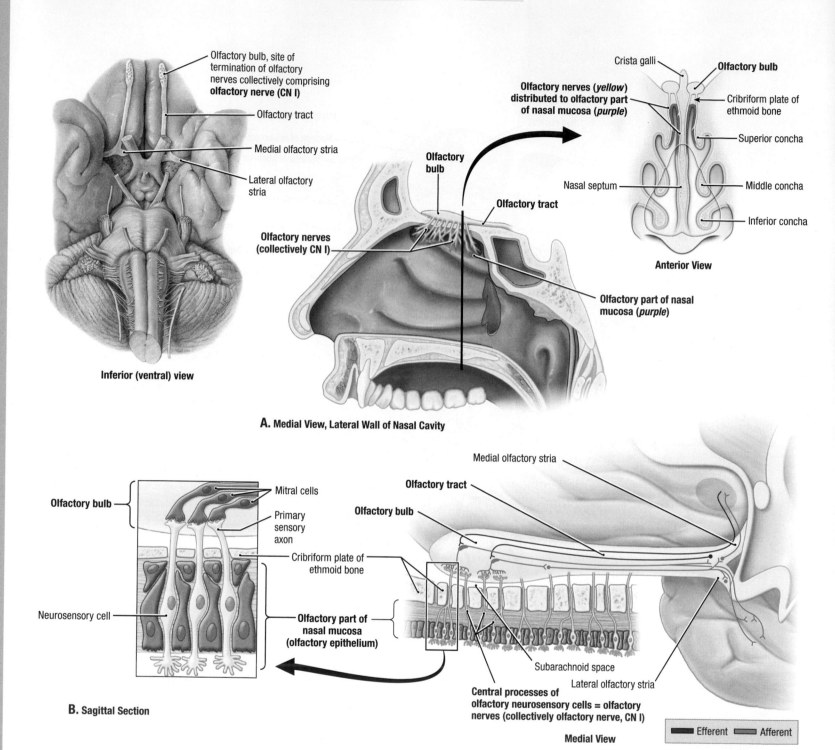

A. Medial View, Lateral Wall of Nasal Cavity

B. Sagittal Section

Medial View

Efferent Afferent

9.5 Olfactory Nerve (CN I)

A. Relationship of olfactory mucosa to olfactory bulb. **B.** Innervation of olfactory epithelium.

TABLE 9.2	Olfactory Nerve (CN I)			
Nerve	**Functional Components**	**Cells of Origin/Termination**	**Cranial Exit**	**Distribution and Functions**
Olfactory	Special sensory	Olfactory epithelium/olfactory cells/olfactory bulb	Foramina of cribriform plate of ethmoid bone	Smell from nasal mucosa of roof and superior sides of nasal septum and superior concha of each nasal cavity

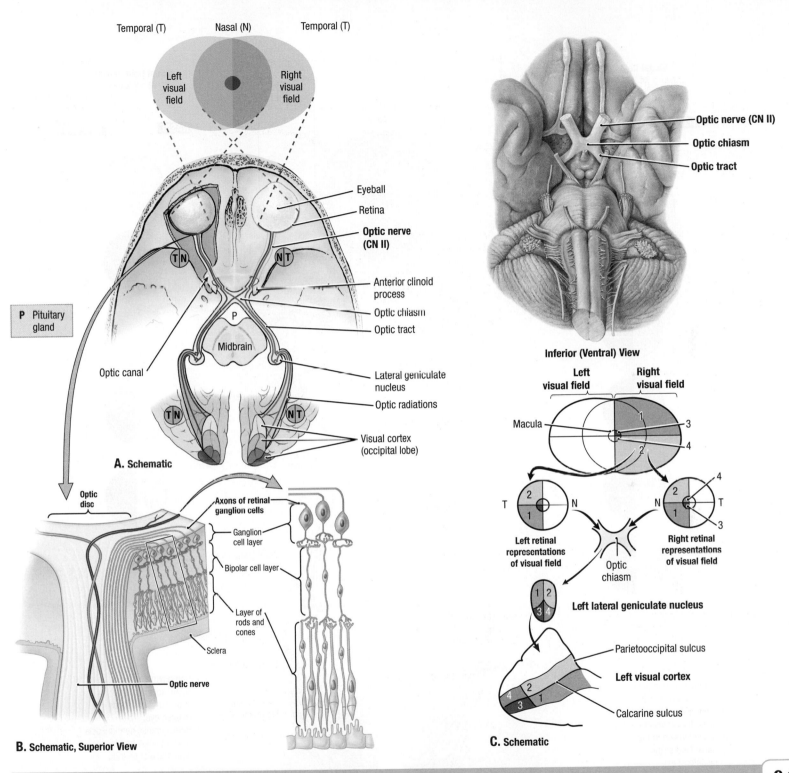

Temporal (T)   Nasal (N)   Temporal (T)

Left visual field   Right visual field

Eyeball
Retina
Optic nerve (CN II)

Anterior clinoid process
Optic chiasm
Optic tract

P   Pituitary gland

Midbrain

Optic canal

Lateral geniculate nucleus

Optic radiations

Visual cortex (occipital lobe)

A. Schematic

Optic disc

Axons of retinal ganglion cells
Ganglion cell layer
Bipolar cell layer
Layer of rods and cones
Sclera
Optic nerve

B. Schematic, Superior View

Optic nerve (CN II)
Optic chiasm
Optic tract

Inferior (Ventral) View

Left visual field   Right visual field

Macula

Left retinal representations of visual field   Optic chiasm   Right retinal representations of visual field

Left lateral geniculate nucleus

Parietooccipital sulcus
Left visual cortex
Calcarine sulcus

C. Schematic

Optic Nerve (CN II)

A. Origin and course of visual pathway. *P,* location of pituitary gland. **B.** Rods and cones in retina. **C.** Right visual field representation on retinae, left lateral geniculate nucleus, and left **visual cortex.** Areas corresponding to (*1*) upper general, (*2*) lower general, (*3*) upper macular, and (*4*) lower macular portions of right visual field. *N,* nasal; *T,* temporal (aspects of visual fields).

9.6

TABLE 9.3	Optic Nerve (CN II)			
Nerve	**Functional Components**	**Cells of Origin/Termination**	**Cranial Exit**	**Distribution and Functions**
Optic	Special sensory	Retina (ganglion cells)/lateral geniculate body (nucleus)	Optic canal	Vision from retina

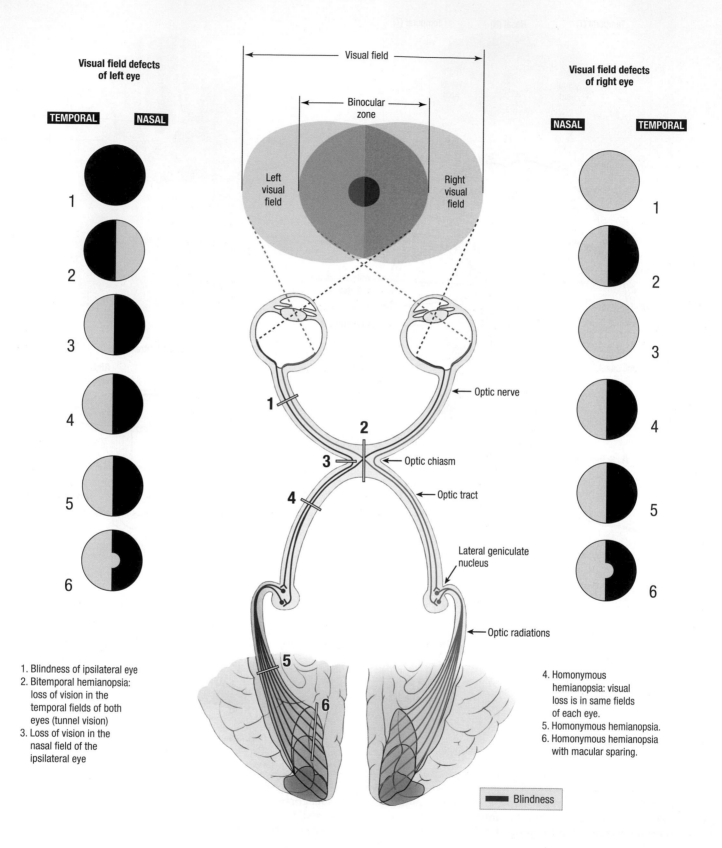

Visual field defects
of left eye

TEMPORAL   NASAL

1. Blindness of ipsilateral eye
2. Bitemporal hemianopsia:
   loss of vision in the
   temporal fields of both
   eyes (tunnel vision)
3. Loss of vision in the
   nasal field of the
   ipsilateral eye

Visual field

Binocular
zone

Left
visual
field

Right
visual
field

Optic nerve

Optic chiasm

Optic tract

Lateral geniculate
nucleus

Optic radiations

Visual field defects
of right eye

NASAL   TEMPORAL

4. Homonymous
   hemianopsia: visual
   loss is in same fields
   of each eye.
5. Homonymous hemianopsia.
6. Homonymous hemianopsia
   with macular sparing.

Blindness

9.7   Visual Field Defects (CN II)

Visual field defects may result from a large number of neurologic diseases. It is clinically important to be able to link the defects to a likely location of the lesion.

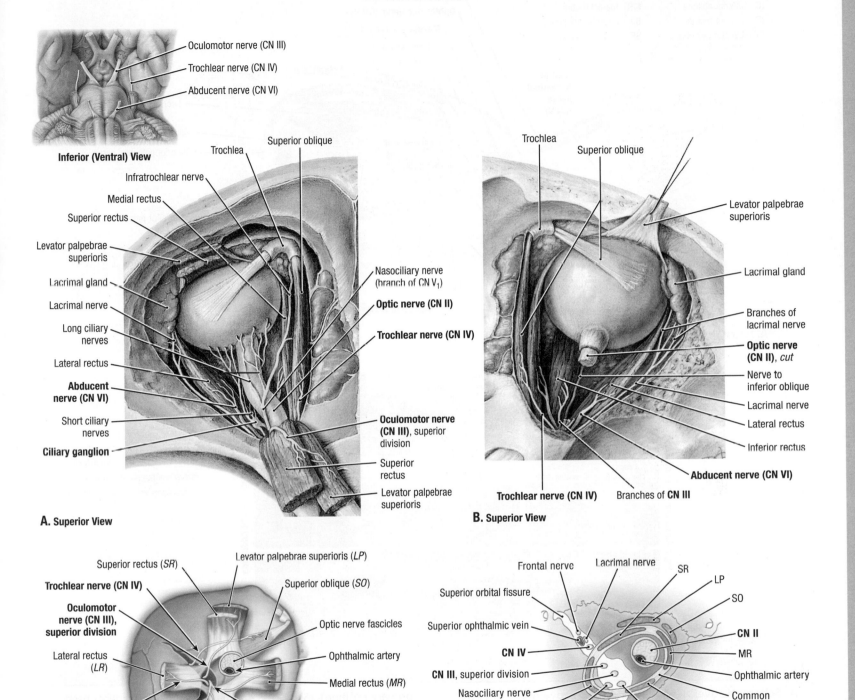

Inferior (Ventral) View

Oculomotor nerve (CN III)
Trochlear nerve (CN IV)
Abducent nerve (CN VI)

A. Superior View

Trochlea
Superior oblique
Infratrochlear nerve
Medial rectus
Superior rectus
Levator palpebrae superioris
Lacrimal gland
Lacrimal nerve
Long ciliary nerves
Lateral rectus
Abducent nerve (CN VI)
Short ciliary nerves
Ciliary ganglion

Nasociliary nerve (branch of CN V₁)
Optic nerve (CN II)
Trochlear nerve (CN IV)
Oculomotor nerve (CN III), superior division
Superior rectus
Levator palpebrae superioris

B. Superior View

Trochlea
Superior oblique
Levator palpebrae superioris
Lacrimal gland
Branches of lacrimal nerve
Optic nerve (CN II), cut
Nerve to inferior oblique
Lacrimal nerve
Lateral rectus
Inferior rectus
Abducent nerve (CN VI)
Trochlear nerve (CN IV) Branches of **CN III**

C. Anterior View

Superior rectus (*SR*)
Levator palpebrae superioris (*LP*)
Superior oblique (*SO*)
Trochlear nerve (CN IV)
Oculomotor nerve (CN III), superior division
Optic nerve fascicles
Lateral rectus (*LR*)
Ophthalmic artery
Medial rectus (*MR*)
Abducent nerve (CN VI)
Oculomotor nerve (CN III), inferior division
Ciliary ganglion
Inferior rectus (*IR*)
Inferior oblique

D. Anterior View

Frontal nerve
Lacrimal nerve
SR
LP
SO
Superior orbital fissure
Superior ophthalmic vein
CN II
CN IV
MR
CN III, superior division
Ophthalmic artery
Nasociliary nerve
Common tendinous ring
LR
IR
CN VI
CN III, inferior division
Inferior ophthalmic vein

Overview of Muscles and Nerves of Orbit

9.8

A. and **B.** Orbital cavities, dissected from a superior approach. **C.** and **D.** Relationship of muscle attachments and nerves at

apex of orbit. The optic nerve is intact (*Part A*) and cut away (*Part B, Part C,* and *Part D*).

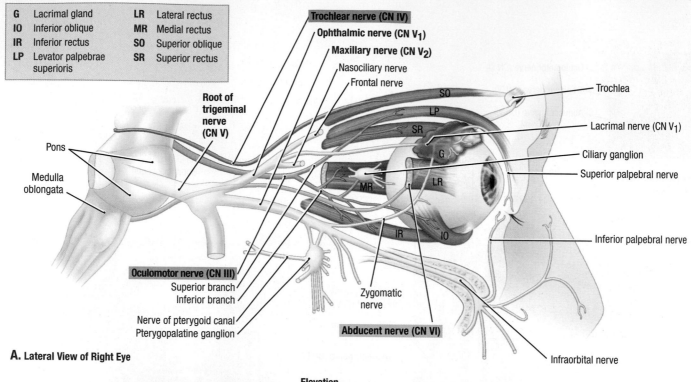

G	Lacrimal gland	LR	Lateral rectus
IO	Inferior oblique	MR	Medial rectus
IR	Inferior rectus	SO	Superior oblique
LP	Levator palpebrae superioris	SR	Superior rectus

A. Lateral View of Right Eye

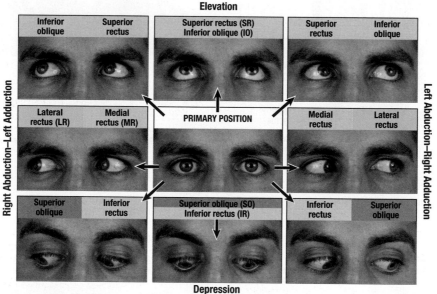

B. Anterior Views

9.9   Oculomotor (CN III), Trochlear (CN IV), and Abducent (CN VI) Nerves

A. Schematic overview. B. Anatomical movements of extra-ocular muscles. Single movements start from the center (rest of primary position). (See Fig. 8.43E for sequential movements used for clinical testing of extraocular muscles and cranial nerves.)

TABLE 9.4   Oculomotor (CN III), Trochlear (CN IV), and Abducent (CN VI) Nerves

Nerve	Functional Components	Cells of Origin	Cranial Exit	Distribution and Functions
Oculomotor	Somatic motor	Nucleus of CN III	Superior orbital fissure	Motor to superior, inferior, and medial recti, inferior oblique, and levator palpebrae superioris muscles; raises upper eyelid, directing gaze superiorly, inferiorly, and medially
	Visceral motor (parasympathetic)	Presynaptic: midbrain (Edinger-Westphal nucleus) Postsynaptic: ciliary ganglion		Motor to sphincter pupillae and ciliary muscle that constrict pupil and accommodate lens of eyeball
Trochlear	Somatic motor	Nucleus of CN IV		Motor to superior oblique that assists in directing gaze inferolaterally
Abducent	Somatic motor	Nucleus of CN VI		Motor to lateral rectus that directs gaze laterally

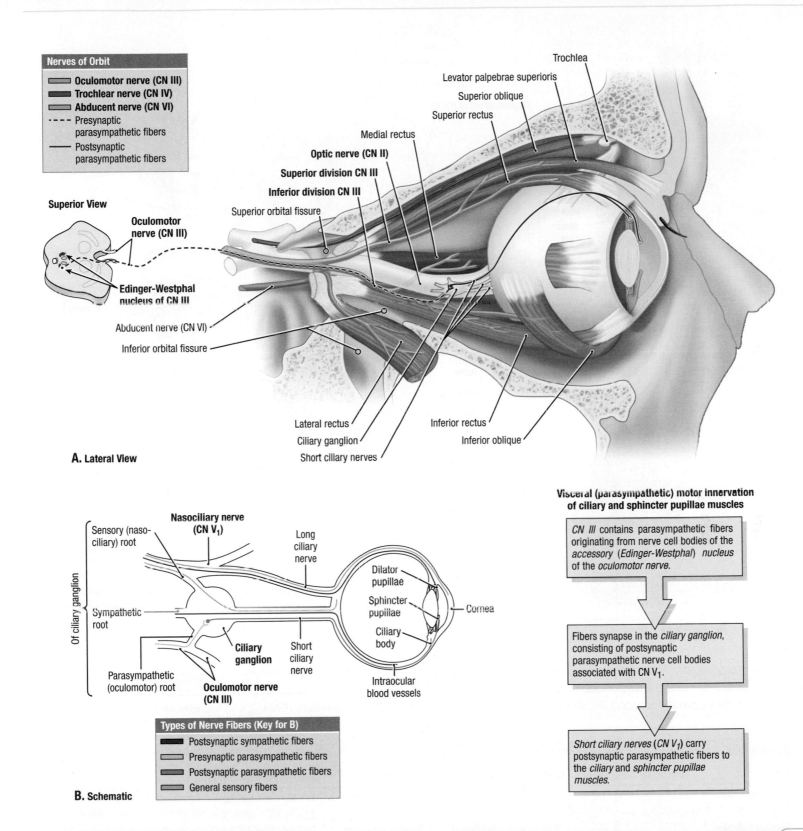

Nerves of Orbit

- Oculomotor nerve (CN III)
- Trochlear nerve (CN IV)
- Abducent nerve (CN VI)
- - - Presynaptic parasympathetic fibers
- —— Postsynaptic parasympathetic fibers

Superior View

Oculomotor nerve (CN III)

Edinger-Westphal nucleus of CN III

Abducent nerve (CN VI)

Inferior orbital fissure

Trochlea

Levator palpebrae superioris

Superior oblique

Superior rectus

Medial rectus

Optic nerve (CN II)

Superior division CN III

Inferior division CN III

Superior orbital fissure

Lateral rectus

Ciliary ganglion

Short ciliary nerves

Inferior rectus

Inferior oblique

A. Lateral View

Nasociliary nerve (CN V₁)

Sensory (naso-ciliary) root

Sympathetic root

Parasympathetic (oculomotor) root

Oculomotor nerve (CN III)

Of ciliary ganglion

Ciliary ganglion

Long ciliary nerve

Short ciliary nerve

Dilator pupillae

Sphincter pupillae

Ciliary body

Cornea

Intraocular blood vessels

Types of Nerve Fibers (Key for B)

- Postsynaptic sympathetic fibers
- Presynaptic parasympathetic fibers
- Postsynaptic parasympathetic fibers
- General sensory fibers

B. Schematic

Visceral (parasympathetic) motor innervation of ciliary and sphincter pupillae muscles

CN III contains parasympathetic fibers originating from nerve cell bodies of the *accessory (Edinger-Westphal) nucleus* of the *oculomotor nerve.*

Fibers synapse in the *ciliary ganglion*, consisting of postsynaptic parasympathetic nerve cell bodies associated with CN V₁.

Short ciliary nerves (*CN V₁*) carry postsynaptic parasympathetic fibers to the *ciliary* and *sphincter pupillae muscles.*

Innervation of Eyeball

9.10

A. Nerves of orbit. **B.** Somatic and autonomic innervation of eyeball.

Orbital tumors. Because of the closeness of the optic nerve to the sphenoidal and posterior ethmoidal sinuses, a malignant tumor in these sinuses may erode the thin bony walls of the orbit and compress the optic nerve and orbital contents. Tumors in the orbit produce exophthalmos (protrusion of eyeball). Tumors in the middle cranial fossa enter the orbital cavity through the superior orbital fissure. Tumors in the temporal or infratemporal fossae enter the orbit through the inferior orbital fissure.

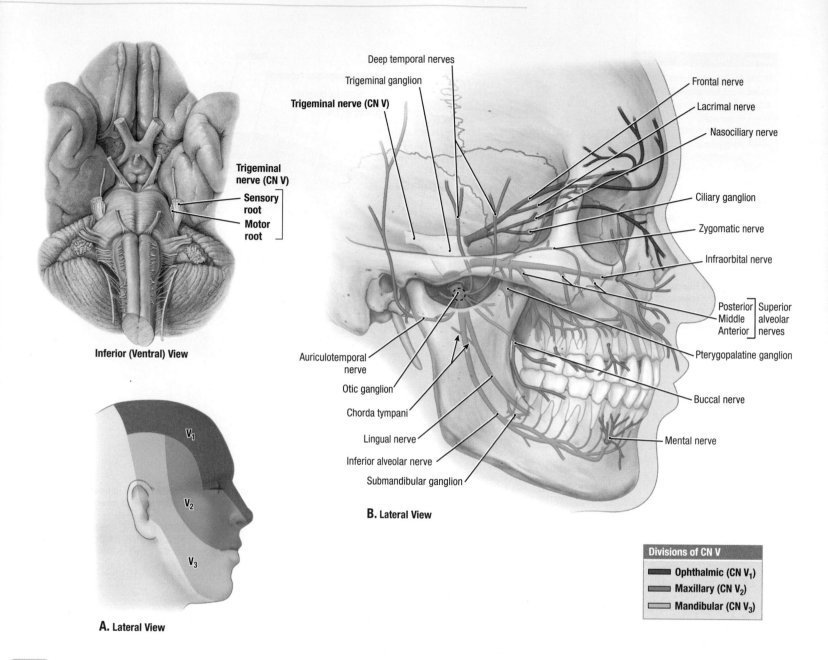

Inferior (Ventral) View

A. Lateral View

B. Lateral View

Deep temporal nerves
Trigeminal ganglion
Trigeminal nerve (CN V)
Frontal nerve
Lacrimal nerve
Nasociliary nerve
Ciliary ganglion
Zygomatic nerve
Infraorbital nerve
Posterior / Middle / Anterior — Superior alveolar nerves
Pterygopalatine ganglion
Buccal nerve
Mental nerve
Submandibular ganglion
Inferior alveolar nerve
Lingual nerve
Chorda tympani
Otic ganglion
Auriculotemporal nerve
Trigeminal nerve (CN V) — Sensory root / Motor root

Divisions of CN V
- Ophthalmic (CN V₁)
- Maxillary (CN V₂)
- Mandibular (CN V₃)

9.11   Trigeminal Nerve (CN V)

A. Cutaneous (somatic sensory) distribution. **B.** Branches of ophthalmic (CN V₁), maxillary (CN V₂), and mandibular (CN V₃) divisions.

TABLE 9.5   Trigeminal Nerve (CN V)

Nerve	Functional Components	Cells of Origin/Termination	Cranial Exit	Distribution and Functions[a]
Ophthalmic division (CN V₁)	Somatic (general sensory)	Trigeminal ganglion/spinal, principal and mesencephalic nucleus of CN V	Superior orbital fissure	Sensation from cornea, skin of forehead, scalp, upper eyelid, nose, and mucosa of nasal cavity and paranasal sinuses; supratentorial dura
Maxillary division (CN V₂)			Foramen rotundum	Sensation from skin of face over maxilla including upper lip, maxillary teeth, mucosa of nose, maxillary sinuses, and palate
Mandibular division (CN V₃)			Foramen ovale	Sensation from the skin over mandible, including lower lip and side of head, mandibular teeth, temporomandibular joint, and mucosa of mouth and anterior two thirds of tongue
	Somatic (branchial) motor	Motor nucleus of CN V		Motor to muscles of mastication, mylohyoid, anterior belly of digastric, tensor veli palatini, and tensor tympani

[a]See following pages for greater detail.

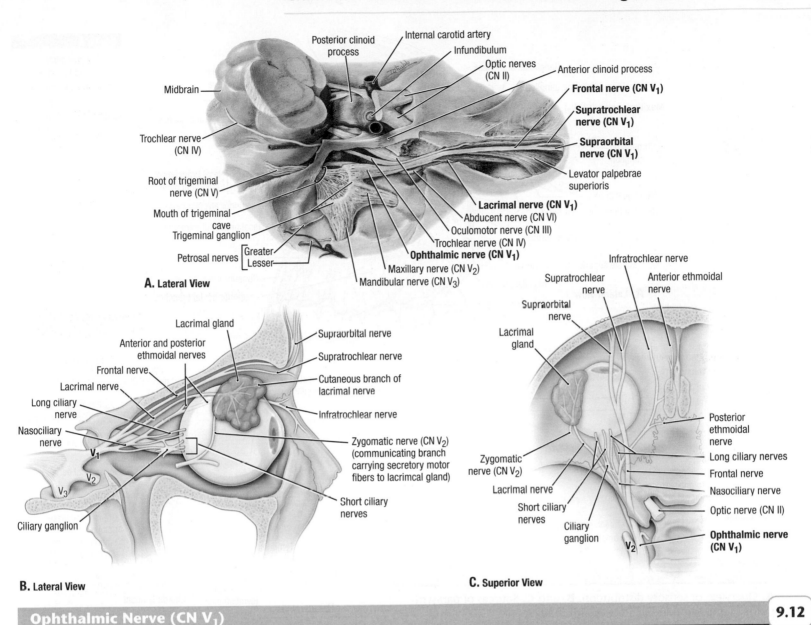

A. Lateral View

B. Lateral View

C. Superior View

Ophthalmic Nerve (CN V₁)

9.12

A. Course through cavernous sinus. **B.** and **C.** Overview.

TABLE 9.6	Branches of Ophthalmic Nerve (CN V₁)	
Function		**Branches**
Ophthalmic nerve (CN V₁)	Somatic sensory CN V₁	*Somatic sensory branches:*
Somatic sensory only at origin from trigeminal ganglion		Tentorial nerve (an intracranial meningeal branch)
Visceral motor: extracranially, conveys (1) postsynaptic parasympathetic fibers from ciliary ganglion to ciliary body and sphincter of pupillae; (2) postsynaptic parasympathetic fibers from communicating branch of zygomatic nerve (CN V₂) to lacrimal gland; and (3) postsynaptic sympathetic fibers from internal carotid plexus to dilator pupillae and intraocular blood vessels		Lacrimal nerve (terminal portion also receives postsynaptic parasympathetic fibers from zygomatic nerve [CN V₂] and conveys them to lacrimal gland)
		Frontal nerve
		Supraorbital nerve
		Supratrochlear nerve
		Nasociliary nerve
		Sensory root of ciliary ganglion
Passes through superior orbital fissure to enter orbit		Long and short ciliary nerves (also convey postsynaptic sympathetic fibers from internal carotid plexus to eyeball additionally, short ciliary nerves convey postsynaptic parasympathetic fibers from ciliary ganglion to eyeball)
Supplies general sensory innervation to cornea; superior bulbar and palpebral conjunctiva; mucosa of anterosuperior nasal cavity; frontal, ethmoidal, and sphenoidal sinuses; anterior and supratentorial dura mater; skin of dorsum of external nose; superior eyelid; forehead; and anterior scalp		Anterior and posterior ethmoidal nerves
		Anterior meningeal nerves
		Internal and external nasal branches
		Infratrochlear nerve

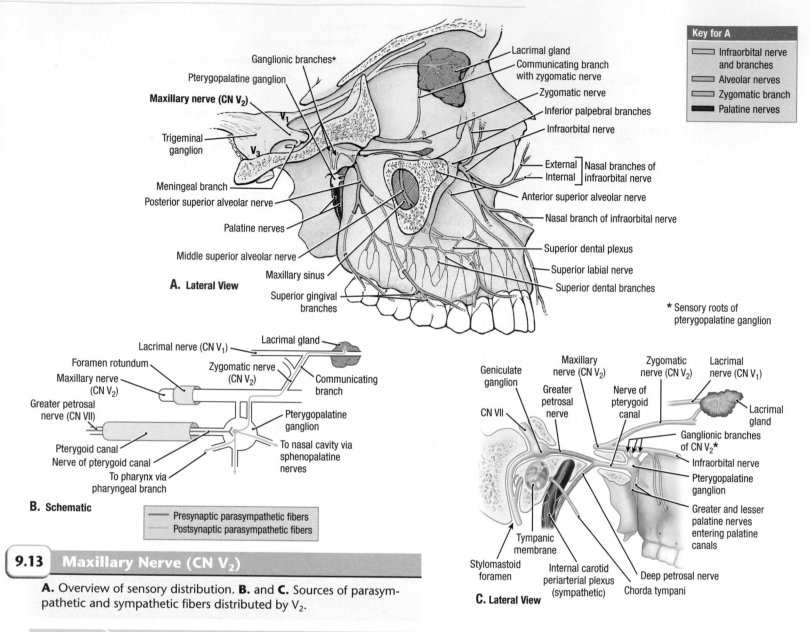

A. Lateral View

Ganglionic branches*
Pterygopalatine ganglion
Maxillary nerve (CN V₂)
V₁
Trigeminal ganglion
V₃
Meningeal branch
Posterior superior alveolar nerve
Palatine nerves
Middle superior alveolar nerve
Maxillary sinus
Superior gingival branches

Lacrimal gland
Communicating branch with zygomatic nerve
Zygomatic nerve
Inferior palpebral branches
Infraorbital nerve
External ⎱ Nasal branches of
Internal ⎰ infraorbital nerve
Anterior superior alveolar nerve
Nasal branch of infraorbital nerve
Superior dental plexus
Superior labial nerve
Superior dental branches

Key for A
- Infraorbital nerve and branches
- Alveolar nerves
- Zygomatic branch
- Palatine nerves

* Sensory roots of pterygopalatine ganglion

B. Schematic

Lacrimal nerve (CN V₁)
Foramen rotundum
Maxillary nerve (CN V₂)
Zygomatic nerve (CN V₂)
Lacrimal gland
Communicating branch
Greater petrosal nerve (CN VII)
Pterygoid canal
Nerve of pterygoid canal
To pharynx via pharyngeal branch
Pterygopalatine ganglion
To nasal cavity via sphenopalatine nerves

Presynaptic parasympathetic fibers
Postsynaptic parasympathetic fibers

C. Lateral View

Geniculate ganglion
CN VII
Greater petrosal nerve
Maxillary nerve (CN V₂)
Nerve of pterygoid canal
Zygomatic nerve (CN V₂)
Lacrimal nerve (CN V₁)
Lacrimal gland
Ganglionic branches of CN V₂*
Infraorbital nerve
Pterygopalatine ganglion
Greater and lesser palatine nerves entering palatine canals
Tympanic membrane
Stylomastoid foramen
Internal carotid periarterial plexus (sympathetic)
Deep petrosal nerve
Chorda tympani

9.13   Maxillary Nerve (CN V₂)

A. Overview of sensory distribution. **B.** and **C.** Sources of parasympathetic and sympathetic fibers distributed by V₂.

TABLE 9.7   Branches of Maxillary Nerve (CN V₂)

Function		Branches

Maxillary nerve (CN V₂)
Somatic sensory only (proximally, at origin from trigeminal ganglion)
Visceral motor: distally, conveys (1) postsynaptic parasympathetic fibers from pterygopalatine ganglion (presynaptic fibers are from CN VII via greater petrosal nerve and nerve of pterygoid canal); and (2) postsynaptic sympathetic fibers from superior cervical ganglion via internal carotid plexus (presynaptic fibers are from intermediolateral column of gray matter, spinal cord segments T1–T3)
Passes through foramen rotundum to enter pterygopalatine fossa
Supplies dura mater of anterior aspect of lateral part of middle cranial fossa; conjunctiva of inferior eyelid; mucosa of posteroinferior nasal cavity, maxillary sinus, palate, and anterior part of superior oral vestibule; maxillary teeth; and skin of lateral external nose, inferior eyelid, anterior cheek, and upper lip
	Somatic sensory CN V₂
	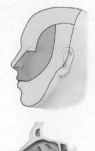
	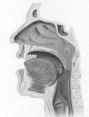
		Meningeal branch
		Zygomatic branch
		  Zygomaticofacial branch
		  Zygomaticotemporal branch
		  Communicating branch to lacrimal nerve
		Ganglionic branches to (sensory root of) pterygopalatine ganglion
		Infraorbital nerve
		  Posterior, middle, and anterior superior alveolar branches
		    Superior dental plexus and branches
		    Superior gingival branches
		  Inferior palpebral branches
		  External and internal nasal branches
		  Superior labial branches
		Greater palatine nerve
		  Posterior inferior lateral nasal nerves
		Lesser palatine nerves
		Posterior superior lateral and medial nasal branches
		Nasopalatine nerve
		Pharyngeal nerve

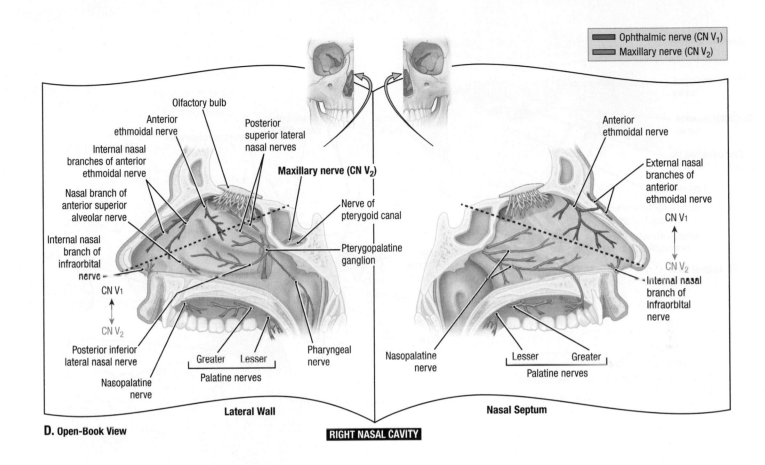

Ophthalmic nerve (CN V₁)
Maxillary nerve (CN V₂)

Olfactory bulb

Anterior ethmoidal nerve

Posterior superior lateral nasal nerves

Internal nasal branches of anterior ethmoidal nerve

Maxillary nerve (CN V₂)

Nasal branch of anterior superior alveolar nerve

Nerve of pterygoid canal

Internal nasal branch of infraorbital nerve

CN V₁

CN V₂

Pterygopalatine ganglion

Posterior inferior lateral nasal nerve

Nasopalatine nerve

Greater   Lesser

Palatine nerves

Pharyngeal nerve

Lateral Wall

Anterior ethmoidal nerve

External nasal branches of anterior ethmoidal nerve

CN V₁

CN V₂

Internal nasal branch of infraorbital nerve

Nasopalatine nerve

Lesser   Greater

Palatine nerves

Nasal Septum

D. Open-Book View

RIGHT NASAL CAVITY

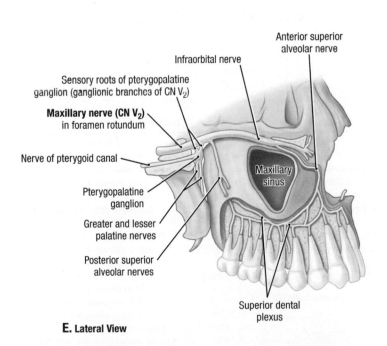

Infraorbital nerve

Anterior superior alveolar nerve

Sensory roots of pterygopalatine ganglion (ganglionic branches of CN V₂)

Maxillary nerve (CN V₂) in foramen rotundum

Nerve of pterygoid canal

Pterygopalatine ganglion

Maxillary sinus

Greater and lesser palatine nerves

Posterior superior alveolar nerves

Superior dental plexus

E. Lateral View

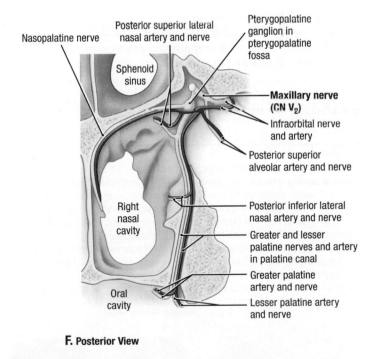

Nasopalatine nerve

Posterior superior lateral nasal artery and nerve

Pterygopalatine ganglion in pterygopalatine fossa

Sphenoid sinus

Maxillary nerve (CN V₂)

Infraorbital nerve and artery

Posterior superior alveolar artery and nerve

Right nasal cavity

Posterior inferior lateral nasal artery and nerve

Greater and lesser palatine nerves and artery in palatine canal

Greater palatine artery and nerve

Oral cavity

Lesser palatine artery and nerve

F. Posterior View

Maxillary Nerve (CN V₂) *(continued)*

9.13

D. Innervation of lateral wall and septum of right side of nasal cavity and palate. **E.** Relationship of nerves to maxillary sinus.

F. Coronal section showing course of nasopalatine and greater and lesser palatine nerves.

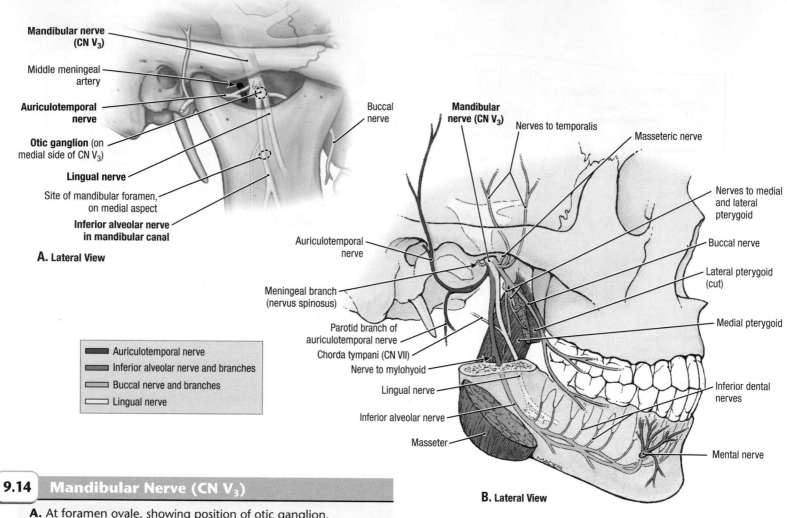

A. Lateral View

Mandibular nerve (CN V₃)
Middle meningeal artery
Auriculotemporal nerve
Otic ganglion (on medial side of CN V₃)
Lingual nerve
Site of mandibular foramen, on medial aspect
Inferior alveolar nerve in mandibular canal

Buccal nerve
Mandibular nerve (CN V₃)
Nerves to temporalis
Masseteric nerve
Nerves to medial and lateral pterygoid
Buccal nerve
Lateral pterygoid (cut)
Medial pterygoid
Auriculotemporal nerve
Meningeal branch (nervus spinosus)
Parotid branch of auriculotemporal nerve
Chorda tympani (CN VII)
Nerve to mylohyoid
Lingual nerve
Inferior alveolar nerve
Masseter
Inferior dental nerves
Mental nerve

B. Lateral View

- Auriculotemporal nerve
- Inferior alveolar nerve and branches
- Buccal nerve and branches
- Lingual nerve

9.14   Mandibular Nerve (CN V₃)

A. At foramen ovale, showing position of otic ganglion.
B. Overview of distribution of CN V₃.

TABLE 9.8	Branches of Mandibular Nerve (CN V₃)
Function	**Branches**

Mandibular nerve (CN V₃)
Somatic sensory and somatic (branchial) motor
Special sensory: extracranially, conveys taste fibers (from CN VII via chorda tympani nerve) to anterior two thirds of tongue
Visceral motor: extracranially, conveys (1) presynaptic parasympathetic fibers to submandibular ganglion (presynaptic fibers are from CN VII via chorda tympani nerve), (2) postsynaptic parasympathetic fibers from submandibular ganglion to submandibular and sublingual glands, and (3) postsynaptic parasympathetic fibers from otic ganglion to parotid gland
Passes through foramen ovale to enter infratemporal fossa
Supplies general sensory innervation to mucosa of anterior two thirds of tongue, floor of mouth, and posterior and anterior inferior oral vestibule; mandibular teeth; and skin of lower lip, buccal and temporal regions of face, and external ear (anterior superior auricle, upper external auditory meatus, and tympanic membrane)
Supplies motor innervation to all four muscles of mastication, mylohyoid, anterior belly of digastric, tensor tympani and tensor veli palatini
	Somatic sensory branches:
	Meningeal branch (nervus spinosum)
	Buccal nerve
	Auriculotemporal nerve (also conveys *visceral motor fibers*)
	   Superficial temporal branches
	   Parotid branches
	Lingual nerve (also conveys *visceral motor* and *special sensory fibers*)
	Inferior alveolar nerve
	   Nerve to mylohyoid
	   Inferior dental plexus
	      Inferior dental branches
	      Inferior gingival branches
	   Mental nerve
	Somatic (branchial) motor branches:
	Masseteric nerve
	Medial and lateral pterygoid branches
	Deep temporal nerves
	Nerve to mylohyoid
	Nerve to tensor tympani
	Nerve to tensor veli palatini

Somatic sensory CN V₃

Somatic motor CN V₃

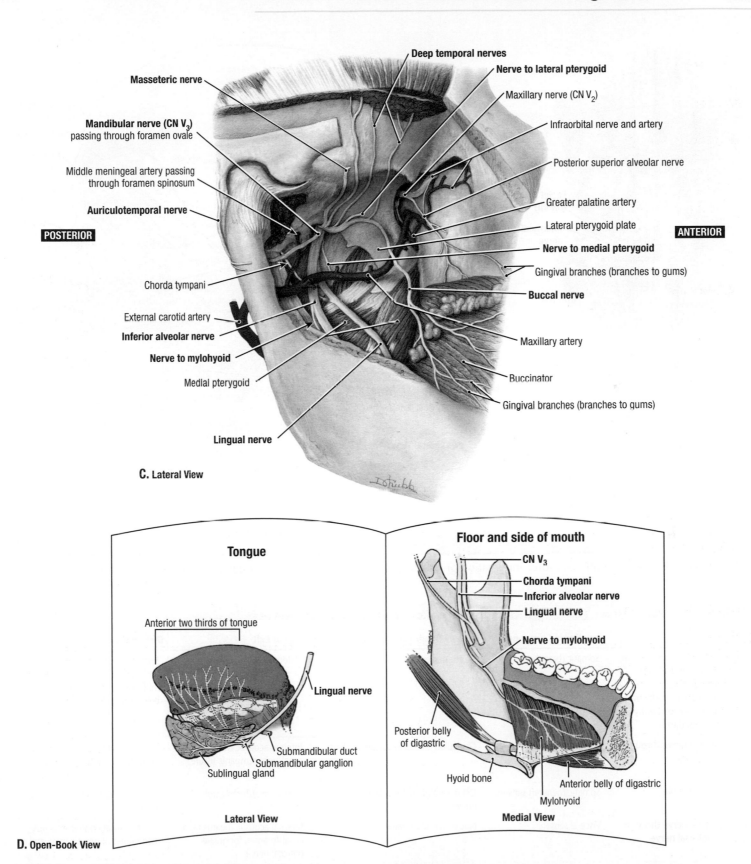

C. Lateral View

Deep temporal nerves

Nerve to lateral pterygoid

Masseteric nerve

Maxillary nerve (CN V₂)

Mandibular nerve (CN V₃) passing through foramen ovale

Infraorbital nerve and artery

Posterior superior alveolar nerve

Middle meningeal artery passing through foramen spinosum

Greater palatine artery

Auriculotemporal nerve

Lateral pterygoid plate

POSTERIOR

ANTERIOR

Nerve to medial pterygoid

Gingival branches (branches to gums)

Chorda tympani

Buccal nerve

External carotid artery

Inferior alveolar nerve

Maxillary artery

Nerve to mylohyoid

Buccinator

Medial pterygoid

Gingival branches (branches to gums)

Lingual nerve

Tongue

Anterior two thirds of tongue

Lingual nerve

Submandibular duct
Submandibular ganglion
Sublingual gland

Lateral View

Floor and side of mouth

CN V₃

Chorda tympani
Inferior alveolar nerve
Lingual nerve

Nerve to mylohyoid

Posterior belly of digastric

Hyoid bone

Anterior belly of digastric

Mylohyoid

Medial View

D. Open-Book View

Mandibular Nerve (CN V₃) *(continued)*

9.14

C. Deep dissection of CN V₃ and branches at foramen ovale.
D. Lateral aspect of tongue and medial aspect of mandible

displayed as pages in an open book; that is, the tongue has been reflected from the mandible.

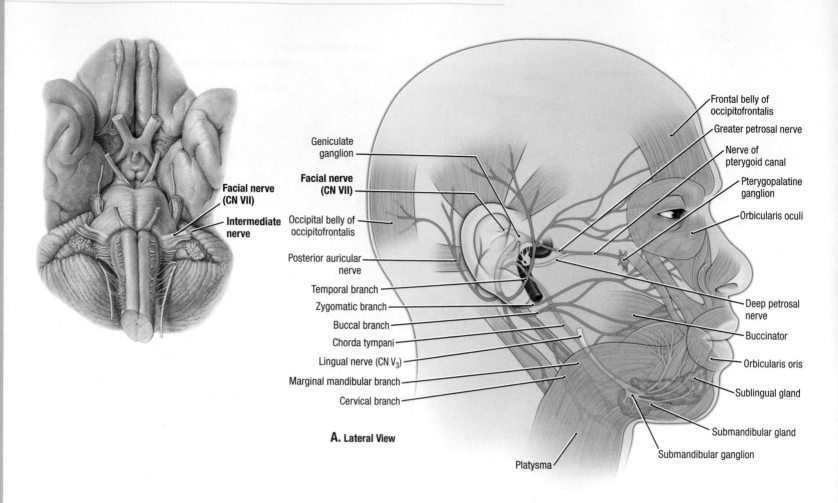

Geniculate ganglion

Facial nerve (CN VII)

Occipital belly of occipitofrontalis

Posterior auricular nerve

Temporal branch

Zygomatic branch

Buccal branch

Chorda tympani

Lingual nerve (CN V₃)

Marginal mandibular branch

Cervical branch

Facial nerve (CN VII)

Intermediate nerve

Frontal belly of occipitofrontalis

Greater petrosal nerve

Nerve of pterygoid canal

Pterygopalatine ganglion

Orbicularis oculi

Deep petrosal nerve

Buccinator

Orbicularis oris

Sublingual gland

Submandibular gland

Submandibular ganglion

Platysma

A. Lateral View

9.15 Facial Nerve (CN VII)

A. Overview. **B.** Parasympathetic motor innervation of lacrimal, submandibular, and sublingual glands. **C.** Nerve of pterygoid canal.

TABLE 9.9 Facial Nerve (CN VII), Including Motor Root and Intermediate Nerve[a]

Nerve(s)	Functional Components	Cells of Origin/Termination	Cranial Exit	Distribution and Functions
Temporal, zygomatic, buccal, mandibular, cervical, and posterior auricular nerves, nerve to posterior belly of digastric, nerve to stylohyoid, nerve to stapedius	Somatic (branchial) motor	Motor nucleus of CN VII	Stylomastoid foramen	Motor to muscles of facial expression and scalp, also supplies stapedius of middle ear, stylohyoid, and posterior belly of digastric
Intermediate nerve through chorda tympani	Special sensory	Geniculate ganglion/solitary nucleus	Internal acoustic meatus/facial canal/petrotympanic fissure	Taste from anterior two thirds of tongue, through chorda tympani floor of mouth, and palate
Intermediate nerve	Somatic (general) sensory	Geniculate ganglion/spinal trigeminal nucleus	Internal acoustic meatus	Sensation from skin of external acoustic meatus
Intermediate nerve through greater petrosal nerve	Visceral sensory	Nuclei of solitary tract	Internal acoustic meatus/facial canal/foramen for greater petrosal nerve	Visceral sensation from mucous membranes of nasopharynx and palate
Greater petrosal nerve Chorda tympani	Visceral motor	Presynaptic: superior salivatory nucleus Postsynaptic: pterygopalatine ganglion (greater petrosal nerve) and submandibular ganglion (chorda tympani)	Internal acoustic meatus/facial canal/foramen for greater petrosal nerve (greater petrosal nerve) petrotympanic fissure (chorda tympani)	Parasympathetic innervation to lacrimal gland and glands of the nose and palate (greater petrosal nerve); submandibular and sublingual salivary glands (chorda tympani)

[a]See Table 9.15.

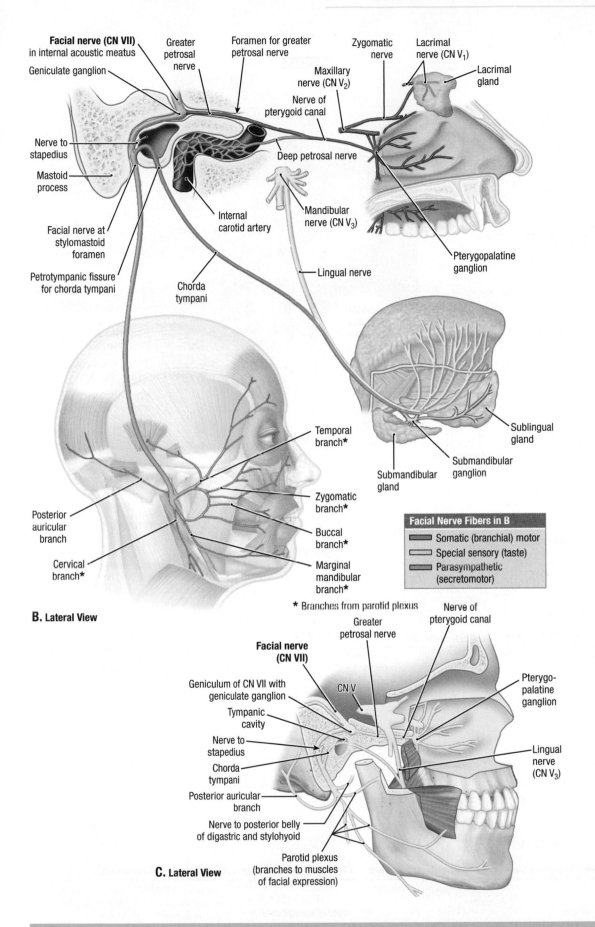

Facial nerve (CN VII) in internal acoustic meatus

Geniculate ganglion

Greater petrosal nerve

Foramen for greater petrosal nerve

Zygomatic nerve

Lacrimal nerve (CN V₁)

Lacrimal gland

Maxillary nerve (CN V₂)

Nerve of pterygoid canal

Nerve to stapedius

Mastoid process

Deep petrosal nerve

Internal carotid artery

Mandibular nerve (CN V₃)

Facial nerve at stylomastoid foramen

Petrotympanic fissure for chorda tympani

Chorda tympani

Lingual nerve

Pterygopalatine ganglion

Temporal branch*

Sublingual gland

Zygomatic branch*

Submandibular ganglion

Submandibular gland

Posterior auricular branch

Buccal branch*

Cervical branch*

Marginal mandibular branch*

B. Lateral View

* Branches from parotid plexus

Facial Nerve Fibers in B
- Somatic (branchial) motor
- Special sensory (taste)
- Parasympathetic (secretomotor)

Facial nerve (CN VII)

Geniculum of CN VII with geniculate ganglion

Tympanic cavity

Nerve to stapedius

Chorda tympani

Posterior auricular branch

Nerve to posterior belly of digastric and stylohyoid

Parotid plexus (branches to muscles of facial expression)

Greater petrosal nerve

Nerve of pterygoid canal

CN V

Pterygo-palatine ganglion

Lingual nerve (CN V₃)

C. Lateral View

Visceral motor (parasympathetic) to lacrimal gland

Greater petrosal nerve arises from CN VII at the geniculate ganglion and emerges from the superior surface of the petrous part of the temporal bone to enter the middle cranial fossa.

Greater petrosal nerve joins the *deep petrosal nerve* (sympathetic) at the foramen lacerum to form the nerve of the pterygoid canal.

Nerve of the pterygoid canal travels through the pterygoid canal and enters the pterygopalatine fossa.

Parasympathetic fibers from the nerve of pterygoid canal in pterygopalatine fossa synapse in the *pterygopalatine ganglion*.

Postsynaptic parasympathetic fibers from this ganglion innervate the *lacrimal gland* via the zygomatic branch of CN V₂ and the lacrimal nerve CN V₁.

Visceral motor (parasympathetic) to submandibular and sublingual glands

The *chorda tympani* branch arises from CN VII superior to stylomastoid foramen.

The chorda tympani crosses tympanic cavity medial to handle of malleus.

The chorda tympani passes through the petrotympanic fissure between the tympanic and petrous parts of the temporal bone to join the lingual nerve (CN V₃) in infratemporal fossa; parasympathetic fibers of the chorda tympani synapse in the *submandibular ganglion*; postsynaptic fibers follow arteries to glands.

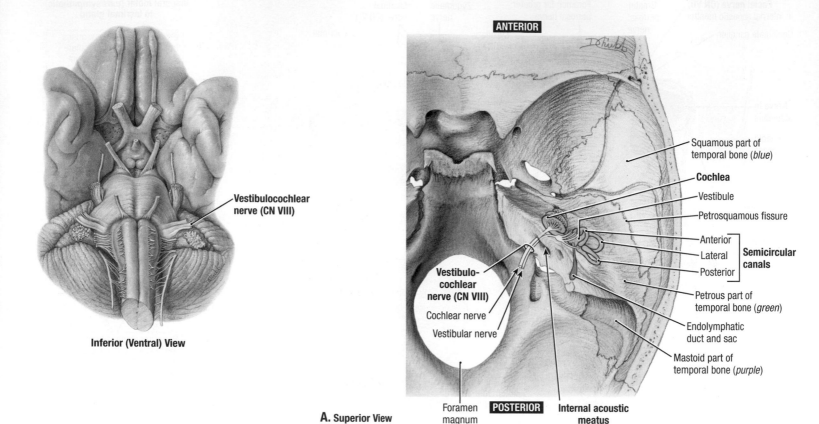

ANTERIOR

Vestibulocochlear nerve (CN VIII)

Inferior (Ventral) View

Squamous part of temporal bone (*blue*)

Cochlea

Vestibule

Petrosquamous fissure

Anterior
Lateral
Posterior
Semicircular canals

Petrous part of temporal bone (*green*)

Endolymphatic duct and sac

Mastoid part of temporal bone (*purple*)

Vestibulo-cochlear nerve (CN VIII)

Cochlear nerve

Vestibular nerve

Foramen magnum **POSTERIOR** **Internal acoustic meatus**

A. Superior View

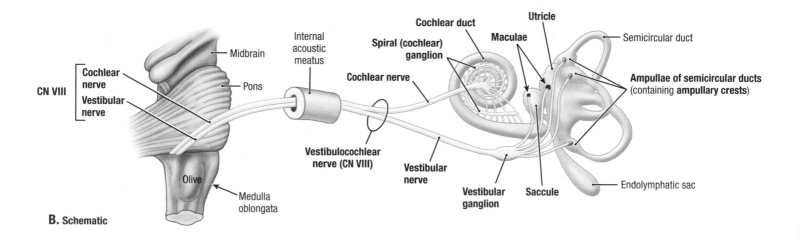

Midbrain

Internal acoustic meatus

Cochlear duct

Utricle

Spiral (cochlear) ganglion

Maculae

Semicircular duct

Cochlear nerve

Cochlear nerve

Vestibular nerve

CN VIII

Pons

Ampullae of semicircular ducts (containing **ampullary crests**)

Vestibulocochlear nerve (CN VIII)

Vestibular nerve

Olive

Medulla oblongata

Vestibular ganglion

Saccule

Endolymphatic sac

B. Schematic

9.16 **Vestibulocochlear Nerve (CN VIII)**

A. Cochlea and semicircular canals in cranium. **B.** Schematic overview of distribution.

TABLE 9.10	Vestibulocochlear Nerve (CN VIII)			
Part of Vestibulocochlear Nerve	**Functional Components**	**Cells of Origin/Termination**	**Exit from Cranial Cavity**	**Distribution and Functions**
Vestibular nerve	Special sensory	Vestibular ganglion/vestibular nuclei	Internal acoustic meatus	Vestibular sensation from semicircular ducts, utricle, and saccule related to head position and movement
Cochlear nerve		Spiral ganglion/cochlear nuclei		Hearing from spiral organ

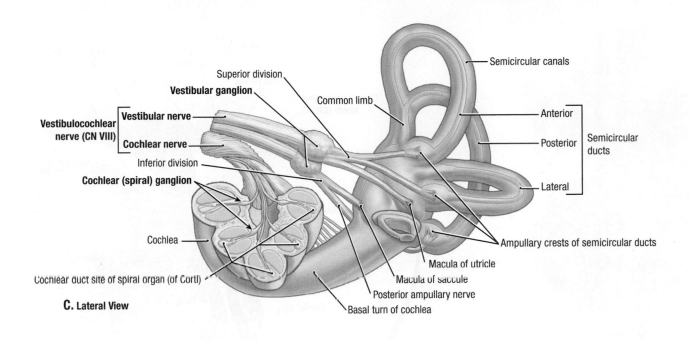

Vestibulocochlear nerve (CN VIII)
- **Vestibular nerve**
- **Cochlear nerve**

Superior division

Vestibular ganglion

Common limb

Semicircular canals

Anterior

Posterior } Semicircular ducts

Lateral

Inferior division

Cochlear (spiral) ganglion

Cochlea

Ampullary crests of semicircular ducts

Macula of utricle

Macula of saccule

Cochlear duct site of spiral organ (of Corti)

Posterior ampullary nerve

Basal turn of cochlea

C. Lateral View

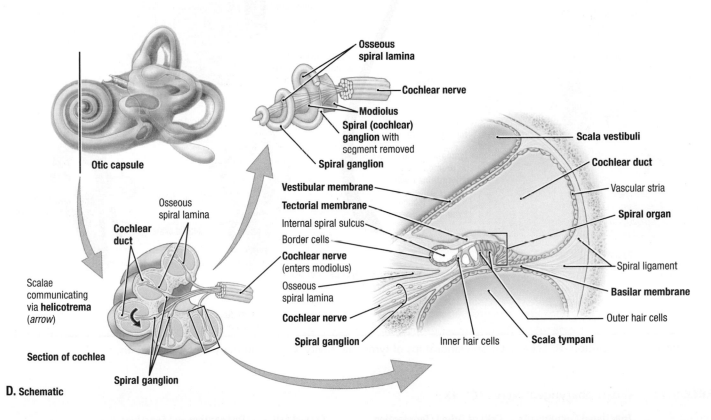

Otic capsule

Osseous spiral lamina

Cochlear nerve

Modiolus

Spiral (cochlear) ganglion with segment removed

Spiral ganglion

Scala vestibuli

Cochlear duct

Vascular stria

Spiral organ

Vestibular membrane

Tectorial membrane

Internal spiral sulcus

Border cells

Cochlear nerve (enters modiolus)

Osseous spiral lamina

Cochlear nerve

Spiral ganglion

Spiral ligament

Basilar membrane

Outer hair cells

Inner hair cells

Scala tympani

Osseous spiral lamina

Cochlear duct

Scalae communicating via **helicotrema** (*arrow*)

Section of cochlea

Spiral ganglion

D. Schematic

Vestibulocochlear Nerve (CN VIII) (*continued*)   **9.16**

C. Labyrinthine and cochlear apparatus, nerves and ganglia.
D. Structure of cochlea. Observe:
- The triangular cochlear duct is a spiral tube between the osseous spiral lamina and the external wall of the cochlear canal (spiral ligament).
- The roof of the cochlear duct is formed by the vestibular membrane and the floor by the basilar membrane and osseous spiral lamina.
- The receptor of auditory stimuli is the spiral organ (of Corti), situated on the basilar membrane; it is overlaid by the gelatinous tectorial membrane.
- The spiral organ contains hair cells that respond to vibrations induced in the perilymph by sound waves.
- The fibers of the cochlear nerve are axons of neurons of the spiral ganglion; the peripheral processes enter the spiral organ (of Corti).

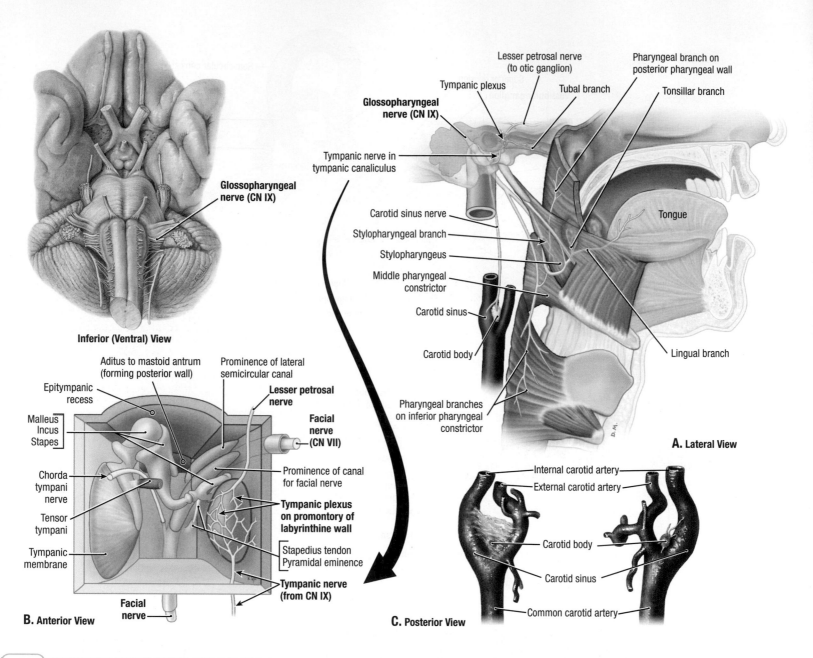

9.17   Glossopharyngeal Nerve (CN IX)

A. Overview of distribution. **B.** Schematic of relationships of tympanic cavity. **C.** Carotid body and carotid sinus.

TABLE 9.11	Glossopharyngeal Nerve (CN IX)[a]			
Nerve	**Functional Components**	**Cells of Origin/Termination**	**Cranial Exit**	**Distribution and Functions**
Glossopharyngeal	Somatic (branchial) motor	Nucleus ambiguus	Jugular foramen	Motor to stylopharyngeus that assists with swallowing
	Visceral motor	Presynaptic: inferior salivatory nucleus Postsynaptic: otic ganglion		Parasympathetic innervation to parotid gland for secretion
	Visceral sensory	Nuclei of solitary tract, spinal trigeminal nucleus/inferior ganglion		Visceral sensation from carotid body and carotid sinus
	Special sensory	Nuclei of solitary tract/inferior ganglion		Taste from posterior third of tongue
	General sensory	Spinal trigeminal nucleus/superior and inferior ganglia		External ear, posterior third of tongue, tympanic cavity and membrane, pharyngotympanic tube, isthmus of fauces, and pharynx

[a]See Table 9.15.

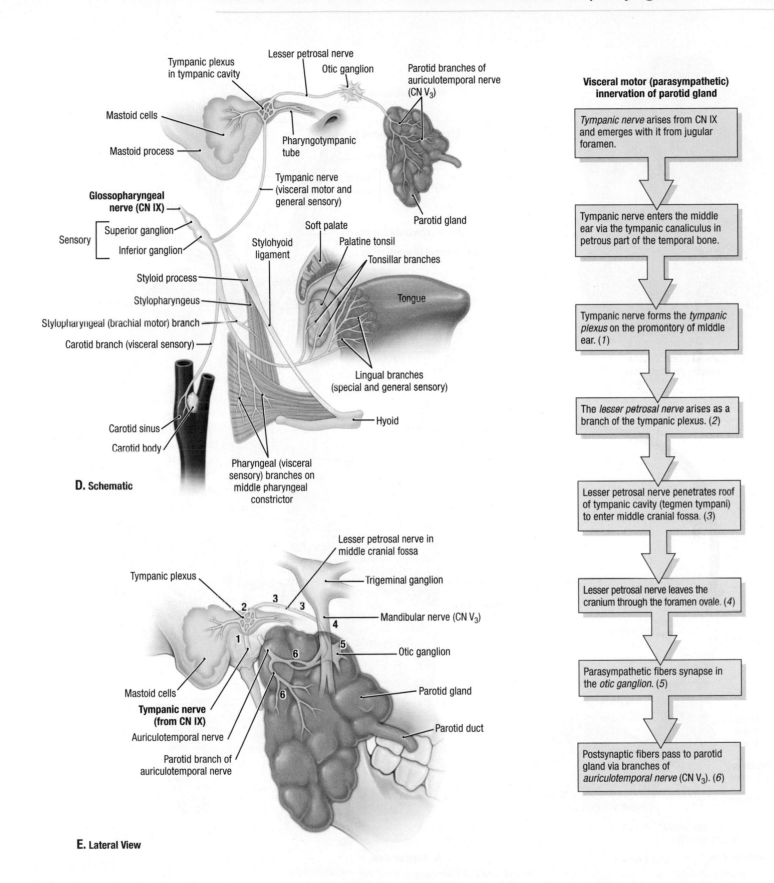

D. Schematic

E. Lateral View

Visceral motor (parasympathetic) innervation of parotid gland

Tympanic nerve arises from CN IX and emerges with it from jugular foramen.

Tympanic nerve enters the middle ear via the tympanic canaliculus in petrous part of the temporal bone.

Tympanic nerve forms the *tympanic plexus* on the promontory of middle ear. (*1*)

The *lesser petrosal nerve* arises as a branch of the tympanic plexus. (*2*)

Lesser petrosal nerve penetrates roof of tympanic cavity (tegmen tympani) to enter middle cranial fossa. (*3*)

Lesser petrosal nerve leaves the cranium through the foramen ovale. (*4*)

Parasympathetic fibers synapse in the *otic ganglion*. (*5*)

Postsynaptic fibers pass to parotid gland via branches of *auriculotemporal nerve* (CN V$_3$). (*6*)

D. Overview of distribution. **E.** Parasympathetic distribution to parotid gland.

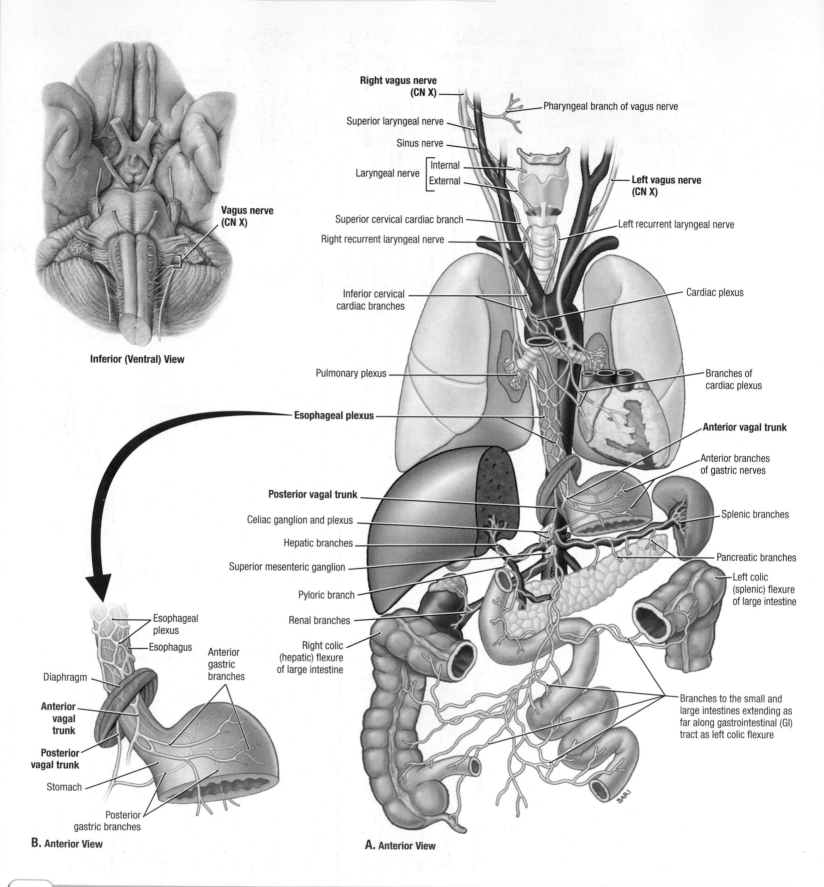

Inferior (Ventral) View

Vagus nerve (CN X)

Right vagus nerve (CN X)

Pharyngeal branch of vagus nerve

Superior laryngeal nerve

Sinus nerve

Laryngeal nerve   Internal / External

Superior cervical cardiac branch

Right recurrent laryngeal nerve

Left vagus nerve (CN X)

Left recurrent laryngeal nerve

Inferior cervical cardiac branches

Cardiac plexus

Pulmonary plexus

Branches of cardiac plexus

Esophageal plexus

Anterior vagal trunk

Anterior branches of gastric nerves

Posterior vagal trunk

Splenic branches

Celiac ganglion and plexus

Hepatic branches

Pancreatic branches

Superior mesenteric ganglion

Left colic (splenic) flexure of large intestine

Pyloric branch

Renal branches

Right colic (hepatic) flexure of large intestine

Branches to the small and large intestines extending as far along gastrointestinal (GI) tract as left colic flexure

A. Anterior View

Esophageal plexus

Esophagus

Anterior gastric branches

Diaphragm

Anterior vagal trunk

Posterior vagal trunk

Stomach

Posterior gastric branches

B. Anterior View

9.18   Vagus Nerve (CN X)

A. Course in neck, thorax, and abdomen. **B.** Anterior and posterior vagal trunks.

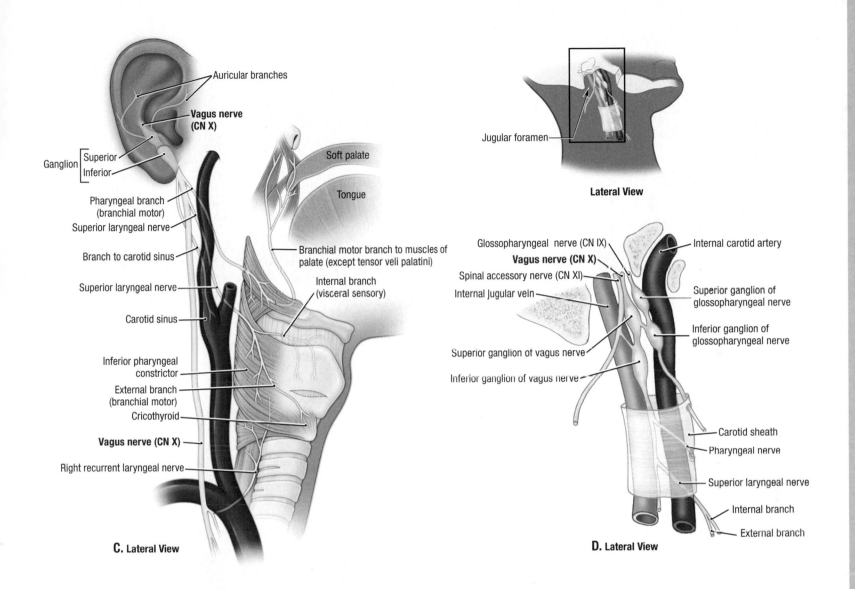

C. Lateral View

D. Lateral View

Vagus Nerve (CN X) *(continued)* **9.18**

C. Branches in neck. D. Superior and inferior sensory ganglia of vagus and glossopharyngeal nerves.

TABLE 9.12	Vagus Nerve (CN X)			
Nerve	**Functional Components**	**Cells of Origin/Termination**	**Cranial Exit**	**Distribution and Functions**
Vagus	Branchial motor	Nucleus ambiguus		Motor to constrictor muscles of pharynx, intrinsic muscles of larynx, muscles of palate (except tensor veli palatini), and striated muscle in superior two thirds of esophagus
	Visceral motor	Presynaptic: posterior (dorsal) nucleus of CN X Postsynaptic: neurons in, on, or near viscera	Jugular foramen	Parasympathetic innervation to smooth muscle of trachea, bronchi, and digestive tract, cardiac muscle
	Visceral sensory	Nuclei of solitary tract, spinal trigeminal nucleus/inferior ganglion		Visceral sensation from base of tongue, pharynx, larynx, trachea, bronchi, heart, esophagus, stomach, and intestine; carotid body and sinus
	Special sensory	Nuclei of solitary tract/inferior ganglion		Taste from epiglottis and palate
	General sensory	Spinal trigeminal nucleus/superior ganglion		Sensation from auricle, external acoustic meatus, and dura mater of posterior cranial fossa

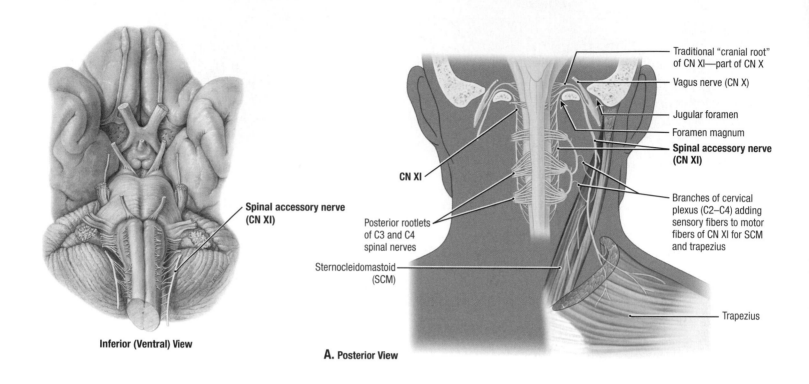

Inferior (Ventral) View

Spinal accessory nerve (CN XI)

CN XI

Posterior rootlets of C3 and C4 spinal nerves

Sternocleidomastoid (SCM)

Traditional "cranial root" of CN XI—part of CN X

Vagus nerve (CN X)

Jugular foramen

Foramen magnum

Spinal accessory nerve (CN XI)

Branches of cervical plexus (C2–C4) adding sensory fibers to motor fibers of CN XI for SCM and trapezius

Trapezius

A. Posterior View

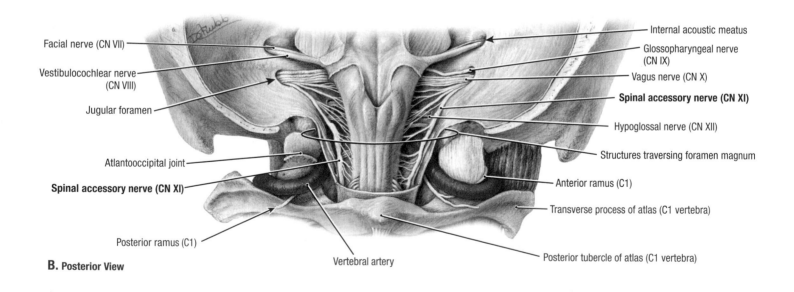

Facial nerve (CN VII)

Vestibulocochlear nerve (CN VIII)

Jugular foramen

Atlantooccipital joint

Spinal accessory nerve (CN XI)

Posterior ramus (C1)

Vertebral artery

Internal acoustic meatus

Glossopharyngeal nerve (CN IX)

Vagus nerve (CN X)

Spinal accessory nerve (CN XI)

Hypoglossal nerve (CN XII)

Structures traversing foramen magnum

Anterior ramus (C1)

Transverse process of atlas (C1 vertebra)

Posterior tubercle of atlas (C1 vertebra)

B. Posterior View

9.19 **Spinal Accessory Nerve (CN XI)**

A. Schematic of distribution. **B.** Intracranial course.

TABLE 9.13 Spinal Accessory Nerve (CN XI)

Nerve	Functional Components	Cells of Origin/Termination	Cranial Exit	Distribution and Functions[a]
Spinal accessory	Somatic motor	Accessory nucleus of spinal cord	Jugular foramen	Motor to sternocleidomastoid and trapezius

[a]General sensory fibers carried by distal branches to muscles are not present in the proximal spinal accessory nerve; these fibers from spinal nerves C2–C4 are transferred from the cervical plexus in the neck.

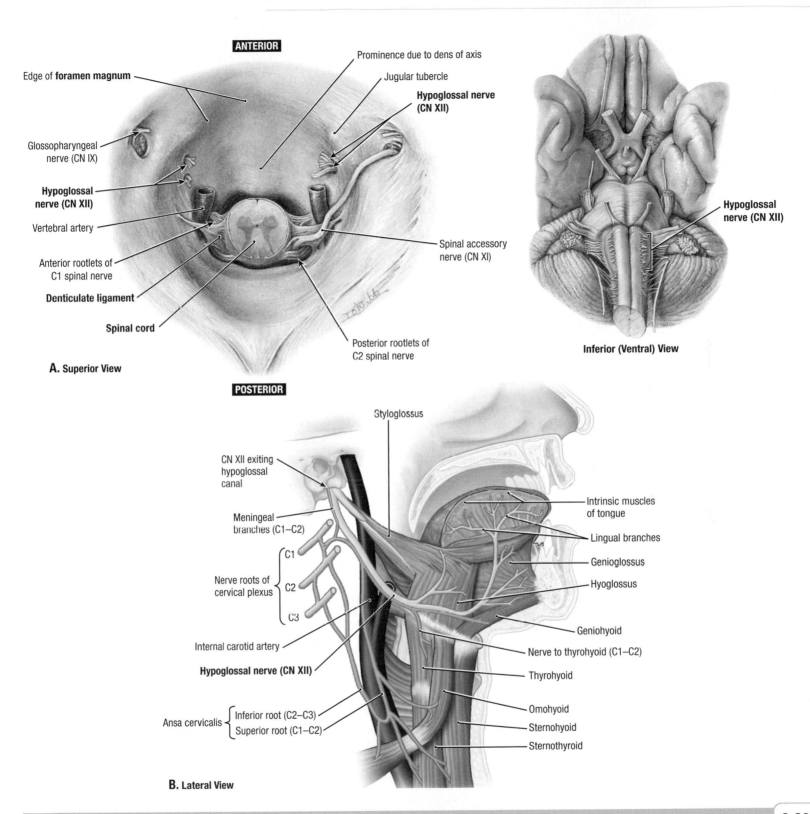

A. Superior View

Edge of **foramen magnum**

Glossopharyngeal nerve (CN IX)

Hypoglossal nerve (CN XII)

Vertebral artery

Anterior rootlets of C1 spinal nerve

Denticulate ligament

Spinal cord

ANTERIOR

Prominence due to dens of axis

Jugular tubercle

Hypoglossal nerve (CN XII)

Spinal accessory nerve (CN XI)

Posterior rootlets of C2 spinal nerve

POSTERIOR

Hypoglossal nerve (CN XII)

Inferior (Ventral) View

B. Lateral View

Styloglossus

CN XII exiting hypoglossal canal

Meningeal branches (C1–C2)

Nerve roots of cervical plexus

C1
C2
C3

Internal carotid artery

Hypoglossal nerve (CN XII)

Ansa cervicalis { Inferior root (C2–C3)
Superior root (C1–C2)

Intrinsic muscles of tongue

Lingual branches

Genioglossus

Hyoglossus

Geniohyoid

Nerve to thyrohyoid (C1–C2)

Thyrohyoid

Omohyoid

Sternohyoid

Sternothyroid

Hypoglossal Nerve (CN XII)   9.20

A. Intracranial exit from cranium into hypoglossal canal. **B.** Schematic of distribution.

TABLE 9.14   Hypoglossal Nerve (CN XII)

Nerve	Functional Components	Cells of Origin/Termination	Cranial Exit	Distribution and Functions
Hypoglossal	Somatic motor	Nucleus of CN XII	Hypoglossal canal	Motor to muscles of tongue (except palatoglossus)

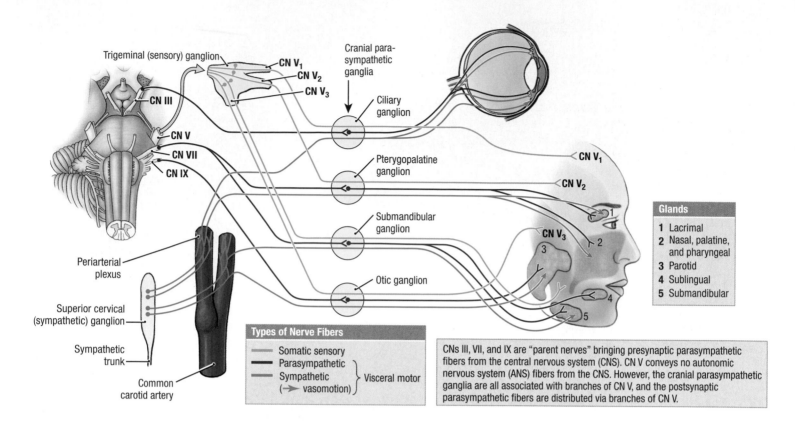

Trigeminal (sensory) ganglion

Cranial para-sympathetic ganglia

CN V₁
CN V₂
CN V₃

CN III
CN V
CN VII
CN IX

Ciliary ganglion

Pterygopalatine ganglion

Submandibular ganglion

Periarterial plexus

Otic ganglion

CN V₁
CN V₂
CN V₃

Superior cervical (sympathetic) ganglion

Sympathetic trunk

Common carotid artery

Glands
1 Lacrimal
2 Nasal, palatine, and pharyngeal
3 Parotid
4 Sublingual
5 Submandibular

Types of Nerve Fibers
— Somatic sensory
— Parasympathetic
— Sympathetic (→ vasomotion) } Visceral motor

CNs III, VII, and IX are "parent nerves" bringing presynaptic parasympathetic fibers from the central nervous system (CNS). CN V conveys no autonomic nervous system (ANS) fibers from the CNS. However, the cranial parasympathetic ganglia are all associated with branches of CN V, and the postsynaptic parasympathetic fibers are distributed via branches of CN V.

9.21 **Summary of Cranial Parasympathetic Ganglia and Related Visceral Motor and Sensory Fiber Distribution**

TABLE 9.15 **Autonomic Ganglia of Head**

Ganglion	Location	Parasympathetic Root (Nucleus of Origin)[a]	Sympathetic Root[b]	Main Distribution
Ciliary	Between optic nerve and lateral rectus, close to apex of orbit	Inferior branch of oculomotor nerve (CN III) (Edinger-Westphal nucleus)	Postsynaptic fibers from superior cervical ganglion branch from periarterial plexus on internal carotid artery in cavernous sinus	Parasympathetic postsynaptic fibers from ciliary ganglion pass to ciliary muscle and sphincter, pupillae of iris; sympathetic postsynaptic fibers from superior cervical ganglion pass to dilator pupillae and blood vessels of eye
Pterygopalatine	In pterygopalatine fossa, where it is attached by pterygopalatine branches of maxillary nerve; located immediately anterior to opening of pterygoid canal and inferior to CN V₂	Greater petrosal nerve from facial nerve (CN VII) (superior salivatory nucleus)	Deep petrosal nerve, a branch of internal carotid plexus that is continuation of postsynaptic fibers of cervical sympathetic trunk; fibers from superior cervical ganglion pass through pterygopalatine ganglion and enter branches of CN V₂	Parasympathetic postsynaptic fibers from pterygopalatine ganglion innervate lacrimal gland through zygomatic branch of CN V₂; sympathetic postsynaptic fibers from superior cervical ganglion accompany branches of pterygopalatine nerve that are distributed to the nasal cavity, palate, and superior parts of the pharynx
Otic	Between tensor veli palatini and mandibular nerve; lies inferior to foramen ovale	Tympanic nerve from glossopharyngeal nerve (CN IX); tympanic nerve continues from tympanic plexus as lesser petrosal nerve (inferior salivatory nucleus)	Fibers from superior cervical ganglion travel via plexus on middle meningeal artery	Parasympathetic postsynaptic fibers from otic ganglion are distributed to parotid gland through auriculotemporal nerve (branch of CN V₃); sympathetic postsynaptic fibers from superior cervical ganglion pass to parotid gland and supply its blood vessels
Submandibular	Suspended from lingual nerve by two short roots; lies on surface of hyoglossus muscle inferior to submandibular duct	Parasympathetic fibers join facial nerve (CN VII) and leave it in its chorda tympani branch, which unites with lingual nerve (superior salivatory nucleus)	Sympathetic fibers from superior cervical ganglion travel via the plexus on facial artery	Postsynaptic parasympathetic fibers from submandibular ganglion are distributed to the sublingual and submandibular glands; sympathetic fibers supply sublingual and submandibular glands

[a]For location of nuclei, see Figure 9.3.
[b]Sympathetic fibers traverse ganglia en route to blood vessels and dilator pupillae muscle but do not synapse in the cranial parasympathetic ganglia.

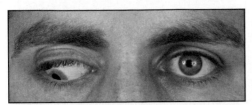

Right eye: Downward and outward directed pupil, dilated pupil, ptosis of eyelid

Left

Gaze directed anteriorly

A. Right Oculomotor (CN III) Nerve Palsy

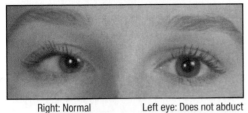

Right: Normal   Left eye: Does not abduct

Direction of gaze →

B. Left Abducent (CN VI) Nerve Palsy

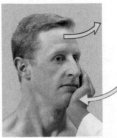

C. Test for Sternocleidomastoid Function

Key for C and D
⇨ Direction of attempted movement
⇨ Direction of resistance applied by examiner

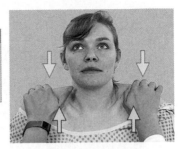

D. Test for Trapezius Function

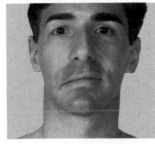

E. Right Facial (CN VII) Nerve Palsy (Bell Palsy)

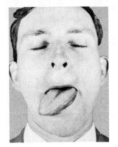

F. Right CN XII Lesion

Cranial Nerve Lesions

9.22

TABLE 9.16 Summary of Cranial Nerve Lesions

Nerve	Lesion Type and/or Site	Abnormal Findings
CN I	Fracture of cribriform plate	Anosmia (loss of smell); cerebrospinal fluid (CSF) rhinorrhea (leakage of CSF through nose)
CN II	Direct trauma to orbit or eyeball; fracture involving optic canal	Ipsilateral dilation of pupil (loss of pupillary constriction)
	Pressure on optic pathway; laceration or intracerebral clot in temporal, parietal, or occipital lobes of brain	Visual field defects
	Increased CSF pressure	Protrusion of optic disc (papilledema)
CN III	Pressure from herniating uncus on nerve; fracture involving cavernous sinus; aneurysms	Dilated pupil, ptosis, eye rotates inferiorly and laterally (down and out), pupillary reflex on the side of the lesion will be lost (**Part A**)
CN IV	Stretching of nerve during its course around brainstem; fracture of orbit	Inability to rotate adducted eye inferiorly
CN V	Injury to terminal branches (particularly CN V₂) in roof of maxillary sinus; pathologic processes (tumors, aneurysms, infections) affecting trigeminal nerve	Loss of pain and touch sensations/paresthesia on face; loss of corneal reflex (blinking when cornea touched); paralysis of muscles of mastication; deviation of mandible to side of lesion when mouth is opened
CN VI	Base of brain or fracture involving cavernous sinus or orbit	Inability to rotate eye laterally; diplopia on lateral gaze (**Part B**)
CN VII[a]	Laceration or contusion in parotid region	Paralysis of facial muscles; eye remains open; angle of mouth droops; forehead does not wrinkle (**Part C**)
	Fracture of temporal bone	As above, plus associated involvement of cochlear nerve and chorda tympani; dry cornea and loss of taste on anterior two thirds of tongue
	Intracranial hematoma ("stroke")	Weakness (paralysis) of lower facial muscles contralateral to the lesion, upper facial muscles are not affected because they are bilaterally innervated
CN VIII	Tumor of nerve	Progressive unilateral hearing loss; tinnitus (noises in ear); vertigo (loss of balance)
CN IX[b]	Brainstem lesion or deep laceration of neck	Loss of taste on posterior third of tongue; loss of sensation on affected side of soft palate; loss of gag reflex on affected side
CN X	Brainstem lesion or deep laceration of neck	Sagging of soft palate; deviation of uvula to unaffected side; hoarseness owing to paralysis of vocal fold; difficulty in swallowing and speaking
CN XI	Laceration of neck	Paralysis of sternocleidomastoid and superior fibers of trapezius; drooping of shoulder (**Part D**)
CN XII	Neck laceration; basal skull fractures	Protruded tongue deviates toward affected side; moderate dysarthria, disturbance of articulation (**Part E**)

[a]Tumors of CN VIII (e.g., acoustic neuroma) within internal acoustic meatus may result in symptoms of a CN VII lesion.
[b]Isolated lesions of CN IX are uncommon; usually, CNs IX, X, and XI are involved together as they pass through the jugular foramen.

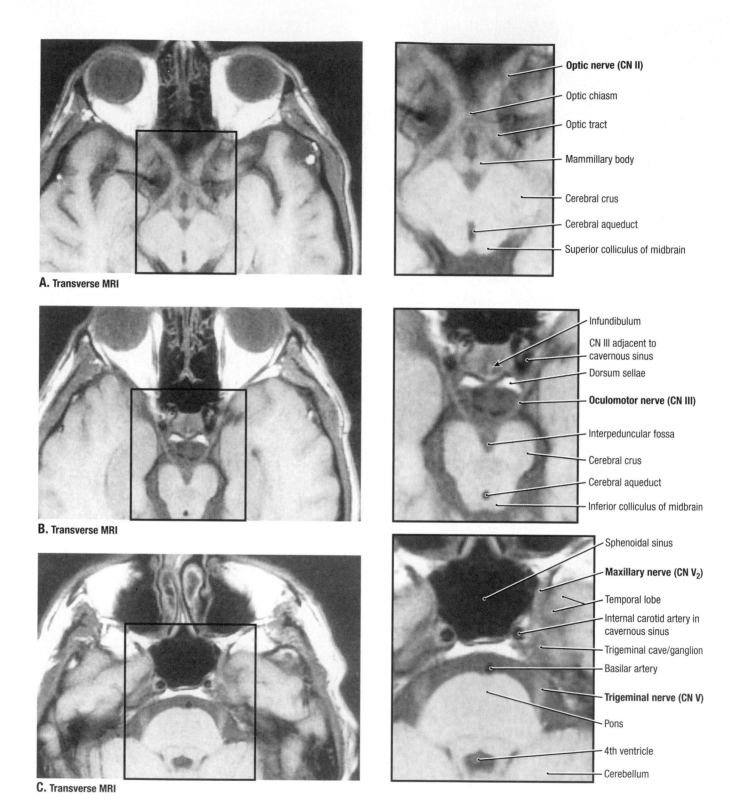

A. Transverse MRI

Optic nerve (CN II)

Optic chiasm

Optic tract

Mammillary body

Cerebral crus

Cerebral aqueduct

Superior colliculus of midbrain

B. Transverse MRI

Infundibulum

CN III adjacent to cavernous sinus

Dorsum sellae

Oculomotor nerve (CN III)

Interpeduncular fossa

Cerebral crus

Cerebral aqueduct

Inferior colliculus of midbrain

Sphenoidal sinus

Maxillary nerve (CN V₂)

Temporal lobe

Internal carotid artery in cavernous sinus

Trigeminal cave/ganglion

Basilar artery

Trigeminal nerve (CN V)

Pons

4th ventricle

Cerebellum

C. Transverse MRI

9.23   Transverse MRIs through Head, Showing Cranial Nerves

A. Optic nerve (CN II). **B.** Oculomotor nerve (CN III). **C.** Trigeminal nerve (CN V).

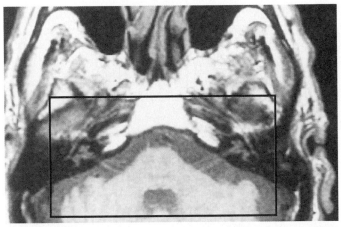

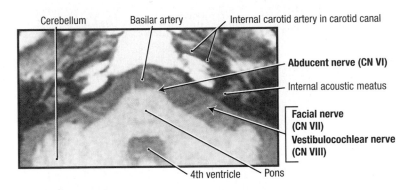

D. Transverse MRI

Cerebellum   Basilar artery   Internal carotid artery in carotid canal

Abducent nerve (CN VI)

Internal acoustic meatus

Facial nerve (CN VII)
Vestibulocochlear nerve (CN VIII)

4th ventricle   Pons

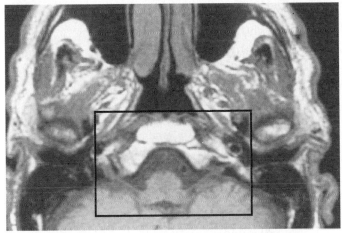

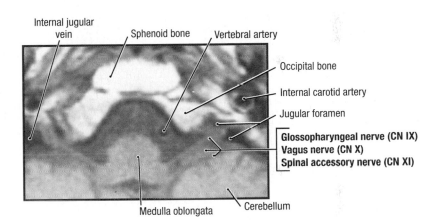

E. Transverse MRI

Internal jugular vein   Sphenoid bone   Vertebral artery

Occipital bone

Internal carotid artery

Jugular foramen

Glossopharyngeal nerve (CN IX)
Vagus nerve (CN X)
Spinal accessory nerve (CN XI)

Medulla oblongata   Cerebellum

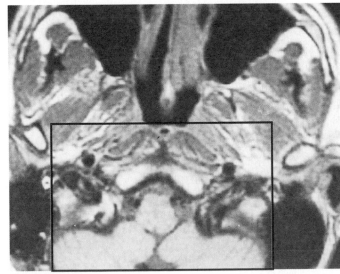

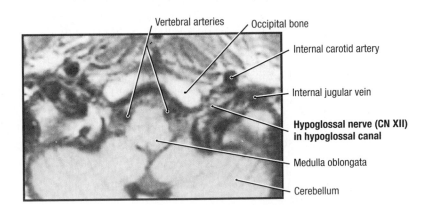

F. Transverse MRI

Vertebral arteries   Occipital bone

Internal carotid artery

Internal jugular vein

Hypoglossal nerve (CN XII) in hypoglossal canal

Medulla oblongata

Cerebellum

Transverse MRIs through Head, Showing Cranial Nerves (continued)   **9.23**

D. Abducent (CN VI), facial (CN VII), and vestibulocochlear (CN VIII) nerves. **E.** Glossopharyngeal (CN IX), vagus (CN X), and spinal accessory (CN XI) nerves. **F.** Hypoglossal nerve (CN XII).

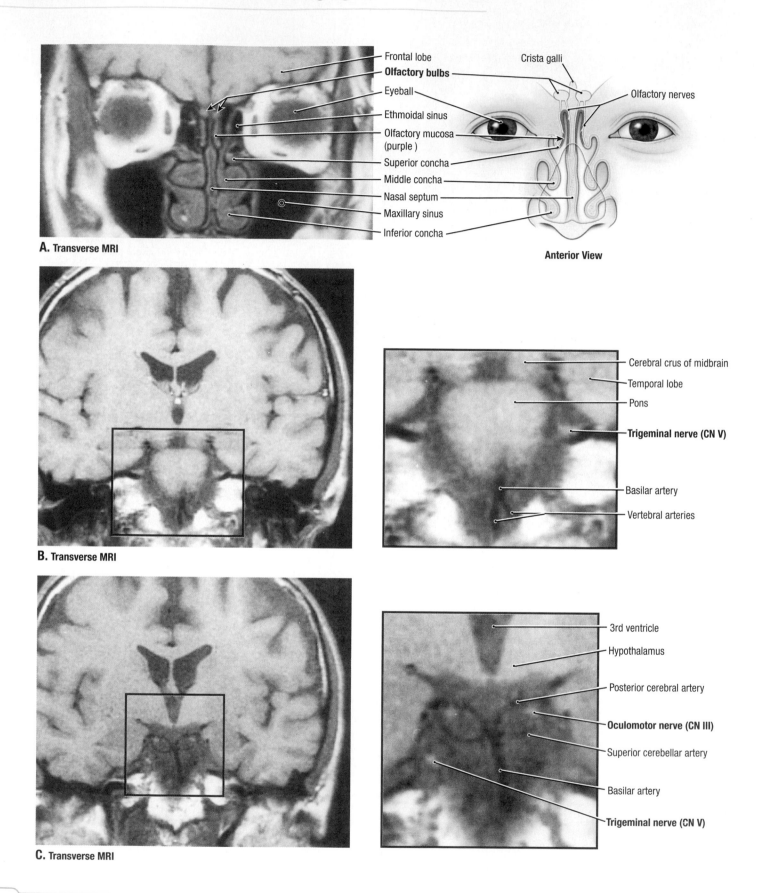

A. Transverse MRI

Frontal lobe
Olfactory bulbs
Eyeball
Ethmoidal sinus
Olfactory mucosa (purple)
Superior concha
Middle concha
Nasal septum
Maxillary sinus
Inferior concha

Crista galli
Olfactory nerves

Anterior View

B. Transverse MRI

Cerebral crus of midbrain
Temporal lobe
Pons
Trigeminal nerve (CN V)
Basilar artery
Vertebral arteries

C. Transverse MRI

3rd ventricle
Hypothalamus
Posterior cerebral artery
Oculomotor nerve (CN III)
Superior cerebellar artery
Basilar artery
Trigeminal nerve (CN V)

9.24   Coronal MRIs through Head, Showing Cranial Nerves

A. Olfactory bulb. **B.** Trigeminal nerve (CN V). **C.** Oculomotor (CN III) and trigeminal (CN V) nerves.

Page numbers followed by "t" denote tables.